# Expert Techniques in Ophthalmic Surgery

# Expert Techniques in Ophthalmic Surgery


***Editors***

**Parul Ichhpujani** MS MBA (HA)
Assistant Professor
Department of Ophthalmology
Government Medical College and Hospital
Chandigarh, India

**George L Spaeth** MD
Louis J Esposito Research Professor
Wills Eye Hospital/Jefferson Medical College
Director, Medical Research and Education
Glaucoma Service, Wills Eye Hospital
Philadelphia, Pennsylvania, USA

**Myron Yanoff** MD
Professor and Chairman
Department of Ophthalmology
Drexel University College of Medicine
Philadelphia, Pennsylvania, USA



JAYPEE *The Health Sciences Publisher*
New Delhi | London | Philadelphia | Panama

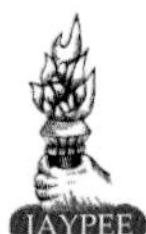

**Jaypee Brothers Medical Publishers (P) Ltd**

**Headquarters**
Jaypee Brothers Medical Publishers (P) Ltd.
4838/24, Ansari Road, Daryaganj
New Delhi 110 002, India
Phone: +91-11-43574357
Fax: +91-11-43574314
E-mail: jaypee@jaypeebrothers.com

**Overseas Offices**
J.P. Medical Ltd.
83, Victoria Street, London
SW1H 0HW (UK)
Phone: +44-20 3170 8910
Fax: +44(0)20 3008 6180
E-mail: info@jpmedpub.com

Jaypee-Highlights Medical Publishers Inc.
City of Knowledge, Bld. 237, Clayton
Panama City, Panama
Phone: +1 507-301-0496
Fax: +1 507-301-0499
E-mail: cservice@jphmedical.com

Jaypee Medical Inc.
The Bourse
111, South Independence Mall East
Suite 835
Philadelphia, PA 19106, USA
Phone: +1 267-519-9789
E-mail: jpmed.us@gmail.com

Jaypee Brothers Medical Publishers (P) Ltd.
17/1-B, Babar Road, Block-B, Shaymali
Mohammadpur, Dhaka-1207
Bangladesh
Mobile: +08801912003485
E-mail: jaypeedhaka@gmail.com

Jaypee Brothers Medical Publishers (P) Ltd.
Bhotahity, Kathmandu, Nepal
Phone: +977-9741283608
E-mail: kathmandu@jaypeebrothers.com

Website: www.jaypeebrothers.com
Website: www.jaypeedigital.com



**Inquiries for bulk sales may be solicited at:** jaypee@jaypeebrothers.com

***Expert Techniques in Ophthalmic Surgery***

*First Edition:* **2015**

ISBN: 978-93-5152-500-4

*Printed at* Replika Press Pvt. Ltd.

**Dedicated to**

*Where would I be without you?*
*Nowhere.*

*To Mom and Dad:*
*It's impossible to thank you adequately*
*for everything you've done for me.*

# Section Editors

**Section 1.** **Basic Principles of Ophthalmic Surgery**
*Parul Ichhpujani*

**Section 2.** **Cataract Surgery**
*Alan S Crandall*

**Section 3.** **Corneal Surgery**
*Walter E Beebe*

**Section 4.** **Vitreoretinal Surgery**
*Allen Ho, Sunir J. Garg*

**Section 5.** **Glaucoma Surgery**
*Ronald Leigh Fellman, Davinder S Grover*

**Section 6.** **Oculoplastic, Orbital, and Lacrimal Surgery**
*Santosh G Honavar*

**Section 7.** **Oncology Surgeries**
*Bertil Damato*

**Section 8.** **Extraocular Muscle Surgery**
*Aparna Ramasubramanian, Deborah K Vanderveen*

**Section 9.** **Open Globe Injuries**
*Rupesh Agrawal*

**Section 10.** **The Practice of Ophthalmic Surgery**
*George L Spaeth*

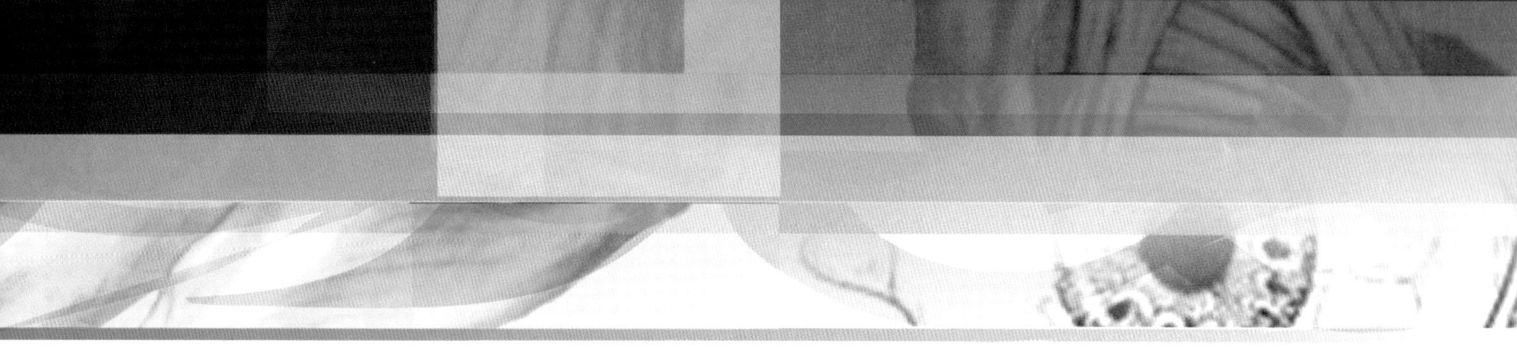

# Contributors


**Jean-Paul Abboud** MD PhD
Ophthalmologist
San Diego, California, USA

**Nathan Abraham** MS
Department of Ophthalmology
Keck School of Medicine of USC
Los Angeles, California, USA

**Isabelle Aerts** MD
Pediatric Department
CLCC Institut Curie
Paris, France

**Rupesh Agrawal** FRCS FAMS MMed
Associate Consultant
National Healthcare Group Eye Institute
Tan Tock Seng Hospital
Singapore

**Mary Anne Ahluwalia** DO
Chief Resident
Department of Ophthalmology
Oklahoma State University
Tulsa, Oklahoma, USA

**Baseer U Ahmad** MD
Vitreoretinal Fellow
The Retina Institute
St. Louis, Missouri, USA

**Iqbal Ike K Ahmed** MD
Assistant Professor
Department of Ophthalmology
University of Toronto
Toronto, Ontario, Canada

**Oscar Albis-Donado** MD
Professor
Department of Glaucoma
Instituto Mexicano de Oftalmolgia
Queretaro, Queretaro, Mexico

**Marcus Ang** MBBS MCI FRCSED
Consultant
Cornea and External Eye
Diseases Service
Singapore National Eye Centre
Singapore

**Tin Aung** FRCS (Ed) PhD
Professor
Department of Ophthalmology
Yong Loo Lin School of Medicine
National University of Singapore
Singapore

**Augusto Azuara-Blanco** PhD FRCS(Ed) FRCOphth
Professor
School of Medicine, Dentistry
and Biomedical Sciences
Queen's University Belfast
Belfast, UK

**Samuel Baharestani** MD
Attending Oculoplastic Surgeon
North Shore Eye Care
Smithtown, New York, USA

**Sally L Baxter** MD
University of California
San Diego, California, USA

**Nicholas P Bell** MD
A.G. McNeese, Jr. Professor of
Ophthalmology
Clinical Associate Professor
Ruiz Department of Ophthalmology and
Visual Science
The University of Texas Medical School
at Houston
Robert Cizik Eye Clinic
Chief of Ophthalmology Service
Lyndon B. Johnson General Hospital
Houston, Texas, USA

**Shibal Bhartiya** MD
Research Associate
Dr RP Center for Ophthalmic Sciences
All India Institute of Medical Sciences
New Delhi, India

**Christopher J Brady** MD
Retina Fellow
Department of Ophthalmology
Wills Eye Hospital
Philadelphia, Pennsylvania, USA

**Cat Nguyen Burkat** MD FACS
Faculty
University of Wisconsin School of
Medicine and Public Health
Madison, Wisconsin, USA

**Sonia Callejo** MD PhD
Montreal General Hospital
Montreal, Quebec, Canada

**Giovanna Casale-Vargas** MD
Asociacion Para Evitar La Ceguera En
Mexico
Guadalupe, Zacatecas
Mexico

**Nathalie Cassoux**
Oftalmología (Tratamiento del
Glaucoma)
Zacatecas, Zacatecas, Mexico

**Clara C Chan** MD FRSC FACS
Faculty
Department of Ophthalmology and
Vision Sciences
University of Toronto
Toronto, Ontario, Canada

**Anny Cheng** MD
Ocular Surface Center and Tissue Tech
Miami, Florida, USA

**James Chodosh** MD MPH
David G Cogan Professor
Department of Ophthalmology
Harvard Medical School
Boston, Massachusetts, USA

**Kelvin KL Chong** MBChB (Hon) FCOphth FHKAM (Ophth)
Assistant Professor
Department of Ophthalmology and Visual Sciences
The Chinese University of Hong Kong
Hong Kong

**Jocelyn L Chua** MBBS (S'pore) MRCS (Ed), MMed (Ophth) FRCS (Ed)
Consultant
Glaucoma Service
Singapore National Eye Centre
Singapore

**Robert Cionni** MD
The Eye Institute of Utah
Department of Ophthalmology
Adjunct Clinical Professor
University of Utah
Salt Lake City, Utah, USA

**Colin I Clement** BSc (Hon) MBBS PhD FRANZCO
Clinical Senior Lecturer and Staff Specialist
Glaucoma Unit, Sydney Eye Hospital
The University of Sydney
Sydney, Australia

**Marcus Colyer** MD
Walter Reed National Military Medical Center
8901 Rockville Pike
Bethesda, Maryland, USA

**Steven M Couch** MD
Assistant Professor, Ophthalmology and Visual Sciences
Center for Advanced Medicine
St. Louis, Missouri, USA

**Sarah E Coupland** MBBS PhD FRCPath
Department of Molecular and Clinical Cancer Medicine
University of Liverpool
Institute of Translational Medicine
Liverpool, UK

**Alan S Crandall** MD
Professor
Department of Ophthalmology
Moran Eye Center
University of Utah
Salt Lake City, Utah, USA

**Philip L Custer** MD
Professor
Department of Ophthalmology and Visual Sciences
Washington University School of Medicine
St. Louis, Missouri, USA

**Bertil Damato** MD PhD FRCOphth
Professor
Department of Ophthalmology
University of California, San Francisco
San Francisco, California, USA

**Sima Das** MS
Consultant
Oculoplasty and Ocular Oncology Services
Dr Shroff's Charity Eye Hospital
New Delhi, India

**Laurence Desjardins** MD
Department d'Ophtalmologie
Institut Curie, Paris, France

**Sorcha Ní Dhubhghaill** MB PhD FEBO
Anterior Segment Fellow
Department of Ophthalmology
University of Antwerp
Edegem, Antwerp, Belgium

**Michael Dollin** MD
Assistant Professor
Department of Ophthalmology
University of Ottawa
Ottawa, Ontario, Canada

**Jonathan J Dutton** MD PhD
Professor Emeritus
Department of Ophthalmology
University of North Carolina
Chapel Hill, North Carolina, USA

**Lucy Eakle Franklin** MD
University of Kentucky College of Medicine
Lexington, Kentucky, USA

**Nicholas Engelbrecht** MD
The Retina Institute
Saint Louis, Missouri, USA

**Ghasem Fakhraie** MD
Department of Ophthalmology
Director, Glaucoma Service
Farabi Eye Hospital
Tehran University of Medical Sciences
Tehran, Iran
Associate Professor of Ophthalmology
Wills Eye Hospital, Thomas Jefferson University, Philadelphia, PA, USA

**Christopher M Fecarotta** MD
Clinical Assistant Professor
Department of Ophthalmology
SUNY Downstate Medical Center
Brooklyn, New York, USA

**Ronald Leigh Fellman** MD
Clinical Associate Professor Emeritus
Department of Ophthalmology
University of Texas Southwestern Medical Center
Dallas, Texas, USA

**Michael Feilmeier** MD
University of Nebraska Medical Center
Omaha, Nebraska, USA

**Mitchell S Fineman** MD
Associate Professor
Department of Ophthalmology
Thomas Jefferson University
Philadelphia, Pennsylvania, USA

**Alexander Foster** MD
Consultant Ophthalmologist
Torrance, California, USA

**Brian A Francis** MD MS
Professor
Doheny Eye Institute
UCLA Department of Ophthalmology
Los Angeles, California, USA

**Lucy E Franklin** MD
Resident Physician
Department of Ophthalmology
University of Kentucky
Lexington, Kentucky, USA

**Adrian T Fung** MBBS MMed FRANZCO
Australian School of Advanced Medicine
Macquarie University Hospital
Save Sight Institute
Central Clinical School
University of Sydney, Sydney, Australia

**Sunir J Garg** MD FACS
The Retina Service of Wills Eye Hospital
Associate Professor of Ophthalmology
Thomas Jefferson University
Philadelphia, Pennsylvania, USA

**Steven J Gedde** MD
Professor
Department of Ophthalmology
University of Miami
Miller School of Medicine
Miami, Florida, USA

**Shubhra Goel** MD
Ophthalmic and Facial Plastic Surgeon
Ocular Oncology Service
Centre for Sight, Banjara Hills
Hyderabad, India

**Roger A Goldberg** MD MBA
Vitreorethal Surgeon
Walnut Creek, California, USA

**Patrick Gooi** MD FRCSC
Department of Ophthalmology
University of Toronto
Toronto, Ontario, Canada

**Carl Groenewald** MD
Consultant Ophthalmologist
St. Paul's Eye Unit
Royal Liverpool University Hospital
Liverpool, UK

**Davinder S Grover** MD MPH
Attending Clinician and Surgeon
Glaucoma Associates of Texas
Clinical Assistant Professor
Department of Ophthalmology
University of Texas, Southwestern
Medical School, Dallas, Texas, USA

**Omesh P Gupta** MD MBA
Assistant Professor
Department of Ophthalmology
Thomas Jefferson University and Wills
Eye Hospital Retina Service
Philadelphia, PA, USA

**Roshmi Gupta** FRCS
Consultant and Head
Ophthalmic Plastics, Orbital Surgery
Ocular Oncology
Narayana Nethralaya Eye Hospital
Bengaluru, India

**Doris Hadjistilianou** MD
Head, Unit of Ophthalmic Oncology
Santa Maria alle Scotte Clinic
Siena, Italy

**Mark S Hansen** MD
Duke Eye Center
Durham, North Carolina, USA

**Aravind Haripriya** MD
Chief, Cataract and IOL Services
Aravind Eye Hospital
Madurai, Tamil Nadu, India

**Heinrich Heimann** MD
Professor
Liverpool Ocular Oncology Centre
The Royal Liverpool Hospital
Liverpool, UK

**Christoph Hintschich** MD
Head of Oculoplastic and
Orbital Service
Munich University Eye Hospital
Munich, Germany

**Edward J Holland** MD
Director
Cornea Services
Cincinnati Eye Institute
Professor of Clinical Ophthalmology
University of Cincinnati
Cincinnati, Ohio, USA

**Santosh G Honavar** MD FACS
Ocular Oncology Service
Centre for Sight Superspeciality
Eye Hospital
Hyderabad, Andhra Pradesh, India

**Jason Hsu** MD
Assistant Professor of Ophthalmology
Thomas Jefferson University
The Retina Service of
Wills Eye Hospital
Philadelphia, Pennsylvania, USA

**Parul Ichhpujani** MD MBA (HA)
Assistant Professor
Department of Ophthalmology
Government Medical College
and Hospital
Chandigarh, India

**Andrew G Iwach** MD
Associate Clinical Professor of
Ophthalmology
University of California, San Francisco
San Francisco, California, USA

**Richard S Kaiser** MD
Mid Atlantic Retina
Lansdale, Pennsylvania, USA

**Douglas I Katz** MD
Professor of Neurology
Braintree Rehabilitation Hospital
Braintree, Massachusetts, USA
Department of Neurology
Boston University Medical Center
Boston, Massachusetts, USA

**Melanie Kazlas** MD
Instructor
Department of Ophthalmology
Harvard Medical School
Boston, Massachusetts, USA

**Nihal Kenawy** MD FRCOphth
Doctor
Liverpool Ocular Oncology Centre
Royal Liverpool University Hospital
Liverpool, UK

**Don O Kikkawa** MD
Professor of Clinical Ophthalmology
Vice-Chairman
Department of Ophthalmology
Chief, Division of Oculofacial
Plastic and Reconstructive Surgery
Shiley Eye Center
University of California San Diego
San Diego, California, USA

**Charles Kim** MD
Fellow, Ophthalmic Plastic and
Reconstructive Surgery
Wills Eye Hospital
Philadelphia, Pennsylvania, USA

**Terry Kim** MD
Cornea Specialist
Duke Medicine
Durham, North Carolina, USA

**Lazaros Konstantinidis** MD
Consultant Ophthalmic Surgeon
Jules Gonin University Eye Hospital
Lausanne, Switzerland

**Bobby S Korn** MD PhD FACS
Associate Professor of Clinical Ophthalmology
Board Certification in Ophthalmology
Fellowship in Ophthalmic Plastic and Reconstructive Surgery
Shiley Eye Center
University of California San Diego
San Diego, California, USA

**Livia Lumbroso Le-Rouic**
The Eye Cancer Network
New York, New York, USA

**Bradford W Lee** MD
Shiley Eye Center
LaJolla, California, USA

**Thomas C Lee** MD
Pediatric Retina Surgeon
Appointed Division Head for The Vision Center at Children's Hospital Los Angeles
Los Angeles, California, USA

**Richard A Lehrer** MD
Assistant Clinical Professor
Department of Ophthalmology
NE Ohio College of Medicine
Rootstown, Ohio, USA

**Gary J Lelli Jr.,** MD
Ophthalmologist
Weill Cornell Physicians
New York, New York, USA

**Richard L Levy** MD
Assistant Professor
Department of Ophthalmology
Weill Cornell Medical College
New York, New York, USA

**Christine Levy-Gabriel** MD
Department of Ophthalmology
Institut Curie
Paris, France

**Andre S Litwin** FRCOphth
Corneoplastic Unit
Queen Victoria Hospital NHS Foundation Trust
East Grinstead, West Sussex, UK

**Nikolas JS London** MD
Retina Consultants San Diego
La Jolla, California, USA

**Taylor Lukasik**
Medical Student
Royal College of Surgeons, Ireland
Dublin, Ireland

**Ashley Lundin** MD
Resident
Department of Ophthalmology and Visual Sciences
University of Wisconsin School of Medicine and Public Health
Madison, Wisconsin, USA

**Joseph I Maguire** MD
Assistant Professor
Department of Ophthalmology
Wills Eye Hospital
Thomas Jefferson University Hospital
Philadelphia, Pennsylvania, USA

**Raman Malhotra** FRCOphth
Corneoplastic Unit
Queen Victoria Hospital
East Grinstead, West Sussex, UK

**Ashwin Mallipatna** MBBS MS DNB
Consultant
Department of Pediatric Ophthalmology and Strabismus
Narayana Nethralaya
Bengaluru, Karnataka, India

**Fairooz P Manjanadavida** MD
Consultant, Ophthalmic Plastic Surgery
Orbit and Ocular Oncology
C-MER (Shenzhen) Dennis Lam Eye Hospital, Shenzhen, China

**Kimberly A Mankiewicz** PhD
Technical Writer III
Ruiz Department of Ophthalmology and Visual Science
The University of Texas Medical School at Houston
Houston, Texas, USA

**Vikas Menon** DNB
Consultant
Department of Oculoplasty and Ocular Oncology
Center for Sight
New Delhi, India

**John R Minarcik** MD
Commander, Medical Corps, USN
Department of Ophthalmology
Vitreoretinal Service
Fort Belvoir Community Hospital
Fort Belvoir, Virginia, USA

**Marlene R Moster** MD
Professor of Ophthalmology
Thomas Jefferson University School of Medicine
Wills Eye Hospital
Philadelphia, Pennsylvania, USA

**Francis Munier** MD
Jules-Gonin Eye Hospital
Lausanne, France

**Sudha Nallasamy** MD
Kellogg Eye Center
Ann Arbor, Michigan, USA

**Jeffrey Nerad** MD
Ophthalmic Plastic and Reconstructive Surgery
Cincinnati Eye Institute
Cincinnati, Ohio, USA

**Donna Nguyen** MD
Glaucoma Fellow
Ruiz Department of Ophthalmology and Visual Science
The University of Texas Medical School at Houston
Robert Cizik Eye Clinic
Houston, Texas, USA

**Bharti Nihalani-Gangwani** MD
Staff Physician, Department of Pediatric Ophthalmology and Strabismus
Boston Children's Hospital
Harvard Medical School
Boston, Massachusetts, USA

**Monisha E Nongpiur** MD
Singapore Eye Research Institute
Singapore

**Mohammed Hosein Nowroozzadeh** MD
Assistant Professor
Penstchi Eye Research Center
Department of Ophthalmology
Shiraz University of Medical Sciences
Shiraz, Iran

**Alexander K Nugent** MD
Glaucoma Fellow
Doheny Eye Institute
UCLA Department of Ophthalmology
Los Angeles, California, USA

**Brett O'Donnell** MD
Ophthalmic Plastic and Reconstructive Surgeon
North Shore Medical Centre
Leonards, Australia

**Jane Olver** MD
Clinica London
London, UK

**Sotiria Palioura** MD PhD
Ophthalmology Resident
Department of Ophthalmology
Massachusetts Eye and Ear Infirmary
Harvard Medical School
Boston, Massachusetts, USA

**Joseph F Panarelli** MD
Assistant Professor
Department of Ophthalmology
Icahn School of Medicine at Mount Sinai
New York, New York, USA

**Jonathan Pargament** MD
Department of Ophthalmology
University of Cincinnati
Cincinnati, Ohio, USA

**Carl Park** MD
Assistant Surgeon, Retina Service
Wills Eye Hospital
Clinical Assistant Professor of Ophthalmology
Thomas Jefferson University
Philadelphia, Pennsylvania, USA

**Manoj V Parulekar** MS FRCS FRCOphth
Consultant Ophthalmologist and Honorary Senior Lecturer
Birmingham Children's Hospital
University of Birmingham
Birmingham, West Midlands, UK

**Rakesh M Patel** MD
Oculofacial and Plastic Reconstructive Surgery
Department of Ophthalmology
University of Illinois at Chicago
Chicago, Illinois, USA

**Sumita Phatak** MD
Ophthalmologist
Mumbai, India

**John D Pitcher, III** MD
Ophthalmologist
Wills Eye Hospital Retina Services
Philadelphia, Pennsylvania, USA

**Sal Porbandarwalla** MD
Retina Fellow
Department of Ophthalmology
University of Washington
Seattle, Washington, USA

**Christina R Prescott** MD PhD
Assistant Professor
Department of Ophthalmology
Johns Hopkins University
Baltimore, Maryland, USA

**Allen M Putterman** MD FACS
Professor of Ophthalmology and Codirector of Oculofacial Plastic Surgery
Department of Ophthalmology
University of Illinois College of Medicine
Chicago, Illinois, USA

**Sunita Radhakrishnan** MD
Research Director
Glaucoma Center of San Francisco
San Francisco, California, USA

**Aparna Ramasubramanian** MD
Assistant Professor
Moran Eye Center
University of Utah
Salt Lake City, Utah, USA

**Naz Raoof** BA BM ChB
Department of Ophthalmology
Royal Hallamshire Hospital
Sheffield, UK

**M Reza Razeghinejad** MD
Professor, Department of Ophthalmology
Shiraz University of Medical Sciences
Shiraz, Iran

**Carl D Regillo** MD FACS
Professor of Ophthalmology
Director, Wills Eye Hospital Retina Service
Thomas Jefferson University
Philadelphia, Pennsylvania, USA

**Daniel B Rootman** MD MS
Doheny Eye Center University of California Los Angeles—Pasadena
Pasadena, California, USA

**Geoffrey E Rose** BSc MBBS MS DSc MRCP FRCS FRCOphth
Professor, Orbital and Adnexal Service
Moorfields Eye Hospital
London, UK

**Iwona Rospond-Kubiak** MD PhD
Ocular Oncology Service
Department of Ophthalmology
Poznań University of Medical Sciences
Poznań, Poland

**Sanduk Ruit** MD
Professor
Tilganga Institute of Ophthalmology
Gaushala, Bagmati Bridge
Kathmandu, Nepal

**Andrea Russo** MD
University Cardiology Group
Cherry Hill, New Jersey, USA

**Steven J Ryder** MD
Ophthalmology Resident
Department of Ophthalmology
Weill Cornell Medical Center
New York, New York, USA

**Mohammad Ali A Sadiq** MD
Assistant Professor
Ophthalmology
King Edward Medical University
Lahore, Pakistan

**Sachin Salvi** FRCOphth
Department of Ophthalmology
Royal Hallamshire Hospital
Sheffield, UK

**Jonathan H Salvin** MD
Nemours Pediatric Specialists
Alfred I. duPont Hospital for Children
Wilmington, Delaware, USA

**Louis Savar** MD
General Surgeon
Beverly Hills, California, USA

**Emil Anthony T Say** MD
Adult/Pediatric Retina and
Ocular Oncology
Wills Eye Hospital
Thomas Jefferson University
Philadelphia, Pennsylvania, USA

**Richard L Scawn** MBBS
Specialist Registrar
Moorfields Eye Hospital NHS Trust
London, UK

**Michael I Seider** MD
Clinical Instructor and
Fellow in Ocular Oncology
Department of Ophthalmology
University of California San Francisco
San Francisco, California, USA

**Stuart R Seiff** MD
Pacific Eye Associates
San Francisco, California, USA

**Ankoor S Shah** MD PhD
Instructor
Department of Ophthalmology
Harvard Medical School and Boston
Children's Hospital
Boston, Massachusetts, USA

**Chirag P Shah** MD MPH
Attending Vitreoretinal Surgeon
Ophthalmic Consultants of Boston
Boston, Massachusetts, USA

**Gaurav Shah** MD
Fellowship Director, Attending Surgeon
The Retina Institute
St. Louis, Missouri, USA

**Rajiv Shah** MD
Assistant Professor
Department of Ophthalmology
Wayne State University School of
Medicine
Kresge Eye Institute
Detroit, Michigan, USA

**Sajani Shah** MD
Surgeon
Assistant Professor
Tufts University School of Medicine
Boston, Massachusetts, USA

**Hosam Sheha** MD PhD
Ocular Surface Center and Tissue Tech
Miami, Florida, USA

**Fabiana Q Silva** MD
Department of Ophthalmology
Weill Cornell Medical College
New York, New York, USA

**Bradley T Smith** MD
Center for Advanced Medicine at
Barnes Jewish Hospital
St. Louis, Missouri, USA

**Scott D Smith** MD
Ophthalmologist
Cleveland Clinic
Cleveland, Ohio, USA

**Abhilasha Solanki** MD
Harvard University
Boston, Massachusetts, USA

**Marc J Spirn** MD
Ophthalmologist
Thomas Jefferson University
Wills Eye Hospital
Philadelphia, Pennsylvania, USA

**Paul J Stewart** MD
Ophthalmology
Eye Center of Texas
Pasadena, Texas, USA

**Michael D Straiko** MD
Associate Director of Corneal Services
Dever's Eye Institute
Portland, Oregon, USA

**Oana Stirbu** MD FEBO
Consultant Ophthalmologist
Glaucoma Service
Institut Comtal d'Óftalmologia ICO
Barcelona, Spain

**George L Spaeth** MD
Louis J Esposito Research Professor
Wills Eye Hospital/Jefferson
Medical College
Director, Medical Research and
Education
Glaucoma Service, Wills Eye Hospital
Philadelphia, Pennsylvania, USA

**Gangadhara Sundar** DO FRCSEd FAMS
Head and Senior Consultant for
Oculoplastic Services
Assistant Professor
Department of Ophthalmology
National University of Singapore
Singapore

**Geoffrey Tabin** MD
Moran Eye Center
University of Utah Health Care
Salt lake City, Utah, USA

**Julia C Talajic** MDCM
Clinical Associate Professor
Department of Ophthalmology
University of Montreal
Montreal, Quebec, Canada

**Donald TH Tan** FRCS(G) FRCS(Ed) FRCOphth FAMS
Professor
Medical Director
Singapore National Eye Centre
Singapore

**Marie-José Tassignon** MD Phd Febo
Professor
Department of Ophthalmology
University of Antwerp and
Antwerp University Hospital
Edegam, Antwerp, Belgium

**Mark A Terry** MD
Corneal Services
Devers Eye Institute
Portland, Oregon, USA

**Aristomenis Thanos** MD
Resident in Ophthalmology
Department of Ophthalmology
Harvard University
Boston, Massachusetts, USA

**Benjamin Thomas** MD
General Adult Neurologist
Board Certified in Neurology
Wilson Neurology
Wilson, North Carolina, USA

**Matthew Thomas** MD
Ophthalmology
Retina Institute
St. Louis, Missouri, USA

**Sean Tighe** MS
Scientist
Tissue Tech Inc
Miami, Florida, USA

**Andrew Tsai** MBBS MMed (Ophth)
Ophthalmology
Singapore National Eye Centre
Singapore

**Scheffer G Tseng** MD PhD
Director, Ocular Surface Center
Miami, Florida, USA

**Nicole C Tsim** MD MBBS
Department of Ophthalmology and
Visual Sciences
Chinese University of Hong Kong
Hong Kong

**James Vander** MD
Clinical Professor of Ophthalmology
Thomas Jefferson University
School of Medicine
Attending Surgeon
Wills Eye Hospital
Philadelphia, Pennsylvania, USA

**Deborah K VanderVeen** MD
Associate Professor
Department of Ophthalmology
Harvard Medical School
Boston, Massachusetts, USA

**Woodford S Van Meter** MD
Ophthalmology
University of Kentucky
Lexington, Kentucky, USA

**Abhay R Vasavada** MD MS FRCS (England)
Director
Iladevi Cataract and IOL Research Centre
Raghudeep Eye Hospital
Ahmedabad, India

**G Atma Vemulakonda** MD
Associate Professor
Department of Ophthalmology
University of Washington
Seattle, Washington, USA

**Rengaraj Venkatesh** MD
Chief Medical Officer
Aravind Eye Hospital
Pondicherry, India

**David H Verity** MD
Adnexal Department
Moorfields Eye Hospital
London, UK

**Steven D Vold** MD
Vold Vision
Fayetteville, Arkansas, USA

**Charles H Weber** MD
The Eye Institute of Utah
Salt Lake City, Utah, USA

**Eric Weichel** MD
Assistant Clinical Professor
Georgetown University
Washington, DC, USA

**Andre J Witkin** MD
Assistant Professor
Department of Ophthalmology
Tufts University School of Medicine
Boston, Massachusetts, USA

**S Chien Wong** MD
Ophthalmology
Los Angeles, California, USA

**Marielle P Young** MD
Assistant Professor
Department of Ophthalmology
University of Utah
Moran Eye Center
Salt Lake City, Utah, USA

**Martin Zehetmayer** MD
Professor (extraord.)
Department of Ophthalmology
University of Vienna
Vienna, Austria

**Christopher I Zoumalan** MD FACS
Clinical Assistant Professor
Department of Ophthalmology
Keck School of Medicine of USC
Los Angeles, California, USA

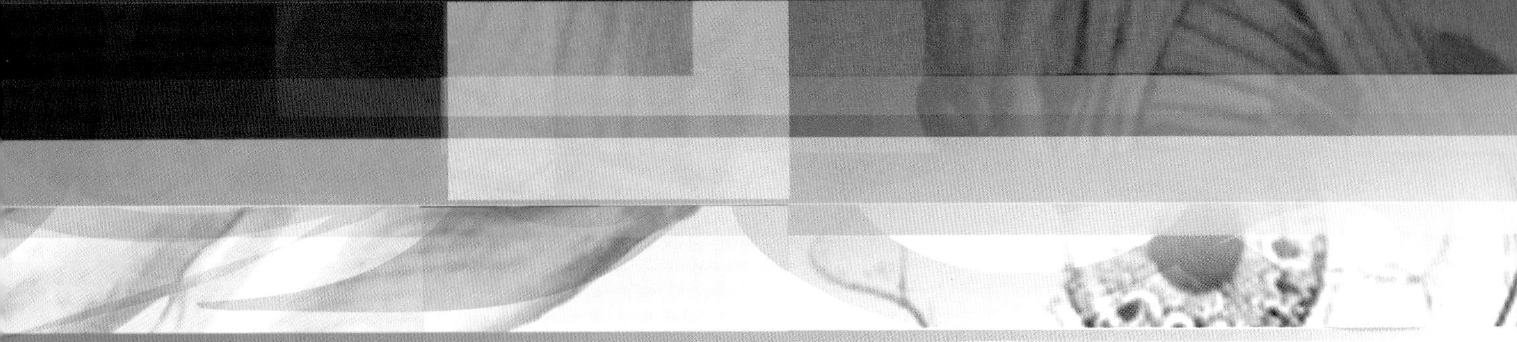

# Preface

The earliest documented reference to the most commonly performed ocular surgery, cataract surgery, has been found in Sanskrit manuscripts dating from the fifth century BC. It was attributed to the Indian surgeon, Susruta. According to Herodotus, the historian of ancient Greece, surgery was practiced by "chirorgos", which combines the words "hand" and "work" and means "surgeon". The early 17th century BC papyrus papers of Edwin Smith also mentioned advanced level of ophthalmic surgery practiced by Egyptians. The mid-nineteenth century saw major developments of surgical practices inherited from the ancient masters. The twentieth century was a century of dramatic advances. Surgeons across the globe have been constantly putting their creative thinking into action for devising novel ways for cutting, reshaping, reforming, bypassing, and fixing ocular anomalies.

This volume is a comprehensive textbook-atlas. It has a highly visual format that includes illustrations and images, as well as features that align with current ophthalmology training. The content has been organized in such a way to facilitate quick access of information, with abundant bullet point lists and boxes, and fewer denser passages of text than found in a traditional textbook. Each section is color-coded for easy cross-referencing and "navigation". In all the sections, operative techniques and surgical strategies are explained step-by-step to increase surgical knowledge and anatomy. A section on ethics and medicolegal aspects of surgical practice is an additional highlight of the book.

This book is the product of almost three years of hard work. It has a global perspective, with the participation of renowned international contributors. It includes a variety of topics of interest to a wide-ranging audience, including operating in areas with limited resources. It has been an honor to work with the section editors and contributors of this book.

I would especially like to thank Mr Joe Rusko and Mr Marco Ulloa, the publishers, for their expert assistance in all the issues concerning this book. I also thank Ms Chetna Malhotra Vohra (Associate Director), for her useful assistance. My gratitude also goes to the technical editors for arranging the book in a uniform format. I am thankful to Jaypee Brothers Medical Publishers (P) Ltd. New Delhi, India, for undertaking this mission.

Newer surgical advances challenge the existing trends. The future of ophthalmic surgery seems as dynamic as its history. We are grateful to all the great ophthalmic surgeons of the past and look forward to the operating room of the future through learning new techniques, understanding and adapting to new technologies, maintaining surgical competencies, and applying the same to our practices.

Thanks for choosing this volume for your collection. If you have any comments, feel free to email me at the address below.

**Parul Ichhpujani**
parul77@rediffmail.com

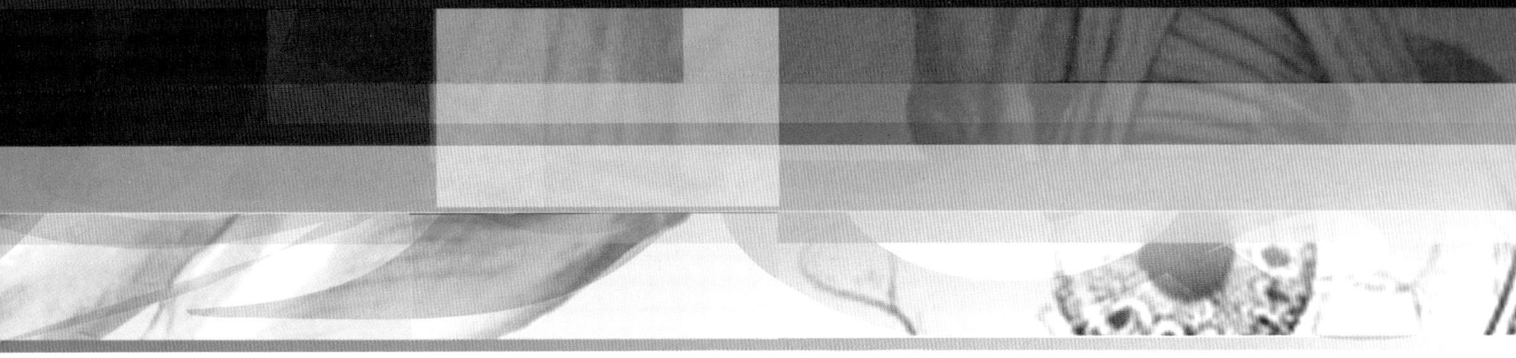

# Acknowledgments

A book of this nature requires the cooperation of many different authors. I am grateful to all the contributors of the book, but some stand out, going well above and beyond the call of duty.

First, I wish to earnestly thank Dr George L Spaeth, my co-editor and Louis J Esposito Research Professor at the Wills Eye Institute, Philadelphia, Pennsylvania, USA. He has been my mentor and has been quite instrumental in adding a unique dimension to my practice of Ophthalmology. I was quite honored, when he asked me to be the chief editor.

Dr Aparna Ramasubramanian for being a great friend, helping in recommending other potential authors and editing her section as per the timeline.

The staff of the Philadelphia office, USA, bent over backwards to make the production of this manuscript pleasant, professional, and fast.

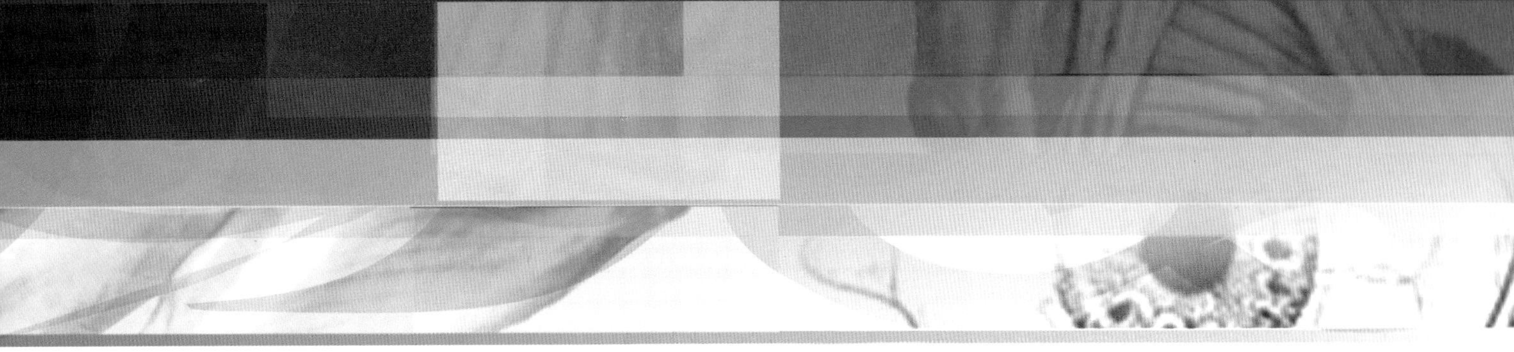

# Contents

## Section 2: Cataract Surgery

*Alan S Crandall*

## Section 3: Corneal Surgery

*Walter E Beebe*

## Section 6: Oculoplastic, Orbital and Lacrimal Surgery

*Santosh G Honavar*

## Section 7: Oncology Surgeries

*Bertil Damato*

## Section 8: Extraocular Muscle Surgery

*Aparna Ramasubramanian, Deborah K Vanderveen*

# Section 1

# Basic Principles of Ophthalmic Surgery

*Section Editor* Parul Ichhpujani

CHAPTER

1

# Asepsis in the Operating Room

Oana Stirbu

## INTRODUCTION

The chain of asepsis obeys the theory of constraints, ruled by the paradigm stating that a chain is no stronger than its weakest link; therefore, discipline and continuous strive of each team member to reduce the incidence of infection to a minimum are mandatory.[1] This systematic effort to prevent infection includes periodic checks, which must be carried out to ensure the continued effectiveness of current practices. Therefore, the Association of peri-Operative Registered Nurses (AORN) have developed standards and recommended practices, which are guidelines to be used by the surgical team to achieve the optimal level of technical and aseptic practice when caring for their patients in the perioperative setting. Pathogenic microorganisms are found in two different reservoirs: the animate environment (infected or colonized personnel and patient) and the inanimate environment [operating room (OR) air and equipment, anesthesia, and surgical instruments].

## PATIENT CARE

The conjunctiva, contaminated mostly with eyelid margin microbes, constitutes a repository of potentially infectious agents and patient's own external bacterial flora present in conjunctiva, eyelid or nose represents the main source of postoperative infection.[2] Patients with advanced age, local risk factors (chronic use of topical medications, contact lens wear, blepharitis, chronic eyelid or conjunctival inflammation), and systemic risk factors (immunosuppression, diabetes, rosacea, autoimmune conditions, and asthma) present a higher rate of bacterial conjunctival contamination before intraocular surgery.[3]

The most strongly recommended technique of preoperative patient prophylaxis based on the current clinical evidence consists of povidone-iodine irrigation.[4,5] Patient prophylaxis consists in periocular skin scrubbing with 5% or 10% povidone-iodine ophthalmic solution, including eyelashes, eye lids, inner canthus, and surrounding area, allowed to act for a minimum of 3 minutes and one drop of 5% povidone-iodine to the cornea and in the inferior conjunctival sac immediately preoperatively.[6-8] Povidone-iodine concentration inferior to 5% and eyelid eversion during conjunctival decontamination are not the recommended agent.[9,10]

Other prophylactic interventions, such as postoperative subconjunctival antibiotic injection, preoperative lash trimming, preoperative saline irrigation, preoperative topical antibiotics, or antibiotic-containing irrigating solutions are not supported by the available literature.[11] Patient preoperative showering or bathing with chlorhexidine or other wash products were not found to reduce surgical site infection.[12]

## PERSONNEL DISCIPLINE

Surgical attire is worn to promote cleanliness, surgical consciousness, and professionalism within the surgical environment and personnel entering the OR complex should strictly obey a dress code, as the human body is a major source of microbial contamination.[13] Personnel working in the OR should be free from overt, active infection. The surgical team is made up of sterile and nonsterile members. Sterile members or "scrubbed" personnel work directly in the surgical field while the nonsterile members work in the periphery of the sterile surgical field.

### Surgical Attire

All surgical team members wear scrub attire. Surgical attire, including scrub clothes, hair coverings, mask, protective eyewear, and other protective garments, provide a barrier to contamination that may pass from personnel to patient as well as from patient to personnel.[14] All persons should change into freshly laundered clothing and must wash their hands thoroughly before entering the OR. Scrub clothes home laundering is a debated issue.[15] Head, hair, and beards should be fully covered by caps and masks. Surgical mask should fully cover mouth and nose.[16] Other personnel in the operating theater should wear surgical masks if an operation is being performed or if sterile instruments are exposed. Hand washing or hospital-approved disinfectant is required between patients and whenever they become soiled. Fingernails should be kept clean and short. Traditionally, nail polish, artificial, and long natural fingernails are not permitted for those providing direct patient care. Presently, there is insufficient evidence to determine whether wearing nail polish or finger ring affects the number of bacteria on the skin postscrub.[17]

## Scrubbing

The surgical team in direct contact with the sterile area should scrub their hands and arms till above the elbows twice for 1–2 minutes each with povidone-iodine or chlorhexidine solution in the scrub area, with sponge or nailbrush. Chlorhexidine-based scrubs seem to be more effective than povidone-iodine scrubs in terms of bacteria colony forming units on the hands, are less irritating, and have more persistent effect.[18,19] An option to traditional hand scrubbing is hand rubbing with alcohol-based hand preparations.[20-22] Approved in some countries as equivalent to traditional hand scrubbing in preventing surgical site infections, the procedure of hand rubbing consists of 1-min hand and forearms wash with nonantiseptic soap and tap water, rinsed with nonsterile tap water, and wiped carefully with nonsterile paper, followed by 3 or 5 minutes of hand rubbing with enough aqueous alcoholic solution to fully cover the hands and forearm, applied twice for 2 minutes 30 seconds (for a total of 5 minutes) without drying.[23] Most alcohol-based hand preparations for surgical antisepsis contain either isopropanol, n-propanol, or ethanol at different concentrations or a combination of these agents, with or without supplements such as quaternary ammonium compounds, octenidine, triclosan, or chlorhexidine.

## Donning Gloves

After hand rub/scrub, sterile gloves should be donned in a sterile manner. The technique is based on the premise that the skin of the surgical team member must remain exclusively in contact with the inner surface of the glove and any error in the performance of this technique requires a change of gloves.[24] Between surgeries, hands should be washed with balanced salt solution or Ringer's lactate to remove the talc, as inadvertent perforations in the gloves are not infrequent, with the lowest perforation rate found in cataract and intraocular lens surgery and the highest rate in oculoplastic surgery.[25]

*Closed donning*:

- Outer pack is peeled open from the corners. The pack is gripped through the gown and opened to display the gloves
- With the gown covering the fingers, right hand is used. to remove the left glove. Left hand is held palm up with fingers straight. The glove is laid on left wrist, and the cuff is gripped with left thumb.
- Right thumb is then placed inside the top cuff edge. A fist is made with right hand, and the glove is stretched over left fingertips.
- The glove is pulled down keeping the left fingers straight.
- The above procedure is repeated to don the other glove, that is, gloved left hand is used to lay the right glove on the right wrist. Left thumb is slid inside the top of the cuff, a fist is made, and the cuff is stretched over right fingertips. Sleeve and glove are pulled down together (Figs. 1-1A to D).

*Open donning:*

- The cuff of the right glove is picked with the left hand. Slide right hand into the glove and ensure a snug fit over the thumb joint and knuckles. The bare left hand should only touch the folded cuff.
- Right fingertips are then slid into the folded cuff of the left glove. The glove is pulled to fit right hand into it.
- The cuffs are unfolded down the gown sleeves, making sure that gloved fingertips do not touch bare forearms or wrists (Figs. 1-2A to C).

## Maintaining Sterility of Supplies and Packages

When opening wrapped supplies or packages, the nonsterile person or the circulating nurse should open the top wrapper flap away from them first, then open the flaps to each side. The last wrapper flap is pulled toward the nonsterile person opening the package. All wrapper edges should be secured to prevent flipping the wrapper and contaminating the contents of the sterile package or field. When a package is double wrapped, each institution has its own policies and procedures, which determine if one or both wrappers have to be opened before presentation to the sterile field. When opening a peel package, the nonsterile person opens the package by rolling the wrapper over his or her hands and presenting the inner contents of the package to the scrubbed person.

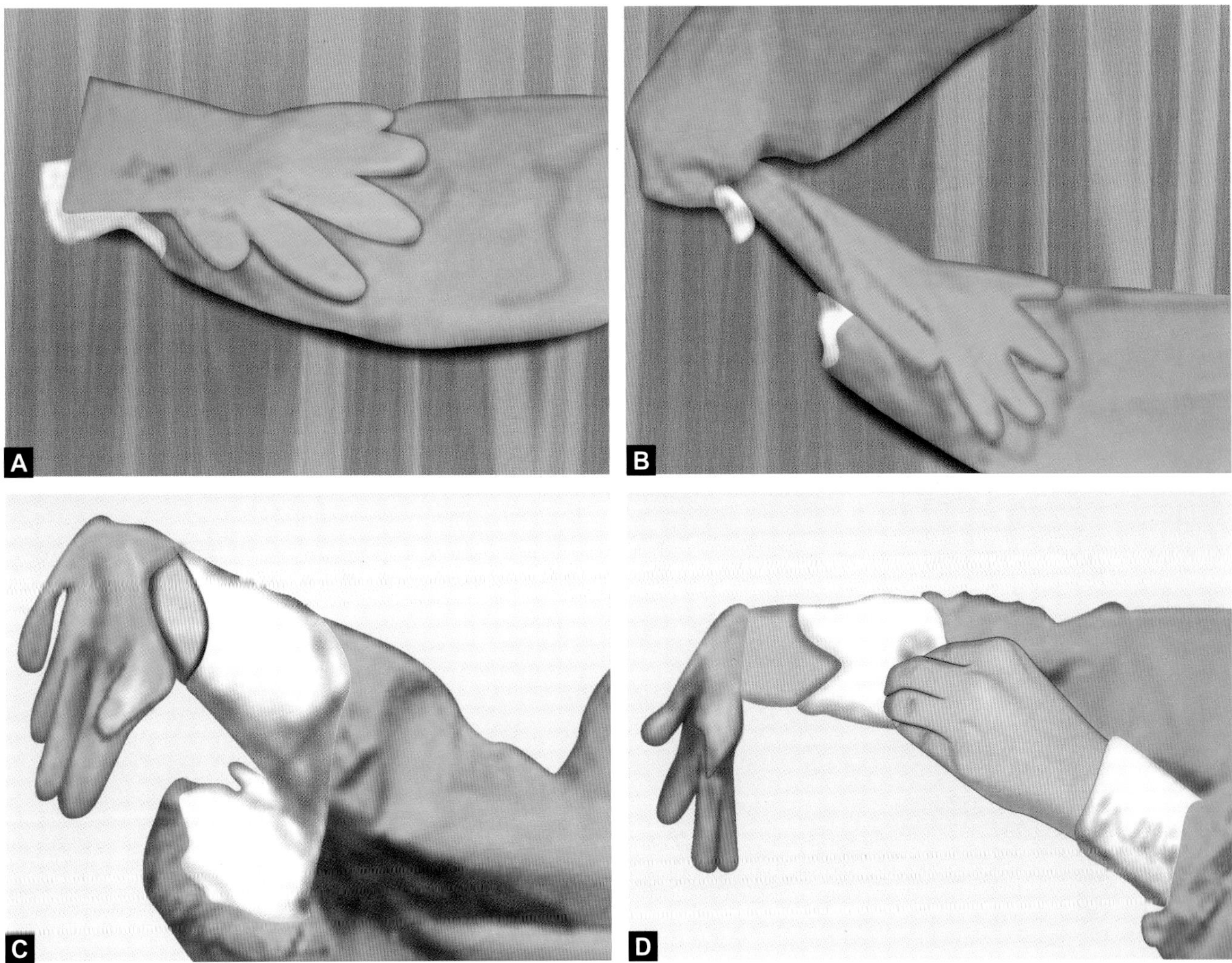

**Figures 1-1A to D** Closed donning.

When opening a solution container, the nonsterile person should lift the cap straight up and pour the contents of the bottle into a sterile container. When solutions are poured onto the sterile field, they should be poured slowly to prevent contamination and fluid strikethrough from splashing.

## OR COMPLEX

While most common source of infecting organisms seems to be the patient and the surgical staff,[26] environmental contamination plays an important role in surgical infections. The OR complex needs to fulfill the criteria of a clean room, an environment with a controlled level of contamination (dust, airborne microbes, particles, chemical vapors, etc.), ensured by OR complex design and architecture, ventilation and cleaning procedures, and care of instruments.

### OR Complex Design and Architecture

Asepsis in the OR starts long before the surgery is actually performed, at the moment when the OR is designed by strict regulatory standards of location and architecture. One of the functions of the OR complex modules is to control varying degrees of cleanliness through scientifically planned traffic flow and differential decreasing positive pressure ventilation gradient. The surgical area is isolated from the rest of the hospital, and the OR is further isolated from other parts of the surgical area.[27]

#### *Zoning*

The OR complex should be located either on the top or on the bottom floor, preferably in a separate or blind wing and

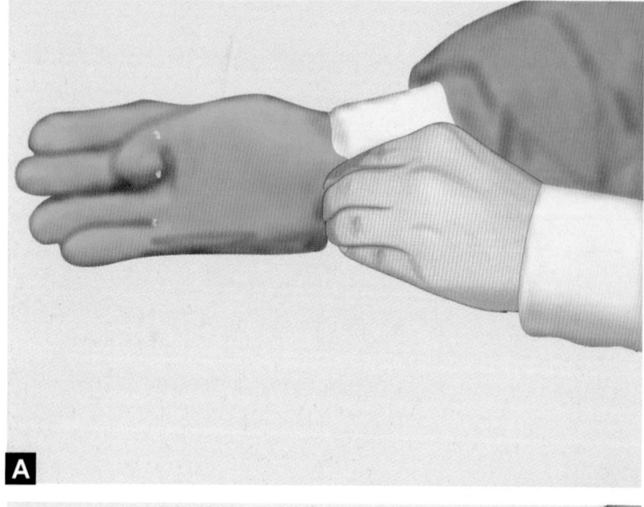

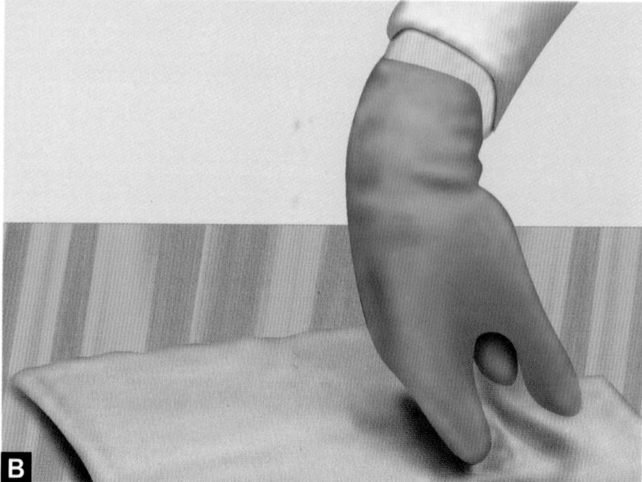

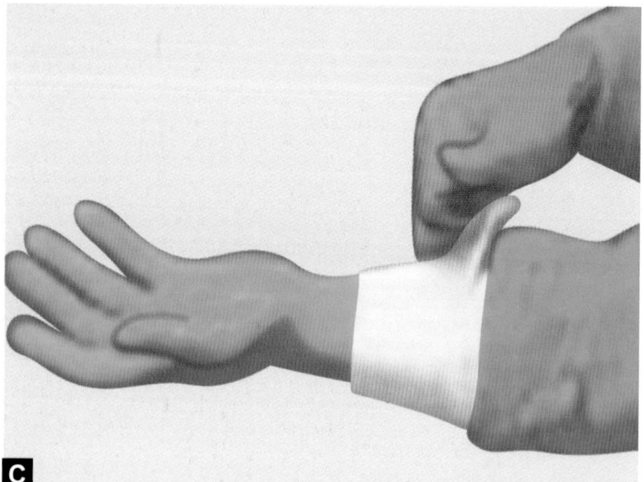

**Figures 1-2A to C** Open donning.

consists of four modules (zones): outer, clean (restricted), aseptic, and disposal zone. The bacteriological count diminishes progressively from the outer to the inner zone.[28]

- *Outer zone*: Reception area with administrative function, patient relative's waiting room, toilets, accessible to all persons and supplies.
- *Clean (restricted) zone*: Staff changing room, patient transfer area, staff lounge, and anesthetist/recovery room. The changing room, located at the entrance of the OR complex, should have a separate entrance (street clothes) and exit (surgical attire), lockers, and washbasin. Showers are not mandatory in the changing room. The patient transfer area includes the patient changing room and a corridor where the patient is transferred from an outside trolley to an inside trolley.
- *Aseptic zone*: Scrub area, OR, and area used for instrument packing and sterilization. The scrub area should be located just outside the OR, wide enough for two to scrub simultaneously without touching the other's elbow. Taps in the scrub area should be foot/elbow operated or preferably infrared sensor electronically controlled taps. The OR is the most critical area of the OR complex, and all design protocols should be duly observed.[29]
  - Minimum recommended size of 325 square feet (30 $m^2$) and rectangular shape.
  - *Floor*: Slip resistant, suitably hard, nonporous, fireproof material, with minimum joints, no floor drains installed.
  - *Doors*: Minimum width of 1.2 m, hermetically sealed surface sliding doors (not recessed into the walls) that eliminate air turbulence caused by swinging doors, kept closed all the time except for the passage of patients and essential equipment and personnel.
  - *Operating table*: The head end directed away from the entrance, enough circulating space around all its sides.

- *Walls and ceiling*: Nonporous fire resistant material, seamless, stain resistant, easy to clean, no artificial ceiling, and minimum of 10 feet high (3.05 m).
- *Lights*: General OR lights recessed into the ceiling to prevent dust collection.

- *Disposal zone*: Area where used equipments are cleaned and biohazardous waste is disposed.

Cleaning the OR on a regular basis represents an often neglected but fundamental step in environmental asepsis. The process of cleaning consists in mechanic elimination of foreign matter from specific surfaces, by means of water, scrubbing, and detergents. If a surface is not mechanically clean, the following step of disinfection is hindered, as dust, soil, and organic debris prevent thorough contact between the surface to be disinfected and the decontaminating agent. Items recommended to be cleaned after each patient include OR table mat and sides, floor, trash buckets, instrument stands, whereas OR walls should be cleaned once a week and whenever directly splashed with contaminated material.

## OR Ventilation and Cleaning Procedures

Proper ventilation in and near the OR is fundamental in halting the spread of infection.[30] The standards for ventilation ensure good indoor air quality and establish limits for the following aspects: air flow, air filters, rate of air change, temperature, pressure relationship to adjacent areas and relative humidity.[31]

The type of ventilation system recommended is the laminar unidirectional vertical airflow with a primary degree of turbulence of < 5% and high-efficiency particulate-air filter.[32]

The air filter, consisting of a mat of randomly arranged glass-reinforced plastic fibers, should be placed in the ceiling and provide a constant vertical stream directed to the floor.

The rate of air change mainly dilutes the pollutants concentration. The minimum requirements for OR air change are 20–25 changes/h, with 4 changes/h of outdoor air. The OR must be maintained at a positive pressure with respect to all adjacent spaces.

The recommended air temperature is 21°C ± 3°C, with the possibility of control to optimize the comfort of the surgical team. While temperatures below 21°C put the patient in risk of becoming hypothermic and increase the chance of a postoperative infection, a temperature above 23°C is usually intolerable for the surgical team.

The relative humidity standards range from 30% to 60%, ideally set at 50–55%, considering the fact that lower relative humidity may result in sensation of dryness and irritation of skin and mucous membranes and increase human electric conductivity, whereas high relative humidity is related to microbial growth, especially fungal genera.

### *OR Sterilization*

Floor of the OR should be cleaned after each operative session with a phenolic solution. After contamination with material/fluids from an infected patient, wet mopping with phenolic detergent may be followed by wiping all equipment surfaces with 70% alcohol. Daily cleaning of shelves, ledges, and lights should be carried out. Anesthetic equipment must be disinfected after each use. Walls should be washed 3–6 monthly.

OR sterilization can be effectively done by using formaldehyde. About 10–15 oz of 40% formalin diluted with equal amount of water is added to 5 ounces of potassium permanganate for every 1000 ft$^3$ of space placed in a jar. The contact of reagents results in violent effervescence and release of formaldehyde. A vaporizer can also be used with 1:20 dilution of 40% formalin is vaporized over an hour.

## Care of Instruments

Instruments pass through a chain of procedures directed to ensure surgical asepsis, consisting of cleaning, disinfection, and sterilization performed within strict guidelines.[33]

### *Cleaning*

Thorough cleaning is an obligatory step before high-level disinfection and sterilization because inorganic and organic remains on the surfaces of instruments interfere with the effectiveness of these processes. Cleaning is also a good time to inspect each instrument for proper function and condition. Surgical instruments should be cleaned as soon as possible after their use. After separating delicate from regular instruments, ultrasonic or manual cleaning is performed.

*Ultrasonic cleaning:* The ultrasonic cleaner contains liquids through which sound waves disrupt the bonds that hold particulate matter to surfaces and clean every part of the instrument, including cannulae lumen. Dissimilar metals (such as aluminium and stainless) should not be mixed in the same cycle to prevent cross-plating. Chrome-plated instruments should not be cleaned in an ultrasonic cleaner. Upon completion of the cycle, instruments should be immediately removed, rinsed, and thoroughly dried, as trapped moisture produces corrosion.

*Manual cleaning:* Manual cleaning of delicate instruments is based on drench, friction, and fluidics. The instruments are soaked for half an hour in a neutral pH7 detergent, because low pH detergents cause breakdown of stainless protective surface and high pH detergent causes surface deposit of brown stain, which interferes with smooth operation of the instruments. The soiled area is afterward scrubbed with a soft brush and finally, fluids under pressure remove the debris. Gloves must be worn while handling the instruments to avoid infective material and cuts. Other forms of cleaning include washer/decontaminators, washer/disinfectors, and washer/sterilizers.

## *Disinfection and Sterilization*

Disinfection implies elimination of most pathogenic microorganisms (excluding bacterial spores) on surfaces and objects and sterilization refers to destruction of all living microorganisms, including spores. The effective use of disinfectants and sterilization procedures in the OR is critical for the prevention of postoperative infections. Medical devices that have contact with sterile body tissues or fluids are considered critical items and should be sterile when used because any microbial contamination could result in disease transmission.

Sterilization can be accomplished by physical or chemical methods.

- *Physical methods*: Of all the methods available for sterilization, moist heat under pressure (autoclaving) is the most widely used because it is nontoxic, dependable, and inexpensive. Saturated steam at a required temperature and pressure for a specified time in an autoclave is microbicidal and sporicidal, producing irreversible coagulation and denaturation of enzymes and structural proteins. The two common steam-sterilizing temperatures are 121°C (250°F) and 132°C (270°F). Recognized minimum exposure periods for sterilization of heat stable critical items are 30 minutes and 121°C in a gravity displacement sterilizer or 4 minutes at 132°C in a prevacuum sterilizer.[34] The process can be hastened by increasing the pressure from 15 psi to 30 psi.
- *Flash sterilization*: It is a method of emergency sterilization. The equipments to be decontaminated are kept at 132°C at 30 lbs of pressure for 3 minutes.
- *Chemical methods*: These are used for the sterilization of heat labile materials, include ethylene oxide (ETO), glutaraldehyde 2%, acetone, and plasma sterilization.
- *ETO*: ETO is a colorless gas that is flammable and explosive. The four operationals are gas concentration (450–1200 mg/L); temperature (37 °C–63 °C), relative humidity (40–80%), and exposure time (1–6 hours). The main disadvantages associated with ETO are the lengthy cycle time, the cost, and its potential hazards to patients and staff.
- *Glutaraldehyde 2%*: It is suitable for instruments that cannot be autoclaved like sharp cutting instruments, plastic and rubber items, and endoscopes. It is effective against vegetative pathogens in 15 minutes and resistant pathogenic spores in 3 hours. It is not recommended for lumen containing instruments such as irrigating cannulae as the residual glutaraldehyde, even after rinsing, causes corneal edema, endothelial cell damage, and uveitis. The recommended time period for effective sterilization is 8–10 hours. Articles can then be stored in a covered sterile container for up to 7 days.
- *Radiation*: Gamma irradiation is a method for cold sterilization with high penetrating power, which is lethal to DNA.
  - Sterilization control can be performed using physical, chemical, or biological methods.
    - Physical monitoring involves independent temperature, pressure, and vacuum, measurements performed automatically by the sterilizer by gauges and data loggers, throughout its cycle. Temperature and pressure readings should be taken at least three or four times during the sterilizing cycle, and the records kept until all tests are completed. Gauges and recorders should be calibrated at regular intervals against standard instruments.
    - Chemical indicators for steam sterilization are printed inks on packaging materials, or paper strips on which the chemical indicator is printed, placed inside packs being sterilized.
    - Biological indicators are the most accepted means of monitoring the sterilization process because they directly determine whether the most resistant microorganisms (e.g. spores of *Bacillus stearothermophilus* in autoclave and spores of Bacillus subtilis in ETO sterilization) are present rather than merely determine whether the physical and chemical conditions necessary for sterilization are met.

Disinfection is achieved using alcohols (ethyl alcohol, isopropyl alcohol, and methyl alcohol), aldehydes (formaldehyde, glutaraldehyde), phenols (5% phenol, hexachlorophene, chlorhexidine, chloroxylenol), halogens (chlorine, bleach, hypochlorite, tincture iodine, iodophors), heavy metals (mercuric chloride, silver nitrate, copper sulfate, organic mercury salts), surface active agents (anionic and cationic detergents), hydrogen peroxide, and dyes (aniline and acridine dyes).

### *Microbiological Monitoring of an OR*

Microbiology department plays a pivotal role in identifying the pathogens and monitoring the antibiotic regimen used. They should be updated with information on the antibiogram patterns from time to time. Swabs are collected from various locations in the OT and cultured for aerobic (chocolate agar) and anaerobic (Robertson's cooked meat medium) growth.

The areas swabbed include:

- Operation table at the head end
- Over head lamp
- Four Walls
- Floor below the head end of the table
- Instrument trolley
- AC duct
- Microscope handles

Asepsis in the OR complex is an issue regulated by local health authorities, and there might be slight differences between countries or even regions within the same country. Although OR complex design and architecture observe general guidelines, ventilation standards present different values in different countries; therefore, it is difficult to know the ideal limits of the individual requirements.

Asepsis in the OR is not a static concept.[35] It starts with constant following the recommended local regulations, passes through a relentless team effort involving nurses, surgeons, and anesthesiologists and continues with conscientious periodic monitoring and educational sessions to reinforce sterile technique.[36]

## REFERENCES


1. Allen HF. Aseptic technique in ophthalmology. Trans Am Ophthalmol Soc. 1959;57:377-472.
2. Speaker MG, Milch FA, Shah MK, et al. Role of external bacterial flora in the pathogenesis of acute postoperative endophthalmitis. Ophthalmology. 1991;98(5):639-49; discussion 650.
3. Miño De Kaspar H, Ta CN, Froehlich SJ, et al. Prospective study of risk factors for conjunctival bacterial contamination in patients undergoing intraocular surgery. Eur J Ophthalmol. 2009;19(5):717-22.
4. Ciulla TA, Starr MB, Masket S. Bacterial endophthalmitis prophylaxis for cataract surgery: an evidence-based update. Ophthalmology. 2002;109(1):13-24.
5. Speaker MG, Menikoff JA. Prophylaxis of endophthalmitis with topical povidone-iodine. Ophthalmology. 1991;98(12):1769-75.
6. Endophthalmitis Study Group, European Society of Cataract & Refractive Surgeons. Prophylaxis of postoperative endophthalmitis following cataract surgery: results of the ESCRS multicenter study and identification of risk factors. J Cataract Refract Surg. 2007;33(6):978-88.
7. Wu PC, Li M, Chang SJ, et al. Risk of endophthalmitis after cataract surgery using different protocols for povidone-iodine preoperative disinfection. J Ocul Pharmacol Ther. 2006;22(1):54-61.
8. Isenberg SJ. The ocular application of povidone-iodine. Community Eye Health. 2003;16(46):30-1.
9. Ferguson AW, Scott JA, McGavigan J, et al. Comparison of 5% povidone-iodine solution against 1% povidone-iodine solution in preoperative cataract surgery antisepsis: a prospective randomised double blind study. Br J Ophthalmol. 2013;57(1):74-9.
10. Inagaki K, Yamaguchi T, Ohde S, et al. Bacterial culture after three sterilization methods for cataract surgery. Jpn J Ophthalmol. 2013;57(1):74-9.
11. Ciulla TA, Starr MB, Masket S. Bacterial endophthalmitis prophylaxis for cataract surgery: an evidence-based update. Ophthalmology. 2002;109(1):13-24.
12. Webster J, Osborne S. Preoperative bathing or showering with skin antiseptics to prevent surgical site infection. Cochrane Database Syst Rev. 2012 Sep 12;9:CD004985. doi: 10.1002/14651858.CD004985.pub4.
13. Ritter MA, Eitzen H, French ML, et al. The operating room environment as affected by people and the surgical face mask. Clin Orthop Relat Res. 1975;111:147-50.
14. Bell RM. Surgical procedures, techniques and skills. In: Lawrence PF, Bell RM, Dayton MT, (eds), Essentials of general surgery, 4th edn. Philadelphia: Lippincott Williams & Wilkins, 2006 pp. 521-3.
15. Belkin NL. Home laundering of soiled surgical scrubs: surgical site infections and the home environment. Am J Infect Control. 2001;29(1):58-64.
16. Doshi RR, Leng T, Fung AE. Reducing oral flora contamination of intravitreal injections with face mask or silence. Retina. 2012;32(3):473-6.
17. Arrowsmith VA, Taylor R. Removal of nail polish and finger rings to prevent surgical infection. Cochrane Database Syst Rev. 2012 May 16;5:CD003325. doi: 10.1002/14651858.CD003325.pub2.
18. Jarral OA, McCormack DJ, Ibrahim S, et al. Should surgeons scrub with chlorhexidine or iodine prior to surgery? Interact Cardiovasc Thorac Surg. 2011;12(6):1017-21.
19. Tanner J, Swarbrook S, Stuart J. Surgical hand antisepsis to reduce surgical site infection. Cochrane Database Syst Rev. 2008 Jan 23;(1):CD004288. doi: 10.1002/14651858.CD004288.pub2.
20. Boyce JM, Pittet D. Guideline for hand hygiene in health-care settings. Recommendations of the healthcare infection control practices advisory committee and the HICPAC/SHEA/APIC/IDSA hand hygiene task force. MMWR—Morbidity & Mortality Weekly Report. 2002;51:1–45.
21. Lai KW, Foo TL, Low W, et al. Surgical hand antisepsis—a pilot study comparing povidone iodine hand scrub and alcohol-based chlorhexidine gluconate hand rub. Ann Acad Med Singapore. 2012;41(1):12-6.
22. Widmer AF. Surgical hand hygiene: scrub or rub? J Hosp Infect. 2013;83 Suppl 1:S35-9.

23. Parienti JJ, Thibon P, Heller R, et al. Hand-rubbing with an aqueous alcoholic solution vs traditional surgical hand-scrubbing and 30-day surgical site infection rates: a randomized equivalence study. JAMA. 2002;288(6):722-7.
24. Pittet D, Allegranzi B, Boyce J. The World Health Organization guidelines on hand hygiene in health care and their consensus recommendations. Infect Control Hosp Epidemiol. 2009;30(7):611-22.
25. Miller KM, Apt L. Unsuspected glove perforation during ophthalmic surgery. Arch Ophthalmol. 1993;111(2):186-93.
26. Drake CT, Goldman E, Nichols RL, et al. Environmental air and airborne infections. Ann Surg. 1977;185(2):219-23.
27. Ram J, Kaushik S, Brar GS, et al. Prevention of postoperative infections in ophthalmic surgery. Indian J Ophthalmol. 2001; 49:59-69.
28. Harsoor SS, Bashkar SB. Designing an ideal operating room complex. Indian J Anaesth. 2007;51(3):193-9.
29. Sharma S, Bansal AK, Gyanchand R. Asepsis in ophthalmic operating room. Indian J Ophthalmol. 1996;44(3):173-7.
30. Allo MD, Tedesco M. Operating room management: operative suite considerations, infection control. Surg Clin North Am. 2005;85(6):1291-7, xii.
31. Melhado MA, Jensen JLM, Loomans M, et al. Review of operating room ventilation standards. Proceedings of the 17th International air-conditioning and ventilation conference. Prague, 2006.
32. Center for Disease Control (CDC) and the Healthcare Infection Control Practices Advisory Committee (HICPAC). Guidelines for environmental infection control in health-care facilities. Atlanta, 2003. http://www.cdc.gov/hicpac/pubs.html. (Retrieved January 6, 2013).
33. Recommended practices for the care and cleaning of surgical instruments and powered equipment. AORN J. 1997;6:124-28 (Retrieved February 26, 2013).
34. Rutala WA, Weber DJ, and the Healthcare Infection Control Practices Advisory Committee (HICPAC). Guideline for disinfection and sterilization in healthcare facilities. Atlanta, 2008. http://www.cdc.gov/hicpac/pubs.html.
35. McWilliams RM. Divided responsibilities for operating room asepsis: the dilemma of technology. Med Instrum. 1976;10: 300-1.
36. Roesler R, Halowell CC, Elias G, et al. Chasing zero: our journey to preventing surgical site infection. AORN J. 2010;9:224-35.

C H A P T E R

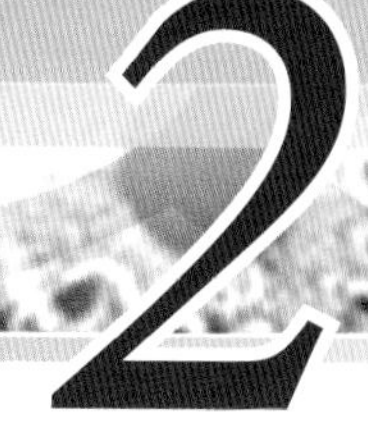

# Anesthesia for Ophthalmic Surgery

Abhilasha Solanki

## INTRODUCTION

Ophthalmic surgery presents unique set of challenges to anesthesiologists. The patient population varies from pediatric patients, often premature with multiple congenital anomalies to elderly patients with significant comorbidities. Patients with poor vision are especially apprehensive prior to surgery, and a detailed discussion of the anesthetic plan and expectations can be extremely valuable in their care. In this chapter, we will be reviewing the most relevant anesthetic concerns in ophthalmology, preoperative evaluation and preparation, regional and general anesthetic options, and anesthetic considerations for specific pediatric and adult ophthalmic procedures.

Ophthalmic anesthesia has come a long way. Mid-19th century saw the introduction of general anesthesia for ophthalmic surgery. In 1884, Koller introduced topical cocaine while Knapp pioneered retrobulbar anesthesia. In the beginning of 19th century, orbicularis block was introduced by Van Lint, O'Beriens, and Alkinson. Past 25 years have seen local anesthesia techniques progress from posterior peribulbar to 'no anesthesia' techniques for cataract extraction.

## RELEVANT ANATOMY, PHYSIOLOGY, AND PHARMACOLOGY

An anesthesiologist should have good working knowledge about the anatomy of the eye to be able to perform ophthalmic regional nerve blocks and to evaluate and manage any complications that arise from these.

### Anatomic Considerations

Adipose tissue forms the bulk of the orbit with the globe suspended in its anterior part. Four rectus muscles delimit the retrobulbar cone (with no intermuscular membrane). Sensory innervation of the globe is supplied by the ophthalmic nerve, the first branch of the trigeminal nerve, which passes through the muscular cone (Fig. 2-1). Motor extraocular nerves except the trochlear nerve pass through the muscular cone. Therefore, injecting local anesthetics inside the cone results in anesthesia and akinesia of the globe and of the extraocular muscles. Only the motor command of the orbicularis muscle of the eyelids has an extraorbital course as it arises from the superior branch of the facial nerve. Optic nerve with its meningeal sheaths; most of the arteries of the orbit; and the autonomic, sensory, and motor innervation of the globe are located in the muscular conus and are therefore vulnerable to the risk of needle injury.

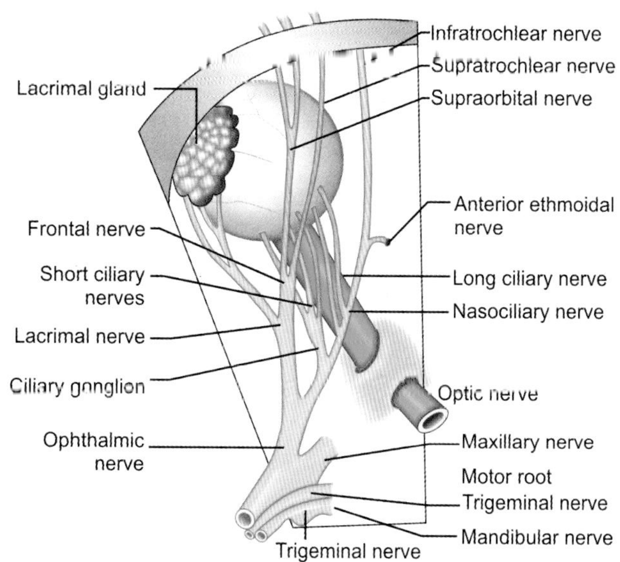


**Figure 2-1** Sensory innervation of the globe.

Tenon's capsule, a fibroelastic layer that surrounds the entire scleral portion of the globe, delimits the episcleral space or sub-Tenon space, a potential space with minimal volume.

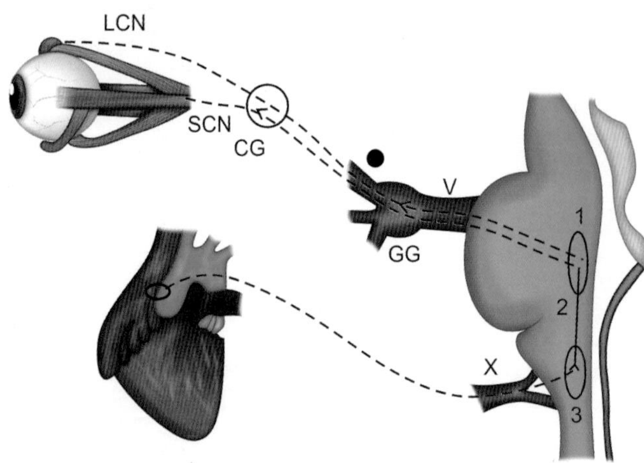


**Figure 2-2** Pathway for Oculocardiac reflex.
(LCN: Long ciliary nerve; SCN: Short ciliary nerve; CG: Ciliary ganglion; GG: Geniculate ganglion; V: Fifth cranial nerve; X: Tenth cranial nerve); (1) Main sensory nucleus of the trigeminal nerve; (2) Short internuncial fibers in the reticular formation (3) Motor nucleus of the vagus nerve).

Near the equator, the tendons of the oblique muscles and rectii perforate the Tenon's capsule before they insert into the sclera. At this point, there is continuity between the Tenon's capsule and the fascial sheath of the muscles. Anteriorly, the Tenon's capsule merges with the bulbar conjunctiva before both insert together into the corneal limbus.

Apart from this, knowledge of some physiology concepts is also imperative in ophthalmic anesthesia.

## Anesthesia and Oculocardiac Reflex (OCR)

Oculocardiac reflex is more common with general anesthesia than regional anesthesia. It is caused by traction on the extra-ocular muscles, manipulation of the globe, and increase in intra-ocular pressure (IOP). It is most often described in strabismus surgery, but it is also prevalent in retinal detachment repair and enucleation. It can manifest as arrhythmias such as bradycardia, ectopics, bigeminy, nodal rhythms, atrioventricular block, and asystole. These may persist as long as the stimulus persists and often times, repeated stimuli cause fatigue with diminished vagal effects.

- *Pathway of OCR*: Its afferent pathway is via the ciliary ganglion to the ophthalmic division of the trigeminal nerve, through the gasserion ganglion to the trigeminal nucleus in the fourth ventricle. The efferent pathway is via the vagus nerve (Fig. 2-2).
- *Diagnosis of OCR*: This requires continuous monitoring of the electrocardiogram.
- *Treatment of OCR*: The severity of the OCR determines the treatment needed. If the patient is hemodynamically stable despite having a bradycardia or any other rhythm disturbance, no treatment is warranted. However, is the patient becomes unstable due to these dysrhythmias, treatment is warranted. First and foremost, cessation of surgical stimulus is indicated. If symptoms persist despite this, treatment with an anticholinergic agent such as atropine or glycopyrrolate is indicated. Caution must be exercised with large doses of atropine since this may on rare occasions result in long lasting severe tachyarrhythmias.

## Other Oculomedullary Reflexes

- *Oculorespiratory reflex*: This may cause shallow breathing, reduced respiratory rate, and even full respiratory arrest. The afferent pathways are similar to OCR and it is thought that a connection exists between the trigeminal sensory nucleus and the pneumotaxic center in the pons and medullary respiratory center. This reflex is also commonly seen in strabismus surgery, and atropine has no effect
- *Oculoemetic reflex*: This reflex is likely responsible for the high incidence of vomiting after squint surgery (60–90%). This is also a trigeminovagal reflex with traction on the extraocular muscles stimulating the afferent arc. Although antiemetics may reduce the incidence, a regional block technique provides the best prophylaxis

## Anesthesia and IOP

Intraocular pressure is exerted by the contents of the eye and is mainly determined by the aqueous humor and blood vessels especially of the choroid. Choroidal vessels constrict as a result of hyperventilation or hypocapnia and hence decrease IOP. In contrast, they dilate as a result of hypoventilation or hypercapnia and hence increase IOP. Similarly, hypoxia causes vasodilation of choroidal vessels causing an increase in IOP.

Normal IOP is 16 + 5 mm Hg in the sitting position and is generally maintained in this range. IOP undergoes minor fluctuations as a result of:

- Changes in body position (+1 mm Hg when supine).
- Diurnal rhythm (2–3 mm Hg).
- Blood pressure oscillations. Hypertension increases and hypotension decreases IOP.
- Respiration (deep inspiration can decrease IOP up to 5 mm Hg).

Possible causes of increase in IOP during anesthesia:

- Acute venous congestion obstructing aqueous outflow (straining, bucking, breath holding or obstructed airway during induction of emergence from general anesthesia).
- Valsalva maneuvers.
- Endotracheal intubation.

- External pressure on the eye from face mask, fingers, tumor, bleed.
- *Side effects of anesthetic medications*: Inhalational and intravenous agents have the most pronounced effect on IOP. Deep inhalational anesthesia or thiopental and propofol reduce the IOP by 30–40% in a dose-related fashion.[1] Narcotics cause a small decrease in IOP. Ketamine may cause an increase in IOP as result of an increase in blood pressure.[2] Succinylcholine causes a 6–12 mm Hg increase in IOP, which can be sustained for 5–10 minutes.[3] This increase has been ascribed to contraction of the extraocular muscles leading to globe compression. This can cause extrusion of orbital contents in a patient with open globe injury. Hence, succinylcholine is avoided in patients with open globe injuries.

## Anesthetic Implications of Ophthalmic Medications

Ophthalmic drugs given topically are absorbed slowly from the conjunctival sac. They are rapidly absorbed via the mucosal surfaces of the nasolacrimal duct and can hence manifest systemic effects.

- Topical beta-blockers such as timolol are commonly used in the treatment of glaucoma. Systemic effects include cardiovascular symptoms like palpitations, syncope, or signs of congestive heart failure.[4] They may also cause central nervous system depression and manifest light headedness and fatigue. Rare cases of apnea in neonates receiving these eye drops have been reported.
- Topical alpha-2 adrenergic agonists such as apraclonidine is used in the treatment of glaucoma. Systemic effects include sedation, drowsiness, and hypotension. Like other alpha-2 agonists, acute withdrawal of this may result in severe hypertension.
- Topical anticholinesterase drugs like echothiophate are used in the treatment of glaucoma. Echothiophate has a long duration of action varying between 4 and 6 weeks. Three weeks after cessation of treatment with this drug, plasma cholinesterase activity is 50% of normal. Hence, administration of usual doses of drugs metabolized by plasma cholinesterase (succinylcholine, ester type local anesthetics like procaine, chloroprocaine, cocaine) results in overdose and prolonged duration of action. Amide-type local anesthetics would hence be a better choice of local anesthetic for regional nerve blocks.
- Topical muscarinic drugs such as atropine and scopolamine are used to produce mydriasis. Systemic side effects include tachycardia, dryness of mouth, eyes, skin, and flushing. Elderly patients may manifest central nervous system side effects including central nervous system excitement and agitation, which requires treatment with physostigmine
- Topical adrenergic agonists such as phenylephrine and epinephrine are used in the treatment of glaucoma can produce systemic effects such as hypertension, dysrhythmias, myocardial infarction, and syncope.[4]
- Carbonic anhydrase inhibitors such as acetazolamide used in the treatment of glaucoma cause alkaline diuresis resulting in potassium depletion. Serum electrolytes should therefore be checked preoperatively in these patients.

**TABLE 2-1:** Basic preoperative assessment

| |
|---|
| • History of presenting illness and indication for surgery |
| • Past medical history |
| • Past surgical history |
| • Family history |
| • Social history, especially smoking and alcohol consumption |
| • Allergies |
| • List of current medications |
| • Physical examination—Vital signs, heart sounds, and breath sounds |

## Preanesthetic Evaluation

All patients must provide a complete history and undergo a complete physical examination before any surgical procedure. Ophthalmic surgeries although considered low-risk procedures are no exception to this (Table 2-1).

Ideally, this assessment should be performed by an anesthesiologist or a certified practitioner and should be available for review a day or two prior to the procedure.

The most common ophthalmic surgery done worldwide is cataract surgery. If a patient is undergoing this under local anesthesia and has no medical issues, no laboratory testing is needed. However, there are certain criteria that should be met (Table 2-2).

In other words consider general anesthesia, in cases of:

- Patient refusal
- Local sepsis
- Perforated globe
- Grossly abnormal coagulation
- Severe reaction, allergy, or other complications associated with local anesthesia
- Inability to communicate or to comply with instructions
- Uncontrolled tremor
- Inability to adopt acceptable positioning.

It is a well-known fact that routine laboratory testing has no value unless indicated by physical examination. The American Society of Anesthesiologists task Force on Preoperative Evaluation has come up with some suggestions listed in Table 2-3.[5]

**TABLE 2-2:** Patient criteria to be fulfilled prior to cataract surgery under local anesthesia

| |
|---|
| • Able to lie flat for 45 minutes |
| • No history of or controlled gastroesophageal reflux |
| • Absence of neuropsychiatric disturbances such as dementia, claustrophobia |
| • Absence of head and neck tremors |
| • Absence of chronic uncontrollable cough |
| • Ability to communicate well in English or some other language |

**TABLE 2-3:** Preoperative evaluation

| |
|---|
| • *Electrocardiogram*: Signs of new or unstable cardiac disease; none within the last year in a patient with diabetes, hypertension, angina, heart failure, smoking, poor functional capacity, peripheral vascular disease |
| • *Serum electrolytes*: Long standing diuretics, digoxin, diuretics, or diarrhea |
| • *Serum glucose*: Polydipsia, polyuria, or weight loss |
| • *Hematocrit*: History of bleeding, anemia, fatigue, or poor oral intake |
| • *Coagulation studies*: History of coagulopathy or use of anticoagulants |

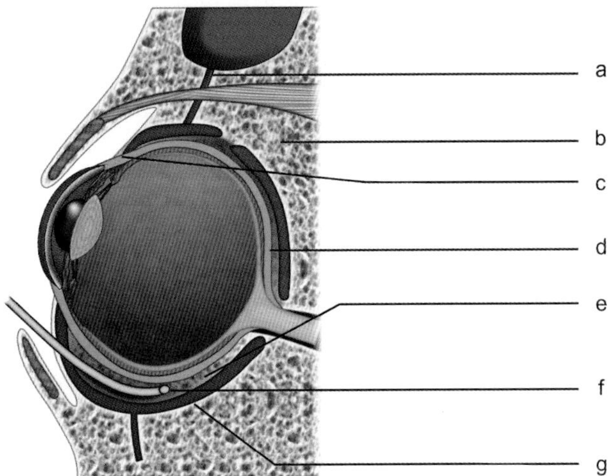

**Figure 2-3** Schematic diagram of Sub-Tenon's space, with the cannula (f) positioned to deliver local anaesthetic agent posterior to the globe, into the base of the retro-orbital cone.
(a: Orbital septum; b: Superior rectus perforating Tenon's capsule; c: Conjunctiva; d, sclera; e: Sub-Tenon's space; f: Cannula; g: Tenon's capsule).

## Types of Regional Anesthesia for Ophthalmic Surgery

- *Subconjunctival block*: Also known as perilimbal block. This block is not preferred much as there is anesthesia with no akinesia.
- *Sub-Tenon's block*: Most popular technique for regional anesthesia in eye surgery, now-a-days. This block is also known as parabulbar block, pinpoint anesthesia, and medial episcleral block. Under topical anesthesia, a buttonhole is made into the conjunctiva and Tenon's capsule about 5–10 mm from the limbus. A blunt cannula is then inserted in the episcleral space and the anesthetic mixture injected (Fig. 2-3).[6] As per the literature, the inferonasal quadrant is the most common site of access, as the placement of cannula in this quadrant allows good fluid distribution superiorly while avoiding the area of access for surgery and damage to the vortex veins. The patient is asked to look upward and outward.

Injection of local anesthetic agent under the Tenon's capsule blocks sensation from the eye by action on the short ciliary nerves as they pass through the Tenon's capsule to the globe. Akinesia is obtained by direct blockade of anterior motor nerve fibers as they enter the extraocular muscles. Vision may be affected by direct action on the optic nerve as the anesthetic solution diffuses along its anterior portion.

- *Peribulbar block (extraconal block)*: Suitable for those patients in whom a sub-Tenon's block is relatively contraindicated. These include patients with previous scleral banding and detachment surgery, medial rectus, or pterygium surgery, and care must also be taken in high myopes because of the occasional presence of staphylomata and/or scleral thinning.[7] The most common sites for needle insertion are medial canthus, lacrimal caruncle, and inferior and temporal peribulbar injections.
- *Topical and intracameral anesthesia*: Use of topical anesthesia should be limited to uncomplicated procedures performed by experienced surgeons in cooperative patients
- *Retrobulbar block (intraconal block)*: Obsolete.

The choice of technique will depend on a balance between the patient's wishes, the operative needs of the surgeon, the anesthetist, and the place where such surgery is being performed.

## Complications of Regional Blocks

Complications may result either from the agents used or the block technique itself.[8]

- *Intravascular injection and anaphylaxis*: Although rare, this complication may occur, hence resuscitation facilities must always be readily available.
- *Retrobulbar hemorrhage*: This is characterized by rapid orbital swelling and proptosis along with a sudden rise of IOP and usually requires surgery to be postponed. The surgeon should be informed immediately, and the pulsation of the central retinal artery assessed. A lateral canthotomy can be performed to alleviate the rise in IOP.

- *Perforation of the globe (< 0.1%)*: This is more likely to occur in myopic eyes. A diagnosis of perforation is made in the presence of excruciating pain at the time of the block associated with sudden loss of vision, hypotonia, a poor red reflex or vitreous hemorrhage. For orbital injections, the risk may be minimized by avoiding injection into the highly vascular orbital apex and normally using fine (25- or 26-gauge) and short needles (not longer than 25 mm) and carefully inserting the needle tangentially and by not going "up and in" until the needle tip is clearly past the equator of the globe.[9]
- *Central spread of local anesthetic*: This is due to either direct injection into the dural cuff, which accompanies the optic nerve to the sclera or to retrograde arterial spread. Symptoms may range from drowsiness, vomiting, contralateral blindness caused by reflux of the drug to the optic chiasma, convulsions, respiratory depression or arrest, neurological deficit, and even cardiac arrest.
- *Injury to optic nerve or central retinal artery*: Injection should be given in the less vascular orbital compartments such as the inferotemporal or nasal sites with the eye in the straight-ahead position.
- *Allergy*: Although uncommon, allergy to hyaluronidase injected during ophthalmic blocks should be considered in the differential diagnosis of patients who present with acute postoperative orbital swelling and inflammation.
- *"Mobile" eye*: Seen mostly with topical anesthesia; may result in surgical difficulty; this can be minimized by careful preoperative selection, appropriate preoperative and intraoperative measures.

## CONCLUSION

The scope of anesthesia practice in the field of ophthalmology has been expanding. Decreased operating times and increasing complex eye surgeries rely on well-administered anesthesia. There is hence a constant need for newer innovations in anesthetic medications and techniques. Best practice dictates that in all cases an intravenous cannula is inserted to allow immediate venous access in case of emergency. The ultimate goal is to provide high quality, safe, and comprehensive patient care.

## REMEMBER[10]

- Patients need not fast prior to local anesthesia for eye surgery without sedation.
- Patients should have their normal medication on the day of surgery.
- Hypoglycemia must be avoided in diabetic patients. Local protocols must be developed to cater for patients having surgery later in the day.
- The minimum monitoring (e.g. for a fit person having routine surgery under topical anesthesia) is clinical observation, communication, and pulse oximetry.
- Electrocardiogram and blood pressure should be monitored in sedated patients and those who are at risk of cardiovascular complications (e.g. hypertensives, patients with pacemaker, diabetes).
- Sedation should only be used to allay anxiety and not to cover inadequate blocks.
- All patients are advised to have a friend or relative to accompany them to surgery and at discharge, and this is essential for those who are frail and elderly.
- All theater personnel should have regular training in Basic Life Support.

## REFERENCES


1. Deramoudt V, Gaudon M, Malledant Y, et al. Effect of propofol on IOP in strabismus surgery in children. Ann FrAnesthReanim. 1990; 9:1.
2. Nagdeve NG, Yaddanapudi S, Pandav SS. The effect of different doses of ketamine on intraocular pressure in anesthetized children. J Pediatr Ophthalmol Strabismus.2006;43(4):219-23.
3. Khosravi MB, Lahsaee M, Azemati S, et al. Intraocular pressure changes after succinylcholine and endotracheal intubation: a comparison of thiopental and propofol on IOP. Indian J Ophthalmol. 2007;55(2):164.
4. Coppens G, Stalmans I, Zeyen T, et al. The safety and efficacy of glaucoma medication in the pediatric population. J Pediatr Ophthalmol Strabismus. 2009;46(1):12-8.
5. American Society of Anesthesiologists Task Force on Preanesthesia Evaluation. Practice advisory for preanesthesia evaluation: a report by the American Society of Anesthesiologists Task Force on Preanesthesia Evaluation. Anesthesiology. 2002; 96:485-96.
6. Davison M, Padroni S, Bunce C, et al. Sub-Tenon's anaesthesia versus topical anaesthesia for cataract surgery. Cochrane Database Syst Rev. 2007;18:CD006291.
7. Ryu JH, Kim M, Bahk JH, et al.: A comparison of retrobulbar block, sub-Tenon block, and topical anesthesia during cataract surgery. Eur J Ophthalmol. 2009; 19:240-6.
8. Eke T, Thompson JR. The National Survey of Local Anaesthesia for Ocular Surgery. II. Safety profiles of local anaesthesia techniques. Eye. 1999;13:196-204.
9. Edge R, Navon S. Scleral perforation during retrobulbar and peribulbar anesthesia: risk factors and outcome in 50,000 consecutive injections. J Cataract Refract Surg. 1999;25:1237-44.
10. Kumar CM, Eke T, Dodds C, et al. Local anaesthesia for ophthalmic surgery. Joint guidelines from the Royal College of Anaesthetists and the Royal College of Ophthalmologists. Eye (Lond). 2012;26(6):897-8.

CHAPTER 3

# Operating Microscopes and Surgical Loupes

Mohammad Hosein Nowroozzadeh, M Reza Razeghinejad

## INTRODUCTION

Operating microscopes have become an essential tool in ophthalmic surgery. Their development has revolutionized eye surgery from historical intracapsular cataract surgery (that used to be done without magnification) toward the current standard of small incision phacoemulsification. The microscopes also offer high magnification and detail recognition that are fundamental to most sophisticated vitreoretinal surgeries. Modern operating microscopes are optically superb, provide effective illumination sources, and highly accommodate the surgeon's ergonomics.[1,2] Surgical loupes are less frequently used magnifiers, with advantages and disadvantages compared with the operating microscopes, making them suitable for distinct situations.

## OPERATING MICROSCOPES

Operating microscopes are either ceiling or floor mounted.[3] Ceiling-mounted microscopes are useful when an operating room is dedicated to ophthalmic microsurgery. They do not pose physical obstacle in the operating room and are easily positioned over the patient's head. On the other hand, floor-mounted microscopes have the great advantage in that they can be moved from room to room. Both types share most other technical features.[1]

### Optical Components

An operating microscope is composed of the following optical components. Astronomical telescope incorporated within the eyepiece and is the main source of magnification. Inverting prism compensates for the inverted image produced by the astronomical telescope (e.g. Porro–Abbe prism). Galilean telescope is a magnification changer in which different lenses can be introduced. Zoom lens is incorporated in most microscopes and smoothly varies magnification without changing the focus. Objective lens adjusts the working distance. Binocular viewing system composed of two parallel optical systems, each a mirror image of the other, to offer a stereoptic view of the patient's eye.[4] Illumination sources are discussed in the following sections.

### Optical Characteristics

#### *Apochromatic Optics*

Modern operating microscopes incorporate apochromatic lenses to correct chromatic and spherical aberrations, allowing a superb optical performance and excellent image quality.[3] In addition, exposed lenses (such as the objective lens and oculars) are equipped with antistain and water shedding coatings to warrant a consistent and durable optical quality.[5]

#### *Magnification and Field of View*

The total magnification of a particular system is the product of the magnification of its optical subsystems.[4] Eyepieces are usually available at 8.33×, 10×, and 12.5× magnifications.[6] The most popular eyepiece for ophthalmic operating microscopes is 12.5×.[4] Based on the other optical components of the operating microscope, it (12.5×) can offer a range of magnification of 6× to 40×.[4] Zoom Galilean telescopes (smoothly variable magnification changers) are incorporated into many operating microscopes, allowing continuous change in the magnification.[4] The zoom ratio is usually set at around 1:6,[3,6] and the focusing range is approximately 50 mm.[3,6]

To accomplish a good focus, the microscope positioning handles (gross focusing) or the motorized system (fine focusing) can be used through Z-axis. The motorized X–Y coupling system allows moving the center of focus in the X–Y axes, and usually ranges from 25 × 25 mm to 61 × 61 mm.[3,6] It, therefore, facilitates the compensation for minor patient movements and changing the operating axis toward different targets to bring the image of interest into the central field during high magnification surgeries.

Increasing the magnification is accompanied by inevitable decrease in the field of view and vice versa. Based on the chosen magnification, the field diameter ranges between approximately 7–80 mm.[6] Although high magnifications offer better discrimination of details, the large field of view allows better appreciation of the surgical field as a whole. Therefore, the surgeon should choose an optimal equilibration between these two parameters to accomplish an optimal qualification for a particular step of the surgery. The most comfortable position is achieved by allowing the target tissue being on both the center of the field and optimal point of focus.

### *Depth of Field*

Depth of field describes a layer that is relatively in focus. In other words, depth of field is the distance between the nearest and farthest object plane with a focused image. Objects located outside the depth of field are unacceptably blurred.[4] In operating microscopes, depth of field is primarily determined by the amount of magnification. Depth of field grows thinner with increased magnification and vice versa. Besides the effect of magnification, depth of field is also influenced by the accommodative reserve of the surgeon and the diameter of the aperture that the light passes through.[4] Young surgeons usually have better accommodative reserve and enhanced depth of field in a given magnification than the senior surgeons who may need multiple focus readjustments while doing surgery under high magnification. However, young beginner surgeons tend to accommodate through the microscope. Sustained accomodation through the microscope is not ideal because it results in fatigue. It could be partially overcome by a defocusing/refocusing maneuver.[1] Decreasing the size of the aperture that light travels through will increase depth of field via the pinhole effect, in exchange for decreasing contrast secondary to lower light transmission.[4] The depth of field management system used in some devices allows the surgeon to choose between maximum depth of field or optimum light transmission.[3]

As a practical point of view, depth of field is not very important when the surgery is performed on a thin plane (e.g. capsulorrhexis, or internal limiting membrane peeling) while it is of utmost importance when the surgery involves a relatively thick plain (e.g. sculpting or removal of vitreous strands). As a result, the former procedures are best performed under high magnification, whereas the latter ones require a better depth of field, and hence, a relatively lower magnification should be applied.

### *Working Distance*

The working distance is the distance from the objective lens to the patient's eye. It is equal to the focal length of the objective lens.[4] For ophthalmic operating microscopes, the working distance is usually set at 150, 175, 200, or 225 mm.[3,4,6] It is important to note that even a 25-mm difference in working distance between different systems can greatly influence the operating surgeon ergonomics.[4]

## Constituents

Each modern operating microscope is composed of several sophisticated constituents that offer its optimal functionality for all purpose ocular surgeries. Operating microscopes are generally composed of a head (which includes optical constituents, Figure 3-1), a trunk (usually with an interactive touch screen), a positioning arm, and a stand (either ceiling mounted or floor stand). Most important constituents with important implications for proper use by the operating staff are discussed here.

### *Positioning Arms and Handles*

The head of the microscope is placed on a swinging positioning arm. The arm has various pivot points that can be released or tightened to allow flexibility and stability in positioning the microscope head. The counterweight setting is an important control on the microscope arm that determines the vertical excursion of the head of microscope when positioned and released.[1] Each microscope has two positioning handles usually covered with slide-on covers that can be sterilized (Fig. 3-1).[3,5,6] In some systems, magnetic brakes are incorporated that make positioning the surgical microscope very easy when released.[3,6]

### *Foot Pedals*

Foot pedals (Fig. 3-2) generally consist of a joystick to maneuver the scope in the X–Y axis, a tab to control the magnification, and a tab to control the fine focus. Some also have a switch to turn the light on and off and even buttons to gauge

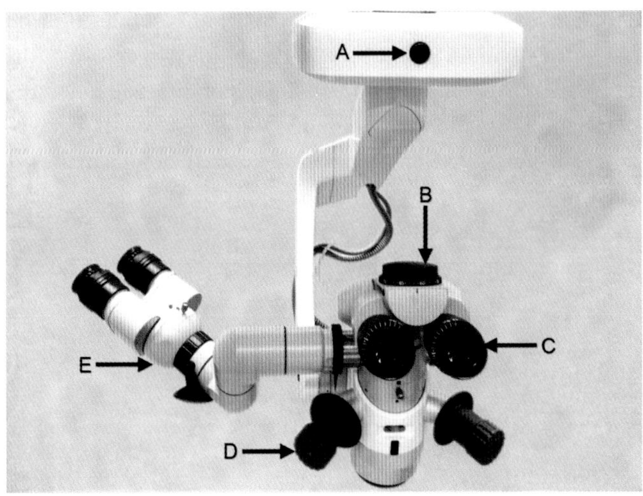


**Figure 3-1** Microscope head, (A) centering button, (B) scale to adjust the pupil distance of the oculars, (C) oculars with built-in scale to adjust the surgeon's refractive error, (D) positioning handles with autoclavable covers, and (E) the assistant arm.

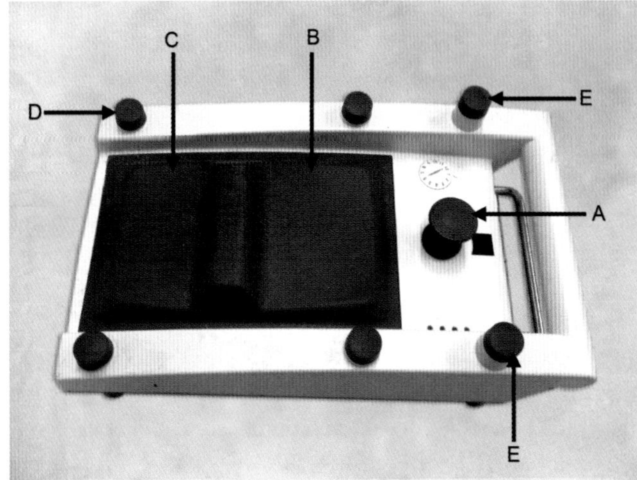


**Figure 3-2** A typical wireless microscope foot pedal. (A) X–Y joystick, (B) focus tab, (C) zoom tab, (D) light on/off switch, and (E) illumination intensity adjustment tabs. The tabs are reprogrammable based on specific surgeon preferences.

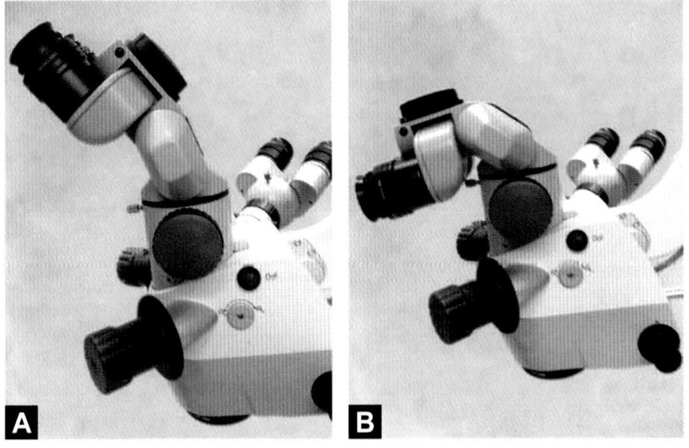


**Figures 3-3A and B** An operating microscope with a tiltable eyepiece. (A) The eyepiece placed in an oblique position (approximately 45° position). (B) The eyepiece dropped downward to assume a near-parallel position (approximately –10° position).

the illumination intensity. These options inhibit unnecessary interruptions (i.e. focusing by hand) during surgery and enhance the versatility of the microscope. Newer devices have a reprogrammable foot pedal in which the buttons can be customized according to surgeon's personal requirements or preferences.[1-3,5,6]

## Centering Button

The centering button is placed on the head of microscope and is used to center the X–Y axes, magnification, and focus. It should be pressed at the beginning of each operation to give full excursion ability in all directions during operation.[2,3,5,6]

## Eyepieces

Microscope eyepieces (oculars) have three important parameters to be set at the start of surgery. Pupil distance (PD) needs to be adjusted based on the surgeon's PD. Diopter setting of ocular lenses, most oculars have a range of +/- 5.00 diopters, and each ocular can be set independently to accommodate the surgeon's anisometropia.[1,6] Alternatively, the surgeon can wear his or her spectacle and set oculars on zero.[1] In addition, surgeons with symmetric low refractive error (e.g. -1.00 diopter in both eyes) can take off their spectacles and set oculars on zero and compensate for their refractive error by changing the working distance of the microscope at the start of surgery, or do focusing during surgery. The latter approach is acceptable when the surgeon has no assistant/trainee at the assistant arm, because an emmetropic assistant will be driven defocused. The third parameter is tilt. Conventional microscopes have oculars inclined approximately 45°. Newer devices provide oculars that can be tilted even up to 180°,[3] to provide the optimal ergonomics for different surgeons (Figs. 3-3A and B). A near parallel position is usually preferred for lengthy operations such as vitreoretinal surgeries.[3] The ocular may be dropped or lifted slightly from the parallel position to help achieve the best position in a short or tall surgeon, respectively.

## Illumination Source

Traditionally, light source was provided with a halogen lamp. Although, halogen bulbs (single or dual) are still frequently used,[3,5,6] some newer systems offer xenon or light emitting diode (LED) light sources as their main illumination system.[3,6] Xenon light allows the surgeon to see the anatomic structure of the eye in its natural colors and highly accurate details.[3] LED light sources are claimed to have lower energy consumption and longer lifespan (about 60,000 hours).[6] Integrating various light sources in a single system, as provided in some modern devices, is particularly beneficial when several surgeons with different preferences regarding the light source use one microscope.[3,6] Alternatively, other devices use only one light source (Xenon or LED), but integrated specialized filters offer a halogen like illumination when flipped in.[3,6] Modern operating microscopes use cold light by fiber-optic delivery system that reduce heat at the microscope head and allows easier change of bulbs during surgery.[3,4] New systems with halogen bulbs have the facility of automatically changing the burned bulb with the backup one, allowing an uninterrupted surgery.[3]

The sophisticated optics within the illumination systems offer the flexibility to project the light to the eye in different directions.[3,5,6] The most well-known illumination system is coaxial illumination, in which the microscope light is emitted vertically to the eye, thus highlighting intraocular structures with retroillumination (red reflex).[4] This type of illumination is especially useful to view the hardly visible structures such as posterior capsule, the vitreous, and fluid interfaces such as the presence of residual viscoelastic in the eye.[3,4,7] Traditional microscopes used near coaxial illuminations (e.g. approximately 2° off a truly coaxial viewing alignment) to offer both retroillumination and enough oblique lighting angle to induce minor shadows around structures, important to highlight depth and contrast.[7] Newer systems have two distinct illumination beam angles that can be switched on or off separately, an oblique field illumination (approximately 4°–6° off-axis),[3,5] and a truly coaxial illumination beam.[3,5,7] Providing separate illumination paths offers full benefits of both oblique- and retroillumination. The so-called stereo coaxial illumination (SCI) system uses two separate coaxial light paths that are individually aligned with each microscope ocular, maximizing the retroillumination even with strongly pigmented, decentered, and ametropic eyes.[3] The SCI is claimed to allow having an acceptable retroillumination with very little light that may decrease the risk of retinal light toxicity in lengthy operations.[3]

Coaxial illumination is particularly useful when the lens capsule need to be visualized as in capsulorrhexis step or checking out a posterior capsule tear.[7] In the presence of corneal opacities, the oblique field illumination can render large amount of backscatter light that could visually wash out the red reflex, then it is useful to turn the oblique light off to enhance red reflex.[7] Nearly, in all steps of phacoemulsification (including sculpting, chopping, and segment removal), the combination of coaxial and oblique options will offer the optimal illumination to highlight contrast and depth perception. The oblique field option could be used alone when working on ocular surface (e.g. corneal suturing) to decrease the transmission of light to the retina.

Besides the above-mentioned characteristics, the illumination system should be adequately intense at maximum power, adjustable, and have special filters to absorb unnecessary ultra violet (UV) and infrared (IR) lights and subsequently protect the patient and surgeon from phototoxic damage.[3,5,6]

### *Retinal Light Toxicity*

Nowadays, with the sophisticated components of modern microscopes, retinal light toxicity is encountered quite rarely. Newer microscopes with apochromatic lenses render such advanced optics that reduces the need for high illumination to achieve a good visualization. But it is important to know that some situations increase the risk, and coincidence of a number of such situations may render a remarkable risk.

The most important risk factors for retinal light toxicity are (1) clear media, the presence of cataract is somehow protective against phototoxicity at the start of the cataract surgery, the risk increases after cataract removal (aphakia) and is maximized after intraocular lens placement (emmetropia combined with clear media), (2) full dilated pupil, (3) lengthy operation, (4) constant exposure, and (5) setting up the microscope light at the maximum (higher energy), as most beginning surgeons do.[7,8] The retinal light transmission could be minimized by covering the pupil or using target shape light with central dark circle while working on the sclera or conjunctiva.

## Accessories

Several accessories to the ophthalmic microscopes have been developed. Based on the type of the accessories attached to a system, it may be specialized for a particular purpose such as teaching, anterior segment and cataract surgery, or vitreoretinal surgery.[6]

### *Stereoscopic Assistant (Teaching) Arm*

Stereoscopic teaching arms help the assistant to see exactly what is going on during the surgery and is essential when the assistant should perform surgical maneuvers such as scleral depression.[2] Most microscopes use a beam splitter that splits the light usually in a 70:30 ratio between the surgeon and assistant.[6] Newer systems, however, use independent light sources for the surgeon and the assistant providing 100% stereo and 100% illumination to both. Some systems offer the advantage of a separate focusing ability for the teaching arm, which is extremely useful where a presbyopic surgeon is accompanied by a young trainee (who has much more accommodation).[2,3]

### *Camera and Monitor*

The availability of a high-quality camera linked to a recording apparatus, helps document surgical procedures (image or video). Some devices also show the video image on a built-in monitor.[3] These options are especially useful where the trainees are involved. Some devices have the advantage of a foot-operated pedal for capturing image during procedure.[2]

### *Vitreoretinal Viewing Systems*

They typically use a front loupe that is aligned coaxially with the operating microscope and a specialized integrated inverter, which rectifies the inverted image provided by the front loupe.[3,5,6] These systems incorporate the principle of indirect ophthalmoscopy in the operating microscope.[9] The concept is similar to using a noncontact fundus lenses to view the fundus through the slit-lamp. However, during surgery an inverted image is not acceptable and should be rectified with the associated inverter of vitreoretinal viewing systems. These systems originally referred as Binocular Indirect Ophthalmo Microscope that obviates the use of retinal contact lenses during vitreoretinal surgery.[9] Usually, multiple lenses with different available powers to offer both the high magnification and wide-angle view are available.[5,6,9]

### *Motorized Fiber Slit Illuminator*

It is an ideal illumination system for bimanual vitreoretinal surgery, allowing great visualization of membranes and vitreous strands. With the standard wide illumination systems, it is difficult to appreciate the clear vitreous or operate on epiretinal membranes. The slit illumination provides both direct and indirect illuminations and also spread shadows of intraocular structures and instruments. With this, sophisticated vitreoretinal procedures can be performed more easily and safely. In fact, depth perception is maximized with a slit light source. When using this option as the light source for vitreoretinal surgery, an endoillumination is unnecessary and the nondominant hand is freed to hold second instrument for intricate maneuvers. The angle of illumination usually travels +/- 23–30°, the slit beam rotates 180°, and the slit width adjusts from 0.01 to a maximum of 15–20 mm.[3,5,6]

### *Filters*

Heat-absorbing, IR, and UV cut filters are usually built in to reduce light toxicity and improve the quality of image.[3,5,6] Other accessory filters that may be useful in particular situations often could be flip-in/out. The most popular filters are (1) laser filters, (2) fluorescence filter, used for intraoperative fluorescein observation,[3] (3) blue blocking filter, [3,6] (4) yellow filter, to allow full protection against retinal phototoxicity,[5] (5) halogen mode filter, incorporated in some systems and set the original xenon light to halogen wavelength, if the surgeon is more convenient with traditional halogen lights,[3] and (6) color temperature filter, enhances visibility and provides a more natural color tone.[5]

### *Others*

As the ongoing development in technology is combined with new demands of novel surgical techniques, new accessories are unceasingly evolved. The toric eye piece provided by some systems is an eyepiece incorporated with a built-in rotatable scale, the image of which is superimposed over the microscope image and helps the surgeon to find the correct toric intraocular lens positioning angle.[6] The keratoscope is mounted onto some ophthalmic microscopes and helps assess the shape of the anterior surface of the cornea intraoperatively.[6] The head-up data display allows that images from digital sources be projected directly into the surgeon's eyepiece, thus showing data exactly where the surgeon needs it.[6]

## Ergonomics

The surgeon, assistant, and patient should be set up properly and comfortably before the procedure starts. This is of particular importance in the setting of local or topical anesthesia. Good positioning is fundamental to both patient and surgeon safety.[1,2]

### *Patient Positioning*

Whether the surgical approach is temporal or superior, the patient's head should be positioned in such a way that the corneal surface of the operative eye is paralleled to the floor. Surgical beds with separate headrest (with its own adjustment system) and upper and lower body parts are ideal for this purpose. Also, these beds have the flexibility to maintain

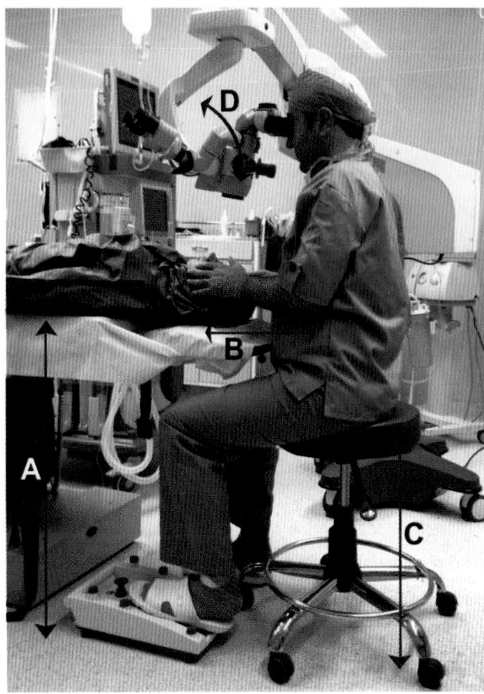


**Figure 3-4** Surgeon positioning at the superior position. Four parameters that should be adjusted are (a) height of the bed, (b) distance of the surgeon from patient's head (note that the head is placed over the surgeon's thigh), (c) height of the surgeon's chair, and (d) microscope head tilt. In a correct positioning as shown here, the surgeon is comfortably seated with the legs adequately cleared of the table, almost erect torso and head position, and dropped shoulder and elbow allowing optimal ergonomics.

the correct position even in special situations such as spinal kyphosis. Dangling the patient's head in midair above the headrest decreases the room below the table for the surgeon and interferes with the foot-pedal maneuvers. A shoulder roll is sometimes necessary, particularly in infants and small children, to maintain the head in a proper position.[1]

### *Surgeon Positioning*

Most ophthalmic surgeries are performed using an ophthalmic microscope with the surgeon sitting at superior or temporal positions. At either position, the patient's eye should be paralleled with the floor. The surgeon should be placed close enough to the table in such a way that the surgeon neither has to lean too far forward or back to view through the microscope oculars. While the surgeon is at an optimal position, his or her legs should easily slide below the table to control the foot pedal. The surgeon should not feel strain in the back or neck, and the hands should be in the most ergonomically favorable position (Fig. 3-4).[1]

With the surgeon at the superior position, placing the foot pedals on either side of the operating table gives more room under the table for foot maneuvers. This approach prevents inadvertent bumping the surgical table by the surgeon's knee during foot maneuvers. When the surgeon uses both feet, one for controlling the microscope and the other for controlling other instruments such as a phacoemulsification or vitrectomy machines, it is more convenient to place the microscope foot pedal under the nondominant leg (left leg for right-handed individuals). The microscope pedal could be placed under the dominant leg when there is no other foot pedal.

The temporal approach is more challenging for proper and comfortable surgeon position. Always one leg of the surgeon (e.g. the right leg in the temporal approach for operating on the right eye of the patient) will be directly under the surgical bed, with difficulty keeping the leg clear of the table. This challenge is more prominent for tall surgeons. Compared with the superior position, the bed must be more raised to accommodate the surgeon's leg, whereas the chair should be left at the same height. To allow proper focus, the microscope must be raised, and the surgeon has to assume an erect torso position to reach the oculars. Alternatively, the surgeon can drop the oculars without significant change in torso position, as long as the hands are left in comfortable position. If all above maneuvers fails to achieve the necessary clearance of the bed over the legs (usually for surgeons with a relatively long legs, or short torso) two additional maneuvers can be tried. One maneuver involves flaring of the knee out slightly and controlling the foot pedal with outside of the foot,[1] the other maneuver is placing both pedals of the microscope under the free leg. In the latter maneuver, using continuous irrigation mode of phacoemulsification machine is recommended, because the surgeon should interrupt the surgery while gauging the microscope pedal.

## Advantages and Disadvantages

The advantages of operating microscopes are far greater than their disadvantages, making them unparalleled for intraocular ophthalmic procedures.

### *Advantages*

Operating microscopes include built-in sophisticated illumination systems that are precisely accustomed to their optical capabilities. The motorized system and foot control allows controlling the microscope intuitively during surgery while operating with both hands. The high and adjustable magnification provides excellent visualization of fine tissues and enables delicate maneuvers. A variety of useful accessories can be mounted on the operating microscope.

### Disadvantages

Higher magnification is only possible at the expense of a decrease in depth of field. High magnification derived by the operating microscope places greater demands on the surgeon. For example, a hand tremor is magnified along with the surgical field. In addition, the highly magnified view could be easily disturbed by the vibrations from construction or maintenance works in the adjacent room or floors; hence, the operating rooms must be constructed to very high vibration-dampening standards.[1]

Procedures in which the surgical field is required to be viewed from different angles are not easily attainable.[1] Being in a single position, treated continuously with the light source, along with high concentration required for operation in high magnification setting, drive the surgeon tired in long lasting operations. Although rare, the risk of light toxicity is preserved for both the patient and surgeon.

## SURGICAL LOUPES

Surgical loupes are ideal for extraocular surgeries such as strabismus, oculoplastic, and scleral buckling operations. The magnification provided by the loupes fits the surgical demand and also offers the surgeon the flexibility to view the surgical field rapidly from several angles.[1] Surgical loupes are usually used by senior surgeons who have presbyopia and cannot enhance the magnification of the surgical field by decreasing the working distance.

Although surgical loupes offer the versatility to change the angle of view during operation, it is important to maintain a constant working distance and keep the head still to have a proper focus. The surgeon should keep his or her sight on the surgical field while asking for an instrument, and the scrub nurse must hand it over to the surgeon.[1] Good light in the surgical field is essential for performing surgery with loupes. Unlike operating microscopes, surgical loupes do not support built-in illumination source. The light can be provided by either a ceiling-mounted source or the overhead surgical lights. Headlamps are usually preferred because the light is always centered on the line of sight, particularly useful when operating on the nasal cavity or orbit.[1]

### Characteristics

#### Magnification

Unlike the operating microscopes, surgical loupes could offer a fixed magnification in a particular operative setting. The magnification is usually ranging from 2× to 6×. Most surgeries need at least 2.5× and usually 3.5× magnification.

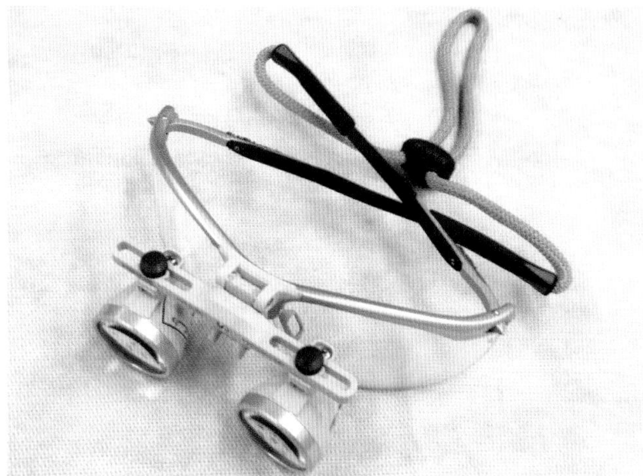

**Figure 3-5** A typical surgical loupe with a spectacle frame and mounted oculars.

As the magnification increases, the field of view and depth of field decrease.[1]

#### Working distance

For a particular loupe, the working distance is fixed. For loupes with lower magnifications (2.5× or less), manufacturers usually offer different working distances ranging from about 10–20 inches. For loupes with magnifications of 3.5× and higher, the optical demands of the loupe hinders such flexibility and often only one working distance is offered by the manufacturer.[1]

#### Field of View

Field of view is influenced by the magnification and the working distance. The higher magnification and shorter working distance tend to have a smaller field of view. For lower magnification levels, manufacturers can offer different fields of view (e.g. 4–10 inches for 2× magnification level). For higher magnifications, however, the field of view is often set.[1]

Based on the surgical demands and the surgeon comfort, the loupe with appropriate magnification, field of view, and working distance should be chosen. Since the depth of field decreases in higher magnification levels, a senior surgeon with low accommodation reserve should keep the head very still to maintain focus while using a loupe with high magnification.[1]

### Constituents

A surgical loupe is composed of a spectacle frame and a pair of eyepieces mounted on a frame (Fig. 3-5). Corrective or protective lenses could be added to the frame. The oculars provide the magnification. PD of the oculars is adjustable.[10]

## Advantages and Disadvantages

### *Advantages*

The viewing angle is flexible, letting the surgeon easily change his position around the patient. The provided magnification is well suited to most extraocular and lid surgeries.[1]

### *Disadvantages*

A surgical loupe has a fixed magnification and focal length, and hence, a fixed working distance for the surgeon.[1]

## REFERENCES

1. Zabriskie N. The operating microscope and surgical loupes. In: Arnold A (ed.), Basic principles of ophthalmic surgery. San Francisco, CA: American Academy of Ophthalmology, 2006: 29-56.
2. Benjamin L.Tools, facilities, and the operating team. In: Benjamin L (ed.), Cataract surgery. Amsterdam, the Netherlands: Saunders, Elsevier, 2007:12-13.
3. Carl Zeiss Meditec. Surgical microscopes. http://www.meditec.zeiss.com/c125679e0051c774/Contents-Frame/c20fe52b-4ca37c7dc12575910048c2fd. (Retrieved 15 March 2013)
4. Atebara N, Asbell P, Azar D, et al. Clinical optics. In: Skuta G, Cantor L, Weiss J, (eds), Basic and clinical science course, vol 3. San Francisco, CA: American Academy of Ophthalmology, 2011-2012.
5. Topcon connecting visions. Operation microscopes. http://www.topcon-medical.eu/eu/categories/42-surgical/#products/eu/categories/42-surgical/43-operation-microscopes/. (Retrieved March 15, 2013)
6. Leica microsystems. Surgical microscopes. http://www.leica-microsystems.com/products/surgical-microscopes/. (Retrieved 15 March 2013)
7. Chang D. Improving the red reflex and surgical outcomes with the Lumera microscope. Cataract & refractive surgery today. March 2009. http://bmctoday.net/crstoday/2009/03/article.asp?f=CRST0309_04.php. (Retrieved 13 March, 2013)
8. Michels M, Sternberg P, Jr. Operating microscope-induced retinal phototoxicity: pathophysiology, clinical manifestations and prevention. Surv Ophthalmol. 1990;34:237-52.
9. Oculus. SDI 4/BIOM 4. www.oculus.sk/sdi_biom/sdi_biom.pdf. (Retrieved 17 March 2013)
10. Oculus. Binocular loupes. http://www.oculus.de/en/sites/detail_ger.php?page=334. (Retrieved 17 March 2013)

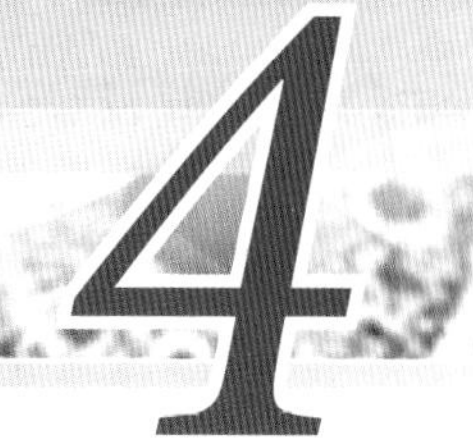

CHAPTER 4

# Sutures and Needles in Ophthalmology

Oscar Albis-Donado, Shibal Bhartiya, Giovanna Casale-Vargas

## INTRODUCTION

Basic knowledge of suture materials and of the needles used with them is an essential part of becoming a successful ophthalmic surgeon. Modern ocular surgeries rely on using the most appropriate instruments and materials for the task in hand.

Needles in common ophthalmic use come in a variety of alloys that are patented by the manufacturer. The alloy should be resistent to breaking or bending, smooth to reduce drag, and should maintain its sharpness despite repetitive passes through tissues.

Suture materials come in absorbable and nonabsorbable types, and they can also be monofilaments or braided (Table 4-1). Depending on the task for which we need them, we might want them to maintain their tensile strength for a few days or permanently. We also need to choose the material depending on the flexibility, elasticity, tying and handling properties, visibility of the material but also on the biomechanical features of the tissue to be sutured (Table 4-2).

## SUTURES

### Size and Calibration

Suture size refers to the diameter of the suture strand and is denoted as zeroes. The more zeroes characterizing a suture size, the smaller the resultant strand diameter. The smaller the suture, the less the tensile strength of the strand.

Sutures are calibrated according to thickness, and the sizes that are commonly in use in ophthalmology go from 5-0 to 11-0, as defined by the United States Pharmacopeia (USP) and chosen depending on the structure to be sutured and the material used.[1] Sutures can withstand different amounts of force based on their size; this is quantified by the USP Needle Pull Specifications.

### Choice of Suture Material

The choice of material will often depend on the tissue, but it can also be chosen by other criteria. As an example, conjunctival closure is often performed with a nonabsorbable suture, with the plan of removing it once sufficient scarring is obtained, 1 week for a pterygium surgery, or 3–4 weeks for trabeculectomies when water tightness is important (Fig. 4-1). But in children we want to avoid having to use general anesthesia if possible, so it makes sense to use a thin, absorbable suture instead (Fig. 4-2). In contrast, using an absorbable suture for a corneal transplant is not a very good idea, since we want the tissue to remain avascular and in place for months, and absorbable sutures will induce vascularization and lose their tensile strength too soon, inducing irregular astigmatism or wound dehiscence.

#### *Absorbable Sutures*

The duration of a suture in a tissue is relevant only while it still maintains its tensile strength. Remaining material might

**TABLE 4-1 Classification of suture materials**

| According to absorption | According to origin | According to the number of fibers |
|---|---|---|
| • *Absorbable*: e.g. Polyglycolic acid | *Natural*: e.g. silk | *Monofilament*: e.g. polyglycolic acid |
| • *Nonabsorbable*: e.g. Nylon, braided silk, stainless steel, polyester | *Synthetic*: e.g. polyglycolic acid | *Multifilament*: e.g. polyglycolic acid |

**TABLE 4-2 Properties of suture materials**

| |
|---|
| • Caliber |
| • *Tensile strength*: Measure of the ability of a material or tissue to resist deformation and breakage |
| • *Capillarity*: Extent to which absorbed fluid is transferred along the suture |
| • *Memory*: Inherent capability of suture to return to or maintain its original gross shape |
| • *Absorption properties*: Progressive loss of mass and/or volume of suture material |
| • Friction coefficient |
| • Extensibility |
| • *Tissue reaction*: Nonelectrolytic, noncapillary, nonallergenic, noncarcinogenic |
| • *Number of fibers:* Monofilament, Multifilament |

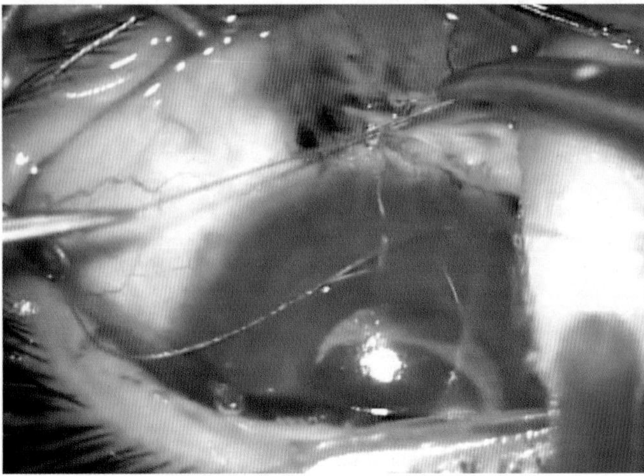

**Figure 4-2** 8-0 Vicryl is used for closing the conjunctiva in a child with congenital glaucoma to avoid returning to the operating room for removing the sutures later.

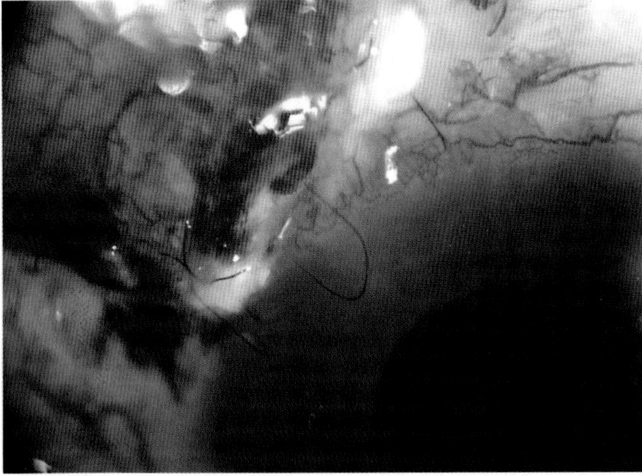

**Figure 4-1** A case of conjunctival advancement for a leaking bleb; 10-0 nylon is holding the conjunctiva with a running mattress suture with bites through cornea and episclera.

still produce inflammatory reactions months after the tensile strength is lost, and sometimes we seek this delayed response, in the hopes that final resilience of the tissue will be greater than at the beginning. The amount of time a given suture will retain its tensile strength and then be degraded will depend on the material, the diameter of the suture, and the vascularity of the tissue.

Absorbable sutures are usually made of polyglactin, polyglycolic acid, polydioxanone, or chromic gut. Surgical gut sutures are made from either bovine or sheep purified connective tissue obtained from their intestines. They are made mostly of collagen, and they can be either plain or chromic. The role of chromic salts is to reduce the enzymatic activity that will make plain gut disappear in a flare of inflammation within a week, so the tensile strength can be maintained for about 2–3 weeks, with less inflammatory reaction.

Polyglactin 910 sutures (e.g. Vicryl Ethicon Inc, Somerville, New Jersey, USA, *see* Figure 4-3) are made from a copolymer of 90% glycolic acid and 10% lactic acid, the coated version (polyglactin 370 and calcium stearate) is the one available for ophthalmic use, having less tissue drag despite it being braided and mounted on spatulated or reverse-cutting needles. Absorption occurs through hydrolytic degradation.[2]

Polyglycolic acid sutures are made from braided or monofilament glycolic acid only, so their absorption is dependent on hydrolysis, an advantage when compared with enzymatic degradation, which tends to cause more inflammation. The tensile strength of both glycolic acid types will last for 2–3 weeks, but the material will remain in the tissue for about 2 or 3 months.

Another type of absorbable suture is made from polydioxanone, and it is designed to retain its tensile strength for up to 6 weeks, so it can be a better option for suturing inner tissues requiring mechanical support, such as a muscle in eyes with poor scarring, or for keeping the position of either an Ahmed or a Baerveldt valve until the fibrous tissue grows through their holes and keeps them in place.

### *Nonabsorbable Sutures*

The most common materials used for nonabsorbable sutures are silk, nylon (polyamide), polypropylene, and polyester, all of them are in current ophthalmic use.

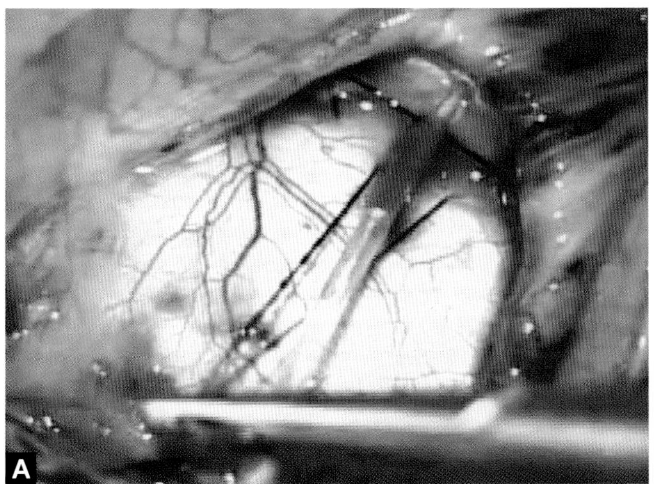


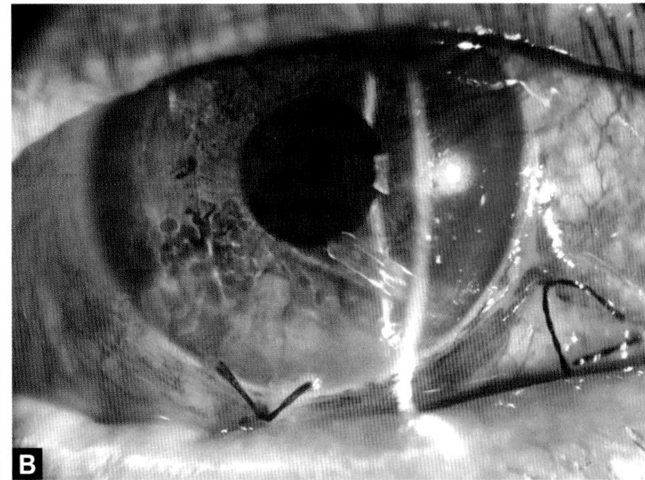


**Figures 4-3A and B** (A) 7-0 silk being used for suturing an Ahmed valve to the sclera, its flexibility avoids deformation or cheese wiring of the sclera. (B) In an adult patient, the same suture is used for conjunctival closure and will be removed 8–10 days later.

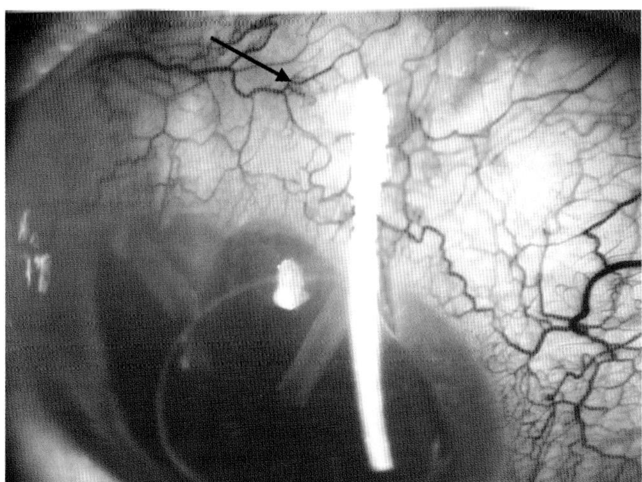

**Figure 4-4** A polypropylene suture holding an intraocular lens in place 4 years, no conjunctival erosion is present.

*Silk:* Surgical grade silk is usually braided, pigmented, and degummed fibroin, with natural waxes removed and coated with several mixtures of waxes for smoothness. It is considered a nonabsorbable suture since it retains its tensile strength for about 3–6 months, although residues of the suture may be found up to a couple of years later. It is the most flexible of the nonabsorbable sutures, a feature that makes it ideal for suturing glaucoma devices to the sclera without cheese wiring through the tissue (Figs. 4-3A and B). Its braided nature needs some getting used to, to avoid breaking it while tying it down. Another problem with silk suture is the acute inflammatory reaction triggered by this material. Host reaction leads to encapsulation by fibrous connective tissue, seen commonly in limbus-based trabeculectomies.

*Polyamide (nylon):* Polyamide is probably the most commonly used material in ophthalmic surgery; it is a relatively flexible monofilament, basically inert, and only loses about 10–15% of its tensile strength per year. This makes it ideal for suturing avascular, slow-healing tissues, such as the cornea, with a very low chance of cutting through the tissue. It is also ideal for adjusting the curvature of the cornea in a more or less predictable way or closing trabeculectomy flaps, since surgeons can easily train themselves in calculating the tension on the tissue.

*Polypropylene:* Polypropylene is also a monofilament that is capable of maintaining its tensile strength for extended periods of time, it is relatively rigid, so it can easily cheese-wire through sclera if handled improperly, but it is the best material for suturing intraocular lenses to the sclera or repairing sector iridectomies (Fig. 4-4).

*Polyester:* Polyester is composed of poly (ethylene terephthalate) and comes as a braided, flexible suture for ophthalmic use. It essentially never loses its tensile strength, so it is suitable for tying down canthal tendons or fixing scleral bands.[3] Although the material is inert, it may become contaminated, causing occasional granulomas, or it can also erode through the conjunctiva with time (*see* Figure 4-5). This is why we prefer to avoid it for glaucoma implants, especially since both Baerveldt and the new Ahmed devices will remain in place once the fibrous bands grow through the plates.

## NEEDLES

Ophthalmic surgery was probably the first speciality that benefited from the development of swaged or atraumatic needles

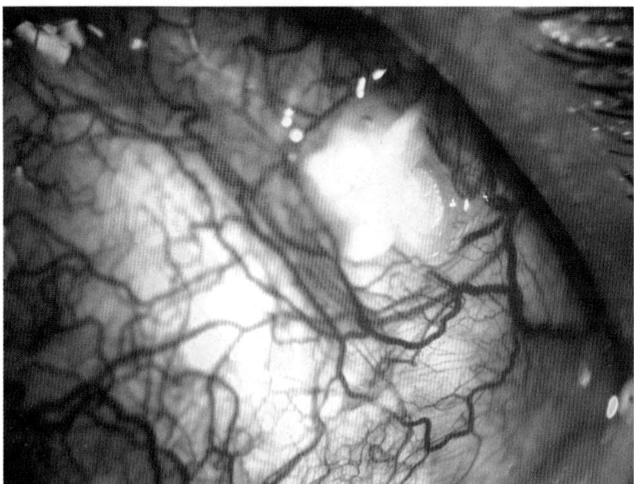

**Figure 4-5** A section of exposed scleral band and polyester suture, 8 years after original surgery.

at the beginning of the 20th century. Initially, intracapsular cataract extraction incisions had been closed with eyed needles and virgin silk or left unsutured, and once swaged needles became available suturing became more commonplace, and patients began to have less risk of complications during and after surgery.

The best surgical needles should have these important characteristics:

- High-quality stainless steel.
- As thin as possible without losing resistance.
- Stability in the needle holder, so a portion that will lie flat against its surface will avoid rotation.
- Capable of threading the suture material through the tissue with the least possible trauma.
- Sharp enough to enter the tissue with minimal resistance.
- Rigid enough to avoid bending but flexible enough to keep it from breaking during surgery.
- Sterile and corrosion resistant to avoid introducing microorganisms or leaving strange materials in the wound.

## Anatomy of a Needle

A needle has three parts, the point, body, and swage (Fig. 4-6).

The point portion of the needle extends from the tip to the maximum cross section of the body. The body part of the needle incorporates most of the needle length and is important for interaction with the needle holder and the ability to transmit the penetrating force to the point. The swage is the point where the suture material joins with the eyeless needles, to prevent damage as the needle and suture thread pass through the wound.

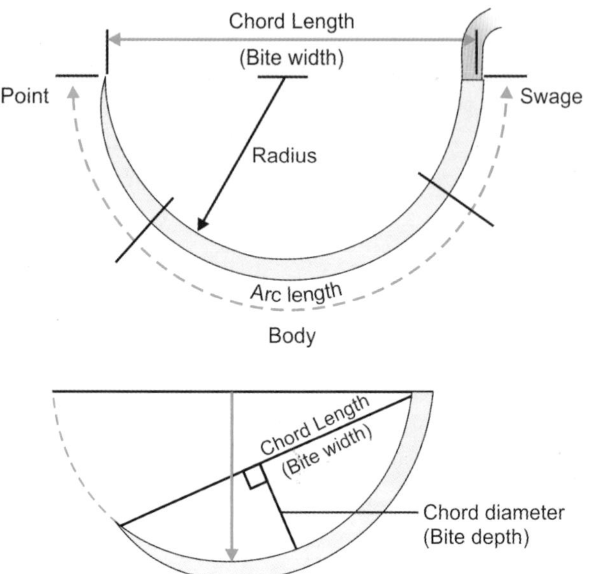


**Figure 4-6** Parts of a needle.

The chord length, or bite width, is the linear distance from the point of the curved needle to the swage (bite width). The needle length is the distance measured along the needle from the point to the swage. Needle length, not chord length, is the measurement supplied on suture packages. The radius is the distance from the body of the needle to the center of the circle along which the needle curves (bite depth), and the diameter is considered the gauge or thickness of the needle wire.

## Classification of Needles

Needles are classified according to shape and to the geometry of the tip. Every variation has its own advantages and disadvantages.[4,5]

### *Based on Shape*

According to shape needles can be (Fig. 4-7)

- Straight
- Half-circle
- 1/4 circle
- 3/8 circle
- 5/8 circle
- Compound curve.

Compound curve needles were developed for anterior segment surgery, allowing the surgeon to take precise and uniform portions of tissue. The curve near the tip has a smaller radius of curvature and occupies about 80° of curvature; the remaining 45° have a flatter curve. The first curvature

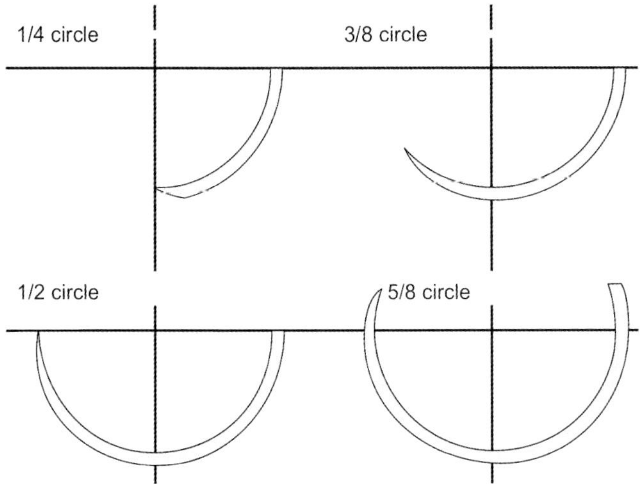


Figure 4-7 Shapes of a needle.

allows reproducible short and deep bites into the tissue. The remaining curvature forces the needle to leave the tissue, everting the borders of the wound and allowing for viewing inside the wound. This ensures that the same amount of suture material will be at both sides of the wound, an important issue when distributing forces for minimizing astigmatism when closing corneoscleral wounds.

### *Based on Configuration of the Point*

The four main types of needles used in ophthalmic surgery may be classified on the basis of the configuration of the point[6] (Fig. 4-8). These include:

- *Cutting*: The point is triangular in cross section, with the cutting edge at the top. It cuts from the tip and the edges. A drawback of this needle is that it may pull out tissue during the creation of the needle track, which is just superficial to its tip. When used to tie down to the sclera extraneous materials that need to remain in place, the tract will be weaker on the outer portion, precisely toward the implant, which will increase chances of the suture cheese wiring through the sclera and freeing the implant.
- *Reverse cutting*: The point is triangular in cross section, with the cutting edge at the bottom, and like the cutting needle, it also cuts from both the tip and the edges. The suture canal, however, is deep to the needle tip. This makes the needle ideal for full thickness sutures through epidermis and skin. A drawback is that accidental perforations may result when partial thickness sutures are placed, a real drawback for suturing through the sclera since it may cut the choroid and/or cause suprachoroidal bleeding.

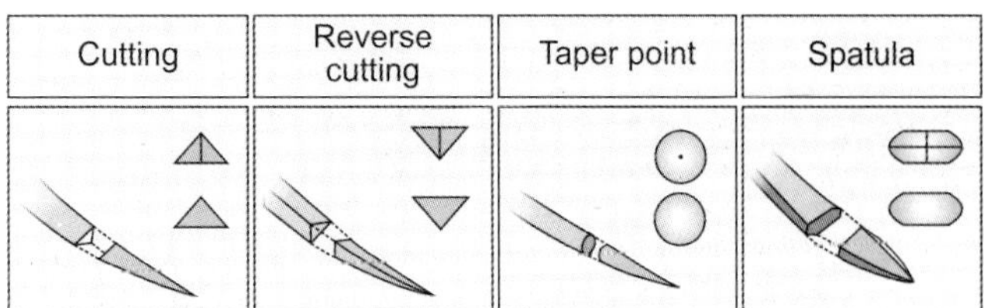


Figure 4-8 Diagrammatic representation of tips of needles.

- *Taper point*: The point is circular in cross section, with the cutting edge at the tip only and therefore creating the smallest needle track of all the available needles. It is relatively atraumatic and is the preferred choice for iris and vascular repair. It is also useful for closing conjunctival advancements and bleb repairs when aqueous leaks are present. The drawback is the greater resistance to passing through the tissues, which can make the thinnest needles (e.g. 10-0 nylon) bend after a few passes.
- Spatulated The spatulated needle is the most versatile, with 4 –6 cutting edges to the point, in cross section. It therefore cuts at the sides and at the tip, parallel to the tissue plane in which it is passed through, avoiding any accidental perforations. It will also provide the surgeon with propioceptive feedback when going through the parallel stacked fibers of both the cornea and sclera, something unique to ophthalmic surgery.

## ALTERNATIVE MATERIALS AND SPECIFIC SUTURES FOR TISSUE APPROXIMATION

### Tissue Adhesives

Topical tissue adhesives have been in use for the past few decades for closing wounds (Table 4-3). One of the most commonly used is cyanoacrylate, a fast-acting compound, which can be used for skin repair, and will also form a barrier to microbial contamination while intact. It is not very useful for nonskin surfaces, but it may be used for closing small ocular perforations in combination with a soft-contact lens to avoid the foreign-body sensation from its hardened active surface.

Fibrin-forming adhesives are more commonly used for the ocular surface and have recently been used successfully for closing the conjunctiva after glaucoma implants or for fixing in place a free conjunctival graft for pterygium surgery.

### Adhesive Tapes

Adhesive tapes such as steri-srips (3M, US) can be used over a skin wound to keep the sides united while it heals. They

TABLE 4-3 USP suture designation and dimensions

| USP designation | Collagen diameter (mm) | Synthetic absorbable diameter (mm) | Nonabsorbable diameter (mm) | American wire gauge |
|---|---|---|---|---|
| 11-0 | | | 0.01 | |
| 10-0 | 0.02 | 0.02 | 0.02 | |
| 9-0 | 0.03 | 0.03 | 0.03 | |
| 8-0 | 0.05 | 0.04 | 0.04 | |
| 7-0 | 0.07 | 0.05 | 0.05 | |
| 6-0 | 0.1 | 0.07 | 0.07 | 38–40 |
| 5-0 | 0.15 | 0.1 | 0.1 | 35–38 |
| 4-0 | 0.2 | 0.15 | 0.15 | 32–34 |
| 3-0 | 0.3 | 0.2 | 0.2 | 29–32 |
| 2-0 | 0.35 | 0.3 | 0.3 | 28 |
| 0 | 0.4 | 0.35 | 0.35 | 26–27 |
| 1 | 0.5 | 0.4 | 0.4 | 25–26 |
| 2 | 0.6 | 0.5 | 0.5 | 23–24 |
| 3 | 0.7 | 0.6 | 0.6 | 22 |
| 4 | 0.8 | 0.6 | 0.6 | 21–22 |
| 5 | | 0.7 | 0.7 | 20–21 |
| 6 | | | 0.8 | 19–20 |
| 7 | | | | 18 |

TABLE 4-4 Surgical adhesives and sealants

- Fibrin sealants
- Cyanoacrylates
- Gelatin and thrombin products
- Polyethylene glycol polymers
- Albumin and glutaraldehyde products

can replace stitches in small wounds sometimes, obtaining a better appearance of the scar, protecting the wound, and allowing for easy removal. They can also help cover sutured wounds to help protect them from infections, reduce stress on the sutures, and avoid external trauma (Table 4-4).

Tissues need to be held in proximity until adequate healing occurs to withstand stress without mechanical support, so choose the suture material accordingly.

## REFERENCES


1. Lai SY, Becker DG. Sutures and needles. eMedicine specialities > otolaryngology and facial plastic surgery > wound healing and care. 2006. http://www.emedicine.com/ent/topic38.htm. (Last accessed April 2013)
2. Hunter P. 10-0 Vicryl suture offers alternative to no stitch. Ocular Surg News. 9(16): August 15, 1991.
3. Lo Piccolo M (ed.). Mersilene suture results found comparable to nylon. Ophthalmology Times, 18 August 15, 1998.
4. Bendel L, Reynolds E, Stoffel F. Ophthalmic needles. An engineering analysis. Ophthalmology. 1986;93(9 Suppl):61-4.
5. McClung WL, Thacker JG, Edlich RF, et al. Biomechanical performance of ophthalmic surgical needles. Ophthalmology. 1992;99(2):232-7.
6. Unknown authors, http://www.mrcophth.com/needles/needle type.htm (Last accesed april 24th, 2013).

CHAPTER

5

# Suturing and Knot Tying

Ghasem Fakhraie

## INTRODUCTION

In this chapter, we discuss about the basic principles of placing surgical sutures and tying knot along with describing how to put some basic and most important surgical sutures especially in the field of ophthalmology.

## BASIC PRINCIPLES OF SUTURE PLACEMENT

Correctly holding the needle by the needle holder is the first step in perfect suture placement. The surgeon uses his/her dominant hand to hold the needle holder. The needle should be grasped by near the distal end (tip) of needle holder at a point on the needle between the middle and one third from the swaged end (where the thread is loaded) (Fig. 5-1). Although grasping the needle more close to the proximal end (hinge) of needle holder (Fig. 5-2) provides more power for passing the needle through the tissue and placing the suture, it decreases the fine pass of the needle through the wound, hence reducing the fineness of the suture. Grasping the needle near its tip or at the end where the thread is loaded (end of the needle) can adversely affect its penetration and cause the needle to break. Also, grasping the needle closerto the tip of the needle may lead to early and unnecessary dulling of the needle and might not provide enough length of the needle for passing through both sides of the wound. Grasping the needle closer to the swaged end of the needle might lead to the rotation or tilting of needle during its pass through the tissue.

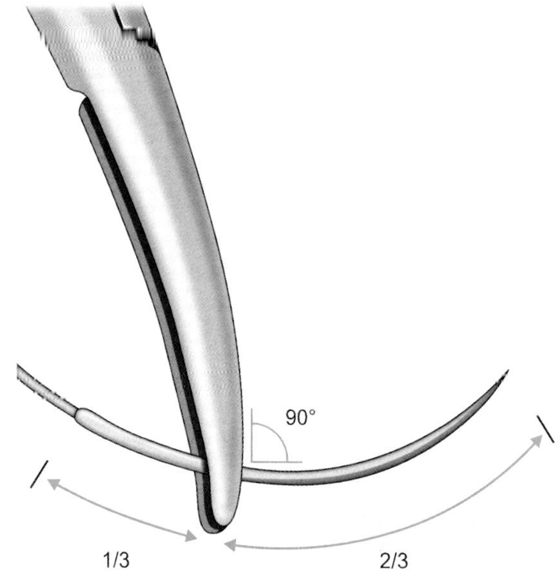


**Figure 5-1** Correct way of grasping the needle: the needle should be grasped by near the distal end (tip) of needle holder at a point on the needle between the middle and one third from the swaged end (where the thread is loaded).

Since the sutures typically come with semicircular needles, they create circular paths when they are passed through tissue. Linear pushing should be avoided with these needles; otherwise, they will bend and distort the tissues. The entry angle of the suture plays a major role in determining the depth of the suture. Because the needle creates a circular path, if the needle entry angle is 90°, then the circular path of the needle will result in a depth equal to the radius of curvature of the needle. Entry angle of < 90° results in a shallow pass, whereas entry angle of > 90° results in a deeper pass. So, it is recommended that the needle enters perpendicular to the tissue (Fig. 5-3) and gently slide forward by rotating the wrist. For this reason, the surgeon should hold his/her hand in a straight position.

As the needle passes through the tissue, the wound lips should be grasp gently by a forceps with the nondominant hand until the needle passes through both sides of the wound

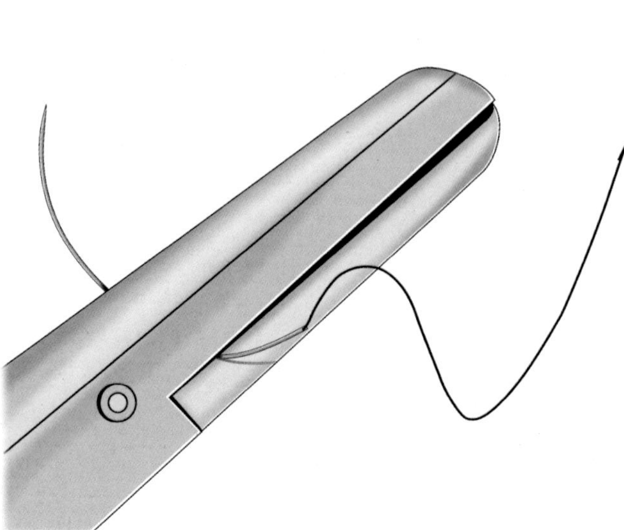

**Figures 5-2** Grasping the needle close to the hinge of the needle holder.

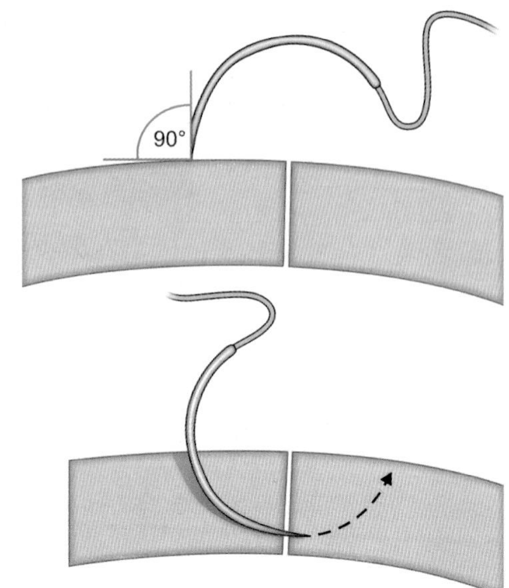


**Figure 5-3** The entry angle of the needle determines the depth of the suture placement. Perpendicular entry results in normal depth, equal to the radius of the needle.

and emerges from the opposite side. The needle should not be released from the needle holder until it comes out from the other side of the wound so that it could be regrasped by the needle holder. Regrasping the tip of the needle should be avoided since it could lead to early needle dulling. This is a common mistake when the surgeon wants to regrasp the needle early upon its exit from the other side of the wound.

In most situations, sutures should be placed symmetrically so that an even amount of tissue on either side of the incision is captured by the suture.

If touched at all, suture material should only be held by forceps or needle holders at the end of the thread. Each time it is held, the suture is damaged – and this is considerably more serious with monofilament threads. Any damage has an effect on the tensile strength of the suture.

In most cases, the surgeon faces a paradox, which should be dealt with meticulously. From one side, the suture should be tight enough so that it could approximate two edges of the wound properly. From the other side, he/she would have to avoid applying overtension on the suture that, in turn, could lead to cheese wiring and tissue necrosis or distortion of the tissue.[1]

## SIMPLE SQUARE KNOT

Square knot is considered the first and basic skill of suturing, and all surgeons should be skilled in tying a square knot. As illustrated in Figure 5-4 the following stages should be followed trying to place a square knot:

- Needle is passed through both sides of the wound, and once it is regrasped it is pulled until the tail of the suture become short enough.
- Needle is then released, and the suture is grasped with a forceps on its long arm at about 3–4 cm (depending on the type of needle holder and forceps, and on suture material) from the exit site.
- While the needle holder is pointed away from the surgeon and its jaws is closed, it is hold on the same side of the wound as the surgeon's dominant hand is.
- The square knot is performed in a similar fashion to shoe lace tying: a right-over-left wrap, followed by a left-over-right wrap. For instrument ties, the tying forceps should stay inside the loop being created (Fig. 5-4A). The approximating loop is followed by two or three throws for additional friction. After the approximating loop is completed, the suture should lie flat across the wound surface, with enough tension to just bring the wound edges together (Fig. 5-4B).
- For making a second throw the suture is released from the needle holder and the needle holder is hold again at the center of the wound this time its tip pointing toward the surgeon. While the jaws of needle holder are closed, the longer end of the suture grasped by forceps is again wrapped around the needle holder tip. The second loop is thrown in the opposite direction (Figs. 5-4C and D), and the securing loop is tightened at right angles to the suture plane. The final securing loop is again thrown in

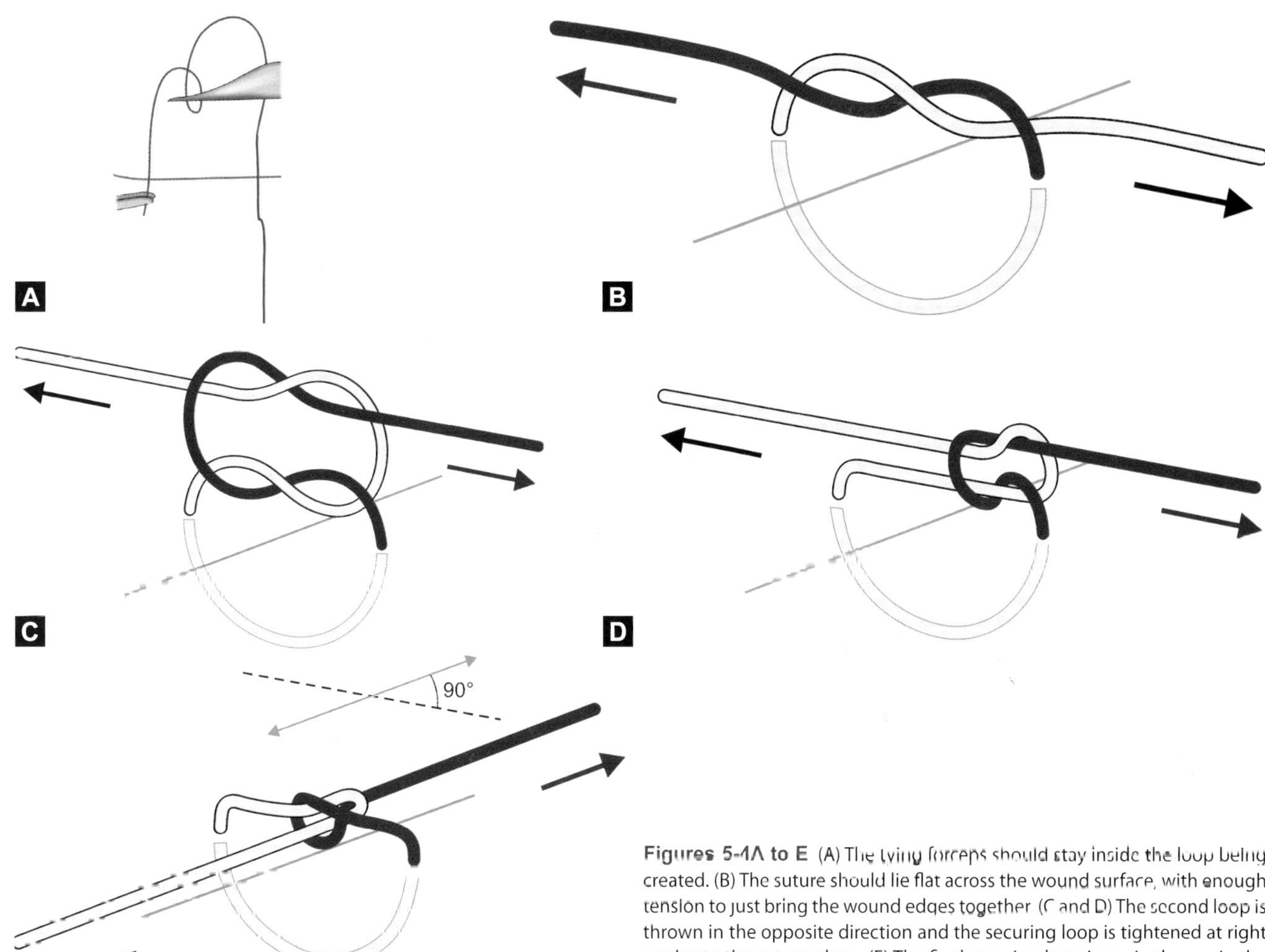


**Figures 5-4A to E** (A) The tying forceps should stay inside the loop being created. (B) The suture should lie flat across the wound surface, with enough tension to just bring the wound edges together. (C and D) The second loop is thrown in the opposite direction and the securing loop is tightened at right angles to the suture plane. (E) The final securing loop is again thrown in the original direction and tightened at right angles to the suture plane.

the original direction and tightened at right angles to the suture plane (Fig. 5-4E).[2]

- Since it might lead to excessive eversion and also tissue necrosis, the surgeon must be cautious about applying overtension on the suture.

### Surgeon's Knot

The ligature knot, (surgeon's knot or the 3-2-1 knot) is a square knot with an additional half knot placed in the approximating loop (Fig. 5-5).[2]

## SUTURING TECHNIQUES

Several types of sutures are commonly used in wound closure. The surgeon's choice of suture type depends on a number of considerations. Sutures can generally be divided into two basic types: namely: individual (interrupted) and continuous sutures. Each of these has its advantages and disadvantages. Interrupted sutures permit very precise adaption of the wound edges. The risk of wound dehiscence is less than that with continuous sutures. The advantage of continuous sutures is that they permit more even approximation of the two sides of the wound. They are also considered for wounds that must prevent the passage of gas and fluids.

### Simple Interrupted Suture

- *Application*: Simple interrupted suture is the basic tool of wound closure and is the most commonly used suturing technique.
- *Technique*: For placing interrupted sutures, first, the wound length is divided into two equal parts, and the first suture is generally placed in the middle of the wound. For this

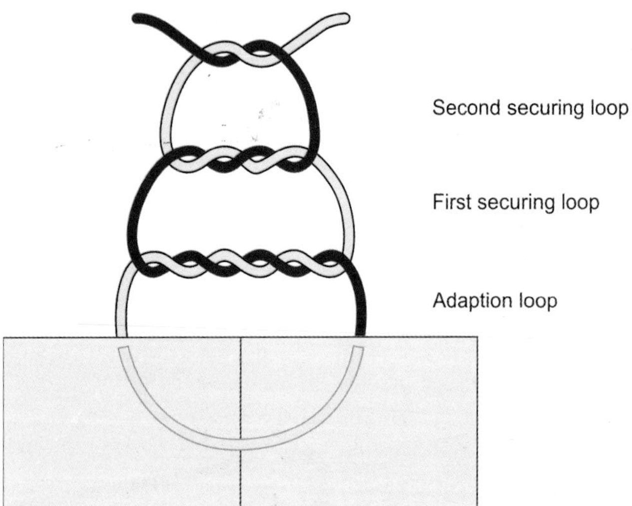


**Figure 5-5** The ligature knot, surgeon's knot or the 3-2-1 knot, is a square knot with an additional half knot placed in the approximating loop.

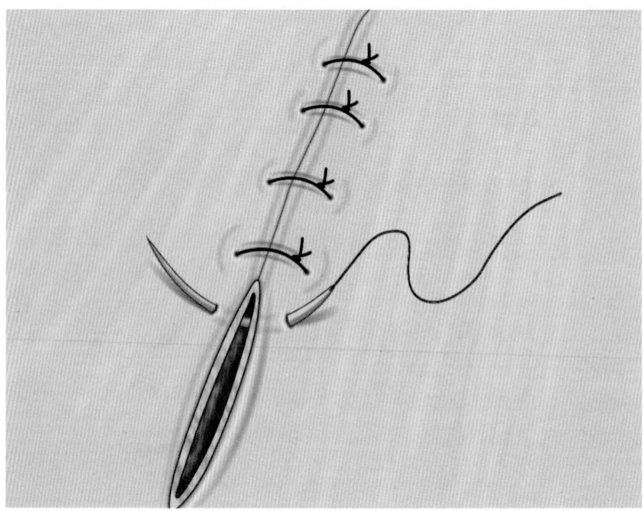

**Figure 5-6** Enough interrupted sutures are placed to create adequate strength for secure wound closure.

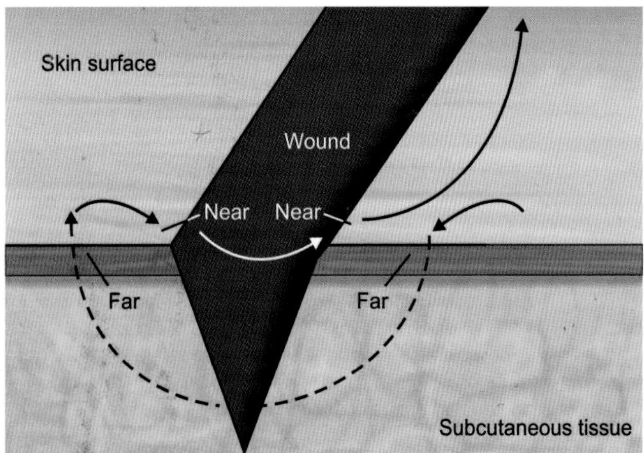


**Figure 5-7** On the second passage, the needle is passed more superficially to the opposite side, exiting closer to the wound margin (near-near passage).

reason, the needle is passed from one side of the wound to the other side of the wound through the underlying tissue. As mentioned earlier, for proper placement of a suture, the needle should enter the tissue perpendicularly and travel in a circular path and at equal depths on both sides of the wound. It is also important that the entrance and exit sites of the suture be the same distance from the wound line. After regrasping the needle from the opposite side of the wound, a square knot is placed and the ends of the suture are cut down. The distance between the two suture penetrations on each side of the wound should be identical, and the suture should be wider at the bottom. Each subsequent suture splits the remaining portions of the wound in half until complete wound closure is achieved. Enough interrupted sutures are placed to create adequate strength for secure wound closure (Fig. 5-6).

- *Advantage*: It is versatile and is easy to use.
- *Disadvantage*: The major disadvantage of this technique is that it tends to leave a series of cross-hatched linear scars resembling railroad tracks.

## Vertical Mattress (far-far near-near) Suture

- *Application*: This is one of the best available suturing techniques to ensure eversion of wound and minimize significant wound tension. Compared with simple interrupted suture, it provides more support for wound closure.
- *Technique*: The vertical mattress suture uses the far-far, near-near system. For placing a vertical mattress suture, the needle is inserted from one side of the wound and driven to the depth of the wound to close the dead space. The needle is then passed to the opposing wound edge, where it exits the tissue equidistant to the insertion (far-far passage). The needle is then reversed in the needle holder, and the tissue is penetrated again on the side through which the suture just exited but closer to the wound line. On the second passage, the needle is passed more superficially to the opposite side, exiting closer to the wound margin (near-near passage) (Fig. 5-7). The distance between the two suture penetrations on each side of the wound should be identical. Finally, the suture ends are tied on the same side of the wound, and the suture ends are cut down (Fig. 5-8).
- *Advantage*: This suturing technique is useful in maximizing the wound eversion, reducing dead space, and minimizing

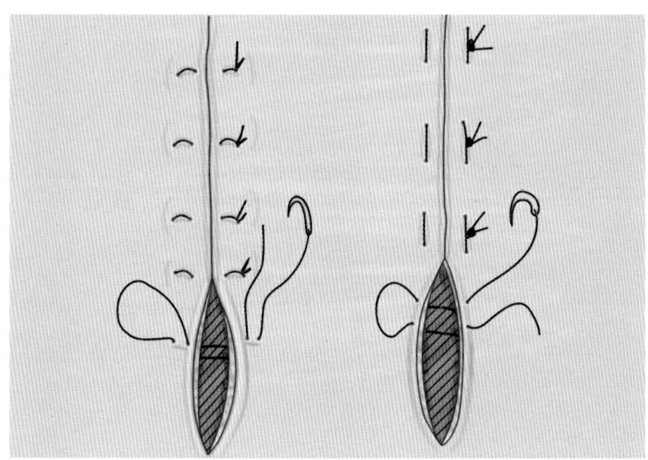

**Figure 5-8** The suture then exits in the same position on the first side of the wound and creating a "rectangle" out of the suture. The ends of the suture are then tied on the same side of the wound.

tension across the wound. This specificity makes the vertical mattress suture a good choice for lid margin laceration repair.

- *Disadvantage*: Since the vertical mattress suture is highly susceptible to wound eversion, one should be cautious about exerting overtension on the suture, which, in turn, could lead to severe eversion of the wound edges and impaired wound healing.

## Near-far Vertical Mattress Suture

- *Application*: This is a modification of standard vertical mattress suture. It is used when tissue expansion and closure of wound, which is under tension, is desired.
- *Technique*: The technique is largely the same as the standard vertical mattress, but the needle goes deeper and exits this time farther from the entry site on its second passage, making a "figure eight" pattern inside the tissue. The ends of the suture are then tied on the same side of the wound.
- *Advantage*: This technique helps elevate the deeper tissues of the wound.

## Horizontal Mattress Suture

- *Application*: Horizontal mattress suture technique is effective in minimizing the wound tension, closing the dead space, and facilitating wound edge eversion. Horizontal mattress suture is useful for closing the palpebral fissure in blepharorrhaphy, securing the conjunctival flap on the cornea or limbus in trabeculectomy, and closing the sclera tunnel incision in conventional cataract surgery. This suture may also be used as a stay stitch to temporarily approximate wound edges.
- *Technique*: For placing a horizontal mattress suture, the needle is introduced on one side of the wound and exited on the opposite side equidistant from the wound edge. The needle is then reintroduced on the second side of the wound lateral to the exit point again at the same distance from the wound edge. The suture then exits in the same position on the first side of the wound and creating a "rectangle" out of the suture. The ends of the suture are then tied on the same side of the wound (Fig. 5-8).
- *Advantage*: This suture is especially good for distributing wound tension across larger wounds particularly for the initial sutures.
- *Disadvantage*: The disadvantage of this suture is the risk of strangulation of tissue and disturbing the blood supply to the wound and subsequent wound necrosis.

## Simple Continuous Suture (Simple Running Stitch)

- *Application*: Using a continuous suture rather than multiple interrupted sutures permits the surgeon to close the wound much more rapidly and offers a significant time saving.
- *Technique*: For placing a running suture, first a simple interrupted suture is placed. Then instead of cutting both ends of the suture, only its free end is cut and the end attached to the needle is saved. The needle is then passed diagonally across the wound and reintroduced to exit the wound on the other side. This cycle is repeated until the surgeon reaches the end of the wound (Fig. 5-9). A single knot is then placed, using the last loop as a suture end. It is important to space each interval of the running suture evenly.
- *Disadvantage*: Continuous suture is not as strong as interrupted sutures and is more prone to strangulation and tissue necrosis. Furthermore, it has the risk of wound dehiscence after the suture break.

## Running Locked Suture

The running locked suture is a variation of the simple running suture. Before beginning each new suture, the needle is looped under the previous external segment of suture crossing the wound. This process is repeated until the end of the wound where a single knot is placed, using the last loop as a suture end (Fig. 5-10).

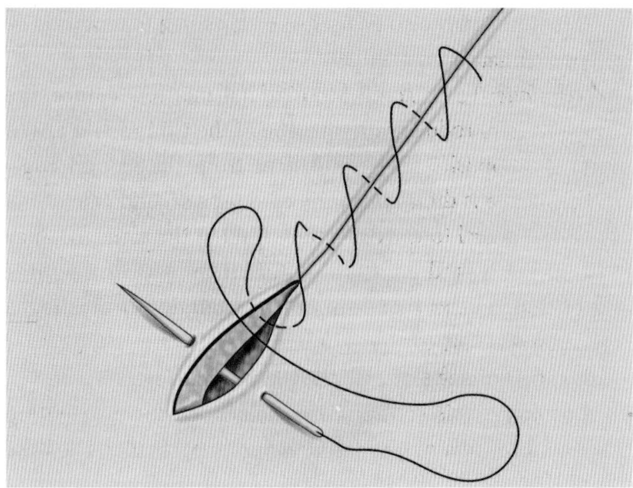

**Figure 5-9** This cycle is repeated until the surgeon reaches the end of the wound.

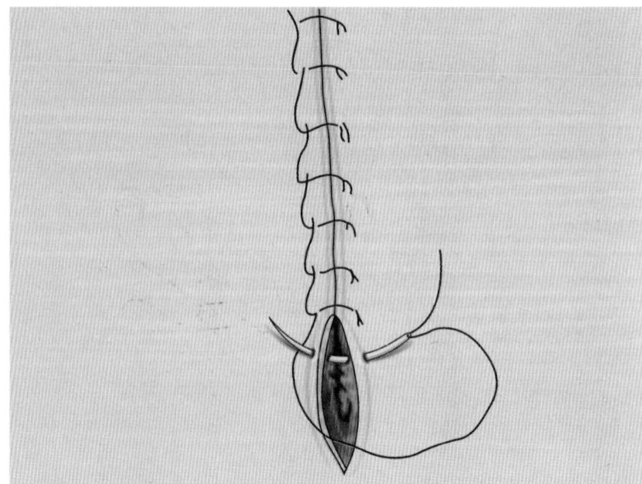

**Figure 5-10** This process is repeated until the end of the wound where a single knot is placed, using the last loop as a suture end.

## Running Horizontal Mattress Suture

It is a combination of simple running and horizontal mattress sutures. For placing a running horizontal mattress suture, first an interrupted horizontal mattress suture is placed. Then instead of tying the two ends of the suture, the needle is passed laterally and re-enters the tissue on the same side through which the suture is exited and passed back to the opposite side to start a second mattress suture. This cycle is repeated until the end of the wound is reached. As in simple running suture, a single knot is then placed, using the last loop as a suture end.

## Buried Interrupted Suture

- *Application*: Buried suture is primarily used to close any dead space, which may have been produced by the wound or surgical excision, to reapproximate the wound edges.
- *Technique*: For placing a buried interrupted suture, first the wound edges should be everted with a forceps. Then the needle mounted on an absorbable suture is entered to the deeper tissue near the base of the wound and moved vertically to exit from more superficial tissue underneath the wound edge at the same side. The needle is then passed to the opposite side and entered the superficial tissue underneath the wound edges at a depth equal to the depth where the needle emerged from the initial side. The needle is then travelled vertically to exit from the deeper tissue at the same level as it was initially entered into on the first side of the wound. The suture ends are then tied. In this manner, all knots will be buried in the deep tissue when the whole wound is closed.
- *Advantage*: It provides longer term support to the healing wound and improves the cosmetic result.

## Running Subcuticular Suture

- *Application*: This suturing technique is actually a subcuticular type of running mattress suture in which only two points of skin surface are penetrated. This technique is useful to enhance the cosmetic result and for closing wounds with equal tissue thickness and in which virtually no tension exists.
- *Technique*: Running subcuticular suture is initiated by introducing the needle into the skin several millimeters farther from one end of the wound. The needle is then driven toward the wound end and brought out inside the apex of the wound within the dermis. The free end of suture is tied off on itself. Then the needle is entered in the dermis at one side of the wound and passed laterally parallel to the surface to emerge from the same side of the wound at the same level as it was entered. The needle is then passed to the opposite side of the wound and is introduced into the dermis at a point directly opposite where the needle just exited from the first side and driven laterally to emerge from the same level as it was introduced. Care should be taken to put the bites of each side with the same length. This process is repeated until the suture reaches the other end of the wound and wound closure is complete. The needle then enters the dermis at the wound apex and passed subcutaneously to exit on the skin surface several millimeters farther from the wound end. Finally, the second free end should be secured in the same way as

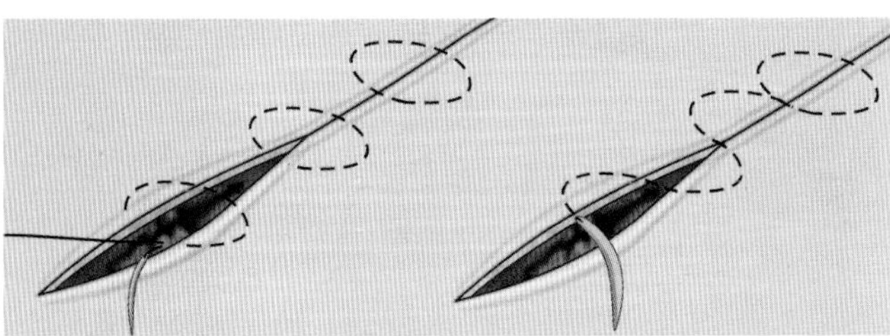

**Figure 5-11** Subcuticular suture (interrupted and continuous).

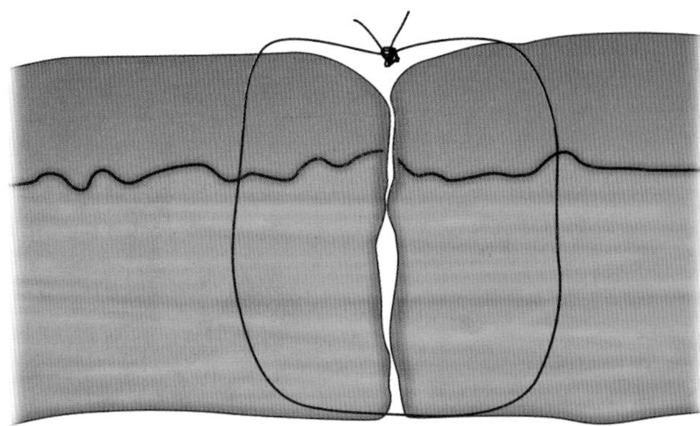

**Figure 5-12** A knot sitting on the wound can cause wound depression, so wound edge should be slightly everted to avoid wound depression.

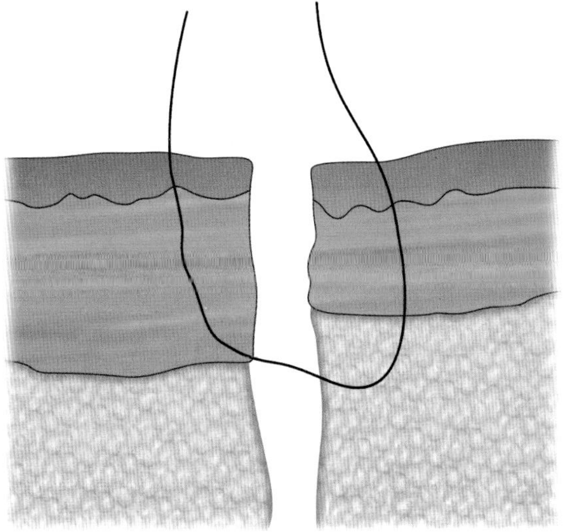

**Figure 5-13** Take a deeper bite on the thin side and a more superficial bite on the thick side to have a better alignment.

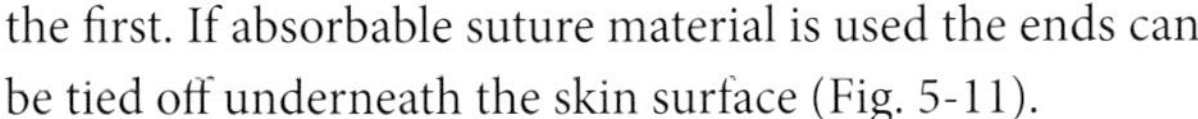

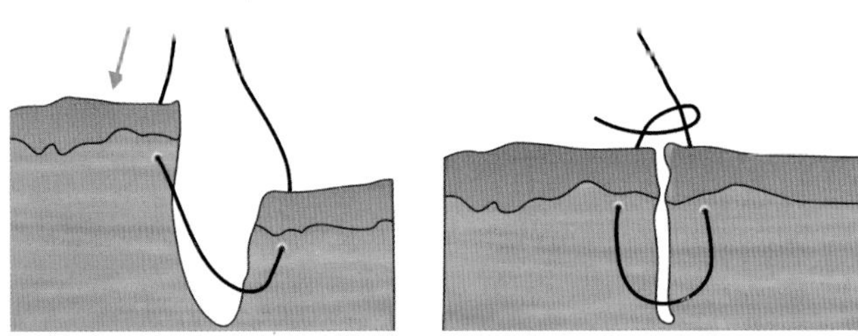

**Figure 5-14** Passing the suture from a higher to lower edge causes the suture to come out easily on the low side and when the long suture limb is pulled with the first throw of the knot it will lift the lower wound edge up to a matching level with the opposite side.

the first. If absorbable suture material is used the ends can be tied off underneath the skin surface (Fig. 5-11).

- *Advantage*: Running subcuticular suture can be placed using both absorbable and nonabsorbable sutures. Since this technique penetrates the wound only at two points, in case of using nonabsorbable suture, it can be left in place for a longer period of time without having concern about excessive scar formation.

Choosing the right suturing technique, placing the appropriate suture at a good depth, maintaining symmetry, spacing and length with the correct tensile forces is both a science and an art.

## CONCLUSIONS

- A knot sitting on the wound can cause wound depression, so wound edge should be slightly everted to avoid wound depression (Fig. 5-12).
- The suture should not constrict the tissue.
- Wound edges should be joined loosely as there is always some postoperative edema.
- When suturing a thin edge to a thick edge, take a deeper bite on the thin side and a more superficial bite on the thick side to have a better alignment (Fig. 5-13).
- When the wound edges are of unequal height, take a superficial bite on the high side superficially and then a deeper bite is taken on the lower side. Passing the suture from a higher to lower edge causes the suture to come out easily on the low side, and when the long suture limb is pulled with the first throw of the knot it will lift the lower wound edge up to a matching level with the opposite side (Fig. 5-14).
- Dead space should be closed to reduce the risk of infection, hematoma and wound depression.

## REFERENCES

1. Roy FH, Arzabe CW. Master techniques in ophthalmic surgery. Thorofare, NJ: SLACK Incorporated, 2004.
2. Macsai MS. Ophthalmic microsurgical suturing techniques. New York, NY: Springer, 2007.

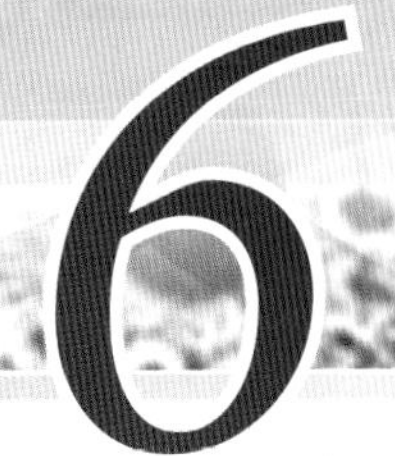


# Hemostasis

Colin I Clement, Adrian T Fung, Brett O'Donnell

## INTRODUCTION

The term "hemostasis" refers to the normal response of a blood vessel to injury by forming a clot that serves to limit hemorrhage. Vessel injury leads to vasoconstriction, platelet aggregation, and activation of the blood coagulation cascade that, in turn, contribute to the development of a stable hemostatic plug (Flowchart 6-1). Excessive activation of this response in the absence of bleeding leads to thrombosis. In contrast, deficiency of this response will result in hemorrhage.

Intraoperative bleeding may obscure the operative field leading to prolonged surgical times, compromise quality of surgery, increase the risk of complication and may lead to longer hospital admission. In severe cases, it may lead to anemia and the requirement for blood product transfusion that exposes the patient to further risk.

**Flowchart 6-1** Algorithm showing the factors that contribute to hemostasis and the development of a stable hemostatic plug. Factors listed in italics indicate the location of action in the hemostasis pathway. NSAIDS, nonsteroidal anti-inflammatory drugs.

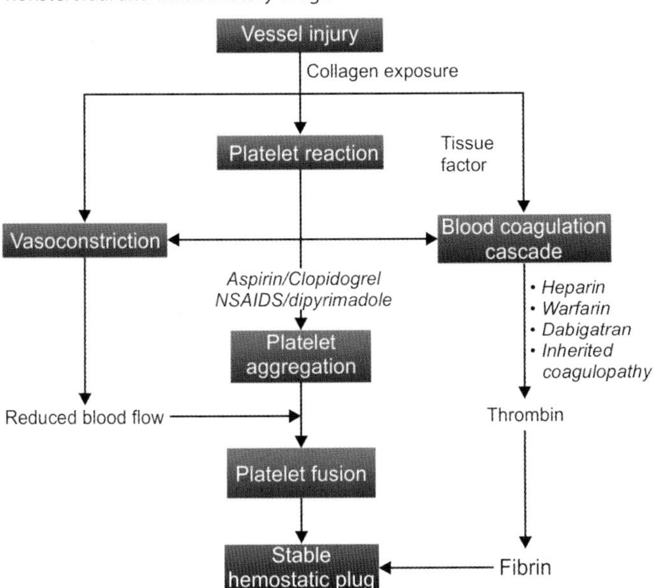


**TABLE 6-1** Factors contributing to operative bleeding

| |
|---|
| • Anticoagulant medication |
| • Antiplatelet medication |
| • High blood pressure |
| • Hypervascular tissue |
| • Unseen sources |
| • Exposed bone |
| • Inflamed tissues |
| • Coagulopathy |
| • Platelet dysfunction |

This chapter aims to review the factors that contribute to intraoperative bleeding (Table 6-1), how to plan surgery to best minimize bleeding, and the intraoperative management of bleeding. Special consideration is given to glaucoma surgery, vitreoretinal surgery, and orbital/oculoplastic surgery where surgical bleeding may be particularly problematic or require special management.

## FACTORS CONTRIBUTING TO INTRAOPERATIVE BLEEDING

All patients should be screened for antithrombotic use, history of spontaneous bruising, known bleeding tendency, problems with previous surgery or conditions that predispose to bleeding (thrombocytopenia, liver disease, inherited coagulopathy).

**TABLE 6-2** Supplemental treatments that may impair hemostasis

| Herb/vitamin/supplement | Usual indication |
|---|---|
| • St John's wort | • Anxiety, depression |
| • Ginkgo biloba | • Memory, glaucoma |
| • Garlic | • Antimicrobial, cardiovascular disease, cancer |
| • Ginger | • Dyspepsia, gastroparesis, constipation |
| • Ginseng | • Aphrodisiac, stimulant |
| • Vitamin E | • Immunity, skin |
| • Feverfew | • Headaches, fever, digestive problems |

It is important to specifically ask about the use of aspirin, warfarin, clopidogrel, dipyridamole, dabigatran, or systemic nonsteroidal anti-inflammatory drugs, and the indications for their use. In certain situations, it may be safe to stop their use in the perioperative period; however, the risk of stopping antithrombotic treatment must be weighed against the risk of continued use during surgery. In many cases, the risk of a serious adverse event does not permit withdrawal of antithrombotic treatment, and the surgeon instead must plan surgery in the presence of such treatment.

It is also important to enquire about the use of supplementary health products as many are associated with increased bleeding risk (Table 6-2). Often, patients do not consider these medications and will not volunteer their use unless questioning is targeted. It is, therefore, important to be familiar with supplements that can potentially interfere with hemostasis.

If possible, coagulopathies should be managed preoperatively in conjunction with a hematologist. Occasionally, blood products may need to be given, but the decision is dependent on the type of surgery. For example, Fabian et al.[1] have shown it is quite safe to perform clear corneal cataract surgery with topical anesthesia in individuals with factor XI deficiency without the need for prophylactic use of inhibitor antibodies. Similar patients having a peribulbar/retrobulbar block or undergoing more invasive surgery [(e.g. dacryocystorhinostomy (DCR)] are likely to fair less well.

## PLANNING SURGERY

*When planning surgery, two key issues arise in relation to risk of intraoperative hemorrhage:*

1. Should antithrombotic medication be stopped?
2. What type of anesthesia is best?

We have already mentioned that withdrawal of antithrombotic medication should be considered to mitigate against intraoperative bleeding, but in many cases this can be harmful. Many patients take systemic antithrombotics because they are at risk of life-threatening conditions, such as pulmonary, coronary, or cerebral thrombosis. In fact, the continued use of antithrombotic medication is generally safe.[2] The decision on continued use should be made on a case-by-case basis and involves the input of the treating physician where possible.

Type of anesthesia may influence the risk of intraoperative bleeding, either from the anesthesia itself or from the surgery. Careful consideration should be given to the best type of anesthesia and whether it is suitable for a given patient. Some studies have provided guidance on the issue of anesthesia and hemostasis. For example, meta-analysis shows subconjunctival hemorrhage and periorbital hematoma are statistically more common in eyes that received retrobulbar or peribulbar anesthesia compared with topical anesthesia for cataract surgery. There is no difference in intraoperative complications from each anesthetic technique. However, topical anesthesia was associated with higher pain perception during surgery.[3] Similarly, in a large series, no significant difference in hemorrhagic complications was seen between eyes undergoing peribulbar block in the presence or absence of systemic clopidogrel. The incidence of low-risk hemorrhagic complications (focal lid or conjunctival ecchymosis) was low (2–3%).[4]

### Glaucoma Filtration Surgery

Not only is hemostasis important during glaucoma surgery for the reasons outlined in the introduction, it can also have a significant effect on the success of surgery. This is because bleeding releases red blood cells, leukocytes, serum, and cytokines into surrounding tissues and induces an acute inflammatory response that ultimately leads to wound repair. The development of subconjunctival scar tissue can block egress of aqueous into the bleb and failure of the surgery. Strategies that limit this response are, therefore, likely to improve outcomes.

Two retrospective studies of similar size (approx 350 trabeculectomies) suggest concurrent use of anticoagulants, but not antiplatelets, is associated with an increased risk of hemorrhagic complication and surgery failure.[4,5] These findings suggest anticoagulant therapy should be suspended perioperatively to limit complications and improve outcomes. However, neither study provides guidance on whether there is a therapeutic range for which it is safe to proceed to surgery with concurrent anticoagulant use. Furthermore, both studies did not evaluate whether suspension of anticoagulation was associated with nonocular complications.

Despite the above findings, evidence suggests most glaucoma surgeons do not stop anticoagulants or antiplatelets before filtration surgery.[6] In a survey of UK glaucoma specialists, 32.8 and 31.2% routinely stopped warfarin and aspirin before surgery. Of those that operated without stopping warfarin, 81.25% were only happy to do so if the INR was < 3.0. The remaining 18.75% were happy to operate at higher INRs.

A correlation between postoperative bleeding and the use of multiple glaucoma medications before surgery has been documented.[7] This is possibly because of the conjunctival hyperemia caused by long-term use of medications such as brimonidine and apraclonidine. Consideration to reduction of topical medications before surgery should be given but only if it is safe to do so.

Sub-Tenon's anesthesia versus general anesthesia have been compared in eyes undergoing glaucoma filtration surgery. There was no significant difference between groups.[7]

## Vitreoretinal Surgery

Most vitreoretinal surgery is performed under peribulbar or retrobulbar anesthesia. In patients who are more likely to bleed, retrobulbar anesthesia should be avoided to minimize the chance of intraconal hemorrhage. Evidence regarding antithrombosis in the setting of vitreoretinal surgery is conflicting. Most studies show no increase in hemorrhagic rates despite perioperative maintenance of antithrombosis.[8-12] Others have shown higher rates of potentially sight threatening complications with antiplatelet therapy;[13] hemorrhage with warfarin therapy (Narendran) or persistent postoperative vitreous cavity hemorrhage after vitrectomy for nonclearing diabetic vitreous hemorrhage.[14]

Proliferative diabetic retinopathy is the single most important predictive risk factor for intraoperative hemorrhage in patients undergoing vitrectomy.[15] If possible and appropriate, preoperative intravitreal bevacizumab should be given 1-week prior.[16] This minimizes intra- and early postoperative hemorrhage.[17] Bevacizumab should be avoided if there is retinal neovascularization associated with fibrovascular traction, as regression of vessels can worsen this traction leading to retinal detachment. If the vitreous hemorrhage is dense, B-scan ultrasonography will be required to look for traction.

## Orbital/Oculoplastic Surgery

The benefits of the surgery need to be weighed against the risks of intra- or postoperative bleeding and technical difficulties associated, e.g. the risk of blindness with orbital hemorrhage, postoperative swelling in ptosis surgery with delayed recovery of final lid height stabilization.

The anesthetic and surgical technique may need to be modified, e.g. in patients needing to continue anticoagulants or requiring orbital surgery on vascular malformations, hypotensive anesthetic agents can be used. In blepharoplasty, fat cauterization in a warfarinized patient may be the only alternative instead of fat removal when anticoagulation has to be continued.

Some eyelid procedures can be done, and the patient remains on warfarin, e.g. canthoplasty and wedge excisions, with a low risk of postoperative bleeding. Skin grafting is better avoided and flap repair preferable if postoperative bleeding likely.

External and endonasal DCR are both difficult when there is significant bleeding. Assisted local anesthetic in external surgery may be safer for the patient's airway; however, the smaller rhinostomy in endonasal surgery may bleed less.

In patients with known bleeding diathesis, consultation with a hematologist is usually required to arrange for the preoperative administration of fresh frozen platelets or desmopressin acetate, overnight admission for observation

# INTRAOPERATIVE MANAGEMENT OF HEMOSTASIS

Application of direct pressure or compression at a bleeding site is often the surgeon's first choice to assist in the control of bleeding. Other mechanical methods such as sutures, staples, and ligating clips have limited use in ophthalmology (Table 6-3). Compression or other mechanical methods may have limited success if the source of bleeding occurs in the context of prior administration of antiplatelet or anticoagulant medications. In recent years, thermal techniques, such as electrocautery, hemostatic scalpels, and lasers, have become viable surgical options to reduce bleeding; however, the frequent use of cautery and other thermal techniques can have its drawbacks. Depending on the procedure and location of the bleeding tissue, it may be impractical or impossible to effectively stop blood loss via mechanical or thermal hemostatic techniques. For example, in bony orbital surfaces, inflamed or friable vessels, or tissues containing multiple and diffuse capillaries, it is extremely difficult to maintain hemostasis with these methods.

The application of pharmacological agents to reduce bleeding has been used to good effect. For example, topical phenylephrine at the commencement of pterygium surgery is associated with significantly reduced need for intraoperative

**TABLE 6-3** Techniques for controlling intraoperative bleeding

| Technique | Options |
|---|---|
| Mechanical | • Direct pressure<br>• Sutures<br>• Staples<br>• Ligating clips<br>• Fabric pads<br>• Gauzes<br>• Sponges<br>• Blood component/replacement therapy |
| Thermal | • Electrocautery<br>• Hemostatic scalpel<br>• Laser |
| Chemical | • Hypotensive anesthesia<br>• Epinephrine<br>• Vitamin K<br>• Protamine<br>• Desmopressin<br>• Aminocaproic acid<br>• Tranexamic acid<br>• Topical hemostats<br>• Collagen<br>• Cellulose<br>• Gelatins<br>• Thrombins<br>• Topical sealants and adhesives<br>• Fibrin sealants<br>• Synthetic glues |

cattery and reduced operative time.[18] Similar results are achieved when vasoconstrictors are used topically in glaucoma surgery and DCR (*see* below).

## Glaucoma Filtration Surgery

The main strategies for the control of intraoperative bleeding in glaucoma surgery are vasoconstriction, minimal tissue handling, and electrocautery.

Risk of bleeding may be minimized by inducing conjunctival vasoconstriction with topical application of apraclonidine or phenylephrine immediately prior to surgery. Additional benefit may be gained from inclusion of epinephrine in a subconjunctival lignocaine at the site of surgery.

Minimal tissue handling may also reduce bleeding risk. Conservative conjunctival peritomy, blunt tissue dissection, and handling of the Tenon's capsule rather than conjunctiva are all helpful strategies. Blind retrieval of subconjunctival pledgets containing antifibrotic medication is sometimes a high-risk maneuver that results in bleeding from a source that is difficult to view and control. Attaching the pledgets to a retrieval suture is one way of preventing this.

Electrocautery is frequently employed to control bleeding. Gentle cattery has the advantage of limiting bleeding without causing excessive tissue damage. Aggressive cattery may lead to contraction of scleral collagen that, in turn, can result in poor scleral flap closure and postoperative hypotony. The induced tissue necrosis may also produce a more pronounced inflammatory response leading to subconjunctival fibrosis and surgical failure.

Surgical iridectomy can be another source of intraoperative bleeding, and large iridectomies may be at greater risk. A small iridectomy is preferred for this reason and in an eye at risk; a procedure where iridectomy is not needed (e.g. deep sclerectomy, Express shunt, viscocanalostomy) may be the surgery of choice.

## Vitreoretinal Surgery

A significant degree of hemorrhage may be associated with scleral buckling. When isolating the rectus muscles, care must be taken to avoid perforating their associated vessels. The sclera should be inspected for vortex veins to avoid puncture during suture passes. Inadvertent full thickness scleral suture passes may lead to subretinal hemorrhage. Scleral perforation is suspected if there is egress of subretinal fluid or acute ocular hypotony. If this occurs, the fundus should be immediately examined by indirect ophthalmoscopy. Small extramacular hemorrhages can be managed conservatively, especially if inferior. Small submacular hemorrhages can be managed by pneumatic displacement and 40° gaze down posturing.[19] Large submacular hemorrhages may require conversion to vitrectomy with subretinal tissue plasminogen activator, intravitreal gas, and gaze down posturing.

During a combined vitrectomy and encirclement, the scleral buckle is often performed before the vitrectomy. Hemostasis of limbal vessels with external diathermy should be performed prior to the vitrectomy. This prevents blood seeping onto the cornea, obscuring the view for vitrectomy.

*Hemotasis during vitrectomy can be achieved by two means:* Iatrogenically elevating the intraocular pressure or with endodiathermy. Tamponade with intraocular pressures up to 60 mm Hg may be required in some instances to stop bleeding. The pressure should be lowered as soon as bleeding has been controlled to minimize the risk of iatrogenic central retinal vein occlusion or progression of any pre-existing glaucoma. Lowering of the intraocular pressure should be done in a step-wise manner, watching for rebleeding. In cases where profuse bleeding is expected (such as during a chorioretinal biopsy), the anesthetist may be able to provide assistance by pharmacologically lowering the patient's systemic blood pressure. Endodiathermy can be applied to bleeding points. Ensure that the endodiathermy tip is clean to allow for effective cauterization. On newer vitrectomy machines linear endodiathermy is possible with the foot pedal. Endodiathermy should be applied at the first sign of hemorrhage to maintain fundus visualization. Once vitreous hemorrhage is extensive, this needs to be cleared with further vitrectomy or aspiration, which lowers the intraocular pressure and can lead to a cycle of further bleeding. Endodiathermy of bridging vessels at sites of retinal tears is important to prevent future vitreous hemorrhage. Suturing of sclerostomies should be performed in patients with intraoperative hemorrhage whenever there is concern about sclerostomy integrity to prevent postoperative hypotony and further hemorrhage.

The posterior hyaloid should be elevated in all diabetic patients undergoing vitrectomy. This removes the physical scaffold for growth of neovascular vessels into the vitreous. Diabetic patients usually have an adherent posterior hyaloids—this should be truncated at the equator, isolating the anterior and posterior vitreous and allowing for safer elevation of the posterior hyaloid at the optic disk. Postoperative hemorrhage can be minimized by the use of intravitreal silicone oil.

### Orbital/Oculoplastic Surgery

Generally, intraoperative cutting with coagulation is considered to reduce intra- and postoperative bleeding and swelling, whether done with cattery, radiofrequency, or laser. These methods have limited use in external DCR surgery but are useful and should be routine in eyelid and orbital surgery. They should be avoided if the patient wears a pacemaker; however, monopolar devices may be used if the patient is monitored, an anesthetist present, and the patient not being paced. Bipolar cattery is safe in the presence of a pacemaker. In some types of surgery, cattery must be very carefully applied and even avoided such as in optic nerve sheath fenestrations.

Eyelid surgery routinely can be performed with stronger epinephrine than is commercially available. For nonptosis or lid recession procedures, I have routinely prepared bupivacaine with 1:80,000 epinephrine for approximately 20 years without problem. Other authors use 1:50,000. Application of iced sterile water or saline can also be performed during ptosis and blepharoplasty surgery and is a quick and simple method of reducing general ooze in these cases that does not interfere with the eyelid height.

*In DCR surgery, there are many techniques that can assist the surgeon when operating including*: Elevation of the head of bed, intranasal cocaine with careful packing to avoid mucosal damage using neuropatties rather than gauze as well as direct nasal mucosal injection of local anesthetic with 1:80,000 epinephrine. Hypotensive anesthetic agents can be requested. Intraoperative injection of the nasal mucosa, application of neuropatties soaked in local anesthetic with adrenalin, and packing at end with expanding pack to prevent adhesions intranasally.

Application of some of the techniques for DCR surgery is limited in orbital surgery, e.g. the use of strong vasoconstrictors should be avoided in proximity to the optic nerve or retinal circulation in case of vasospasm and ischemia. Bone wax is usually difficult to apply in DCR surgery but is very useful for bleeding from the lateral orbital wall in an orbital decompression.

Drain insertion is a simple procedure to perform at the end of orbital surgery and rarely need to be left in longer than 24 hours. Generally, a small vacuum drain is preferable but a Penrose drain is an alternative.

## POSTOPERATIVE MANAGEMENT

Management of operative bleeding does not stop at the end of surgery as complications from impaired hemostasis may present in the postoperative period. Understanding of the potential complications and how to limit them will help reduce the likelihood of their occurrence.

### Glaucoma Surgery

Suprachoroidal hemorrhage is a serious postoperative complication of glaucoma surgery with an incidence of approximately 1% (range: 0.5–8.3%).[20] It typically presents within 7 days of the surgery and occurs most frequently after nonvalved glaucoma drainage device (GDD) implantation but also following valved GDD implantation, trabeculectomy (with or without antimetabolite) cyclodestructive procedures and trabeculectomy bleb needling.[20-22] Ocular risk factors for its development include aphakia, postoperative hypotony, and a prior history of intraocular surgery (penetrating keratoplasty, vitrectomy). Systemic hypertension, anticoagulant use, cardiovascular disease, and respiratory disease are also associated with increased risk.

Identification of risk factors for suprachoroidal hemorrhage may help minimize the risk, but when confronted with this clinical situation treatment will depend on severity, the factors contributing to it and the likelihood of spontaneous improvement. Those that are peripheral, not enlarging rapidly, occurring in the setting of a normal coagulation profile and in the absence of hypotony may be monitored closely as spontaneous resolution is possible. Large or rapidly progressing suprachoroidal hemorrhage, in setting of coagulopathy and/or hypotony require invention. Strategies include treatment of the coagulopathy, intervention to correct hypotony (e.g. intracameral viscoelastic, bridle suture of the bleb, bleb revision), suprachoroidal drainage or vitrectomy with or without gas, heavy liquid, or oil tamponade.

## Vitreoretinal Surgery

Postoperative hemorrhage is usually dependent on intraoperative technique. It is not uncommon for some dispersed postoperative vitreous cavity hemorrhage to occur. If there is no visualization of the fundus, B-scan ultrasonography is required to exclude a retinal tear or detachment. In most cases this can be treated conservatively, although persistent hemorrhage lasting longer than one month may require reoperation with washout. Rarely, recurrent delayed postoperative hemorrhage may occur secondary to neovascularization at internal sclerostomy sites. If this is suspected, endoscopic vitrectomy may be required for diagnosis and treatment with endolaser.

## Orbital/Oculoplastic Surgery

Intraorbital hemorrhage is a risk of any orbital surgery even when there are no unusual risk factors. Much orbital surgery is now day only, e.g. orbital fractures and anterior orbital biopsy. In day case surgery, pupil or functional endoscopic sinus surgery (FESS) observations are limited in duration unless the patient stays overnight. This is not routine practice for many surgeons after simple orbital. ptosis and blepharoplasty surgery, as the risk of postoperative loss of vision from bleeding is so small. Patients may be best advised to check their vision every few hours regularly after day only orbital and lower eyelid blepharoplasty surgery.

Although grafts are best left 4–5 days with a tie over bolster for graft compression, flaps can be checked at any time for development of hematoma and drained if fluctuant.

Postoperative blindness following surgery continues to occur but is rare. Blindness after blepharoplasty is estimated at 1:10,000 cases. Risk factors include hypertension, preoperative aspirin, increased physical activity, dependent head position, nonsteroidal anti-inflammatories, and coexistent vascular disease. Most cases follow lower lid blepharoplasty and 50% occur within 6 hours. The surgeon needs to be contactable for initial 24-hour period.

Any patient with loss of vision and pain must be assessed immediately. The time for onset of schemia from central retinal artery compression is not known but is in the vicinity of 90 minutes.

*If hemorrhage follows blepharoplasty or orbital surgery*: Urgent opening of the wound is required to release any haematoma. If this is not possible then lateral cantholysis is the important initial step and elevate the patient's head. Other options include intravenous corticosteroids. Continuing increased orbital pressure may require removal of the medial orbital wall to decompress the orbit, preferable to removing the floor due to the lower risk of postoperative diplopia.

Early postoperative DCR bleeding usually settles with ice packs, head elevation, and avoidance of bending. In later postoperative DCR bleeding, nasal packing is usually required. Insertion of Vaseline-coated gauze or preferably Rapid Rhino dressing (Arthro Care ENT, 7000W William Cannon Dr, Austin, TX 78735) and injecting air or fluid to expand the balloon. After waiting a few minutes and inspecting the throat for continuing bleeding, leave the balloon for 24–48 hours. If the mucosa is very swollen, the nose can be prepacked to shrink the mucosa initially, then remove the initial pack and repack. The procedure can be done in an operating theatre, ward, or emergency department.

## REFERENCES

1. Fabian ID, Sachs D, Moisseiev J, et al. Cataract extraction without prophylactic treatment in patients with severe factor XI deficiency. Am J Ophthalmol. 2009;148:920-4.
2. Lip GY, Durrani OM, Roldan V, et al. Peri-operative management of ophthalmic patients taking antithrombotic therapy. Int J Clin Pract. 2011;65:361-71.
3. Zhao LQ, Zhu H, Zhao PQ, et al. Topical anesthesia versus regional anesthesia for cataract surgery: a meta-analysis of randomized controlled trials. Ophthalmology. 2012;119:659-67.
4. Calenda E, Lamothe L, Genevois O, et al. Peribulbar block in patients scheduled for eye procedures and treated with clopidogrel. J Anesth. 2012;26:779-82.
5. Cobb CJ, Chakrabarti S, Chadha V, et al. The effect of aspirin and warfarin therapy in trabeculectomy. Eye (Lond). 2007;21: 598-603.
6. Law SK, Song BJ, Yu F, et al. Hemorrhagic complications from glaucoma surgery in patients on anticoagulation therapy or antiplatelet therapy. Am J Ophthalmol. 2008;145:736-46.
7. Alwitry A, King AJ, Vernon SA. Anticoagulation therapy in glaucoma surgery. Graefes Arch Clin Exp Ophthalmol. 2008; 246:891-6.
8. Dietlein TS, Moalem Y, Schild AM, et al. Subconjunctival or general anesthesia in trabeculectomy – a retrospective analysis of the bleeding risk from a glaucoma surgeon's point of view. Klin Monbl Augenheilkd. 2012;229:826-9.
9. Dayani PN, Grand MG. Maintenance of warfarin anticoagulation for patients undergoing vitreoretinal surgery. Arch Ophthalmol. 2006;124:1558-65.
10. Fu AD, McDonald HR, Williams DF, et al. Anticoagulation with warfarin in vitreoretinal surgery. Retina. 2007;27:290-5.

11. Brown JS, Mahmoud TH. Anticoagulation and clinically significant postoperative vitreous hemorrhage in diabetic vitrectomy. Retina. 2011;31:1983-7.
12. Oh J, Smiddy WE, Kim SS. Antiplatelet and anticoagulation therapy in vitreoretinal surgery. Am J Ophthalmol. 2011;151: 934-9.
13. Ryan A, Saad T, Kirwan C, et al. Maintenance of perioperative antiplatelet and anticoagulant therapy for vitreoretinal surgery. Clin Experiment Ophthalmol. 2013;41(4):387-95.
14. Fabinyi DCA, O'Neill EC, Connell PP, et al. Vitreous cavity haemorrhage post-vitrectomy for diabetic eye disease: the effect of perioperative anticoagulation and antiplatelet agents. Clin Experiment Ophthalmol. 2011;39:878-84.
15. Passemard M, Koehrer P, Juniot A, et al. Maintenance of anticoagulant and antiplatelet agents for patients undergoing peribulbar anesthesia and vitreoretinal surgery. Retina. 2012;32: 1868-73.
16. Ahmadieh H, Shoeibi N, Entezari M, et al. Intravitreal bevacizumab for prevention of early postvitrectomy hemorrhage in diabetic patients. A randomized clinical trial. Ophthalmology. 2009;116:1943-8.
17. Smith JM, Steel DHW. Anti-vascular endothelial growth factor for prevention of postoperative vitreous cavity haemorrhage after vitrectomy for proliferative diabetic retinopathy. Cochrane Database System Rev. 2011; (5). Art. No.: CD008214.
18. Villegas Becerril E, Pérula de Torres L, Bergillos Arillo M, et al. Evaluation of topical vasoconstrictors in pterygium surgery and their role in reducing intraoperative bleeding. Arch Soc Esp Oftalmol. 2011;86:54-7.
19. Lincoff H Kreissig I, Stopa M, et al. 40° Gaze down position for pneumatic displacement of submacular hemorrhage: clinical application and results. Retina. 2008;28:56-9.
20. Jeganathan VSE, Ghosh S, Ruddle JB, et al. Risk factors for delayed suprachoroidal haemorrhage following glaucoma surgery. Br J Ophthalmol 2008;92:1393–6.
21. Gressel MG, Parrish RK, Heuer DK. Delayed nonexpulsive suprachoroidal hemorrhage. Arch Ophthalmol. 1984;102: 1757-60.
22. Howe LJ, Bloom P. Delayed suprachoroidal haemorrhage following trabeculectomy bleb needling. Br J Ophthalmol. 1999 83:753.

CHAPTER

# 7

# Surgical Field: Asepsis and Preparation

Parul Ichhpujani, Shibal Bhartiya

## INTRODUCTION

Both antisepsis and asepsis of the operating field are essential for infection control. Antisepsis refers to prevention of infection by inhibiting the growth of pathogenic microorganisms, while asepsis means a condition in which living pathogenic organisms are absent. In ocular surgeries, the main source of infection is the patient's own ocular flora: *S aureus, S epidermidis, B coagulase, E coli, Corynebacteria, Pseudomonas aerugnosa* and *Streptococci*, both alpha- and beta-hemolytic.[1] Hence, it is imperative that all patients undergoing surgery get a meticulous preparation of the surgical field. The techniques of preoperative patient preparation vary from institution to institution, but basic principles are common.

### Basic Principles

- To decrease the resident and transient microbial counts at the surgical site
- To minimize the growth of microbes in the postoperative period
- To reduce the risk and rates of infection postsurgery.

## ANTISEPTIC AGENTS

Antiseptic agents are classified as aqueous-based or alcohol-based solutions.

### Aqueous-Based Solutions

#### *Povidone-Iodine*

Traditional aqueous-based iodophor, povidone-iodine (PVP-I; referred also as "tamed iodine"), contains iodine complexed with a solubilizing agent that allows for the release of free iodine when in solution.[2] Iodine acts in an antiseptic fashion by destroying microbial proteins and DNA. The mechanism of bactericidal action is not fully understood but thought to be by oxidation and substitution/iodination of amino acids and fatty acids.

Iodophor-containing products have broad-spectrum antimicrobial properties, efficacy and safety on nearly all skin surfaces in patients regardless of age. There has been no reported microbial resistance to PVP-I. Studies have shown that more dilute formulations of PVP-I demonstrate greater and more rapid killing efficacy than more concentrated ones, while also being less irritating to mucosal surfaces.[3]

Typically, a 10% PVP-I solution yields 1% iodine and iodide. The concentration of free iodine, $I_2$, is not stated and is difficult to quantify, also changing from batch to batch.

Ruptured globes or those at risk of rupture should not be prepared with PVP-I as with a pH of 3–5, it is well tolerated by corneal epithelium but not endothelium.[4]

#### *Chlorhexidine Gluconate*

Another agent, chlorhexidine gluconate (CHG), works by disrupting bacterial cell membranes. Aqueous solutions must be prepared with distilled sterile water. Dilution of CHG with saline solutions results in the precipitation of chlorhexidine salts which are not only irritant but do not exhibit any antimicrobial activity. Bacterial uptake of chlorhexidine has been shown to be very rapid, with maximum bioavailability reached in less than 20 seconds. CHG has more sustained antimicrobial activity and is more resistant to neutralization by blood products than the iodophors.[5]

### Alcohol-Based Agents

Ethyl and isopropyl alcohol are two of the most effective antiseptic agents available. When used alone, alcohol is fast- and short-acting and has broad-spectrum antimicrobial activity. Alcohol-based solutions that contain CHG or iodophors have sustained and durable antimicrobial activity that lasts long after alcohol evaporation. A limitation to the use of alcohol in the operating room is its flammability on skin surfaces prior to evaporation.[6]

## PREOPERATIVE USE OF TOPICAL ANTIBIOTICS

Prophylactic antibiotics instilled topically have been shown to reduce postoperative infection.[7] Loading doses of topical antibiotics and frequent application (every 15–30 minutes) have been found to provide prolonged therapeutic levels in the cornea and aqueous humor. Topical antibiotics should begin 24 hours before surgery and should be used 6–8 times during the day. Instillation of topical antibiotics for more than 24 hours may lead to replacement of the patients' own flora by more virulent microorganisms.

## PREPARATION OF THE SURGICAL FIELD

The importance of a scrub bath with a head wash on the day of surgery or the night prior to the surgery should be emphasized to the patient.[8] Thorough facial washing with a medicated soap on the day of surgery further helps to ensure that the eye and surrounding area is clean and there is no contamination. These days, cilia are not trimmed rather lashes are isolated with sterile adhesive drapes. As the hairline is considered to be a contaminated area, the hair should be neatly tucked in under a surgical cap or a towel.

Preparing the surgical field commences with instillation of a drop of PVP-I solution (5%) into the inferior conjunctival fornix. PVP-I is bactericidal in 30 seconds and need not be irrigated out of the eye before surgery. Cleaning the lids, lid margins and adjacent skin with PVP-I 5% is an effective method of eliminating microbes. Following this, a cotton swab/ball soaked in PVP-I solution (10%) is used to prepare the surgical field. The skin is painted in progressively larger concentric circles, starting from the medial canthus and proceeding laterally. The eye to be operated, the ipsilateral cheek, forehead and nose should be painted using semicircular strokes (Figs. 7-1A to C).

Care should be taken not to touch the previously cleaned area a second time. The process is repeated thrice with fresh soaked cotton balls. The prepared area is then blotted with a sterile towel without wiping off the PVP-I (which is a contact disinfectant) and allowed to air-dry. To prevent the agent from entering the patient's ears, they may be temporarily plugged using cotton pledgets.

## DRAPING

*Principles of draping are*: Isolation of clean from dirty; provision of a barrier; creation of a sterile field; equipment cover and fluid control. A variety of surgical drapes or towels are available to isolate the periorbital area from rest of the face. Regardless of which materials are used, all surgical drapes should possess the following traits:

- *Abrasion resistance*: Should not abrade under normal, wet and dry conditions
- *Barrier properties*: Should resist the penetration of liquids and/or microbes
- *Biocompatibility*: Free of toxic ingredients
- *Drapeability*: Ability to conform to the shape of the object over which it is placed
- *Electrostatic properties*: Ability of the material to accept or dissipate an electrical charge
- *Nonflammability*: Should not support open combustion
- *Nonlinting*: Should not contain or generate free fiber particles
- *Tensile strength*: Should be strong enough to withstand the stresses encountered during typical use when wet or dry.

There is no one material that meets all the entire criteria. Each material has characteristics that make it either more or less suited for draping specific surgical procedures. A material characteristic that makes a material an excellent choice for an ophthalmic drape might make it a poor choice for an orthopedic drape.

### Types of Drapes

#### *Nondisposable Drapes*

Most commonly used nondisposable drape is a cloth drape made of loosely woven cotton cloth (100 × 100 cm) with an oval opening allowing adequate exposure of the eye to be operated, while covering the head and neck. The main disadvantage of these cotton drapes is that they are not waterproof and get soaked by the irrigating fluid. This may potentially contaminate the underlying skin, predisposing to infections. Also, these require meticulous autoclaving. With fabric drapes, it is difficult to bring the edge of the sterile field in close proximity to the operative site because of the

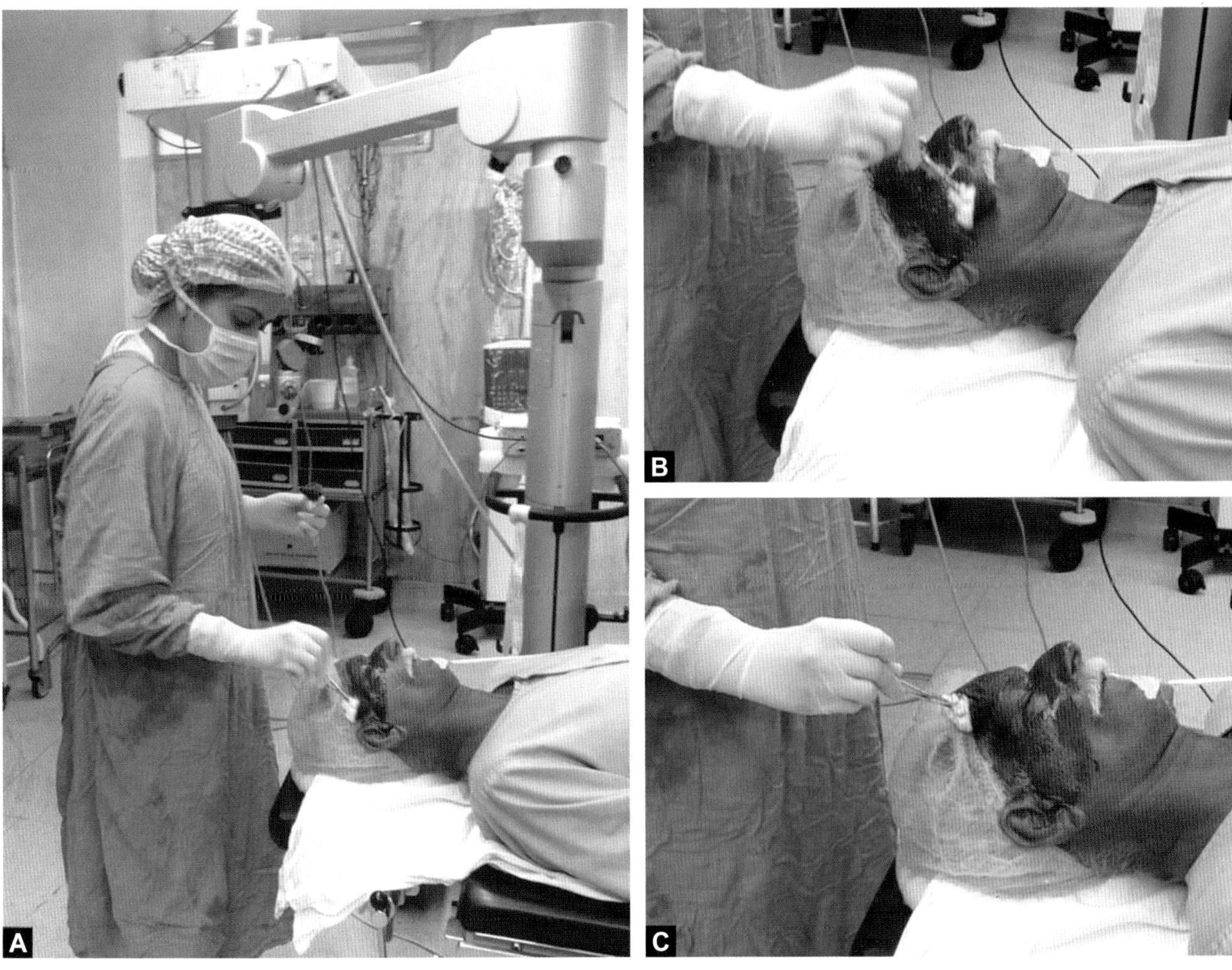

**Figures 7-1A to C** Painting with povidone-iodine.

contour around the eye. The fabric drapes may not stay in a fixed position during the surgical procedure and if towel clips are used to secure the drapes to the patient›s skin, they further limit the already restricted area in which the surgeon must work. The advantage of these drapes is that they are eco-friendly, reusable, biodegradable and cost-effective.

### *Disposable Drapes*

Disposable drapes may be made of water-repellent paper or plastic/trilaminate fabric.[9] These are usually three-ply, absorbent drapes ranging from 60 × 60 cms to 150 × 200 cms, with an integrated oval adhesive fenestration which constitutes the incision area. This fenestration may vary from 5 × 7 cms to 10 × 15 cms. One or two self-adhesive fluid collection pouches are available with each drape. These drapes are ethylene oxide (ETO)-sterilized.

## Technique of Draping

Draping can be done using four-quarter drapes, whereby four drapes are laid down to achieve exposure of the surgical site (Figs. 7-2A to G).

A sterile, nondisposable drape is folded in half and slipped under the patient's head and this serves as a rest for the surgeon's wrist during the surgical procedure. Another drape, folded lengthwise is slipped under the patient's head. Both the ends are then swathed over the patient's forehead to ensure that all the hair is covered with the towel. A towel clip may be used to secure the drape, or the ends tucked under the head of the patient to ensure that the drape does not slip.[2] In case a nondisposable drape with a precut hole or "eye" is used, ensure the correct positioning of the "eye" for exposing the area of surgical interest. At some centers, an additional disposable plastic drape is used over the nondisposable ones, while some choose to use only the disposable drape.

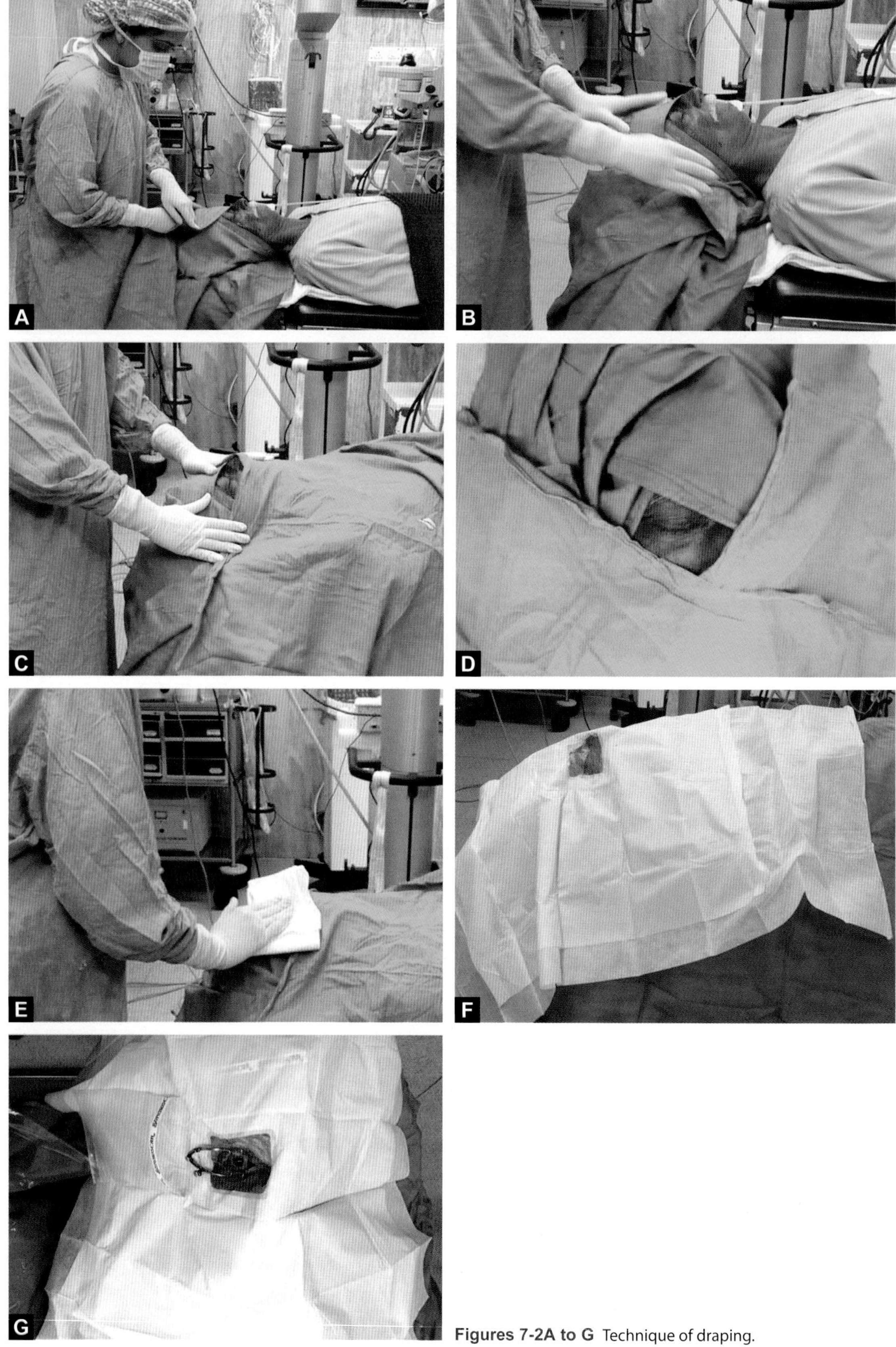

**Figures 7-2A to G** Technique of draping.

The disposable plastic drape must be placed directly over the open eye to cover the eyelashes and the meibomian gland orifices. The patient is asked to open eyes as wide as possible during this process. In case a peribulbar/facial block has been administered, a sterile cotton tip applicator or a swab stick may be used to keep the eyelids open.

The plastic drape is then cut. The incision commences at the medial canthus and extends laterally to the lateral canthus. Relaxing incisions may be placed if more exposure is desired, and the cut ends of the drape tucked into the fornices.

Alternatively, the H-shaped incision has also been described and consists of two parallel vertical limbs, 10–12 mm high. Then the horizontal limb, equal in length to the palpebral aperture, is incised.[10]

Additionally, the sterile adhesive strips which are available with the drape may be used to further expose the surgical site. A surgical speculum is then inserted ensuring that the cut ends of the drape rest within the fornices, and any jagged ends may be trimmed at this point.

The fluid collection pouch is then attached to the lateral side of the drape to act as a receptacle for irrigating fluid. A cellulose or cotton wick may be placed at the lateral canthus to prevent pooling of fluid within the operating field. Lengthy procedures may lead to the accumulation of irrigation fluids within the pouch that can result in the distortion of the surgical site, due to the weight of the fluid within the pouch. Suction apparatus may be used to allow for continued aspiration of fluids during a lengthy procedure; as a last resort, an incision may be made into the pouch and fluid is drained into an appropriately placed receptacle.

### Modifications While Draping

*In case the patient is claustrophobic or asthmatic, the following modifications will ensure greater patient comfort during surgery*:

- A nasal cannula connected to oxygen/fresh air source may be attached beneath the drape under the patient's chin. An instrument stand may be placed over the patient's chest in order to create a "tent", minimizing the feeling of being cloistered.
- Alternatively, a bridge may be used at the level of the patient's chin in order to keep the drape off the patient's face, thereby facilitating breathing.[11]

## PEARLS AND PITFALLS

- Use lint-free drapes, sponges and applicators.
- Care should be taken not to transfer microbes from the "unclean" site to the site that has already been cleaned.
- Cotton used for each pass should be fresh in order to minimize chances of contamination of the cleaning solution.
- Area that is prepared must leave ample room for potential shifting of the drape fenestration as well as extension of the proposed incision.
- Povidone-iodine should not be wiped off but should be allowed to air-dry.
- In case a patient is allergic to iodine, the protocol for preparation of the surgical field remains the same. Instead of PVP-I for skin preparation, 2% chlorhexidine should be used, making sure that it does not touch the conjunctiva or the cornea. The fornices should be thoroughly irrigated with balanced salt solution (BSS).

## REFERENCES


1. Capriotti JA, Pelletier JS, Shah M, et al. Normal ocular flora in healthy eyes from a rural population in Sierra Leone. Int Ophthalmol. 2009;29(2):81-4.
2. Digison MB. A review of antiseptic agents for pre-operative skin preparation. Plast Surg Nurs. 2007;27:185-9. quiz 190-1.
3. Berkelman RL, Holland BW, Anderson RL. Increased bactericidal activity of dilute preparations of povidone-iodine solutions. J Clin Microbiol. 1982;15(4):635-9.
4. Alp BN, Elibol O, Saragon MF, et al. The effect of povidone-iodine on the corneal endothelium. Cornea. 2000;9(4):546-50.
5. Apt L, Isenberg S. Chemical preparation of skin and eye in ophthalmic surgery: an international survey. Ophthalmic Surg. 1982;13(12):1026-9.
6. Ram J, Kaushik S, Brar GS, et al. Prevention of postoperative infections in ophthalmic surgery. Indian J Ophthalmol. 2001;49(1):59-69.
7. Christy NE, Sommer A. Antibiotic prophylaxis of postoperative endophthalmitis. Ann Ophthalmol. 1979;11:1261-65.
8. Mangram AJ, Horan TC, Pearson ML, et al. Hospital Infection Control Practices Advisory Committee. Guideline for prevention of surgical site infection, 1999. Infect Control Hosp Epidemiol. 1999;20(4):250-78.
9. Surendran TS, Bhaskaran S, Badrinath SS. Disposable drapes used in ocular surgery. Indian J Ophthalmol. 1983;31:499-501.
10. Atchoo P, Hionis M, Cinotti AA. A practical drape for eye surgery. Arch Ophthalmol. 1966;75(4):508-9.
11. Schlager A. New support for ophthalmic drapes. Arch Ophthalmol. 1999;117(10):1441-2.

# Section 2

# Cataract Surgery

*Section Editor* Alan S Crandall

CHAPTER 8

# Introduction

Alan S Crandall

Cataract is the number one cause of curable blindness in the world. Everyone is destined to have them, but not all need to have surgical correction. This section will deal with many of the techniques available to manage the surgery from the pediatric team approach, to "routine" cataracts, combined surgeries, the new Femtosecond technology as well as techniques for small incision extracapsular, the in-the-bag innovation and the use of adjunctive devices for surgery in eyes with zonular problems.

There has been a tremendous amount of innovation that has lead to cataract surgery becoming one of the safest, reliable, and cost-effective major surgeries. It improves the quality of life and in developing countries where blindness removes not only the blind person but also their care giver from productivity cataract surgery is very effective by restoring their sight thus returning both to a productive and meaningful life.

## SUGGESTED READING

1. http://one.aao.org/preferred-practice-pattern/cataract-in-adulteye-ppp–october-2011.

CHAPTER

9

# Technique for a Routine Cataract Surgery

Alan S Crandall

## INTRODUCTION

Cataract extraction is generally a safe, outpatient, and a highly gratifying procedure. It is important that the surgery is performed for the correct indications to achieve the desired outcome. The planning and decision-making process for cataract surgery involves judgment about appropriate treatment, surgical techniques including appropriate antibiotic, prophylaxis, intraocular lens (IOL) selection, ophthalmic viscosurgical devices, and prevention of complications. This chapter discusses the commonly followed cataract surgery techniques.

## INDICATIONS

As per the American Academy of Ophthalmology, Preferred Practice Pattern for Cataract surgery in an adult, the primary indication is visual acuity that no longer meets the patients' needs. The patient's history of visual disturbance along with the question as to how these symptoms impact this/her pertinent daily tasks, such as walking, driving, maintaining an occupation, and personal chores. Visual acuity causing impaired participation in social activities and/or the reduction of ocular imbalance and troublesome refractive states also warrant cataract surgery.

## CONTRAINDICATIONS

Surgery should not be considered under the following circumstances:

- Patient does not desire surgery
- Spectacles or visual aids provide functional vision satisfactory to the patient's needs
- Surgery not likely to improve visual function to patients' expectations
- Patient is known to be medically unfit for safe surgical intervention
- Surgery may compromise patient's lifestyle.

## PREOPERATIVE EVALUATION

The ophthalmic examination must be comprehensive enough to establish that the cataract without concomitant ophthalmic (e.g. glaucoma and/or macular degeneration) or medical considerations (e.g. neurological, diabetes) explains the visual disturbances in the patient.

Preoperative evaluation should include Snellen visual acuity (unaided and aided) but may also include Brightness Acuity tests (for glare disability) and/or contrast sensitivity testing.

Once it is established that the cataract formation is commensurate with the functional visual problems then cataract surgery can be entertained. It is important that the patient understands that they have the final say as to the timing of the surgery.

Majority of patients undergoing cataract surgery are elderly and likely to have concurrent multiple medical conditions such as coronary artery disease, hypertension, diabetes mellitus, chronic obstructive pulmonary disease, and thromboembolic disease requiring anticoagulant therapy problems. Hence, a thorough preoperative medical examination and appropriate testing/imaging should be done in all patients planned for cataract surgery.

## ANESTHESIA

Anesthesia techniques for cataract surgery have also gone through a number of changes, but the minimally invasive procedures have allowed us to reuse topical anesthesia (the use of topical Cocaine in the 1800s for cataract surgery was the standard). We will review the different modalities that are presently used.

## General Anesthesia

General anesthesia in cataract surgery is reserved for special situations. Indications for general anesthesia include:

- Children (congenital/pediatric cataract)
- Extremely anxious patient
- Uncooperative patient
- Known allergy to local or topical anesthetic medications
- Mentally challenged individuals
- Patients with involuntary kinetic neurological movements, or psychological issues
- Patients with severe back pain, postural problems, etc.

General anesthesia is now safer, but there are still significant risks such as malignant hyperthermia or patients with cardiac or respiratory situations that must be considered.

## Retrobulbar Anesthesia

The use of retrobulbar anesthesia for routine cataract surgery has decreased over the past few decades, but it still remains a common technique in some centers. In recent American Society of Cataract and Refractive Surgery surveys, the percentage of surgeons using injection techniques has continued to drop, but in 1998 it still was 32% with retrobulbar, 27% using peribulbar, and 37% using topical and intracameral variations. Now, it is around 55% topical with a mixture of the injection techniques accounting for the rest. Most residency programs teach a variation of the Atkinson technique.

Originally, the needle was introduced into the retrobulbar space by having the patient look up and nasally; however, this was shown to actually rotate the optic nerve toward the needle entrance thus increasing the risk for penetration. Now most surgeons keep the patient in a primary gaze and use slightly shorter needles (31 mm).

## Peribulbar Anesthesia

The technique usually involves four injections. The first injection is made a few centimeters medial to the lateral canthus through the lower lid. Anesthetic is injected both subcutaneously and into the orbicularis muscle. Moving just above the orbital rim and into the anterior portion of the orbit, a 1–2 mL is injected. Next, moving superiorly to the region below the supraorbital notch, a similar set of injections is done. These injections can be done with sharp short needles. Then using a retrobulbar needle, the third injection, which may be either superior or inferior, is injected more deeply into the orbit. Inferiorly, one starts approximately one third of the distance from the lateral to the medial canthus (about 12 mm medial to the lateral canthus), the needle is advanced next to the equator of the globe and advanced superiorly and medially. Two milliliter is injected and then superiorly an injection is administered in the superior nasal region just below the supraorbital notch. Usually, 10 mL is enough. Different surgeons use variations of this technique.

Both peribulbar and retrobulbar anesthesia should be administered to properly monitored patients with an intravenous access established and oxygen mask available. The following monitoring techniques are essential:

- Electrocardiogram
- Pulse oximetry
- Blood pressure
- Respiration.

## Parabulbar (Sub-Tenon's) Anesthesia

Tenon's capsule fuses with the conjunctiva near the surgical limbus. Therefore, it can provide access to the retrobulbar space. Hansen et al.[1] reported the use of sub-Tenon's anesthesia in 1990, and multiple cannulas have been designed since then to facilitate the technique. In this technique, a dissection is made through both conjunctiva and Tenon's capsule down to bare sclera. With a blunt cannula the anesthetic agent is forced posteriorly.

## Topical Anesthesia

Topical anesthesia was re-introduced by Fichman in the 1990s (it had been in common use in the 1800s–cocaine drops).[2] With the addition of intracameral lidocaine most patients are quite comfortable using topical anesthetics only. There are a few contraindications (mostly relative) to the use of topical anesthesia. Proparacaine 0.5% is the commonly used topical agent.

### *Technique for Topical Anesthesia*

- In the outpatient room, drops of 0.5% proparacaine are started. Dilating drops if used can be started as well
- Usually, two more sets of topical drops are given, I prefer 0.75% bupivacaine, which lasts longer than 0.5% proparacaine
- Two to 4 drops of half-strength Betadine (Purdue Frederick Co, Norwalk, CT, USA) are instilled into the cul-de-sac
- Many surgeons also instill an antibiotic and an anti-inflammatory (although only the Betadine has evidence-based data)

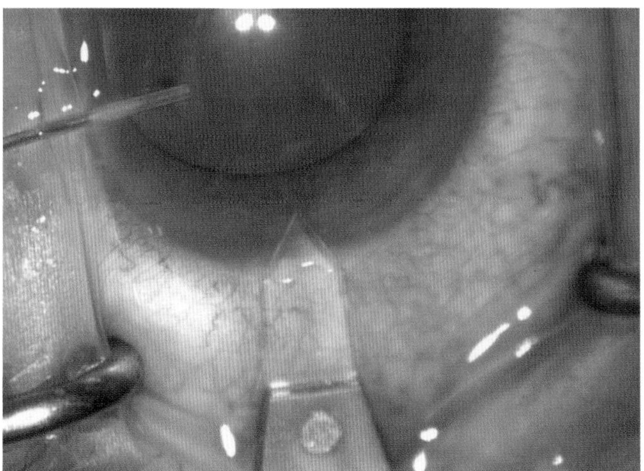

Figure 9-1 Entry point for a clear corneal incision for phacoemulsification.

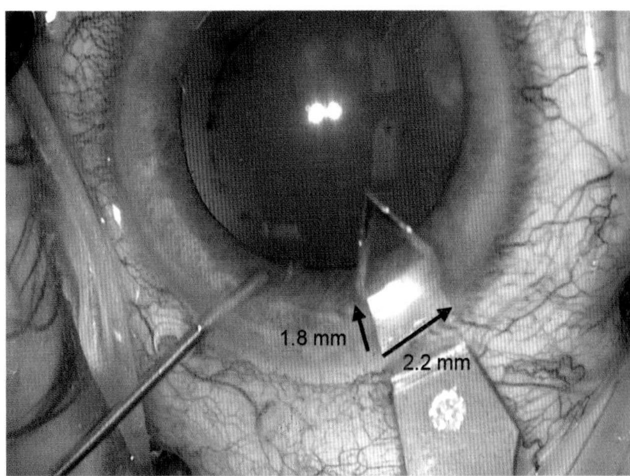


Figure 9-2 Dimensions of a clear corneal incision for phacoemulsification.

- Just prior to entering the operating room viscous lidocaine is instilled in the cul-de-sac, and the patient is instructed to maintain lid closure
- After the standard prep the eyelids are dried. The patient is asked to look down and the sterile drape can be applied. It is important to cover the lashes especially for patient's comfort with placing the lid speculum.

### Intracameral Anesthesia

Dilation for cataract surgery is important, and the standard technique usually consists of three sets of dilating drops (1% tropicamide, 1% cyclopentolate, and 10% phenylephrine hydrochloride) over a 15-minute period. Although this does work occasionally, there are problems with the epithelium, and if a patient has narrow angles, the pressure can be high to start the surgery.

To avoid this, Cionni et al.[3] reported using 1% unpreserved lidocaine, which paralyzes the sphincter muscle. After 30 seconds, adequate dilation occurred. To improve the speed and obtain slightly greater dilation, we now add 1:1000 of unpreserved bisulfate-free epinephrine.

There are a number of advantages to the use of the intracameral anesthesia:

- Patients are moved through the system quicker
- The corneas remain pristine since they receive much fewer drops–helpful in patients with diabetes or patients with corneal diseases
- Patients are less light sensitive to start the case
- One can easily identify the pupil center, which can be helpful in premium lenses
- No risk to induce a narrow angle attack.[4]

## SURGICAL TECHNIQUE

Modern cataract surgery includes a number of different approaches, which range from intracapsular technique requiring a large incision to phacoemulsification procedures that, even with coaxial surgery, can be done through incisions as small as 1.8 mm. Smaller incisions reduce chances of wound dehiscence, allow more rapid healing, and reduce postoperative astigmatism.

### Cataract Incisions

Cataract incisions are important as they influence the fluidic balance, infection resistance, and astigmatic outcome. The incision can be placed in the peripheral clear cornea, at the limbus, or in the sclera.

1. *Scleral incisions*: The scleral incisions may be linear, frown, or parallel to the cornea (smile). An initial groove is set at 50% depth with a blade (Fig. 9-1). A crescent-shaped blade is then used to dissect into clear cornea. The entrance into the eye is similar in concept to a clear corneal incision to be described (Fig. 9-2)
2. *Clear corneal incisions*: Construction of the clear corneal wound is extremely important. One should realize that the wound architecture determines wound strength. Due to the natural asymmetry of the eye, the superior limbus is closer to the central visual axis than the temporal limbus and hence has more of an astigmatic effect given the same size incision. The length should be at least 1.8 mm, the entrance into the anterior chamber should be parallel to the limbus. The width depends on the tip and sleeve that is used, but care must be taken to avoid stretching and damaging the wound during phacoemulsification. A near clear incision may be more stable

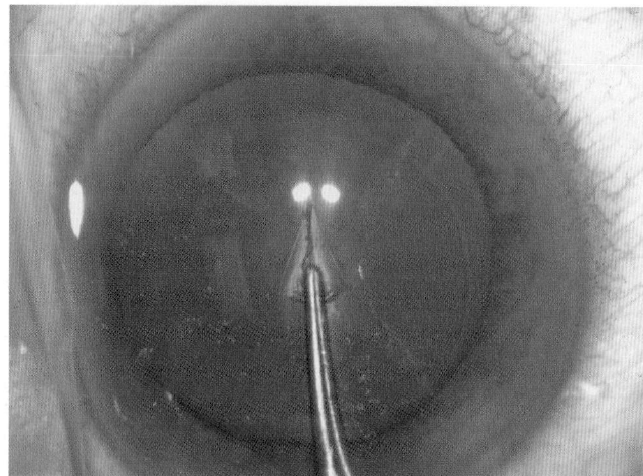

**Figure 9-3** Initiating the continuous curvilinear capsulorhexis with Utrata's forceps.

3. *"Near clear" corneal incisions*: in a "near clear" corneal incision, one identifies an area 0.5 mm near the limbus that does not have Tenon's capsule, so starting here results in a clean wound without ballooning the conjunctiva. Hydrating the wound at the end of the case and checking carefully for any potential leak is important. If there is any question, one should place a suture to prevent infection

## Capsulorhexis

A continuous curvilinear capsulorhexis is ideal to allow the maneuvers to make phacoemulsification safe. It facilitates the hydrodissection, allows rotation of the nucleus, and makes divide and conquer and chopping techniques easier. While there are a variety of ways to make the tear, all are based on the understanding of vector forces. Generally, the tear is initiated in the center of the capsule. It can be started with a cystitome, bent needle, or a forceps with a sharp tip such as Utrata's forceps (Fig. 9-3). One then grasps the edge and folds it so the epithelial (inner side) faces the cornea. By watching the edge, it can be torn in a circular (which uses a shearing mechanism) manner by influencing the tear vectors (Figs. 9-4A to C). When first learning, most use a multiple grasp technique and lead the capsule around. Once the principles are understood, one can reduce the number of grasps and one can also use a centripetal pull technique (mechanically this is a ripping motion), which is not only faster but also has the advantage of using smaller incisions with a forceps (Figs. 9-5A to C). Using a needle, one can do the tear through a side port or the main incision, although most surgeons prefer to use a forceps. The size of the capsulorhexis should be large enough to facilitate the cataract removal, but it should also cover the entire optic of the lens. A corneal marker can be used to aid in sizing the rhexis. Since for most of the IOLs optic is 6.0 mm, a well centered, 360° overlapping capsulorhexis of 5.5 mm works well in most cases.

## Hydrodissection and Hydrodelineation

Hydrodissection and hydrodelineation are two hydromaneuvers utilized to allow for rotation, reducing capsular, and zonular stress. Hydrodissection creates a wave of fluid that separates the cortex from the capsule, which allows the nucleus to rotate easily, whereas hydrodelineation creates a space between the nucleus and the epinucleus, which creates a buffer zone to prevent posterior capsule tears. It is important to use a 3-cm$^3$ syringe with a Luer–Lok syringe to prevent the possibility of the cannula releasing and tearing the capsule. The use of a 25- or 27-gauge blunt cannula such as a Chang cannula allows one to ensure proper flow and control of the fluid waves. The cannula is placed just under the edge of the capsulorhexis, and the wave is directed toward the lens equator (Figs. 9-6A to C). The wave should be slow, gentle, and steady. Once you see the wave slowly cross the posterior surface, the lens may move forward slightly. I usually depress the nucleus gently to disperse the fluid and then move 180° and duplicate the wave to ensure the nucleus is free (Fig. 9-6C). If one is using a dispersive viscoelastic such as Healon V [AMO(Abbott Medical Optics), Chicago, Illinois USA] or DiscoVisc (Alcon Laboratories, Dallas, TX, USA) it is helpful to burp a small amount out to prevent a pressure rise and possible zonular tear or capsule rupture.

Hydrodelineation is helpful in posterior polar cataracts (just in case there is a preexisting hole in the posterior capsule), and many surgeons like the buffer created by the epinuclear shell. This can be done directing the fluid wave slightly posteriorly to separate the epinucleus from the denser endonucleus. The nucleus can be harder to rotate with this maneuver so it is important to gently check and slowly rotate the nucleus.

In cases where there is evidence of zonular weakness and the surgeon anticipates using capsule devices, I find viscodissection with a cohesive viscoelastic [some prefer a dispersive agent to maintain the viscoelastic especially if it is used to move nuclear pieces in cases with zonule weakness such as pseudoexfoliation (PXE) or trauma] is helpful to create space and help maintain the space during the phacoemulsification.

## Nuclear Disassembly Technique

Nuclear disassembly techniques fall into many different forms.[5] The most commonly taught and still used by >50% of

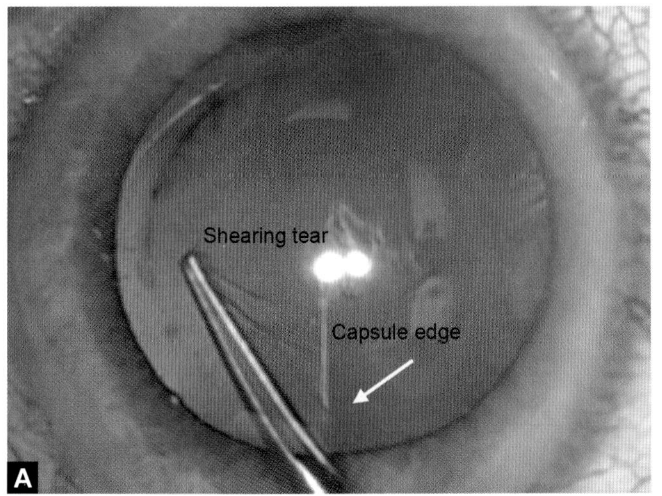


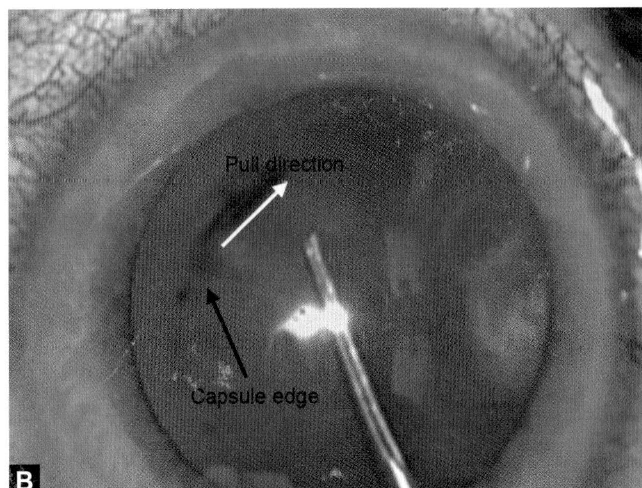


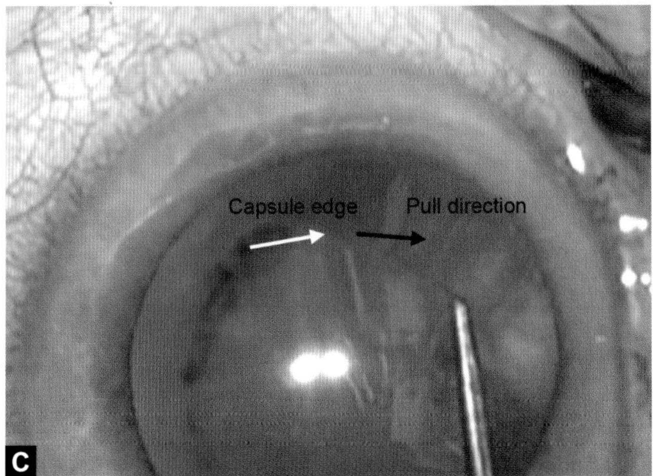


**Figures 9-4A to C** Shearing techniques for continuous curvilinear capsulorhexis.

cataract surgeons is the "divide and conquer" method followed by chopping techniques.

## *Divide and Conquer*

In this technique, the nucleus is divided, usually into quadrants.

- *Sculpting*: The nucleus is grooved along two orthogonal axes creating a cruciform pattern. The important factor to understand is that the grooving is a nonocclusion phase so it can be done with low vacuum and slowly remove nuclear material. It is critical to understand the anatomy of the lens and go deep centrally (using the Y sutures and red reflex to ensure good depth) but avoid going too deep peripherally.
- Once the grooves are done then the quadrants can be separated mechanically using the phaco tip in foot position 1 and a second instrument, T.
- Then switch to a quadrant removal mode, which has more vacuum and aspiration flow rate so that the pieces can be brought to the "safe" zone in the center of the rhexis just above the iris hence less likely to damage iris, capsule, or the cornea.

This technique is the most commonly used because it allows most of the nucleus to be removed within the capsular bag reducing potential corneal endothelial damage. The sculpting of the nucleus allows for a reliable technique and can be mastered fairly easily. It can be used in a variety of nuclear densities, although it can be difficult to use in soft cataracts and is not efficient for denser cataracts. It can be used to achieve a crack to rescue a case if another technique is not working.

## *Chop Techniques*

Chopping techniques fall into two broad categories, vertical and horizontal. They are more efficient than divide and conquer and are zonular friendly. They can be used in harder cataracts but demand a real understanding of the physics of

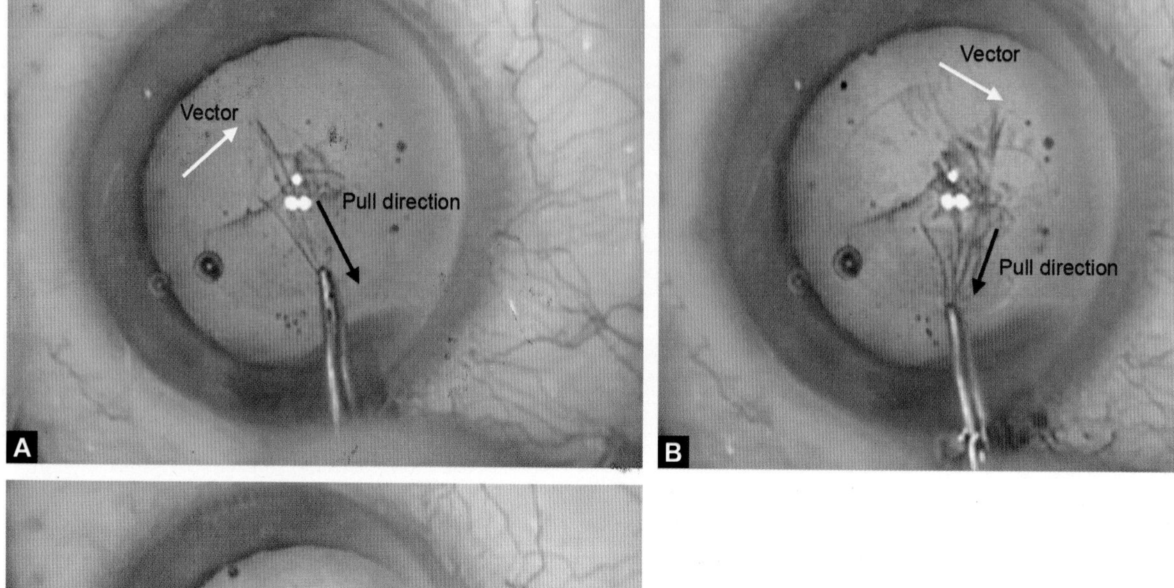


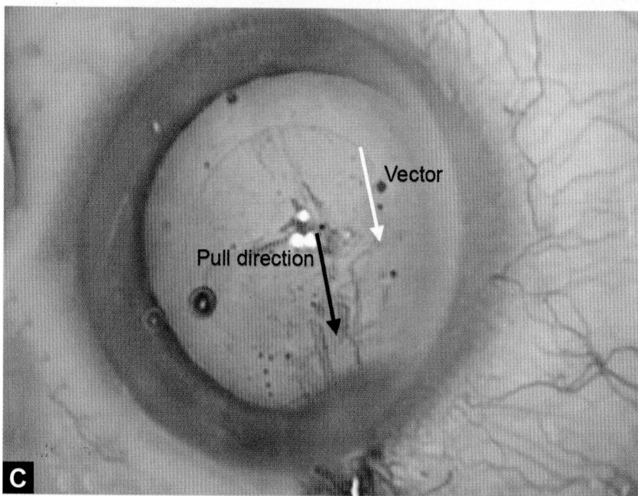


**Figures 9-5A to C** Capsulorhexis technique using a centripetal (ripping motion).

phacodynamics as well as understanding the anatomy of the nucleus itself.

- Vertical chop:
  - The phacoemulsification tip is buried deep in the nucleus by first using phacoemulsification foot position 3 and then holding the nucleus in foot position 2 (Figs. 9-7A and B)
  - Once the vacuum builds and the nucleus is held then a second instrument is brought in front of the phaco tip, and the nucleus is chopped by finding cleavage planes.

This maneuver can be repeated to obtain quadrants or even ≥6 pieces, which can be brought up and safely emulsified similar to the divide and conquer technique.

- Horizontal chop:
  - In this technique, the phaco tip is once again buried in the nucleus. The second instrument is then introduced under the capsule and drawn toward the phaco tip splitting the nucleus
  - The nucleus is rotated and the maneuver is repeated multiple times
  - Once the nucleus has been divided into pieces, they can be safely brought to the "safe" zone where it can be emulsified at a safe distance from both the cornea and the posterior capsule (Fig. 9-8).

With the newer phacoemulsification machines (which can include torsional or elliptical movement as well as traditional longitudinal), there is less chance of complete occlusion and thus help prevent surge.

- *Prechop*: There are a number of ways to divide the nucleus and the prechop technique is a versatile method to mechanically divide cataracts where the nuclear grade is 1–3. Dr Taka Akahoshi from Japan has been a major force in promulgating this procedure, and it has become a favorite maneuver for me.
  - After the hydrodissection the prechopper (many companies make them I use AISCO number- 4192) is used

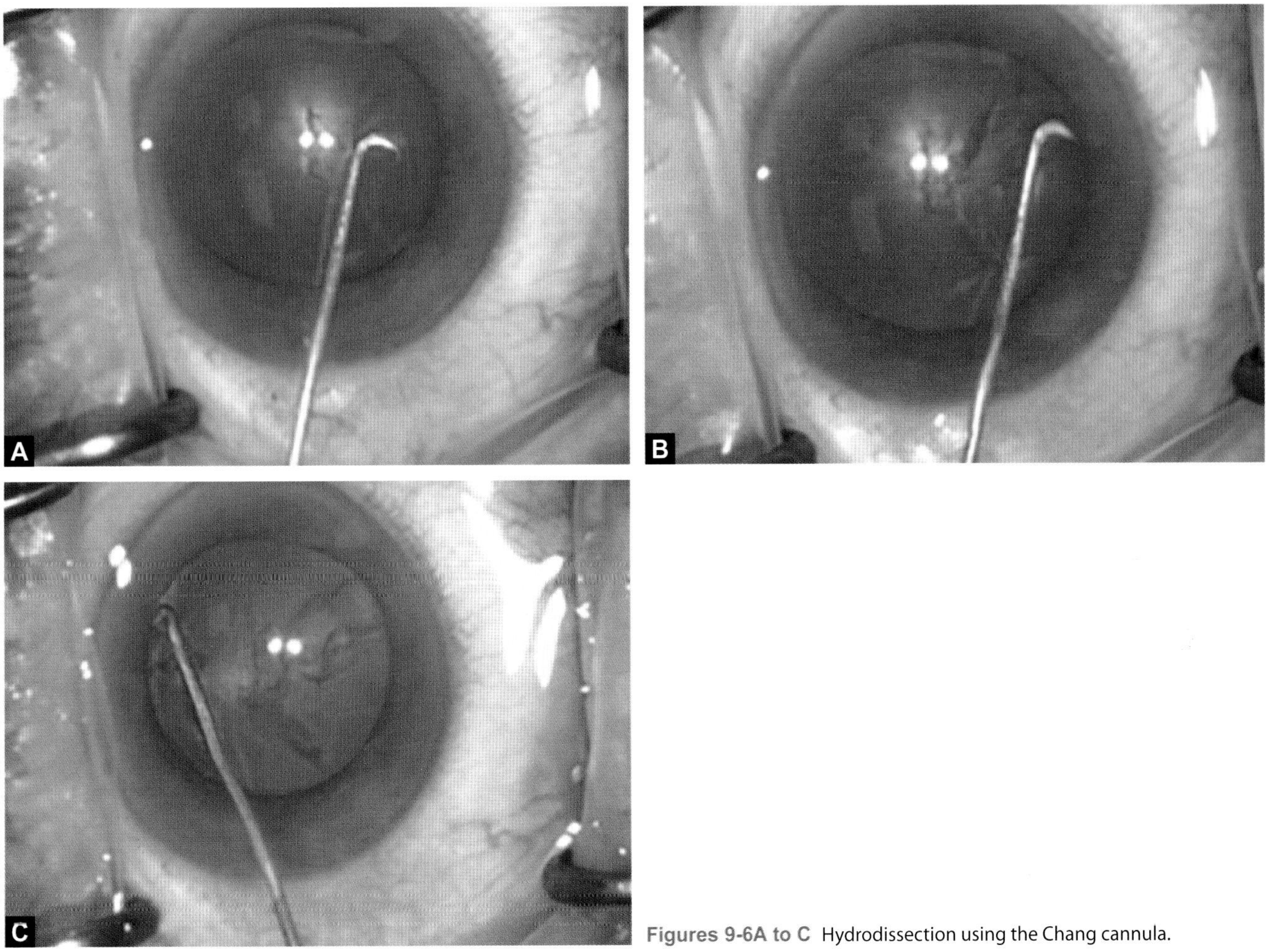

**Figures 9-6A to C** Hydrodissection using the Chang cannula.

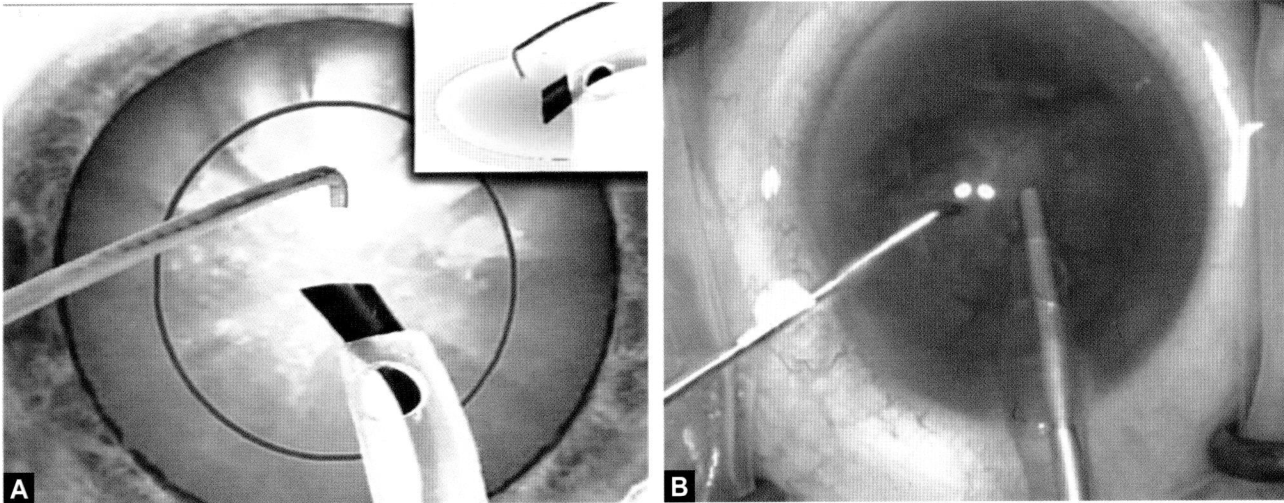

**Figures 9-7A and B** Vertical chop.

to enter the nucleus and by opening the blades the nucleus is divided into halves, the nucleus is rotated 90°, and the blade re-enters the nucleus to divide the halves into quadrants

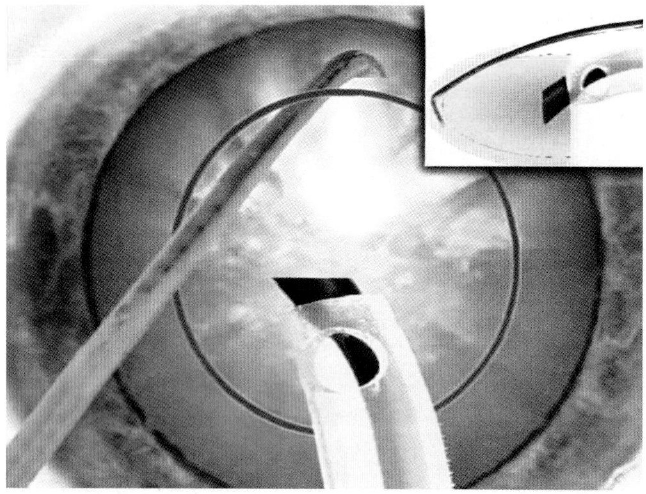

**Figure 9-8** Horizontal chop.

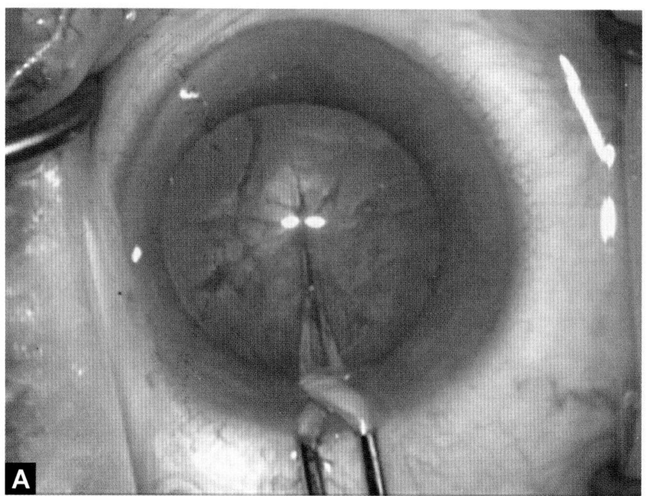


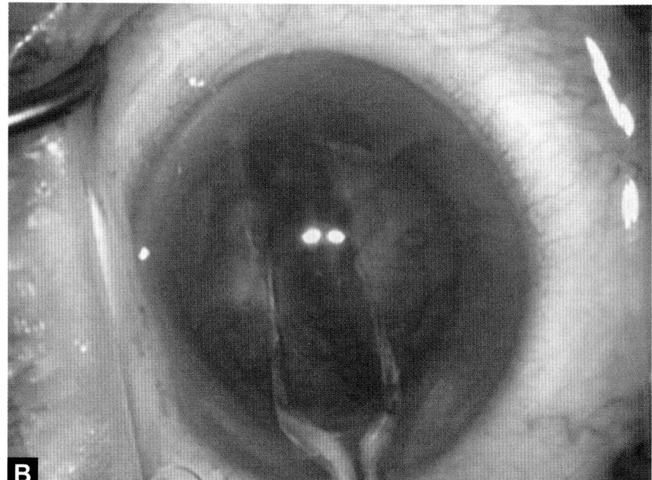


**Figures 9-9A and B** Pre-chopper used to divide the nucleus.

- The quadrants can then be removed by a standard quadrant removal.

The advantage of this maneuver is the nucleus can be divided without fluid and with no ultrasound. However, it does not work well with soft or with denser nuclei.

- *Ultrachopper*: Harder cataracts [LOCS (Lens Opacities Classification System, copyright by Leo Chylack)] grade 4 or higher] can still be difficult to manage. An additional aid is the Ultrachopper. It is designed similar to a standard phaco tip except the tip is sharp and angled similar to Kelman tips. It can be used on all Alcon machines. It has both longitudinal and torsional movements at ultrasonic speeds. It is used to score the nucleus similar to divide and conquer then a prechopper instrument is used to complete the cracks and allowing the pieces to be removed (Figs. 9-9A and B).

### *Phaco Flip*

In this technique, the nucleus is either partially or totally tumbled out the capsule. This is done by using the hydrodissection wave to bring the nucleus up. I usually tilt the nucleus thus leaving some of the material still in the bag. This technique is very helpful for soft cataracts, patients with high myopia and postvitrectomy eyes (these eyes tend to have deep chambers, and this can make standard approaches more difficult). It is important to have an adequate capsulorhexis opening, and make sure that there are no tears that could extend.

## Management of a Small Pupil

There are a number of situations, which require management of a small pupil. Although with modern cataract techniques especially with chop techniques one can consider removing the cataract without enlarging the pupil but the complication rate increases with small pupils and completing the cortical cleanup can be problematic. This can lead to increased inflammation, Sommering's rings, and possibly capsule phimosis.

Small pupils are seen in patients with:

- PXE syndrome
- Uveitis
- Narrow angle glaucoma
- Diabetes
- Older age
- Patients who are taking alpha 1 inhibitors [used in patients with prostate enlargement, classically tamsulosin as well nutritional supplements that contain Saw Palmetto all of which induce the intraoperative floppy iris syndrome (IFIS)].

The surgical approach to the patients will vary with the cause as well as with comorbidities (e.g. glaucoma).

Patients with PXE often have small pupils along with brittle capsules and zonular weakness. The small pupil is more frequently associated with the zonular problems, and therefore, it is important to have a large enough pupil to allow for a decent rhexis size (5.5 mm), which allows one to use capsule devices (Malyugin ring or MacKool hooks) if needed and decrease the risk for capsule phimosis, which may be a factor involved in the late spontaneous subluxations.

Patients with chronic uveitis will often have posterior synechiae, and these must be mechanically broken (a cyclodialysis spatula or other blunt instrument will suffice). Once the adhesions are broken, the pupil may still not dilate well (discussion on pupil management techniques to follow).

With the introduction of Tamsulosin, it soon became obvious (with the wonderful detective work of Campbell and Chang)[6] that this drug affected the iris enough to induce the new condition, IFIS. In patients with IFIS there is a triad of floppy iris that billows with normal flow, the iris tends to prolapse into the phaco tip and wounds and then, most problematic, is progressive pupil constriction. IFIS presents a new set of surgical issues.[7]

As always, the surgical plan should include back-up strategies for the different etiologies. The tools that we have available for managing small pupils include:

- *Preservative-free intracameral solutions (e.g. epi-Shugarcaine):*[8] The intracameral injections by themselves will often open the pupil enough to proceed and when used in conjunction with viscoelastics one can usually manage most cases of IFIS
- *Viscoelastics*: One needs to understand the various properties of the different viscoelastics (cohesive/dispersive/adaptive). The two that are very useful for small pupils are Healon V (AMO) and DiscoVisc (Alcon). With IFIS the main problems occur with high aspiration flow rates and with high inflow. With the pupil maintained the viscoelastics will remain in the eye with a low bottle height and with aspiration flow rates ≤25. Both agents will maintain the pupil size
- *Iris hooks and rings*: If viscoelastics do not maintain the pupil size or the iris is extremely flaccid then I prefer to use a Malyugin ring (MicroSurgical Technology), which gives eight points of contact rather than the four or five from iris hooks and decreases the risk for iris bombe and iris incarceration into wounds

**Table 9-1** Epi-Shugarcaine

| | |
|---|---|
| • 1:1000 epinephrine (American Reagent) | pH 3.133 |
| • 4% nonpreserved lidocaine (Abbott Labs) | pH 6.333 |
| • BSS Plus (Alcon Labs) | pH 7.197 |
| • Shugarcaine is 4% lidocaine mixed with BSS | |
| • Plus 1:3, which makes the lidocaine 1% | pH 6.97 |
| • 3:1 shugarcaine /epinephrine | pH 6.899 |

Knowing the disadvantages of a small pupil, I have certainly changed my approach to small pupils and have a tendency to use pupil expanding devices. Although there are a number of devices available, my preference for ease of use is the Malyugin ring.

Try the aforementioned measures along with decreasing flow (asp flow rate <25 $cm^3$/min), lowering bottle height and using viscoadaptive agents, such as Healon V (AMO) or DiscoVisc (Alcon) (Table 9-1).

## Irrigation and Aspiration

Classically, irrigation and aspiration of residual cortex has been a maneuver that gets little attention (the "hard work" is over!?), but it is a very important part of the procedure and a time that problems can easily happen. Attention to details and correct instruments are important. If one is using a metal tip make sure that it does not have a small defect in the bore that could tear the capsule. For this reason, I prefer either a silicone or ceramic tip that is gentle on the capsule. It is also important to reduce the risk for zonular stress. This is done by making sure one has only cortex in the tip and we now know that tangential stripping of the cortex causes less zonular stress and is the preferred technique (Figs. 9-10A and B) than the radial stripping maneuver.

Another technique that is commonly used is bimanual in which the irrigation and aspiration are separated and two small (usually approximately ≤1 mm) incisions are used with

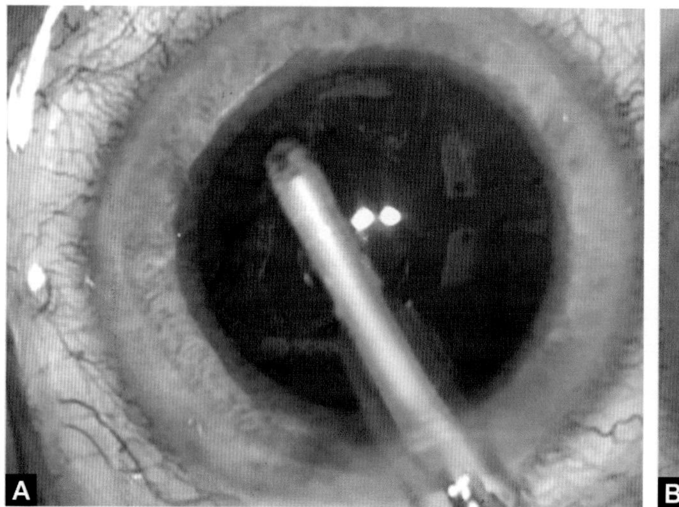


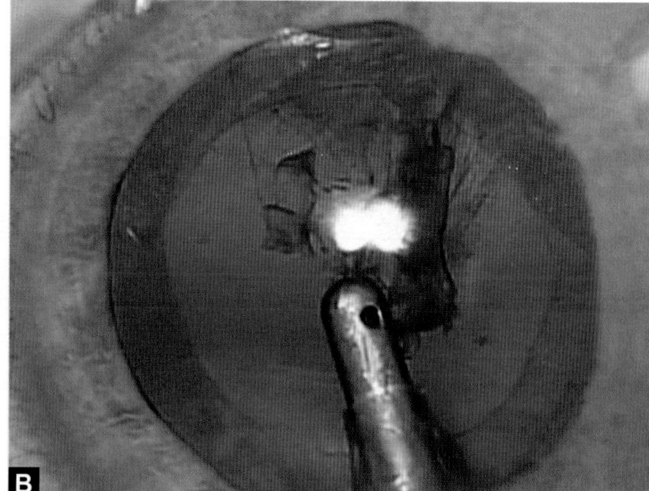


**Figures 9-10A and B** Tangential stripping of cortex.

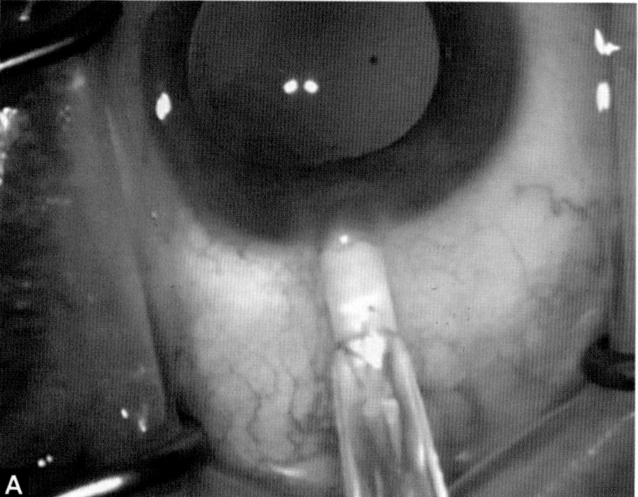


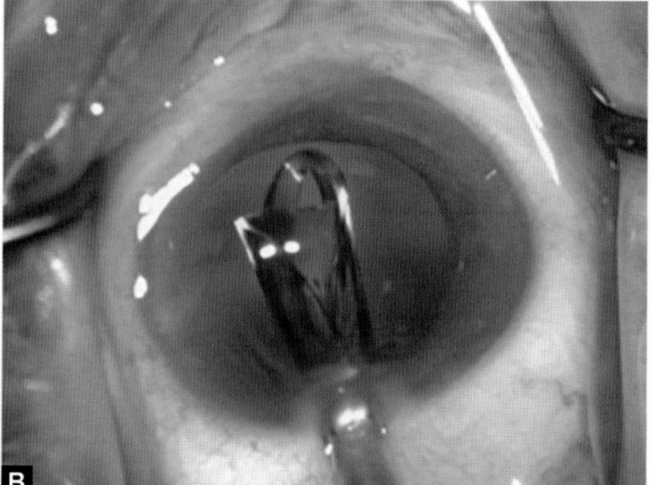


**Figures 9-11A and B** (A) Intraocular lens (IOL) injection; (B) Unfolding of IOL.

an irrigation cannula in one and an aspiration cannula through the other. The advantage of this technique is that by using the two incisions one is not as restricted addressing cortex (there is no area such as subincisional that is difficult to approach).

## IOL Implantation

Once the cortex has been removed, the chamber is filled with viscoelastic, one may proceed to implantation of the IOL (Figs. 9-11A and B); however, it is also common to use a sweep instrument (such as a Singer sweep) to remove anterior epithelial cells to potentially reduce the incidence of capsule phimosis (Fig. 9-12).

## Wound Closure

Most clear corneal wounds are 3.0 mm or less. If the wound is designed correctly (nearly square incision) it will close with hydration of the wound edges (Figs. 9-13A and B) the wound is checked to ensure it will not leak. If there is any question then 10-0 nylon suture can be used.

## Special Condition: Combined Glaucoma and Cataract

The decision to combine a glaucoma procedure with cataract is based on a number of factors. In general, it is related to the extent of damage to the patients' optic nerve as well as to the control of the intraocular pressure on the present regimen.

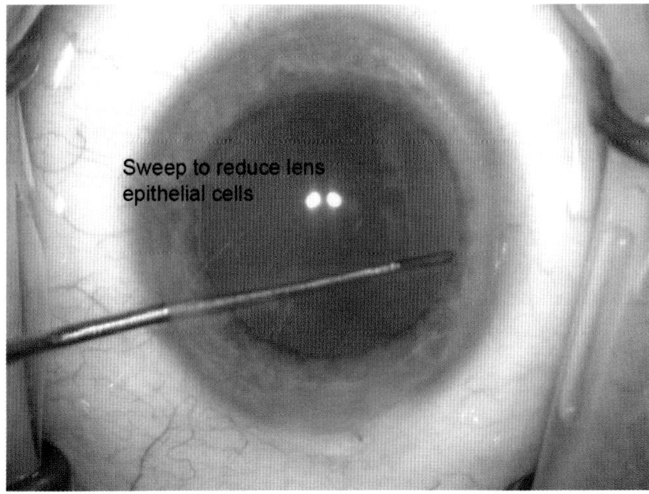


Figure 9-12 A sweep instrument (such as a Singer sweep-ASICO) to remove anterior epithelial cells to reduce the incidence of capsule phimosis.

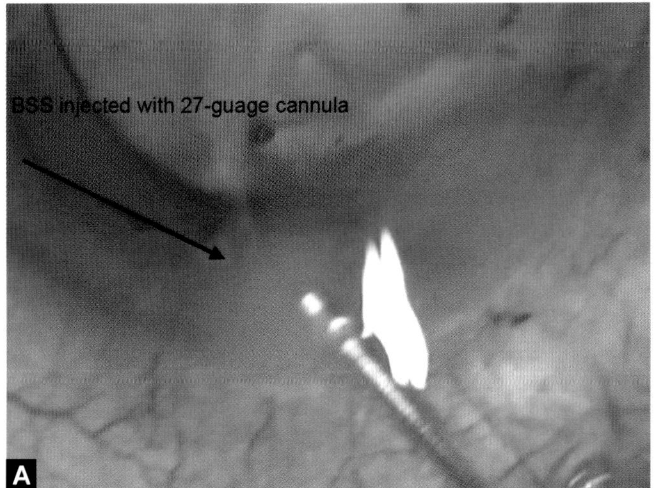


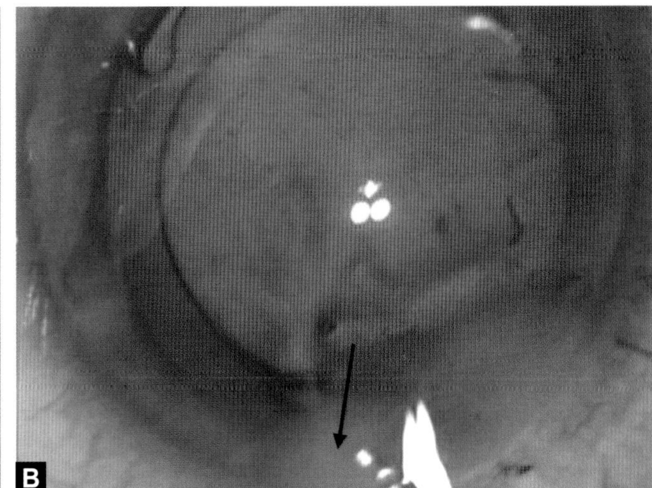


Figures 9-13A and B Hydrating the clear corneal incision with a 27-guage cannula.

There have been multiple recent studies that have shown that an uncomplicated phacoemulsification with IOL implantation is usually associated with a pressure decrease of approximately 4–6 mm Hg. Therefore, if a patient has good control and mild to moderate damage, one can consider the cataract procedure as adjunctive to the medications and avoid the potential complications of the glaucoma procedure. If needed a glaucoma procedure can be done later. This of course means a second procedure.

If the decision is to proceed with a combined surgery, there are a number of options available.

- *Phacoemulsification with trabeculectomy*: One can do a single-site trabeculectomy with the cataract, but most surgeons now prefer a temporal clear corneal cataract with a superior trabeculectomy. In this setting, one can first do the cataract then rotate the microscope superiorly and do their standard trabeculectomy (refer to glaucoma chapter). The patient must be aware of the probability that the visual recovery will be delayed by the glaucoma procedure
- *Phacoemulsification with ExPress glaucoma filtration device (Alcon)*: ExPress implantation has been shown to have similar results to standard trabeculectomy with slightly less hypotony and a quicker visual recovery along with slightly fewer number of postoperative visits
- *Phacoemulsification with endocyclophotocoagulation*: After the IOL has been implanted the diode laser is placed through the cataract wound and using the optical probe to find the ciliary processes then under direct visualization, the energy is increased to whiten the pigment on the processes. Usually, I prefer to do as many degrees as I can, at least 230°. There is increased inflammation from the laser, and the pressure takes some time to reduce

- *Phacoemulsification with canaloplasty*: Canaloplasty is technically harder and more time consuming. The procedure allows for quicker visual recovery and fewer bleb-related problems
- *Phacoemulsification with MIGS (micro invasive glaucoma surgery) procedures*: At present, only the I-Stent (Glaucos, Irvine, California, USA) has Food and Drug Administration (FDA) approval and may be used with phacoemulsification in the United States. It has been shown to add approximately additional 2–3 mm Hg drop in intraocular pressure when compared with phacoemulsification alone, which may be significant in management of the glaucoma. There are other devices in FDA clinical trials that are promising, but there are no data available yet concerning safety or efficacy.

## PEARLS AND PITFALLS

- A temporal incision induces about 0.5 D of flattening at that meridian, whereas a superior clear corneal incision may cause as much as 1 D of flattening at its axis. Therefore, keep preoperative keratometry in mind when choosing the incision site.
- For an eye with pre-existing against the rule astigmatism, have a wider temporal incision with short tunnel length.
- Malyugin ring helps stabilize iris tissue in IFIS.

## REFERENCES


1. Hansen EA, Mein CE, Mazzoli R. Ocular Anesthesia for Cataract Surgery: a direct sub-Tenon's Approach. Ophthalmic Surg. 1990;21(10):696-9.
2. Fichman R. Use of Topical Anesthesia alone is cataract Surgery J Cataract Refract Surg. 1996;22(5):612-4.
3. Cionni, RJ, Barrow M, Kaufman AH, et al. Cataract Surgery without pre-operative dilation. J Cataract Refract Surg. 2003;29: 2281-3.
4. Nouvellon E, Cuvillon P, Ripart J, et al. Anaesthesia for cataract surgery. Drugs Aging. 2010;27(1):21-38.
5. Devgan U. Surgical techniques in phacoemulsification. Curr Opin Ophthalmol. 2007;18(1):19-22.
6. Chang D, Campbell J, Intraoperative floppy iris syndrome associated with tamsulosin. J Cataract Refract Surg. 2005;31(4): 664-73.
7. Tint NL, Dhillon AS, Alexander P. Management of intraoperative iris prolapse: stepwise practical approach. J Cataract Refract Surg. 2012;38(10):1845-52.
8. Shugar JK. Use of epinephrine for IFIS prophylaxis. J Cataract Refract Surg. 2006;32(7):1074-5.

CHAPTER

# 10

# Manual Small Incision Cataract Surgery

Rengaraj Venkatesh, Geoffrey Tabin, Michael Feilmeier, Benjamin Thomas, Sanduk Ruit

## INTRODUCTION

Cataract is the leading cause of blindness [as defined by the World Health Organization, best corrected visual acuity (BCVA) in the better eye of < 20/400] throughout the world and is responsible for approximately 50% of blindness in the developing world, affecting nearly 20 million people. As this number continues to grow, the need for a high-quality, cost-effective cataract surgical technique becomes more obvious.

It is well established that the combination of continuous curvilinear capsulorhexis (CCC), phacoemulsification, and in-the-bag placement of an intraocular lens (IOL) is the standard of care in developed nations for the treatment of most visually disabling cataracts. Phacoemulsification allows the removal of cataracts through small (< 3.0 mm) self-sealing incisions, resulting in minimal surgically induced astigmatism and rapid visual rehabilitation. However, the high cost of purchasing and maintaining a phacoemulsification machine, the dependence on unreliable amenities, such as electricity, and the limited availability of appropriate training for technicians and surgeons are significant obstacles currently limiting the widespread use of this technique in the developing world, where 90% of cataract blindness exists.

Manual small incision cataract surgery (MSICS)–a remarkable technique first described by Blumenthal in 1994–has received significant international attention as a low-cost, low-technology, high-quality alternative to phacoemulsification. MSICS is similar to extracapsular cataract extraction (ECCE) in that it involves removal of an intact crystalline lens from the eye while maintaining the integrity of the posterior capsule. However, in contrast to traditional ECCE, in MSICS the lens is explanted through a 6.0- to 7.0-mm wedge-shaped, multiplanar, self-sealing sclerocorneal tunnel that is large enough to allow removal of the nucleus and insertion of a rigid posterior chamber IOL. A major advantage of this innovative technique is the self-sealing nature of the incision, effectively eliminating the need for suturing of the wound. This allows for less surgically induced astigmatism, more rapid visual rehabilitation, and improved long-term wound stability. In addition, surgeons properly trained in MSICS can routinely perform surgeries in < 5 minutes, with outcomes comparable with phacoemulsification in the setting of advanced cataracts. In this chapter, we describe the different MSICS techniques and their employment throughout the world (Table 10-1).

**TABLE 10-1** List of instruments necessary for the manual small incision cataract surgery procedure

| | | |
|---|---|---|
| Dish for gauze pads | Toothed forceps (0.12 or 0.3) | Cautery (low-temp or wet-field) |
| Gauze pads | Bevel-up crescent blade | 25–27 gauge needle |
| 5% betadine | Microkeratome blade | 1-mL syringe |
| Eyelid speculum | Viscoelastic | 3-mL syringe |
| 4–0 silk | 27-gauge cannula | Sinskey hook |
| Needle driver | Simcoe I/A cannula | Rigid posterior chamber intraocular lens |
| Superior rectus forceps | Tying forceps | |
| Wescott scissors | Vannas scissors | |

# GENERAL SURGICAL TECHNIQUE OF MSICS

## Placing a Bridle Suture

Manual small incision cataract surgery can be performed through either a superior or a temporal scleral tunnel. When using a superior tunnel, a bridle suture may be placed beneath the tendon of the superior rectus muscle to facilitate surgical exposure. In cases with a temporal approach, the lateral rectus muscle can be used. The bridle suture is useful in the following ways:

- To maneuver and fixate the globe during certain steps of surgery, such as tunneling
- To provide counter-tractional force during procedures such as nucleus removal and epinucleus delivery, thereby making these procedures easier and less traumatic.

## Creating a Scleral Tunnel

### *Site*

The size of the external incision is approximately 6–7 mm and, hence, substantially larger than that required for instrumental phacoemulsification. A temporal tunnel is preferred over a superior tunnel for the following reasons:

- It tends to counteract the pre-existing against-the-rule astigmatism, which is predominantly present in the elderly
- It minimizes the crowding effect of the brow, especially in deep sockets, and facilitates intraoperative exposure
- It permits the globe to remain parallel to the axis of the microscope, allowing the red reflex to be better appreciated, providing better visibility.

### *Initial Incision*

A fornix-based conjunctival flap of around 7 mm is made. After Tenon's capsule is dissected off, light cautery is applied. A 30–50% thickness external scleral groove of around 6–7 mm in width is made approximately 2 mm posterior to the surgical limbus. The incision should be tangential to the limbus (or frown-shaped) to limit postoperative astigmatism and improve wound stability. The size of the wound is determined by the size of the nucleus, and accurate estimation of nuclear size will improve with experience. However, as a rule, beginning surgeons should begin with a 7-mm external incision (Fig. 10-1).

### *Sclerocorneal Tunneling*

A sclerocorneal tunnel is created using an angled, bevel-up crescent blade. The blade is gently advanced parallel to the ocular surface to create a single plane tunnel of uniform thickness approximately 1.5 mm into the clear cornea (Figs. 10-2 and 10-3). The wound should be trapezoidal in appearance, with the internal portion of the tunnel extending limbus to limbus. The anterior chamber should not be entered at this point.

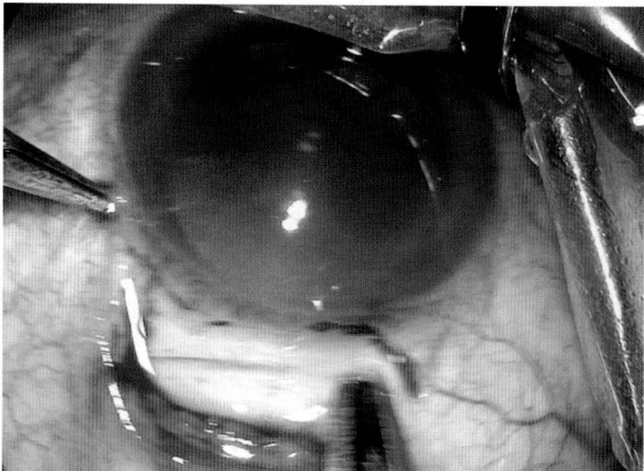

**Figure 10-1** External 7.0-mm scleral incision.

The depth of the incision is the single most important aspect of the tunnel. A tunnel that is too shallow will result in buttonholes and an unstable wound. A tunnel that is too deep can result in early entry into the anterior chamber, difficulty in anterior chamber stability, iris prolapse, and an unstable wound.

## Creating a Side Port Entry

One side port entry can be made using a #15 super blade at the 10 o'clock position or perpendicular to the tunnel in the clear cornea. It is useful (but not required) for:

- Injection of viscoelastic
- Subincisional cortical aspiration and
- Injection of balanced saline solution (BSS) into anterior chamber at the end of the procedure to adjust the intraocular pressure to a physiologic level.

## Making the Internal Corneal Incision

A sharp 3.2-mm-angled keratome is used to enter the anterior chamber after viscoelastic has been injected. The heel of the keratome is raised until the blade becomes parallel to the iris plane, resulting in a dimple on the corneal surface. The keratome is then advanced anteriorly in the iris plane until the anterior chamber is entered and the internal wound is visualized as a straight line (Fig. 10-4). The initial incision is then extended from side to side for the full extent of the tunnel. During extension of the incision, care should be taken to keep the internal incision in the same plane.

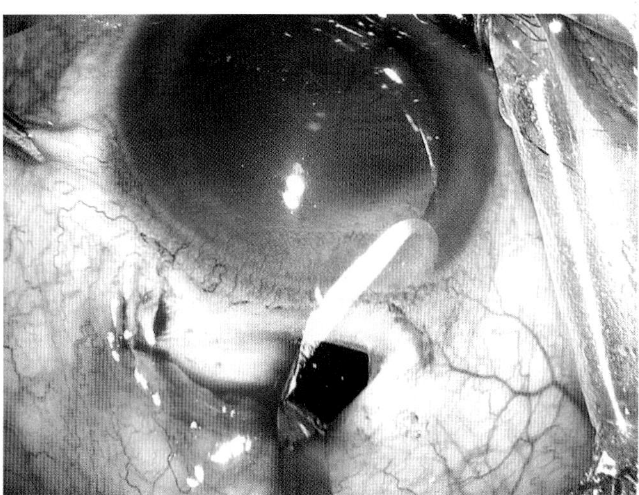

Figure 10-2 Sclerocorneal tunnel.

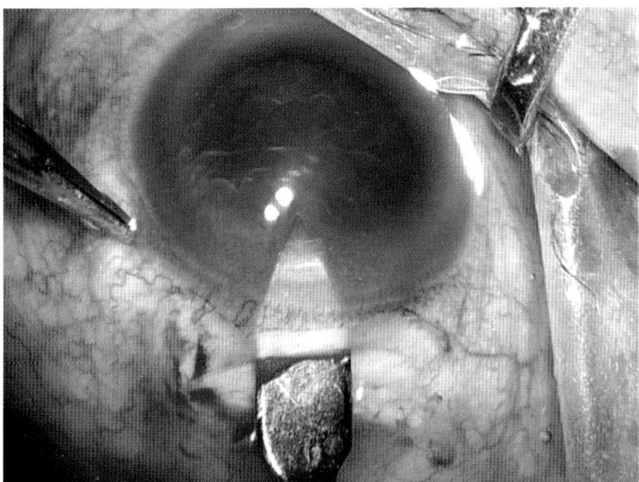

Figure 10-4 Creation of the internal corneal incision using a microkeratome blade.

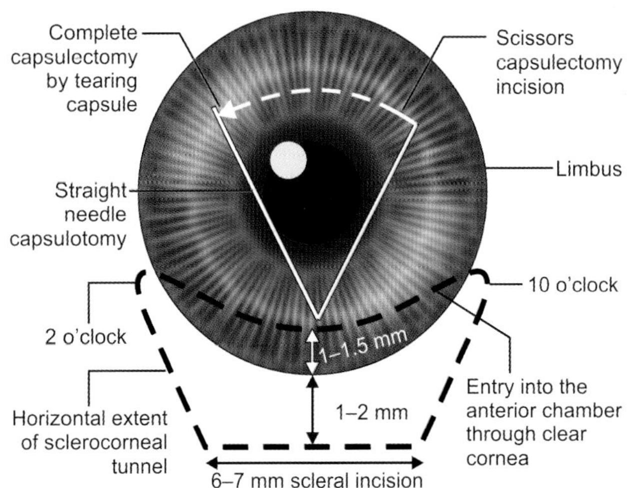


Figure 10-3 Manual small incision cataract surgery diagram with a triangular (V-shaped) capsulotomy. With permission from Ruit S, Paudyal G, Gurunq R, Tabin G, Moran D, Brian G. An innovation in developing world cataract surgery: suture less extracapsular cataract extraction with intraocular lens implantation. Clin Experiment Ophthalmol. 2000;28(4):274-9.

## Performing the Capsulotomy

Several different capsulotomy techniques are possible with MSICS surgery. CCC may provide optimal IOL positioning but can be difficult in the setting of large mature, hypermature, or morgagnian cataracts, and in the setting of poor surgical visibility due to corneal scars, pterygium, and suboptimal operating microscopes, all of which are common circumstances in the developing world. The triangular capsulotomy and can-opener capsulotomy can be particularly useful in these suboptimal surgical settings, especially when capsular staining techniques are not available (*see* Fig. 10-3).

If performing a CCC, the size of the capsulorhexis should be based upon the size and density of the cataract. It should have a minimum diameter of 5–6 mm and may need to be as large as 7–8 mm in diameter for more mature cataracts. If the CCC is too small for prolapse of the lens into the anterior chamber, the surgeon can make eight or more radial relaxing incisions or convert to "canopener" capsulotomy.Capsular staining is helpful in cases with white or dense browncataracts.

However, if performing a CCC is not feasible, MSICS can also be safely performed using a "can opener" or triangular (V-shaped) capsulotomy. In cases of mature and hypermature cataracts, a "can opener" or triangular capsulotomy is actually preferred, because it facilitates prolapse of the nucleus into the anterior chamber.

If the surgeon uses a triangular capsulotomy, this step can be performed prior to creation of the internal corneal incision and entry into the anterior chamber. A straight 25- to 27-gauge needle attached to a 1-mL syringe filled with BSS is advanced into the sclerocorneal tunnel just posterior to the limbus, angled parallel to the iris plane, and then advanced into the anterior chamber. Using the bevel tip of the needle, a linear cut is made from 4 o'clock to 12 o'clock and then from 8 o'clock to 12 o'clock so the two incisions meet at 12 o'clock (assuming a superiorly placed sclerocorneal tunnel, *see* Figure 10-3). Thus, a triangular, or V-shaped, flap of anterior lens capsule is created with its base still attached. The apex of the 'V' should be oriented toward the surgeon, and the base of the capsulotomy away from the surgeon.[1] Each point of the triangle should be approximately 3 mm from the center of the pupil. Next, the apex is lifted with the tip of the needle and peeled away from the surgeon. This confirms the capsulotomy incisions are connected at the apex.

## Performing Hydrodissection

Hydrodissection is performed using a 27-gauge bent-tip cannula attached to a syringe filled with BSS. In the presence of a CCC, this procedure is completed in one smooth step by injecting the fluid beneath the anterior capsular rim (Fig. 10-5). However, in the presence of a "can opener" or triangular capsulotomy, small amounts of fluid can be injected in multiple areas so as to "unshackle" the nucleus from the confines of the cortical but one must be careful not to cause an extension which could lead to posterior nuclear loss. At the end of a successful hydrodissection, the nucleus should be freely mobile within the capsular bag. Alternatively, hydrodissection can be performed with an irrigating Simcoe cannula. This low-pressure system is ideal in the setting of a triangularcapsulotomy.

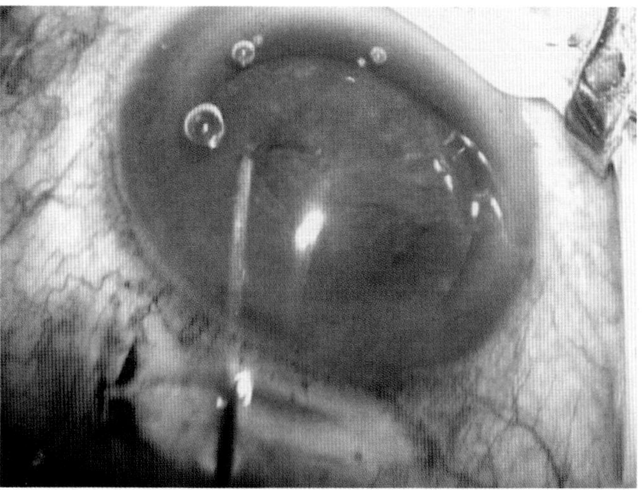

**Figure 10-5** Hydrodissection of the lens nucleus.

## Prolapsing the Nucleus into the Anterior Chamber

Oftentimes when hydrodissection is performed, one pole of the nucleus will prolapse into the anterior chamber along with the fluid wave. At the sight of this prolapse, further hydrodissection can be stopped and under the cover of an adequate amount of viscoelastics, the remainder of the nucleus can be delivered by rotating the prolapsed pole with a Sinskey hook. If the nucleus does not prolapse with hydrodissection alone, then a combination of careful fluid infusion and lens rotation using a Simcoe cannula or a viscoelastic cannula can be employed.

### *Prolapsing the Nucleus: Particular Techniques for Specific Types of Cataract*

*Mature cortical cataracts:* White cataracts can be managed by doing a capsulorhexis after staining the capsule with 0.1 mL of 0.06% trypan blue dye. The nucleus can be levered out of the bag using a Sinskey hook, often without hydroprocedures, if the cortical attachments to the nucleus are loose. It is also worthwhile to debulk the cortical matter using a Simcoe cannula prior to prolapsing the nucleus. The capsular staining helps in performing the difficult step of nucleus prolapse through an intact capsulorhexis, as the dye-stained capsular rim is distinctly visible throughout the surgery. A Sinskey hook is first used to retract the stained capsulorhexis, then to engage the equator of the nucleus, and to lever one pole outside the capsular bag, after which the rest of the nucleus is rotated into the anterior chamber. During this maneuver, any compromise to the capsular bag can be detected easily and relaxing incisions can be made at any point of the process.[2]

### *Hypermature Cataracts and Phacolytic Glaucoma*

With this technique, after staining the capsule with trypan blue, a small nick is made in the anterior capsule using a bent 26-G needle mounted on a syringe, and the liquid cortex is aspirated. The capsular bag is inflated with viscoelastic and the capsulorhexis is completed using Utrata Capsulorhexis Forceps or equivalent. A Sinskey hook is then used to lever one pole of the nucleus outside the capsular bag, and the rest of the nucleus is then rotated out into the anterior chamber.[3]

*Hard brown/black cataracts:* In these cases, the safest technique will be to perform a "can opener" or triangular capsulotomy and prolapse the nucleus, as described earlier. If the surgeon is keen to perform a capsulorhexis, it is safer to stain the capsule and perform a larger capsulorhexis (6.0–7.5 mm) followed by a less forceful hydrodissection. As the capsule is stained, it will be easy to retract the capsule and lever out a part of the nucleus with a Sinskey hook (as described above). The nucleus is then gently rotated out, watching the movement of the capsular bag throughout the procedure. If the capsular bag seems to be compromised, a few relaxing incisions in the capsule can avoid intracapsular extraction of the nucleus. Alternatively, a bimanual technique can be tried, which is described later.

*Small pupils:* In patients with small pupils, one can resort to procedures such as stretch pupilloplasty using Kuglen hooks or make sphincterotomies. This allows greater visualization for performing capsulotomy and hydrodissection and makes easing the nucleus into the anterior chamber a much safer maneuver. In certain high-risk cases, such as pseudoexfoliation with a small rigid pupil and an associated hard nucleus, it would be prudent to go in for a small sector iridectomy or a "keyhole" iridectomy. If the small pupil is pliable, an alternative–and more aesthetically pleasing, bimanual technique is possible. This technique is useful if one has failed to prolapse the nucleus by the mechanical method, or in cases of small pupils with hard cataract.

*Bimanual technique:* In cases with zonular compromise, a bimanual prolapse technique is employed: in this technique, a cyclodialysis spatula and a Sinskey hook are used for the prolapse. The nucleus is retracted to one side (temporal in right eye or nasal in left eye, assuming a superior position) with a Sinskey hook through the sclerocorneal tunnel (Fig. 10-6). Following this, the spatula is introduced through the side port incision and placed under the nucleus. Using the spatula as a fulcrum, the nucleus is rotated with the Sinskey hook out of the capsular bag. With proper use of this technique, the cyclodialysis spatula absorbs the rotational forces, minimizing stress on the zonules.[4]

*Subluxated cataracts:* The MSICS can be done in selected cases of subluxated cataracts wherein the pupil is well dilated, and the nucleus is not very dense. Here also, staining of the capsule with trypan blue facilitates the capsulorhexis, helps with implanting a capsular tension ring (CTR), and aids safe prolapsing of the nucleus. After assessing the extent of subluxation and the density of nucleus, the capsule is stained and the capsulorhexis is performed. This is followed by cortical-cleaving hydrodissection and manual insertion of the CTR through the paracentesis. The nucleus is then hydrodelineated, and irrigation is continued until one pole of the nucleus prolapses out of the capsular bag. The rest of the nucleus is wheeled into the anterior chamber using a Sinskey hook.[5]

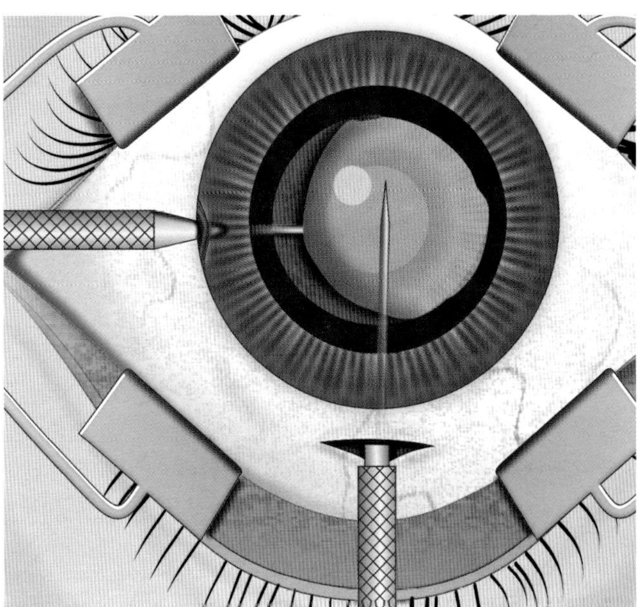

**Figure 10-6** Bimanual nuclear prolapsed technique.

## Extracting the Nucleus

Once the nucleus is prolapsed into the anterior chamber, it can be extracted through the tunnel by one of the following techniques:

- Irrigating vectis technique
- Phacosandwich technique
- Phacofracture technique
- Modified Blumenthal technique
- Fish hook technique, or
- Simcoe technique.

Each will be discussed here in turn.

### *Irrigating Vectis Technique*

This technique makes use of a combination of mechanical and hydrostatic forces to extract the nucleus. An irrigating vectis is, of course, necessary for this procedure (Figs. 10-7A and B). This vectis is 8-mm long, 4-mm wide, and has an anterior and posterior surface. The anterior surface has a slight concavity and has two ends, with the anterior end bearing three small irrigating ports, each 0.3 mm in size. The posterior end is continuous with the main body of the vectis and is attached to a syringe containing lactated Ringer's solution or BSS.

After the nucleus is prolapsed into the anterior chamber, viscoelastics are liberally injected, first above and then below the nucleus. The upper layer shields the endothelium, whereas the lower layer pushes the posterior capsule and iris diaphragm posteriorly. This maneuver creates adequate space in the anterior chamber for atraumatic nuclear delivery.

A good superior rectus bridle suture is necessary for the success of the next step. To perform, the bridle suture is first held loosely in the left hand. After checking the patency of the ports, the vectis is then inserted under the nucleus with the anterior surface facing up. If it is an immature cataract, one will be able to see the margins of the vectis under the nucleus in place. It is extremely important to visualize the tip of the vectis lying anterior to the iris, for if iris tissue is pinched between the lens nucleus and the vectis; a large (or complete) iridodialysis may result upon attempted removal of the nucleus.

As the superior rectus bridle suture is pulled tight, the irrigating vectis is slowly withdrawn without irrigating, until the superior pole of the nucleus is engaged in the tunnel. Gentle irrigation is then started and the vectis is slowly withdrawn while pressing down gently on the posterior lip of the sclerocorneal tunnel. The force of irrigation must be reduced when the maximum diameter of the nucleus just crosses the inner lip of the tunnel. This decreases the likelihood of

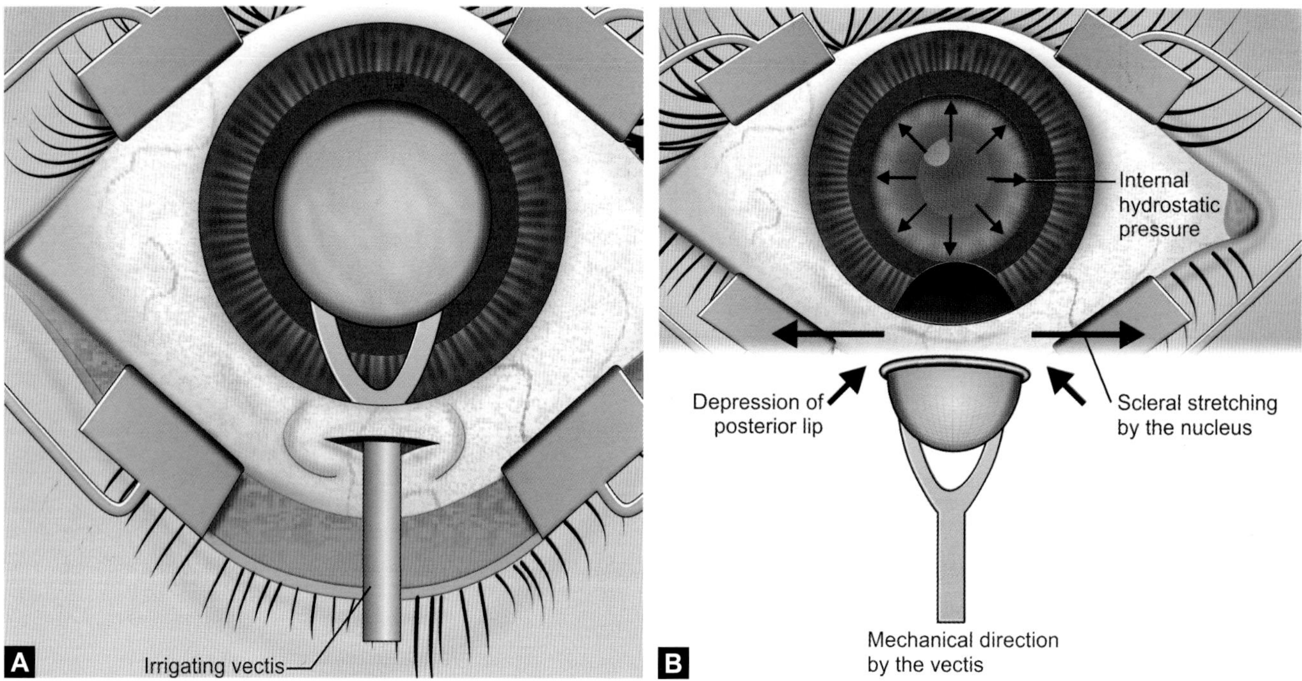


**Figures 10-7A and B** Nucleus extraction using the irrigating vectis technique.

forcefully expelling the nucleus from the anterior chamber. A high-pressure evacuation of the lens from the anterior chamber can result in sudden anterior chamber decompression, shallowing of anterior chamber, and extrusion of ocular contents, including lens capsule and vitreous.

Of note, if the wound is placed temporally, a pull on the nasal conjunctiva by the surgical assistant can aid in nucleus extraction, as the bridle effect of the lateral rectus is usually not sufficient.

Potential complications of nucleus extraction with an irrigating vectis and their causes are listed in Table 10-2.

### *Phacosandwich Technique*

In this technique, a Sinskey hook is used in addition to the vectis. The key requirement is that the anterior chamber is adequately filled with viscoelastics. Once the vectis is placed beneath the nucleus, the Sinskey hook is carefully introduced and placed on top of the nucleus, effectively "sandwiching" it between the vectis and the Sinskey hook. The tip of the Sinskey hook is placed beyond the central portion of the lens, enabling a more secure grip on the nucleus with this two-handed technique. With the Sinskey hook in the dominant hand and the vectis in the other, the nucleus is "sandwiched" and extracted. While extracting the nucleus, the assistant should pull the superior rectus suture and simultaneously pull the globe inferiorly by grasping the conjunctiva at the 6 o'clock position near the limbus with toothed forceps. The outer portion of the nucleus, the epinucleus, and a portion of the cortex will be sheared off in this technique and can be removed with the irrigating vectis immediately after nucleus delivery (Figs. 10-8A and B).

### *Phacofracture Technique*

This is the technique of manual nuclear fragmentation for removing a large nucleus through a small incision. A bisector or trisector can be used instead of a Sinskey hook, which is used to cleave its way through the nuclear substance. Steady, constant pressure on the bisector or the trisector, combined with the posterior pressure of gently lifting with the vectis, will split the nucleus. The split nuclear fragments can then be removed one at a time using the irrigating vectis.

### *Modified Blumenthal Technique*

This technique uses an "anterior chamber maintainer" (ACM) throughout the procedure. An ACM is a hollow tube with a 0.9-mm outer diameter and 0.65-mm inner diameter. The tube of the ACM is attached to a bottle of BSS, suspended 50–60 cm above the patient's eye.

Two small beveled entries are made in the cornea; the first is 1.5-mm long, placed between the 5 and 7 o'clock position (assuming a superior wound position), for inserting the ACM. The second port is 1-mm wide, placed at the 11 o'clock position, for the entry of various instruments. The fluid flow from the ACM is stopped only during the capsulotomy. After

TABLE 10-2 Potential complications of nucleus extraction with an irrigating vectis and their causes

| Potential complications | Cause |
|---|---|
| Corneal endothelial damage | • Misjudged nuclear size leading to disproportion between nucleus and wound size<br>• Inadequate use of viscoelastics<br>• Improper technique in handling the vectis<br>• Iatrogenic: Surgeon's ego leading to repeated attempts at forceful extraction |
| Trapped nucleus | • Improper bridle suture<br>• Misjudged nuclear size<br>• Improperly designed vectis, i.e. not having sufficient concavity<br>• Poor technique |
| Iris trauma/iris stretching/iridodialysis | • Premature entry causing iris to be washed out through the weak site<br>• Premature injection of fluid<br>• Vectis incarceration of the iris opposite the sclerocorneal tunnel<br>• Vectis not pressed down sufficiently on the posterior scleral lip |
| Posterior capsular rent with vitreous loss | • Sharp edges of the vectis<br>• Forceful extrusion of the nucleus<br>• Enlargement of a pre-existing zonular dialysis caused while prolapsing the nucleus |

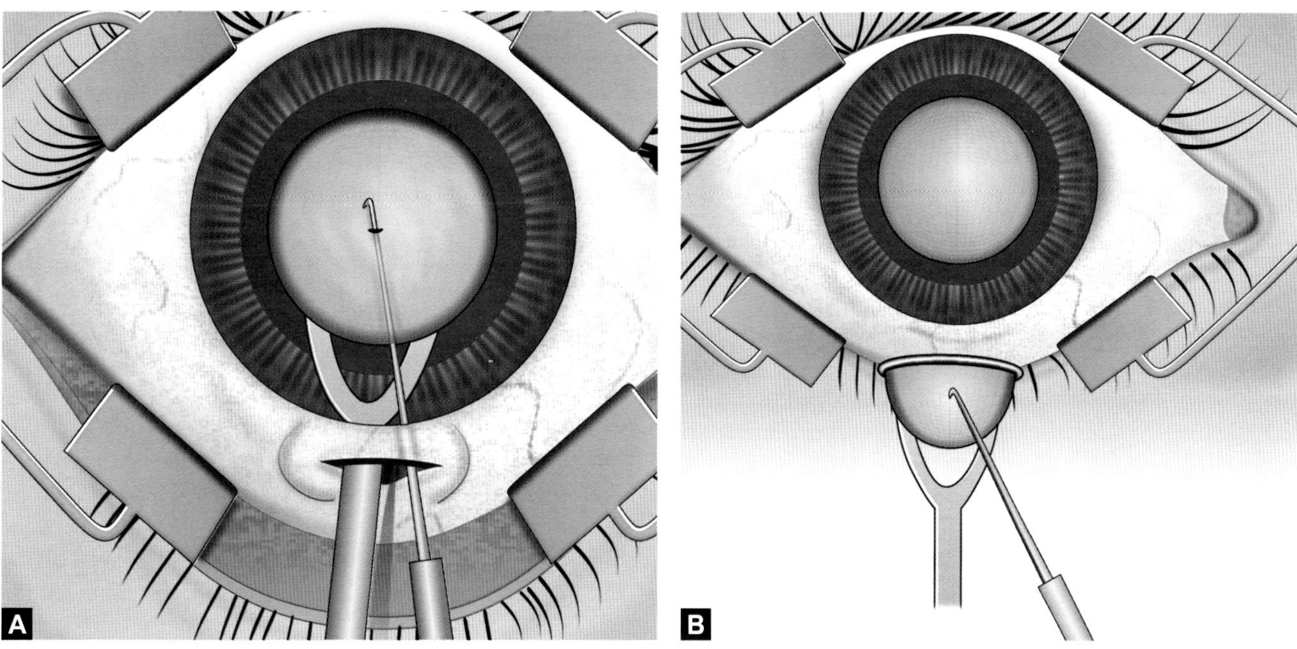


**Figures 10-8A and B** Nucleus extraction using the phacosandwich technique.

a good hydrodissection, the nucleus is prolapsed into anterior chamber. The freed nucleus, extremely mobile in a deep anterior chamber, is ready for being propelled out by the hydropressure generated by an ACM system.

A plastic glide 3–4-mm wide, 0.3-mm thick, and 3-cm long is subsequently inserted under the nucleus, one-third to one-half width nucleus distance. The bottle height is then raised to 60–70 cm above the patient's head, and slight pressure is applied over the lens glide on the scleral side. Intermittent pressure then propels the nucleus out of the sclerocorneal tunnel. Finally, a few more taps should enable the epinucleus and cortex to easily flow out of the anterior chamber.

*If the nucleus is not engaging the inner lip of the tunnel despite the full volume of ACM flow, the reasons may be*:

- A tunnel that is small, irregular, or incomplete
- Improperly fashioned or leaky side ports
- Premature entry of the tunnel, or
- Vitreous in the anterior chamber.

### *Fish hook Technique*

In this technique, a 30-gauge disposable needle is bent in the form of a fishhook and used in the nucleus extraction. After a thorough hydrodissection or hydrodelineation, the anterior chamber is filled with viscoelastic and only the superior pole of the nucleus is brought into the anterior chamber. Viscoelastic is injected in front of and behind the nucleus again to protect the surrounding structures.

The 30-gauge "fish hook" needle is then advanced into the anterior chamber with a sideways tilt to prevent endothelial injury. It is then maneuvered behind the nucleus to hook the undersurface of the lens. At this point, viscoelastic can be reinjected if there is any difficulty in traversing the fishhook. Once the nucleus is hooked, it is delivered out of the eye by applying slight downward pressure on the posterior lip of the tunnel. The nucleus is thus delivered without performing extensive maneuvers in the anterior chamber.

### *Simcoe Technique*

The Simcoe technique uses the same principles as the Blumenthal technique, combining mechanical and hydrostatic forces to allow extraction of the nucleus. After delivery of the lens into the anterior chamber and injection of viscoelastic anterior and posterior to the lens, the sclera or Tenon's capsule is grasped with 0.12 toothed forceps, and the globe is rotated away from the surgeon. The Simcoe is introduced into the anterior chamber through the sclerocorneal tunnel and is centered posterior to the lens and anterior to the iris. The irrigation is then turned on. The tip of the cannula should be visualized distal to the nucleus. The hydrostatic forces will bring the nucleus to the internal incision. Once the nucleus engages in the tunnel, slight downward pressure is applied to the external lip of the wound using the cannula while slowly withdrawing the cannula at the same time. Upon nuclear delivery, the Simcoe can be used immediately for cortical cleanup.

## Performing the Epinucleus Removal, Cortex Aspiration, and IOL Implantation

After the extraction of the endonucleus from the anterior chamber, a mixture of epinucleus and viscoelastic materials remains in the anterior chamber. It is easier to remove this mixture with the help of an irrigating vectis, although either of the following two methods can be employed:

- The epinucleus can be flipped out of the bag by introducing the Simcoe cannula under the anterior capsular rim and lifting out the epinucleus into the anterior chamber. The prolapsed epinucleus can then be extracted by depressing the inferior scleral lip with the Simcoe cannula and pulling the superior rectus bridle suture at the same time
- The epinucleus can also be manipulated by doing viscodissection. Viscoelastic is injected under the capsular rim, between the capsule and cortex, to lift this material out of the bag and into the anterior chamber, where it can be extracted through the sclerocorneal tunnel. The remainder of the cortical matter can then be aspirated using a Simcoe cannula.

The IOL is then placed through the tunnel into the intact capsular bag. As the size of the wound is above 6 mm, it is preferable to place a rigid Poly(methyl methacrylate) (PMMA) IOL with a 6 mm optic, especially in the setting of a "can opener" capsulotomy. In case where a capsulorhexis has been performed, then the option of implanting a foldable lens into the bag is available.

Smooth placement of the IOL is imperative to prevent anterior chamber collapse, iris trauma, and zonular dehiscence. If there is vitreous loss or prior zonular dehiscence, this is even more critical. Viscoelastic should be used to inflate the capsular bag, and a small amount should be injected over the subincisional iris, effectively creating a "viscoelastic ramp" for passage of the IOL and preventing inadvertent iris trauma or prolapse. (In straightforward cases, some experienced surgeons use air instead of viscoelastic to maintain the anterior chamber). The IOL is then inserted through the sclerocorneal tunnel in a two-step maneuver: using the nontoothed forceps, the leading haptic and optic are inserted, assuring that the leading haptic begins to enter the capsular bag. At this point, the surgeon's other hand can use forceps to stabilize the wound and prevent retraction of the IOL from out of the anterior chamber. Then, the trailing haptic is grasped by the nontoothed forceps and pushed toward the left aspect of the anterior chamber, rotating the leading haptic and optic fully into the capsular bag and allowing placement of the trailing haptic safely after. Any remaining viscoelastic can then be removed with the Simcoe cannula, and the wound can be tested for stability.

In select cases, the IOL may be strategically placed earlier in the procedure. For example, for cases of hypermature or morgagnian cataracts in which the capsular bag is extremely weak and collapsible, the IOL can be inserted pre-emptively between the nucleus and the posterior capsule, where it

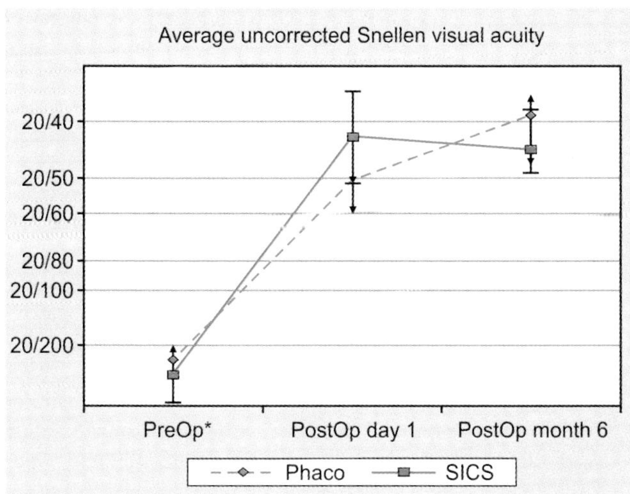


**Figure 10-9** Mean uncorrected visual acuity for the phacoemulsification (Phaco; dashed line) and manual sutureless small incision extracapsular cataract surgery groups. Vision recorded at preoperative testing (PreOp) and postoperative (PostOp) day 1 and month 6. Error bars denote 95% confidence interval. With permission from Ruit S, Tabin G, Chang D, et al. A prospective randomized clinical trial of phacoemulsification vs manual sutureless small incision. Extracapsular cataract surgery in Nepal. Am J Ophthalmol. 2007;143(1):32-38.e2.

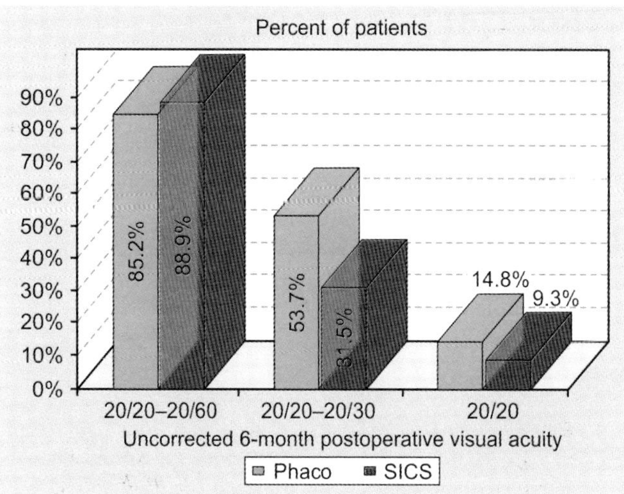


**Figure 10-10** Uncorrected visual acuity (UCVA) by functional level at 6 months after operation. Stratified into groups with visual acuity of 20/20, better than or equal to 20/30, and better than or equal to 20/60 in the phacoemulsification group (Phaco; black) versus the manual sutureless small incision extracapsular cataract surgery (SICS; gray) group. With permission from Ruit S, Tabin G, Chang D, et al. A prospective randomized clinical trial of phacoemulsification vs manual sutureless small-Incision. Extracapsular cataract surgery in Nepal. Am J Ophthalmol. 2007;143(1): 32-38.e2.

serves as a makeshift CTR. This allows for safe removal of the hypermature nucleus from a stabilized capsular bag, without subsequent tearing of the zonules or vitreous loss.

### Assuring Wound Closure

The anterior chamber is reformed by injecting BSS through the side port incision, or through the tunnel if no side port has been created. If the wound is constructed properly, a watertight closure is observed, and no sutures are necessary. One should be able to press down moderately on the central cornea without noting wound distortion or collapse of the anterior chamber.

After watertight closure is ensured, the conjunctiva should be placed to cover the external scleral incision. This can be performed on both superior and temporal incisions using cautery. Alternatively, the conjunctiva can be closed using a single interrupted suture.

## OUTCOMES: PHACOEMULSIFICATION VERSUS MSICS

As discussed above, phacoemulsification is considered the gold standard for cataract extraction in developed nations. But, undoubtedly, phacoemulsification is disadvantaged (particularly in the developing world setting) by being significantly more expensive than intracapsular cataract extraction, ECCE, or MSICS. Still, cost aside, how do outcomes with phacoemulsification compare with MSICS?

Three randomized controlled studies have measured and compared patient outcomes in phacoemulsification and MSICS in the developing world.[6–8] All these studies have reported similar uncorrected visual acuity (UCVA) and BCVA ≥ 20/60 at 6 weeks (2 studies) and 6 months (1 study) postoperatively. A recent randomized prospective study from Nepal evaluated 6-month outcomes of 108 patients randomized to phacoemulsification or MSICS for the treatment of advanced cataracts (average VA ≤ 20/300). The two techniques demonstrated equal rates of UCVA ≥ 20/60 and BCVA ≥ 20/60 at 6 months (Figs. 10-9 and 10-10). In the Nepal study setting, phacoemulsification was less efficient, requiring 15.5 minutes on average for completion compared with 9 minutes for MSICS. In addition, complication rates, including endophthalmitis rates, were shown to be similar between the two procedures.

Thus, in summary, the BCVA and UCVA ≥ 20/60 at 6 months after surgery was similar between the phacoemulsification and MSICS groups. However, MSICS was more efficient, more economical, and resulted in faster visual rehabilitation compared with phacoemulsification in treating advanced cataracts in the developing world.

## CONCLUSION

The MSICS technique provides a low cost, highly efficient surgical option for the developing world, with outcomes comparable with the most advanced surgical techniques used throughout the developed world. The high speed and low cost with which the surgery can be performed, even in the setting of very mature cataracts, make this technique ideal for decreasing the burden of cataract blindness in the developing world.

## REFERENCES


1. Ruit S, Tabin GC, Nissman SA, et al. Low-cost high-volume extracapsular cataract extraction with posterior chamber intraocular lens implantation in Nepal. Ophthalmology. 1999; 106:1887-92.
2. Venkatesh R, Tan CSH, Kumar TT, et al. Safety and efficacy of manual small incision cataract surgery for phacolytic glaucoma. Br J Ophthalmol. 2007; 91:279-81.
3. Venkatesh R, Tan CSH, Singh GP, et al. Safety and efficacy of manual small incision cataract surgery for brunescent and black cataracts. Eye. 2009;23(5):1155-7.
4. Venkatesh R, Das MR, Prashanth S, et al. Manual small incision cataract surgery in eyes with white cataracts. Indian J Ophthalmol. 2005; 53:173-6.
5. Venkatesh R. Use of capsular tension ring in phacoemulsification: indications and technique. Indian J Ophthalmol. 2003;51: 197.
6. Ruit S, Tabin G, Chang D, et al. A prospective randomized clinical trial of phacoemulsification vs. manual sutureless small-incision extracapsular cataract surgery in Nepal. Am J Ophthalmol. 2007;143:32-8.
7. Gogate PM, Kulkarni SR, Krishnaiah S, et al. Safety and efficacy of phacoemulsification compared with manual small-incision cataract surgery by randomized controlled clinical trial. Ophthalmology. 2005;112:869-74.
8. Gogate P, Deshpande M, Nirmalan PK. Why do phacoemulsification? Manual small-incision cataract surgery is almost as effective, but less expensive. Ophthalmology. 2007;114: 965-8.

CHAPTER

11

# Capsular Tension Segments

Patrick Gooi, Taylor Lukasik, Iqbal Ike K Ahmed

## INTRODUCTION

Cataract surgery in the setting of severe zonular weakness represents some of the most challenging cases faced by ophthalmic surgeons. Zonular weakness varies in etiology, ranging from trauma to genetic diseases such as Marfan's syndrome (Fig. 11-1) and Weill–Marchesani syndrome.[1,2] Previous methods for intraocular lens (IOL) insertion in the setting of zonular weakness include capsular tension rings (CTRs), modified capsular tension rings (M-CTRs), lensectomy with scleral fixation of a posterior chamber intraocular lens (PCIOL), and placement of an anterior chamber intraocular lens (ACIOL).[3-5] The capsular tension segment (CTS) designed by Ahmed in 2002 has shown to be effective in providing intraoperative capsular support during surgery as well as continued centration of the IOL postoperatively (Fig. 11-2).[6] Using an endocapsular support device such as the CTS allows for phacoemulsification with placement of a PCIOL in the capsular bag, which is presently the favored approach in modern cataract surgery. Placement of the PCIOL in the bag reduces the risk of chafing of uveal structures by the IOL edge, thus reducing the incidence of uveitis-glaucoma-hyphema syndrome. Furthermore, there is less risk of damage to the corneal endothelium and trabecular meshwork compared with ACIOLs. This chapter will describe the implantation technique for capsular tension segments in cataract surgery.

The CTS is a 120° ring segment with a radius of 5 mm that is made of polymethylmethacrylate with an anteriorly placed eyelet that hooks around the capsulorrhexis and is positioned anterior to the surface of the peripheral capsule

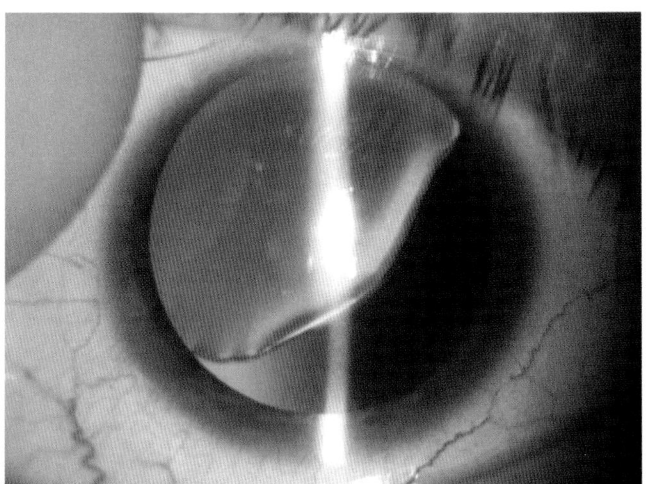

Figure 11-1 Slit lamp photograph preoperatively of a dislocated crystalline lens in a patient with Marfan's syndrome.

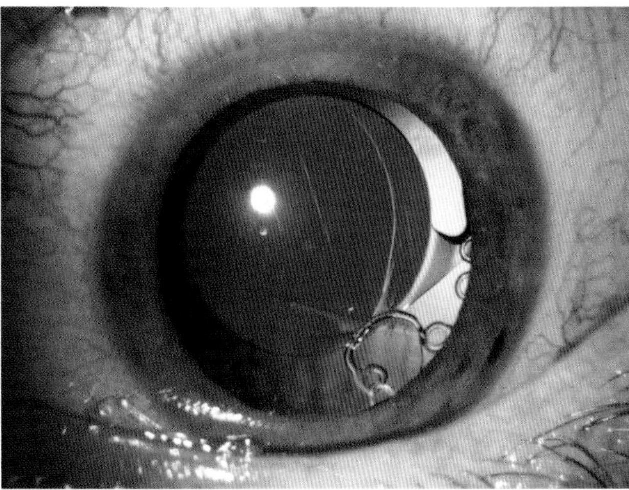

Figure 11-2 Slit lamp photograph postcataract extraction with a posterior chamber intraocular lens inserted in the bag stabilized by a capsular tension ring and capsular tension segment.

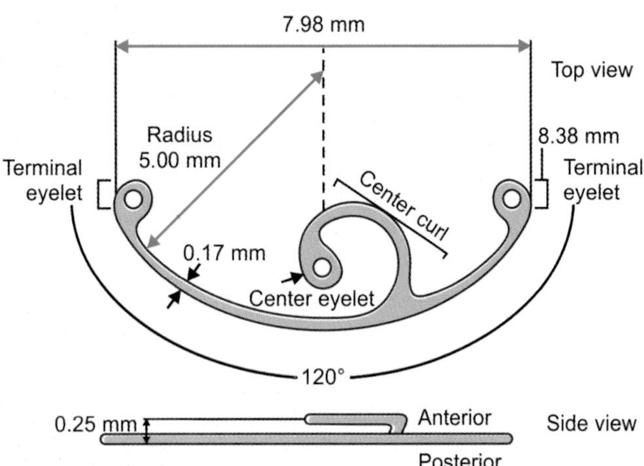


**Figure 11-3** Schematic diagram of the capsular tension segment with dimensions.

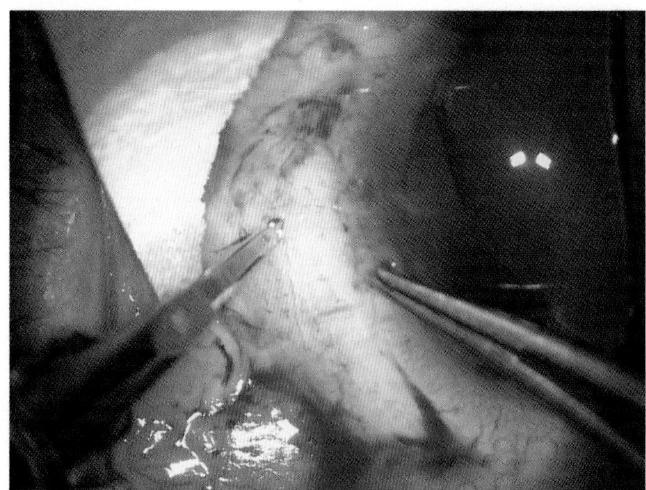

**Figure 11-4** Intraoperative photograph showing the scleral groove where the capsular tension segment will be sutured to the sclera.

(Fig. 11-3). The CTS may be atraumatically inserted prior to phacoemulsification and is stabilized with an iris hook through the anterior eyelet to provide intraoperative capsular support. The anterior eyelet allows for scleral fixation providing lasting capsular stability. Multiple capsular tension segments may be used depending on the extent of zonular instability.[4,5,7,8]

Capsular tension segments provide tension in the transverse plane and therefore can be used in conjunction with a CTR, which provides circumferential support around the equator of the capsular bag.[5] Placement of the CTS in the bag prevents the device from interacting with the corneal endothelium and angle structures.

## PREOPERATIVE CONSIDERATIONS

For a first case, choose one without vitreous in the anterior chamber. We would recommend booking about 2 hours for a CTS case early in the learning curve. With time, CTS cases can be done within an hour. General anesthesia or a retrobulbar block is also advisable.

## AVOIDING VITREOUS AND A VITRECTOMY

Combining the case with a vitrectomy considerably increases the surgical challenge. To avoid the need for a vitrectomy, dispersive ophthalmic viscosurgical devices (OVD) is applied to the area of zonulodialysis to keep the vitreous compartmentalized. Anterior chamber shallowing should be prevented at all costs, as this will encourage vitreous to migrate forward. To prevent anterior chamber shallowing, inject balanced salt solution on a 27-gauge cannula into the anterior chamber during instrument exchanges. OVD can be injected as well if it is to be used in the next step.

## SURGICAL TECHNIQUE

### Peritomy and Incisions

A peritomy for 4 clock hours is centered on the intended site for the scleral suture of the CTS. Subconjunctival local anesthetic is infiltrated in this area. After cautery, a scleral groove is fashioned, length 3-mm long, following the curvature of the limbus. It is positioned 1 mm posterior to the anatomical scleral spur (Fig. 11-4).

Two paracentesis are made in a "knife and fork" fashion (Fig. 11-5); these must be able to accommodate 23-gauge microtyers and iris microforceps. Short, narrow, and steeper paracentesis are made for iris hooks.

### Stabilizing Anterior Chamber with OVD/Iris Hooks/Capsulorrhexis

Dispersive OVD is injected first in the area of zonulodialysis to prevent vitreous migration anteriorly and then is used to coat the endothelium, followed by cohesive OVD to maintain the anterior chamber in a "soft shell technique."[9] The anterior capsule is often painted with vision blue prior to initiation of the capsulorrhexis. Vision blue is not injected freely into the anterior chamber, or it may diffuse posteriorly around the zonules to stain the retina and obliterate the red reflex. To initiate the capsulorrhexis, a 27gauge needle may be required to puncture the capsule, or one can use the iris microforceps on the anterior capsule to provide countertraction. Iris hooks may be placed on the rhexis edge in areas of the dialysis to stabilize the capsule (Fig. 11-6), but it is important to release the hooks prior to finishing the rhexis to avoid a radial tear.

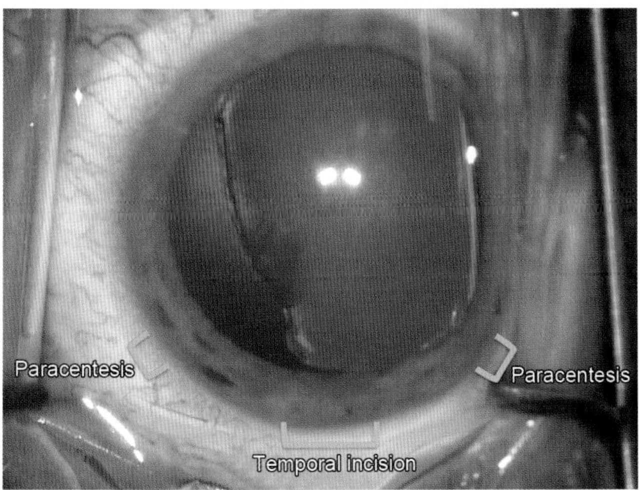


**Figure 11-5** Intraoperative photograph showing the "knife and fork" configuration of paracentesis, as well as the main incision.

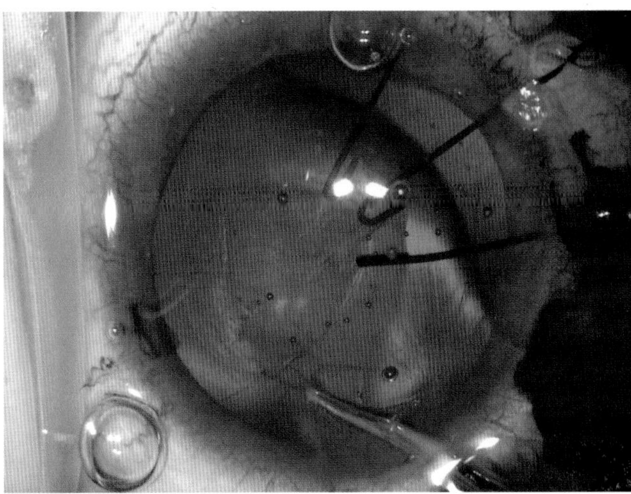

**Figure 11-6** Intraoperative photograph of iris hooks engaging capsulorrhexis edge to provide stability during capsulorrhexis.

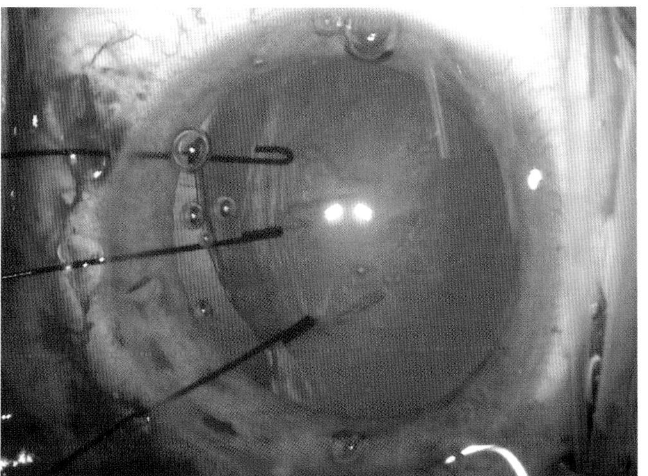

**Figure 11-7** Intraoperative photograph of iris hooks used to "tent up" on the capsule to make space to receive the capsular tension segment.

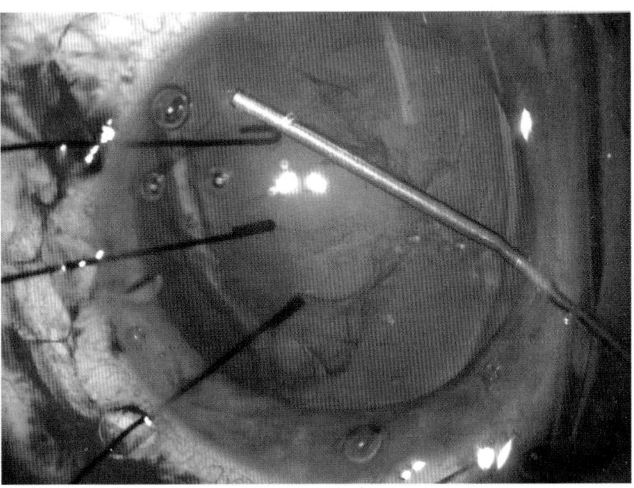

**Figure 11-8** Intraoperative photograph of cohesive OVD used to further open the pocket for the capsular tension segment.

## Insertion of CTS

The space for the CTS is prepared by placing the iris hooks on the rhexis edge to "tent up" on the capsule (Fig. 11-7). Furthermore, cohesive OVD can viscodissect a local area to create a pocket for the CTS (Fig. 11-8). It is important to avoid stirring up cortex during these maneuvers. One iris hook may be positioned along the same meridian of the intended scleral suture for the CTS. This iris hook is positioned with the opening facing anteriorly, as it will engage the eyelet of the CTS during phacoemulsification.

The CTS is grasped with curved tyers around the center of the CTS. Colibri forceps are used in the other hand to hold open the main wound for CTS insertion. A Sinskey hook engages an eyelet of the CTS for manipulation in the anterior chamber (Fig. 11-9). Iris microforceps can then grasp the center "curl" of the CTS to direct it into the bag. The iris hook engages the center eyelet of the CTS to give stability to the capsular bag in preparation for phacoemulsification (Fig. 11-10).

## Early CTR Insertion

At this point, the decision is made whether or not to insert a CTR. Advantages with an early CTR insertion are that it will stabilize the bag and facilitate phacoemulsification, and it will also expand the bag to prevent vitreous from coming anteriorly. A disadvantage is that cortex can easily become trapped behind the CTR. Furthermore, suturing the CTS to sclera is more difficult with a CTR expanding the bag, with a greater risk of nicking the bag with the needle.

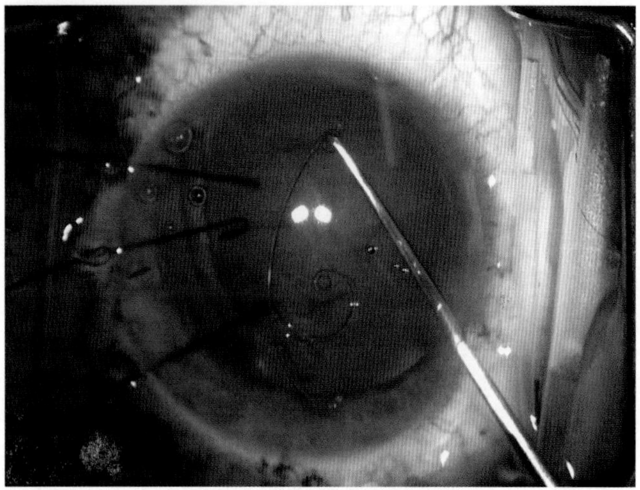

Figure 11-9 Intraoperative photograph of a Sinskey hook positioning the capsular tension segment in the anterior chamber.

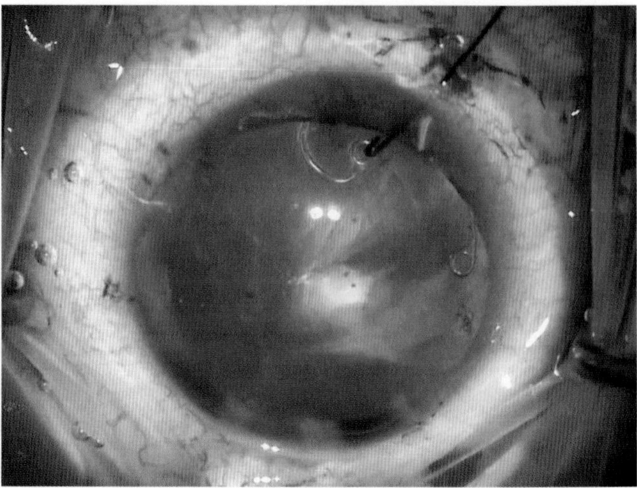

Figure 11-10 Intraoperative photograph of an iris hook engaging the central eyelet of capsular tension segment to provide stability during phacoemulsification.

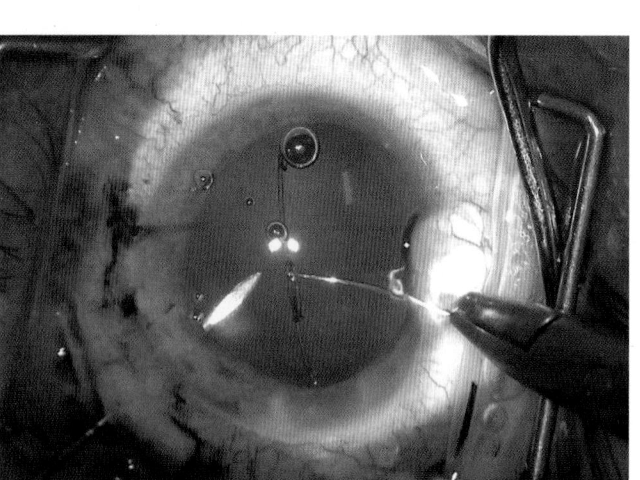

Figure 11-11 Intraoperative photograph showing the vertical orientation of capsular tension segment perpendicular to suture passes.

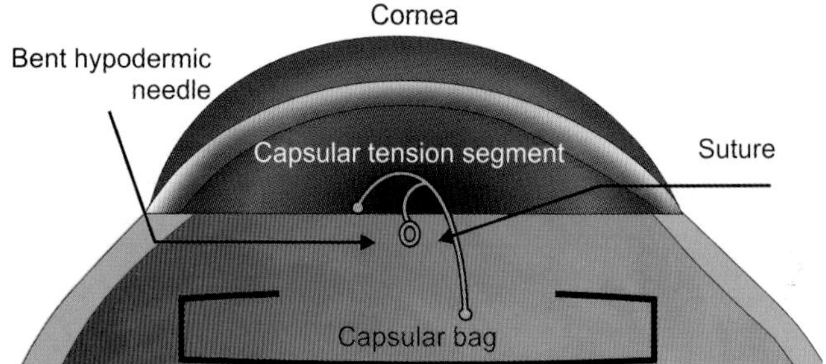


Figure 11-12 Schematic diagram showing the trajectory of the 25G hypodermic needle as well as the 7-0 Gore-Tex suture.

## Phacoemulsification

Hydrodissection is performed with balanced salt solution. The capsular bag can be stabilized with the CTS on an iris hook alone. Phacoemulsification is then completed in the usual fashion. Cortex removal with the irrigation/aspiration handpiece is first performed around the area of the CTS, followed by the subincisional area.

## Suturing of CTS

Initially, dispersive OVD is injected around the area of dialysis. The bag is topped up with cohesive OVD. If necessary a paracentesis for passing the suture is made 180° from the scleral groove. The iris hook is disengaged from the CTS, and the iris hook then maximally retracts the iris in the area of the future scleral suture. Iris microforceps reposition the CTS out of the capsular bag, as this will keep the capsule away from the needle passes. The CTS is positioned at the center of the anterior chamber, with the plane of the CTS vertically, and approximately perpendicular to the axis of the placement of the suture passes (Fig. 11-11). The double-armed, curved 7-0 GORE-TEX® sutures are straightened out with two locking needle drivers using a hand over hand technique. The tip of the 7-0 GORE-TEX® suture is placed into the anterior chamber, just past the paracentesis while wiggling the suture from side to side within the wound. This will ensure that the suture does not engage the corneal stromal fibers.

The trajectory of the 25-gauge needle for docking with the GORE-TEX® suture is outlined in (Fig. 11-12). OVD is topped up to firm the globe to facilitate needle entry. A 25 gauge hypodermic needle is bent at the hub with the bevel facing up and placed on an OVD syringe. It enters the sclera 1 mm posterior to the anatomical scleral spur and then follows the

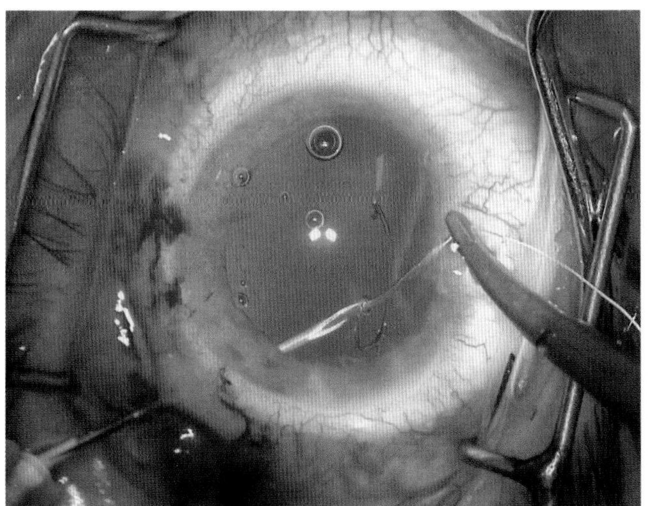

**Figure 11-13** Intraoperative photograph showing the suture docked with the hypodermic needle.

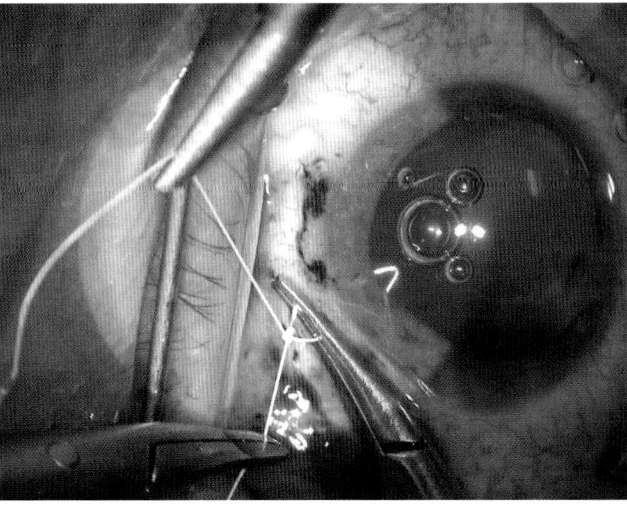

**Figure 11-14** Intraoperative photograph showing our method for tying the slipknot.

iris plane, posterior to the iris, but anterior to the lens capsule. Scleral entry is perpendicular to the sclera and facilitated with Colibri forceps. Once the needle has passed through sclera, the Colibri forceps are quickly switched to a Kuglen hook, which may be used to further retract the iris for improved visualization, facilitate entry of the needle through the sclera, as well as retract the capsular bag from the needle. While holding the hypodermic needle steady in the anterior chamber, the needle driver grabs the 7-0 GORE-TEX® suture, threads it though the anterior eyelet of the CTS, and docks the suture into the 25-gauge needle (Fig. 11-13). Previous positioning of the CTS so it is centered and vertically oriented facilitates this step. It is important to firmly dock the suture in the needle. As the 25-gauge needle and docked suture are pulled from the eye, a Kuglen hook may be needed for countertraction on the CTS. Microtyers can be used to direct the suture through the eyelet. Once the suture is externalized, the redundant suture is pulled through, paying close attention to the position of the CTS in the eye, to ensure that the CTS is not displaced in any direction, using iris microforceps as needed for stabilization. GORE-TEX® sutures are very adherent to the instruments; to prevent sudden movements of the CTS, instruments must be slowly disengaged from the GORE-TEX® material.

Prior to the second suture pass, additional OVD may be needed to firm the globe, and additional dispersive OVD may be injected around the area of zonulodialysis. Iris microforceps and a Sinskey hook replace the CTS into the bag. The second 25-gauge needle entry is made along the scleral groove 2 mm away from the previous site. This separation facilitates rotation of the suture to bury the knot later on. As the 7-0 GORE-TEX® is pulled though, the Sinskey and Kuglen hooks can help direct the suture to ensure that the suture does not get caught on the wrong side of the central eyelet.

## Tying the Slipknot for the CTS/Adjusting Tension/IOL Insertion

The slipknot is tied loosely so it is easier to adjust tension to center the CTS—bag complex. Prior to tightening the second throw of the slipknot, the surgeon holds the base of the knot with a needle driver. This allows cinching of the knot without excess movement of the CTS. The second throw is then cinched down with the surgeon holding the short end of the knot with a needle driver, and the assistant holding the long end (Fig. 11-14). The bag is filled with cohesive OVD, and a CTR is injected into the bag. Prior to insertion of the IOL, the wound is slightly enlarged to ensure the injector can fully enter the anterior chamber. The IOL is injected directly into the bag. If the capsulorrhexis is on the small side, iris hooks may be employed to stretch open the capsulorrhexis to facilitate IOL insertion. We recommend leaving the slipknot with a slight amount of slack to prevent the CTS from being pulled out of the bag. The final throw locks the slipknot in place. The knot is rotated into the sclera with curved tyers. A Sinskey hook may be used to push the final parts of the knot into the sclera.

## Closing

Manual OVD removal is performed with a 27-gauge Rycroft cannula on a syringe filled with balanced salt solution. This gentle method keeps a stable anterior chamber compared

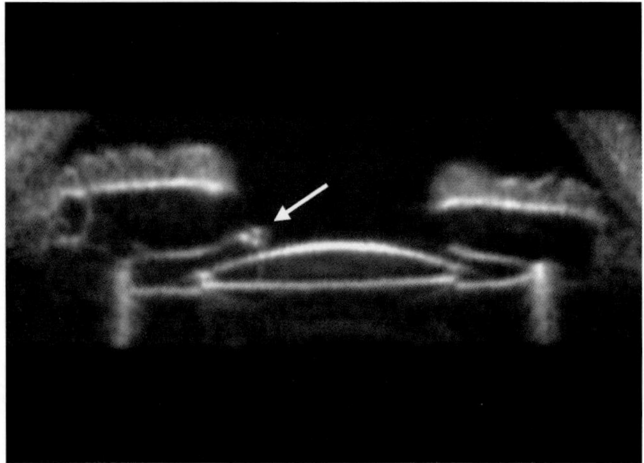

**Figure 11-15** Postoperative ultrasound biomicroscopy showing the capsular tension segment with the eyelet anterior to the capsule (arrow), with the intraocular lens centered and flat.

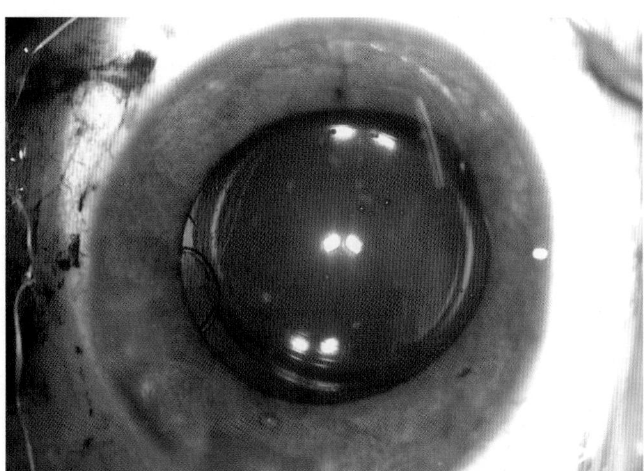

**Figure 11-16** Intraoperative photograph showing a toric intraocular lens used in conjunction with a capsular tension segment.

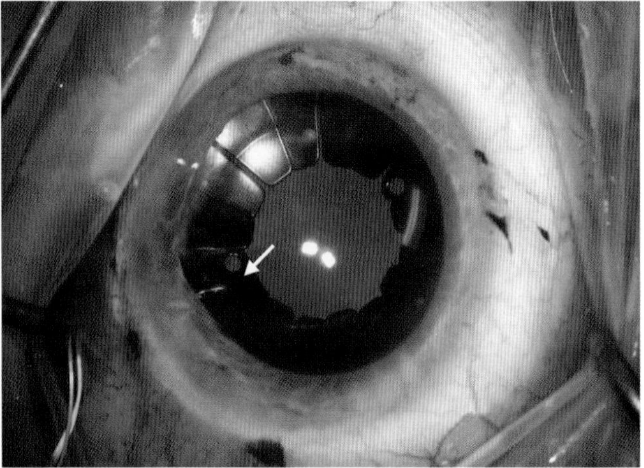

**Figure 11-17** Intraoperative photograph of two Morcher 50E iris prosthesis used in conjunction with a capsular tension segment (arrow).

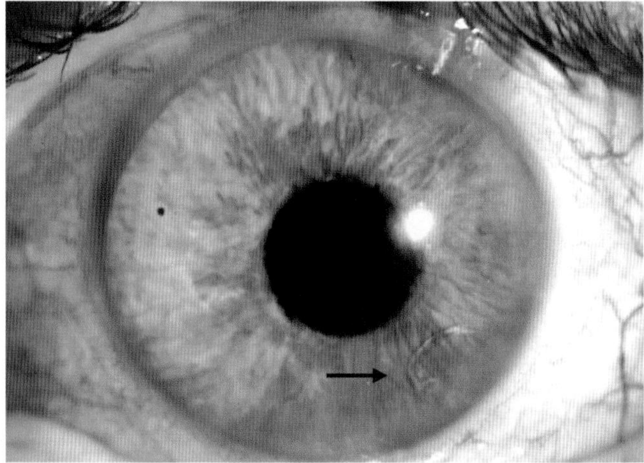

**Figure 11-18** Postoperative slit lamp photograph of a custom-made artificial iris prosthesis (human optics) implanted in the bag, stabilized with a capsular tension segment (arrow).

with the automated irrigation/aspiration handpiece, although the patient should be placed on oral acetazolamide postoperatively for a couple of days. Michol is injected into the anterior chamber to constrict the pupil. We often suture the main wound and paracentesis with 10-0 nylon, to prevent any anterior chamber shallowing and vitreous migration anteriorly. The peritomy is closed with 10-0 vicryl.

## POSTOPERATIVE MANAGEMENT

Patients are seen 1 day and 1 week postoperatively. Usually, we obtain ultrasound biomicroscopic imaging of the IOL approximately 2 months after surgery (Fig. 11-15) to check for IOL centration and tilt. If a small capsulorrhexis appears to be tilting the IOL, it is possible to perform radial relaxing incisions with the Nd: YAG (Neodymium-doped Yttrium Aluminium Garnet) laser applied to the anterior capsule. This is performed any time after 1 month postoperatively. If posterior capsular opacification occurs, a YAG capsulotomy is performed in the usual fashion.

## ADVANCED ANTERIOR SEGMENT RECONSTRUCTION

Advanced anterior segment reconstruction often calls for dislocated cataract extraction and iris reconstruction. Since the capsular bag is preserved, it is possible to implant advance technology IOLs, such as toric and multifocal IOLs (Fig. 11-16), which are often only available in a 1 piece platform. Endocapsular iris prosthesis can be used (Figs. 11-17 and 11-18). These can be implanted through small incisions, which reduce the surgically induced astigmatism and also increase the safety of surgery. The iris prosthesis is particularly useful in cases where there is insufficient quantity or quality of iris tissue to perform a sutured pupilloplasty.

## CONCLUSION

Capsular tension segments are an excellent tool for cataract extraction with severe zonulopathy and allow for in the bag PCIOL implantation. We feel this is the safest position for the IOL, as it is less likely to chafe iris structures and is well away from the corneal endothelium and angle structures. With a preserved capsular bag, advance technology IOLs can be used. Furthermore, iris reconstruction with endocapsular iris prosthesis may be performed through small incisions. Small incision surgery offers a better safety profile to prevent anterior chamber shallowing and vitreous prolapse. Capsular tension segments are an excellent addition to the armamentarium of the ophthalmic surgeon. It provides a platform for advance anterior segment reconstruction in a highly customizable, modular fashion.

## REFERENCES


1. Kohnen T, Baumeister M, Buhren J. Scheimpflug imaging of bilateral foldable in-the-bag intraocular lens implantation assisted by a scleral – sutured capsular tension ring in Marfan's syndrome. J Cataract Refract Surg. 2003;29:598-602.
2. Groessi SA, Anderson CJ. Capsular tension ring in a patient with Weill-Marchesani syndrome. J Cataract Refract Surg. 1998; 24:245-9.
3. Mark H. Blecher MH, Matthew R. Kirk. Surgical strategies for the management of zonular compromise. Curr Opin Ophthalmol. 2008;19:31-5.
4. Hasanee K, Ahmed II. Capsular tension rings: update on endocapsular support devices. Ophthalmol Clin North Am. 2006;19(4):507-19.
5. Hasanee K, Butler M, Ahmed II. Capsular tension rings and related devices: current concepts. Curr Opin Ophthalmol. 2006;17(1):31-41.
6. Chee SP, Jap A. Management of traumatic severely subluxated cataracts. Am J Ophthalmol. 2011;151(5):866-71.
7. Blecher MH, Kirk MR. Surgical strategies for the management of zonular compromise. Curr Opin Ophthalmol. 2008;19(1):31-5.
8. Ahmed II, Chen SH, Kranemann C, et al. Surgical repositioning of dislocated capsular tension rings. Ophthalmology. 2005;112(10):1725-33.
9. Arshinoff SA. Dispersive-cohesive viscoelastic soft shell technique. J Cataract Refract Surg. 1999;25(2):167-73.

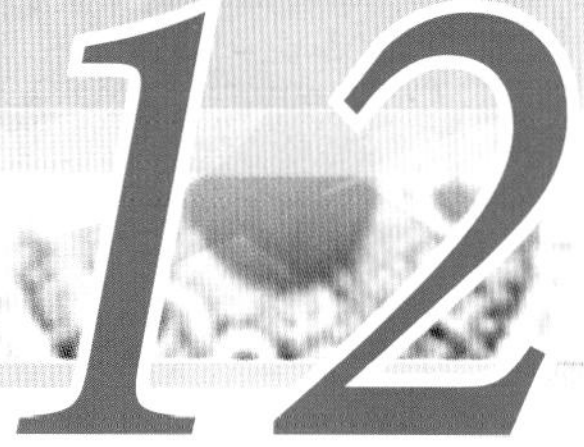


# Femtosecond Laser Cataract Surgery

Robert Cionni, Charles H Weber

## INTRODUCTION

Femtosecond laser cataract surgery may provide superior refractive outcomes by providing a more stable intraocular lens (IOL) position[1-10] while requiring reduced phacoemulsification energy[7,9,11-14] after laser lens fragmentation. Femtosecond capsulotomies and clear corneal incisions are more reproducible and stable,[1,4,5,15-18] and laser corneal relaxing incisions promise improved accuracy in the treatment of preexisting astigmatism.[17]

## INDICATIONS

- Astigmatism
- Visually significant cataract
- Refractive lens exchange

## CONTRAINDICATIONS

- Corneal disease, opacity, or implant that precludes transmission of laser light at 1030-nm wavelength or applanation of the cornea
- Conditions that would cause inadequate clearance between the intended capsulotomy depth and the corneal endothelium (applicable to capsulotomy only)
- Presence of blood or other material in the anterior chamber
- Corneal thickness requirements that are beyond the range of the system in use
- Glaucoma filtering blebs
- Hypotony
- Any contraindication to cataract or keratoplasty surgery
- Noncooperative patient

Relative contraindications:

- White cataract (able to complete capsulorhexis and corneal incisions, but not lens fragmentation).
- Poorly dilating pupil, such that the iris is not peripheral to the intended diameter for the capsulotomy (able to perform corneal incisions but not capsulotomy or lens fragmentation).

## SURGICAL TECHNIQUE

### Patient Selection

The femtosecond laser may be used for any patient undergoing cataract extraction or refractive lens exchange provided there are no contraindications as outlined above. A cooperative patient is required for successful positioning and docking, with the patient preferably capable of locating and following the fixating light. Patients should have an adequate palpebral fissure, without conjunctival symblepharon or other notable lid pathology. Pupillary dilation should ideally be >6.0 mm; however, it has been our experience that pupils down to 5.0 mm in diameter may be acceptable with adjustments made for capsulorhexis size and area of lens fragmentation. If the pupil is <5.0 mm, the surgeon may choose to perform corneal incision but defer capsulotomy and lens fragmentation.

### Billing and Reimbursement

- A complete discussion of billing for use of the femtosecond laser is beyond the scope of this book, but there are a few aspects of reimbursement worth mentioning.[19]
- The allowable Medicare reimbursement for cataract surgery does not change according to the surgical methods

used, and Medicare beneficiaries cannot be charged an additional fee for services that would otherwise be reimbursed, regardless of technique.

- Medicare patients can be charged for services beyond standard medically necessary cataract extraction with a conventional IOL, which may include additional charges related to femtosecond laser astigmatic keratotomy performed for refractive indications.
- Medicare patients may also be charged for use of the imaging portion of the femtosecond laser during cataract surgery when using an advanced technology IOL to achieve an anticipated refractive result.
- A refractive lens exchange is not medically necessary and therefore is not covered under Medicare, and a surgeon and the facility may bill the patient for any services related to the surgery, including use of the femtosecond laser.

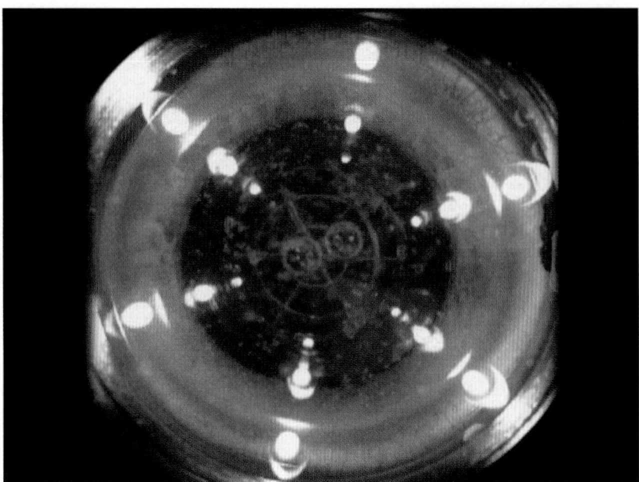

**Figure 12-1** Femtosecond laser energy produces gas, which forms bubbles in the capsular bag and in the anterior chamber.

## Laser Parameters: Capsulotomy Size and Fragmentation Profile

Femtosecond laser energy results in the formation of gaseous bubbles as it photodisrupts tissue (see section "Mechanism of action" below),[20] and thus bubbles are formed during creation of corneal incisions, capsulotomy, and lens fragmentation with the femtosecond laser when used for cataract surgery. Factors that can affect the degree of bubble formation include the following: energy level, spot size, spot spacing, degree of lens/eye tilt with docking, capsulotomy size, chop diameter, number of chops, cylinder diameter, number of cylinders, lens thickness, and depth of lens fragmentation treatment.

Bubbles formed during femtosecond laser lens fragmentation may increase intralenticular pressure and decrease visualization (Fig. 12-1). These bubbles tend to remain within the capsular bag and overaggressive hydrodissection combined with an already pressurized capsular bag could encourage a posterior capsule rupture. One goal for the surgeon, therefore, is to minimize bubble formation while, at the same time, maximizing laser fragmentation effect, which can be achieved by limiting laser treatment to zones where effect is most needed as well as utilizing the minimum power level needed to achieve the desired effect. For example, with typical Grade 2 to Grade 3 cataract densities, a two-chop program (four segments) may have utility equal to that of a three or four chop setting. Reducing lens chop diameter to 4.7 from 6.0 mm further diminishes bubble formation, yet the lens chop effect is not decreased. In addition, as long as the capsulotomy diameter is set larger than the chop or cylinder settings, the forward extent of lens fragmentation can be brought quite anteriorly so that fragmentation-induced bubbles escape into the anterior chamber rather than remaining within the capsular bag.

We typically have utilized a three-chop (six segments) program combined with two central small cylinders. For dense cataracts, four cylinders are preferred. With the current software, we use the following settings: a lens three chop diameter of 4.7 mm and a lens two cylinder diameter of 2.5/3.5 mm. The capsulotomy diameter is set at 4.9 mm to be slightly larger than the lens fragmentation.

More recently, we have implemented a columnar fragmentation. The nuclear columnar fragments can be further fragmented in halves or thirds. We have found this pattern to be extremely effective in softening the central hardest portion of the cataract, often allowing for removal of the cataract with little or no ultrasound energy (Fig. 12-2).

As we gain more and more experience with femtosecond laser cataract surgery, we will also learn to optimize energy levels and fragmentation patterns based on cataract grade and type to more efficiently fragment the nucleus while minimizing bubble formation.

## Laser Parameters: Astigmatic Keratotomy

For corneal arcuate incisions, we currently program an 8.5-mm optical zone and a cut of 85% corneal depth, as determined by the laser's optical coherence tomography (OCT) device. We use the Donnenfeld nomogram but reduce it by one third. In other words, if the nomogram calls for a 60° arc, we make a 40° arc (Figs. 12-3 and 12-4).

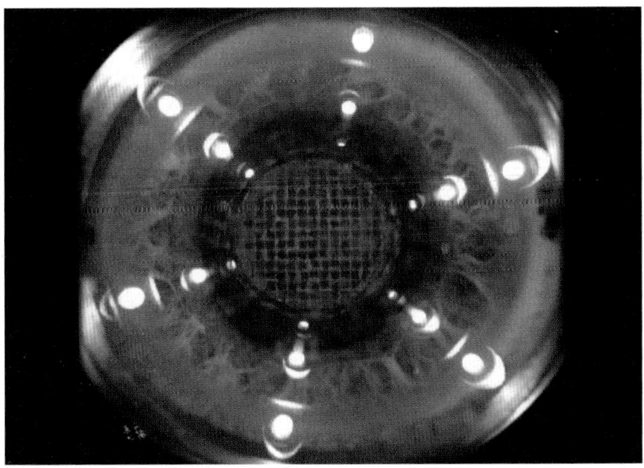

Figure 12-2 LenSx Laser columnar lens fragmentation pattern.

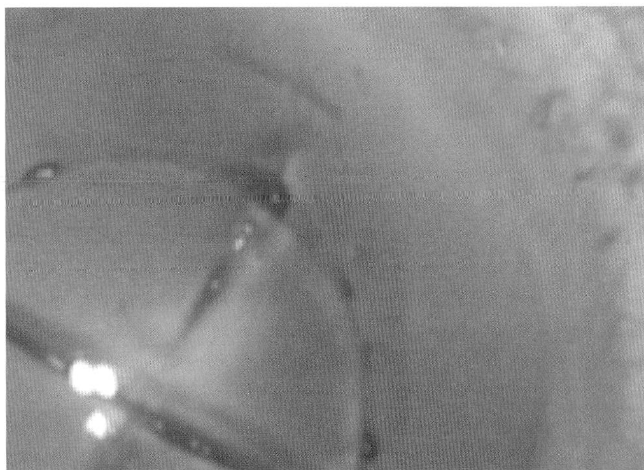

Figure 12-3 Optical coherence tomography and microscopic photo of an arcuate corneal incision made by the LenSx Laser.

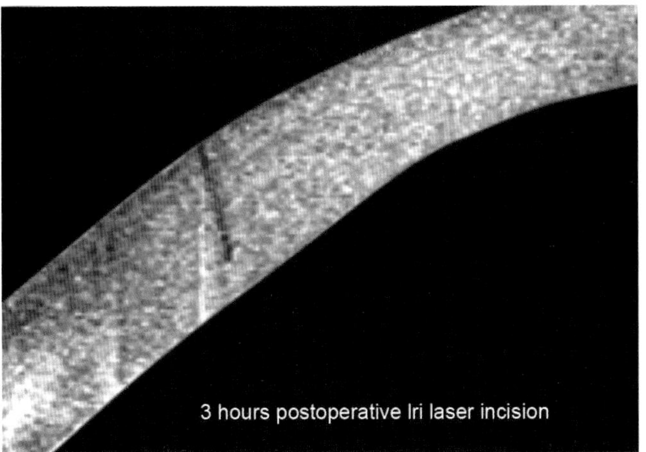


Figure 12-4 Optical coherence tomography photo showing the precision of an 85% depth arcuate corneal incision made by the LenSx Laser.

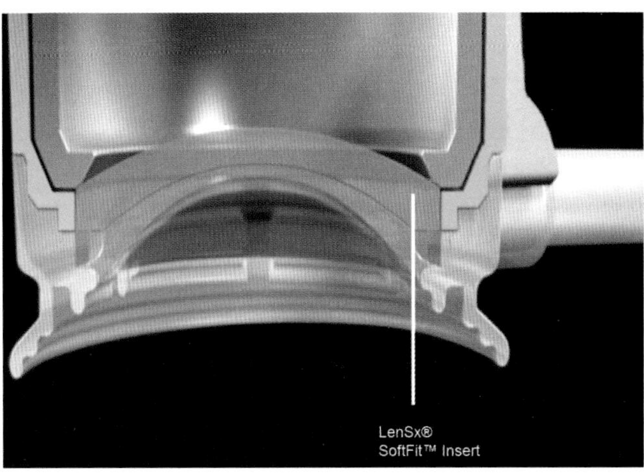


Figure 12-5 Illustration of the LenSx Laser, SoftFit patient interface. The soft curved interface minimizes corneal folds and IOP rise.

## Patient Positioning and Docking

During application of the femtosecond laser, the patient's eye must remain stable, which is provided through a patient interface. Femtosecond laser manufacturers have variations in their method of patient docking, but all achieve stabilization of the eye with limited intraocular pressure (IOP) rise.[21-23] The process of docking with the Alcon LenSx Laser with SoftFit patient interface will be demonstrated here (Fig. 12-5).

With the patient placed supine under the docking apparatus, and a topical anesthetic applied to the operative eye, a lid speculum is placed. The patient interface is then docked to the patient's eye, taking care to center the patient's visual and pupillary axis at the center of the patient interface. Sensors in the delivery system detect eye position and the applanation force, which is indicated on the screen. A flat dock allows for maximal lens fragmentation, whereas a tilted dock limits the anterior and posterior extent of lens fragmentation to avoid damaging the anterior and posterior capsules (Figs. 12-6A and B).

## Anterior Segment Visualization and Customization of Treatment Parameters

It is critical for any femtosecond laser cataract system to accurately identify ocular structures to complete the laser treatment safely. For example, identification of the posterior lens surface is required to maintain a safe distance for laser application to prevent posterior capsule rupture, and precise corneal thickness measurement is essential for accurate depth of corneal relaxing incisions.

Manufacturers vary in their approach to anterior segment visualization. Alcon's LenSx, Bausch & Lomb's Victus, and OptiMedica's Catalys utilize Fourier-domain OCT for

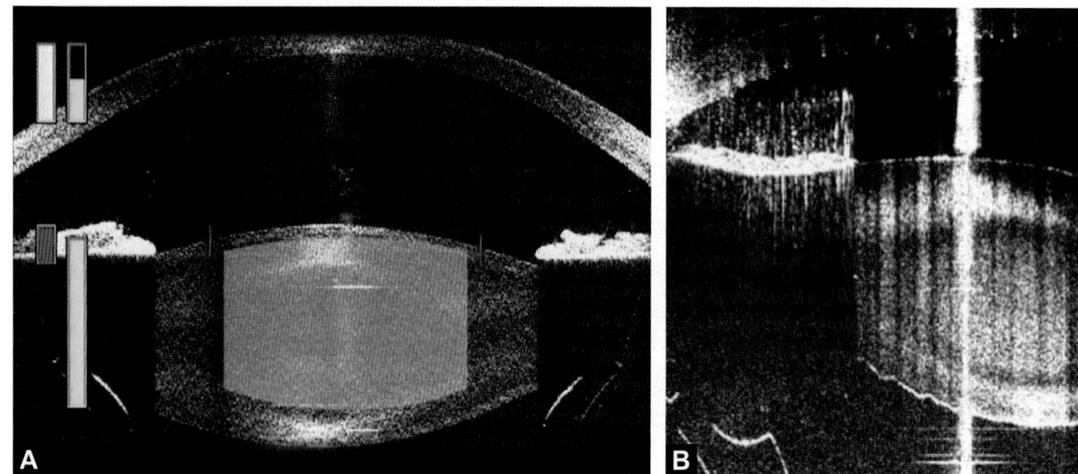


Figures 12-6A and B (A) A flat dock results in the ability to create a maximum fragmentation pattern. Notice the absence of corneal folds provided by the SoftFit patient interface; (B) A tilted dock resulting from use of a rigid curved interface limits the ability to achieve maximal lens fragmentation.

three-dimensional, high-resolution viewing of ocular structures, whereas LensAR uses a three-dimensional confocal structured illumination-scanning transmitter very similar to Scheimpflug technology. Anterior segment visualization with these technologies allows for high-resolution measurements of lens position, corneal thickness, and pupillary margin.

Once the patient's eye has been properly docked with the patient interface, the above-mentioned anterior segment imaging is utilized to view ocular structures and the surgeon is directed in customizing the location and dimension of laser incisions and zones of lens fragmentation. The LenSx laser provides a point-and-click computer interface with a live microscopic OCT image to make necessary adjustments to incision size and location as well as depth and diameter of the capsulotomy and lens fragmentation (Figs. 12-1 to 12-3, 12-6A and 12-8).

## Treatment

Once the laser parameters have been customized for the individual patient, the treatment is begun by depression of the laser footswitch. Each pattern of the laser is applied from posterior to anterior to maintain focus and minimize laser scatter. Once the laser treatment is complete, the patient is undocked from the patient interface. Delivery of laser energy can be stopped at any point by releasing the footswitch. Currently, the laser procedure typically takes about 30–60 seconds of treatment time and about 3–4 minutes of surgeon time in the laser room.

## Cataract Extraction

After laser treatment, the patient is prepped and draped in a typical fashion for cataract surgery. A variety of instruments have been developed to bluntly open the laser-created corneal incisions. Occasionally, incomplete incisions may require the use of a sharp blade for completion.

Ideally, a free-floating capsulotomy will be present, ensuring completion of the capsulotomy. Injecting a dispersive ophthalmic viscoelastic device through the side-port incision anterior to the capsulotomy button is advised to avoid displacing the button into the angle. The ophthalmic viscosurgical devices can also be used to displace any bubbles that may have come forward during femtosecond laser application (Fig. 12-7). If capsular attachments remain, a capsulorhexis forceps or cystotome is used to tangentially tear the remaining connections in the same method as done for a traditional capsulorhexis.

With a hydrodissection cannula, gentle hydrodissection is performed with care taken not to overexpand the capsular bag that has likely already inflated somewhat with gas formed by femtosecond laser fragmentation of the lens. Bubbles present within the capsular bag can be evacuated by gently depressing one pole of the nucleus as a partial fluid wave is directed under the anterior capsule rim until it reaches the bubbles located along the posterior capsule. Gentle yet firm pressure on the opposite pole of the nucleus dissects the bubble and fluid around the remainder of the lens, allowing both to escape into the anterior chamber. The lens nucleus can then be rotated freely.

As phacoemulsification begins, the central nucleus is emulsified and aspirated first. Clearing the central nucleus creates a generous space in which the phaco tip and a nucleus chopper/manipulator can be placed to grasp and propagate the fragmented segments peripherally and posteriorly. Each segment, one at a time, is thus separated and brought centrally

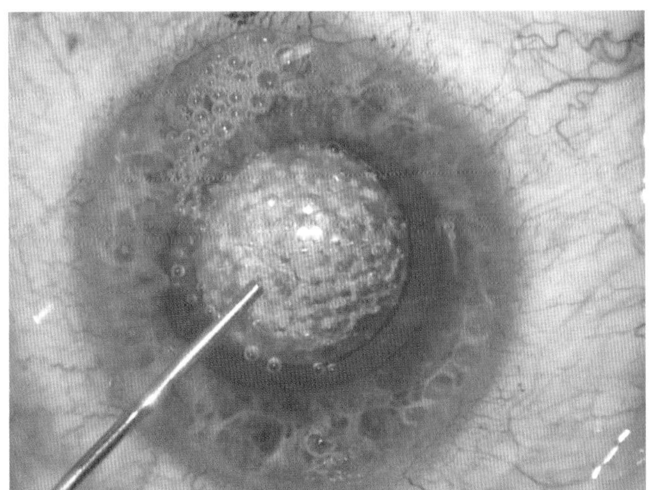

Figure 12-7 Ophthalmic viscosurgical device is injected anterior to the capsule button as the air bubbles are displaced for better visualization.

within this space for easy emulsification. Alternatively, a prechop technique can be employed to propagate the lens fragmentation into segments before inserting the phacoemulsification handpiece. The epinucleus typically follows the last segment into the phacoemulsification tip.

Phacoemulsification typically requires lower total energy than required for a cataract of similar density that has not undergone femtosecond fragmentation.[7,9,11-14]

## MECHANISM OF ACTION

Femtosecond lasers use a shorter pulse time of $10^{-15}$seconds compared with $10^{-9}$ seconds used by photocoagulation (argon), photoablation (excimer), and photodisruption (Nd:YAG) lasers.[20] Laser power is a function of energy per unit time, and decreasing the pulse time increases the power generated by a given energy, or conversely decreases the energy needed to create a given effect (power). In addition, the near-infrared wavelength femtosecond laser can be focused at any point within a target tissue, where the laser energy can be set to a plasma-generating threshold, which when applied creates a shock wave, followed by cavitation and gas bubble formation.[20] Thus, the femtosecond laser uses low energy to create a high-power photodisruption of small volumes of tissue with tight focus. These characteristics make the femtosecond laser an ideal choice for use in cataract surgery, as it is able to exert its effect with precision and avoid disruption of surrounding nontargeted tissues.

## POSTOPERATIVE CARE

The postoperative care after femtosecond laser cataract surgery is the same as with conventional cataract surgery.

## SPECIFIC INSTRUMENTATION

### Operating Room Furniture

Our femtosecond laser resides in a separate operating room (OR) from where the phacoemulsification of the procedure takes place. We use rolling chairs/beds that function as the OR bed, and the patient remains supine in the rolling bed when transferred from the laser OR to the phacoemulsification OR. Several companies manufacture beds that work well for this purpose. Some femtosecond laser platforms utilize beds that are fixed to the laser.

### Intraoperative Instruments

As stated above, a number of different instruments have been developed for the purpose of opening the femtosecond-created corneal incisions. Our current preference is to use Cionni Femtosecond Spatula/Nucleus Manipulator (Duckworth and Kent, St Louis, MO). No additional intraoperative equipment is required.

## COMPLICATIONS

Complications, both intraoperative and postoperative, of femtosecond laser cataract surgery are overall much the same as those with traditional cataract surgery.[7,11,24] Complications include:

- Pupillary constriction
- Anterior capsule radial tears
- Posterior capsule tears
- Posterior lens dislocation
- Corneal abrasion or defect
- Subconjunctival hemorrhage
- Capsular block syndrome[25]
- Endophthalmitis

## SURGICAL OUTCOMES: SCIENTIFIC EVIDENCE

### Surgical Outcomes and Safety of Femtosecond Laser Cataract Surgery: A Prospective Study of 1500 Consecutive Cases

In this prospective, single-center study, Roberts et al.[25] evaluated the safety and surgical outcomes of femtosecond laser cataract surgery in 1500 consecutive eyes undergoing femtosecond laser cataract and refractive lens exchange surgery in a single group private practice. The cases underwent anterior capsulotomy, lens fragmentation, and corneal incisions with the Alcon LenSx femtosecond laser. The cases were divided into two groups with group 1 consisting of the first 200 cases and group 2 being the subsequent 1300 cases performed by the same surgeons.

In the study, anterior capsule tears occurred in 4 and 0.31% of eyes, posterior capsule tears in 3.5 and 0.31% of eyes, and posterior lens dislocation in 2 and 0% of eyes in groups 1 and 2, respectively ($P < 0.001$ for all comparisons). In addition, the number of docking attempts per case (1.5 vs 1.05), incidence of postlaser pupillary constriction (9.5 vs 1.23%), and anterior capsular tags (10.5 vs 1.61%) were significantly lower in group 2 ($P < 0.001$ for all comparisons).

In summary, they found that greater surgeon experience, development of modified techniques, and improved technology were associated with a significant reduction in complications. The group went on to state that, in their opinion, most complications are now predictable and largely preventable with a complication rate in group 2 comparable with the largest published reports of manual phacoemulsification surgery.

## Comparison of IOL Power Calculation and Refractive Outcome after Laser Refractive Cataract Surgery with a Femtosecond Laser Versus Conventional Phacoemulsification

In this prospective study, Filkorn et al.[2] compared IOL power calculation and refractive outcome between 77 eyes of 77 patients who underwent laser refractive cataract surgery with a femtosecond laser (Alcon LenSx) and 57 eyes of 57 patients who underwent conventional cataract surgery. Biometry was done with optical low coherence reflectometry (Lenstar LS900, Haag-Streit AG) and IOL calculation performed using third-generation IOL formulas (SRK/T, Hoffer Q, and Holladay). At least 6 weeks after surgery, their main refractive outcome, mean absolute error, was significantly lower in the femtosecond laser group (0.38 ± 0.28 diopters) than in the conventional group (0.50 ± 0.38 D) ($P = 0.04$).

In this study, they concluded that femtosecond laser cataract surgery resulted in a significantly better predictability of IOL power calculation than manual phacoemulsification surgery.

## PLACE OF THE TECHNIQUE IN SURGICAL ARMAMENTARIUM

Femtosecond laser cataract surgery is a viable alternative to manual phacoemulsification cataract surgery, being as safe and effective.[24] The improvement in surgical precision[1,4,5,8,9,15,16,18] and refractive outcomes[1-3,5,6,10] as well as the decrease in phacoemulsification time[7,9,11-14] during femtosecond cataract surgery can benefit all patients. We have found femtosecond cataract surgery useful in patients ranging from those undergoing refractive lens exchange to those with dense cataract. We have also found utility in the femtosecond's ability to safely create a round capsulotomy in subluxed crystalline lenses and those with generalized zonular compromise such as patients with pseudoexfoliation syndrome (Fig. 12-8).

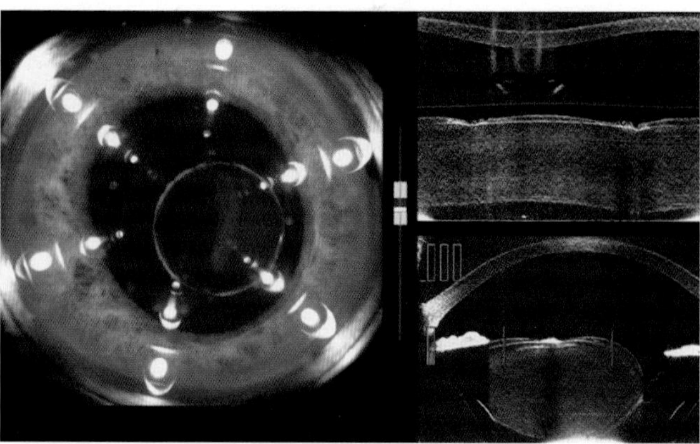

**Figure 12-8** LenSx Laser optical coherence tomography of a traumatic cataract with zonular dialysis and anterior capsular fibrosis. Notice that the capsulotomy is manually positioned "off-center" of the dilated pupil but centered on the subluxed capsule.

## PEARLS AND PITFALLS

- Do not select patients that are uncooperative; have corneal opacity precluding adequate laser delivery; have advanced glaucoma (due to IOP rise during the procedure); or have small interpalpebral fissures preventing proper docking.
- Communicate with the patient during docking and the procedure to reinforce the impact of their eye position and cooperation on the success of the surgery.
- The clear corneal incision should be made as peripherally as possible but not so peripheral as the sclera or limbal vessels. Otherwise, even if created manually, it will not seal as well as a limbal incision and will induce corneal folds during phacoemulsification, limiting visualization and likely leading to more postoperative corneal edema than desired.
- Check that the capsulotomy is completely free of any microadhesions or an area of uncut capsule. Failure to notice this could result in anterior capsular tears.
- Resist aggressive hydrodissection to avoid capsular block syndrome.[26]

- The femtosecond laser capsulotomy cuts the anterior cortex flush with the edge of the capsulorhexis, resulting in the absence of irregular tags beneath the capsulorhexis' edge to grab during cortical aspiration. We recommend a tangential sweep 'hurricane' technique with the irrigation–aspiration handpiece under the anterior capsule.[27]

## REFERENCES


1. Colas E, Abrieu M, Laayoun J, et al. Improving effective lens position: comparison of femtosecond laser vs manual capsulotomy. Acta Ophthalmologica. 2012;90:0-0. (Abstracts from the 2012 European Association for Vision and Eye Research Conference).
2. Filkorn T, Kovacs I, Takacs A, et al. Comparison of IOL power calculation and refractive outcome after laser refractive cataract surgery with a femtosecond laser versus conventional phacoemulsification. J Refract Surg. 2012;28(8):540-4.
3. Hill WE. Effective lens position following laser anterior capsul otomy. Paper presented at the Annual Meeting of the American Academy of Ophthalmology, Orlando, FL: October 2011.
4. Kranitz K, Takacs A, Mihaltz K, et al. Femtosecond laser capsulotomy and manual continuous curvilinear capsulorrhexis parameters and their effects on intraocular lens centration. J Refract Surg. 2011;27(8):558-63.
5. Kranitz K, Mihaltz K, Sandor GL, et al. Intraocular lens tilt and decentration measured by Scheimpflug camera following manual or femtosecond laser-created continuous circular capsulotomy. J Refract Surg. 2012;28(4):259-63.
6. Mihaltz K, Knorz MC, Alio JL, et al. Internal aberrations and optical quality after femtosecond laser anterior capsulotomy in cataract surgery. J Refract Surg. 2011;27(10):711-6.
7. Nagy ZZ, Takacs A, Filkorn T, et al. Initial clinical evaluation of an intraocular femtosecond laser in cataract surgery. J Refract Surg. 2009;25(12):1053-60.
8. Nagy ZZ, Kranitz K, Takacs AI, et al. Comparison of intraocular lens decentration parameters after femtosecond and manual capsulotomies. J Refract Surg. 2011;27(8):564-9.
9. Roberts TV, Lawless M, Chan CC, et al. Femtosecond laser cataract surgery: technology and clinical practice. Clin Experiment Ophthalmol. 2013;41(2):180-6.
10. Uy H, Hill WE, Edwards K. Refractive results after laser anterior capsulotomy. Invest Ophthalmol Vis Sci. 2011; 52 [E-abstract 5695].
11. Abell RG, Kerr NM, Vote BJ. Catalys femtosecond laser-assisted cataract surgery compared to conventional cataract surgery. Clin Experiment Ophthalmol. 2012. Oct 19.
12. Abell RG, Kerr NM, Vote BJ. Toward zero effective phacoemulsification time using femtosecond laser pretreatment. Ophthalmology. 2013;120(5):942-8.
13. Conrad-Hengerer I, Hengerer FH, Schultz T, et al. Effect of femtosecond laser fragmentation of the nucleus with different softening grid sizes on effective phaco time in cataract surgery. J Cataract Refract Surg. 2012;38(11):1888-94..
14. Conrad-Hengerer I, Hengerer FH, Schultz T, Dick HB. Effect of femtosecond laser fragmentation on effective phacoemulsification time in cataract surgery. J Refract Surg. 2012;28(12):879-83.
15. Friedman NJ, Palanker DV, Schuele G, et al. Femtosecond laser capsulotomy. J Cataract Refract Surg. 2011;37(7):1189-98.
16. Masket S, Sarayba M, Ignacio T, et al. Femtosecond laser-assisted cataract incisions: architectural stability and reproducibility. [letter]. J Cataract Refract Surg. 2010;36(6):1048-9.
17. Palanker DV, Blumenkranz MS, Andersen D, et al. Femtosecond laser-assisted cataract surgery with integrated optical coherence tomography. Sci Transl Med. 2010;17;2(58):58ra85.
18. Tackman RN, Kuri JV, Nichamin LD, Edwards K. Anterior capsulotomy with an ultrashort-pulse laser. J Cataract Refract Surg. 2011;37(5):819-24.
19. ASCRS. Guidelines for billing Medicare beneficiaries when using the femtosecond laser. 2012
20. Sugar A. Ultrafast (femtosecond) laser refractive surgery. Curr Opin Ophthalmol. 2002;13(4):246-9.
21. Data on file. Alcon Labs, Inc. Presented at ACOS 2013 Deer Valley Femtosecond Leadership Summit.
22. Kerr NM, Abell RG, Vote BJ, et al. Intraocular pressure during femtosecond laser pretreatment of cataract. J Cataract Refract Surg. 2013;39(3):339-42.
23. Schultz T, Conrad-Hengerer I, Hengerer FH, et al. Intraocular pressure variation during femtosecond laser-assisted cataract surgery using a fluid-filled interface. J Cataract Refract Surg. 2013;39(1):22-7.
24. Talamo JH, Gooding P, Angeley D, et al. Optical patient interface in femtosecond laser-assisted cataract surgery: contact corneal applanation versus liquid immersion. J Cataract Refract Surg. 2013;39(4):501-10.
25. Roberts TV, Lawless M, Bali SJ, et al. Surgical outcomes and safety of femtosecond laser cataract surgery: a prospective study of 1500 consecutive cases. Ophthalmology. 2013;120(2): 227-33.
26. Roberts TV, Sutton G, Lawless MA, et al. Capsular block syndrome associated with femtosecond laser-assisted cataract surgery. J Cataract Refract Surg. 2011;37(11):2068-70.
27. Nakano CT, Hida WT, Motta AFP, et al. The Hurricane I/A Technique [Video]. 2012

CHAPTER

13

# Pediatric Cataract

Abhay R Vasavada, Sajani Shah

## PEDIATRIC CATARACT

Pediatric cataract is the most common cause of treatable childhood blindness, accounting for 5–20% of blindness in children worldwide.[1-3] The incidence has been reported as 2.5/10,000 by the age of 1 year, increasing to 3.5/10,000 by age 15.[4] It is estimated that > 2,00,000 children are blind from disorders of the lenses. Although blindness in most cases can be principally attributed to unoperated cataract, dense amblyopia after delayed surgery, complications of surgery, or associated ocular abnormalities may also be other causes of blindness.

Pediatric cataract surgery is a complex issue best left to surgeons who are familiar with its long-term complications and lengthy follow-up. Cataract surgery in children is the first stepping stone in the long road to visual rehabilitation. Treatment is often difficult and tedious, requiring a dedicated team effort, the most important members of the team being the parents. Maintaining a clear visual axis while correcting the eye for a changing residual refractive error requires careful observation, sound judgment, and diligent follow-up.

## TIMING OF SURGERY

Visually significant cataract in children calls for prompt surgical intervention to clear the ocular media and provide a focused retinal image. Indications for cataract surgery include visually significant central cataracts, dense nuclear cataracts, cataracts obstructing the examiner's view of the fundus, and cataracts associated with strabismus. The timing of treatment is crucial to the visual development and successful rehabilitation of children, especially during early infancy. In case of a unilateral dense cataract diagnosed at birth, the surgeon can wait until the patient is 4–6 weeks of age. This decreases anesthesia related complications and facilities the surgical procedure. Waiting beyond this time, however, adversely affects the visual outcome. In the case of bilateral cataract diagnosed at birth, a good visual outcome can be achieved if the child is operated before 10 weeks of age. It is important to keep the time interval between the surgeries performed on the two eyes to a minimum.

Simultaneous cataract surgery on both the eyes is performed only when anesthesia poses a higher than average risk, or if the patient lives for away and a visit for a surgery on the second eye would be difficult.

## PREOPERATIVE EVALUATION

The preoperative examination includes age appropriate vision testing and details of strabismus and nystagmus. Visual function in older children can be assessed with charts such as preferential looking charts (Teller Acuity Card, Keeler, Berkshire, SL4 4AA), Lea gratings and symbols (Precision Vision, Lasalle, IL, USA), Sheridan–Gardiner tests, and 'E' charts or Snellen's charts. In very young children, who cannot co-operate for vision tests, the ability to fixate or follow light or objects should be assessed. The presence of squint or nystagmus should be noted.

A preoperative examination with fully dilated pupils, if necessary under anesthesia, is mandatory in both the eyes. It includes examination under the operating microscope or slit lamp biomicroscope to assess the cataract and tonometry to rule out any association of glaucoma. The examination also helps in the measurement of corneal diameter, posterior segment evaluation, keratometry, biometry, and gonioscopy.

During the examination, the surgeon must look for the type and severity of cataract including pre-existing posterior capsule defect.

Clinical examination of the child should include a complete examination of all systems, including respiratory, nervous, and cardiovascular systems. Supportive laboratory investigations should include hemogram, blood sugar, titers for antibodies to TORCH [toxoplasmosis, other infections, rubella, cytomegalovirus (CMV), and herpes simplex virus (HSV)] agents, HIV, HBsAg, and X-rays or echocardiography if required. Special tests to rule out metabolic diseases should be ordered whenever necessary.

## Biometry: Intraocular Lens (IOL) Power Calculation

Implantation of a fixed-power IOL into an eye that is still growing makes it difficult to choose the IOL power. The child's growing eye is expected to develop a myopic shift in refraction. IOL implantation at the calculated emmetropic power helps fight amblyopia during childhood, but there is the risk of developing significant myopia at ocular maturity. On the other hand, too much undercorrection of the IOL power will lead to immediate postoperative hypermetropia with the possibility of amblyopia. An ideal IOL power should aim at prevention of amblyopia in childhood with the least possible residual refractive error in adulthood.

Most surgeons tend to undercorrect the IOL power at the time of surgery in anticipation of the postoperative myopic shift. Several monograms on IOL power selection have been published in literature.[5-7] However, these tables are only meant to help as a starting point toward appropriate IOL power selection, which is a multifactorial decision customized for each child based on many variables [including age, laterality (one eye or both), amblyopia status (dense or mild), compliance with glasses, and family history of myopia].The axial length increases faster in the first few years of life. If the decision regarding IOL implantation needs to be changed, e.g. in cases of ciliary sulcus, appropriate adjustment may need to be done. The residual refractive error needs to be corrected with spectacles or contact lens that are adjusted throughout the growing period according to refractive development.

However, even after undercorrection, refractive surprises can occur. The long-term outcome will certainly remain an open question for years to come.

# SURGICAL TECHNIQUE

Pediatric cataract needs a special surgical strategy as these eyes have greater elasticity of the capsule, lower scleral rigidity, higher incidence of inflammation and posterior capsule opacification (PCO), a thick vitreous gel, and a small, growing eye. The surgeon should strictly adhere to the principles of the closed chamber technique, such as valvular incision, injection of ophthalmic viscosurgical devices (OVD) before removing any instrument from the eye, and bimanual irrigation/aspiration.

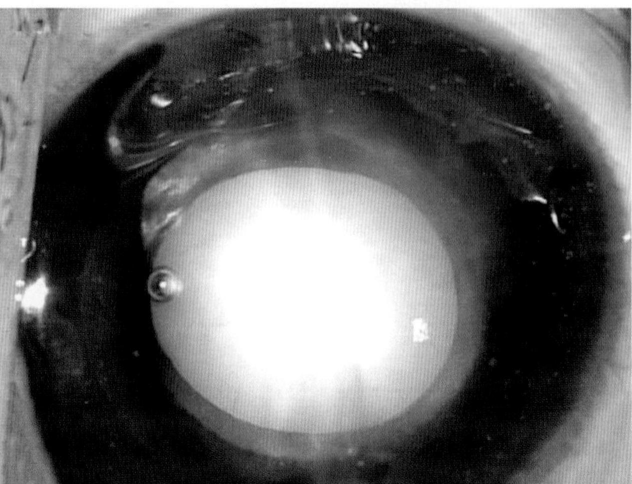

**Figure 13-1** Dye enhanced primary manual anterior capsule continuous curvilinear capsulorhexis.

## Anterior Capsule Management

The anterior capsule in children is very elastic, and therefore, it may be difficult to perform a controlled manual continuous curvilinear capsulorhexis (CCC). However, a manual CCC is the gold standard in terms of maintaining the integrity of the capsular edge. The shape, size, and edge integrity of anterior capsulotomy are very important for long-term centration of the IOL.[8-10] Capsulorhexis is usually performed with Kraff–Utrata forceps (Fig. 13-1). Care is taken to frequently grasp and regrasp the capsule to avoid peripheral extension of the CCC.

Alternatives to manual CCC currently available include vitrectorhexis, radio frequency diathermy with a Fugo plasma blade,[11,12] the two incision push pull technique, and the four incision technique.[13,14]

Vitrectorhexis is easier to perform as compared with manual CCC, and it is often the preferred approach. In contrast, a diathermy-cut capsulotomy, even when performed perfectly, shows coagulated capsular debris along the edge. The Fugo blade is a unique cutting instrument that employs plasma for ablating tissue. It helps make a perfectly controlled anterior capsulotomy of any size, without the risk of radial tear. Radio frequency diathermy with a Fugo blade is recommended when fibrotic capsules are encountered or in white cataract the absence of red reflex.

High viscosity OVDs[15] aid in performing anterior CCC (ACCC) approximately 5.0 mm in diameter. Capsular staining with trypan blue[16-18] is a useful adjunct in pediatric cataract surgery, especially in cases where there is a poor glow. Localized capsular staining is performed with 0.0125% trypan blue.

## Cortical Cleaving Hydrodissection

After making the incision and carrying out capsulorhexis, multiquadrant hydrodissection is preferred, in all cases except in eyes with a white mature cataract or when a pre-existing posterior capsule defect is suspected. It is documented that multiquadrant cortical-cleaving hydrodissection in pediatric cataract surgery facilitates lens substance removal and also reduces removal time.[19]

## Management of the Posterior Capsule and Anterior Vitreous Face in Children

The most frequent and significant problem after pediatric cataract surgery is visual axis opacification (VAO).[20-22] The younger the child, the higher the incidence and the earlier the onset of VAO. Maintenance of a clear visual axis remains a high priority when planning management of the posterior capsule in the amblyogenic age range. Posterior capsulotomy can be performed with various approaches including manual posterior CCC (PCCC), vitrectorhexis, radio frequency diathermy, and Fugo plasma blade.[23] Manual PCCC is performed before IOL implantation, whereas, if a pars plana vitrectorhexis is performed, it is done after the IOL is implanted.

The size of the posterior capsulorhexis should be large enough to provide a clear central visual axis, but smaller than the IOL optic, so as to allow stable in-the-bag IOL fixation. Manual PCCC offers the advantage of a controlled size and strong edges but is more difficult to perform (Fig. 13-2). Many investigators have observed that performing manual PCCC is technically difficult. A potential complication associated with this procedure is the disruption of the anterior vitreous face (AVF). However, AVF disruption often goes unnoticed because anterior vitrectomy is a part of the surgical strategy in younger children. The signs of AVF disruption vary from subtle to obvious. These are (1) the presence of vitreous strands in the anterior chamber. (2) The attachment of the vitreous to the capsular flap. (3) Distortion of the capsulorhexis margin.[24] Some surgeons prefer pars plicata vitrectorhexis after performing IOL implantation in the bag. When a pars plicata approach is chosen, the IOL should be inserted into the capsular bag using OVD while the posterior capsule is still intact. While the irrigation cannula remains in the anterior chamber an MVR (Microvitroretinal) blade is used to enter pars plana 2–3 mm (1.5–2 mm in patients < 1 year of age, 2.5 mm in patients of 1–4 years of age, and 3 mm in patients > 4 years of age) and posterior to the limbus. The vitrector is then inserted through this incision and used to open the center of the posterior capsule.[25]

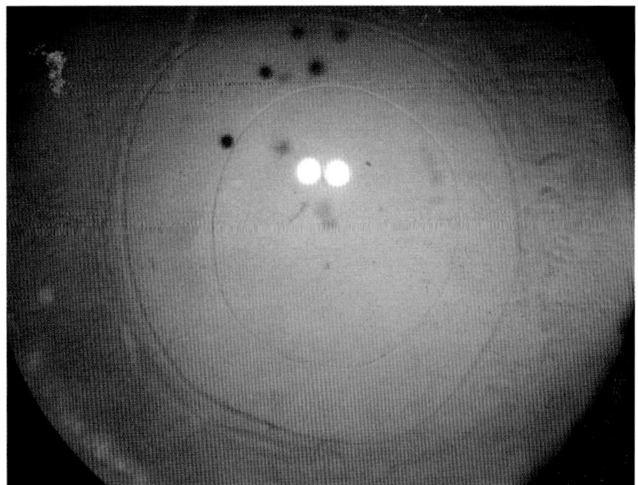

**Figure 13-2** Primary manual anterior and posterior continuous curvilinear capsulorhexis (ACCC, PCCC) showing a smooth and regular edge.

The PCCC alone may delay the onset of VAO but cannot eliminate it completely.[26] The AVF may act as a scaffold for the proliferating lens epithelial cells. Moreover, since the inflammatory response in small children is severe, fibrous membranes may form on the intact AVF, resulting in VAO. Hence, anterior vitrectomy along with posterior capsulotomy is advocated in infants and children < 6–7 years of age.[26] Most surgeons prefer manual anterior limbal vitrectomy over pars plana vitrectomy. The adequacy of anterior vitrectomy may be confirmed by injecting triamcinolone to aid visualization of the vitreous. We have described a technique to render the vitreous visible and ensure a thorough, complete anterior vitrectomy in pediatric cataract surgery after a manual PCCC with or without IOL implantation using preservative-free triamcinolone acetonide[27] (Fig. 13-3).

However, considering the implications of vitrectomy, especially in children with a family history of myopia, diabetes mellitus, and possibility of cystoid macular edema, posterior capsule management has been stratified according to the age of the child.[28,29] Children < 3 years of age are subjected to PCCC

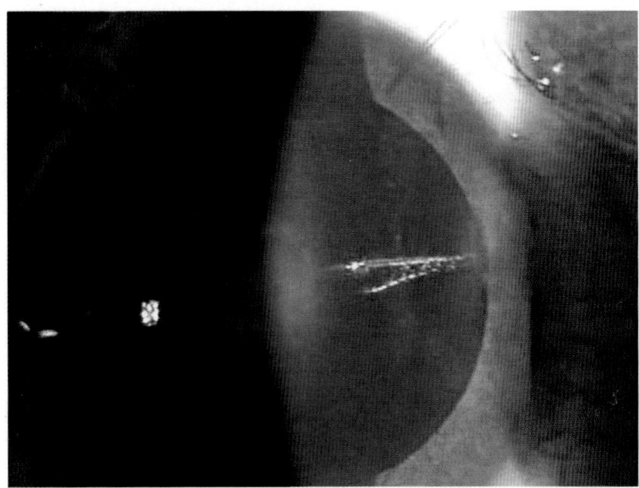

Figure 13-3 Vitreous strands extending towards the incision, clearly seen with triamcinolone staining.

and anterior vitrectomy. Children between 3 and 6 years of age are subjected to PCCC but no vitrectomy. In children > 6 years of age, PCCC is not performed.

### IOL Implantation

Options for optical correction after pediatric cataract surgery are primary IOL implantation, aphakic glasses, and contact lenses. Primary IOL implantation has become a preferred approach in children >2 years.[30,31] IOL implantation is still controversial in children < 2 years, especially those < 1 year, as the safety of IOL implantation in these eyes is not proven. Eyes with juvenile rheumatoid arthritis, microcornea, microphthalmos, and severe persistent fetal vasculature maybe considered as contraindications for IOL implantation.

IOL implantation in children has the benefit of providing at least partial optical correction, which aids in visual development especially in eyes prone to amblyopia. Advances in surgical techniques and instrumentation, combined with implantation of better quality IOLs, have now resulted in fewer IOL-related complications in children. This encourages more and more surgeons to use IOLs even in very young children. For bilateral cataract during this first year, aphakic glasses and/or contact lens use may be a reasonable option. However, for unilateral cataract, it is still controversial whether to offer primary IOL implantation at the time of infantile cataract surgery. A large randomized clinical trial—the Infant Aphakia Treatment Study is currently underway to compare primary IOL implantation to contact lens correction in children undergoing unilateral cataract surgery in the first 6 months of life.

Both polymethyl methacrylate and hydrophobic acrylic foldable IOLs have been widely used in pediatric eyes. However, several studies have now shown that hydrophobic acrylic IOLs are preferable as they offer better uveal biocompatibility and decreased incidence of VAO,[32] with hydrophobic acrylic IOLs causing a delayed onset of PCO. In-the-bag fixation is the most preferred site of IOL implantation, although IOL may also be implanted in the ciliary sulcus in cases of inadequate posterior capsular support.

## COMPLICATIONS OF PEDIATRIC CATARACT SURGERY

### Visual Axis Opacification (VAO)

VAO still remains the most frequent complication of pediatric cataract surgery. The most critical factor influencing the occurrence of VAO is age at surgery. While opacification is nearly universal in infantile eyes, the incidence decreases with increasing age. Primary management of the posterior capsule and anterior vitrectomy is effective in preventing reopacification of visual pathways. The type and material of IOL also is a very important factor affecting the incidence of VAO.

### Glaucoma

Glaucoma is a recognized complication of pediatric cataract surgery. Despite improved surgical techniques, the incidence of glaucoma after successful cataract removal remains high.[33,34] A significant number of surgeons regard aphakia as a cause of glaucoma. However, the glaucoma occurring postoperatively may be better described as "glaucoma in aphakia" and "glaucoma in pseudophakia". The most common type of glaucoma that develops after congenital cataract surgery is open-angle glaucoma. The risk factors include age at the time of surgery; pre-existing ocular abnormalities; type of cataract; and the effect of lens particles, lens proteins, inflammatory cells, and retained lens material. In addition, microcornea, secondary surgery, chronic postoperative inflammation, the type of lensectomy procedure or instrumentation used, pupillary block, and the duration of postoperative observation have been found to influence the likelihood of glaucoma after pediatric cataract surgery. It has been suggested that the immaturity of the developing infant's angle leads to increased susceptibility to secondary surgical trauma. Hence, some surgeons feel that it is prudent to consider delaying surgery until the infant is 4 weeks old in bilateral cases. Glaucoma can occur at any time after congenital cataract surgery. Therefore, patients who have undergone congenital cataract surgery should be monitored for glaucoma throughout their lives.

### Uveal Inflammation

Intense uveal inflammation or severe fibrinoid reaction is a concern particularly in infants and young children. In our opinion, a traumatic surgical technique and ciliary sulcus, or asymmetrical fixation of the IOL are other contributing factors, which may be responsible for producing an exaggerated inflammatory response.

### Other Complications

Retinal detachment and cystoid macular edema are infrequent after aphakia in pediatric cataract surgery. The reasons for this low incidence of postoperative retinal complications are not very well known.

## NEWER APPROACHES

Bag-in-the-lens implantation: Tassignon et al. reported the outcome of a surgical procedure they called 'bag-in-the-lens' in pediatric cataractous eyes. In this technique, the anterior and posterior capsules are placed in the groove of a specially designed IOL after a capsulorhexis of the same size is created in both capsules. The principle behind this IOL design is to ensure a clear visual axis by mechanically tucking the two capsules into the IOL, thereby preventing any migration of proliferating lens epithelial cells. For more information on this technique, please refer to Dr Tassignon's Chapter: How to successfully perform the bag in the lens technique in cataract surgery.

Posterior capsulorhexis combined with optic buttonholing: Recently R. Menapace introduced posterior optic buttonholing a safe and effective technique, which not only excludes retro-optical opacification, but also withholds capsular fibrosis by obviating direct contact between the anterior capsular leaf and the optic surface.[35]

## SUMMARY

Although dramatic advances have occurred in this field over the past 10 years, some technical aspects of surgery, changing refraction, and functional outcome continue to pose significant problems. Primary management of the posterior capsule is mandatory depending on the age of the child at surgery. With refinements in surgical techniques, improvisation of IOLs and better understanding of growth of the pediatric eye, in the coming years, IOL implantation is likely to become an established mode of treatment of children even in the youngest age group.

## REFERENCES


1. Foster A, Gilbert C, Rahi J. Epidemiology of cataract in childhood: a global perspective. J Cataract Refract Surg. 1997;23:601-4.
2. Cetin E, Yaman A, Berk A. Etiology of childhood blindness in Izmir, Turkey. Eur J Ophthalmol. 2004;14:531-7.
3. Thakur J, Reddy H, Wilson ME, Jr, et al. Pediatric cataract surgery in Nepal. J Cataract Refract Surg. 2004;30:1629-35.
4. Rahi JS, Dezateaux C, British Congenital Cataract Interest Group. Measuring and interpreting the incidence of congenital ocular anomalies: lessons from a national study of congenital cataract in the UK. Invest Ophthalmol Vis Sci. 2001;42(7):1444-8.
5. Dahan E. Intraocular lens implantation in children. Curr Opin Ophthalmol. 2000;11(1):51-5. Review
6. Nihalani BR, VanderVeen DK. Comparison of intraocular lens power calculation formulae in pediatric eyes. Ophthalmology. 2010;117(8):1493-9.
7. Kekunnaya R, Gupta A, Sachdeva V, et al. Accuracy of intraocular lens power calculation formulae in children less than two years. Am J Ophthalmol. 2012;154(1):13-19.
8. Wilson ME. Anterior capsule management for pediatric intraocular lens implantation. J Pediatr Ophthalmol Strabismus. 1999;36:314-9.
9. Wilson ME, Jr. Anterior lens capsule management in pediatric cataract surgery. Trans Am Ophthalmol Soc. 2004;102:391-422.
10. Guo S, Wagner RS, Caputo A. Management of the anterior and posterior lens capsules and vitreous in pediatric cataract surgery. J Pediatr Ophthalmol Strabismus. 2004;41:330-7.
11. Singh D. Use of the Fugo blade in complicated cases. J Cataract Refract Surg. 2002;28(4):573-4.
12. Wilson ME, Jr, Bartholomew LR, Trivedi RH. Pediatric cataract surgery and intraocular lens implantation: practice styles and preferences of the 2001 ASCRS and AAPOS memberships. J Cataract Refract Surg. 2003;29(9):1811-20.
13. Mohammadpour M. Four-incision capsulorhexis in pediatric cataract surgery. J Cataract Refract Surg. 2007;33(7):1155-7.
14. Nischal KK. Two-incision push-pull capsulorhexis for pediatric cataract surgery. J Cataract Refract Surg. 2002;28(4):593-5.
15. Gimbel H. High viscosity viscoelastic eases pediatric cases. Ocular Surg News. 1992;10:16.
16. Pandey SK, Werner L, Escobar-Gomez M, et al. Dye enhanced cataract surgery. Part 1: anterior capsule staining for capsulorhexis in advanced/white cataracts. J Cataract Refract Surg. 2000;26:1052-9.
17. Saini JS, Jain AK, Sukhija J, et al. Anterior and posterior capsulorhexis in pediatric cataract surgery with or without trypan blue dye: randomized prospective clinical study. J Cataract Refract Surg. 2003;29:1733-7.
18. Brown SM, Graham WA, McCartney DL, et al. Trypan blue in pediatric cataract surgery. J Cataract Refract Surg. 2004;30:2033.

19. Vasavada AR, Trivedi RH, Apple DJ, et al. Randomized, clinical trial of multiquadrant hydrodissection in pediatric cataract surgery. Am J Ophthalmol. 2003;135(1):84-8.
20. Parks MM. Posterior lens capsulectomy during primary cataract surgery in children. Ophthalmology. 1983;90:344-5.
21. Knight-Nanan D, O' Keefe M, Bowell R. Outcomes and complications of intraocular lenses in children with cataract. J Cataract Refract Surg. 1996;22:730-6.
22. BenEzra D, Cohen E. Posterior capsulectomy in pediatric cataract surgery; the necessity of a choice. Ophthalmology. 1997;104:2168-74.
23. Vasavada AR, Praveen MR, Tassignon MJ, et al. Posterior capsule management in congenital cataract surgery. J Cataract Refract Surg. 2011;37(1):173-93.
24. Praveen MR, Vasavada AR, Koul A, et al. Subtle signs of anterior vitreous face disturbance during posterior capsulorhexis in pediatric cataract surgery. J Cataract Refract Surg. 2008;34(1):163-7.
25. Vasavada AR, Shah SK, Praveen MR, et al. Pars plicata posterior continuous curvilinear capsulorhexis. J Cataract Refract Surg. 2011;37(2):221-3.
26. Vasavada A, Desai J. Primary posterior capsulorhexis with or without anterior vitrectomy in congenital cataract. J Cataract Refract Surg. 1997;23:645-51.
27. Shah SK, Vasavada V, Praveen MR, et al. Triamcinolone-assisted vitrectomy in pediatric cataract surgery. J Cataract Refract Surg. 2009;35(2):230-2.
28. Vasavada AR, Nath VC, Trivedi RH. Anterior vitreous face behaviour with AcrySof in pediatric cataract surgery. J AAPOS. 2003;7:384-8.
29. Vasavada AR, Trivedi RH, Nath VC. Visual axis opacification after AcrySof intraocular lens implantation in children. J Cataract Refract Surg. 2004;30:1073-81.
30. Basti S, Ravishankar U, Gupta S. Results of a prospective evaluation of three methods of management of pediatric cataracts. Ophthalmology. 1996;103:713-20.
31. Wilson ME. Intraocular lens implantation: has it become the standard of care for children? Ophthalmology. 1996;103:1719-20.
32. Wilson ME, Jr, Trivedi RH, Buckley EG, et al. ASCRS white paper. Hydrophobic acrylic intraocular lenses in children. J Cataract Refract Surg. 2007;33(11):1966-73.
33. Mandal AK, Netland PA. Glaucoma in aphakia and pseudophakia after congenital cataract surgery. Indian J Ophthalmol. 2004;52:185-98.
34. Chen TC, Walton DS, Bhatia LS. Aphakic glaucoma after congenital cataract surgery. Arch Ophthalmol. 2004;122:1819-25.
35. Menapace R. Posterior capsulorhexis combined with optic buttonholing: an alternative to standard in-the-bag implantation of sharp-edged intraocular lenses? A critical analysis of 1000 consecutive cases. Graefes Arch Clin Exp Ophthalmol. 2008;246(6):787-801.

CHAPTER

14

# Phacoemulsification in Hard Cataracts

Aravind Haripriya, Rengaraj Venkatesh

## INTRODUCTION

Phacoemulsification is the surgery of choice for cataract extraction.[1] Nowadays, apart from immature cataracts, it is widely practiced for extraction of almost all kinds of cataractous lenses[2] including brown and white cataracts,[3] complicated cataracts, subluxated lenses,[4] and pediatric cataracts.[5] However, performing safe and successful phacoemulsification remains a challenge in brunescent cataracts (Fig. 14-1). Many would turn to extra capsular cataract surgery or manual small incision cataract surgery[6,7] to handle them. However, better phaco machines, phaco techniques, and OVDs (ophthalmic viscosurgical devices) available today makes it possible to have consistently good outcomes and clear cornea day post-op day 1. Most patients with a dense cataract present late for surgery as they do not notice a reduction in visual acuity, which hinders their routine activities. They might also not note the reduced contrast, which is gradually decreasing.

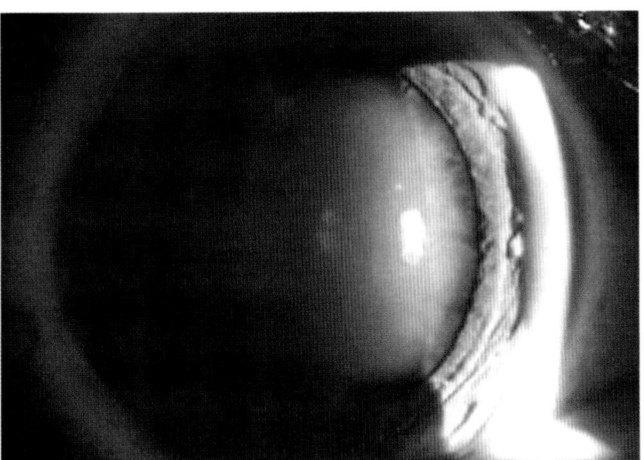

Figure 14-1 Dense brunescent cataract.

The lens consists of a central hard nucleus surrounded by the epinucleus cushion. With advancing age endonucleus volume increases with a corresponding decrease in epinucleus cushion. Use of the Lens Opacities Classification System III (LOCS III) cataract classification system[8] is recommended to grade the cataract.[9] Nuclear color, or the level of brown color, is the key feature relevant to phacoemulsification energy in this cataract grading system of 0.1 to 6.9 in increments of 0.1 unit.[9] The amount of energy required to emulsify increasingly hard lenses as graded on this linear scale is, in fact, exponential.

## CHALLENGES IN HANDLING BROWN CATARACTS

- None to poor red reflex makes capsulorhexis challenging.
- Despite a complete capsulorhexis, the margins are difficult to visualize during nuclear emulsification, which increases the risk of damaging the rhexis margin.
- Incisional burns, particularly with a clear corneal incision.
- The disassembly of a hard nucleus is very difficult because the nuclear fibers are strong and densely packed. Higher ultrasound energy, higher vacuum, and stronger forces for nuclear separation may be needed.
- As hard nuclear fragments do not mould well to the phaco tip, poor followability and greater chatter occur at the phaco tip. Excessive turbulence within the anterior chamber can lead to increased endothelial damage. Dense cataracts are more typically seen in older people who might also have fewer endothelial cells to begin and therefore as increased chance of postoperative stromal edema.
- Brown cataracts often have weak zonules, especially when the nucleus is very dense.

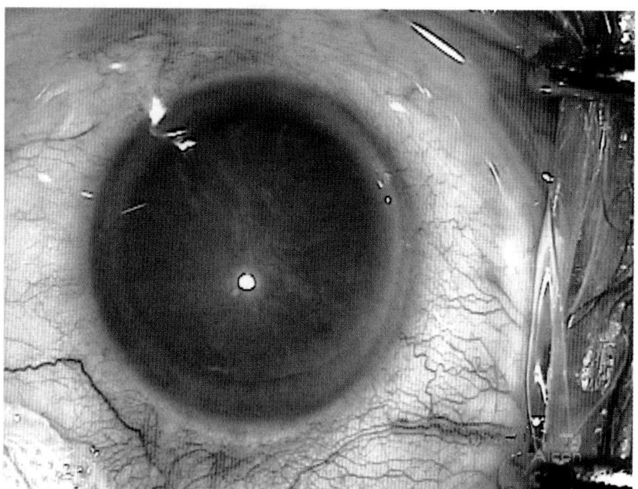

Figure 14-2 Brunescent cataract with minimal red reflex.

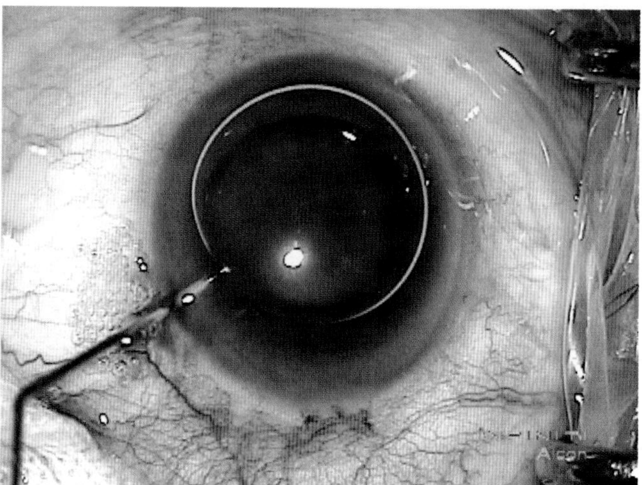

Figure 14-3 Injection of trypan blue dye under air.

- Higher chances of posterior capsule rupture – more endonucleus and less epinucleus cushion exist with brunescent cataracts. The phaco tip has to work closer to the posterior capsule, as a deep central trough is required to split the leathery posterior plate. Also with the thinner posterior capsule and absence of epinuclear bowl, the exposed posterior capsule tends to dome toward the phaco tip further increasing the risk of capsular rupture

## ANESTHESIA

Local anesthesia should be considered in eyes with brown cataracts as in case the patient is uncooperative, this may complicate an already difficult surgery. Moreover, the surgery time may be prolonged in which case the effect of topical anesthesia may wear out. Local anesthesia will allow the surgeon to enjoy a more comfortable and relaxed procedure.

## PREREQUISITES

A clear corneal tunnel is safe for phaco in brunescent cataracts but for someone who is just beginning to handle these cases, a scleral pocket incision is preferred. With the scleral pocket incision, the chance of wound burn is minimized and also permits extension of the tunnel in case the need to convert arises because of a posterior capsular tear.

The viscoelastic of choice is a dispersive viscoelastic with chondroitin sulfate, which coats the endothelium and reduces endothelial cell loss. The authors believe that using the right viscoelastic along with in the bag phaco goes a long way in achieving clear cornea postop day 1. The soft shell technique recommended by Steve Arshinoff[10] is invaluable in dealing with hard nuclei, which is a combination of dispersive and cohesive viscoelastic, the former for endothelial protection and the latter to create and retain space. The dispersive viscoelastic is injected first, followed by the cohesive such that the dispersive viscoelastic coats the endothelium. In eyes with shallow anterior chamber and hard nucleus, the soft shell is an invaluable technique.

Make a large capsulorhexis of about 5.5–6 mm, which will give more working space to trench, crack, and elevate the pieces to the pupillary plane for emulsification. This is easier to achieve in hard lenses as typically the capsule is thinner and well stretched around the large nucleus. A large capsulorhexis also reduces chances of capsular–lenticular block and unnecessary pressure on the posterior capsule. If one has to convert mid-way, the entire or remaining nucleus can be prolapsed out into the anterior chamber if the capsulorhexis is large. If the red reflex is poor, trypan blue dye (0.06%) is used to provide better contrast during capsulorhexis, hydrodissection, and phacoemulsification. The dye is typically injected beneath air to get uniform staining of the anterior capsule (Figs. 14-2 to 14-4).

Ensure adequate hydrodissection and nucleus mobility before commencing phaco so as to minimize zonular stress. To avoid capsular–lenticular block, hydrodissection should be terminated as soon as the solid nucleus elevates against the capsulorhexis. The temptation to continue injecting until the migrating fluid wave completely crosses behind the nucleus should be avoided. Instead, the center of the elevated nucleus is tapped to dislodge it posteriorly before resuming hydrodissection from the opposite quadrant. A right-angled hydrodissection cannula facilitates the latter step. Unlike soft cataracts, the adhesions between the capsule and nucleus are not very strong, and so nucleus mobility is achieved early.

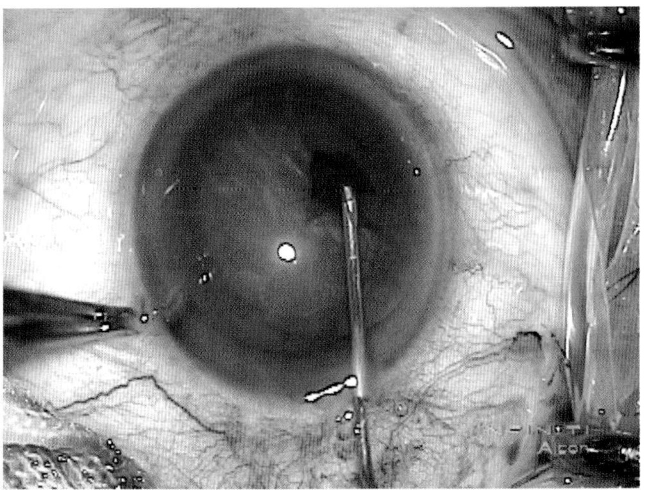

Figure 14-4 Good visualization of advancing edge of anterior capsule due to the stain.

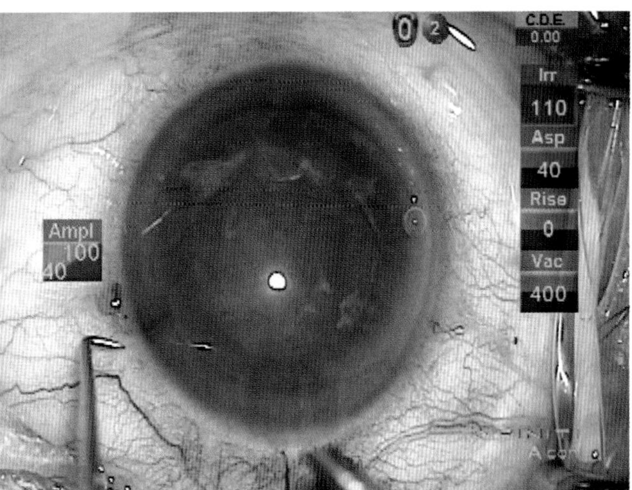


Figure 14-5 Use of a long chopper with a sharp pointed edge is preferred while handling brown cataracts.

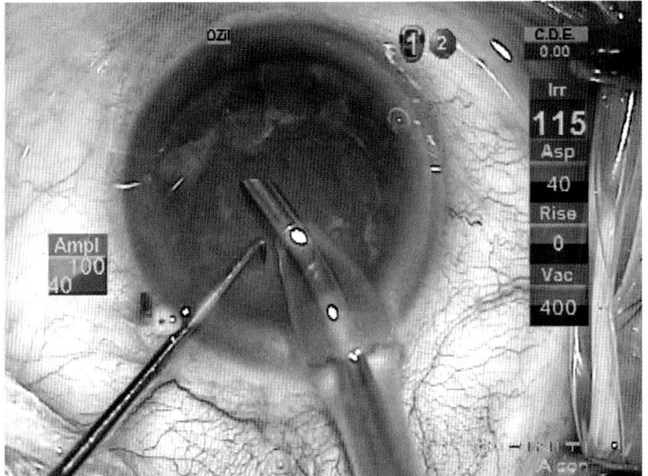


Figure 14-6 Sleeve is retracted such that about 2 mm of the tip is exposed.

## PHACOEMULSIFICATION OF A BROWN CATARACT

During phacoemulsification always attempt to have infusion on, except for brief seconds needed to inject viscoelastic so as to avoid fluctuation in intraocular pressure. If the surgery time is prolonged, viscoelastic is reintroduced periodically to ensure endothelial protection. If divide and conquer or stop and chop is the preferred technique, adequate power is to be used with low vacuum and flow rate so as to achieve a deep trench. Initial phaco sculpting should be very slow and shallow to ascertain the stability of the bag and zonules and density of nucleus. In the presence of a wobbly lens, a capsule tension ring with or without capsule retractors is useful to stabilize the bag prior to other maneuvers. Once the zonular integrity is ascertained, the trench is deepened following the curve of the posterior capsule. In many instances the surgery becomes difficult because of the insufficient depth rather than going too deep, so it is imperative to groove deep enough. To achieve a deep trench, the sleeve is retracted so that about 1.5 mm of the tip is exposed. A trench of two tip widths is created so that the sleeve can also be accommodated in the trench as it goes deep. Once the trench is deep enough, the posterior plate of the nucleus is cracked so as to achieve complete separation of the nucleus into two heminuclei. If the crack is incomplete in the center, it is important to trench further and then reattempt cracking. While removing the quadrants the vacuum and the flow rates are increased. Paused ultrasound such as the pulse mode reduces chatter thereby increasing followability. The pulse mode also helps conserve the amount of phaco energy used thus reducing the incidence of wound burn.

Although the divide and conquer can be successfully used to handle the brunescent cataract, the authors strongly believe that a phaco chop technique is better as the amount of phaco energy used is minimal and the pressure on the posterior capsule is lesser compared with the four quadrant technique. A vertical chop technique is preferred over the horizontal chop in hard cataracts. A long chopper (1.75–2 mm) with a sharp tip is recommended to pierce the dense nuclear fibers (Fig. 14-5). While dealing with hard cataracts, the sleeve is retracted such that about 2 mm of the phaco tip is exposed (Fig. 14-6). Cutting is enhanced with a 45° Kelman, 0.9-mm mini-flare tip in brunescent cataracts. It will also make a difference to use a new or sharp phaco tip to handle these cataracts. With the chop technique, the first challenge is to achieve a complete chop of the central leathery posterior plate, and the second is to release the first nuclear piece.

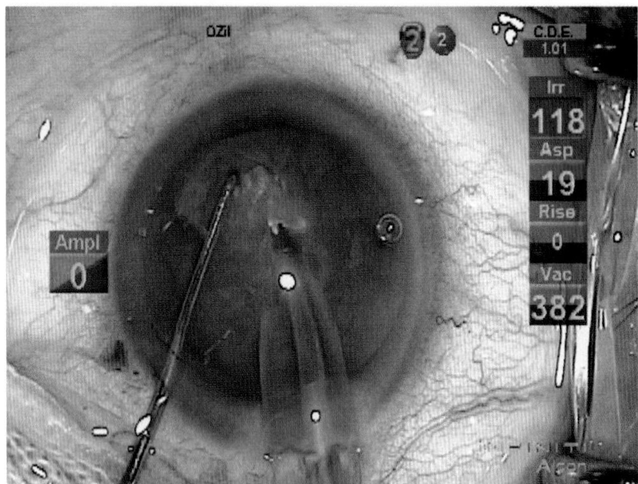


**Figure 14-7** Phaco tip is impaled deep in the nucleus at the pupillary center followed by the chopper, which is introduced about 2 mm away.

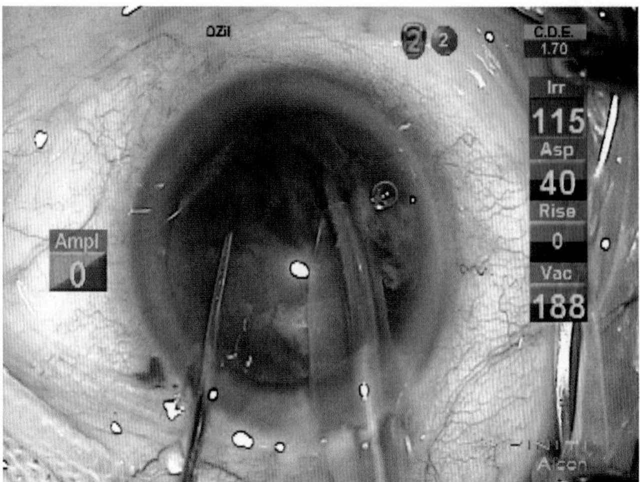


**Figure 14-8** Split of nucleus by lateral movement of phaco tip and chopper.

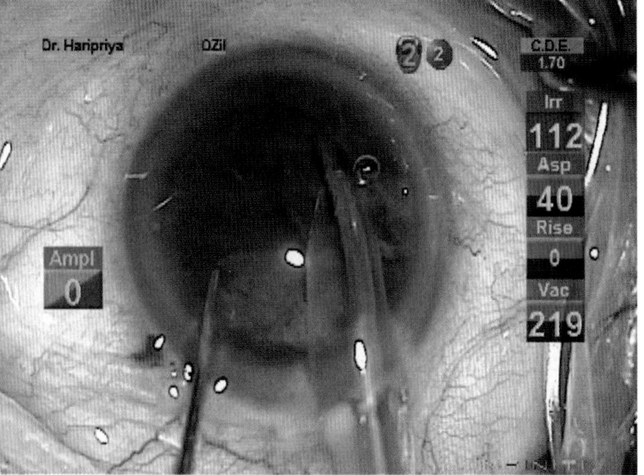


**Figure 14-9** Complete split of posterior plate of nucleus at the center.

Nucleus disassembly involves creating an initial short burrow at the center of the nucleus followed by impaling the tip deep in the nucleus until the tip completely occluded. To achieve a complete crack the tip has to be impaled on the lower third of the central nucleus, ensuring complete occlusion. The initial half trench and retracted sleeve help in getting a deep hold on the nucleus. If longitudinal ultrasound is used, the burst mode is recommended to get a good hold on the nucleus during the chop. While the nucleus is stabilized with the phaco tip, the chopper is placed just inside edge of the capsulorhexis and introduced diagonally deep into the nucleus toward the phaco tip (Fig. 14-7). Continuing to use vacuum, the tip and chopper are then moved laterally so as to achieve a complete crack. The important aspects to achieve the primary chop include deep hold on central nucleus with the phaco tip, maintaining vacuum (foot pedal control), placement of the chopper deep into the nucleus and maximum lateral separation of the nucleus with the tip and chopper (Figs. 14-8 and 14-9). If the crack is incomplete, the same maneuver is repeated by impaling deeper so that a complete crack is achieved. The nucleus is then rotated 180° and chop is completed. Each half is then split into 3–4 fragments before they are emulsified. Nucleus disassembly is safer when there is lateral support of the adjacent pieces, thus complete nucleus disassembly is done prior to emulsification of the fragments. Parameters the authors use for a 2.8-mm incision include 100% continuous torsional ultrasound, 40-mL/min flow rate, 400-mm Hg vacuum, and 110-cm bottle height. With a 2.2-mm incision, the flow rate and vacuum are marginally decreased by about 10% to match the smaller sleeve used here. During nucleus disassembly, the torsional ultrasound can be used on panel mode as this ensures a good hold on the nucleus.

Once the pieces are separated, one can switch to linear mode so that there is more control during fragment emulsification. The pieces have to be as small as possible as this minimizes chatter and endothelial damage. In case of a large fragment the pieces are subdivided into smaller pieces. The fragment is elevated by holding the side of the pie with the 45° tip so that there is better holdability (Fig. 14-10). During fragment emulsification the bevel of phaco tip should be at or below the pupillary plane and face sideways so that there is less chance of endothelial damage and at the same time there is good visibility. The vacuum and flow rate are set such that there is maximum followability but negligible surge. The optimum setting would be based on surgeon's preference and phaco machine. While removing the last piece, the chance

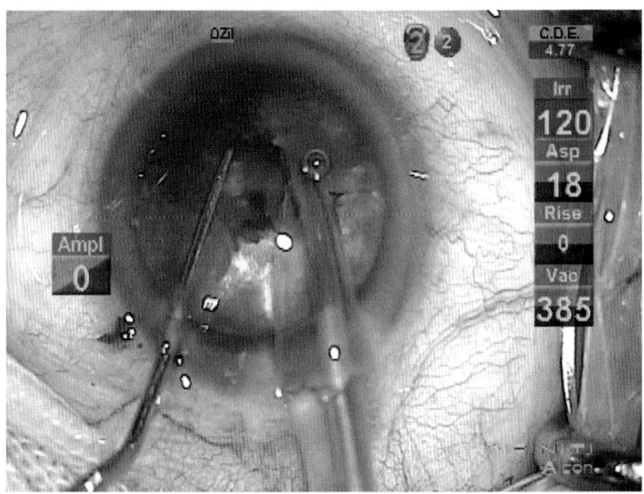


**Figure 14.10** Elevation of the nuclear fragment from the capsular bag by holding the piece from the side.

of posterior capsular rupture is higher as the epinuclear cushion is either very thin or absent. Hence, the flow and the vacuum parameters have to be lowered so that there is better chamber stability and less chance for the posterior capsule to trampoline toward the phaco tip. Keep the phaco times short once the phaco tip is occluded to ensure adequate flow into the eye at all times and prevent build-up. While converting from the four quadrants to the chop technique, it is advisable to first adopt the stop and chop technique. The initial trench created gives adequate space within the capsular bag for manipulation and then the rest of the nucleus is chopped and emulsified.

Typically, the epinucleus and central cortex are absent in hard cataracts. The posterior capsule here may be more friable so ensure the peripheral cortex is removed by holding the anterior leaflet of the cortex.

On the basis of the intraop comfort and postop corneal clarity, we can modify the parameters so as to target clear cornea postop day 1. Postoperative corneal stromal edema indicates an anterior plane of emulsification and probable turbulence in the anterior chamber. It is possible to get a consistently clear cornea even with dense brunescent cataracts if one is meticulous with the technique.

In conclusion, by observing a few precautions as mentioned above, the management of a dense nucleus can be almost routine and very satisfying for both the patient and the surgeon.

## REFERENCES

1. Emery JM. Phakoemulsification–cataract surgery of the future? Int Ophthalmol Clin. 1978;18(2):155-70.
2. Vasavada A, Singh R. Surgical techniques for difficult cataracts. Curr Opin Ophthalmol. 1999;10(1):46-52.
3. Hiles DA. Phacoemulsification of infantile cataracts. Int Ophthalmol Clin. 1977;17(4):83-102.
4. Vajpayee RB, Bansal A, Sharma N, et al. Phacoemulsification of white hypermature cataract. J Cataract Refract Surg. 1999; 25(8):1157-60.
5. Morley MG. Pars plana lensectomy for primary extraction and removal of lens fragments. In: Steinert RF (ed.), Cataract surgery: technique, complications, & management. Philadelphia, PA: WE Saunders, 1995:192-8.
6. Venkatesh R, Tan CS, Singh GP, et al. Safety and efficacy of manual small incision cataract surgery for brunescent and black cataracts. Eye. 2009;23:1155-7.
7. Gonglore B, Smith R. Extracapsular cataract extraction to phacoemulsification: why and how? Eye (Lond). 1998;12 (Pt 6): 976-82.
8. Chylack LT, Jr, Wolfe JK, Singer DM, et al. The Lens Opacities Classification System III. The Longitudinal Study of Cataract Study Group. Arch Ophthalmol. 1993;111(6):831-6.
9. Davison JA. Phacoemulsification of hard cataract. In: Buratto L (ed.), Phacoemulsification principles and techniques, 2nd edn. Thorofare, NJ: Slack Inc, 2003:551-3.
10. Arshinoff SA. Dispersive-cohesive viscoelastic soft shell technique. J Cataract Refract Surg. 1999;25(2):167-73.

CHAPTER

# 15

# How to Successfully Perform the Bag-in-the-Lens Technique in Cataract Surgery?

Marie-José Tassignon, Sorcha Ní Dhubhghaill

## INTRODUCTION

One of the most commonly encountered postoperative cataract complications is posterior capsular opacification (PCO). Developments in intraocular lens (IOL) design have emphasized lens shape and composition, although none of these lens developments have been shown to prevent PCO completely.[1] Even the most optimized lens-in-the-bag technique appears to delay PCO development rather than completely prevent it.[2] It is, therefore, clear that while lens epithelial cells (LEC) can proliferate and transform behind the IOL, there is still a risk of PCO. The bag-in-the-lens (BIL) technique is a unique approach to lens placement and positioning in cataract surgery.[3] Unlike the standard lens-in-the-bag techniques, the BIL implant is kept in place by the formation of equally sized anterior and posterior capsulorhexes. The design of the lens implant allows it to be tightly fitted into the blades of the anterior and posterior rhexes, which support its weight entirely (Figs. 15-1A to D). This positioning confers stability and a high degree of predictability.[4,5] The IOL itself is designed to form a barrier to LEC growth and reduces the chance of the development of PCO to 0% when correctly sited.

In the past, PCO was considered an inevitable, albeit relatively minor complication of cataract surgery. As technology has improved, the optical qualities of the lens implants have similarly developed. Complex optics such as multifocal IOLs confer additional refractive benefits; however, they depend heavily upon a clear optical medium and accurate implant placement. Subsequent PCO development can distort the centration and function of the advanced optical qualities, such as diffractive rings, rendering lenses suboptimal, and, in some cases, intolerable. The BIL implant provides a solution to PCO that may be the optimal platform for complex lens optics.

## GENERAL INDICATIONS

The BIL cataract surgery approach is indicated and appropriate in all cases where a standard cataract surgery is considered. Situations where there is a high risk of PCO or visual axis reopacification are particularly suited to the BIL approach, i.e.

- Congenital cataract
- Pediatric cataract
- Uveitis associated Cataract
- Diabetic cataract

## SPECIAL INDICATIONS

The only absolute contraindications to BIL surgery are cases where there is no capsular material in which to implant the lens. Research is currently ongoing into the development of an artificial capsule. In addition, there are particular cases that require special consideration and additional equipment.

- High myopia is a consideration (> 26-mm axial length)
- Weak zonnular suspension
- Complicated phacoemulsification, inadvertent posterior capsular (PC) rupture, dropped nucleus

Some cases may require the insertion of a CTR to support the suspension of the lens.

## SURGICAL TECHNIQUE

The BIL surgery is performed with the surgical incision in the temporal position. The limbus incision is made with a 2.8-mm keratome. One milliliter of the Adrenaline/Xylocaine solution, described below, is injected into the anterior chamber followed by the viscoelastic. We recommend the use of Healon GV for this stage. The creation of an accurately sized anterior continuous curvilinear capsulorhexis (CCC) is

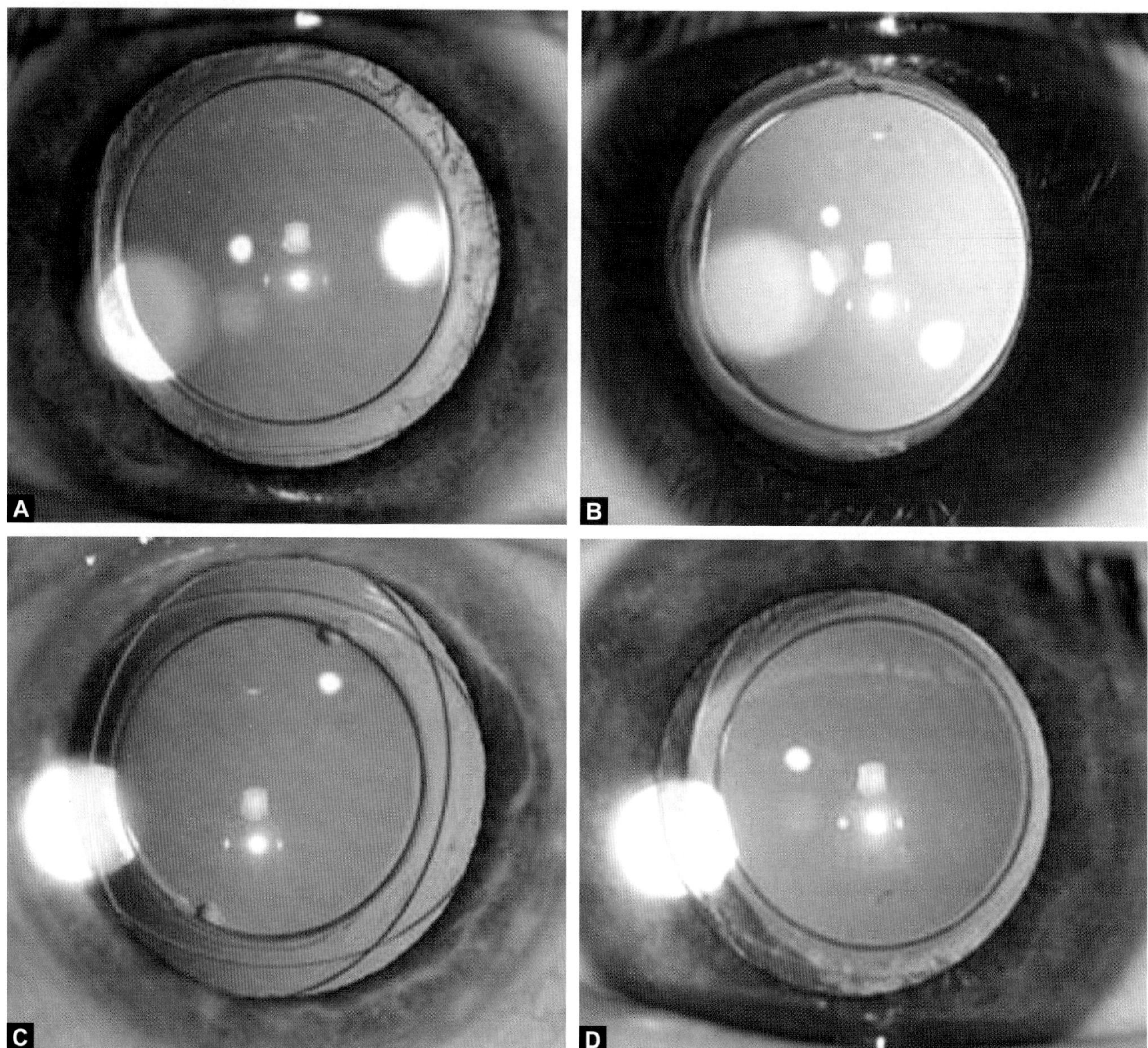

**Figures 15-1A to D** Image of lenses in position in (A) an adult case, (B) a pediatric case, (C) an astigmatic patient with a toric correction, (D) 10-year follow-up case.

a crucial step in the procedure. This is greatly assisted by the use of a 5-mm ring-shaped caliper (Type 4L Morcher), which is used as a guide (Fig. 15-2).[6] The ring caliper is positioned on the surface of the anterior capsule, and the central alignment is confirmed with Purkinje light reflexes 1 and 4 augmented with the use of the Eye Cage alignment device (ECT100 Technop) (Fig.15-3).

Once the alignment and centration of the caliper is confirmed, the anterior rhexis is performed. Hydrodissection and phacoemulsification may then be performed based on the surgeon's preferred technique. Once the lens material and the residual cortex are removed, the capsule may be further cleaned with balanced salt solution using a Helsinki cannula (1273E Steriseal). The anterior chamber, in front of the anterior capsule, is then refilled with Healon GV. It is essential that the injected viscoelastic be confined to the area above the level of the anterior capsule. Filling the capsular bag separates the anterior and posterior capsules and greatly hinders the insertion of the BIL implant. The capsular bag should therefore NEVER be filled with viscoelastic, as this will greatly hinder the insertion of the capsular blades into the interhaptic groove (Fig. 15-4A).

The residual cortical fibers are gently aspirated manually with a syringe and Helsinki cannula. The vacuum has the

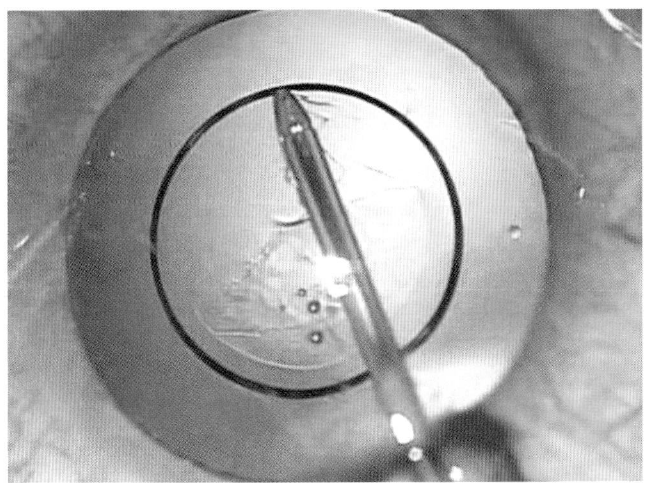
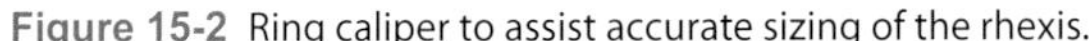

Figure 15-2 Ring caliper to assist accurate sizing of the rhexis.

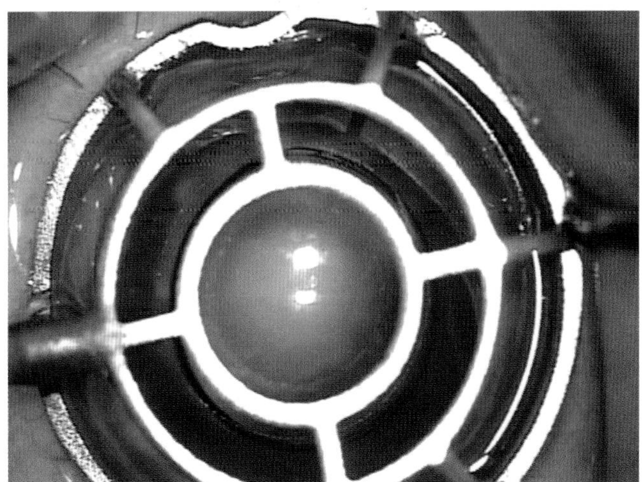

Figure 15-3 Eye cage device to center the caliper placement.

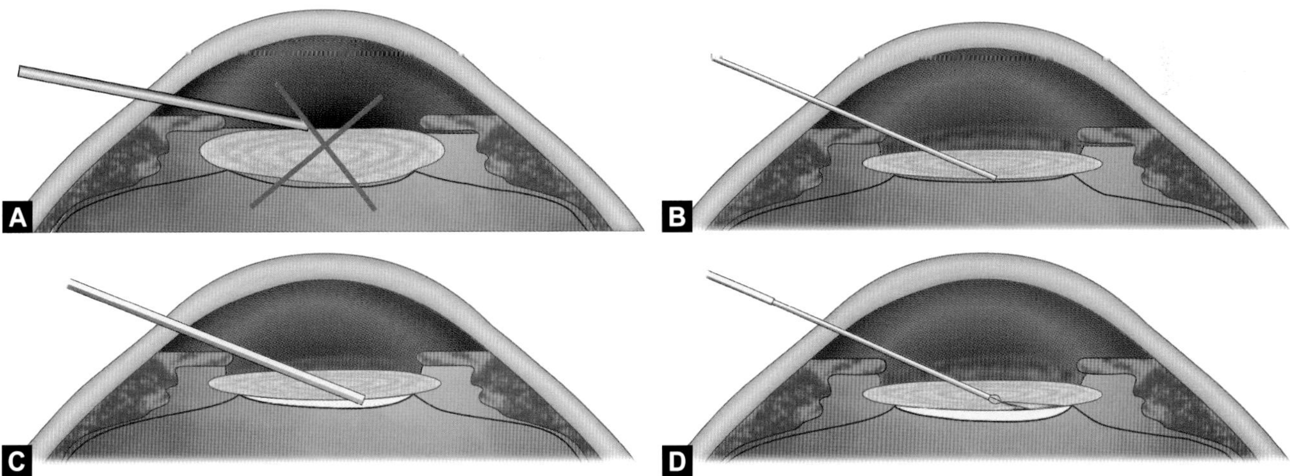


Figures 15-4A to D (A) Never fill the bag with viscoelastic; (B) Puncture made in the posterior rhexis; (C) Viscoelastic injected into the space of Berger; (D) Posterior rhexis is performed with microforceps.

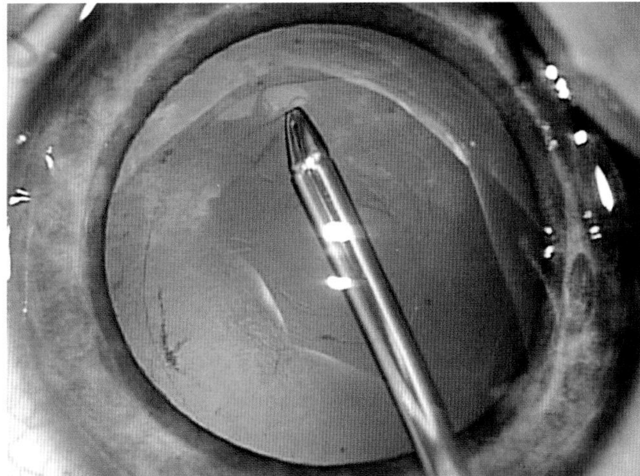

Figure 15-5 Image of performing posterior continuous curvilinear capsulorhexis.

additional effect of drawing the anterior capsular blades down to the posterior capsule, apposing them in preparation for the lens insertion. A primary posterior CCC (PPCCC) is then begun with a small incision into the posterior capsule with a tuberculin or a 30-ga needle (Fig. 15-4B). Healon ophthalmic viscosurgical device (OVD) is then injected through this small perforation and behind the capsule into the space of Berger (Fig. 15-4C). The OVD collects within the Berger's space, and injection should continue until a blister slightly larger than the anterior rhexis is formed.

The posterior rhexis is performed using an Ikeda forceps (Fr 2268 EyeTech) (Fig. 15-4D). The size of the PCCC is gauged using the view of the anterior rhexis as a guide (Fig. 15-5). The BIL is then folded into the cartridge and placed into the anterior chamber with an injector (MedicelLp 604410). The implant is maneuvered into a position on top

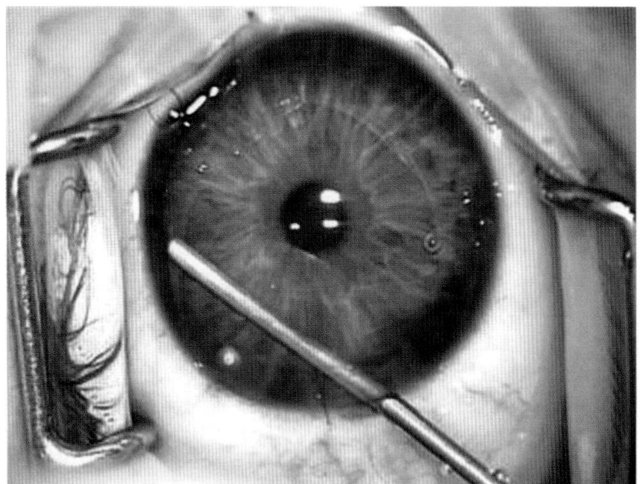

Figure 15-6 Peripheral iridectomy in a child at the 12 o'clock position.

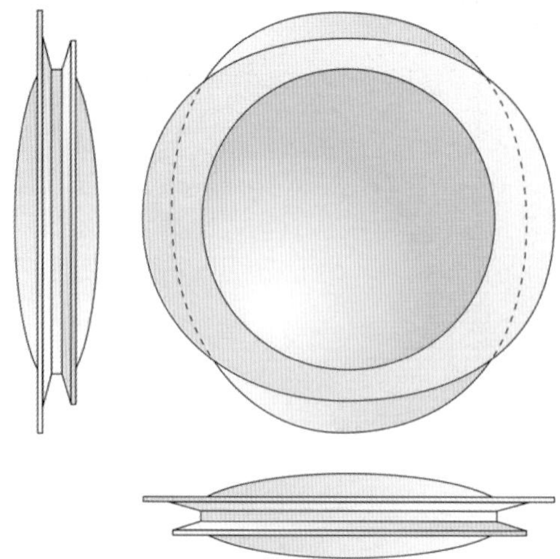

Figure 15-7 Structure and profile of the bag-in-the-lens intraocular implant.[18]

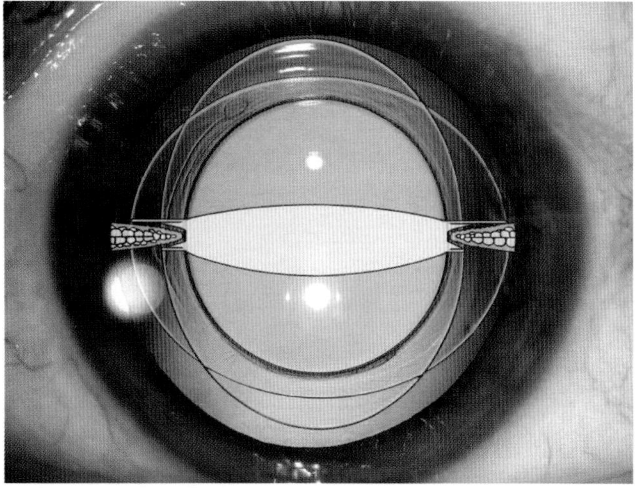

Figure 15-8 Centrally sited intraocular lens with side-on schematic view.

of the anterior capsule with the lens apposed to the rhexis edge at the 6 o'clock position. The lens may be stabilized with additional Healon and then manipulated temporally and nasally to engage both blades of the capsular bags. The edges will become engaged in the interhaptic groove as the posterior haptics slide under the posterior rhexis. The position and width of the anterior haptics prevent subluxation of the lens into posterior chamber. After the lens placement, the iris may be captured within the haptics of the implant. To prevent this, Miostat (carbachol/carbamylcholine) is injected into the anterior chamber to constrict the pupil, ensuring correct placement of the lens. The residual OVD is aspirated and the corneal wound is hydrated or sutured as standard. Routine intracameral cefuroxime is used at the end of each case based on best practice recommendations.[7]

The technique requires modification in cases of pediatric cataract.[8] The ring caliper used is 4.5 mm and two side ports of 1 mm are required for bimanual lens removal. The initial incision is performed as previously described, but the injection of Healon into the posterior capsule is performed with a 41-ga needle (Dorc 1270.0.100). One or both side ports are subsequently enlarged to 2.8 mm to accommodate the injection and positioning of the lens. Children are at a particular risk of iris capture and pupil block so routine intraoperative peripheral iridectomy is recommended (Fig. 15-6).

In patients with weak zonnular fibers a CTR should be placed after the irrigation and aspiration of cortex remnants. A bimanual technique is required to retract both capsules with ones hand and hold the lens in place with the other. A CTR is also recommended in myopic patients (axial lengths ≥ 26.0 mm) to stabilize the larger capsules in these patients. This is recommended because myopic patients are more prone to anterior vitreous schisis and have a very large space of Berger. Consequently, there is very little weak anterior vitreous support. The use of the CTR stabilizes the anterior vitreo–capsular interface facilitating the PPCCC and lens placement.

## MECHANISM OF ACTION

The BIL implant is a monofocal spherical hydrophilic lens, which is composed of a 5-mm biconvex optic with two elliptical flanged haptics (Fig. 15-7).[3] The plane haptics are sited at 90° to one another, with the posterior plate haptic positioned on the horizontal meridian and the anterior plate lies along the vertical meridian (Fig. 15-8). The plate haptics are

Table 15-1 Bag-in-the-lens implantation instruments

| Description | Comments | Ref. No. | Manufacturer |
|---|---|---|---|
| 'Bag-in-the-lens' foldable intraocular lens | 28% hydrophilic acrylic | 89A-D-E-F | Morcher |
| Ring caliper (4.5, 5.0, 6.0) | To caliper the position of the anterior capsulorhexis | Type 4L<br>Type 5 NO | Morcher |
| Tassignon caliper ring positioner | To position the ring caliper over the anterior capsule | sh-7017 | EyeTech |
| Ikeda angled 30° capsulorhexis 23.0 g forceps | To perform the anterior and posterior capsulorhexes | Fr 2268 | EyeTech |
| Straight scissors with curved shaft | To adjust capsulorhexis if needed | Fr 2295c | EyeTech |
| Naviject injector atraumatic/naviglide<br>–cartridge 2.5-IP injector set foldable<br>–cartridge 2.8-IP injector set foldable | <br>Up to +20.0 diopters<br>For all diopters | <br>Lp 604420<br>Lp 604410 | Medicel |
| Rycroft/Helsinki hydrodissection needle 27G | To inject dispersive viscoelastic behind the posterior capsule | 1273E | Steriseal |
| 41-ga Needle | As above but for pediatric surgery | E7370<br>1270.0.100 | Bausch & Lomb Dorc |
| Eye Cage alignment device | To center the caliper based on limbal centration and corneal Purkinje of the microscope light | ECT100 | Technop |
| Eye Cage alignment device | To center the caliper based on limbal centration and corneal Purkinje of the microscope light | ECT100 | Technop |

Table 15-2 Adrenaline/Xylocaine solution instructions

| | |
|---|---|
| Adrenaline/preservative-free Xylocaine solution components | 1 syringe 1.0 mL<br>1 aspiration needle (pink)<br>Adrenaline ampoule 1.0 mL (1:1000)<br>Xylocard ampoule |
| Procedure | Take 0.9-mL xylocard in a 1.0-mL syringe. Fill the additional 0.1 mL with 1:1000 solution of Adrenaline |

Table 15-3 Miostat solution instructions

| | |
|---|---|
| Miostat solution components | 1 syringe 2.0 mL<br>1 aspiration needle (pink)<br>Miostat ampoule (only contents are sterile)<br>Balanced salt solution 15.0 mL |
| Procedure | Take 0.5-mL Miostat in a 2.0-mL syringe. Add 1.5-mL balanced salt solution |

0.15-mm thick with an intervening groove of 0.25 mm. When the lens is correctly sited, the two blades of the anterior and capsular rhexes are tightly apposed in the groove, preventing the access of LECs into the posterior segment. The total diameter of the lens implant varies from 6.5 to 8.5 mm. When performed correctly, the crucial step of forming the PPCCC is a gentle technique, with little disturbance of the anterior vitreous face. We have reported the 1-year follow-up of 60 patients and no case experienced vitreous loss during the PPCCC.[9] The risks of accidental PC rupture include loss of vitreous, disturbance of the anterior hyaloid, and cystoid macular edema. Apprehension in performing a primary PPCCC may stem from a concern of inducing these or similar complications. The technique we describe here, with a particular emphasis on the preservation of the anterior hyaloid face, retains the diffusion properties across the vitreous and aqueous interface of an eye with an intact PC unlike accidental PC rupture.[10] In a long-term follow-up study of patients who underwent PPCCC, postoperative complications were no higher than the standard approach.[11]

## POSTOPERATIVE CARE

Patients do not require any specialized postoperative care. The postoperative cataract care includes overnight patching and 4 weeks of topical antibiotic and corticosteroid treatment. This is tapered off as standard. In patients with quiescent uveitis, no additional postoperative treatment regimen is needed unless the severity of the underlying uveitis merits special consideration.

## SPECIFIC INSTRUMENTATION

Additional instrumentation list for BIL technique (Table 15-1).

*Medication preparation*: Adrenaline/preservative-free Xylocaine solution preparation (Table 15-2).

Miostat solution (Table 15-3).

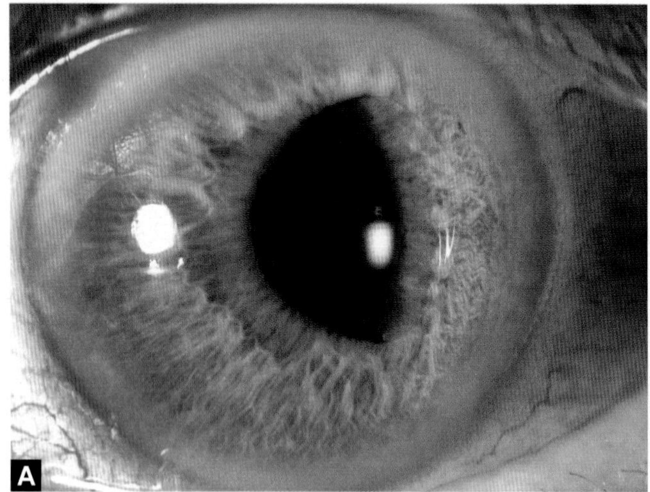


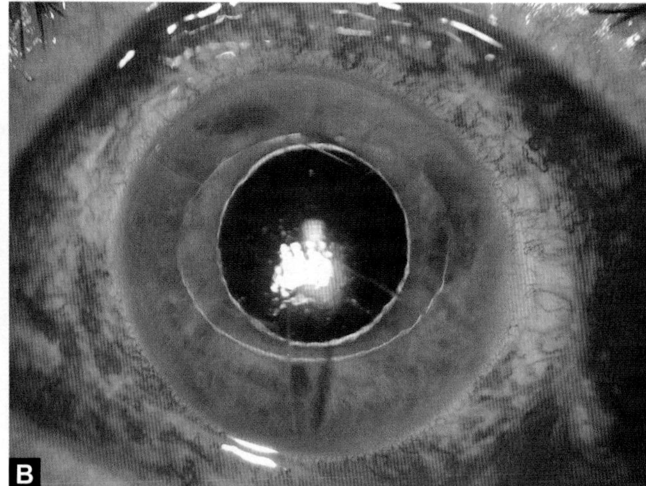


**Figures 15-9A and B** (A) Partial iris capture. (B) Total iris capture.

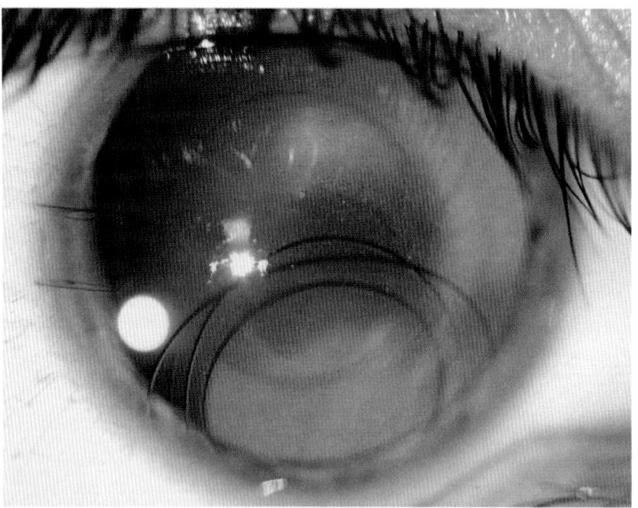

**Figure 15-10** Post-traumatic anterior bag-in-the-lens dislocation.

## COMPLICATIONS

We recently reported the largest cohort of BIL patient outcomes.[12] In this series of 807 cases, there was a rate of retinal detachment of 1.24% (10 eyes), hypopyon in 0.37% (three patients) and toxic anterior segment syndrome in one patient (0.12%). Cystoid macular edema occurred in one patient. A specific complication seen with the use of the BIL is iris capture, where the iris becomes engaged in the interhaptic groove either partially (18/807) or totally (1 case) (Figs. 15-9A and B). In total, this complication occurred in 2.35%.[12] In the acute phase, aggressive dilation can disengage the iris from the haptics. If the iris is unresponsive, surgery may be required to manually remove the iris from the groove. We have also documented two episodes of anterior lens subluxation (Fig. 15-10). In both cases, anterior subluxation was secondary to blunt trauma sustained after lens insertion. Patients were treated by surgically repositioning the lens back into the original rhexis, with a subsequent improvementin vision.

## SURGICAL OUTCOMES: SCIENTIFIC EVIDENCE

Microscopic investigation of the capsular bags has illustrated some fundamental differences between the BIL and standard lens-in-the-bag techniques. An in vitro model of the posterior capsule indicated significant transformation of LECs in culture without a lens (Fig. 15-11A). The standard lens-in-the-bag implant position also resulted in proliferation and shrinkage of the bag (Fig. 15-11B). In contrast, the BIL showed proliferation but not transformation of the LECs with no occlusion of the visual axis (Fig. 15-11C).[13] Even after 6-week culture, the LECs did not proliferate over the anterior or posterior surface of the IOL.[14] Similarly, there was no evidence of LEC proliferation behind lens implant in the rabbit animal model.[15] Analysis of the first postmortem eye with a BIL implant showed that when the lens is in place, the proliferating LECs are confined in the space between the anterior and posterior capsules, sealed by means of a fibrotic plug within the interhaptic groove.[16] Further examples confirm the presence of LEC proliferation in the periphery confined by the lens groove forming the fibrotic part of a Soemmering's ring.[17] At no stage did the LECs gain access to the posterior segment, retaining a clear visual axis in all experimental and histological assessments.

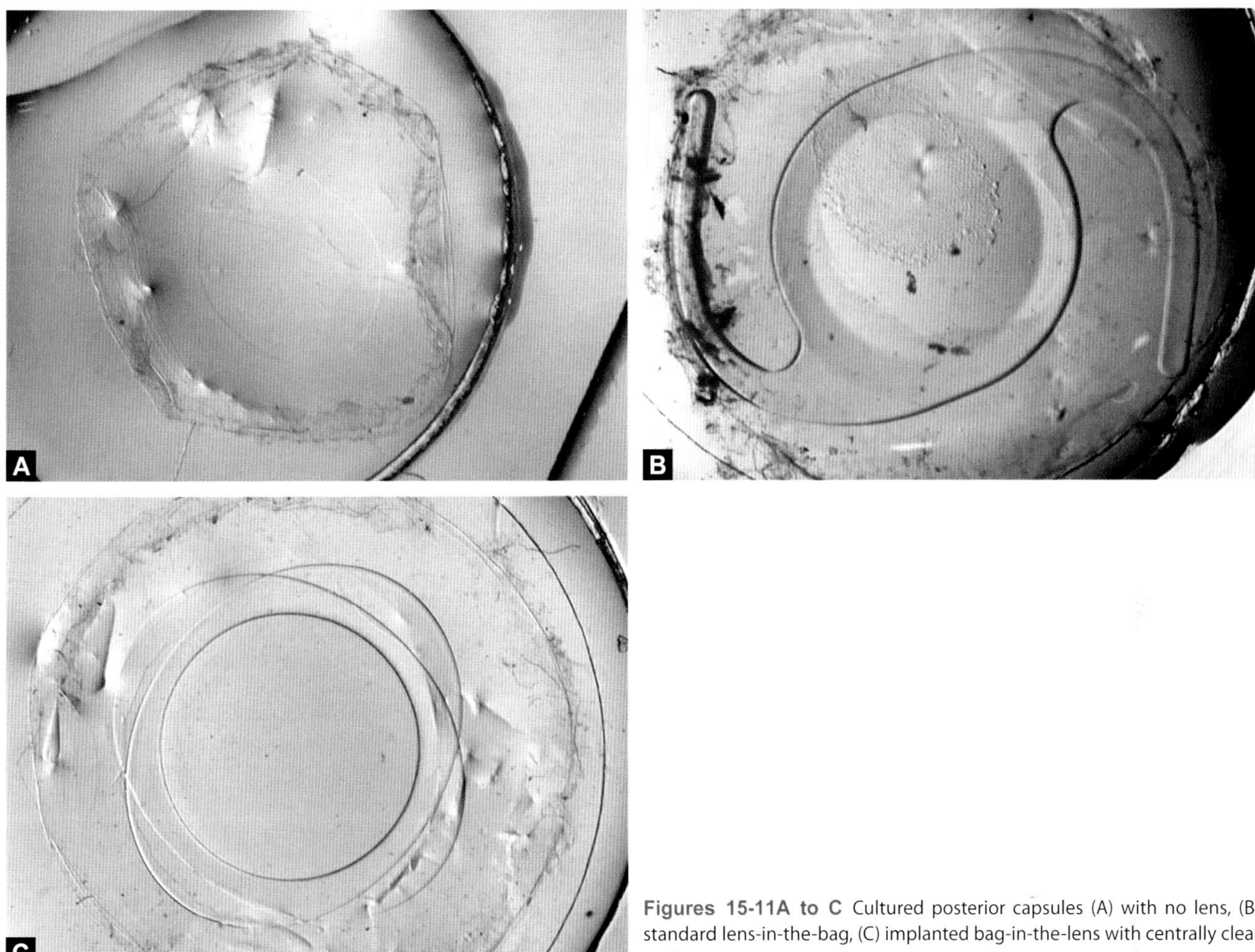


**Figures 15-11A to C** Cultured posterior capsules (A) with no lens, (B) standard lens-in-the-bag, (C) implanted bag-in-the-lens with centrally clear optic.

## PLACE OF THE TECHNIQUE IN SURGICAL ARMAMENTARIUM

As previously mentioned, the BIL cataract surgical approach may be adopted as a primary means of treating all patients with cataract provided some degree of capsule is available. With the correct precautions, the surgery may be used in more difficult cases such as myopic eyes, uveitis, weak zonules, post-trauma, and diabetic retinopathy.

## PEARLS AND PITFALLS

### How can You Stabilize the Ring Caliper?

In the BIL technique, the balance in pressure between the anterior and posterior segment is crucial. When the ring caliper is placed over the anterior capsule, increased anterior chamber pressure stabilizes the position. This is achieved by the use of OVD and we recommend Healon (GV) (AMO, Abbott Medical Optics). Reflux of OVD through the main incision indicates complete filling of the anterior chamber.

### Why Don't We Fill the Capsular Bag with OVD?

Prior to performing the PPCCC, the anterior chamber is filled with OVD though great care must be taken not to allow this into the capsular bag itself. Filling the bag pushes the posterior capsule back and closer to the anterior hyaloid. The capsule then takes a concave shape compared with the previous horizontal position. In the case of low pressure in the anterior chamber, the capsule adopts a slightly convex shape and the vitreous moves forward increasing the likelihood of vitreous prolapsing into the anterior chamber. Both convex and concave positions make the PPCCC more unpredictable and prone to tearing. To prevent this, we recommend some precautions. After the lens material has been removed, the anterior chamber is refilled by injecting the OVD to the periphery over the anterior capsulorhexis. Keep both anterior and posterior capsules in close apposition. Puncture the posterior capsule in the middle and use a microforceps to perform the PPCCC.

## How do You Implant the Lens?

The lens in injected into the anterior chamber. Using the OVD cannula, the lens can be moved to position the posterior haptics horizontally. Injecting OVD over the lens pushes it back onto the surface of the anterior capsule. The OVD cannula can then be used to push the optic to the right and slide the left haptic under the margin of the posterior capsulorhexis on the left side. The right haptic is then inserted by sliding the optic to the left and pushing the optic under the rhexis. Both capsulorhexis blades will automatically glide into the lens groove.

## What is the Tolerance for Anterior and Posterior Rhexis Size?

Tolerance is greater in adults than in children or babies. In adults, at least one of the two rhexis openings must intact and correctly sized between 4.5 and 5.0 mm, so even if one rhexis was made too large, the BIL may still be used. No LEC proliferation will occur over the visual axis. In children, however, the proliferative potential is much higher and so both capsules should be correctly sized and sited. Too small a rhexis may require additional pressure and manipulation, which may stress the zonnular fibers.

## How is the BIL Removed?

Uniquely, the BIL may be easily removed at any time after the initial surgery. This is of a particular advantage in children where refraction might change over time. To remove the lens, the anterior chamber is first filled with viscoelastic to control the anterior and posterior chamber pressures. The blunt viscoelastic cannula can be used to push one of the posterior haptics down to disengage the capsules from the interhaptic groove. The needle is then placed behind the lens, and viscoelastic is injected to push the anterior vitreous face back. The BIL is then luxed into the anterior chamber and freed from the rest of the capsular support. The lens may then be cut and removed as any other BIL.

## REFERENCES

1. Findl O, Buehl W, Bauer P, et al. Intervention for preventing posterior capsule opacification. Cochrane Database Syst Rev. 2010;17(2):doi: 10.1002/14651858.CD003738.pub3.
2. Spalton D. Posterior capsule opacification: have we made a difference? Br J Ophthalmol. 2013;97(1):1-2.
3. Tassignon MJ, DeGroot V, Vrensen GF. Bag-in-the-lens implantation of intraocular lenses. J Cataract Refract Surg. 2002;28(7):1182-8.
4. Verbruggen KHM, Rozema J, Gobin L, et al. Intraocular lens centration and visual outcomes after bag-in-the-lens implantation. J Cataract Refract Surg. 2007;33(7):1267-72.
5. Rozema JJ, Gobin L, Verbruggen K, et al. Changes in rotation after implantation of a bag-in-the-lens intraocular lens. J Cataract Refract Surg. 2009;35(8):1385-8.
6. Tassignon MJ, Rozema JJ, Gobin L. Ring-shaped caliper for better anterior capsulorhexis sizing and centration. J Cataract Refract Surg. 2006;32(8):1253-5.
7. Endophthalmitis Study Group, European Society of Cataract & Refractive Surgeon. Prophylaxis of postoperative endophthalmitis following cataract surgery: results of the ESCRS multicentre study and identification of risk factors. J Cataract Refract Surg. 2007;33(6):978-88.
8. Tassignon MJ, De Veuster I, Godts D, et al. Bag-in-the-lens intraocular lens implantation in the pediatric eye. J Cataract Refract Surg. 2007;33(4):611-7.
9. DeGroot V, Leysen I, Neuhann T, et al. One-year follow-up of bag-in-the-lens intraocular lens implantation in 60 eyes. J Cataract Refract Surg. 2006;32(10):1632-7.
10. DeGroot V, Hubert M, VanBest JA, et al. Lack of fluorophotometric evidence of aqueous-vitreous barrier disruption after posterior capsulorhexis. J Cataract Refract Surg. 2003;29(12): 2330-8.
11. Galand A, van Cauwenberge F, Moosavi J. Posterior capsulorhexis in adult eyes with intact and clear capsules. J Cataract Refract Surg. 1996;22(4):458-61.
12. Tassignon MJ, Goblin L, Mathysen D, et al. Clinical outcomes of cataract surgery after the bag-in-the-lens intraocular lens implantation following ISO standard 11979-7:2006. J Cataract Refract Surg. 2011;37(12):2120-9.
13. De Keyzer K, Leysen I, Timmermans JP, et al. Lens epithelial cells in an in vitro capsular bag model: lens-in-the-bag versus bag-in-the-lens technique. J Cataract Refract Surg. 2008;34(4):687-95.
14. DeGroot V, Tassignon MJ, Vrensen GFJM. Effect of bag-in-the-lens implantation on posterior capsule opacification in human donor eyes and rabbit eyes. J Cataract Refract Surg. 2005;31(2):398-405.
15. DeGroot V, Tassignon MJ, Vrensen GF. Effect of bag-in-the-lens implantation on posterior capsule opacification in human donor eyes and rabbit eyes. J Cataract Refract Surg. 2005;31(2):398-405.
16. Werner L, Tassignon MJ, Gobin L, et al. Bag-in-the-lens: first pathological analysis of a human eye obtained postmortem. J Cataract Refract Surg. 2008;34(12):2163-5.
17. Werner L, Tassignon MJ, Zaugg BE, et al. Clinical and histopathological evaluation of six human eyes implanted with the bag-in-the-lens. Ophthalmology. 2010;117(1):55-62.
18. Tassignon MJBR (inventor), Morcher GmbH (assignee). Intraocular lens and method for preventing secondary opacification. US patent 6 027 531. 2000. http://patftusptogov/netacgi/nph-Parser?Sect1=PTO1&Sect2=HITOFF&d=PALL&p=1&u=%2Fnetahtml%2FPTO%2Fsrchnumhtm&r=1&f=G&l=50&s1=6027531PN&OS=PN/6027531&RS=PN/6027531.

*Section* 3

# Corneal Surgery

*Section Editor* Walter E Beebe

CHAPTER

# 16

# Penetrating Keratoplasty

Lucy Eakle Franklin, Douglas I Katz, Woodford S Van Meter

## INTRODUCTION

Penetrating keratoplasty (PK) is a procedure in which full-thickness host corneal tissue is removed and replaced by donor corneal tissue. Zirm performed the first corneal transplant in 1905; it was the first solid tissue to be successfully transplanted in humans.[1] In 2012, nearly 60,000 corneal grafts performed in the United States with PK accounted for approximately 40% of these procedures (EBAA 2012 Statistical Report).[2]

With advances in surgical technique and corneal tissue preparation, the surgical options for management of corneal disease extend beyond PK. Surgeons have the capability to selectively remove and replace diseased endothelium with procedures such as Descemet's stripping automated endothelial keratoplasty or Descemet's membrane endothelial keratoplasty. The stroma and anterior cornea can be replaced with superficial anterior lamellar keratoplasty or deep anterior lamellar keratoplasty. However, full thickness PK remains an effective procedure for the treatment of corneal pathology involving all or multiple layers of the cornea, patients with failed grafts, and cases requiring extensive anterior segment reconstruction.

Traditional success rates for PK are above 90% when defined by the presence of a clear cornea. Statistics will vary depending on how "success" is defined. Success depends heavily on patient selection, quality of tissue, surgical technique, and adequate postoperative management.[3-4] In addition to a clear cornea, other measures of keratoplasty success include, cosmesis, decreased pain, restoration of an intact globe, and improved function and quality of life.

In the preoperative period, management of comorbid ocular and systemic conditions can help increase success rates. Complicating factors that adversely impact graft survival, include lid and ocular surface abnormalities, hypotony, elevated intraocular pressures, decreased corneal sensation, peripheral anterior synechiae, chemical burns, previous radiation, intraocular inflammation, presence of anterior chamber lens, and younger age. In addition, previous grafts, prior corneal procedures, deep stromal blood vessels, and ABO blood group incompatibility have been shown to confer a worse prognosis.[5]

## INDICATIONS

Penetrating keratoplasty is indicated for any stromal or endothelial corneal pathology; however, as mentioned previously, the most important factor for successful PK is proper patient selection. PK is indicated for patients with corneal pathology in whom improvement can be expected from the procedure. Typically, a combination of the reasons below comprises the indication for PK.[6]

- Optical indications include correction of vision. For example, patients with keratoconus may have a clear cornea yet vision that is uncorrectable with glasses. More commonly, patients with a central corneal opacity from infectious keratitis or trauma may require a PK to replace the central opacity with a clear cornea.
- Tectonic/reconstructive procedures involve restoration or improved structure of the cornea. (Thinning or perforation due to trauma and ulcers are common examples).
- Therapeutic indications involve treatment of corneal disease that diminishes the transparency of the cornea and

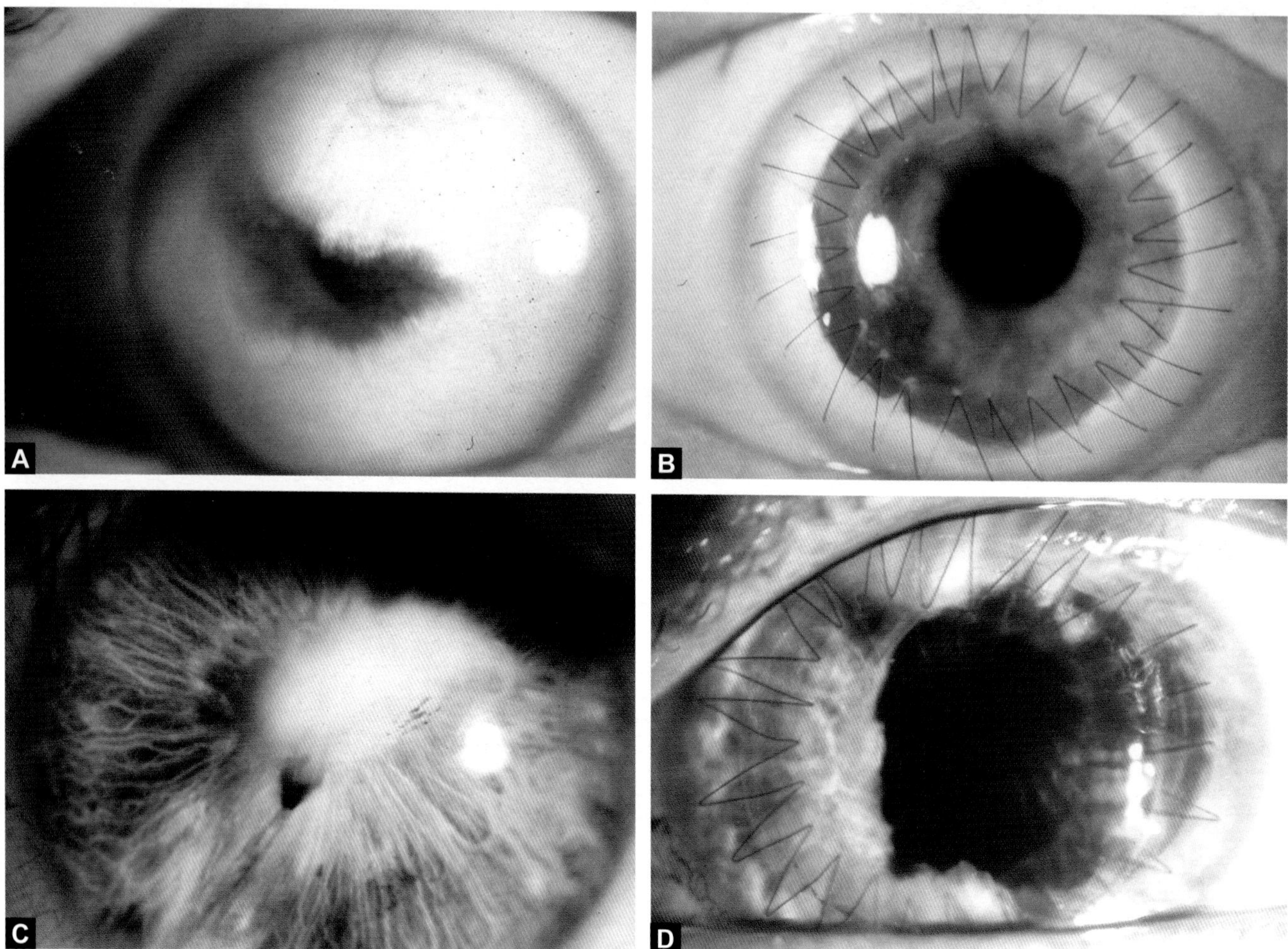


**Figures 16-1A to D** (A) Opaque cornea with lipid deposition involving the central cornea. (B) Clear penetrating keratoplasty graft—the same eye as shown in (A). (C) Central corneal scarring with underlying iris involvement. (D) Clear penetrating keratoplasty graft—the same eye as shown in (C). Note that iris adhesions were released intraoperatively.

comprises the most common indication for PK. Examples include: corneal dystrophies, degenerations, deposits, edema, scarring, and infections unresponsive to medical therapy (Figs. 16-1A to D).

Table 16-1 shows the different indications for penetrating keratoplasty, as reported in the 2013 Eye Bank Association of America Statistical Report.

## CONTRAINDICATIONS

Penetrating keratoplasty should generally be avoided in the following scenarios:

- Neurotrophic corneas
- Corneas with deep and/or extensive vascularization
- Corneas with active inflammation or infection
- Corneas with severe ocular surface disease.

## SPECIFIC INSTRUMENTATION

The choice of instruments used during PK largely depends on surgeon preference, with the goal of maximizing ease and efficiency during the operation. The following discussion will cover commonly used instruments.

### Speculum

The patient should be prepped and draped in a standard sterile fashion with draping placed to cover the lashes.[7-8] Different specula may be used depending on the draping procedure and the patients' anatomy. The lid speculum should not place pressure on the globe. A Barraquer wire speculum is often chosen due to its lightweight and relatively simple design, which avoids sutures getting snagged. There are several

TABLE 16-1 Indications

| Indications for Penetrating Keratoplasty | 2013 | |
|---|---|---|
| A. Post-cataract surgery edema | 3,398 | 9.2% |
| B. Keratoconus | 6,215 | 16.8% |
| C. Fuchs' Dystrophy | 1,229 | 3.3% |
| D. Repeat Corneal Transplant | 4,261 | 11.5% |
| E. Other degenerations or dystrophies | 1,822 | 4.9% |
| F. Post-refractive surgery | 121 | 0.3% |
| G. Microbial changes | 762 | 2.1% |
| H. Mechanical or chemical trauma | 1,127 | 3.0% |
| I. Congenital opacities | 685 | 1.9% |
| J. Pterygium | 14 | 0.0% |
| K. Non-infectious ulcerative keratitis or perforation | 1,080 | 2.9% |
| L. Other causes of corneal dysfunction or distortion (non-endothelial) | 3,162 | 8.5% |
| M. Other causes of endothelial dysfunction | 1,220 | 3.3% |
| Z. Unknown, unreported, or unspecified | 11,902 | 32.2% |
| **Total Penetrating Keratoplasty Procedures** | **36,998** | |

different lid speculums that are available all with different advantages and disadvantages that may be chosen based on the patient's lids, draping technique, or surgeon preference.

## Globe Supporting Rings

Globe supporting rings, such as a Flieringa ring or McNeill–Goldman blepharostat, can be used to help maintain the architecture of the globe.[9] Although not necessary in every case, they may be useful in patients with a previous vitrectomy, planned vitrectomy, patients undergoing combined cataract extraction with PK, and pediatric cases. Flieringa rings are available in numerous sizes; 17 mm or 18 mm are commonly used. Scleral fixation rings should be sized 3–4 mm larger than the limbus to permit suturing. The ring is sutured to the globe in all four quadrants with either 8-0 silk or 8-0 vicryl suture using partial thickness scleral bites. The sutures at 6 o'clock and 12 o'clock may be left long, secured to the drape, and used for globe positioning.

## Needle Holder

Blunt-tipped needle holders are typically used suturing with 7-0 or 8-0 sutures. A finer tipped needle holder is employed for placing stitches with 10-0 suture, such as securing the graft to the host bed.

## Forceps

Castroviejo forceps, with 0.3-mm tips, can be used for tasks, such as suturing globe supporting rings. The 0.12 mm forceps should be used when handling donor tissue to induce as little tissue damage as possible. Colibri 0.12-mm forceps have the advantage of allowing the surgeon to work from many different angles and can increase efficiency when also used as a tying platform. For passage of the initial suture securing the donor tissue to the host bed, many surgeons prefer to use double-fixation forceps as tissue slips easily at this point. An example is the Colibri-style Polack double corneal forceps.

## Scissors

Curved corneal scissors are transplant-specific instruments, which excise the corneal button from the host. The specific curvature of the blades precludes substitution of any other scissors for this task. Paired corneal scissors, which cut to the right and to the left, are designed to aid in tight wound construction. Other scissors that should be available during the procedure include Vannas scissors for cutting corneal sutures or tissues in the anterior chamber and Wescott or tenotomy scissors for cutting larger sutures, drapes, and conjunctival tissues.

## Instruments for Preparation of Host Cornea

The central host cornea can be marked with a round inked optical zone marker to help center the trephine blade. The cornea may subsequently be marked with an inked radial marker such as those used in radial keratotomy to aid in radial and evenly spaced suture placement. A trephine—a cylindrical scalpel blade—creates the circular incision on

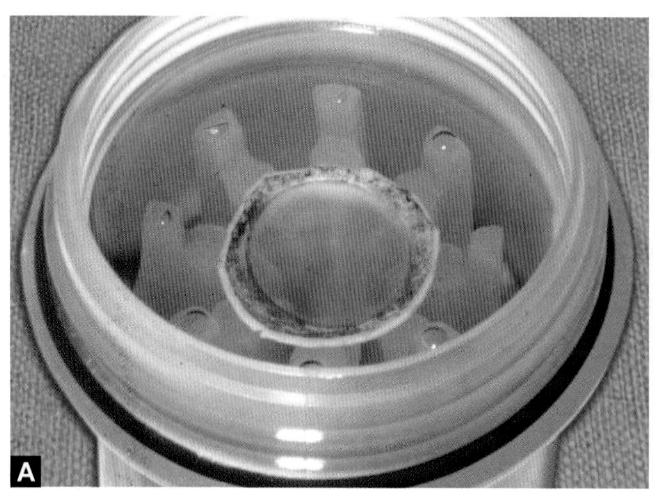


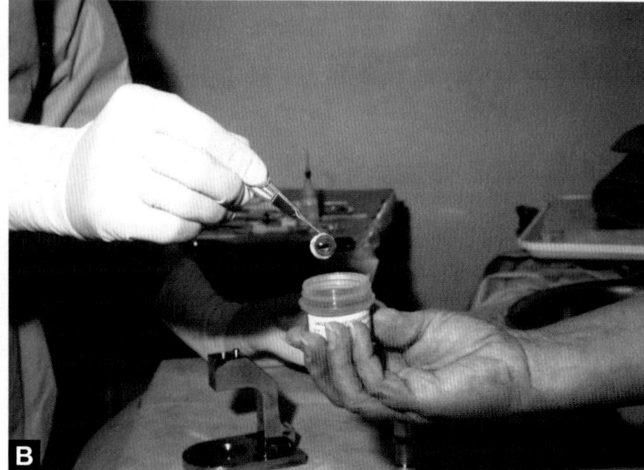


**Figures 16-2A and B** (A) Typical donor cornea, shown in storage medium, including 2–4 mm of sclera. (B) Donor cornea removed from storage medium, prior to trephination.

the host cornea. Trephines come in a range of sizes to allow for a slight oversize of the donor cornea relative to the host cornea. Some trephination systems are vacuum assisted. The trephination procedure ideally cuts down to Descemet's membrane for controlled entry into the anterior chamber with a sharp surgical blade.

## Instruments for Preparation of Donor Cornea

A typical donor cornea includes 2–4 mm of sclera (Figs. 16.2A and B). The donor cornea is cut endothelial side up using a trephine punch instrument, such as the Iowa punch or the Troutman corneal punch. The Barron corneal donor button punches are a disposable system with centration marks to allow centering of the trephine over the donor tissue and a vacuum application to hold the donor securely during trephination. Artificial anterior chamber systems allow both the donor and host to be cut from the anterior surface.

## Spatulas/Hooks

A variety of spatulas and/or hooks can be helpful during the procedure for manipulation of tissues within the anterior chamber, as well as intraocular lenses. Some surgeons use the Paton spatula/spoon for transfer of the donor corneal button to the field, although forceps are an acceptable alternative.

## Blades

A sharp surgical blade may be necessary for entrance into the anterior chamber through the trephination groove during PK, if the trephination does not enter the anterior chamber. Blades are also used to create paracenteses if needed. The 15° blade, 75 blade, and diamond blade are commonly used for entry into the anterior chamber.

## Cannulas

Cannulas can be useful to maintain and reconstitute the anterior chamber during the procedure. They can be introduced either at the interface between host and donor tissue or through a paracentesis.

## Keratometers

Assessing intraoperative corneal astigmatism can be achieved using a keratometer or instrument to qualitatively measure the radial symmetry of the donor cornea. Intraoperative keratometry, with a keratometer mounted on the operating microscope, is ideal but more expensive. More cost-effective options rely on the principle of reflecting a circle from the corneal surface to assess curvature. Intraoperative keratometry allows sutures to be adjusted intraoperatively based on the findings.

# SURGICAL TECHNIQUE

## Preoperative Medications

Preoperative medications for a typical patient having a PK for a central corneal opacity involving multiple layers of the host cornea may be selected to minimize the risk of infection and facilitate additional intraoperative procedures (i.e. dilate or constrict the patient).

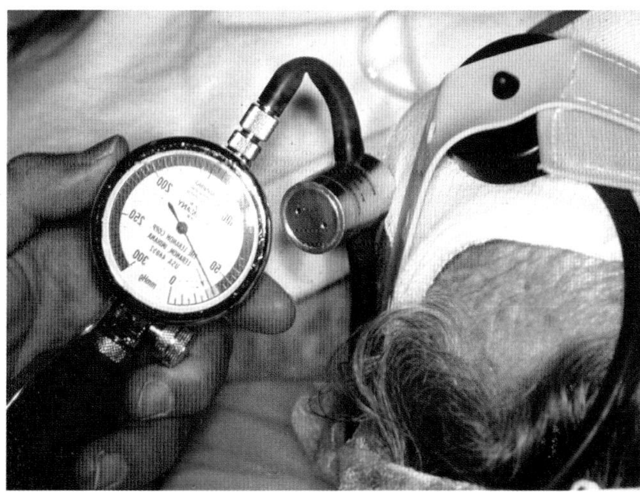

**Figure 16-3** Honan balloon in place for decompression of the vitreous.

- *Topical antibiotics*: Preoperative antibiotics may reduce the incidence of postoperative endophthalmitis that is most commonly caused by periocular flora.[10] Drops may be instilled four times a day for 2–3 days prior to the operation
- *Miotics*: Pilocarpine 1–2% should be used for phakic patients undergoing PK when no vitrectomy or lens exchange is planned
- *Dilating drops*: Cyclopentolate 1%, tropicamide 1%, and/or phenylephrine 2.5% drops are used when cataract extraction is to be performed with PK. Dilation should also be considered when posterior chamber lens removal/exchange is planned, although some prefer not to use the drops if a sutured lens is planned
- *Betadine 5%*: Should be instilled in the cul-de-sac prior to starting the procedure
- *Intravenous Mannitol 20%*: Dosage of 1 g/kg given over 20–30 minutes. This should be considered in patients who are overweight/obese and/or patients undergoing combined cataract/PK procedures

## Anesthesia

Choice of anesthesia is dependent on patient factors and surgeon preference. Below are various options and the rationale for use. PK is generally performed safely as an outpatient procedure. Maintaining control of blood pressure, heart rate, and anxiety during the procedure avoids unnecessary complications.

- *General anesthesia with use of a paralytic agent*: Appropriate for young anxious patients, overweight/obese patients, and patients with low risk for general endotracheal anesthesia (GETA). GETA should also be considered for combined or longer procedures. It is important to avoid "light anesthesia", which may result in unexpected patient movement or 'bucking.'
- *Retrobulbar block with lid block*: Appropriate for patients with good cooperation and/or those who are at risk for undergoing GETA. Long lasting agents, such as bupivacaine, are commonly used. The procedure is typically performed under monitored anesthesia care
- *A Honan balloon or digital pressure*: Used to help decompress the vitreous, lower intraocular pressure prior to the incision, reduce the risk of suprachoroidal hemorrhage, and aid in dispersion of the local anesthetic after a retrobulbar block (Fig. 16-3).[11]

## Patient Preparation in the Operating Room

Patients are prepped and draped in sterile fashion using a drape that isolates eyelashes from the sterile field. The head should be positioned to facilitate suture placement. In some cases, especially with patients under monitored anesthesia care, the head should be secured in position with tape. Placing the patient in a slight reverse Trendelenburg position can help reduce intraocular pressure and reduce the risk of suprachoroidal hemorrhage, which occurs less commonly in patients undergoing GETA. Finally, a lid speculum is placed ensuring that it confers no additional pressure on the globe.

## Procedural Technique

The optical center of central host cornea is marked using an inked optical zone marker. The optical center usually coincides with the center of the pupil and not the center of the cornea. Decentration may be required to encompass corneal pathology. For instance, in cases of keratoconus, grafts may be decentered inferiorly to incorporate the entire cone. Some surgeons then mark the cornea with a radial marker to aid in subsequent suture alignment.[12] An appropriately sized trephine marks the epithelium prior to trephination to assure centration. An 8.0-mm trephine is most commonly used on the host, but other sizes are available and appropriate for this step.

Preparation of donor corneal tissue should be completed prior to trephining the host. The donor button is cut endothelial side up using a trephine loaded punch instrument (Fig. 16-4). The remaining peripheral tissue rim is sent to pathology for culture. Donor grafts should typically be oversized by 0.25 mm compared with the host bed, although

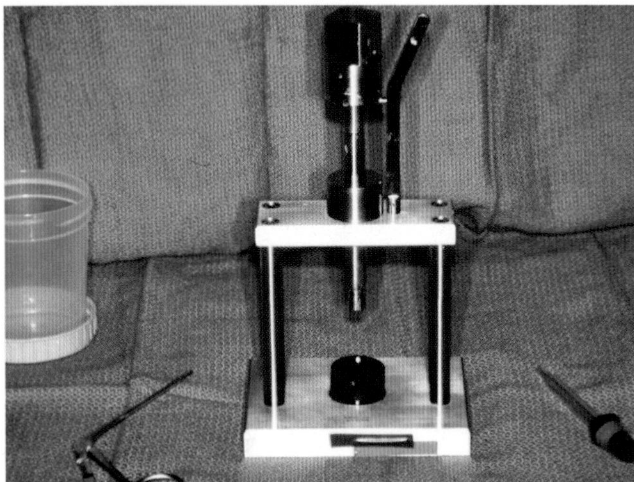

**Figure 16-4** Illustration of a trephination setup employed in cutting the donor corneal tissue.

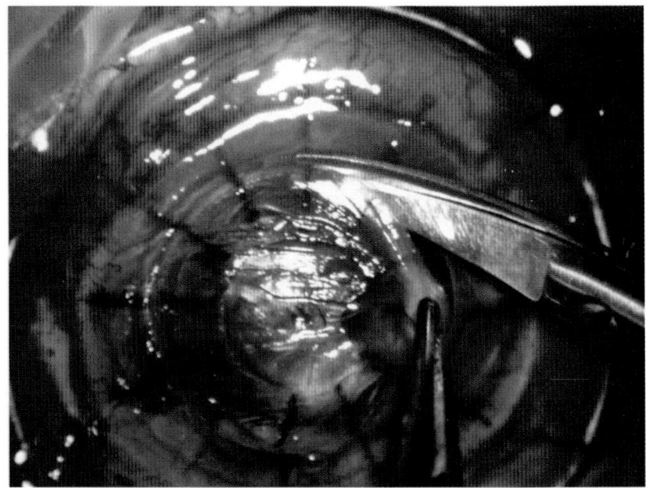

**Figure 16-5** Removal of the host cornea using corneal scissors.

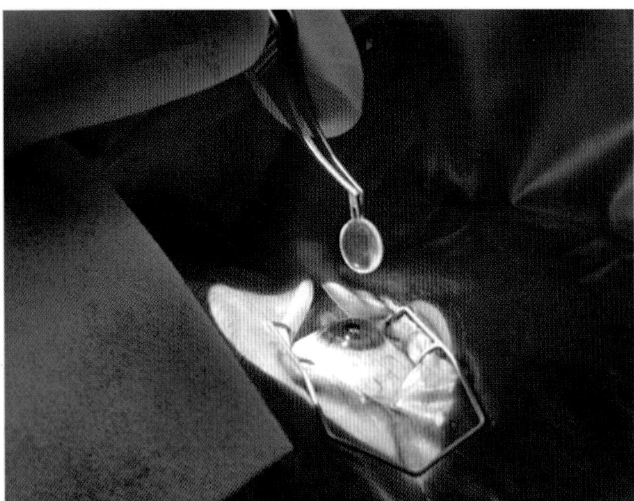

**Figure 16-6** Donor cornea being transferred to the recipient bed.

certain situations necessitate different sizing guidelines. For patients with a shallow anterior chamber or with glaucoma, the graft can be oversized by 0.50 mm. In cases of globe perforation or flat anterior chamber, oversizing the graft by 0.50–0.75 mm may be necessary. For keratoconus patients, the surgeon may consider same size grafting to minimize residual myopia.[13] Once the donor button is cut, the tissue is protected until ready for use.

Once centered, trephination to approximately 90% depth is performed on the host cornea. The anterior chamber enters through the base of the trephination groove using a 75 blade or similar cutting blade. Viscoelastic is instilled to maintain the anterior chamber, providing protection to the iris and lens. The cornea is then carefully removed using corneal scissors to the right and to the left, taking care to avoid placing pressure on the globe, inadvertently cutting the iris, or straying outside of the trephination incision (Fig. 16-5). Some surgeons prefer angling the scissors to leave a small inferior ledge to aid in closure particularly if using same sized grafts. Once the host cornea is removed, additional viscoelastic is applied in the angle and to the anterior chamber in preparation for placement of the graft.

The donor graft is irrigated to remove storage solution and transferred to the recipient bed using double fixation forceps such as the Polack forceps (Fig. 16-6). The host corneal tissue is sent to pathology for evaluation, and the donor rim may be sent for culture.

Suprachoroidal hemorrhage is a dreaded intraoperative complication that occurs more often in patients with advanced age, hypertension, tachycardia, glaucoma, and anticoagulant therapy than in young, healthy patients.[14] Care must be taken to minimize open sky time during the keratoplasty procedure, and instrumentation should be available at all times to quickly suture either the new donor or old host in place if this complication occurs.

## Suturing Techniques

Different suturing techniques for securing the donor tissue to the host bed vary for different patients. The foremost goal of corneal suturing is to achieve a stable wound. Tissue alignment and symmetric suture placement are important irrespective of wound construction. Ideally, the suturing technique should minimize postoperative astigmatism, as well as facilitate rapid visual rehabilitation after PK. Following is a brief overview of the following four categories of suturing techniques[15]:

1. Interrupted sutures
2. Combined interrupted and continuous sutures
3. Single continuous suture
4. Double continuous suture.

The graft is secured to the host initially using at least four interrupted cardinal sutures, which may or may not be removed. Typically, 10-0 nylon suture is used because of its strength, elasticity, and biocompatibility with the cornea.

Double fixation forceps help stabilize the graft for first suture placement at the 12 o'clock position, using the radial markings as a guide. The suture is placed at 90% depth through the donor tissue and then at 90% depth and a similar length through the 12 o'clock position on the host bed. Full thickness bites create postoperative hypotony, a possible tract into the anterior chamber for infection and should be avoided. The suture may be tied with either a traditional or slipknot. Approximation of Bowman's layer of both the host and the graft tissues should be attempted. Good graft apposition aids in epithelialization and wound healing. The second suture is then placed at 6 o'clock with care taken to achieve 90% depth and similar lengths on the donor and host sides. The second cardinal suture is 180° from the initial suture and is the most important determinant of final graft position and corneal astigmatism. There should be equal amounts of donor and host tissue on both sides of the 12-6 suture axis; if not, replacement of the suture is indicated.

The third and fourth cardinal sutures are placed at the 3 o'clock and 9 o'clock positions bisecting the wound on both sides of the 12-6 sutures; this frequently produces a diamond-shaped pattern of corneal striae in the graft. The anterior chamber should be maintained with balanced salt solution to protect the endothelium from trauma, if the anterior chamber collapses. Although the chamber may form at this point, the wound will usually still leak. In many cases, such as pediatric grafts or keratoconus patients where the donor or host is thin or has less rigidity, eight sutures may be necessary before the chamber is secure.

Once the initial cardinal sutures are placed, one of the four above-mentioned suturing techniques can be employed.

### *Interrupted Sutures*

This is a standard method for keratoplasty suturing. Interrupted sutures have the advantage of allowing partial or complete suture removal in one region of a graft. Indications for interrupted suturing include: multiple previous grafts, pediatric cases, vascularization of the host cornea, or inflammatory conditions. Many surgeons prefer this method for all keratoplasties. Single interrupted 10-0 nylon sutures are placed as described previously and tied with either a traditional 3-1-1 closure or as a slipknot (1-1-1-1). Slipknots allow for intraoperative adjustment of astigmatism. Prior to permanently tying the sutures, astigmatism is adjusted using a keratometer.

If a scleral fixation ring was placed, it should be removed prior to final suture adjustment. Once all sutures have been securely tied, loose ends should be cut short using a blade. The knots should be buried. Knots may either be buried in the host or donor tissue. Burying the knots in host tissue reduces the risk of dehiscence when the sutures are removed by lessening the tension on the graft–host interface. Alternatively, burial in the donor tissue reduces inflammation and vascularization by placing the knot further from the limbal vessels.

Eight sutures generally provide a watertight closure, with 16 sutures being the average number for 360° wound closure. In some cases, such as same size donor–host grafts, keratoconus patients, or pediatric grafts, 24 or 32 interrupted sutures may be used to secure the wound (Fig. 16-7).

### *Combined Interrupted and Continuous Sutures*

This technique allows for removal of the interrupted sutures earlier than if interrupted sutures alone were used. Often, 8 to 16 interrupted 10-0 nylon sutures are placed in conjunction with a continuous 12-bite running suture with either 10-0 nylon or 11-0 nylon (Fig. 16-8). Interrupted suture knots should be buried prior to placement of the running suture. Continuous suture bites are placed in between and in close proximity to the interrupted sutures. The suture is knotted and tightened. The continuous suture maintains wound closure when interrupted sutures are removed. The combination of interrupted and a continuous suture allows for mitigation of astigmatism after 6 to 8 weeks. Tight interrupted sutures can be removed, based on keratometry or refraction, to flatten a steep axis. The continuous suture supports the wound when the interrupted sutures are removed.

### *Single Continuous Suture*

Continuous sutures are challenging, because one improper suture pass can impair the closure. The effectiveness of a single continuous suture is compromised by its one least perfect pass. The sutures must be passed with adequate depth and spacing for each bite to hold the wound closed. Twenty-four passes in 360° is generally sufficient to close an 8.0- or 8.5-mm graft. Once the suture is passed, it cannot be removed without removing the entire suture.

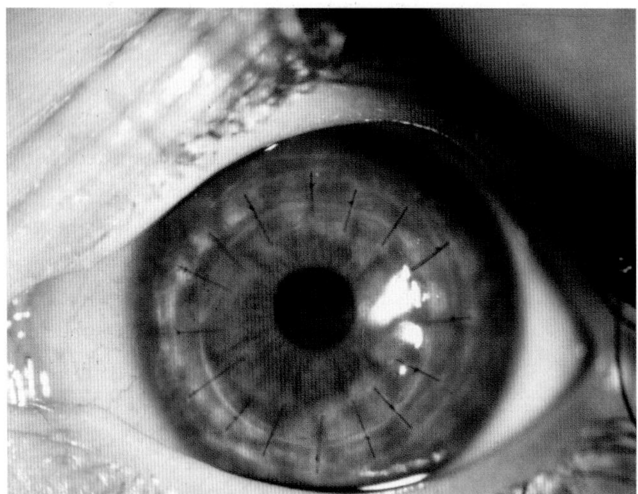

**Figure 16-7** Penetrating keratoplasty with interrupted suture closure using 16, 10-0 nylon single interrupted sutures.

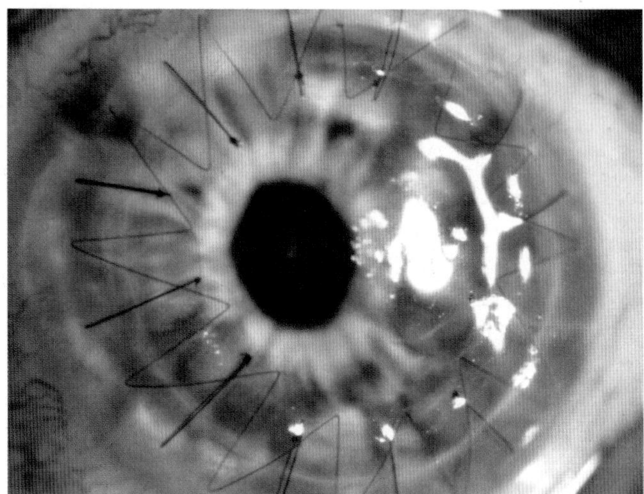

**Figure 16-8** Combined interrupted and continuous suture closure with 12 interrupted 10-0 nylon sutures in conjunction with a 10-0 nylon continuous 12-bite running suture (arrow).

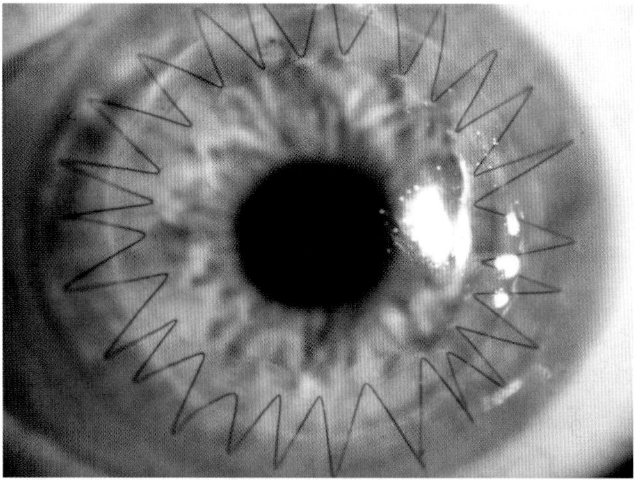

**Figure 16-9** Penetrating keratoplasty with a 24-bite single continuous suture in place.

Typically, four cardinal sutures are placed to secure the wound, followed by a 24-bite continuous suture. Care should be taken to preserve the needle and suture, as the entire suture may need to be repeated if problems arise. A balance must be achieved between ensuring appropriate wound closure with a tight suture and minimizing astigmatism in the graft. After the continuous suture is completed and knotted temporarily at 12 o'clock, the four cardinal sutures are removed. At this point, the anterior chamber is reformed and the suture is tightened and adjusted with the help of a keratometer. Then, the suture is permanently knotted at 12 o'clock, and the knot is buried (Fig. 16-9).

### *Double Continuous Suture*

With this method, the first of the two continuous sutures are placed in a manner similar to that described for a single continuous suture; four cardinal sutures are placed and then a 12-bite 10-0 nylon continuous suture is placed at approximately 80% depth. For the second suture, an 11-0 nylon suture is placed at approximately 50–60% depth. The second continuous suture allows for earlier astigmatism adjustment via removal of the 10-0 nylon suture 2–3 months postoperatively. The second suture is typically left in place for 12–18 months. This technique can be even more challenging than single continuous suture closure, since the surgeon must place symmetric, regular bites for both continuous sutures. In contrast, interrupted sutures can be replaced individually as many times as needed to obtain the desired position and tension (Figs. 16-10A and B).

Once the graft is sutured in place and all knots are buried, a fluorescein strip is used to assure that the wound is watertight. Subconjunctival injections of an antibiotic and a steroid are performed prior to removal of the lid speculum. If ocular surface issues are a concern, a temporary or permanent tarsorrhaphy can be placed. At the conclusion of the procedure, antibiotic ointment with or without a steroid is applied to the ocular surface; a pressure patch and shield are placed for overnight protection of the operative eye.

In cases where a PK is performed in conjunction with other procedures, modifications of the previously described surgical technique are often necessary. For example, a temporary Frost suture tarsorrhaphy may be placed in patients with dry

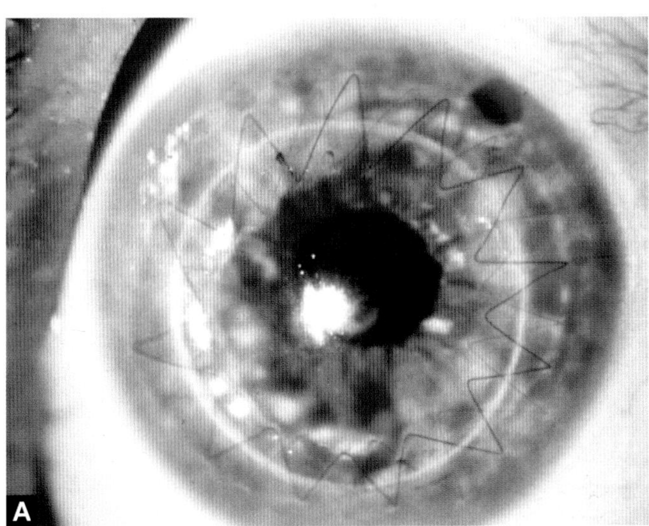


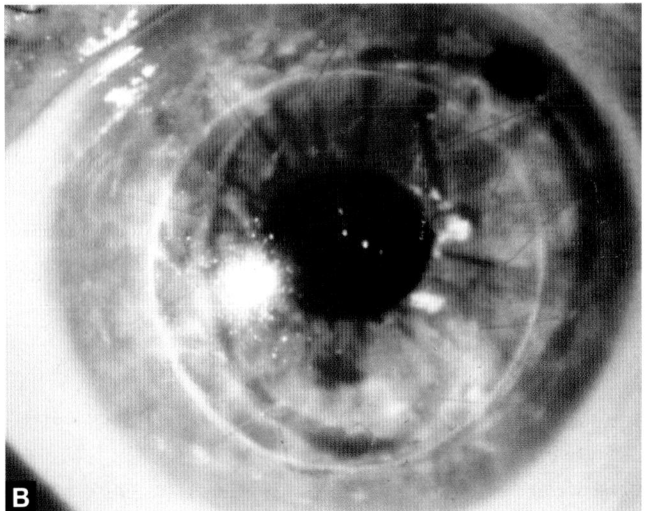


**Figures 16-10A and B** (A) Double continuous suture (DCS) closure for penetrating keratoplasty employing a 10-0 nylon continuous suture at approximately 80% depth and an 11-0 nylon continuous suture at 50–60% depth. (B) The same eye as shown in (A) with the 10-0 nylon suture removed.

eye or ocular surface disease. Other modifications include preoperative pupil treatment for concomitant vitrectomy (no dilating or constricting drops), anterior chamber lenses (constrict), or cataract extraction (dilate). Patients requiring concomitant transclerally sutured posterior lenses will need scleral flaps made during surgery before opening the globe. Surgical modifications in technique are dictated according to the skill and preference of the surgeon and the needs of the individual patient.

## POSTOPERATIVE CARE

In the immediate postoperative period, re-establishment of the ocular surface, confirmation of wound integrity, and prevention of infection are paramount. Additional goals include control of intraocular pressure, maintaining an intact ocular surface, reduction of astigmatism, and patient comfort. Medications, which are used to help control inflammation and prevent infection, may be toxic to the ocular surface. Astigmatism cannot be effectively measured until the ocular surface re-establishes itself and corneal edema resides enough to stabilize suture tension in the wound.

### Postoperative Medications

#### *Antimicrobials*

Patients are treated with topical antibiotics, typically four times daily during the first week. Ideally, the antibiotic should be broad spectrum with low toxicity and allergic potential. Fluoroquinolones are often used.[16] If a tarsorrhaphy is present, patients should use ointment on the stitches and lid margins. If the PK was performed for an infectious cause, antimicrobials should be selected based on cultures; perioperative cultures from the host and donor rim can guide antimicrobial therapy. Oral antibiotics (e.g. fluoroquinolones) or antifungals (e.g. voriconazole) can be added for cases of advanced infections or perforated ulcers. For patients with a history of herpes simplex virus (HSV), oral Acyclovir or Valtrex is used for at least 6 months to 1 year. Acyclovir is dosed prophylactically with a dose of 400 mg twice daily.[17-19]

#### *Immune-modulators*

Patients are also treated with a topical corticosteroid drops, such as difluprednate 0.05% ophthalmic suspension (Durezol, Alcon) or prednisolone acetate 1.0% ophthalmic suspension (Pred Forte, Allergan) four times daily (average; may be more often in younger patients or patients with inflammation or vascularization, less often in rheumatoid or elderly patients). The frequency may be increased for inflamed eyes or decreased for epithelial defects, postinfectious cases, or in patients with a rheumatoid melt. Steroids are tapered depending on the patient. In general, steroids are continued four times daily for several months, followed by three times daily for 2 months, twice daily for 2 months, and daily for at least 4 months. If the patient is phakic and has little inflammation, a more rapid taper may be considered, balancing the risk of complications of the corticosteroid drops with the risk of inflammation or rejection. For pseudophakic patients the steroid is often continued indefinitely as long as it is tolerated. In eyes with a high risk of rejection, topical cyclosporine 1–2% can be added and topical difluprednate can be substituted for prednisolone acetate. Perioperative oral steroids should be started in patients at high risk for rejection. In addition, longer term immunosuppression can also be considered in more extreme cases. These agents require routine blood work and should be given in conjunction with a physician familiar with these medications.

### Intraocular Pressure Lowering Agents

Intraocular pressure should be monitored at each postoperative visit. If significantly elevated, agents for lowering pressure are employed. Topical α-2-adrenergic agonists (e.g. brimonidine), β-adrenergic antagonists (e.g. timolol), and prostaglandin analogs (e.g. latanoprost) are good treatment options. Oral carbonic anhydrase inhibitors, such as acetazolamide decrease aqueous production and can thereby compromise endothelial cell function. Oral osmotics can also be used in the acute setting. The etiology of elevated intraocular pressure needs to be addressed in the context of other examination findings, because a shallow anterior chamber can be indicative of angle closure, phacomorphic glaucoma, aqueous misdirection, or choroidal hemorrhage. Patients with a history of glaucoma are at a higher risk of having ocular hypertension in the early postoperative period and should have their medications adjusted appropriately.

### Ocular Lubricants

Ocular lubricants function to maintain and preserve the corneal epithelium. Nonpreserved artificial tears can be started early in the postoperative period. Additional options to help protect epithelium include placement of a tarsorrhaphy and use of bandage contact lenses—which should be used with caution as it can increase the risk of postoperative keratitis.[20] In the absence of significant ocular surface disease, the tarsorrhaphy is removed around 1–2 weeks postoperatively, or once the epithelium is intact. Reduction of other topical medications is also helpful. In severe cases, autologous serum drops may be of use. Punctal occlusion, either temporary with plugs or permanent with cautery, may be beneficial in the long-term treatment of patients with dry eye or ocular surface disease.

### Pain Medication

Pain following a PK can generally be managed conservatively with over-the-counter medications, such as acetaminophen and nonsteroidal anti-inflammatories. Narcotic pain medications are usually not necessary, but they can be considered on a case-by-case basis.

Patients should avoid eye rubbing, straining, and heavy lifting [no more than 2.3–4.5 kg (5–10) lbs] for the first few weeks after surgery. Glasses should be worn at all times and a shield used while sleeping to minimize the chance of external trauma to the operative eye.

Penetrating keratoplasty patients are routinely seen on postoperative day 1, 1 week, 2–4 weeks, 2 months, 3 months, and then every 2–3 months during the first year. During the first week, focus is placed on re-establishing corneal epithelium, prevention of infection, reducing inflammation, and treating any complications that may arise. Postoperative weeks 1–12 represent the period of greatest change. In this time frame, care should be taken to prevent infection, rejection, and begin early adjustment of astigmatism. During each postoperative visit, visual acuity, intraocular pressure, epithelial status, wound architecture, and suture status should be assessed. Seidel testing can be used to detect problems with wound construction and wound healing. Mild suture tract leaks in the presence of a formed chamber typically self-seal and can be monitored. Wound gape and graft-host override need to be repaired early. The ocular surface and epithelium should be continuously monitored for any signs of breakdown or infection, since an intact epithelium is the best protection against infection. In addition, the patient should always be monitored for the possibility of endophthalmitis, graft rejection, and recurrence of disease.

Once the patient has reached the third postoperative month, care begins to shift to visual rehabilitation. Follow-up examinations can be spaced out to every 2 months depending on the risk factors and the need for suture adjustment. Indications for suture removal include astigmatism, inflammation, vascularization, infection, and loosening or breakage. Any and all loose sutures should be removed immediately because there is a risk of infection/inflammation and a loose suture provides no wound stability. In the earlier postoperative period (< 3 months), loose or broken sutures can be replaced as necessary. Vascularized, inflamed, or infected sutures should be removed immediately and treated as indicated.

Even with the presence of a clear graft, astigmatism is a leading cause of decreased visual acuity after surgery.[21] The average amount of postoperative astigmatism is 4–5 diopters and is influenced by suture depth, tension, and symmetry. Moreover, corneal wound healing is not always symmetric and can contribute to overall astigmatism. Evaluation can be

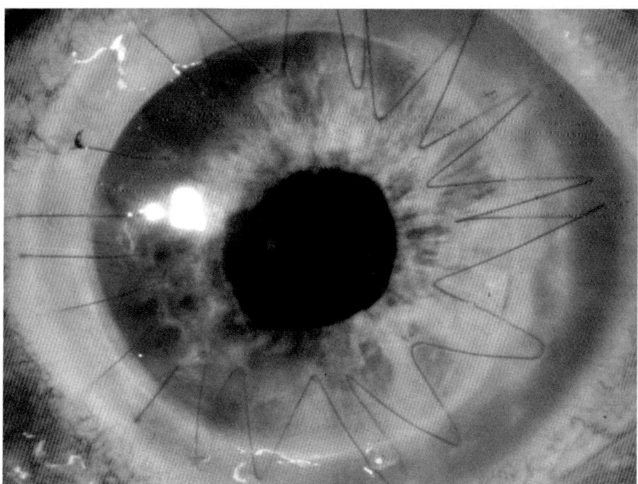

**Figure 16-11** Uneven continuous suture placement resulting in wound leak.

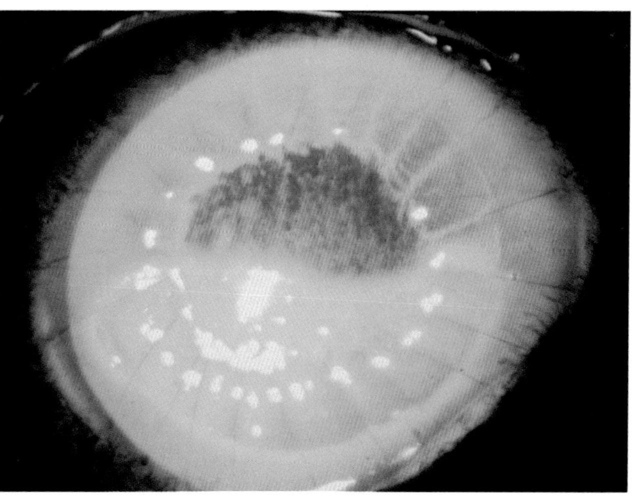

**Figure 16-12** Large persistent epithelial defect following penetrating keratoplasty.

performed using keratometry, keratoscopy, and/or corneal topography. Removal of interrupted sutures can flatten a steep meridian. Elective removal of interrupted sutures begins approximately 3 months postoperatively. With a continuous suture in place, adjustment can flatten a steep meridian and also has the ability to steepen a flat meridian. Once astigmatism has been reduced satisfactorily—with or without sutures still in place—further visual rehabilitation should be attempted with glasses or contact lenses.

Occasionally, select patients may require surgical intervention to achieve the best-corrected visual acuity. Surgical techniques include refractive procedures such as laser-assisted in situ keratomileusis or photorefractive keratectomy, compression sutures, or incisional surgery, such as relaxing incisions. These procedures are beyond the scope of this chapter.

## COMPLICATIONS

Below is a list of complications that can occur after PK.

- *Wound leaks*: These can be indicated by low intraocular pressure and/or a shallow anterior chamber; Seidel testing can help confirm the diagnosis. As noted previously, small suture tract leaks generally self-seal and can be observed. Treatment options include: aqueous suppressants, bandage contact lens placement, patching, or resuturing. Any leak with iridocorneal touch needs repair within 24 hours (Fig. 16-11).
- *Wound displacement*: This is more commonly seen in patients with thin corneas, irregular wounds, or early suture removal. This complication can result in severe astigmatism and should be repaired early. Observation for resolution can be employed initially in cases with mild edema. Full thickness wound dehiscence requires surgical repair and should always be addressed immediately.[22]
- *Persistent epithelial defects*: These may result in infection, scarring, and possibly graft failure. It is important to preserve donor epithelium during the procedure. Epithelium should typically be healed by 1 week postoperatively as it becomes more difficult further out. Risk factors include ocular surface disease, neurotrophic corneas, alkali burns, and eyelid abnormalities. Options for management include decreasing topical medications and use of ocular lubricants or bandage contact lenses. If HSV is suspected, oral antivirals can be employed. Temporary or permanent tarsorrhapies can also aid in epithelialization. Unresponsive patients may benefit from an amniotic membrane patch (Fig. 16-12).
- *Infection*: Risk factors for infection include, but are not limited to, persistent epithelial defects, exposed sutures or suture knots, chronic steroid use, bandage contact lenses, poor patient compliance, poor hygiene, immunodeficiency, and atopy. In addition, eyes grafted for HSV tend to have higher rates of microbial keratitis postoperatively. Visual outcomes after postoperative infectious keratitis tend to be poor; approximately, 70% of patients are 20/200 or worse.[23] Gram-positive organisms are most common followed by gram-negative organisms, fungi, and rarely *Acanthamoeba*.[24-25]

Extensive involvement of the graft places the eye at risk for endophthalmitis. The incidence of postoperative endophthalmitis after PK has been cited as approximately 0.4%.[26]

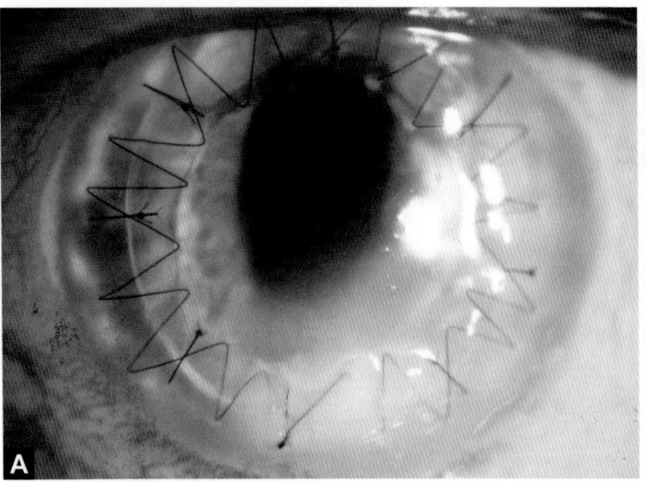

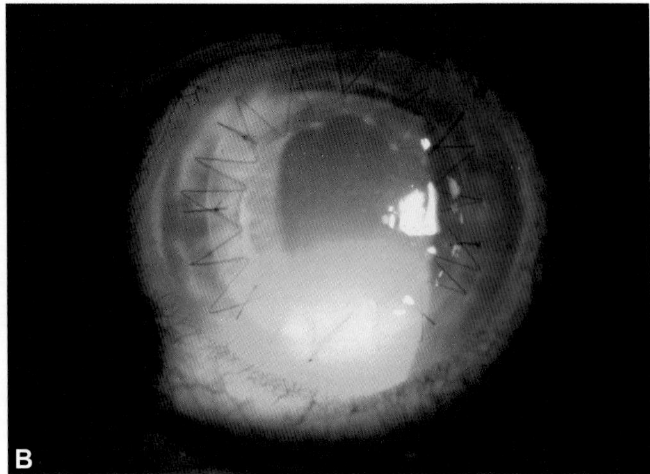

**Figures 16-13A and B** (A) Inferior corneal ulcer with an infiltrate at the host–graft interface. (B) Fluorescein staining pattern of figure ulcer (A), showing an epithelial defect overlying the infiltrate.

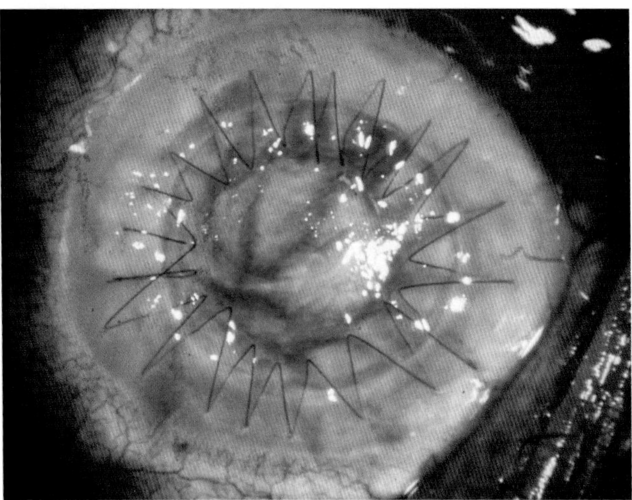

**Figure 16-14** Primary graft failure manifesting as irreversible corneal edema.

Infectious keratitis (Figs. 16-13A and B) should be managed per routine with gram stain, corneal cultures, and appropriate antimicrobial therapy. Steroids should be decreased or discontinued. Some patients may need regrafting to eradicate the infection. In cases of early postoperative keratitis, it is important to check culture results from donor rim tissue, as well as host tissue. Fungal infections have been found to correlate most closely with donor rim cultures.

Another form of postoperative infection is a suture abscess. This can occur as an infectious infiltrate contiguous with a suture – often broken or loose. The suture is removed and should be cultured. Infectious crystalline keratopathy, classically due to α-hemolytic *Streptococcus viridans*, is an intrastromal noninflammatory bacterial colonization of the graft. The epithelium is usually intact in these cases. Treatment involves topical antimicrobials, but it may require regrafting.

- *Primary graft failure*: Primary donor failure occurs in the immediate postoperative period and is manifested by irreversible corneal graft edema (Fig. 16-14). It is due to endothelial cell dysfunction or inadequate endothelial cell counts and is unresponsive to steroids or hypertonic solutions. Primary donor failure requires regrafting.
- *Corneal graft rejection*: Corneal graft rejection remains the leading cause of corneal graft failure.[27] Risks for rejection include young patients, stromal vascularization, history of previous grafts, history of glaucoma or uveitis, and necessity of a large graft.[28] Patients often present with a red eye, light sensitivity, decreased vision, and discomfort. Any of these symptoms persisting more than a few hours should prompt an evaluation. Graft rejection is immune-mediated, often accompanied by inflammatory signs; ciliary flush, anterior chamber flare, cellular infiltration of the anterior segment with associated edema with kerato-precipitates are all signs of graft rejection.

Epithelial rejection manifesting with an epithelial rejection line can occur up to 1 year after surgery. Subepithelial rejection presents with patchy anterior infiltrates. The infiltrates can occur in different patterns and can be specific to the portion of the graft that is rejecting. Although these can be a harmless finding, the infiltrates could be a precursor of impending severe rejection and should be treated with topical steroids. Endothelial rejection is the most severe and presents with edema with underlying keratoprecipitates. They may form an endothelial rejection line that can march across the cornea leaving edema in its wake. This needs to be treated with aggressive topical steroids and possibly oral steroids as well. The patient should be followed closely until resolution occurs.

## REFERENCES


1. Armitage WJ, Tullo AB, Larkin DF. The first successful full-thickness corneal transplant: a commentary on Eduard Zirm's landmark paper of 1906. Br J Ophthalmol.2006;90(10):1222-3.
2. Eye Bank Association of America. Eye banking statistical report, Washington, DC, Eye Bank Association of America, 2009.
3. Thompson RW, Jr, Price MO, Bowers PJ, et al. Long-term graft survival after penetrating keratoplasty. Ophthalmology. 2003;110(7):1396-1402.
4. Ing JJ, Ing HH, Nelson LR, et al. Ten-year postoperative results of penetrating keratoplasty. Ophthalmology. 1998; 105(10): 1855-65.
5. Brightbill FS, Brass RE. Preoperative evaluation of the keratoplasty patient. In: Krachmer JH, Mannis MJ, Holland EJ (eds.), Cornea. 2nd edn. Philadelphia, PA: Elsevier Mosby, 2005:1423-9.
6. Lois N, Kowal VO, Cohen EJ, et al. Indications for penetrating keratoplasty and associated procedures, 1989-1995. Cornea. 1997;16:623-9.
7. Wilbanks GA, Cohen S, Chipman M, et al. Clinical outcomes following penetrating keratoplasty using the Barron-Hessburg and Hanna corneal trephination systems. Cornea. 1996; 15(6):589-98.
8. Stansbury FC. Circular corneal transplants: surgical technic; instruments and sutures; comparison with the use of square transplants. JAMA Ophthalmol. 1949;42(2):155-69.
9. Soong HK. Corneal transplantation. In: Spaeth GL (eds.), Ophthalmic surgery: principles and practice. 3rd edn. Philadelphia, PA: Elsevier Health Sciences, 2003:139-60.
10. Speaker MG, Milch FA, Shah MK, et al. Role of external bacterial flora in the pathogenesis of acute postoperative endophthalmitis. Ophthalmology. 1991;98:639-49.
11. Quist LH, Stapleton SS, McPherson SD, Jr. Preoperative use of the Honan intraocular pressure reducer. Am J Ophthalmol. 1983;95:536-8.
12. Geggel HS. Technique to minimize asymmetric suture placement during penetrating keratoplasty. Cornea. 2002;21:17-21.
13. Olson RJ. Variation in corneal graft size related to trephine technique. Arch Ophthalmol. 1979;97:1323-5.
14. Speaker MG, Guerriero PN, Met JA, et al. A case-control study of risk factors for intraoperative suprachoroidal expulsive hemorrhage. Ophthalmology. 1991;98:202-9.
15. Van Meter WS, Katz DG. Keratoplasty suturing techniques. In: Krachmer JH, Mannis MJ, Holland EJ (eds.), Cornea. 2nd edn. Philadelphia, PA: Elsevier Mosby, 2005:1481-92.
16. Mather R, Karenchak LM, Romanowski EG, et al. Fourth generation fluoroquinolones: new weapons in the arsenal of ophthalmic antibiotics. Am J Ophthalmol. 2002;133(4):463-6.
17. Tambasco FP, Cohen EJ, Nguyen LH, et al. Oral acyclovir after penetrating keratoplasty for herpes simplex keratitis. Arch Ophthalmol. 1999;117(4):445-9.
18. Halberstadt M, Machens M, Gahlenbek K-A, et al. The outcome of corneal grafting in patients with stromal keratitis of herpetic and non-herpetic origin. Br J Ophthalmol. 2003;86:646-52.
19. Van Rooij J, Rijneveld WJ, Remeijer L, et al. Effect of oral acyclovir after penetrating keratoplasty for herpetic keratitis. Ophthalmology. 2003;110(10):1916-9.
20. Smith SG, Lindstrom RL, Nelson JD, et al. Corneal ulcer-infiltrate associated with soft contact lens use following penetrating keratoplasty. Cornea. 1984;3(2):131-4.
21. Perlman EM. An analysis and interpretation of refractive errors after penetrating keratoplasty. Ophthalmology. 1981; 88(1):39-45.
22. Abou-Jaoude ES, Brooks M, Katz DG, et al. Spontaneous wound dehiscence after removal of single continuous penetrating keratoplasty suture. Ophthalmology. 2002;109:1291-6.
23. Wagoner MD, Al-Swailem SA, Sutphin JE, et al. Bacterial keratitis after penetrating keratoplasty: incidence, microbiological profile, graft survival, and visual outcome. Ophthalmology. 2007;114(6):1073-9.
24. Tixier J, Bourcier T, Borderie V, et al. Infectious keratitis after penetrating keratoplasty. J Fr Ophtalmol. 2001;24(6):597-602.
25. Vajpayee RB, Boral SK, Dada T, et al. Risk factors for graft infection in India: a case-control study. Br J Ophthalmol. 2002; 86:261-5.
26. Taban M, Behrens A, Newcomb RL, et al. Incidence of acute endophthalmitis following penetrating keratoplasty: a systematic review. Arch Ophthalmol. 2005;123(5):605-9.
27. Tan DT, Dart JK, Holland EJ, et al. Corneal transplantation. Lancet. 2012;379(9827):1749-61.
28. Boisjoly HM, Tourigny R, Bazin R, et al. Risk factors of corneal graft failure. Ophthalmology. 1993;100(11):1728-35.

CHAPTER

17

# An Overview of Endothelial Keratoplasty

Julia C Talajic, Michael D Straiko, Mark A Terry

## INTRODUCTION

Endothelial keratoplasty (EK) describes selective transplantation of the posterior cornea. This is a burgeoning field. Over the past decade, EK has revolutionized the field of corneal transplantation. It has replaced full-thickness penetrating keratoplasty (PK) as the treatment of choice for pathologies of the corneal endothelium and has become widely adopted by corneal surgeons around the world. There are several different forms of EK, and the field continues to evolve today.

## ADVANTAGES OF ENDOTHELIAL KERATOPLASTY

The advantages of EK over PK are multiple, which explains the exponential rise in the number of EK surgeries performed over time (Fig. 17-1).

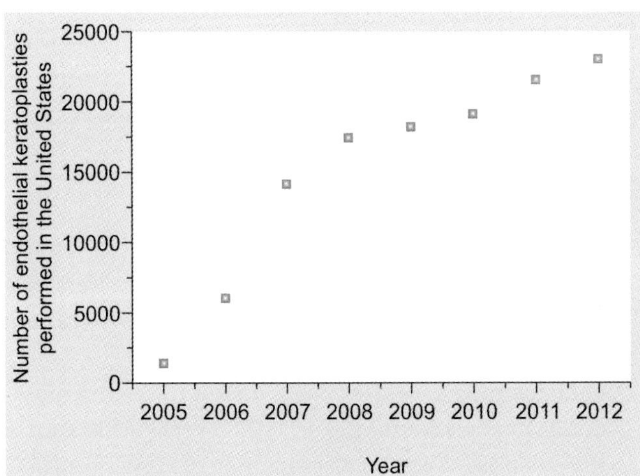


**Figure 17-1** The number of endothelial keratoplasty surgeries performed annually in the United States.[1,2]
*Source* Adapted with permission from Talajic et al, using data from the Eye Bank Association of America.

- EK avoids a 360° penetrating wound
  - The globe maintains its structural integrity, and the risk of globe rupture with ocular trauma is greatly reduced in the long term
  - Expulsive hemorrhage at the time of surgery is avoided.
- EK avoids inducing high levels of astigmatism
  - The normal anterior corneal curvature is preserved in EK because a large corneal incision is avoided; sutures are not needed as the graft is held in place with an anterior chamber air bubble.
- EK allows for rapid visual recovery
  - This is attributable to the preservation of preoperative corneal morphology and avoidance of inducing high degrees of astigmatism
  - Significant visual improvement is obtained in a matter of 4–6 weeks after EK as opposed to months to years following PK.
- EK has a lower rate of graft rejection
  - The long-term rate of rejection after PK is approximately 20%
  - In one series, the 2-year rate of rejection after EK is approximately 9% after Descemet's stripping automated EK (DSAEK) and <1% after Descemet's membrane automated EK (DMAEK).[3]

## HISTORY AND OVERVIEW OF EK TECHNIQUES

### Early EK

- In the mid-20th century, Tillet performed the first human EK when he created an anterior corneal stromal flap and then sutured a posterior corneal graft beneath it[4]
- In 1993, Ko et al. demonstrated that transplantation of the posterior cornea (posterior lamellae, Descemet's

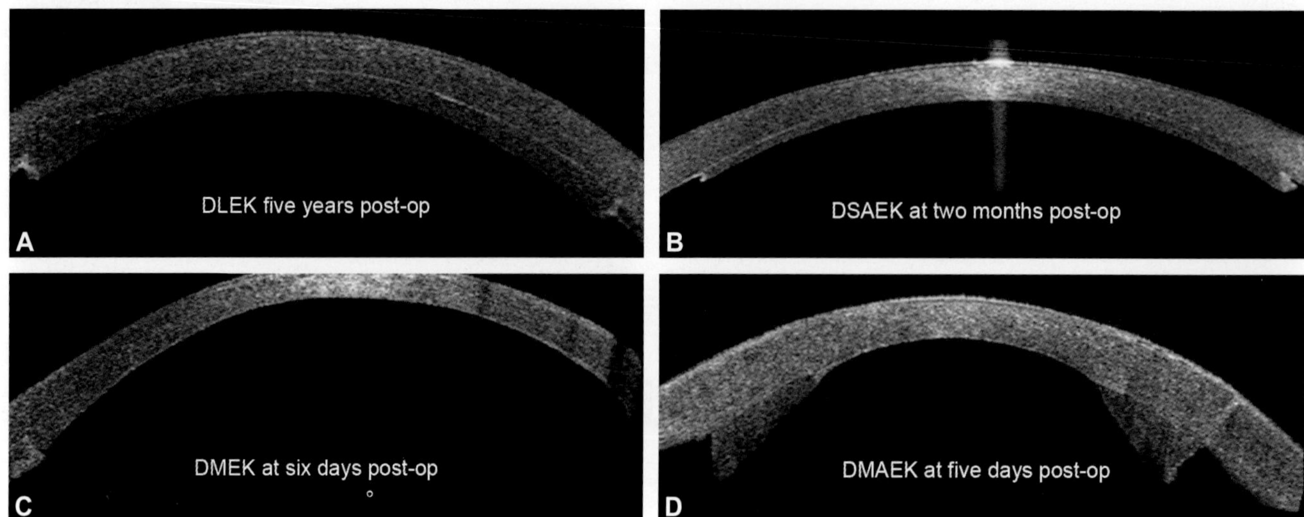


**Figures 17-2A to D** Variations in endothelial keratoplasty: anterior segment optical coherence tomography images. Deep lamellar endothelial keratoplasty (DLEK) (Figure A), Descemet's stripping automated endothelial keratoplasty (DSAEK) (Figure B), Descemet's membrane endothelial keratoplasty (DMEK) (Figure C), and Descemet's membrane automated endothelial keratoplasty (DMAEK) (Figure D). Adapted with permission from Talajic et al.[1]

membrane, and endothelium) could result in a clearer cornea when performed in rabbits with endothelial damage via a limbal incision.[5] These and another early attempt at EK[6] were limited by graft suturing.

## Modern EK

Figures 17-2A to D illustrates various forms of EK.

- Posterior lamellar keratoplasty (PLK)/deep lamellar endothelial keratoplasty (DLEK)
  - Melles et al. performed the first modern posterior corneal transplant in humans in 1998.[7] Their technique, PLK, was novel in that he used air to secure the graft into position rather than sutures. The posterior recipient stroma was manually dissected and excised and then was replaced with donor posterior stroma and endothelium manually dissected from a whole globe
  - In 2001, Terry and Ousley developed DLEK, a modified form of PLK, implementing the use of an artificial anterior chamber, new instruments, and cohesive viscoelastic to more easily accomplish modern EK.[8]
- Descemet's stripping endothelial keratoplasty (DSEK)
  - In 2004, Melles et al. eliminated the need for posterior recipient stromal dissection by performing a "descemetorhexis." This involved creating a 360° circular break in Descemet's membrane of the recipient cornea and then peeling it off.[9]
  - In 2005, Price and Price modified this procedure and named it DSEK. The posterior stromal graft was manually dissected, as in PLK and DLEK.[10]
- Descemet's Stripping Automated Endothelial Keratoplasty (DSAEK)
  - In 2006, Gorovoy described the use of the microkeratome to eliminate manual preparation of posterior corneal donor. This became known as DSAEK.[11]
- Descemet's membrane endothelial keratoplasty (DMEK)
  - In 2002, Melles et al. transplanted Descemet's membrane with its attached endothelium, without any donor stroma, following descemetorhexis of the recipient.[12]
- Descemet's Stripping Automated Endothelial Keratoplasty (DSAEK)
  - McCauley et al. described a hybrid technique in which Descemet's membrane is bared in the central graft while retaining a rim of posterior stroma is in the peripheral graft. This form of EK is not widely practised.[13]

## Current EK Practices

- DSAEK is by far the most commonly practiced form of EK in the United States. 23,049 EK surgeries were performed in the United States in 2012. This number has been steadily increasing every year (*see* Fig. 17-1)[2]
- It is interesting to note that while there is research demonstrating multiple advantages of DMEK over DSAEK, DMEK still comprises a very small proportion of EK performed in the United States (748 of 23,049 EK procedures in 2012). This number, however, has increased 112% from the 344 DMEK surgeries performed in 2011[2]

**TABLE 17-1** The most common indications for endothelial keratoplasty reported by US Eyebanks in 2012[2]

| Indication | Percentage of total EK surgeries (%) |
|---|---|
| Endothelial corneal dystrophies, including Fuchs' | 47 |
| Postcataract surgery edema | 19 |
| Unknown, unreported, or unspecified | 14 |
| Other causes of endothelial dysfunction | 12 |
| Repeat corneal graft | 8 |

EK: (Endothelial keratoplasty)
*Source*: Adapted with permission from The Eye Bank Association of America.[2]

- The following advantages of DMEK over DSAEK have been described:
  - Better visual acuity
  - Faster visual acuity
  - Fewer posterior corneal higher order aberrations
  - Dramatically lower rate of graft rejection (*see* above)
  - Better anatomical replacement of damaged endothelium
  - Greater patient satisfaction

## INDICATIONS FOR EK

- EK is indicated for any corneal pathology arising primarily from endothelial dysfunction:
  - Fuchs endothelial corneal dystrophy
  - Postsurgical bullous keratopathy
  - Posterior polymorphous corneal dystrophy
  - Congenital hereditary endothelial dystrophy
  - Iridocorneal endothelial syndrome
  - Endothelial failure of an existing corneal transplant (whether it be prior PK or EK)
  - Pain control in the setting of corneal edema causing painful bullae
  - Cosmesis in the setting of corneal edema causing corneal whitening
- Table 17-1 outlines the most common indications for EK in the United States in 2012

## CONTRAINDICATIONS TO EK

- Significant anterior corneal scarring
- Abnormal topography. (For example, a failed PK with high irregular astigmatism prior to endothelial decompensation would not be a good candidate for EK).
- Contraindications to DMEK:
  - Previous vitrectomy
  - Inadequate iris support
  - Aphakia
  - Presence of a tube shunt
  - Very large eye, very deep anterior chamber
  - Anterior chamber intraocular lenses
  - Poor visualization of the anterior chamber (and iris details) due to severe corneal edema.

## SURGICAL TECHNIQUE: DSAEK

A number of different DSAEK techniques have been described. The Terry forceps technique[14] has been performed in over 1500 surgeries with excellent published results. The Terry forceps technique is illustrated in Figures 17-3 and is described below:

- A 5-mm-wide temporal corneoscleral tunnel is created
- Two paracenteses are created superotemporally and inferotemporally
- Cohesive viscoelastic is used to fill the anterior chamber. An alternative to using viscoelastic is to fill the anterior chamber with air, or to use an anterior-chamber maintainer with an infusion of balanced salt solution (BSS).
- An optical marker representing the size of the DSAEK graft is used to mark the epithelial surface of the recipient cornea. The graft size is selected relative to the size of the recipient cornea and is generally 8.0–9.0 mm (*see* Fig. 17-3A).
- Descemet's membrane is stripped over the central 8.0–9.0 mm, avoiding overlap with the paracentesis sites, using a Reverse Sinskey hook (Bausch and Lomb Surgical, St. Louis, MO, USA) (*see* Fig. 17-3A to C).
- A Terry scraper (Bausch and Lomb Surgical, St. Louis, MO, USA) is used to roughen the posterior stromal fibers in the 1–2 mm of the peripheral stripped stromal bed, taking care to avoid the visual axis (see Fig. 17-3D).
- The scleral wound is enlarged to 5 mm and the viscoelastic is completely evacuated (*see* Fig. 17-3E).
- The donor cornea is cut using a 300–350-mm head microkeratome. The anterior cap is replaced. This step can be performed either by an eye bank technician or the surgeon. The donor corneoscleral button is then prepared in the operating room under the microscope. While it is laid epithelial-side up, the circular microkeratome cut is marked with ink, as is the center of the cornea (*see* Fig. 17-3F).
- The tissue is then trephinated epithelial-side down using these marks for good centration. It is important to avoid eccentric trephination so as to avoid a full-thickness edge of the graft (*see* Fig. 17-3G).
- A very small strip of cohesive viscoelastic is injected onto the endothelium, and the graft is folded into a 40–60 "underfolded" taco (*see* Fig. 17-3H).

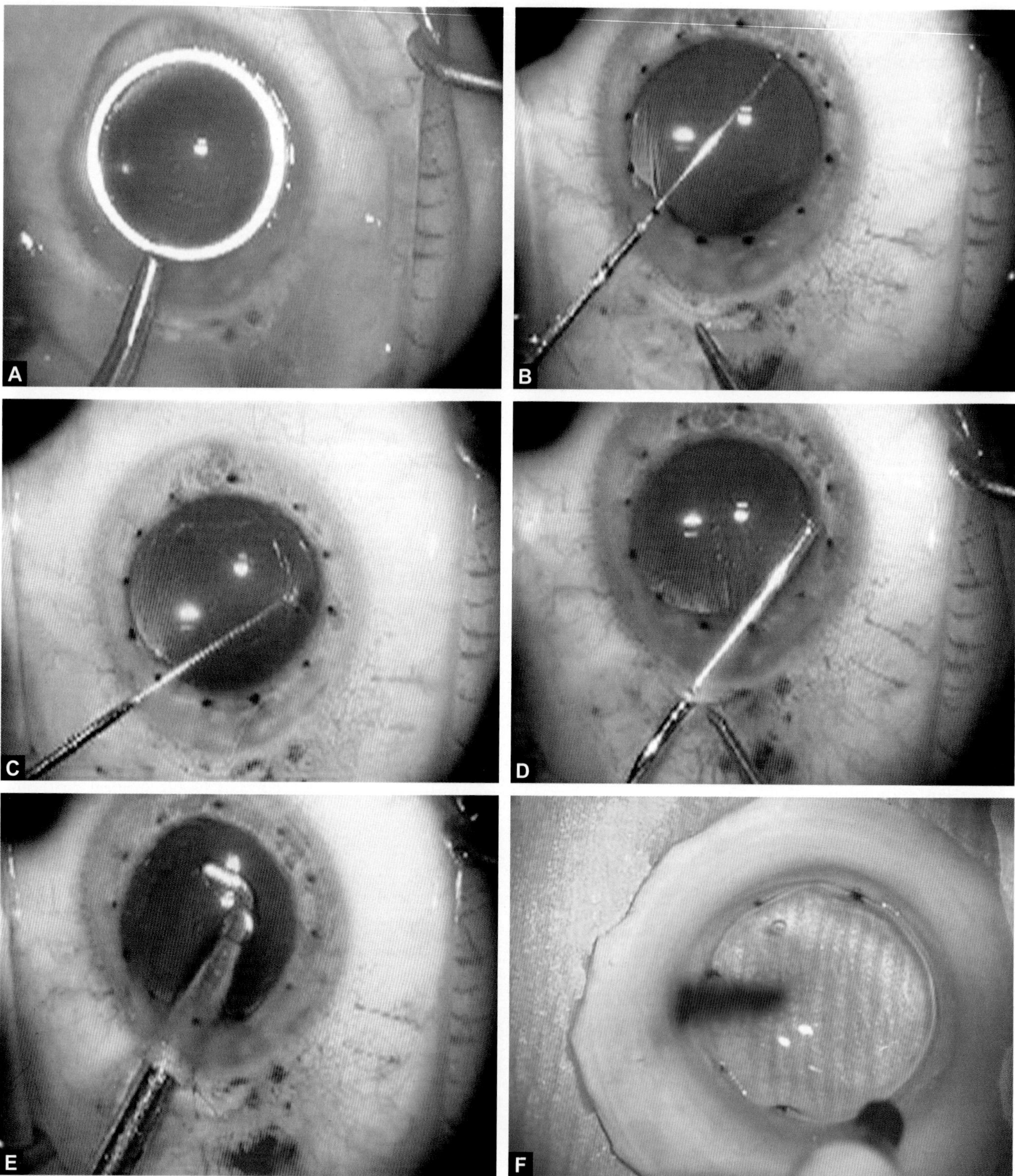


Figures 17-3A to F

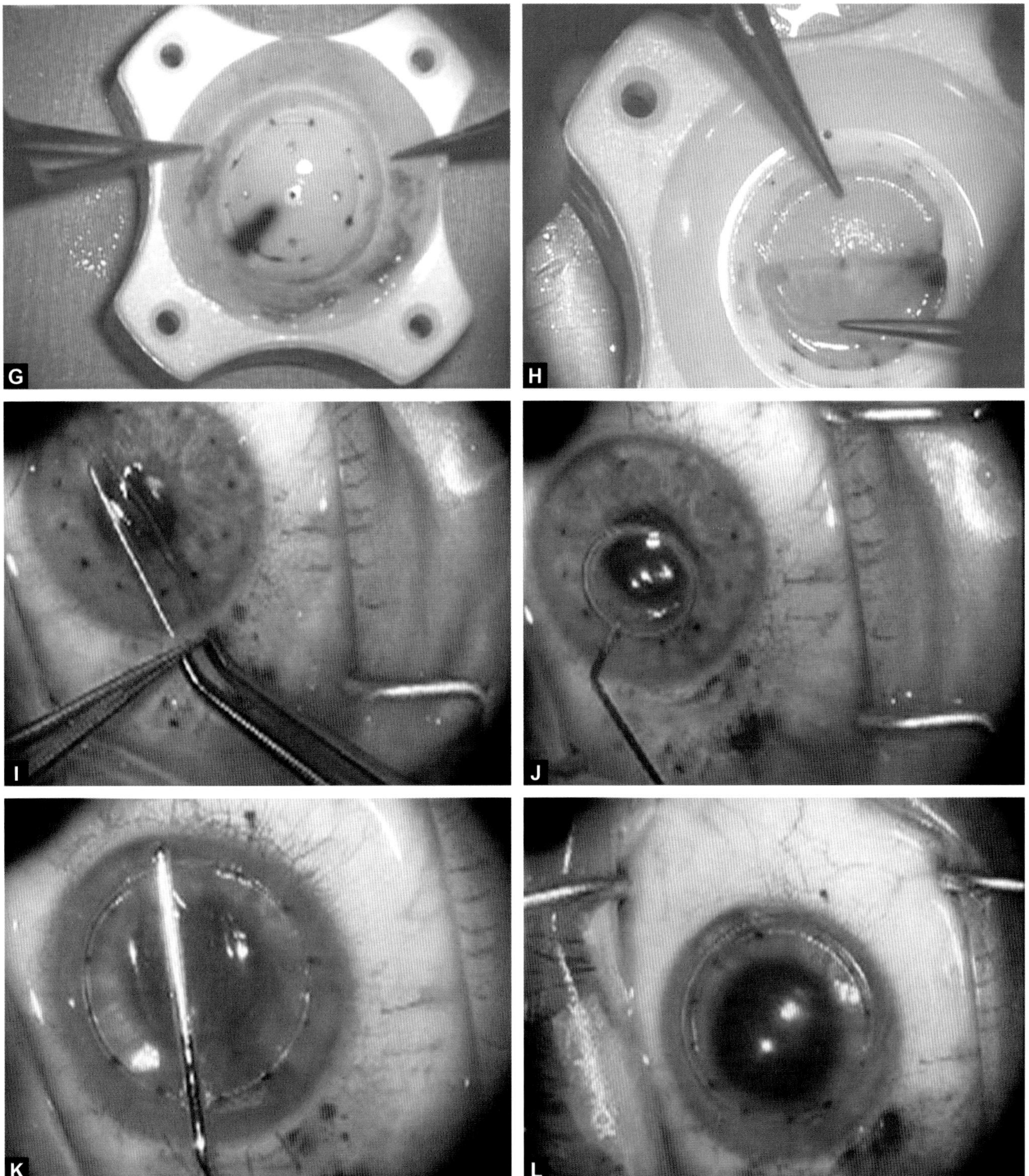


**Figures 17-3A to L** An overview of Descemet's stripping automated endothelial keratoplasty. (A to L): See description in the section "Surgical Technique: DSAEK."

*Source* Adapted with permission from Terry et al.[14]

- The graft is grasped with Charlie II non-coating forceps (Bausch and Lomb Surgical, St. Louis, MO, USA) and inserted with the 60% side facing anteriorly and the 40% side posteriorly (*see* Fig. 17-3I).
- BSS is injected to deepen the anterior chamber and partially unfold the graft. Air is injected to complete the unfolding of the graft endothelial-side down (*see* Fig. 17-3J).
- External compression with the Cindy Sweeper (Bausch and Lomb Surgical, St. Louis, MO, USA) is performed first to center the graft and then to remove interface fluid, by milking the interface from the center to the periphery while the anterior chamber is filled with air (*see* Fig. 17-3K).
- The wound is closed with absorbable sutures.
- The graft is left undisturbed under air for 10 full minutes. The air is then partially exchanged with BSS to prevent pupillary block. At the end of the case, an 8 mm or smaller freely mobile air bubble is left in the anterior chamber. Care is taken to ensure that no air remains posterior to the iris to prevent pupillary block (*see* Fig. 17-3L).

## SURGICAL TECHNIQUE: DMEK

- Inferotemporal and superotemporal paracenteses are created, and cohesive viscoelastic is used to fill the anterior chamber. An alternative to using viscoelastic is to fill the anterior chamber with air, or to use an anterior-chamber maintainer with an infusion of BSS.
- An optical marker representing the size of the DMEK graft is used to mark the epithelial surface of the recipient cornea. The graft size is selected relative to the size of the recipient cornea and is generally 7.75–8.5 mm.
- A 3.0–3.5 mm clear corneal incision is created.
- Descemet's membrane is stripped over the central 8.0–8.5 mm using a reverse Terry-Sinskey hook (Bausch and Lomb Surgical, St. Louis, MO, USA).
- An inferior peripheral iridotomy is created either preoperatively with a YAG laser or at the time of surgery using a bent 30-gauge needle and a Sinskey hook. This is performed to prevent pupillary block in a patient with a near-total intracameral air fill. If the patient is phakic, an inferior surgical iridectomy is created.
- A tissue injector is used in the wound to ensure an appropriate fit. Figures 17-4A to F describes various injectors that have been used for DMEK surgery. The wound size is adjusted as necessary. The viscoelastic is completely evacuated from the anterior chamber and from the tissue injector.
- The DMEK graft is generally stripped from the donor stroma prior to surgery. This avoids last-minute case cancellation should Descemet's membrane tear during graft stripping. Prestripped donor tissue is now available from several eye banks.
- If the pupil is not already miotic, intracameral carbachol is injected to induce miosis before graft insertion. This may offer endothelial protection as it minimizes endothelial contact with the intraocular posterior chamber lens.
- In the operating room, the graft is trephinated, then peeled from the donor stroma, and steeped in a bath of trypan blue.
- When the graft is adequately stained, it is loaded into a DMEK injector and inserted into the anterior chamber. It is of utmost importance that the eye not be overpressurized at the time of graft injection, so as to avoid tissue prolapse through the main wound or a paracentesis site. The wound is immediately sutured after tissue injection.
- The tissue is unfolded endothelial-side down with as little surgical manipulation as possible. Figures 17-5A to C illustrates that the endothelial side of the DMEK scroll is always oriented on the outside of the scroll; therefore, the scroll should be "upward facing" prior to unfolding. Ensuring that the tissue has been unfolded with the endothelium-side down is of paramount importance in DMEK surgery. Failure to do so results in primary iatrogenic graft failure. Figures 17-6A to D shows optical coherence tomography images of DMEK detachment postoperatively and how to determine graft orientation.
- Techniques used to verify correct DMEK graft orientation intraoperatively prior to unfolding are outlined below:
  - *Moutsouris sign*: the insertion of a cannula into one of the double scrolls of the DMEK graft to verify its orientation (*see* Figs. 17-7A to D).
  - Deepening the anterior chamber allows the DMEK graft to become less flattened and improves stereopsis, allowing the surgeon to better identify the orientation of the graft.
  - Injecting a small amount of fluid and inducing movement of graft allows for easier identification of graft orientation.
  - Using a hand-held portable slit beam can help identify the orientation of the DMEK graft.[16]
  - Using tangential light (by holding a light pipe obliquely to the cornea) can help identify the orientation of the DMEK graft.
- Another method to ensure proper graft orientation is the creation of asymmetrical notches in the rim of the DMEK graft (*see* Fig. 17-8). Correct orientation is confirmed after graft unfolding.
- Terry and colleagues have recently introduced the use of a preoperative blue "S" stamp onto the DMEK graft in order to ensure correct graft orientation.
- Unfolding techniques include:

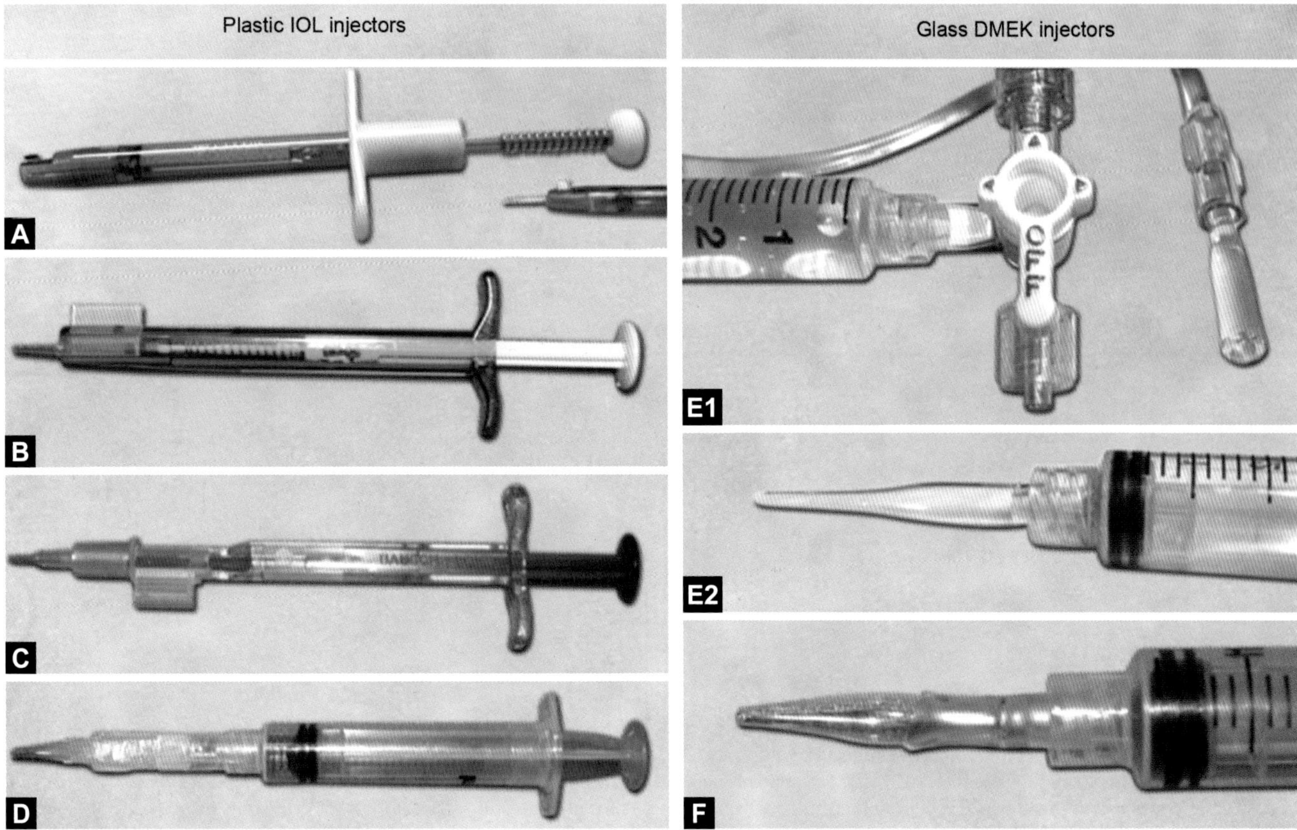


**Figures 17-4A to F** Descemet's membrane endothelial keratoplasty (DMEK) injectors. Various injectors have been used for DMEK tissue injection. (A to D) Intraocular lens (IOL) injectors have been used off-label for DMEK tissue insertion. However, IOL injection devices are not connected to a syringe of balanced salt solution (BSS), which can lead to inadvertent injury to fragile graft tissue. Moreover, the spring present in some injectors can be cumbersome and flimsy for the purpose of graft injection. Injector A requires the use of cohesive viscoelastic, which can interfere with graft unfolding. Injector D has been fashioned by the surgeon using an IOL cartridge, a sterile plastic pipette, tape, and a syringe filled with BSS; assembly is time consuming and the injector can be prone to leaks. (E to F) Glass injectors designed for DMEK surgery. Glass is believed by some to be associated with less endothelial damage as compared to plastic. DMEK injector E has been used in Europe (Geuder AG, Heidelberg, Germany) and connects to a syringe of BSS. The tissue is loaded via the larger end (E1) before the glass tip is attached to a syringe filled with BSS. The tissue is injected via the narrow end (E2). DMEK injector F is a Straiko DMEK modified Jones tube glass tip, made by Gunther Weiss (Portland, Oregon). This glass tube is connected to 14 French tubing, which then creates a watertight seal with a syringe filled with BSS. Both injectors use a continuous stream of BSS that greatly facilitates graft insertion.

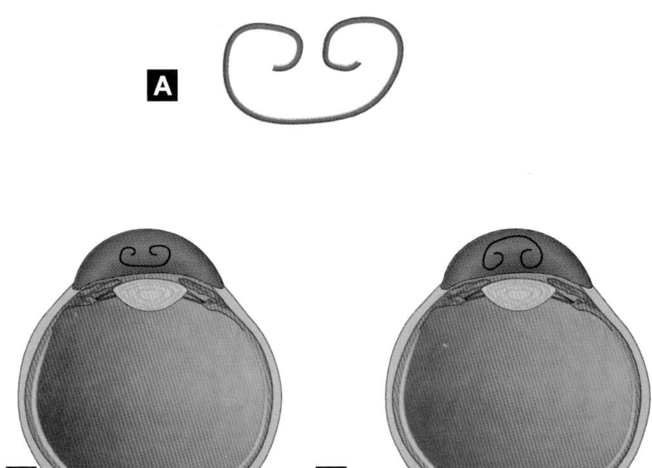


**Figures 17-5A to C** Orientation of the Descemet's membrane endothelial keratoplasty (DMEK) graft. The DMEK graft naturally forms a scroll. The endothelial side of the graft is always found on the outside of the scroll, indicated by the blue line in Figure A. Figure B shows correct orientation of the DMEK graft inside the anterior chamber prior to unfolding, with the scroll facing upward. The scroll must always be upward facing to achieve unfolding of the graft with the endothelium facing downward. Figure C shows incorrect orientation with the scroll facing downward. Unfolding in this position will result in an incorrectly oriented graft with the endothelium facing upward, which will result in primary iatrogenic graft failure.

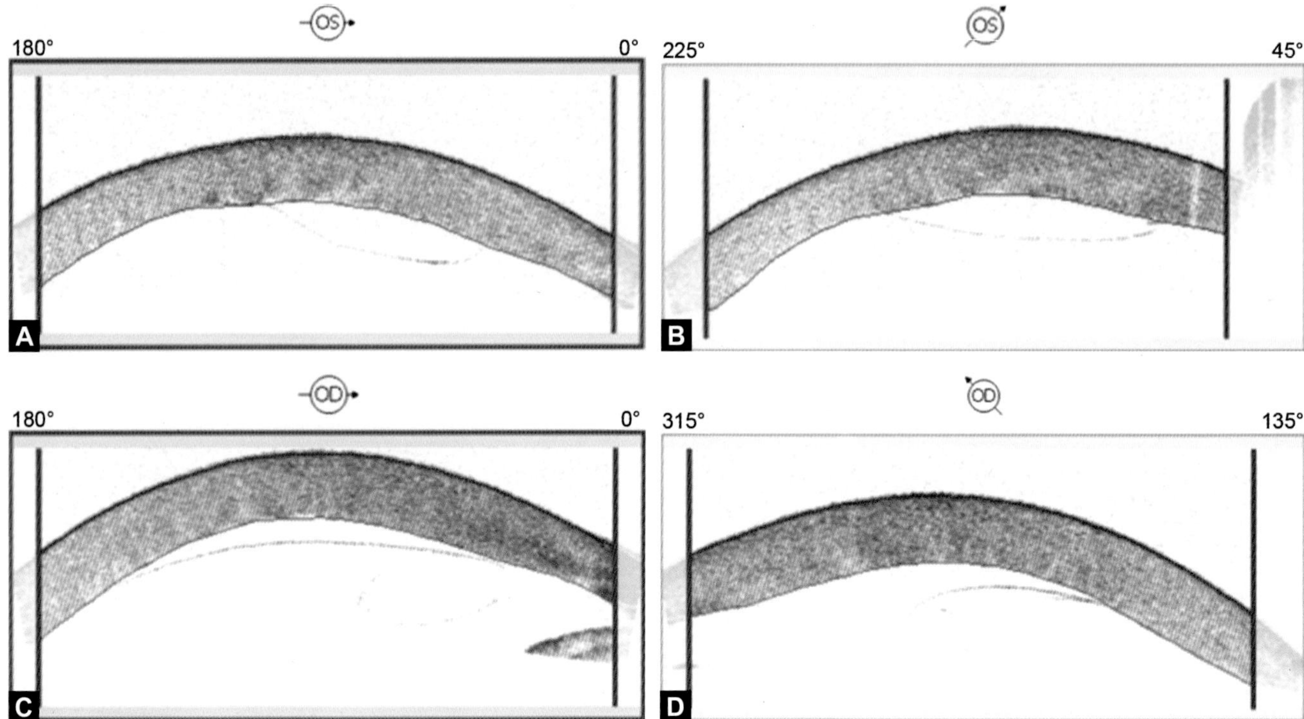


**Figures 17-6A to D** Descemet's membrane endothelial keratoplasty (DMEK) detachment: Determining graft orientation postoperatively. Optical coherence tomography images illustrating partial DMEK graft detachment. Figures A and B show the graft edge curling toward the recipient stroma in one patient. This indicates that the endothelium is correctly oriented, or downward facing, as the endothelium is always located on the outside of the scroll. Figures C and D are images from a different patient's eye, and show the graft edge curling toward the anterior chamber, indicating that the endothelium is oriented toward the recipient stroma—the graft is inverted and results in primary iatrogenic graft failure.

  - Using an air bubble inside the DMEK scroll to help it unfold with directed taps on the surface of the host cornea[15]
  - Using a large air bubble anterior to the DMEK graft to flatten the graft; however, this pushes the endothelium against the iris and IOL[15]
  - Using the Yoeruek tap technique to unfold the tissue in the setting of a shallow anterior chamber, without intracameral air. With this technique, a cannula or spatula is used to deliver directed taps to the surface of the host cornea and digital pressure to the globe, generating an intracameral fluid wave that facilitates DMEK unfolding.[18]
- Once the tissue is unfolded, air or a nonexpansile concentration (20%) of $SF_6$ gas is injected posterior to the graft, in the very center of the pupil to avoid decentration. The graft is left undisturbed under air or gas for 10 minutes. A partial BSS-air (or gas) exchange is performed so as to reduce the intracameral bubble to approximately 9 or 10 mm, ensuring that the peripheral iridotomy will be uncovered in the upright position. It is important to ensure that no air or gas is posterior to the iris at the end of the case.

## COMPLICATIONS AFTER EK

- Primary Iatrogenic graft failure
  - This is defined as failure of the graft to clear within 6 weeks postoperatively and can most often be attributed to endothelial damage secondary to surgical trauma
  - Rates of primary graft failure after DSAEK in the largest published series by Terry are under 1%, with a forceps insertion[14,19,20]
  - New data show that the rate of primary graft failure after DMEK has been improving with surgeons' experience.[21] While initial studies reported failure rates of 8%[22] and 20%,[23] more recent data show a 2–3% failure rate[21,24] and is, therefore, not dramatically different from DSAEK.
- Graft dislocation
  - This complication most commonly arises from endothelial damage secondary to surgical trauma.
  - Other causes can include hypotony, retained viscoelastic, residual interface fluid, eye rubbing, and an unrecognized upside-down graft.
  - "Rebubbling" is performed for significant graft dislocation (*see* Fig. 17-9).

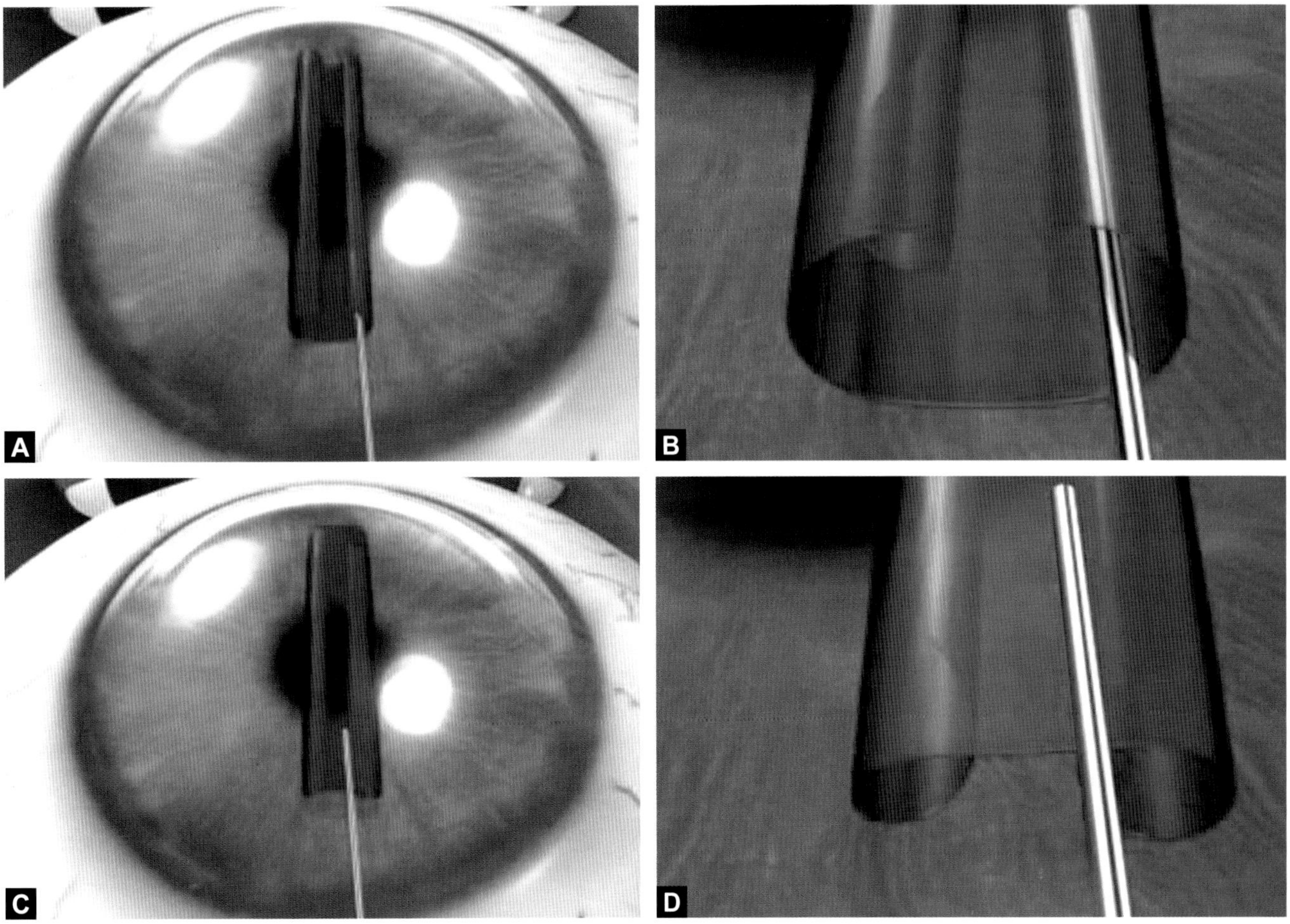

**Figures 17-7A to D** Moutsouris sign. Moutsouris sign occurs when a cannula is inserted into one of the double scrolls of the Descemet's membrane endothelial keratoplasty graft. That is if the scroll edges are facing anteriorly (correct orientation), then moving the cannula from the center into one of the double scrolls will change the color of the cannula tip from silver to blue (positive Moutsouris sign, A and B). If the scroll edges are facing posteriorly (inverted orientation), moving the cannula from the center to one side causes no color change, as the cannula is above the graft edges (C and D).
*Source* Adapted with permission from Dapena et al.[15]

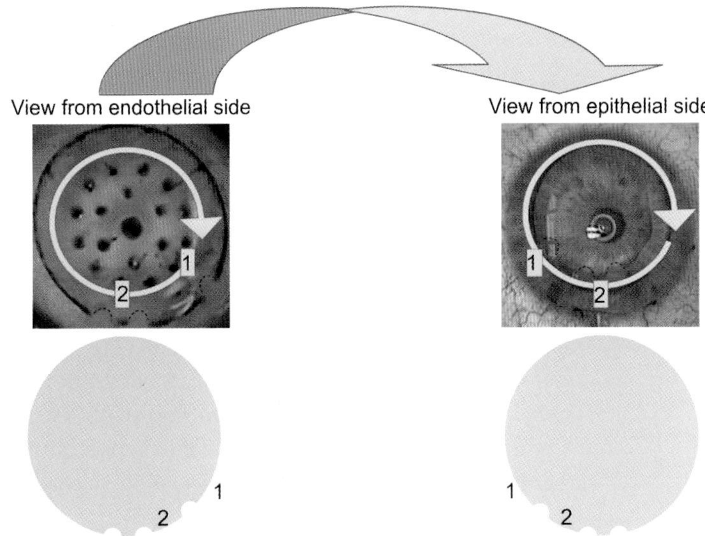


**Figure 17-8** Using asymmetric notches in Descemet's membrane endothelial keratoplasty (DMEK) graft edge to ensure correct orientation intraoperatively. A 1-mm trephine is used to create three asymmetric notches along the DMEK graft edge. View from the endothelial side is shown on the left, whereas view from the epithelial side is shown on the right. Clockwise inspection of the graft shows that the notches 1 and then 2 are perceived from the endothelial side, whereas notches 2 and then 1 are seen from the epithelial side (when the graft is in correct, endothelial-side down position in the anterior chamber).
*Source* Adapted with permission from Bachmann et al.[17]

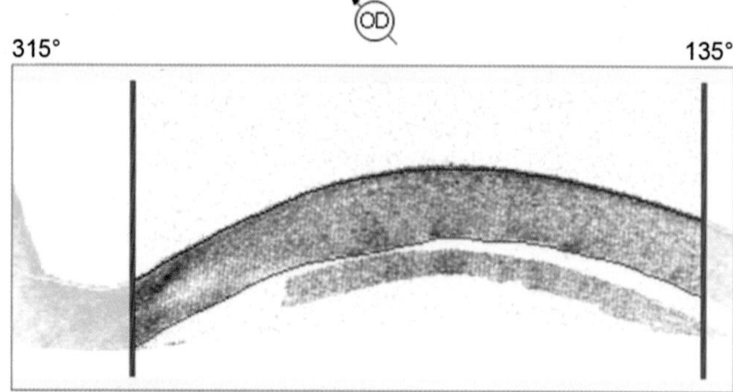


**Figure 17-9** Complete Descemet's stripping automated endothelial keratoplasty detachment as seen with optical coherence tomography.

- Dislocation rates of 2–3% are reported in the largest published DSAEK studies by Goshe et al.[25] and by Anshu et al.[26]
- Dislocation and rebubbling rates in DMEK studies are also reported to improve with surgeons' experience. Guerra et al. reported rebubbling rates that improved from 62% initially[22] to 14% more recently, which they attribute using an inserter that avoids the use of viscoelastic.[21,27] Melles' group once reported a detachment rate of 24%[28] while more recently reporting a detachment rate of 4%.[24,29]

- Glaucoma
  - Pupillary block can arise in the immediate postoperative period due to the presence of an intracameral air bubble without adequate pupillary dilation or without an adequate inferior iridotomy.
  - Steroid-response glaucoma is the most common type of glaucoma following EK.
- Graft rejection
  - Graft rejection is thought to occur in approximately 10% of patients postoperatively in DSAEK.[30]
  - Anshu et al. demonstrated a rejection rate of under 1% within 2 years following DMEK.[3]
- Endophthalmitis
- Dislocation of graft into the posterior segment
- Infectious keratitis
- Epithelial downgrowth into venting incisions

## LONG-TERM OUTCOMES

- Endothelial cell density (ECD) is thought to reflect the long-term health of a corneal transplant.
- Endothelial cell loss (ECL) is calculated as follows:

$$\frac{\text{Preoperative graft ECD} - \text{Current postoperative ECD}}{\text{Preoperative graft ECD}}$$

  - ECL after DSAEK was 23–24% at 6 months, 1 year, and 2 years postoperatively, as reported by Terry et al., using a 40–60 underfolding technique with forceps through a 5-mm scleral tunnel incision.[31]
  - Other large studies by Terry et al. and by Price et al. reported ECL of 31–37% at 1 year.[19,32-35]
  - ECL after DMEK has been reported by Price and Melles' groups to be in the range of 34–36%[22,36] at 1 year, which is comparable to that of DSAEK.
  - There have also been two different studies comparing ECD between DSAEK and DMEK, with neither study finding significant differences between the two.[21,37,38]
- Late endothelial failure is defined as graft failure at least 6 weeks after surgery, after initial corneal deturgescence.

## PEARLS AND PITFALLS

- The use of larger diameter grafts in DSAEK has not been shown to lessen ECL.[26,39]
- There are many different forms of tissue insertion in DSAEK. The method of tissue insertion that causes the least amount of endothelial damage should be employed. Endothelial cell densities using noncoapting forceps techniques have been the most widely validated form of tissue insertion with good published ECD results.[40,41] Other tissue insertion techniques include a pull-through or push-through technique with a suture, needle, Busin glide, and endoglide. Tissue platform injectors such as the endoserter and NCI devices are also now available.
- DSAEK tissue insertion (without injectors) through a 3-mm incision causes more ECL than through a 5-mm incision.[42] Increased cell loss is due to increased endothelial trauma while the graft tissue is compressed to fit through a smaller wound.
- Lens extraction should generally be performed concurrently with EK if a significant cataract is present and endothelial replacement is needed. One study demonstrated that patients >50 years of age at the time of phakic DSAEK were more likely to require cataract surgery within 3 years postoperatively (55%) than those <50 years of age (7%).[43]
- "Ultrathin DSAEK" surgery attempts to achieve a postoperative donor thickness on optical coherence tomography of ≤100 mm, in the hopes of achieving better visual acuity and quality of vision than conventional DSAEK. Some authors have reported improved visual acuity outcomes with this technique,[44,45] whereas other series have not substantiated an association between graft thickness and visual results.[46,47]

## FUTURE HORIZONS FOR ENDOTHELIAL REPLACEMENT

Rho-kinase (ROCK) inhibitor eye drops have been demonstrated to have a beneficial effect on endothelial healing and proliferation.[48,49] It is conceivable that these could play a role in the pharmacological treatment of endothelial dysfunction in years to come.

In addition to this, corneal endothelial cell lines are under active investigation in a laboratory setting.[49,50] The transplantation of cultured endothelial cells may very well replace cadaveric allografts in the future.

## REFERENCES


1. Talajic JC, Straiko MD, Terry MA. Descemet's stripping automated endothelial keratoplasty: then and now. Int Ophthalmol Clin. 2013;53(2):1-20. doi: 10.1097/IIO.0b013e31827eb6ba.
2. EBAA. 2005-2012 Eye Banking statistical reports. Washington, DC: Eye Bank Association of America.
3. Anshu A, Price MO, Price FW Jr. Risk of corneal transplant rejection significantly reduced with Descemet's membrane endothelial keratoplasty. Ophthalmology. 2012;119:536-40.
4. Tillet CW. Posterior lamellar keratoplasty. Am J Ophthalmol. 1956;41:530-33.
5. KoW, Freuh B, Shield C, et al. Experimental posterior lamellar transplantation of the rabbit cornea. Invest Ophthalmol Vis Sci. 1993;34:1102.
6. Barraquer J, Rutlan J (eds), The technique for penetrating keratoplasty. Microsurgery of the cornea. Barcelona, Spain: Scriba; 1984:289-94.
7. Melles GR, Eggink FA, Lander F, et al. A surgical technique for posterior lamellar keratoplasty. Cornea. 1998;17:618-26.
8. Terry MA, Ousley PJ. Deep lamellar endothelial keratoplasty in the first United States patients: early clinical results. Cornea. 2001;20:239-43.
9. Melles GR, Wijdh RH, Nieuwendaal CP. A technique to excise the Descemet membrane from a recipient cornea (descemetorhexis). Cornea. 2004;23:286-8.
10. Price FW, Jr, Price MO. Descemet's stripping with endothelial keratoplasty in 50 eyes: a refractive neutral corneal transplant. J Refract Surg. 2005;21:339-45.
11. Gorovoy MS. Descemet-stripping automated endothelial keratoplasty. Cornea.2006;25:886-9.
12. Melles GR, Lander F, Rietveld FJ. Transplantation of Descemet's membrane carrying viable endothelium through a small scleral incision. Cornea. 2002;21:415-8.
13. McCauley MB, Price FW, Price MO. Descemet membrane automated endothelial keratoplasty: hybrid technique combining DSAEK stability with DMEK visual results. J Cataract Refract Surg. 2009;35:1659-64.
14. Terry MA, Shamie N, Chen ES, et al. Endothelial keratoplasty a simplified technique to minimize graft dislocation, iatrogenic graft failure, and pupillary block. Ophthalmology. 2008;115(7):1179-86.
15. Dapena I, Moutsouris K, Droutsas K, et al. Standardized "no-touch" technique for Descemet membrane endothelial keratoplasty. Arch Ophthalmol. 2011;129(1):88-94.
16. Burkhart ZN, Feng MT, Price MO, et al. Handheld slit beam techniques to facilitate DMEK and DALK. Cornea. 2013;32(5): 722-4.
17. Bachmann BO, Laaser K, Cursiefen C, et al. A method to confirm correct orientation of Descemet membrane during Descemet membrane endothelial keratoplasty. Am J Ophthalmol. 2010;149(6):922-925.e2.
18. Yoeruek E, Bayyoud T, Hofmann J, et al. Novel maneuver facilitating Descemet membrane unfolding in the anterior chamber. Cornea. 2013;32(3):370-3.
19. Terry MA, Shamie N, Chen ES, et al. Endothelial keratoplasty for Fuchs' dystrophy with cataract: complications and clinical results with the new triple procedure. Ophthalmology. 2009;116:631-9.
20. Terry MA, Shamie N, Chen ES, et al. Endothelial keratoplasty: the influence of preoperative donor endothelial densities on dislocations, primary graft failure, and one year cell counts. Cornea. 2008;27:1131-7.
21. Feng MT, Price MO, Price FW, Jr. Update on Descemet membrane endothelial keratoplasty (DMEK). Int Ophthalmol Clin. 2013;53(2):31-45.
22. Guerra FP, Anshu A, Price MO, et al. Descemet's membrane endothelial keratoplasty: prospective study of 1-year visual outcomes, graft survival, and endothelial cell loss. Ophthalmology. 2011;118:2368-73.
23. Dapena I, Ham L, van Luijk C, et al. Back-up procedure for graft failure in Descemet membrane endothelial keratoplasty (DMEK). Br J Ophthalmol. 2010;94:241-4.
24. Dapena I, Ham L, Droutsas K, et al. Learning curve in Descemet's membrane endothelial keratoplasty: first series of 135 consecutive cases. Ophthalmology. 2011;118:2147-54.
25. Goshe JM, Terry MA, Li JY, et al. Graft dislocation and hypotony after Descemet's stripping automated endothelial keratoplasty in patients with previous glaucoma surgery. Ophthalmology. 2012;119:1130-3.
26. Anshu A, Price MO, Price FW, Jr. Descemet stripping automated endothelial keratoplasty for Fuchs endothelial dystrophy-influence of graft diameter on endothelial cell loss. Cornea. 2013;32(1):5-8.
27. Price MO, Price FW, Jr. Effect of preparation-to-use time on DMEK outcomes. Eye Bank Association of America annual meeting, June 23, 2012, Hollywood, FL.
28. Dirisamer M, van Dijk K, Dapena I, et al. Prevention and management of graft detachment in Descemet membrane endothelial keratoplasty. Arch Ophthalmol. 2012;130:280-91.
29. Parker J, Dirisamer M, Naveiras M, et al. Outcomes of Descemet membrane endothelial keratoplasty in phakic eyes. J Cataract Refract Surg. 2012;38:871-7.
30. Lee WB, Jacobs DS, Musch DC, et al. Descemet's stripping endothelial keratoplasty: safety and outcomes: a report by the American Academy of Ophthalmology. Ophthalmology. 2009;116:1818-30. Review.
31. Terry MA, Li J, Goshe J, et al. Endothelial keratoplasty: the relationship between donor tissue size and donor endothelial survival. Ophthalmology. 2011;118:1944-9.

32. Terry MA, Shamie N, Straiko MD, et al. Endothelial keratoplasty: the relationship between donor tissue storage time and donor endothelial survival. Ophthalmology. 2011;118:36-40.
33. Price MO, Price FW. Endothelial cell loss after Descemet's stripping with endothelial keratoplasty: influencing factors and 2-year trend. Ophthalmology. 2008;115:857-65.
34. Terry MA, Chen ES, Shamie N, et al. Endothelial cell loss after Descemet's stripping endothelial keratoplasty in a large prospective series. Ophthalmology. 2008;115:488-96.
35. Price MO, Fairchild KM, Price DA, et al. Descemet's stripping endothelial keratoplasty five-year graft survival and endothelial cell loss. Ophthalmology. 2011;118: 725-9.
36. Ham L, Dapena I, Van Der Wees J, et al. Endothelial cell density after descemet membrane endothelial keratoplasty: 1- to 3-year follow-up. Am J Ophthalmol. 2010;149(6):1016-7.
37. Tourtas T, Laaser K, Bachmann BO, et al. Descemet membrane endothelial keratoplasty versus descemet stripping automated endothelial keratoplasty. Am J Ophthalmol. 2012;153:1082.e2-1090.e2.
38. Guerra FP, Anshu A, Price MO, et al. Endothelial keratoplasty: fellow eyes comparison of Descemet stripping automated endothelial keratoplasty and Descemet membrane endothelial keratoplasty. Cornea. 2011;30:1382-6.
39. Terry MA, Li J, Goshe J, et al. Endothelial keratoplasty: the relationship between donor tissue size and donor endothelial survival. Ophthalmology. 2011;118:1944-9.
40. Price MO, Fairchild KM, Price DA, et al. Descemet's stripping endothelial keratoplasty five-year graft survival and endothelial cell loss. Ophthalmology. 2011;118:725-9.
41. Terry MA, Shamie N, Straiko MD, et al. Endothelial keratoplasty: the relationship between donor tissue storage time and donor endothelial survival. Ophthalmology.2011;118:36-40.
42. Price MO, Bidros M, Gorovoy M, et al. Effect of incision width on graft survival andendothelial cell loss after Descemet stripping automated endothelial keratoplasty. Cornea. 2010;29: 523-7.
43. Price MO, Price DA, Fairchild KM, et al. Rate and risk factors for cataract formation and extraction after Descemet stripping endothelial keratoplasty. Br J Ophthalmol. 2010;94:1468-71.
44. Neff KD, Biber JM, Holland EJ. Comparison of central corneal graft thickness to visual acuity outcomes in endothelial keratoplasty. Cornea. 2011;30:388-91.
45. Dickman MM, Cheng YY, Berendschot TT, et al. Effects of graft thickness and asymmetry on visual gain and aberrations after Descemet stripping automated endothelial keratoplasty. JAMA Ophthalmol. 2013;131(6):737-44.
46. Terry MA, Straiko MD, Goshe JM, et al. Descemet's stripping automated endothelial keratoplasty: the tenuous relationship between donor thickness and postoperative vision. Ophthalmology. 2012;119:1988-96.
47. Phillips PM, Phillips LJ, Maloney CM. Preoperative graft thickness measurements do not influence final BSCVA or speed of vision recovery after Descemet stripping automated endothelial keratoplasty. Cornea. 2013;32(11):1423-7.
48. Okumura N, Koizumi N, Ueno M, et al. Enhancement of corneal endothelium wound healing by Rho-associated kinase (ROCK) inhibitor eyedrops. Br J Ophthalmol. 2011;95:1006-9.
49. Okumura N, Ueno M, Koizumi N, et al. Enhancement on primate corneal endothelial cell survival in vitro by a ROCK inhibitor. Invest Ophthalmol Vis Sci. 2009;50:3680-7.
50. Haydari MN, Perron MC, Laprise S, et al. A short-term in vivo experimental model for Fuchs endothelial corneal dystrophy. Invest Ophthalmol Vis Sci. 2012;53(10):6343-54.

CHAPTER

# 18

# Anterior Lamellar Keratoplasty

Donald TH Tan, Marcus Ang

## INTRODUCTION

Penetrating keratoplasty (PK) is still the predominant form of corneal transplantation today; however, anterior lamellar keratoplasty (ALK) exists as an alternative form of transplantation that involves targeted replacement of the corneal stroma without replacement of the healthy endothelium.[1] ALK obviates the risk of endothelial allograft rejection, leading to better preservation of endothelial cells over time and, subsequently, improved graft survival.[2] Largely a nonpenetrating procedure, ALK results in a tectonically stronger eye with reduced risk of intraoperative complications, such as expulsive hemorrhage, glaucoma, and endophthalmitis, Table 18-1.[3] Due to the reduced need for long-term topical corticosteroids, other steroid-related complications, such as cataract and raised intraocular pressure, may also be reduced.[2]

For decades, few corneal surgeons practiced ALK surgery due to the surgical challenges of lamellar stromal dissection and the potential for reduced visual outcomes in less experienced hands. However, with the onset of surgical advances and the more recent evolution of ALK toward deeper dissection, i.e. deep ALK (DALK), we are achieving better visual outcomes which match PK surgery. Predescemetic DALK involves the subtotal removal of corneal stroma, with the retention of a thin posterior stromal layer, Descemet's membrane (DM), and host corneal endothelium. Newer DALK techniques now allow for complete stromal removal, with the baring of DM (descemetic DALK), Figure 18-1.

Recent studies of DALK now suggest that this procedure may be able to attain visual outcomes equivalent to PK in terms of best-spectacle corrected visual acuity, whereas refractive outcomes remain similar.[2] Although DM baring with descemetic DALK may be more challenging or difficult to achieve, descemetic DALK is associated with a better visual outcome due to lack of a manually dissected stroma-to-stroma interface, which occurs in predescemetic DALK.[4-6]

### Indications for ALK

The indications for ALK are usually limited to conditions affecting only the cornea stroma, such as keratoconus, post-traumatic, infectious or inflammatory stromal scarring, or corneal stromal dystrophies. (Summary of indications in Table 18-2.) Techniques of DALK surgery enable deeper and

**TABLE 18-1** Advantages and disadvantages comparing anterior lamellar keratoplasty (ALK) to penetrating keratoplasty (PK)

| Advantages of ALK | Disadvantages of ALK |
|---|---|
| • Extraocular technique with reduced risks associated with intraocular surgery, such as endophthalmitis, glaucoma, cataract formation, and expulsive hemorrhage<br>• No risk of endothelial rejection, although epithelial and stromal rejection may still occur<br>• Tectonically stronger eye<br>• Corneal donors with low endothelial quality may be utilized for ALK surgery<br>• Lower duration of immunosuppressant therapy required | • Technically demanding, longer surgery<br>• Lamellar interface problems, residual scarring, and irregular recipient stromal bed dissection affect visual outcomes<br>• Perforation of Descemet's membrane during deep ALK surgery may necessitate conversion to PK |

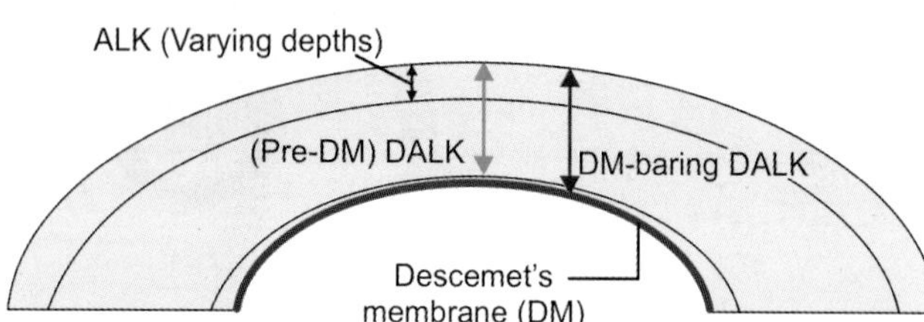


**Figure 18-1** Diagram depicting the spectrum of anterior lamellar keratoplasty (ALK) surgeries. The evolution of ALK from manual dissection techniques to achieve predescemetic deep ALK (DALK) (Malbran1965),[7] intrastromal air injection (Archila 1985),[8] hydrodelamination (Sugita & Kondo)[12] to descemetic DALK techniques, most notably the "big-bubble" technique (Anwar & Teichmann).[4]

**TABLE 18-2** Summary of indications for anterior lamellar keratoplasty

| | |
|---|---|
| Optical indications | • Keratoconus<br>• Pellucid marginal degeneration<br>• Post laser-assisted in situ keratomileusis ectasia<br>• Corneal stromal dystrophies<br>• Anterior stromal scaring |
| Therapeutic indications | • Infectious keratitis |
| Tectonic indications | • Corneal perforations<br>• Corneal thinning disorders, ectasias, and descemetoceles |

more consistent removal of stromal disease down to DM, Figure 18-2.[9] Other optical indications for ALK include other forms of corneal ectasia (pellucid marginal degeneration, post-LASIK, laser-assisted in situ keratomileusis, ectasia) and other postrefractive surgery complications, which cause stromal opacities or scarring. Therapeutic indications for ALK are mainly for unperforated cases of active infectious keratitis not responding to medical therapy. Since ALK is mainly extraocular, there is a reduced risk of intraocular spread of infection (i.e. endophthalmitis) and a lower risk of subsequent endothelial rejection or failure, compared with PK. Deeper dissection using descemetic DALK techniques (described below) has been shown to be useful for infective keratitis and reduced recurrent infection compared with PK, Figures 18-3A to D.[10] Although more technically challenging, ALK is useful for tectonic indications, such as descemetoceles and small corneal perforations, which may be secondary to underlying pathologies such as inflammation, infection, trauma, or ocular surface disease. For these tectonic indications, ALK surgeries have shown better physiological graft survival compared with the traditional PK, and the relative ease of repeat ALK transplantation is an important benefit in many of these relapsing conditions.[11]

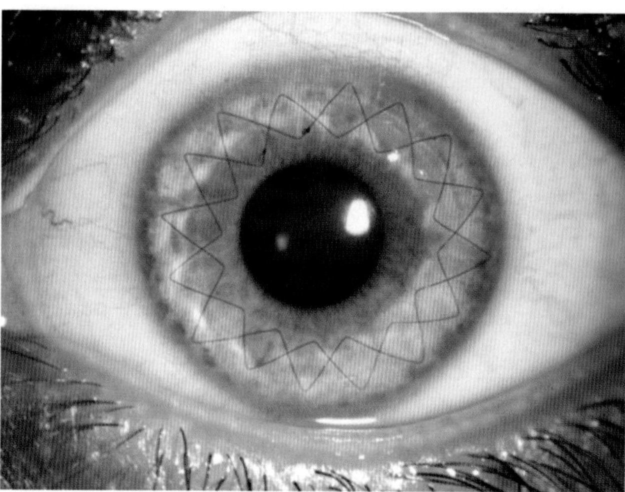

**Figure 18-2** Deep anterior lamellar keratoplasty, postoperative appearance with continuous sutures.

## CONTRAINDICATIONS

Generally, ALK may be considered for all corneal pathologies other than those pathologies affecting the endothelium (such as aphakic and pseudophakic bullous keratopathy, Fuchs' endothelial dystrophy, iridocorneal endothelial syndrome, and posterior polymorphous dystrophy). Although deeper scars or pre-existing defects involving the DM are relative contraindications to DALK by virtue of greater surgical difficulties, it still may be possible to perform predescemetic DALK by leaving a thin layer of posterior stroma in place.

## SURGICAL TECHNIQUES

### Anterior Lamellar Keratoplasty

The original ALK technique was first described using a manual, layer-by-layer dissection, with various modifications described in Table 18-3. In the conventional technique of manual ALK dissection, a partial trephination to the desired corneal depth is first performed, followed by layered stromal dissection and removal using blunt lamellar dissectors or sharper crescent blades, Figures 18-4A and B. This technique is time consuming and technically challenging, with visual outcomes inversely proportional to the depth of dissection achieved. There exists a significant risk of DM perforation when attempting to bare DM, whereas an imperfect recipient stromal bed dissection will affect the final visual outcome.[12] The use of intrastromal air injection to assist in stromal dissection was first described by Achilar; here the corneal stroma was made to appear opaque

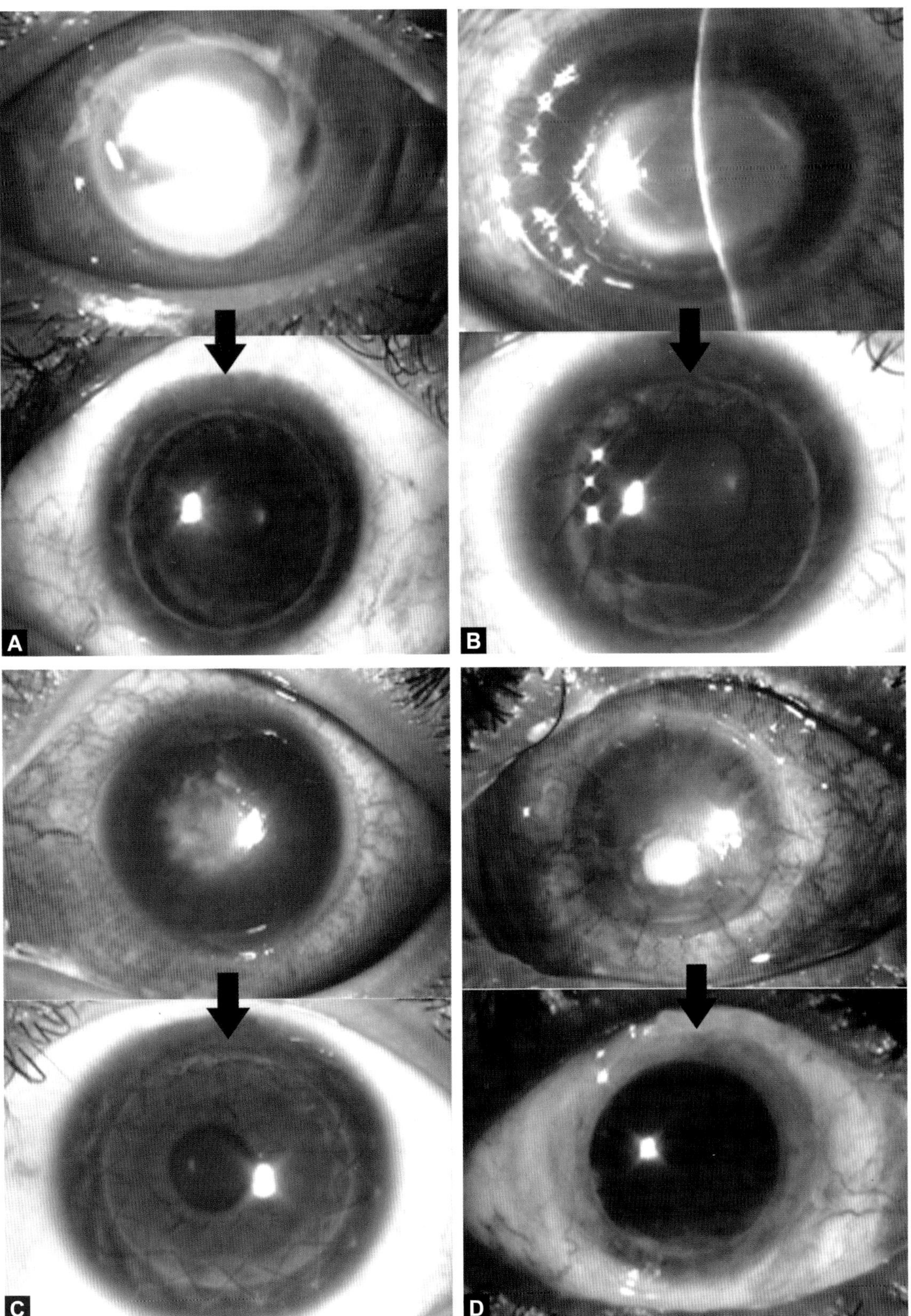


**Figures 18-3A to D** Therapeutic deep anterior lamellar keratoplasty (DALK) to treat infective keratitis: examples of severe infections successfully treated with DALK (preoperative and postoperative photos), which include *Pseudomonas* (A), *Acanthamoeba* (B), Fusarium (C), and Acremonium (D) Infective keratitis.

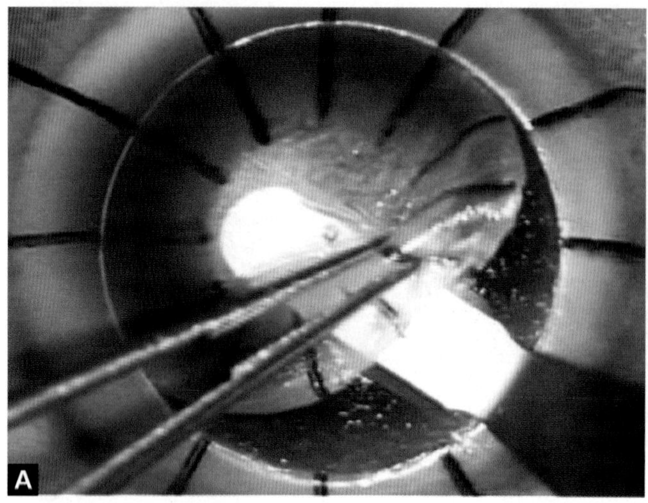

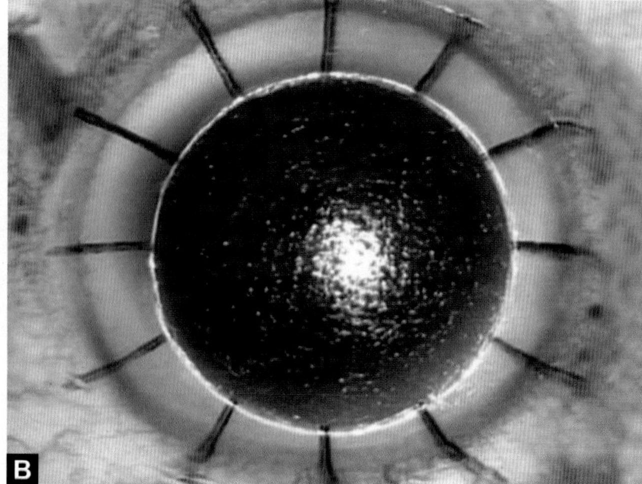

**Figures 18-4A and B** Manual dissection technique used in predescemetic deep anterior lamellar keratoplasty showing (A) the layered corneal dissection and (B) resultant thin stromal bed.

**TABLE 18-3** Summary and classification of anterior lamellar keratoplasty (ALK) techniques

| Type of ALK | Surgical technique |
|---|---|
| ALK | • Manual layer-by-layer dissection<br>• Intrastromal air<br>• Hydrodissection (saline) |
| Deep ALK (DALK)<br>– Predescemetic DALK<br>– Descemetic DALK | • Manual dissection<br>• Air-assisted<br>• Big-bubble technique<br>• Viscoelastic |
| Microkeratome-assisted ALK | • Automated lamellar therapeutic keratoplasty |
| Femtosecond laser-assisted ALK | |

with "microbubbles," followed by a manual dissection of the emphysematous corneal layers.[13] This technique ultimately led to the discovery of the use of air to separate DM from posterior stroma (*see* below). Another use of air during ALK to enhance visualization of the depth of lamellar dissection involves filling the anterior chamber (AC) completely with air to create an air interface. This generates a reflection of DM in relation to the depth of the lamellar dissector within the stromal pocket, helping to achieve as deep a stromal dissection as possible while lessening the risk of direct DM entry.[14] The use of "hydrodelamination" to aid manual dissection has also been described using intrastromal balanced salt solution injection.[12] Saline solution is injected directly into the cornea to enhance identification and removal of the deeper stromal fibers.[12]

## Deep ALK (Predescemetic DALK)

Manual dissection DALK, using the layer-by-layer technique of stromal removal, was first described leaving up to about 10% of the remaining posterior stroma and DM behind (i.e. predescemetic DALK) to avoid the risk of inadvertent perforation; however, the remnant stromal layers could lead to interface irregularities and, thus, poorer visual outcomes. This basic manual technique using a layered corneal dissection is still useful in cases with deeper pre-existing corneal scars with DM adhesions or DM defects, which may preclude baring of the DM. It also remains a very useful back-up technique when big bubble DALK surgery fails (see below) or as a rescue procedure when DM perforation occurs.

## Descemetic DALK – "Big-bubble" Technique

The most recent breakthrough in DALK, which has revitalized anterior lamellar surgery, is the "big bubble" DALK technique first described by Anwar and Teichmann, Figures 18-5A to C. A partial-depth trephine cut is first performed followed by insertion of a 27-gauge needle attached to an air-filled syringe. This is inserted carefully into the deep corneal stroma from the edge of the partial corneal trephination margin until it reaches the mid-periphery of the cornea.[4] A forceful injection of air into the stromal tissue then causes a sudden separation of the DM from the posterior stromal surface. Manual dissection and removal of the overlying stroma above the big bubble is then accomplished.

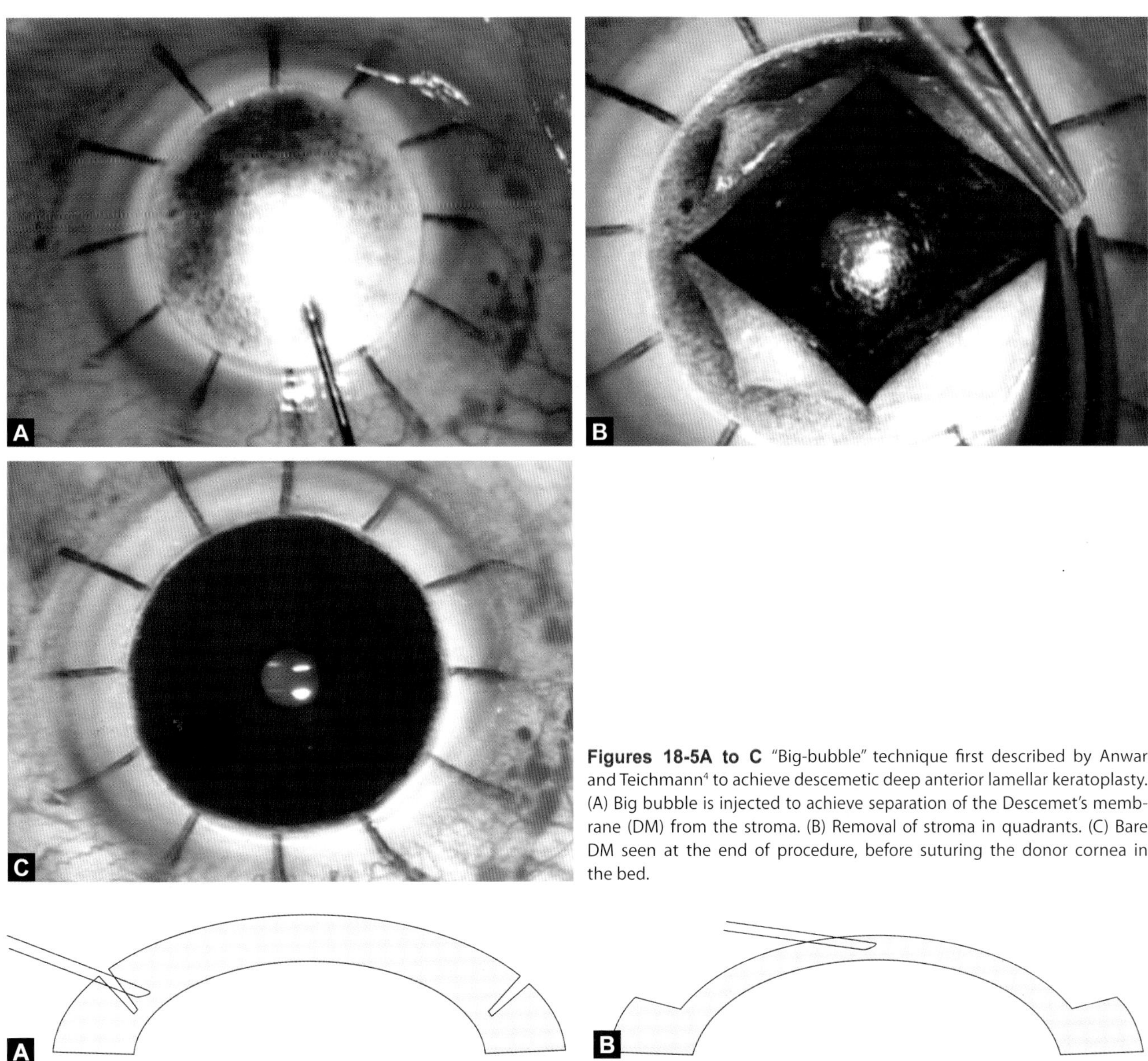

**Figures 18-5A to C** "Big-bubble" technique first described by Anwar and Teichmann[4] to achieve descemetic deep anterior lamellar keratoplasty. (A) Big bubble is injected to achieve separation of the Descemet's membrane (DM) from the stroma. (B) Removal of stroma in quadrants. (C) Bare DM seen at the end of procedure, before suturing the donor cornea in the bed.

**Figures 18-6A and B** Diagram comparing the step of intrastromal air injection in the traditional 'big-bubble' technique (A), compared with the modified "big-bubble" technique (B) after removal of the anterior stromal layer of cornea.

## Air-injection Augmented by Manual Dissection (Modified Big-bubble Technique)

Although big bubble separation of DM appears to be an ideal approach in practice, this procedure remains one of the most challenging surgical procedures for the corneal surgeon to master and has a steep learning curve. Adequate depth of air injection is essential for successful bubble formation, but it also carries a very significant risk of DM perforation (up to 14%).[15] More recent modifications to the big bubble procedure coupled with new DALK instruments have, however, greatly enhanced success in obtaining big bubble separation of DM while significantly reducing needle perforation rates.[16] Tan and Mehta[16] described prior removal of the anterior stromal layers before air needle injections (leaving a residual stroma of approximately 150–250 µm) helping to ensure consistently deep needle insertion, Figures 18-6A and B. Baring of the central stroma also allows for needle entry more parallel to DM (further reducing perforation risk) and a more central needle placement, which allows for more central big bubble formation, Figures 18-7A to F. New DALK instruments are now available in the form of blunt DALK cannulas and

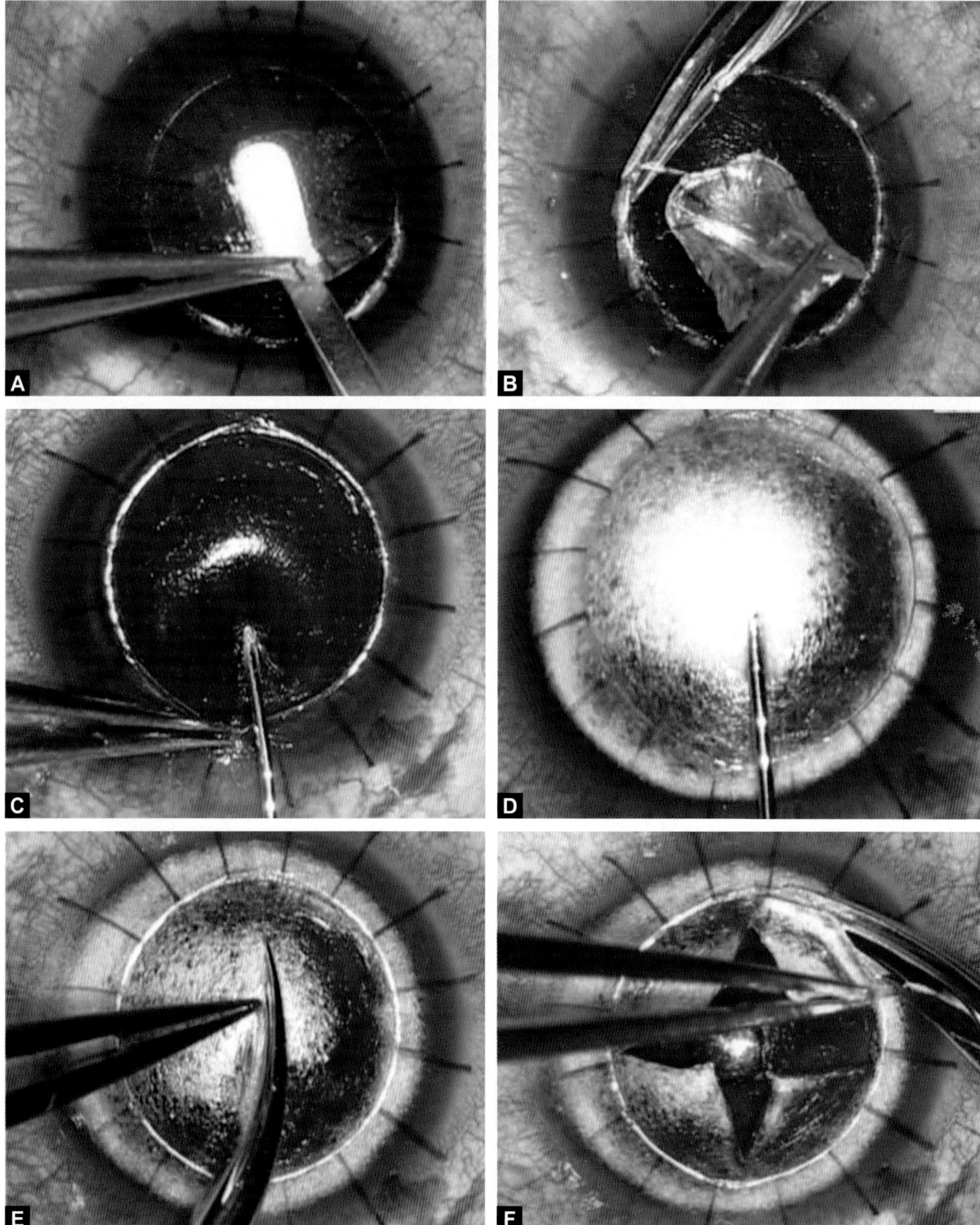


**Figures 18-7A to F** Steps of the modified "big-bubble"technique. (A) Manual dissection. (B) Removal of the anterior stromal layer prior to big-bubble injection allows better central exposure to insert the needle in the correct plane. (C) Insertion with a curved blunt-tipped cannula with a bevel down opening allows a deeper and safer insertion. (D) A large, circular silvery circle with rounded margins denotes successful attainment of the big bubble. (E) The big bubble is then entered with a blade to gain access to Descemet's membrane layer, and the overlying stroma is then carefully exposed in quadrants with corneal scissors. (F) The stroma quadrants are excised with blunt-tipped scissors.

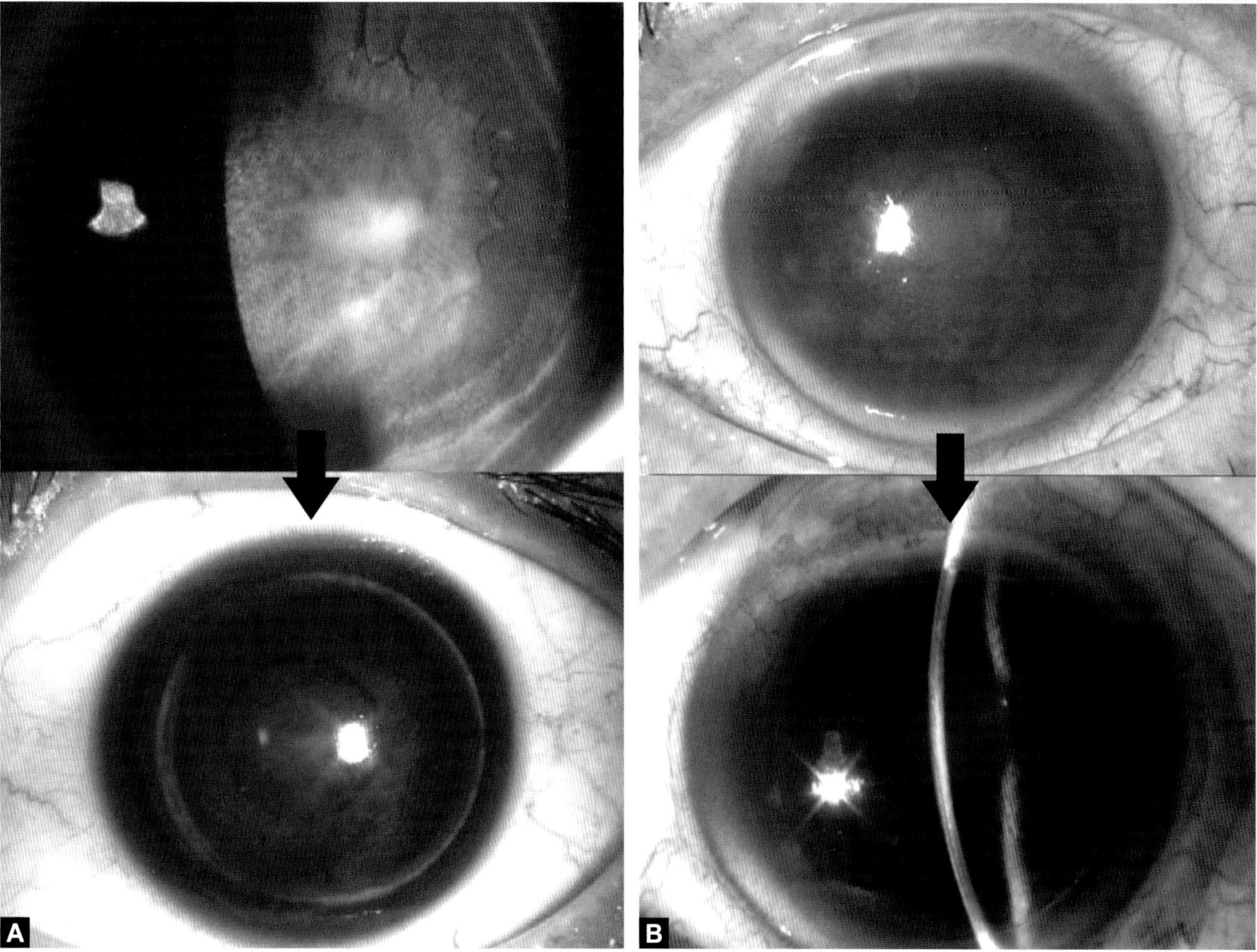


**Figures 18-8A and B** Results of microkeratome-assisted anterior lamellar surgery using the automated lamellar therapeutic keratoplasty technique. (A) Post-photorefractive keratectomy scarring and haze. (B) Scarring due to Reis–Buckler corneal dystrophy. Advantages include higher precision with better refractive accuracy.

probes, blunt-tipped dissectors to clear any final stromal adhesions around the trephination margins, and blunt-tipped DALK scissors with safety platforms to prevent inadvertent DM perforation and rupture.

## Viscoelastic Dissection

Instead of using air to separate the DM, ophthalmic viscoelastic device (OVD) may be incorporated into various stages of DALK techniques described above to remove remaining stromal layers. The use of a combination of OVD and air has also been described for descemetic DALK,[17,18] by first creating a limbal corneal pocket at approximately 95% corneal depth, which is extended up to the limbus over 360°. OVD is then injected to displace the posterior corneal layers toward the iris, followed by corneal trephination to remove the anterior stromal button without damaging the underlying posterior stroma, which is protected by the OVD.[17,18] However, adequate irrigation and removal from the interface is essential as retained OVD in the interface will not easily resorb and can also lead to interface haze.[17]

## Microkeratome-assisted ALK

Surgical microkeratomes used in LASIK surgery may be used in ALK to create a smoother lamellar dissection quality compared with manual dissection, e.g. the automated-lamellar therapeutic keratoplasty (ALTK) (Moria, Antony, France) system. Presently, this system is also utilized for donor preparation in Descemet's stripping automated endothelial keratoplasty, Figures 18-8A and B. However, this may only be performed in corneas with a superficial scar and normal or regular topography, as deeper dissections using this

**TABLE 18-4** Complications of anterior lamellar keratoplasty (ALK) surgery

| | |
|---|---|
| Intraoperative | • Microperforation of the Descemet's membrane (DM)<br>• Macroperforation of the DM leading to conversion to penetrating keratoplasty<br>• Failure to achieve "big-bubble" (deep ALK) |
| Early postoperative | • Double anterior chamber<br>• Pupillary block<br>• Endothelial cell damage |
| Late postoperative | • Recurrence of primary disease<br>• Interface irregularity/ haze or debris<br>• Epithelial ingrowth<br>• Graft rejection (epithelial or stromal)<br>• Ocular surface problems<br>• Infection |

automated system are less predictable and may lead to perforations. It is also unsuitable for very flat or steep corneas with a limited depth of dissection. Diameters of the recipient and donor may, however, vary significantly, and a useful two-stage modification to the standard ALTK procedure has been described. During the first stage, a large recipient flap is dissected and replaced (akin to a large free LASIK flap); a month later, a guarded keratoplasty trephine is used to trephine within the original recipient dissection, and the central layer with vertical edges of the exact intended diameter is peeled away. The donor similarly undergoes large diameter lamellar dissection and secondary central trephination to the exact diameter to match the recipient bed.[19]

## Femtosecond-laser Assisted ALK

The role of femtosecond laser in ALK surgery is still evolving.[20,21] The potential advantages include a smoother graft interface, better wound healing with reduced need for sutures and, thus, faster visual rehabilitation.[20,22] Deeper stromal laser dissection such as the depths required for DALK are not currently able to achieve as smooth a lamellar bed as microkeratome dissection, and visual results have been disappointing. Another interesting use of the femtosecond-laser is to perform the first stage of anterior lamellar bed dissection with the laser at an accurate predefined corneal depth, which will then allow for precise depth placement of the DALK cannula for subsequent "big-bubble" creation.[21,23]

# COMPLICATIONS

Complications for ALK surgery may be divided into intraopera tive, early, and late postoperative, Table 18-4. Intraoperative complications include: inability to attain big bubble separation of DM membrane and micro- or macroperforations or ruptures of DM (11.7%, range 0–39%)[2] and subsequent conversion to PK (2%, range 0–14%).[15] Early postoperative complications include: double AC (3.5%, range 0–16%),[24] pupillary block from air left in the AC, and resultant endothelial cell damage due to air injection or raised intraocular pressure. Late postoperative complications include disease recurrence, interface haze and irregularities, DM folds, interface debris such as blood and blood vessels, epithelial ingrowth, graft rejection (0-14%),[24] infection, poor ocular surface, persistent epithelial defects, and glaucoma.[1,3]

An unsuccessful or incomplete big bubble is technically not a complication, but it is likely to reduce visual outcomes. Alternative techniques to bare DM and the ability to perform high-quality predescemetic deep lamellar dissection remain important. Repeated air injections may result in stromal air greatly limiting a view of the AC or even obscuring the presence of an underlying big bubble. A simple procedure in this situation is the "small bubble test".[25] A small amount of air is injected peripherally into the AC. If the small bubble remains at the periphery of the AC, it confirms that a convex central big bubble must be present. If there are areas of a clear cornea, a second and third attempt for big bubble can be performed. However, if there is a complete white emphysematous cornea, a dry manual layer-by-layer deep dissection can be performed with a crescent blade or with the aid of air, fluid, or an OVD to attempt DM exposure or a resultant thin residual stroma bed.[2]

## Intraoperative Complications

### *Perforation of DM*

Reported rates of microperforation of the DM are higher with manual layer-by-layer dissection (26.3%) compared with the viscodissection (8.3%), hydrodelamination (7.3%), and air "big-bubble" techniques (5.5%).[26] A perforation of DM can occur in any step of the procedure—trephination, lamellar dissection, needle/cannula insertion, air injection, removal of stroma, or even during donor suturing. Early perforations, which result in AC collapse, provide for more challenging residual stromal dissection, which may result in excessive stromal tissue left in place and poorer visual outcomes. A larger perforation could lead to a flat anterior chamber requiring multiple air injections associated with greater endothelial cell damage. Furthermore, a large DM rupture after baring of DM, which is not well repositioned, may result in permanent stromal edema and graft failure.[27]

Management of DM perforation depends on the stage at which it occurs and the location and size of the perforation. If a microperforation occurs early during trephination, the perforation can be sutured, the AC reformed with air, and a manual predescemetic dissection performed.[4] Small microperforations with the air needle are often self-sealing with a layer of stroma; thus, the procedure can proceed in the hands of an experienced surgeon, leaving the predescemetic dissection of the perforated site to the end while maintaining the AC with air.[4] Other methods of maintaining the AC include air injection or sealing the perforation with fibrin glue, cyanoacrylate or using a corneal patch graft.[1] A microperforation that occurs during suturing is often self-sealing or can be easily managed with air injection into the AC. In cases where a macroperforation or large DM tear occurs, conversion to PK is often necessary, although complex surgical techniques have now been described, which enable the continuation of the DALK procedure.[15]

## Early Postoperative Phase

### *"Pseudo" or "double" Anterior Chamber*

This complication usually follows a DM perforation or with retained viscoelastic underneath the donor graft.[15] While a shallow "pseudo-AC" may resolve spontaneously, often intracameral air injection is required for deep or large "pseudo-AC" formations. Other intracameral air mixtures that have been reported include $SF_6$ or $C_3F_8$ gas with air injections.[4] Complications of air injection include: pupillary block, iris atrophy, endothelial cell damage, and cataract formation.[15]

### *Pupillary Block*

Urrets—Zavalia syndrome may occur due to ischemia of the iris from raised intraocular pressure. Complications include iridoplegia, posterior synechia formation, and anterior subcapsular cataract. It is, therefore, important to perform an inferior peripheral iridectomy or ensure wide pupil dilatation postoperatively in cases where a large air bubble is required in the AC after surgery.

## Late Postoperative Phase

### *Interface Folds*

In cases of big bubble DALK for severe keratoconus, there will be a mismatch between the donor button and the recipient ectatic DM, which may result in significant DM folds or creases limiting visual outcomes. In these cases, during placement of the first 4 cardinal sutures of the donor, the central cornea should be examined to ensure that no significant DM folds are present in the pupil area. (Concentric DM folds in the periphery will be present but will not affect visual outcomes). Predescemetic DALK should be avoided in severe keratoconus, as rigid stromal folds in the central visual axis will often be unavoidable and result in reduced best-corrected visual acuity and increased higher order aberrations.[28]

### *Allograft Rejection*

Although the risk of endothelial rejection in ALK is practically obviated, epithelial or stromal rejection may still occur (3–14.3%).[29] In cases with a healthy ocular surface, removal of donor epithelium alone (easily performed when the DM is removed), and the use of a temporary bandage contact lens until complete recipient epithelization of the graft will further obviate any risk of epithelial rejection. Long-term sequelae after graft rejection include vascularization or scarring, which can affect the visual acuity. Nonetheless, the predicted long-term graft survival is significantly better in DALK (big-bubble and manual) compared with PK. Furthermore, most cases of subepithelial or stromal rejection can be reversed successfully with topical steroids.[9]

### *Infection*

Infections can still occur related to the sutures, which may follow sterile inflammatory reactions, early suture loosening, and vascularization around the sutures. Infections can also occur due to organisms such as Candida,[30] which can proliferate within the interface without a host immune response.

# IMAGING IN ALK SURGERY

Anterior segment optical coherence tomography (AS-OCT) allows for rapid, noncontact, high-resolution imaging of the cornea after ALK, Figures 18-9A and B.[31] Preoperatively, AS-OCT may be useful in the evaluation of the depth of corneal scars, as well as in determining corneal thickness. The adjunctive use of the intraoperative AS-OCT during DALK surgery has been described.[32,33] Newer intraoperative real-time imaging, such as the spectral domain AS-OCT (iVue 100-2; Optovue Inc, Fremont, CA), may guide manual dissection depth to achieve successful DM-baring without perforation. The AS-OCT imaging also enables closer study of the interface, such as that after ALTK surgery, Figures 18-10A and B. Postoperatively, AS-OCT imaging may help diagnose double or triple-anterior chamber, DM detachment and interface keratitis, especially if the DALK graft is hazy with a poor view.

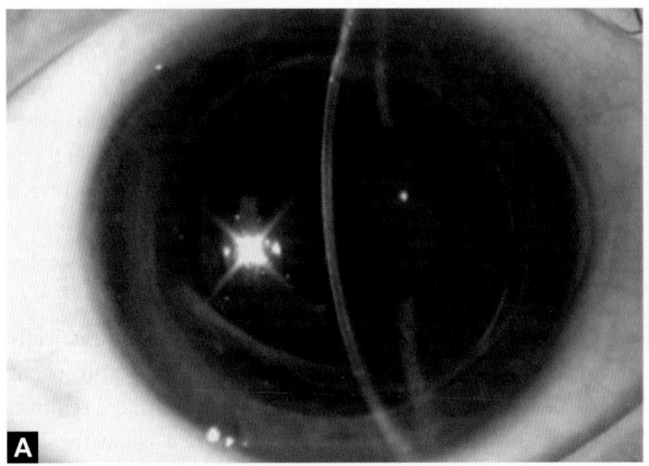

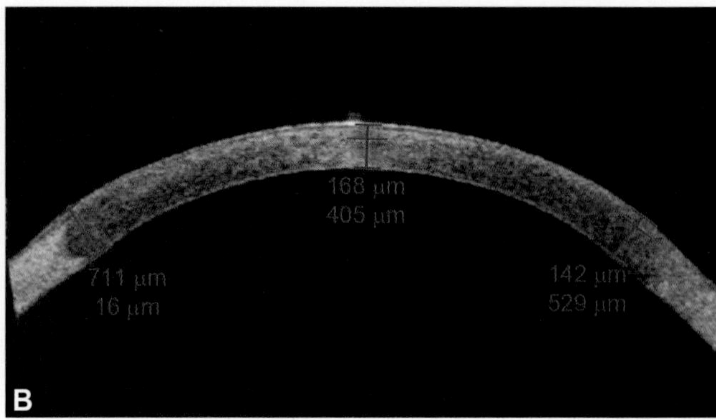


**Figures 18-9A and B** Anterior segment optical coherence tomography after descemetic deep anterior lamellar keratoplasty using the "big-bubble" technique, demonstrating the interface at the descemetic layer.

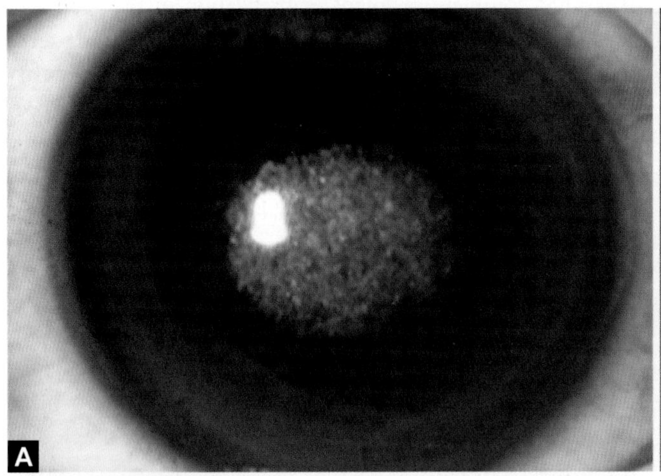

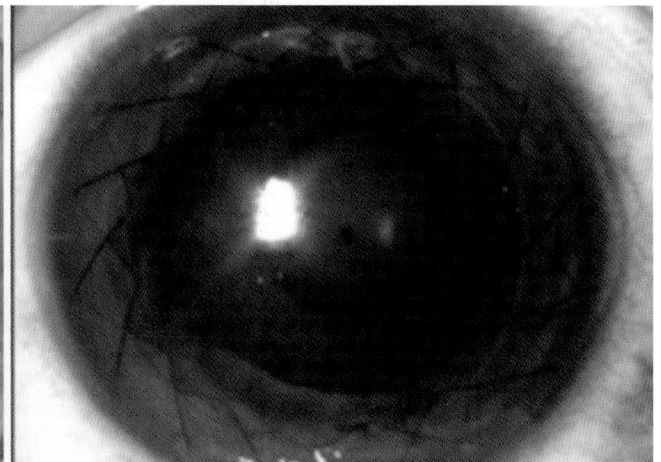

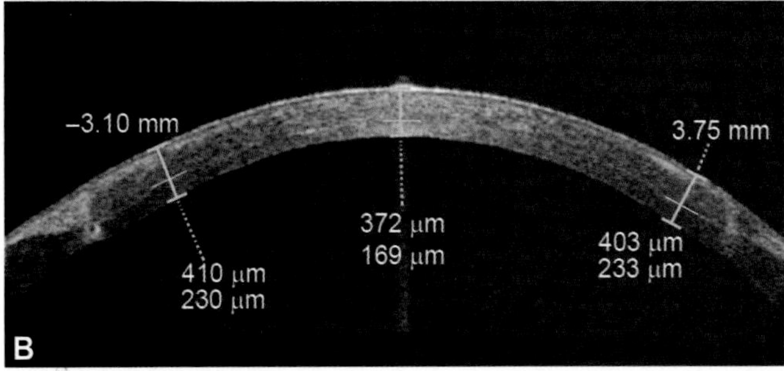


**Figures 18-10A and B** Anterior segment optical coherence tomography after automated lamellar therapeutic keratoplasty technique, demonstrating the regular interface.

## CONCLUSION

The ALK and DALK are emerging surgical alternatives to conventional PK for the treatment of a wide range of corneal stromal disorders. They have clear advantages over PK in terms of enhanced long-term graft survival, reduced risk of endothelial rejection and failure, and other complications of intraocular surgery. The newer approaches to baring DM, such as the big bubble DALK technique and its modifications, now result in visual outcomes matching PK surgery. DALK surgery remains challenging, and further surgical innovations will continue to improve and enhance the field.

## REFERENCES

1. Luengo-Gimeno F, Tan DT, Mehta JS. Evolution of deep anterior lamellar keratoplasty (DALK). Ocul Surf. 2011;9:98-110.
2. Reinhart WJ, Musch DC, Jacobs DS, et al. Deep anterior lamellar keratoplasty as an alternative to penetrating keratoplasty a report by the american academy of ophthalmology. Ophthalmology. 2011;118:209-18.

3. Tan DT, Dart JK, Holland EJ, et al. Corneal transplantation. Lancet. 2012;379:1749-61.
4. Anwar M, Teichmann KD. Deep lamellar keratoplasty: surgical techniques for anterior lamellar keratoplasty with and without baring of Descemet's membrane. Cornea. 2002;21:374-83.
5. Tan DT, Anshu A, Parthasarathy A, et al. Visual acuity outcomes after deep anterior lamellar keratoplasty: a case-control study. Br J Ophthalmol. 2010;94:1295-9.
6. Ardjomand N, Hau S, McAlister JC, et al. Quality of vision and graft thickness in deep anterior lamellar and penetrating corneal allografts. Am J Ophthalmol. 2007;143:228-35.
7. Malbran E. Lamellar keratoplasty in keratoconus. Int Ophthalmol Clin. 1966;6:99-109.
8. Archila EA. Deep lamellar keratoplasty dissection of host tissue with intrastromal air injection. Cornea. 1984;3:217-8.
9. Borderie VM, Sandali O, Bullet J, et al. Long-term results of deep anterior lamellar versus penetrating keratoplasty. Ophthalmology. 2012;119:249-55.
10. Anshu A, Parthasarathy A, Mehta JS, et al. Outcomes of therapeutic deep lamellar keratoplasty and penetrating keratoplasty for advanced infectious keratitis: a comparative study. Ophthalmology. 2009;116:615-23.
11. Ang M, Mehta JS, Sng CC, et al. Indications, outcomes, and risk factors for failure in tectonic keratoplasty. Ophthalmology. 2012;119:1311-9.
12. Sugita J, Kondo J. Deep lamellar keratoplasty with complete removal of pathological stroma for vision improvement. Br J Ophthalmol. 1997;81:184-8.
13. Archila EA. Deep lamellar keratoplasty dissection of host tissue with intrastromal air injection. Cornea. 1984;3:217-8.
14. Melles GR, Rietveld FJ, Beekhuis WH, et al. A technique to visualize corneal incision and lamellar dissection depth during surgery. Cornea. 1999;18:80-6.
15. Tan DT, Anshu A. Anterior lamellar keratoplasty: 'back to the future'– a review. Clin Experiment Ophthalmol. 2010;38: 118-27.
16. Tan DT, Mehta JS. Future directions in lamellar corneal transplantation. Cornea. 2007;26:S21-8.
17. Melles GR, Remeijer L, Geerards AJ, et al. A quick surgical technique for deep, anterior lamellar keratoplasty using viscodissection. Cornea. 2000;19:427-32.
18. van Dooren BT, Mulder PG, Nieuwendaal CP, et al. Endothelial cell density after deep anterior lamellar keratoplasty (Melles technique). Am J Ophthalmol. 2004;137:397-400.
19. Tan DT, Ang LP. Modified automated lamellar therapeutic keratoplasty for keratoconus: a new technique. Cornea. 2006; 25:1217-9.
20. Shousha MA, Yoo SH, Kymionis GD, et al. Long-term results of femtosecond laser-assisted sutureless anterior lamellar keratoplasty. Ophthalmology. 2011;118:315-23.
21. Buzzonetti L, Petrocelli G, Valente P. Femtosecond laser and big-bubble deep anterior lamellar keratoplasty: a new chance. J Ophthalmol. 2012;2012:264590.
22. Yoo SH, Kymionis GD, Koreishi A, et al. Femtosecond laser-assisted sutureless anterior lamellar keratoplasty. Ophthalmology. 2008;115:1303-7, 7 e1.
23. Buzzonetti L, Laborante A, Petrocelli G. Standardized big-bubble technique in deep anterior lamellar keratoplasty assisted by the femtosecond laser. J Cataract Refract Surg. 2010;36:1631-6.
24. Kubaloglu A, Sari ES, Unal M, et al. Long-term results of deep anterior lamellar keratoplasty for the treatment of keratoconus. Am J Ophthalmol. 2011;151:760-7 e1.
25. Parthasarathy A, Por YM, Tan DT. Using a "small bubble technique" to aid in success in Anwar's "big bubble technique" of deep lamellar keratoplasty with complete baring of Descemet's membrane. Br J Ophthalmol. 2008;92:422.
26. Sarnicola V, Toro P, Gentile D, et al. Descemetic DALK and predescemetic DALK: outcomes in 236 cases of keratoconus. Cornea. 2010;29:53-9.
27. Leccisotti A. Descemet's membrane perforation during deep anterior lamellar keratoplasty: prognosis. J Cataract Refract Surg. 2007;33:825-9.
28. Bahar I, Kaiserman I, Srinivasan S, et al. Comparison of three different techniques of corneal transplantation for keratoconus. Am J Ophthalmol. 2008;146:905-12 e1.
29. Watson SL, Tuft SJ, Dart JK. Patterns of rejection after deep lamellar keratoplasty. Ophthalmology. 2006;113:556-60.
30. Kanavi MR, Foroutan AR, Kamel MR, et al. Candida interface keratitis after deep anterior lamellar keratoplasty: clinical, microbiologic, histopathologic, and confocal microscopic reports. Cornea. 2007;26:913-6.
31. Radhakrishnan S, Rollins AM, Roth JE, et al. Real-time optical coherence tomography of the anterior segment at 1310 nm. Arch Ophthalmol. 2001;119:1179-85.
32. Riss S, Heindl LM, Bachmann BO, et al. Pentacam-based big bubble deep anterior lamellar keratoplasty in patients with keratoconus. Cornea. 2012;31:627-32.
33. Lim LS, Aung HT, Aung T, et al. Corneal imaging with anterior segment optical coherence tomography for lamellar keratoplasty procedures. Am J Ophthalmol. 2008;145:81-90.

CHAPTER

19

# Keratoprosthesis

Sotiria Palioura, Christina R Prescott, James Chodosh

## INTRODUCTION

Although the first keratoprosthesis was designed more than 120 years ago,[1] efforts in improving its design and clinical use were at a standstill until the 1960s because of the advances and widespread use of standard allograft surgery. Corneal transplantation, whether penetrating or lamellar, has a success rate as high as 90% after 1 year and > 80% after 5 years (in the USA and Europe) in patients with keratoconus, traumatic corneal scarring, and corneal dystrophies and degenerations.[2,3] The allograft survival rate of standard keratoplasty remains low for patients with autoimmune ocular surface disorders; these include Stevens Johnson syndrome/toxic epidermal necrolysis and mucous membrane pemphigoid; cases of limbal stem cell deficiency or failure, such as in aniridia or after severe chemical burns; severe keratoconjunctivitis sicca; and in the presence of severe corneal vascularization from other causes.[4,5] In such patients, implantation of a keratoprosthesis device may be the only effective option to safely restore vision.

## KERATOPROSTHESIS DESIGNS

Many keratoprosthesis designs have been proposed in the last 20 years, but only three devices are in use in the USA and Europe: (1) the Boston keratoprosthesis, (2) the osteo-odonto-keratoprosthesis (OOKP), and (3) the AlphaCor keratoprosthesis. Only the Boston keratoprosthesis and AlphaCor are approved for marketing by the US Food and Drug Administration (FDA).

### Boston Keratoprosthesis

The Boston keratoprosthesis, previously known as the Dohlman–Doane keratoprosthesis, was developed at the Massachusetts Eye and Ear Infirmary and the Schepens Eye Research Institute in the late 1960s.[6] Unlike the OOKP and the AlphaCor designs described below, the Boston keratoprosthesis is a nonintegrated keratoprosthesis that comes in two forms. The type I device is a collar button-shaped device composed of polymethylmethacrylate (PMMA) and titanium and is placed in a corneal donor graft and covered with a contact lens (Fig. 19-1A); the type II device has an additional anterior extension that allows for implantation through surgically closed eyelids (Fig. 19-1B). The corneal allograft is sandwiched between the front and back PMMA plates and then sutured in place in one stage performed similarly to standard penetrating keratoplasty. Since its FDA approval in 1992, > 8000 type I devices have been implanted, rendering the Boston keratoprosthesis type I the most frequently implanted artificial cornea worldwide.[7-10]

### Osteo-odonto-keratoprosthesis

The OOKP was first developed and used in Italy by Strampelli in the 1960s[11] and then modified by Falcinelli.[12] It is composed of a rigid PMMA optic attached to a peripheral haptic made out of an excised monoradicular tooth root; this is thought to allow for improved biointegration into host tissue (Fig. 19-2A). The device is implanted in a two-stage procedure, then covered with an autologous mucous membrane graft (Fig. 19-2B) (*see* section "Surgical technique" below).

### AlphaCor Keratoprosthesis

The AlphaCor device (Addition Technology Inc, Des Plaines, IL, USA) was designed by Chirila et al. in Australia.[13] It consists of a nonporous optic with a porous peripheral skirt, both made of poly-2-hydroxyethyl methacrylate (pHEMA). Its radius is 7.0 mm, its thickness is 0.5 mm and its refractive index is 1.43.[14] It is designed to be implanted in an

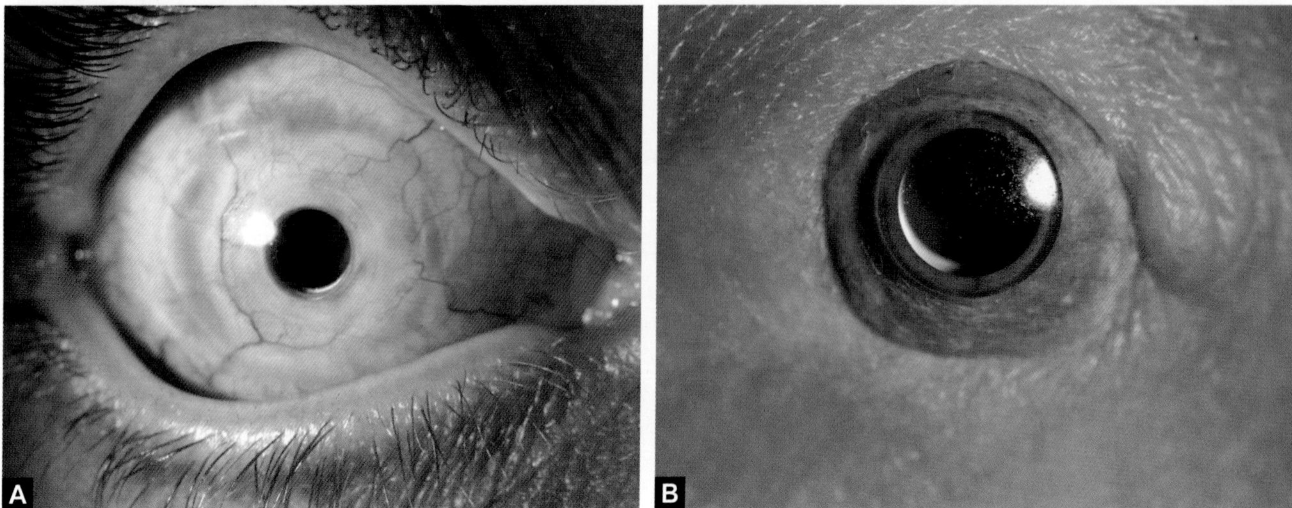

**Figures 19-1A and B** Photomicrographs of the Boston keratoprosthesis type I (A) and II (B) devices several years after implantation. The type I device is constructed around a corneal donor graft, which is sutured in place as with a standard penetrating keratoplasty and covered with a contact lens (A). The type II device has an additional 2 mm anterior nub that allows for implantation through surgically closed eyelids (B). In the patient shown, a ring of keratin has formed around the keratoprosthesis stem. This commonly occurs and is of no consequence to the device or its retention.

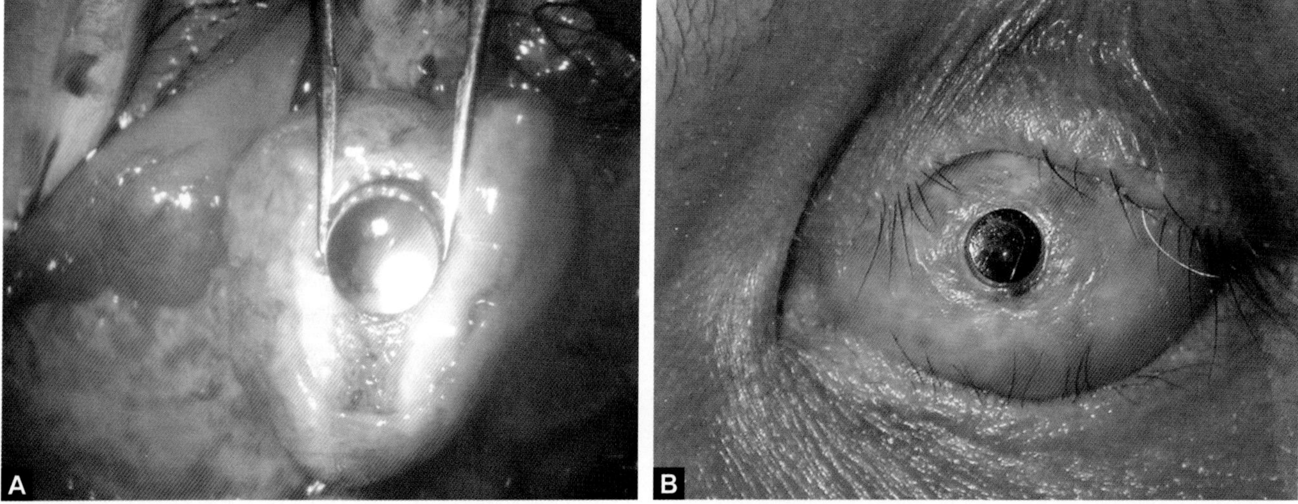

**Figures 19-2A and B** Photomicrographs of an osteo-odonto-keratoprosthesis device, just before implantation into the eye (A), and several years after implantation (b). The polymethylmethacrylate optic is cemented within the tooth, left for 2–3 months in a subdermal pocket to generate a fibrovascular capsule (a), and then implanted beneath a mucous membrane graft (B). Shown here, the mucous membrane graft typically keratinizes over time and becomes fused to the eyelids. Much like the Boston keratoprosthesis type II, the eye is continuously "open".
*Source* Courtesy of Dr Geetha Iyer, Chennai, India.

intrastromal corneal pocket and, like the OOKP, it is inserted in a two-stage procedure (Figs. 19-3A and B) (see section "Surgical technique" below). Similar to the OOKP, the principle behind the design of the AlphaCor is biointegration of the device within the surrounding tissues via cellular ingrowth and collagen deposition.[15] After implantation, the outer skirt is colonized by keratocytes while the central zone remains optically clear. It was first implanted in human eyes in 1998 and became FDA approved in 2003.[16]

## INDICATIONS

Keratoprosthesis surgery is indicated for patients with corneal blindness, in whom penetrating keratoplasty would likely fail or has already failed. The distinct design of each of the three keratoprosthesis devices accounts for the different clinical indications for their use.

- Boston keratoprosthesis type I surgery is indicated for patients with relatively normal eyelids, blink response,

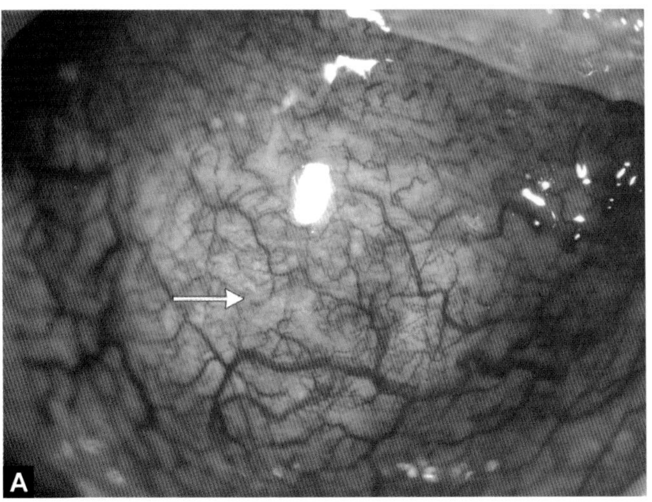


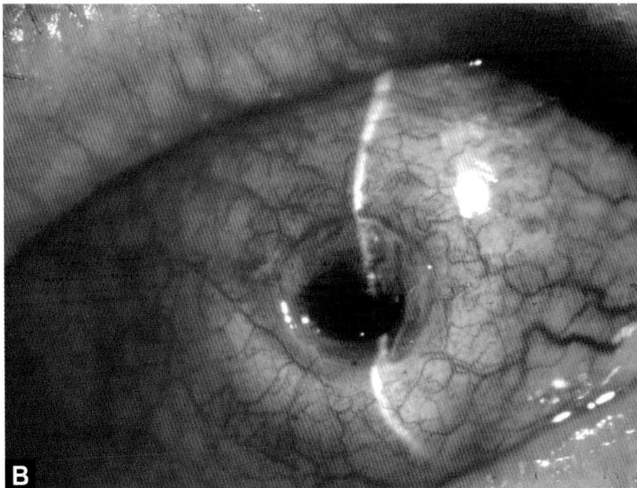


**Figures 19-3A and B** Photomicrographs of the AlphaCor device at stage 1, covered by a conjunctival flap (A), and after stage 2, in this case, months after opening the center of the conjunctival flap (B). In stage 1, the optical center of the device is visible as a bluish clearing (arrow, a) through the conjunctival flap. At stage 2, the optical component of the device is uncovered by surgical excision of conjunctiva over the optic. This AlphaCor device is shown several months after trephination of the central opening over the optic, and early ulceration at the edge of the conjunctival opening is evident (B).
*Source* Courtesy of Dr James V Aquavella Buffalo, New York.

and adequate tear film; this allows for a soft contact lens to be used indefinitely after the procedure, to prevent desiccation and subsequent melting. The most common indications for the Boston keratoprosthesis type I include a history of repeated allograft failure, corneal opacity with extensive neovascularization, and limbal stem cell deficiency in select cases, such as aniridia

- Boston keratoprosthesis type II and OOKP are best suited for patients with corneal blindness and abnormal lid function, diminished tear secretion, forniceal foreshortening, and ocular surface keratinization.[17,18] Thus, the most common indications for the OOKP and the Boston keratoprosthesis type II are severe chemical injuries and severe autoimmune ocular surface diseases, such as mucous membrane pemphigoid, Stevens–Johnson syndrome/toxic epidermal necrolysis, and end-stage keratoconjunctivitis sicca. OOKP implantation is the most invasive and technically challenging of the keratoprosthesis surgeries, followed by the Boston keratoprosthesis type II surgery.

For this reason and because of the poor cosmesis associated with both devices, Boston keratoprosthesis type II and OOKP surgery should only be considered in patients with bilateral corneal blindness. Surgery is typically carried out in only one eye, and the other eye is kept as a "spare" eye. Patients should realize during the preoperative evaluation that the use of tinted spectacle lenses may be the only option for acceptable cosmesis after Boston keratoprosthesis type II implantation or OOKP.

- AlphaCor implantation may be indicated for patients with intact eyelids, normal blink, and healthy tear film, to prevent tissue melting. Occasionally, a Gunderson conjunctival flap is required after implantation; therefore, patients should have adequate and healthy conjunctivae as well. The most accepted indication for the AlphaCor device is a history of repeated corneal allograft failure.[16]

## CONTRAINDICATIONS

- Incomplete eyelid closure and poor quality/low quantity tear film can lead to detrimental evaporative damage and melting of the corneal tissue carrying the AlphaCor or the Boston keratoprosthesis type I device
- OOKP and Boston keratoprosthesis type II surgery should not be considered for patients with vision that allows them to perform their daily activities
- Evidence of poor compliance with medication use and preoperative follow-up appointments should be considered a contraindication for any keratoprosthesis implantation, because it will likely compromise the visual benefits from the initial surgery and result in loss of the keratoprosthesis and/or the eye. The need for life-long follow-up with a qualified cornea specialist is of utmost importance, to recognize and treat indolent infection, corneal perforation, and worsening glaucomatous damage in a timely fashion. Patients with autoimmune inflammatory conditions, such as Stevens–Johnson syndrome and mucous membrane pemphigoid, must understand the possible

need for systemic immunosuppression as guided by a rheumatologist or uveitis specialist. Optimal control of ocular and systemic inflammation is key to the long-term retention of any keratoprosthesis device

- End-stage retinal or optic nerve disease and phthisis bulbi are absolute contraindications to keratoprosthesis implantation, regardless of type.

## SURGICAL TECHNIQUE

### Boston Keratoprosthesis Type I

The optical portion of the device consists of a PMMA front plate (5.0 mm in diameter) and its stem. The front plate is available in different dioptric powers. Use of the appropriate power is determined by the patient's axial length and lens status.[19] The back plate, which is available in an adult size (8.5 mm in diameter) and a pediatric size (7.0 mm in diameter), is connected to the front plate by the stem. In the current commercially available keratoprosthesis version, the back plate is also made of PMMA and has two rows of eight perforations each. This allows for nourishment of the donor corneal graft with aqueous humor, which decreases the risk of keratolysis.[4,20]A titanium back plate has been associated with less retroprosthetic membrane formation[21] and was recently approved for use by the US FDA.

A corneal graft is sandwiched between the two plates, and a titanium locking ring is placed around the posterior stem to prevent disassembly of the device; it is then sutured to the host cornea, as discussed later on in this section. The donor corneal graft should be at least equal or greater in diameter than the keratoprosthesis back plate and at least 0.5 mm greater in size than the host cornea trephination diameter. Thus, for the standard 8.5-mm-diameter back plate, the donor graft should be at least 8.5 mm in diameter, and for the 7.0-mm-diameter back plate, the donor graft should be at least 7.0 mm in diameter. It is important that the donor graft never be < 7.0 mm in diameter with the standard 5.0 mm front plate or the donor corneal rim will be insufficient to allow for suture fixation.

As with standard corneal transplantation, retrobulbar anesthesia is generally adequate. After selection of the respective donor and host diameters (see discussion above), the donor graft is prepared by performing an inner 3.0 mm trephination using a skin biopsy punch (packaged by the manufacturer with the keratoprosthesis) and an outer trephination with a standard trephine. For eccentric keratoprosthesis placement the central corneal trephination should be correspondingly eccentric. Assembly of the keratoprosthesis begins with placing the front plate face down on a double-sided adhesive that is provided by the manufacturer; this secures the device and facilitates its assembly. The donor cornea's 3.0 mm central opening is then placed over the stem with the endothelial side facing up and is slowly slid down the stem of the front plate, so that its epithelial side comes in contact with the back surface of the front plate. A small amount of viscoelastic is placed on the endothelial surface of the donor graft to minimize trauma. The back plate is then pushed down the stem with the concave side up using a manufacturer-provided assembly tool. This is followed by placement of the titanium locking ring behind the back plate so that an audible snap is heard to indicate that the components are secured into place. Proper assembly should always be confirmed by careful inspection of the device under magnification. The assembled device is then immersed into corneal preservation medium until needed.

Host cornea trephination is then performed as traditional penetrating keratoplasty surgery, and the removed tissue is sent for histopathologic examination. An iridoplasty should be done if corectopia results in obstruction of the visual axis by iris tissue. For phakic patients, lens extraction is mandatory at this stage. Implantation of a plano posterior chamber intraocular lens may be undertaken in select cases (e.g. if a glaucoma drainage device will be placed at the time of surgery or may be needed in the future).[22] Preoperative selection of a plano posterior chamber intraocular lens ensures proper power of the keratoprosthesis, even if capsular support is compromised and intraocular lens implantation has to be aborted intraoperatively. If the patient is pseudophakic and the lens is stable, the surgeon may decide to leave the intraocular lens in place and use a pseudophakic powered keratoprosthesis. The assembled type I keratoprosthesis device is brought to the operating field and sutured into the host corneal rim as in a standard penetrating keratoplasty. We typically secure the assembled device with 12 interrupted 9-0 nylon sutures or 16 interrupted 10-0 nylon sutures. Knots are buried in the host tissue, and the wound is checked for leakage.

After implantation of the device, peribulbar vancomycin (25 mg in 0.5 mL), ceftazidime (100 mg in 0.5 mL), and triamcinolone (20 mg in 0.5 mL) are administered, as modified by the patient's medication allergies. It is important to avoid ballooning of the conjunctiva lest subsequent contact lens placement be compromised. A 16-mm diameter, 9.8 base curve Kontur contact lens (Hercules, CA, USA), provided with the device by the manufacturer, is placed over the cornea at the end of the procedure and remains in place postoperatively. Ophthalmic ointment should not be used as it can displace the contact lens. A semipressure patch and a Fox shield are placed at the conclusion of surgery.

## Boston Keratoprosthesis Type II

The Boston keratoprosthesis type II device is similar to the type I, except for an additional anterior extension of the optic that allows for through-the-lid implantation. The optical portion of the device consists of a PMMA front plate, its stem, and a 2-mm anterior nub. Similar to the type I device, the stem connects the front plate with the back plate. The extent of periocular tissue dissection and the duration of the surgery typically mandate general anesthesia in cases of Boston keratoprosthesis type II implantation. Sizing and preparation of the donor corneal graft for implantation of the type II device is similar to type I surgery. Thus after inner and outer trephination of the donor graft, the type II keratoprosthesis device is assembled in a similar fashion as the type I device.

The rest of the procedure is much more extensive than type I implantation. Prior to trephination of the patient's cornea, extensive dissection and removal of all ocular surface epithelium is performed; this will prevent postoperative complications due to epithelial encystment beneath surgically closed eyelids. Symblephara are divided, and bulbar, forniceal, and tarsal conjunctival epithelium are removed with sharp dissection. After infiltration of the eyelid margins with 1% lidocaine with epinephrine, the margins are excised taking care to remove all eyelash follicles. The host cornea is marked with the appropriate trephine, and the limbal and corneal epithelium peripheral to the marked area are removed with sharp dissection prior to trephination. The host cornea is then trephined and removed as in the type I surgery described above.

Additional procedures, such as pars plana vitrectomy or implantation of a glaucoma drainage device, are performed at this stage by a vitreoretinal or glaucoma surgeon, respectively, and placement of a temporary (e.g. Eckhardt's model) keratoprosthesis for wide angle visualization of the peripheral vitreous and retina may be necessary as an intermediate step. Total iridectomy should also be considered at this stage. Total iridectomy is well tolerated since surgical eyelid closure after implantation of the type II device reduces postoperative glare. If the patient is phakic, the crystalline lens must be removed. If the patient is pseudophakic and the intraocular lens is stable, then it may be left in place for some cases and a pseudophakic-powered keratoprosthesis is used.

The assembled type II keratoprosthesis device is then brought to the operating field and sutured into the host corneal rim in a similar fashion to the type I device (with the exception that knots need not be buried). After implantation of the device and prior to surgical closure of the eyelids, peribulbar vancomycin (25 mg in 0.5 mL), ceftazidime (100 mg in 0.5 mL), and triamcinolone (20 mg in 0.5 mL) are given as in the type I surgery. The eyelids are then surgically closed around the optic. The upper and lower tarsi are approximated with two or three interrupted 6-0 vicryl sutures on either side of the keratoprosthesis using partial thickness tarsal bites. The eyelid margins are then closed with 8-0 nylon mattress sutures over plastic bolsters. Finally, with the eye in primary gaze, Vannas scissors are used to fashion a notch in the upper lid and allow the keratoprosthesis nub to protrude through the closed eyelids. Prior to reversal of general anesthesia, a retrobulbar anesthetic may be injected to minimize postoperative pain. Antibiotic ointment is placed over the skin closure, along with a gentle patch and a Fox shield.

## OOKP

Potential candidates for OOKP implantation must undergo a preoperative oral assessment of the buccal mucosa graft donor site, as well as a tooth and its associated alveolar bone that will form the osteo-odonto lamina of the device. Smoking cessation is necessary to improve the chance of buccal graft survival. A monoradicular tooth, most commonly the canine tooth, is chosen after careful clinical and radiographic evaluation to exclude the presence of periodontal disease. If no tooth is deemed suitable, then an allograft from a human leukocyte antigen (HLA)-matched living relative may be considered, albeit with the understanding that the risk of extrusion will be higher.

The OOKP surgery is usually carried out as a two-stage procedure. In patients at risk for delayed mucous membrane graft healing and vascularization, stage I may be subdivided into two separate steps.[17,23,24] Mucous membrane harvesting and placement on the ocular surface is done first (stage Ia); once the graft is mature and well established, tooth extraction and OOKP lamina preparation is then undertaken (stage Ib).

Stage Ia begins with harvesting a full-thickness buccal mucous membrane graft, usually 3 cm in size that is used to cover the entire ocular surface from the medial to the lateral canthus and from the upper to the lower lid fornix. Once obtained, the graft soaks in antibiotic solution until required, and attention is shifted to preparation of the ocular surface. A 360° peritomy, thorough synechiolysis, total debridement of the surface epithelium, and Bowman's membrane from the cornea and reinforcement of areas of significant corneal thinning with a lamellar patch graft are subsequently performed. The buccal mucosal graft is then sutured to the sclera at or beyond the rectus muscle insertions with interrupted 6-0 vicryl sutures. If possible, the graft edges are also sutured to the recessed conjunctivae. Vascularization of this graft will occur in the next 2–4 months and is essential for providing the blood supply to the bone part of the OOKP lamina after the second stage of the procedure is performed.

Stage Ib involves harvesting a monoradicular tooth, its surrounding alveolar bone and the associated mucoperiosteum, to prepare an osteo-odonto-lamina. The bone is sectioned on either side and below the chosen tooth with a fine saw, and the complex is then removed from the mouth. The resulting bony defect is covered with adjacent mucosa or with a mucous membrane graft, but it typically re-epithelializes very rapidly. An optical cylinder of appropriate power (based on preoperative A-scan ultrasonographic measurements), and size is chosen so that there will be at least 1 mm of dentine ring around the central channel. A hole is drilled in the center of the tooth root, it is enlarged with a diamond burr, and then the PMMA optical cylinder is cemented in place. Any periosteum that becomes detached in the process is reattached with fibrin glue. The tooth crown is removed and the assembled tooth-optic lamina is immersed in the patient's own blood before implantation into a submuscular pouch, usually in the lower lid of the fellow eye, for 2–4 months.

Stage II surgery is performed after the mucous membrane graft has matured, usually in 2–4 months. If the lamina stays buried in the lid for a longer period of time, it may undergo significant resorption. The OOKP lamina is first retrieved from the fellow lower lid and thoroughly examined to ensure that the optic is stable and an adequate fibrovascular capsule has formed. Excess tissues are then trimmed to expose the optical cylinder on both sides. A template of the lamina is made, to plan placement of a Flieringa ring and preplaced sutures that will later secure the lamina into place. The cornea is exposed by making an arcuate incision in the mucous membrane graft from 3 o' clock to 9 o'clock and reflecting the mucous membrane graft inferiorly. A Flieringa ring is sutured in place, the center of the cornea is marked, the template is placed on the cornea, and cardinal sutures are preplaced. Corneal trephination is performed using a 5- or 5.5-mm trephine, depending on the diameter of the posterior part of the optical cylinder. Total iridectomy, intracapsular cryoextraction of the lens and anterior vitrectomy are carried out, and the lamina is finally placed onto the corneal opening and sutured in place using 6-0 vicryl sutures. Sterile air is injected through the pars plana to reinflate the eye, and the macula and optic nerve are examined using indirect ophthalmoscopy. Any tilt of the optical cylinder is corrected by adjusting suture tightness in different quadrants. The Flieringa ring is removed, and the mucous membrane is sutured back in place to cover the lamina. Finally, a central hole 3–4 mm in diameter is trephined to expose the optical cylinder anteriorly.

### AlphaCor

The AlphaCor is also implanted in two steps. Depending on the phakic status of the patient, one of two versions of the device is selected. AlphaCor-P has a lower power (about +42.0 D) and is used for phakic or pseudophakic eyes. AlphaCor-A has a refractive power of +58.0 D and is suitable for aphakic eyes.

The first stage of the procedure involves making an intrastromal pocket with a posterior central opening in the following fashion. A 360° conjunctival peritomy is made, the corneal epithelium is debrided, and a superior half-thickness paralimbal incision is made (about 1–1.5 mm posterior to the limbus) and extended for 180°. The incision is extended into the cornea at about 50% depth using a lamellar dissecting blade. After an intralamellar pocket about 7.5 mm in diameter is made, the superior corneal flap is reflected inferiorly. The central posterior corneal lamella is then trephinated with a 3.5-mm trephine until the anterior chamber is entered. The AlphaCor device is then placed within the pocket, sandwiched between the anterior and posterior corneal lamellae, and is centered over the posterior lamellar opening. The superior corneal flap is then placed over the AlphaCor device and sutured at the limbus, with interrupted 10-0 nylon sutures. In cases of significant limbal stem cell deficiency, a Gunderson conjunctival flap is used to cover the corneal surface.[16,25] An IntraLase laser can also be used to create the pocket, and the pocket can also be made within an existing failed corneal transplant.

The device is left within the intrastromal pocket for 2–3 months to allow infiltration into the peripheral porous skirt by surrounding tissue stromal cells and blood vessels. The second stage of the procedure is then undertaken. Using a 3.5-mm skin biopsy trephine, the corneal lamella (and conjunctiva, if present) anterior to the AlphaCor optic is removed to expose the optical component of the prosthesis.

## POSTOPERATIVE CARE

### Boston Keratoprosthesis Type I

Administration of a fourth generation fluoroquinolone and topical prednisolone acetate 1%, both four times daily, is started on the first postoperative day. Both are slowly tapered to once daily over the next 2–3 months. Once a day administration of topical vancomycin 1.4% (14 mg/mL in benzalkonium chloride preservative) may be started within the first postoperative week.[26] Long-term topical steroid use is unnecessary in most cases; however, use of two antibiotics, either Trimethoprim/Polymyxin B or a topical fluoroquinolone and topical vancomycin, is continued once daily indefinitely. In cases where the risk of secondary infection is higher, twice daily administration of both antibiotics is recommended. More frequent use of topical antibiotics in the long-term is not advisable, since it may promote fungal contamination of the contact lens and/or front plate, with subsequent infection.

Frequent follow-up visits are required initially to assess for postoperative infection, inflammation, and elevation in intraocular pressure. Follow-up should be individualized, but typically patients are seen two to three times in the first two postoperative weeks, and then weekly up to the first month after surgery. Monthly examinations are then performed for the first 6 months, and return visits are extended to every 2–3 months after that. Elevation of the intraocular pressure found at any visit should prompt involvement of a glaucoma specialist in the care of the patient.

### Boston Keratoprosthesis Type II

Similar to the type I surgery, antibiotic prophylaxis starts on the first postoperative day and continues indefinitely. Administration of a fourth generation fluoroquinolone four times a day, tapered to twice daily during the following month, is combined with twice daily administration of topical vancomycin 1.4% (14 mg/mL in benzalkonium chloride preservative); the latter begins within the first postoperative week, and both are continued indefinitely.[26] Topical corticosteroids, typically prednisolone acetate 1%, are also started four times a day on the first postoperative day and tapered off over the next month. Use of the antibiotic ointment to the eyelid margins is discontinued about 2 weeks postoperatively, at which time the skin sutures and bolsters are removed.

It is important to realize that once the eyelid skin is fully healed around the keratoprosthesis optic, typically within 2 to 3 weeks after surgery, topical medications no longer penetrate to the ocular surface. Thus, any rise in intraocular pressure should be treated with oral acetazolamide or methazolamide. This also means that the goal of the indefinite administration of a topical fluoroquinolone and vancomycin twice daily is to reduce microbial colonization of the skin around the keratoprosthesis optic, to prevent infection from reaching the eye.

### OOKP

Adequate pain control is essential in the immediate postoperative period, and the patients are admitted for 1 week after each stage of the procedure. After stage I, patients are prescribed oral prednisone 20 mg and lansoprazole 30 mg for 5 days, oral antibiotics for a week, and nystatin and chlorhexidine mouth washes until the oral harvest sites heal. Moreover, a conformer is usually placed over the buccal mucous membrane graft and daily glass rodding is carried out to keep the fornices open. After stage II, oral acetazolamide is prescribed in addition to the oral steroids and antibiotics. The optic is cleaned daily, and the health of the buccal mucous membrane graft is closely monitored. Patients who receive an allograft are placed on long-term immunosuppression with cyclosporin A.

After the first week, patients are seen at weekly intervals for a month, then monthly for 3–6 months, and then every 4–6 months. The intraocular pressure is checked digitally at each visit, and the mucous membrane graft is carefully examined for signs of dryness, thinning, or ulceration. The optical cylinder is tested for tilt, stability, and presence of a retroprosthetic membrane. Bone resorption is assessed both clinically by palpating the mass and dimensions of the lamina and radiographically using spiral computed tomography or magnetic resonance imaging.

### AlphaCor

In the early postoperative period, topical prednisolone acetate 1% and antibiotics are used and are slowly weaned off over the next 4 weeks. Patients are seen two or three times in the first two postoperative weeks, and follow-up is then spaced out more as indicated by the patient's course. Postoperative refractive correction is usually done with high oxygen permeability contact lenses, which also provide protection for the device surface.

## COMPLICATIONS

The most common postoperative complication after keratoprosthesis surgery (Boston keratoprosthesis type I or II) is ongoing ocular inflammation, such as formation of retroprosthetic membrane, vitritis, epiretinal membrane, and retinal detachment. The most common threat to good quality long-term vision after keratoprosthesis surgery is glaucoma, and this is clearly exacerbated by the presence of chronic inflammation. The severity of postoperative inflammation is determined, at least partly, by the degree of preoperative inflammation. Thus, aggressive management of preoperative inflammation with immunomodulatory therapy is indicated in patients with underlying autoimmune diseases such as Stevens–Johnson syndrome or mucous membrane pemphigoid.

Complications associated with any keratoprosthesis implantation include:

- Glaucoma
- Retinal or choroidal detachment
- Infectious endophthalmitis
- Tissue necrosis, melt, and device extrusion
- Retroprosthetic membrane formation.

### Boston Keratoprosthesis

In addition to complications listed above for keratoprosthesis implantation, Boston keratoprosthesis surgery can also be associated with:

- Sterile uveitis–vitritis.

### OOKP

Specific oral and ocular complications associated with OOKP implantation[27,28] include:

- Lamina or mucous membrane infection
- Excess buccal scarring and limitation of mouth opening
- Injury to maxillary sinus
- Facial and jaw bone fractures.

### AlphaCor

Complications specifically associated with AlphaCor implantation include:

- Herpetic eye disease-related keratolysis
- Fibrous reclosure of the posterior lamellar opening
- White intraoptic deposits.

## SURGICAL OUTCOMES: SCIENTIFIC EVIDENCE/META-ANALYSIS

### Boston Keratoprosthesis Type I

Numerous studies have reported outcomes for the Boston keratoprosthesis type I surgery.[8,10,29-42] In the first multicenter study to report outcomes after implantation of 141 Boston keratoprosthesis type I devices in 17 centers, most of the 133 operated patients experienced a significant improvement in visual acuity.[8] Best corrected visual acuity of 20/200 or better was measured in 57% of the operated eyes at 1 year postoperatively compared with 3.6% preoperatively, with 23% of operated eyed attaining vision of 20/40 or better. Failure of the visual acuity to improve after Boston keratoprosthesis type I implantation in this series was commonly secondary to coexisting conditions, such as advanced glaucoma, macular degeneration, and retinal detachment. The anatomical retention rate was 95% at an average follow-up of 8.5 months (range, 0.03–24 months; median, 12 months). Visual and anatomic outcomes were also analyzed based on the preoperative diagnosis and were shown to be better in noncicatrizing graft failure (e.g. in cases of bullous keratopathy, infection, and dystrophies) and chemical burns than in autoimmune diseases (e.g. mucous membrane pemphigoid, Stevens–Johnson syndrome/toxic epidermal necrolysis). The main complications were retroprosthetic membrane formation (25% or 35 eyes), high intraocular pressure (14.8% or 21 eyes), sterile vitritis (4.9% or 7 eyes), and retinal detachment (3.5% or 5 eyes). Thus, the most common postoperative surgical procedures performed were YAG laser membranectomy and glaucoma tube shunt placement. No case of endophthalmitis was encountered in this study.

In a recently published international series of outcomes, analysis after implantation of 113 Boston keratoprostheses type I in 11 centers in Armenia, India, Indonesia, Nepal, Philippines, Russia, and Saudi Arabia, postoperative visual acuity, anatomical retention rate, and incidence of postoperative complications (with the exception of endophthalmitis) were similar to those experienced by North American surgeons.[10] In particular, at 6 months, 1 year and 2 years postoperatively, 70, 68, and 59 of eyes had a best corrected visual acuity of 20/200 or better, compared with 2% of eyes preoperatively. Anatomical retention rate was 80.5% at a mean follow-up of 14.2 months. Although infectious endophthalmitis was more common in the international series (9% of eyes), the incidence of other complications (e.g. retroprosthetic membrane formation) was similar to the North American experience.

In our experience, several improvements in the device design and the postoperative care have improved outcomes of Boston keratoprosthesis surgery over the last 15 years. The addition of eight perforations—1.3 mm each – to the back plate in 1999 and an additional row of back plate holes in 2001 reduced rates of keratolysis by allowing hydration and nourishment of the posterior corneal stroma with aqueous humor.[4,20] The modification from a threaded back plate to a snap-in design with a titanium-locking ring prevents disassmbly of the device in situ. Moreover, a change in the back plate material from PMMA to titanium has been associated with a decreased incidence of retroprosthetic membrane formation.[21] Since the inclusion of vancomycin in the postoperative treatment regimen and the continuous use of low-dose prophylactic antibiotics indefinitely, the rate of acute Gram-positive endophthalmitis among type I keratoprosthesis patients has diminished dramatically.[43] Finally, although unclear whether healthy corneal endothelium is required for successful retention of keratoprosthesis,[44] we do favor the use of a healthy graft when possible.

## Boston Keratoprosthesis Type II

The type II device is used much less commonly than the type I. At the Massachusetts Eye and Ear Infirmary, only 29 eyes received a Boston keratoprosthesis type II over a 10-year period (from January 2000 to December 2009) compared with > 350 that received a type I device in the same time period.[18]

The most comprehensive report on the success rate of Boston keratoprosthesis type II implantation[18] in patients with ocular surface diseases such as mucous membrane pemphigoid, Stevens–Johnson syndrome and severe chemical burns comes from our institution. In this study, out of the 29 eyes that received a type II device over a 10-year period, 50% of eyes (6 eyes) with mucous membrane pemphigoid and 62.5% of eyes (5 eyes) with Stevens–Johnson syndrome achieved and maintained vision of 20/200 or better for > 2 years. Anatomical retention rate was 58.6% (17 out of 29 eyes) during a total follow-up time of 107.9 person-years. In a subsequent report,[42] comparing the outcomes of Boston keratoprosthesis implantation in patients with mucous membrane pemphigoid, postoperative visual acuity and device retention were strikingly better for the type II device. Kaplan–Meier analysis for retention of visual acuity of 20/200 or better was 33% for the mucous membrane pemphigoid eyes that underwent Boston keratoprosthesis type I surgery and 67% for the eyes that received a type II device. At 3 years postoperatively, only 18% of the eyes retained a type I device without revision or replacement compared with 73% of the eyes with a type II device.

Prior studies on the use of Boston keratoprosthesis implantation did not differentiate the outcomes by disease[10] or by the type of the keratoprosthesis device implanted.[31,45] For example, for 16 eyes of patients with Stevens–Johnson syndrome/toxic epidermal necrolysis treated at Massachusetts Eye and Ear Infirmary over a 6-year time period (1997–2003), Sayegh et al.[31] reported that 75% (12 out 16 eyes) had vision equal or better than 20/200 for a mean period of 2.5 ± 2 years after keratoprosthesis (type I or II) implantation.

Due to the small number of type II recipients, it is not possible to accurately evaluate changes in the intraoperative or postoperative management. We know that monitoring the intraocular pressure after type II surgery is very difficult, thus rapidly progressive glaucoma can irreversibly compromise vision before there is time for any intervention to be undertaken.[18,31,40,46-53] Thus, in most cases we favor the implantation of a glaucoma drainage device at the time of the type II keratoprosthesis surgery. We also favor pars plana vitrectomy at the time of the type II keratoprosthesis implantation as a way to decrease the risk of postoperative retinal detachment by releasing vitreous traction. Finally, the role of low-dose long-term prophylactic antibiotics in preventing infections in type II recipients still needs to be formally defined. Because of the well-documented advantage of chronic antibiotic use in type I recipients, we also recommend their use by type II keratoprosthesis recipients.[43]

## OOKP

A relative strength of OOKP implantation in corneal blindness associated with severe ocular surface dryness and keratinization is its projected retention rate of 66–85% at 10–18 years after surgery.[12,54] The underlying principle behind the longer survival and low extrusion rate of the OOKP in a hostile ocular surface environment lies in its ability to be integrated into the surrounding sclera and mucous membrane and thus derive its own blood supply. Falcinelli's modifications to the original Strampelli technique were instrumental in improving visual outcomes and device retention.[12,55,56] These include use of a biconvex larger optic, cryoextraction of the lens and vitrectomy, preservation of the periosteum, use of a buccal rather than a labial mucous membrane graft and of a nonerupted tooth allograft, and implantation of a posterior drainage tube in refractory glaucoma.

Several studies have reported outcomes after OOKP implantation.[12,27,54,57-61] The two most cited studies on the long-term outcomes of OOKP surgery are the reports by Falcinelli et al.[12] and Michael et al.[54] Falcinelli et al.[12] reported the outcomes of 181 patients who underwent OOKP between 1973 and 1999 with a median follow-up of 12 years (range, 1–25 years). The cumulative probability of retaining an intact OOKP 8 years after surgery was 90% and 18 years after implantation was 85% (17 patients). The cumulative probability of retaining the best-corrected postoperative acuity within two lines was > 70% 9 years after the surgery and 55.5% 18 years after implantation. The most common complication after OOKP surgery was glaucoma, which was reported in 10.4% of eyes within 24 months of the stage II procedure. Mucous membrane ulceration was the second most frequent complication, and it occurred in 7% of cases.

Endophthalmitis was reported to occur rarely (4 eyes) and was associated with poor preoperative tooth condition.

Michael et al.[54] reported the results of 145 patients who underwent OOKP implantation between 1974 and 2005. The 10-year anatomical success, defined as retention of the carrier keratoprosthesis lamina, was 66%. Functional success, as defined by best-corrected visual acuity > 0.05 (> 20/400), was 63% at the 2-year follow-up and 38% at the 10-year follow-up. In a subsequent publication, the same group showed that anatomic and functional survival greatly depended on the primary diagnosis.[61] For example, the mucous membrane pemphigoid group had the worst anatomic survival 10 years after the surgery, and the thermal burn group had the worst functional survival at the 10-year follow-up. The most common complications were extrusion of the keratoprosthesis lamina, retinal detachment, and refractory glaucoma.

### AlphaCor

Implantation of the AlphaCor device is technically simpler than the OOKP, but it does require familiarity with corneal lamellar surgical techniques. In particular, corneas that are thinned and scarred can be particularly challenging for AlphaCor implantation. Initial reports on the outcomes of AlphaCor implantation suggested a lower incidence of complications, such as glaucoma, than with other keratoprosthesis devices;[14,16,25,62] however, subsequent studies with longer follow-up showed worse visual results and increased corneal stromal melting.[63] Eyes with prior herpetic eye disease have particularly poor outcomes after AlphaCor implantation.[64] Reactivation of herpes simplex virus is thought to induce chronic inflammation and subsequent melting of the anterior corneal stroma.

The most comprehensive study by Hicks et al.[63] included 322 eyes that underwent AlphaCor implantation by 84 surgeons up to February 2006 with a mean follow-up of 15.5 months (range, 0.5 months to 7.4 years). The reported retention rate was 92% at 6 months, 80% at 1 year, and 62% at 2 years postoperatively. The median preoperative visual acuity was hand movements, and it ranged from light perception to 20/20 postoperatively, depending on the preexisting ocular pathology (e.g. macular disease, glaucoma). Mean functional improvement after surgery was two lines of vision. The most common complications were stromal melting (11.4%), fibrous reclosure of the posterior lamellar opening (5.1%), and white intraoptic deposits due to topical medications (2.6%). Loss of the eye due to complications occurred in 1.3% of cases, and the incidence of endophthalmitis was 0.6%. Topical use of medroxyprogesterone was associated with fewer corneal melts.[63,65]

## PLACE OF THE TECHNIQUE IN SURGICAL ARMAMENTARIUM

Identifying the underlying etiology and fully assessing the condition of the ocular surface is paramount in the selection of appropriate candidates for any type of keratoprosthesis implantation. The best candidates for the OOKP or the Boston keratoprosthesis type II device are patients with history of Stevens–Johnson syndrome, mucous membrane pemphigoid, end-stage keratoconjunctivitis sicca, or severe chemical burns with evidence of significant symblepharon or ankyloblepharon, ocular surface keratinization, and absence of normal blink function and tear production. Ocular surface inflammation should be minimized prior to surgery, especially in patients with underlying autoimmune inflammatory conditions. A normal tear film and healthy conjunctiva are required for a successful AlphaCor or Boston keratoprosthesis type I implantation, which makes patients with repeated allograft failures the best candidates for these devices. Regardless of the keratoprosthesis to be implanted, patient motivation to submit to life-long care and regular follow-up examinations are essential for a successful outcome. Postoperative inflammation and glaucoma remain the most important obstacles in attaining and maintaining functional vision. Thus, preoperative efforts should be focused at minimizing inflammation and optimizing intraocular pressure.

## REFERENCES


1. de Quengsy P. Precis ou cours d'operations sur la chirurgie des yeux. Paris, France: Didot; 1789.
2. Niederkorn JY. Mechanisms of corneal graft rejection: the sixth annual Thygeson Lecture. Cornea. 2001;20:675-9.
3. Rahman I, Carley F, Hillarby C, et al. Penetrating keratoplasty: indications, outcomes, and complications. Eye (Lond). 2009;23: 1288-94.
4. Khan B, Dudenhoefer EJ, Dohlman CH. Keratoprosthesis: an update. Curr Opin Ophthalmol. 2001;12:282-7.
5. Tugal-Tutkun I, Akova YA, Foster CS. Penetrating keratoplasty in cicatrizing conjunctival diseases. Ophthalmology. 1995;102: 576-85.
6. Dohlman CH, Schneider HA, Doane MG. Prosthokeratoplasty. Am J Ophthalmol. 1974;77:694-70.
7. Klufas MA, Colby KA. The Boston keratoprosthesis. Int Ophthalmol Clin. 2010;50:161-75.
8. Zerbe BL, Belin MW, Ciolino JB. Results from the multicenter Boston Type 1 Keratoprosthesis Study. Ophthalmology. 2006; 113:1779 e1-7.
9. Rudnisky CJ, Belin MW, Todani A, et al.. Risk factors for the development of retroprosthetic membranes with Boston keratoprosthesis type 1: multicenter study results. Ophthalmology. 2012;119:951-5.

10. Aldave AJ, Sangwan VS, Basu S, et al. International results with the Boston type I keratoprosthesis. Ophthalmology. 2012;119: 1530-8.
11. Strampelli B. [Osteo-Odontokeratoprosthesis]. Ann Ottalmol Clin Oculist. 1963;89:1039-44.
12. Falcinelli G, Falsini B, Taloni M, et al. Modified osteo-odonto-keratoprosthesis for treatment of corneal blindness: long-term anatomical and functional outcomes in 181 cases. Arch Ophthalmol. 2005;123(10):1319-29.
13. Chirila TV, Vijayasekaran S, Horne R, et al. Interpenetrating polymer network (IPN) as a permanent joint between the elements of a new type of artificial cornea. J Biomed Mat Res. 1994;28:745-53.
14. Chirila TV. An overview of the development of artificial corneas with porous skirts and the use of PHEMA for such an application. Biomaterials. 2001;22:3311-7.
15. Hicks CR, Werner L, Vijayasekaran S, Mamalis N, Apple DJ. Histology of AlphaCor skirts: evaluation of biointegration. Cornea. 2005;24:933-40.
16. Crawford GJ, Hicks CR, Lou X, et al. The Chirila keratoprosthesis: phase I human clinical trial. Ophthalmology. 2002;109: 883-9.
17. Hille K, Grabner G, Liu C, et al. Standards for modified osteo-odonto-keratoprosthesis (OOKP) surgery according to Strampelli and Falcinelli: the Rome-Vienna Protocol. Cornea. 2005;24:895-908.
18. Pujari S, Siddique SS, Dohlman CH, Chodosh J. The Boston keratoprosthesis type II: the Massachusetts Eye and Ear Infirmary experience. Cornea. 2011;30:1298-303.
19. Doane MG, Dohlman CH, Bearse G. Fabrication of a keratoprosthesis. Cornea. 1996;15:179-84.
20. Khan BF, Harissi-Dagher M, Khan DM, Dohlman CH. Advances in Boston keratoprosthesis: enhancing retention and prevention of infection and inflammation. Int Ophthalmol Clin. 2007;47:61-71.
21. Todani A, Ciolino JB, Ament JD, et al. Titanium back plate for a PMMA keratoprosthesis: clinical outcomes. Graefe's Arch Clin Exp Ophthalmol. 2011;249:1515-8.
22. Utine CA, Tzu J, Dunlap K, Akpek EK. Visual and clinical outcomes of explantation versus preservation of the intraocular lens during keratoprosthesis implantation. J Cataract Refract Surg. 2011;37:1615-22.
23. Liu C, Paul B, Tandon R, et al. The osteo-odonto-keratoprosthesis (OOKP). Sem Ophthalmol. 2005;20:113-28.
24. Gomaa A, Comyn O, Liu C. Keratoprostheses in clinical practice—a review. Clin Exp Ophthalmol. 2010;38:211-24.
25. Hicks CR, Crawford GJ, Lou X, et al. Corneal replacement using a synthetic hydrogel cornea, AlphaCor: device, preliminary outcomes and complications. Eye (Lond). 2003;17:385-92.
26. Nouri M, Terada H, Alfonso EC, et al. Endophthalmitis after keratoprosthesis: incidence, bacterial causes, and risk factors. Arch Ophthalmol. 2001;119:484-9.
27. Liu C, Okera S, Tandon R, et al.. Visual rehabilitation in end-stage inflammatory ocular surface disease with the osteo-odonto-keratoprosthesis: results from the UK. Br J Ophthalmol. 2008;92:1211-7.
28. Hughes EH, Mokete B, Ainsworth G, et al. Vitreoretinal complications of osteo-odonto-keratoprosthesis surgery. Retina. 2008;28:1138-45.
29. Bradley JC, Hernandez EG, Schwab IR, Mannis MJ. Boston type 1 keratoprosthesis: the University of California Davis experience. Cornea. 2009;28:321-7.
30. Chew HF, Ayres BD, Hammersmith KM, et al. Boston keratoprosthesis outcomes and complications. Cornea. 2009;28: 989-96.
31. Sayegh RR, Ang LP, Foster CS, et al. The Boston keratoprosthesis in Stevens-Johnson syndrome. Am J Ophthalmol. 2008;145:438-44.
32. Aldave AJ, Kamal KM, Vo RC, et al. The Boston type I keratoprosthesis: improving outcomes and expanding indications. Ophthalmology. 2009;116:640-51.
33. Kang JJ, de la Cruz J, Cortina MS. Visual outcomes of Boston keratoprosthesis implantation as the primary penetrating corneal procedure. Cornea. 2012;31:1436-40.
34. Shihadeh WA, Mohidat HM. Outcomes of the Boston keratoprosthesis in Jordan. Middle East Afr J Ophthalmol. 2012;19:97-100.
35. Al Arfaj K, Hantera M. Short-term visual outcomes of Boston keratoprosthesis type I in Saudi Arabia. Middle East Afr J Ophthalmol. 2012;19:88-92.
36. Hou JH, de la Cruz J, Djalilian AR. Outcomes of Boston keratoprosthesis implantation for failed keratoplasty after keratolimbal allograft. Cornea. 2012;31:1432-5.
37. Patel AP, Wu EI, Ritterband DC, et al. Boston type 1 keratoprosthesis: the New York Eye and Ear experience. Eye (Lond). 2012;26:418-25.
38. Sejpal K, Yu F, Aldave AJ. The Boston keratoprosthesis in the management of corneal limbal stem cell deficiency. Cornea. 2011;30:1187-94.
39. Robert MC, Harissi-Dagher M. Boston type 1 keratoprosthesis: the CHUM experience. Can J Ophthalmol. 2011;46:164-8.
40. Greiner MA, Li JY, Mannis MJ. Longer-term vision outcomes and complications with the Boston type 1 keratoprosthesis at the University of California, Davis. Ophthalmology. 2011;118: 1543-50.
41. Dunlap K, Chak G, Aquavella JV, et al. Short-term visual outcomes of Boston type 1 keratoprosthesis implantation. Ophthalmology. 2010;117:687-92.
42. Palioura S, Kim B, Dohlman CH, Chodosh J. The Boston Keratoprosthesis type I in mucous membrane pemphigoid. Cornea. 2013;32:956-61.
43. Durand ML, Dohlman CH. Successful prevention of bacterial endophthalmitis in eyes with the Boston keratoprosthesis. Cornea. 2009;28:896-901.
44. Robert MC, Biernacki K, Harissi-Dagher M. Boston keratoprosthesis type 1 surgery: use of frozen versus fresh corneal donor carriers. Cornea. 2012;31:339-45.
45. Yaghouti F, Nouri M, Abad JC, et al. Keratoprosthesis: preoperative prognostic categories. Cornea. 2001;20:19-23.
46. Dohlman CH, Grosskreutz CL, Chen TC, et al. Shunts to divert aqueous humor to distant epithelialized cavities after keratoprosthesis surgery. J Glaucoma. 2010;19:111-5.
47. Panarelli JF, Ko A, Sidoti PA, Garcia JP, et al. Angle closure after Boston keratoprosthesis. J Glaucoma. 2012;doi: 10.1097/IJG.0b013e318259b2fc
48. Kamyar R, Weizer JS, de Paula FH, et al. Glaucoma associated with Boston type I keratoprosthesis. Cornea. 2012;31:134-9.
49. Cade F, Grosskreutz CL, Tauber A, et al. Glaucoma in eyes with severe chemical burn, before and after keratoprosthesis. Cornea. 2011;30:1322-7.

50. Talajic JC, Agoumi Y, Gagne S, et al. Prevalence, progression, and impact of glaucoma on vision after Boston type 1 keratoprosthesis surgery. Am J Ophthalmol. 2012;153:267-74.
51. Banitt M. Evaluation and management of glaucoma after keratoprosthesis. Curr Opin Ophthalmol. 2011;22:133-6.
52. Rivier D, Paula JS, Kim E, et al. Glaucoma and keratoprosthesis surgery: role of adjunctive cyclophotocoagulation. J Glaucoma. 2009;18:321-4.
53. Netland PA, Terada H, Dohlman CH. Glaucoma associated with keratoprosthesis. Ophthalmology. 1998;105:751-7.
54. Michael R, Charoenrook V, de la Paz MF, et al. Long-term functional and anatomical results of osteo- and osteoodonto-keratoprosthesis. Graefe's Arch Clin Exp Ophthalmol. 2008;246:1133-7.
55. Falcinelli GC, Barogi G, Caselli M, et al. Personal changes and innovations in Strampelli's osteo-odonto-keratoprosthesis. An Inst Barraquer (Barc). 1999;28:47-8.
56. Liu C, Pagliarini, S. Independent survey of long term results of the Falcinelli osteo-odonto-keratoprosthesis (OOKP). An Inst Barraquer (Barc). 1999;28:91-3.
57. Tan DT, Tay AB, Theng JT, et al. Keratoprosthesis surgery for end-stage corneal blindness in Asian eyes. Ophthalmology. 2008;115:503-10.
58. Caselli M, Colliardo P, Falcinelli G, et al. Falcinelli's osteo-odonto-keratoprosthesis: long term results. An Inst Barraquer (Barc). 1999;28:113-4.
59. Hille K, Landau H, Ruprecht KW. [Osteo-odonto-keratoprosthesis. A summary of 6 years surgical experience]. Ophthalmologe. 2002;99:90-5.
60. Marchi V, Ricci R, Pecorella I, et al. Osteo-odonto-keratoprosthesis. Description of surgical technique with results in 85 patients. Cornea. 1994;13:125-30.
61. De La Paz MF, De Toledo JA, Charoenrook V, et al. Impact of clinical factors on the long-term functional and anatomic outcomes of osteo-odonto-keratoprosthesis and tibial bone keratoprosthesis. Am J Ophthalmol. 2011;151:829-39.
62. Hicks CR, Crawford GJ, Tan DT, et al. AlphaCor cases: comparative outcomes. Cornea. 2003;22:583-90.
63. Hicks CR, Crawford GJ, Dart JK, et al. AlphaCor: clinical outcomes. Cornea. 2006;25:1034-42.
64. Hicks CR, Crawford GJ, Tan DT, et al. Outcomes of implantation of an artificial cornea, AlphaCor: effects of prior ocular herpes simplex infection. Cornea. 2002;21:685-90.
65. Hicks CR, Crawford GJ. Melting after keratoprosthesis implantation: the effects of medroxyprogesterone. Cornea. 2003;22:497-500.

CHAPTER

# 20

# Amniotic Membrane Transplantation

Hosam Sheha, Sean Tighe, Anny Cheng, Scheffer C G Tseng

## INTRODUCTION

Cryopreserved amniotic membrane (AM) is known to have potent anti-inflammatory mediators, a myriad of growth factors and an active matrix that are important to promote regenerative healing of the ocular surface.[1] Hence, amniotic membrane transplantation (AMT) has successfully been used to treat a number of nonhealing corneal epithelial defects caused by diverse etiologies. AMT is considered a standard of care in the United States and has been granted with three Level 1 CPT codes (65778, 65779, and 65780) by the Center of Medicare and Medicaid Services. Cryopreserved AM can be used as a permanent graft or as a temporary biological bandage in order to restore corneal integrity and clarity.[2] The biological bandage can either be self-retained or secured using sutures. The former can be done in the office to eliminate suture-related complications and facilitate the care by interrupting the disease process at an early stage to avert the risk of developing corneal scarring or haze. This chapter focuses on the use of AM as a biological bandage.

## AMNIOTIC MEMBRANE AS A BIOLOGICAL BANDAGE

When AM is used as a temporary biological bandage, the main goal is to suppress acute or chronic host tissue inflammation caused by diseases or surgery, to promote healing and to minimize scarring. AM can be sutured as a bandage or patch to cover the cornea at the site of interest so that the host epithelium heals underneath. Recently, a FDA-cleared medical device, termed PROKERA (Bio-Tissue, Inc., FL, USA) has been introduced to deliver AM biological actions on a temporary manner without sutures (Fig. 20-1). At the present time, the PROKERA family products contain three members, i.e. Classic, Slim, and Plus. Their specifications and proposed indications are listed in Table 20-1.

## INDICATIONS

AM as a biological bandage can be used to treat ocular surface disorders that have delayed healing, uncontrolled inflammation, or the potential of scar formation (Table 20-2).[3]

**TABLE 20-1** PROKERA classifications

| | PROKERA Slim | PROKERA Classic | PROKERA Plus |
|---|---|---|---|
| Design | Single layer of AM totally covering the PROKERA ring | Single layer of AM clipped between 2-ring system | Double layers of AM clipped between 2-ring system |
| Outer/inner diameter | 21.6/17.9 | 21.6/15.5 | 21.6/15.5 |
| Benefits | Maximizes contact with the cornea and limbus | Standardizes contact with the cornea | Maximizes the therapeutic effect and overcomes rapid dissolution |
| Indications based on the severity of the condition | Mild to moderate | Moderate to severe | Severe |

TABLE 20-2 Common indications of AM as a biological bandage

| Defects/delayed healing | Inflammation/infection | Haze/scar formation |
|---|---|---|
| Persistent epithelial defect | Inflammatory/infectious keratitis | Haze after refractive surgery |
| Recurrent corneal erosion | Chemical/thermal burns | Scar (Salzmann nodular degeneration) |
| Delayed epithelial healing | Stevens–Johnson syndrome | Limbal stem cell deficiency |

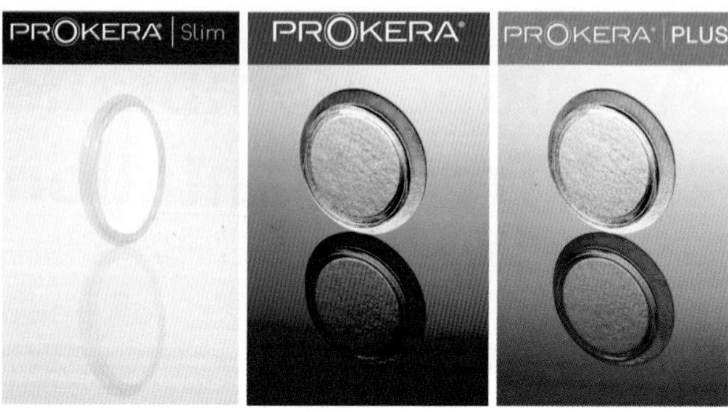


Figure 20-1 PROKERA classification.

TABLE 20-3 Indications for amniotic membrane as a permanent graft

- Pterygia
- Conjunctival tumors
- Conjunctival scarring and symblepharon
- Superior limbal keratoconjunctivitis
- Conjunctivochalasis
- Glaucoma surgery

AM may also be used as a permanent graft in areas with a conjunctival defect. In this setting, AM restores a normal stroma and provides a basement membrane (BM) for epithelial growth (Table 20-3).

## CONTRAINDICATIONS

To the best of our knowledge, there are no known contraindications of AMT; however, the use of self-retained AM via PROKERA is contraindicated in eyes with glaucoma blebs or glaucoma drainage implant to avoid the potential contact and abrasion that can be caused by the ring to the bleb or shunt tube.[4] In these cases, AMT using sutures is recommended to maximize the therapeutic value.

## PROCEDURES

### Amniotic Membrane Patch Graft with Sutures

- Under local anesthesia, secure a single layer of cryopreserved AM (2.5 × 2.0 cm size) by a 10-0 nylon suture at 2–3 mm from the limbus in a purse-string fashion (Figs. 20-2A to D) for a total of 6–8 episcleral bites to cover the corneal surface
- AM can be sutured with the sticky stromal surface facing up or down
- If multiple layers are required or a larger surface area needs to be covered, a larger size AM is needed (3.5 × 3.5 cm size), which can be fashioned to the desired area.

### PROKERA Placement (Fig. 20-3)

- Apply topical anesthesia
- Hold the upper eyelid
- Ask the patient to look down
- Insert the PROKERA into the superior fornix
- Slide the PROKERA under the lower eyelid.

### PROKERA Removal (Fig. 20-4)

- Pull down the lower eyelid
- Ask the patient to look up
- Grab the lower edge of the PROKERA with forceps
- Slide the PROKERA downward and out of the eye.

## CLINICAL APPLICATIONS AND OUTCOMES

### Persistent Epithelial Defect (PED)

PED is usually "neurotrophic", which is characterized by decreased corneal sensation, epithelial breakdown, and poor healing. Coexisting ocular surface diseases such as dry eye, exposure keratitis, and/or limbal stem cell deficiency (LSCD) may worsen the prognosis. The disease progression is often asymptomatic and may lead to infection, corneal melting, or silent perforation. Conventional treatments usually fail to promote healing and tend to leave a corneal scar. On the contrary, AM contains active wound healing components and nerve growth factor (NGF) that not only facilitates epithelial

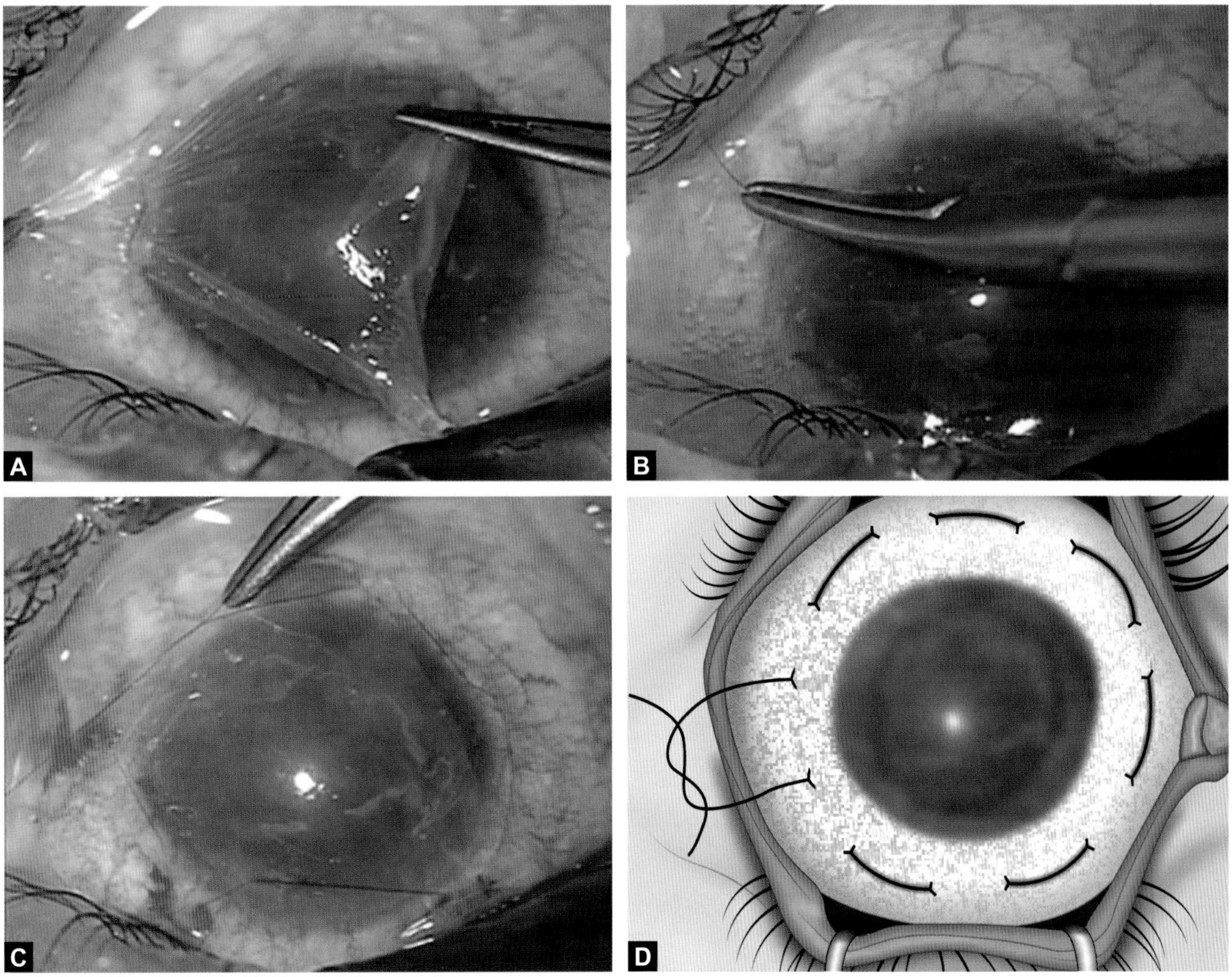

**Figures 20-2A to D** Amniotic membrane patch graft with suture.

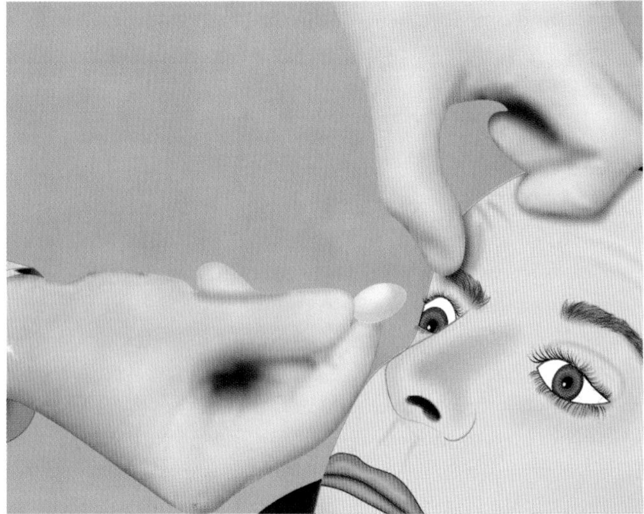

**Figure 20-3** PROKERA placement.

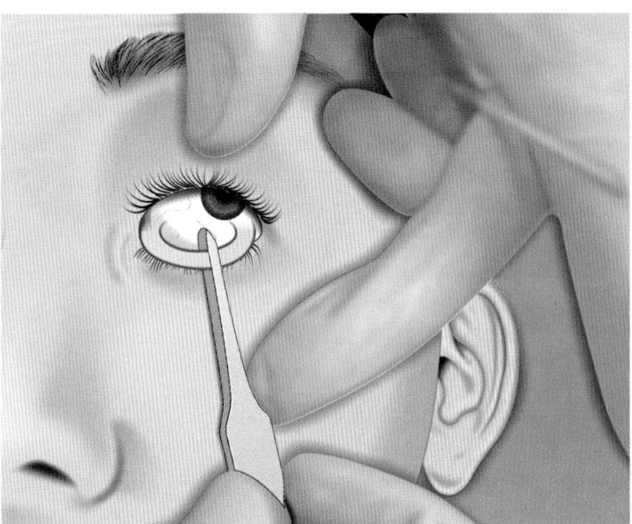

**Figure 20-4** PROKERA removal.

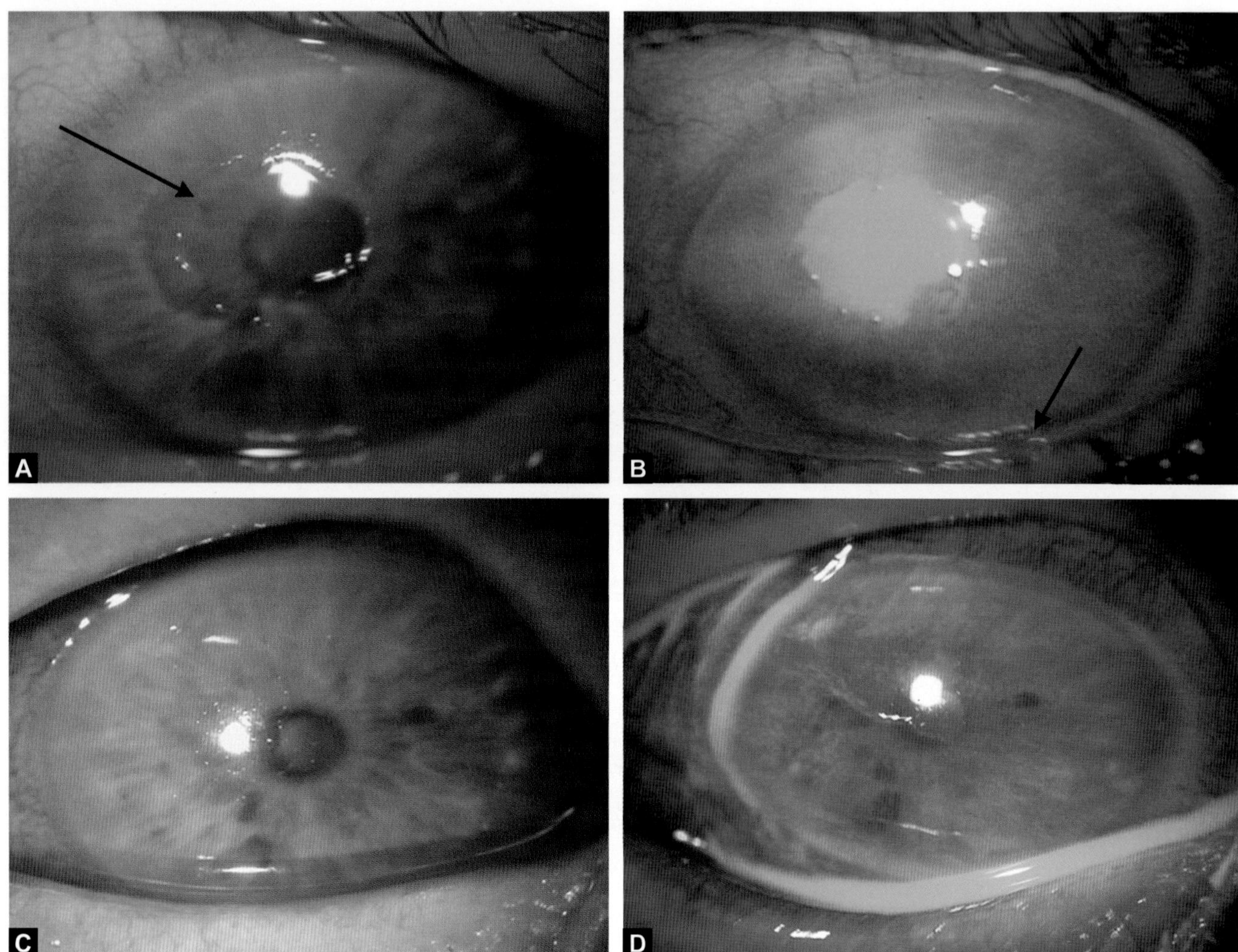


**Figures 20-5A to D** PROKERA for neurotrophic persistent epithelial defect.

healing but also helps recover corneal sensitivity.[5] Treatment of underlying causes or associated disorders should be immediately addressed. Following this, early placement of self-retained AM "PROKERA" is crucial to promote regenerative healing and prevent corneal haze.[6] Corneal surface breakdown may recur if severe neurotrophic keratopathy persists; therefore, it is advised to perform punctual occlusion and/or temporary tarsorrhaphy at the time of AM placement and insert an extended high DK bandage contact lens or permanent tarsorrhaphy after healing.

*Case #1*: A 67-year-old patient had a history of HSV keratitis and dry eye. She presented with mild ocular discomfort and progressive diminution of vision (20/400) for several weeks. Examination revealed a central corneal epithelial defect surrounded by a rim of loose epithelium, stromal edema, and anterior chamber inflammatory reaction (Figs. 20-5A and B). The diagnosis was made as neurotrophic PED. PROKERA was placed along with punctual plugs, tapesorrhaphy, and oral acyclovir. Complete healing occurred within one week, resulting in a clear cornea and 20/20 vision (Figs. 20-5C and D).

## Recurrent Corneal Erosion (RCE)

RCE is a common ocular surface disorder characterized by a disturbance at the level of the corneal epithelial BM, resulting in defective adhesions and recurrent breakdowns of the epithelium. RCE may occur spontaneously or secondary to corneal injury and is more common in diabetes or corneal dystrophy. Patients with RCE often show increased levels of matrix metalloproteinases (MMPs) that dissolve the BM and its anchoring components including integrins, laminin, and type VII collagen.[7]

Current treatments include lubricating agents, patching, bandage contact lens, debridement, anterior stroma puncture,

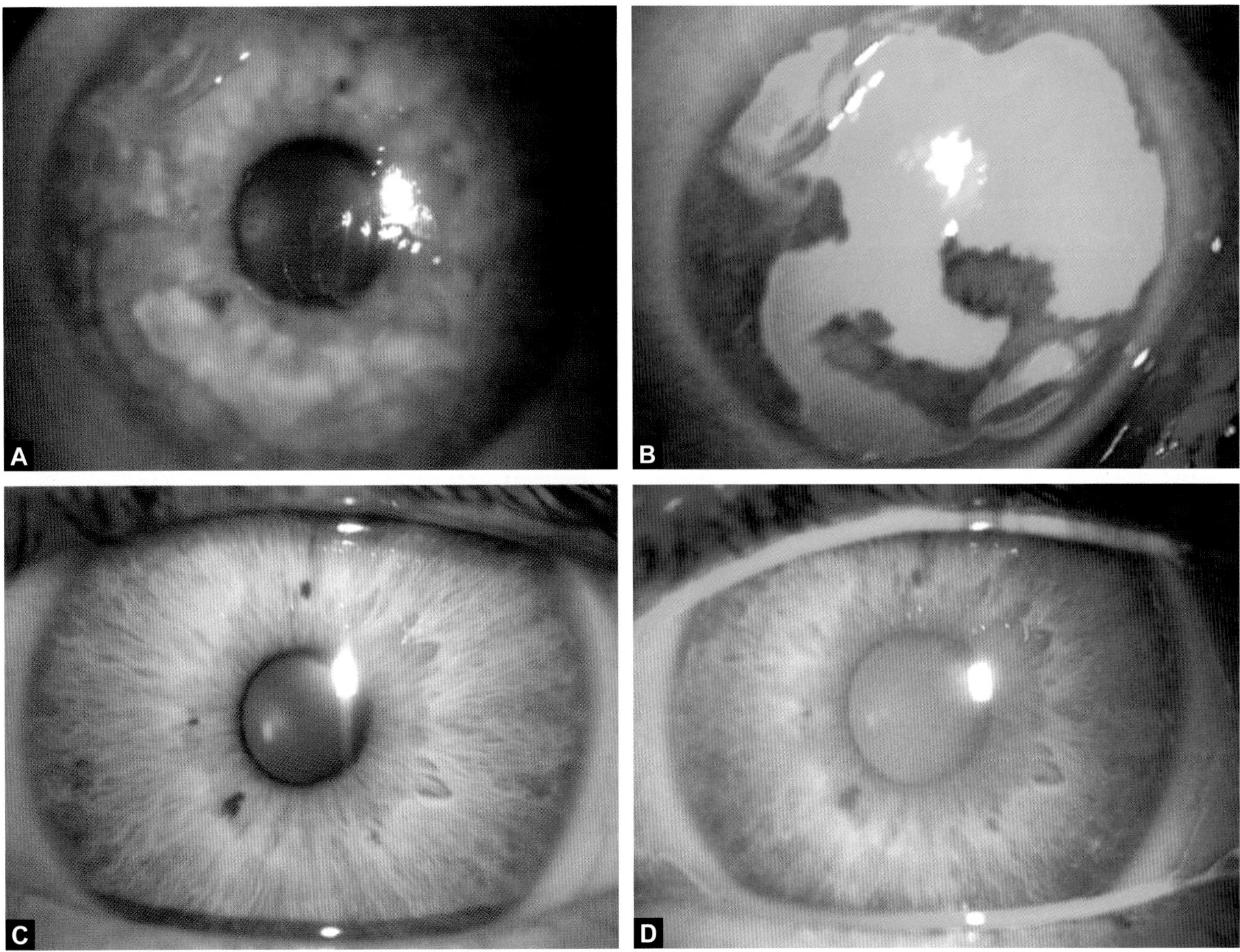


**Figures 20-6A to D** PROKERA for recurrent corneal erosion.

and phototherapeutic keratectomy (PTK). These treatments still have a high recurrence rate and carry the risk of developing haze.[8] AM, however, contains MMPs inhibitors that prevent the breakdown of the BM. It also has active matrix components including collagen type VII and laminin, which are essential for regenerative healing of the BM and its anchoring system. Placement of self-retained cryopreserved AM via PROKERA has achieved rapid healing with reduced recurrence in patients suffering from RCE.[9]

*Case #2*: A 52-year-old female presented with ocular pain and blurred vision (20/200) for 2 weeks. She had a history of similar attacks and was diagnosed with RCE. Epithelial debridement, lubricants, and bandage contact lens failed to relieve pain or halt recurrence. Epithelial debridement to remove loose epithelium (Figs. 20-6A and B) followed by placement of self-retained AM (Fig. 20-6C) resulted in complete healing in 3 days with a clear cornea and 20/20 vision. A smooth surface remained stable with no recurrence for more than 2 years follow-up (Fig. 20-6D).

## Infectious Keratitis

Infectious keratitis may cause corneal destruction directly by the infectious agents and by the associated inflammatory response. The principal therapeutic goals are to eliminate the pathogens and to prevent irreversible corneal structural damage. In order to achieve these goals, immediate treatment with intensive topical fortified antibiotics along with anti-inflammatory agent is required. The fortified topical antibiotics are known to have a potent toxic effect on the corneal epithelium, and the use of steroids in infectious keratitis is controversial because it may flare up the infection and further delay the healing process. AM patch graft has been used as an adjuvant treatment to suppress the inflammation,

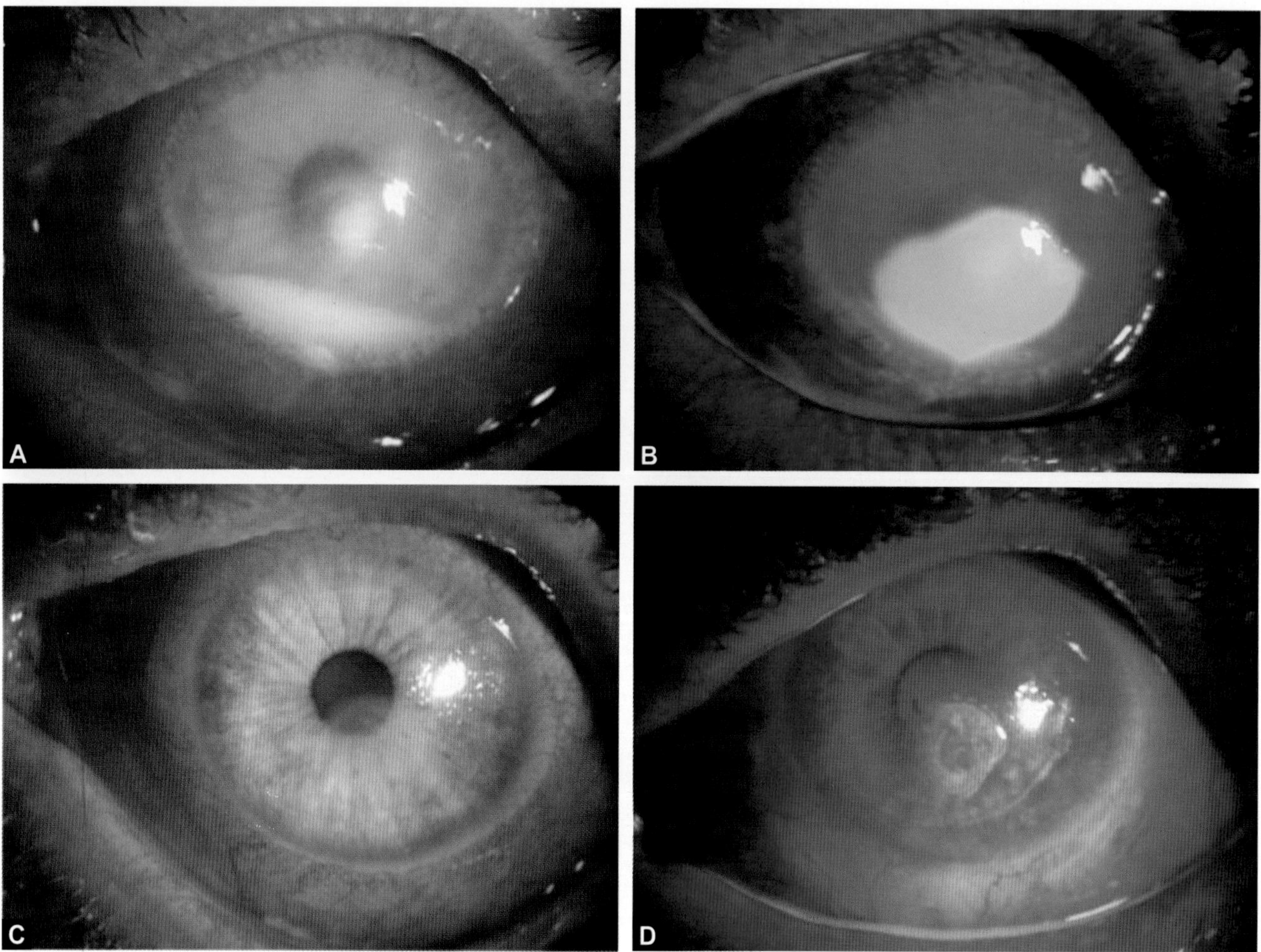


**Figures 20-7A to D** PROKERA for severe bacterial keratitis. Modified from Sheha et al.[12]

promote healing, and counteract the side effects of both steroids and fortified antibiotics.[10,11]

Recently we reported the use of PROKERA in cases with severe microbial keratitis.[12] Pain was significantly relieved, inflammation was markedly reduced, and the corneal ulceration rapidly healed within 2 weeks resulting in visual improvement.

*Case#3*: A 61-year-old contact lens wearer presented with severe left ocular pain and loss of vision. Examination revealed a central corneal ulcer, deep stromal infiltration, hypopyon, and severe ocular surface inflammation (Figs. 20-7A and B). Microbiologic workup confirmed the diagnosis of severe bacterial keratitis. PROKERA was placed shortly after treatment with fortified antibiotics. Two weeks later, the inflammation was markedly reduced, the corneal epithelial defect completely healed (Figs. 20-7C and D), and the patient regained 20/25 vision.

## Delayed Epithelial Healing After Corneal Transplantation

Several factors influence graft re-epithelialization after penetrating keratoplasty. Delayed epithelial healing is commonly seen in diabetic recipients, patients receiving multiple grafts and in association with chronic ocular surface disorders. In general, the use of AM is a beneficial strategy in these patients.

*Case#4*: A 62-year-old single-eyed male presented with rapid loss of vision after multiple corneal graft failures. Examination revealed a total nonhealing corneal epithelial defect (Figs. 20-8A and B). Corneal transplant was performed along with AM patch graft with sutures. Complete healing occurred within 1 week (Figs. 20-8C and D). The AM patch graft was removed, and the cornea was clear with no epithelial defect (Figs. 20-8E and F). The patient regained 20/40 vision and the ocular surface remained stable for 18 months.

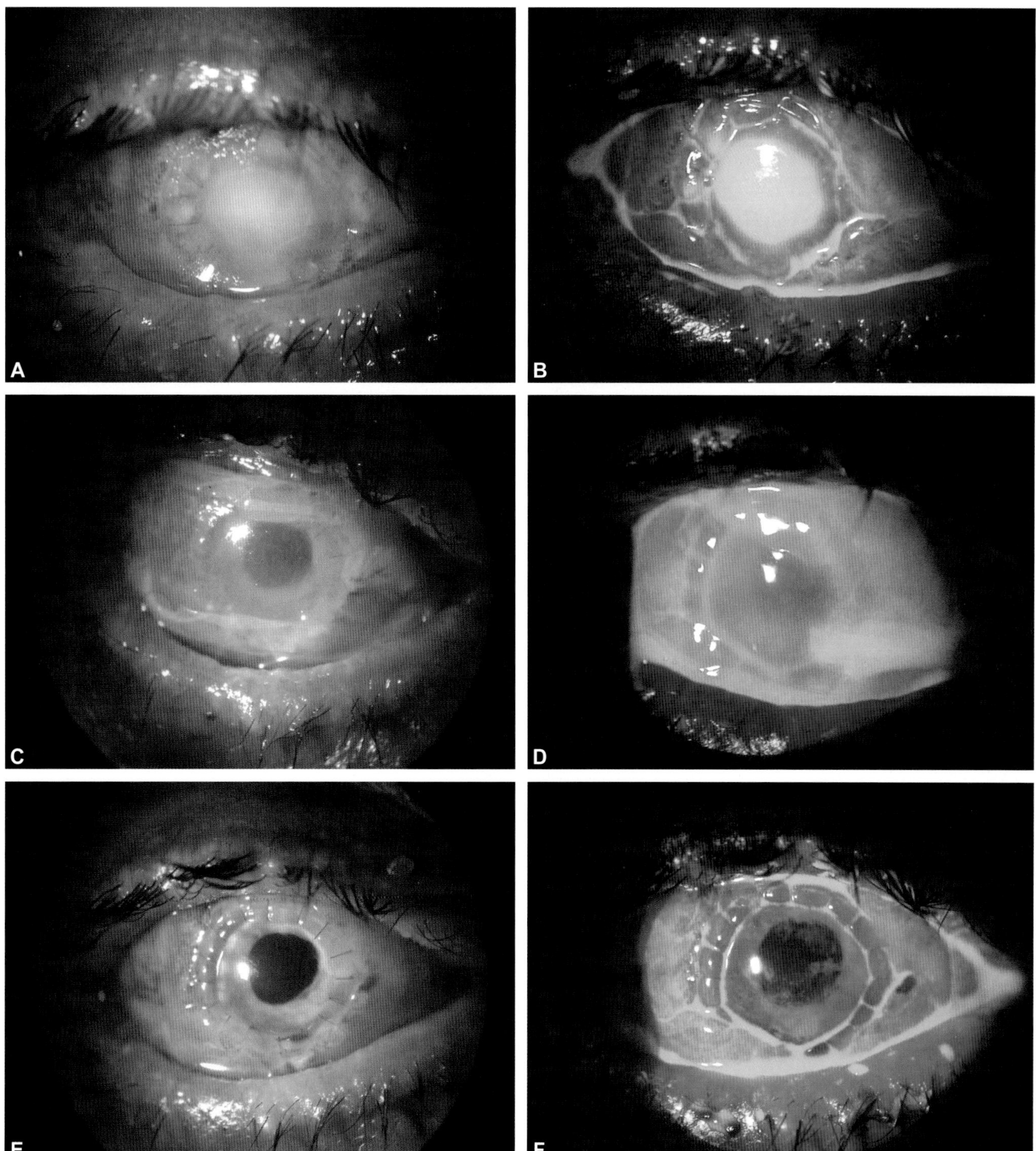


**Figures 20-8A to F** Amniotic membrane-sutured patch graft after repeated corneal graft failure.

## Acute Chemical Burn

Ocular chemical burn injury is a serious ocular emergency in which rapid, devastating, and permanent damage can occur. The severity of the injury correlates directly to exposure, duration, and the causative agent. Treatment of such injuries requires medical and surgical intervention, both acutely and in the long term. Regardless of the underlying chemical

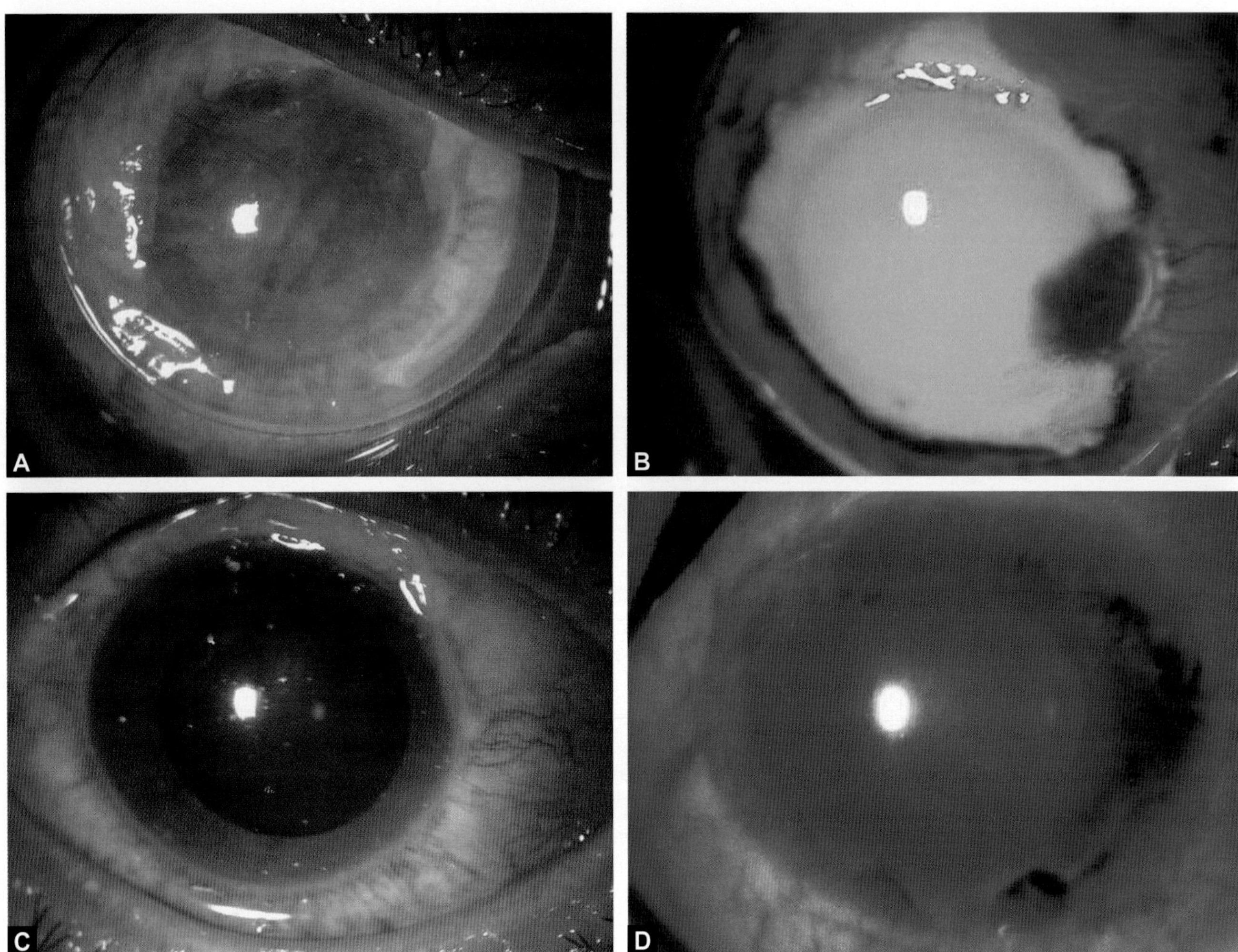


**Figures 20-9A to D** PROKERA for acute chemical burn.

involved, the common goals of management include removing the offending agent, controlling inflammation, and promoting ocular surface healing with maximal visual rehabilitation. Various medical therapies have been used to achieve these objectives including topical and systemic ascorbate, citrate, tetracycline, progesterone, and steroids. Previous studies revealed that early intervention with AMT in mild and moderate chemical burns results in marked reduction in symptoms, rapid restoration of the ocular surface, and improved visual acuities, while preventing cicatricial complications in the chronic stage.[13] However, surgically performed AMT renders a relatively high cost and potentially unnecessary surgical trauma in such compromised eyes. Hence, early application of PROKERA, simultaneously with the conventional treatment, may help break the inflammatory cycle and promote healing as previously reported.[14]

*Case#5*: A 27-year-old female had an ocular alkali burn injury to her right eye. After initial irrigation, she received topical antibiotic steroids, homatropine, and oral vitamin C and doxycycline for 1 week. She was referred to us for further management of delayed epithelialization. Examination of revealed right ocular pain, photophobia, blepharospasm, and decreased vision (20/200). There was a nearly total corneal epithelial defect, corneal edema, limbal ischemia, and diffuse conjunctival inflammation (Figs. 20-9A and B). PROKERA was placed for 1 week, in addition to topical preservative-free steroids. The conjunctival inflammation was reduced, the corneal surface completely healed (Figs. 20-9C and D), and the patient regained 20/25 vision.

## Limbal Stem Cell Deficiency (LSCD)

The hallmark of LSCD is conjunctivalization of the cornea, and it is frequently associated with superficial vascularization.[15] LSCD can be found with a number of corneal diseases such as chemical burn, SJS, aniridia, peripheral keratitis, and severe limbitis. For eyes with partial LSCD, the corneal surface can be reconstructed by debridement of the conjunctivalized epithelium followed by AMT.[16] Previous studies have shown that in eyes with partial LSCD, AM promotes expansion of remaining limbal epithelial stem cells. AMT as a permanent graft was secured with sutures[16] or fibrin glue[17] followed by placement of self-retained AM via PROKERA to enhance the healing process.[17]

For eyes inflicted with total LSCD, transplantation of limbal epithelial stem cells (SCs) is required. AMT has been used as a substrate for the transplanted SCs[18] and as a temporary biological bandage using self-retained PROKERA to enhance the healing as well.[17] These measures can augment AM's therapeutic actions in restoring a healthy limbal stromal niche with less inflammation and scarring that may support the success of transplanted autologous or allogeneic limbal grafts.

## COMPLICATIONS AND LIMITATIONS

Although AMT has been successfully used in different ophthalmic surgeries, the common surgical complications may include infection, bleeding, and graft detachment. The success of AMT can be limited by other factors that may alter the wound healing process. For the ocular surface, the degree of desiccation and exposure are important limiting factors that require simultaneous treatment. Uncontrolled inflammation and ischemia are other risk factors. Furthermore, if the host cells are intrinsically abnormal, e.g. LSCD, AMT alone cannot achieve successful reconstruction without transplanting healthy epithelial or mesenchymal progenitors.

## REFERENCES


1. Tseng SCG, Espana EM, Kawakita T, et al. How does amniotic membrane work? Ocul Surf. 2004;2(3):177-87.
2. Dua HS, Gomes JA, King AJ, et al. The amniotic membrane in ophthalmology. Surv Ophthalmol. 2004;49(1):51-77.
3. Sheha H, Tseng SCG. Amniotic Membrane Transplantation. In: Albert DM, Lucarelli MJ (eds), Clinical Atlas of Procedures in Ophthalmic and Oculofacial Surgery. Atlanta: Oxford University Press; 2012. pp. 155-65.
4. Prasher P, Lehmann JD, Aggarwal NK. Ahmed tube exposure secondary to PROKERA® implantation. Eye Contact Lens. 2008;34(4):244-5.
5. Touhami A, Grueterich M, Tseng SC. The role of NGF signaling in human limbal epithelium expanded by amniotic membrane culture. Invest Ophthalmol Vis Sci. 2002;43(4):987-94.
6. Pachigolla G, Prasher P, Di Pascuale MA, et al. Evaluation of the role of PROKERA® in the management of ocular surface and orbital disorders. Eye Contact Lens. 2009;35(4):172-5.
7. Fini ME, Cook JR, Mohan R. Proteolytic mechanisms in corneal ulceration and repair. Arch Dermatol Res. 1998;290Suppl (S12-S23).
8. Reidy JJ, Paulus MP, Gona S. Recurrent erosions of the cornea: epidemiology and treatment. Cornea. 2000;19(6):767-71.
9. Huang Y, Sheha H, Tseng SC. Self-retained amniotic membrane for recurrent corneal erosion. J Clin Exp Ophthalmol. 2013;(4)2.
10. Kim JS, Kim JC, Hahn TW, et al. Amniotic membrane transplantation in infectious corneal ulcer. Cornea. 2001;20(7): 720-26.
11. Gicquel JJ, Bejjani RA, Ellies P, et al. Amniotic membrane transplantation in severe bacterial keratitis. Cornea. 2007;26(1): 27-33.
12. Sheha H, Liang L, Li J, et al. Sutureless amniotic membrane transplantation for severe bacterial keratitis. Cornea. 2009; 28(10):1118-23.
13. Meller D, Pires RTF, Mack RJS, et al. Amniotic membrane transplantation for acute chemical or thermal burns. Ophthalmology. 2000;107:980-90.
14. Kheirkhah A, Johnson DA, Paranjpe DR, et al. Temporary sutureless amniotic membrane patch for acute alkaline burns. Arch Ophthalmol. 2008;126(8):1059-66.
15. Lavker RM, Tseng SC, Sun TT. Corneal epithelial stem cells at the limbus: looking at some old problems from a new angle. Exp Eye Res. 2004;78(3):433-46.
16. Anderson DF, Ellies P, Pires RT, et al. Amniotic membrane transplantation for partial limbal stem cell deficiency. Br J Ophthalmol. 2001;85(5):567-75.
17. Kheirkhah A, Casas V, Raju VK, et al. Sutureless amniotic membrane transplantation for partial limbal stem cell deficiency. Am J Ophthalmol. 2008;145(5):787-94.
18. Meallet MA, Espana EM, Grueterich M, et al. Amniotic membrane transplantation for recipient and donor eyes undergoing conjunctival limbal autograft for total limbal stem cell deficiency. Ophthalmology. 2003;110:1585-92.

CHAPTER

21

# Tissue Adhesives in Ophthalmic Surgery

Mark S Hansen, Terry Kim

## INTRODUCTION

Tissue adhesives have been used off-label in ophthalmic surgery for decades. Their use was first reported in 1963; the advances in formulation and technique since that time have made them commonplace in the armamentarium of surgical tools for ophthalmologists. Tissue adhesives can be used for structural support, as replacement and/or complement to sutures and as a barrier to facilitate healing.

## OPHTHALMIC USES OF TISSUE ADHESIVES

- Replacement and/or complement to sutures
- Corneal perforations and bleb leaks
- Corneal thinning and descemetocele
- Amniotic membrane grafting
- Glaucoma surgeries
- Oculoplastics procedures
- Sutureless lamellar keratoplasty
- Ocular surface pathology
- *Less common uses*: Strabismus surgery, scleral buckle attachment, postoperative wound leak, and temporary tarsorrhaphy.

## TYPES OF TISSUE ADHESIVES

*There are two classifications of tissue adhesives*: synthetic and biologic.

### Synthetic

Cyanoacrylate is an ester of cyanoacrylic acid that polymerizes with contact to water or a weak base (such as cell membranes). There are a variety of formulations and manufacturers as seen in Table 21-1. Cyanoacrylate is most commonly used for corneal perforations (usually <1–2 mm), corneal thinning, and descemetoceles. Due to its toxic by-products, it is reserved for the ocular surface. Cyanoacrylate has also been shown to have bacteriostatic properties for gram-positive organisms.

**TABLE 21-1** Synthetic adhesives

| |
|---|
| • Indermil (butyl-2-cyanoacrylate; Sherwood, Davis and Geck, St Louis, MO, USA) |
| • Histoacryl (butyl-2-cyanoacrylate; BBraun Melsungen, Germany) |
| • Histoacryl Blue (*N*-butyl-2-cyanoacrylate; BBraun Melsungen, Germany) |
| • Nexacryl (*N*-butyl-cyanoacrylate; Closure Medical, Raleigh, NC, USA |
| • Dermabond (2-octyl-cyanoacrylate; Closure Medical, Raleigh, NC, USA) |

- Advantages:
  - Easy to use
  - High tensile strength with strong bond
  - Rapidly polymerizes with contact.
- Disadvantages:
  - Foreign body sensation
  - Polymerizes into a hard, brittle consistency often necessitating a bandage contact lens and limiting the view through the cornea
  - Irritation that leads to hyperemia, neovascularization, or tissue necrosis.

### *Instructions for Use for Corneal Perforation*

1. *Set-up*: Assemble the following supplies: cyanoacrylate glue, 1-mm syringe, large-gauge filtered needle, small gauge needle (27 or 30 gauge), Weck-Cel sponges, antibacterial eye drops, bandage contact lens (*see* Fig. 21-1).

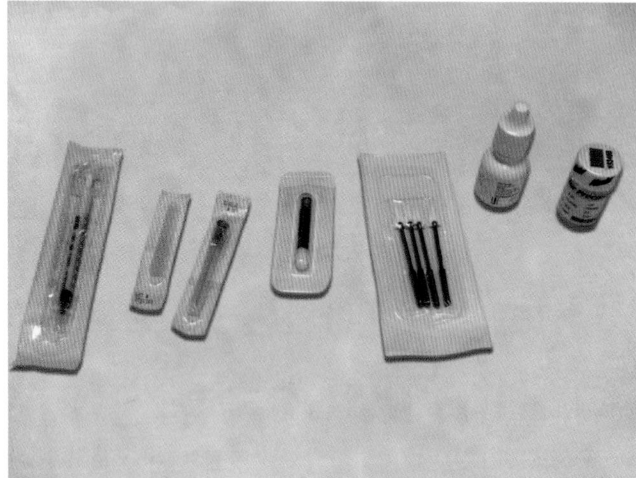

**Figure 21-1** Supplies for gluing the cornea.

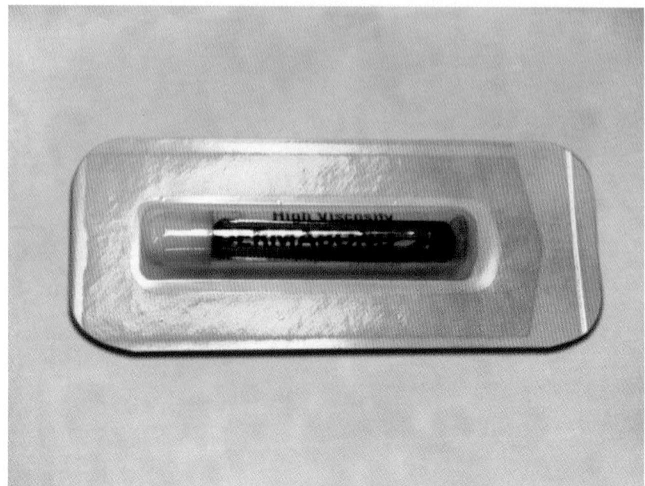

**Figure 21-2** Dermabond.

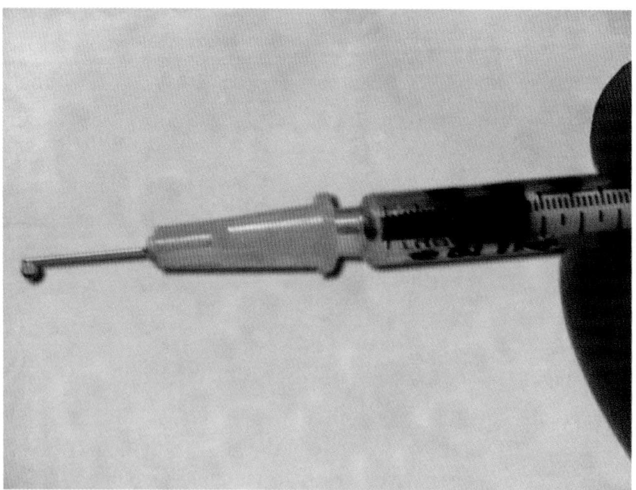

**Figure 21-3** Droplet from syringe.

2. *Prepare the patient*: Lie the patient back and place an anesthetic eyedrop (tetracaine, proparacaine) onto the ocular surface of affected eye.
3. *Prepare the glue*: Dermabond comes backed in a tube for application on the skin (*see* Figure 21-2). The tube can be punctured with a large-gauge filtered needle and liquid contents aspirated into a 1-mm syringe.
4. Replace the large-gauge filtered needle with a 30-gauge needle.
5. *Prepare the tissue*: Using the Weck-Cel sponges, gently debride the epithelium around the area of the perforation. It is critical that the tissue is extremely dry or polymerization will occur before the glue comes in contact with the tissue, preventing adhesion to the tissue.
6. After the tissue has been adequately dried, express a very small droplet of glue from the needle (*see* Figure 21-3) and apply to the center of the perforation. It is very easy to place too much glue, which can extend across the cornea. If more glue is needed after the first application, wait for previously placed glue to dry and then apply another small drop to the area as needed Fig. 21-6.
7. Place a bandage contact lens for comfort and start an antibiotic drop as needed.
8. If the anterior chamber is flat, it may be necessary to perform the procedure in the operating room. Prior to placing glue, inflate the anterior chamber with filtered air to prevent ingress of glue into the anterior chamber.

### *Complications*

1. Poor adhesion of glue to tissue leading to reperforation
2. Inflammation and irritation that may lead to neovascularization
3. Hypotony
4. Keratitis
5. Toxicity due to intraocular glue.

### *Contraindications*

Due to the nature of cyanoacrylate, it is reserved for use on the ocular surface. Defects that are >1–2 mm may be too large to seal with glue and may need a tissue patch graft. Exclusion of active infection is also critical prior to application of cyanoacrylate.

## Biologic

Fibrin-based adhesive is a blood-derived product that is biodegradable and easy to use. It imitates the final stages of the

**TABLE 21-2** Biologic adhesives

| |
|---|
| • Tisseel VH Fibrin Sealant (Baxter Healthcare Corp; Deerfield, IL, USA) |
| • Evicel (Ethicon, Inc, Somerville, NJ, USA) |
| • Beriplast Fibrin Sealant (Hycom Ed, Roskilde, Denmark) |

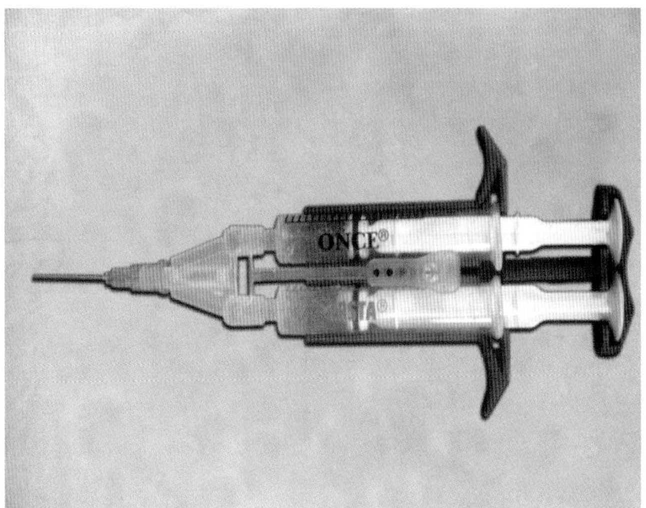


**Figure 21-4** Tisseel Duploject system.

coagulation cascade using a two-component system where mixing converts fibrinogen to fibrin with cross-linking of fibrin monomers to form a strong adhesion. While fibrin-based glue can be manufactured from autologous blood, it is not routinely done due to the time required and the large amount of blood needed to make a small amount of glue. The commercially available product systems are listed in Table 21-2. While Food and Drug Administration approval for use of fibrin glue is hemostasis, there are many useful off-label ophthalmic uses as listed above. Fibrin glue has not been shown to have any antibacterial properties.

- Advantages:
  - Biodegradable nature and elasticity allow it to be used under tissues and not just reserved for the ocular surface
  - Minimal inflammation/irritation
  - Slower polymerization.
- Disadvantages:
  - Lower tensile strength
  - May need repeat applications as it usually degrades within 2 weeks
  - Theoretical chance of viral transmission, although none reported.

## *Instructions for Use*

1. *Set-up*: Assemble the following supplies: fibrin glue components, injector system, tissue (if needed), and antibacterial drops
2. *Prepare the patient*: Depending on the use of the glue, the patient may need to be reclined in the clinic chair or supine in the operating room. For sealing of perforated cornea, a topical anesthetic drop is placed in the affected eye and the area debrided and dried
3. *Prepare the glue*: A double-barreled injection device comes packaged with the commercially available glue (*see* Figure 21-4). The system mixes the two components, thrombin and fibrinogen, as the glue is expressed in the cannula tip. With the injection system it is difficult to control the amount expressed. If multiple applications are needed the cannula tip will need to be replaced, as the glue will plug the tip after the first use. For more precision, each component can be expressed separately with a fine-tip needle on the syringe
4. *Allow the glue to dry*: A bandage contact lens may be placed, and antibiotic drops should be started/continued
5. To use for gluing tissue, such as amniotic membrane (*see* Figures 21-5A to D) or conjunctival graft after pterygium excision: after the glue has been applied to the grafting bed, quickly apply the premeasured and precut tissue to the area. Hold the tissue in place for several minutes.

## *Complications and Contraindications*

Although rare, there are reports of allergic reactions, including anaphylaxis. Fibrin glue is contraindicated in patients who have had prior allergic reactions.

# OTHER TISSUE ADHESIVES IN DEVELOPMENT

Many new, novel adhesives are being explored and tested. Some of these include polyethylene glycol compounds, acrylic copolymer tissue adhesives, biodendrimers, and dendritic macromers. These compounds show promise as tissue adhesives and as an alternate modality to corneal sutures.

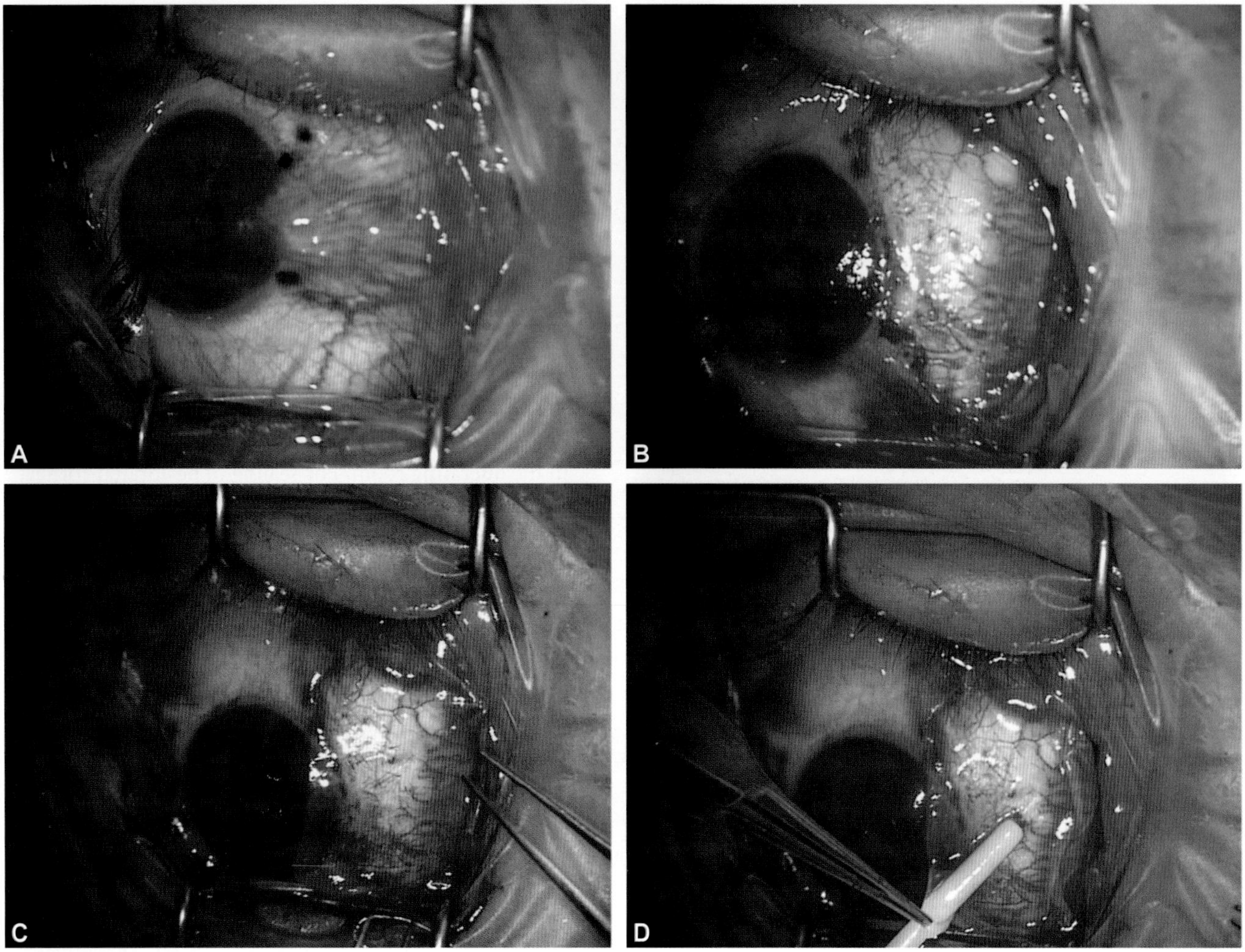

**Figures 21-5A to D** (A) Pterygium. (B) Pterygium excision showing exposed sclera and muscle. (C) Positioning the amniotic membrane over the tissue defect. (D) Amniotic membrane successfully attached with Tisseel glue.

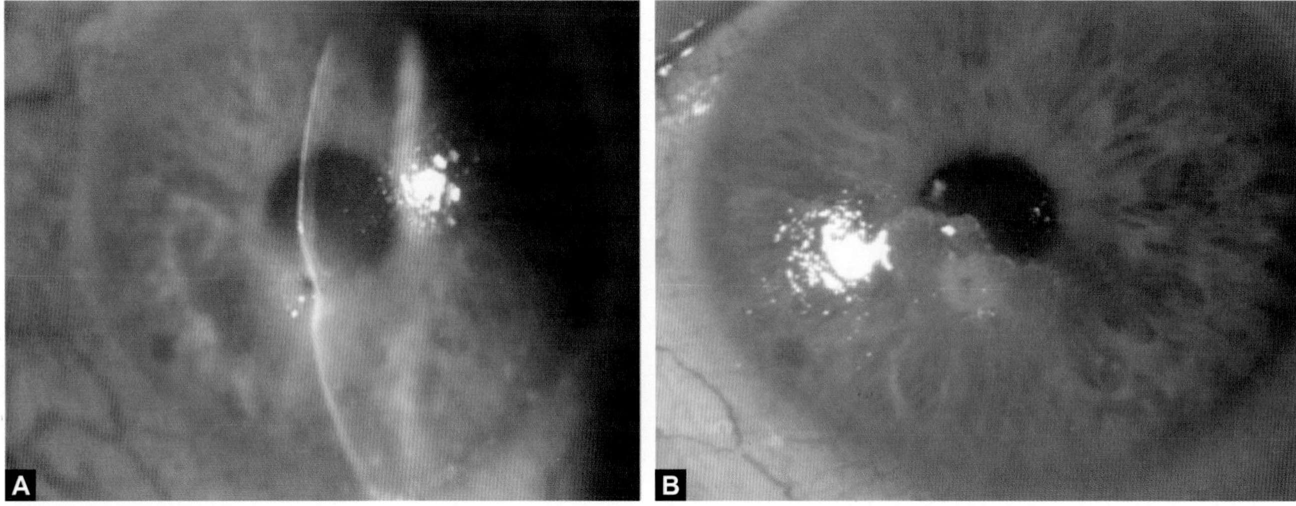


**Figures 21-6A and B** (A) Corneal perforation. (B) Corneal perforation sealed using cyanoacrylate glue.
*Source* Christopher J Rapuano, MD of Wills Eye Hospital.

## SUGGESTED READING


1. Chan SM, Boisjoly H. Advances in the use of adhesives in ophthalmology. Curr Opin Ophthalmol. 2004;15(4):305-10. Review.
2. Bhatia SS. Ocular surface sealants and adhesives. Ocul Surf. 2006;4(3):146-54. Review.
3. Kim T, Kharod BV. Tissue adhesives in corneal cataract incisions. Curr Opin Ophthalmol. 2007;18(1):39-43. 17159446.
4. Panda A, Kumar S, Kumar A, Bansal R, Bhartiya S. Fibrin glue in ophthalmology. Indian J Ophthalmol. 2009;57(5):371-9. doi: 10.4103/0301-4738.55079. Review.
5. Vote BJ, Elder MJ. Cyanoacrylate glue for corneal perforations: a description of a surgical technique and a review of the literature. Clin Experim Ophthalmol. 2000;28(6):437-42. Review.

CHAPTER

# 22

# Ocular Surface Reconstruction and Limbal Stem Cell Transplantation

Clara C Chan, Edward J Holland

## INTRODUCTION

Ocular surface reconstruction requires a systematic and step-by-step approach. The ophthalmologist needs to first make the accurate diagnosis of limbal stem cell deficiency (LSCD) based on patient symptoms and clinical findings. The state of severity of ocular surface disease needs to be taken into consideration. Prior to any limbal stem cell transplantation surgery, control of glaucoma and optimizing the lids, tear film, and conjunctival inflammation must first occur. The three most common forms of surgery will be discussed: (1) conjunctival limbal autograft (CLAU), (2) living-related conjunctival limbal allograft (CLAL), and (3) keratolimbal allograft (KLAL). Once the ocular surface has stabilized, an optical keratoplasty may be needed. Receipt of any form of limbal stem cell allografts necessitates systemic immunosuppression in all patients; principles of managing immunosuppression will be presented in this chapter.

## DIAGNOSIS OF LSCD

- Patient symptoms:
  - Decreased vision
  - Chronic or recurrent discomfort, foreign body sensation
  - Tearing
  - Photophobia.
- Clinical findings can include varying combinations of:
  - Conjunctivalization of the cornea with vascularization and fibrovascular pannus (Figs. 22-1 to 22-3)
  - Corneal scarring or stromal haze (Fig. 22-3)

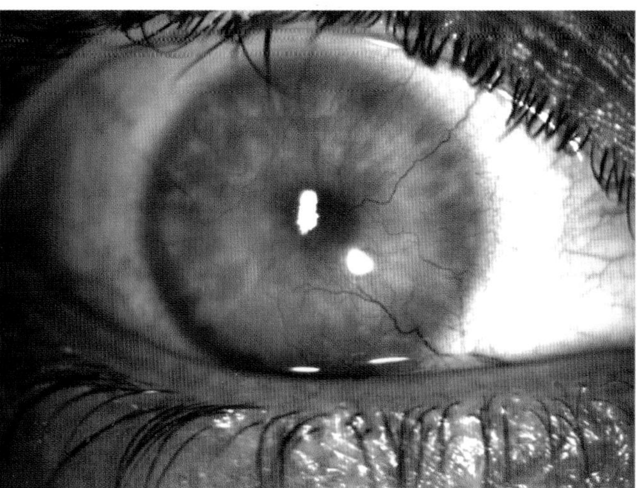

**Figure 22-1** Conjunctivalization of the cornea in a patient with soft contact-lens wear-related limbal stem cell deficiency. The surrounding conjunctiva is not inflamed.

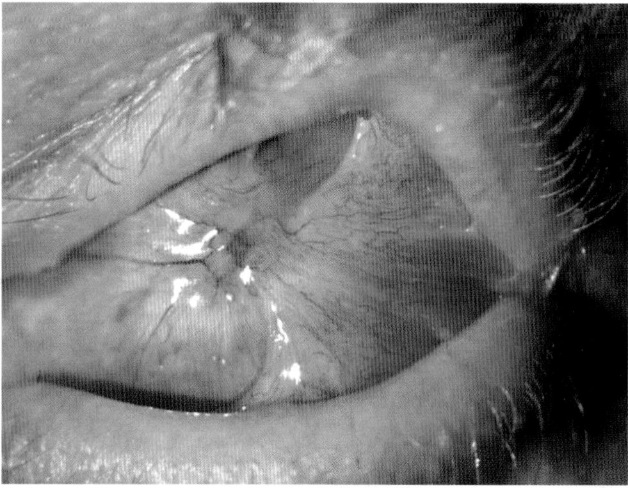

**Figure 22-2** Severe conjunctivalization of the cornea and symblephara in a patient 3 months after a base chemical ocular injury.

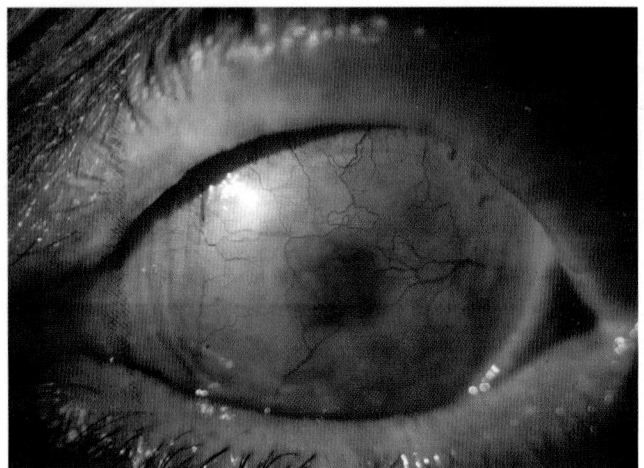

**Figure 22-3** Conjunctivalization, corneal scarring, and stromal haze in a patient with congenital aniridia.

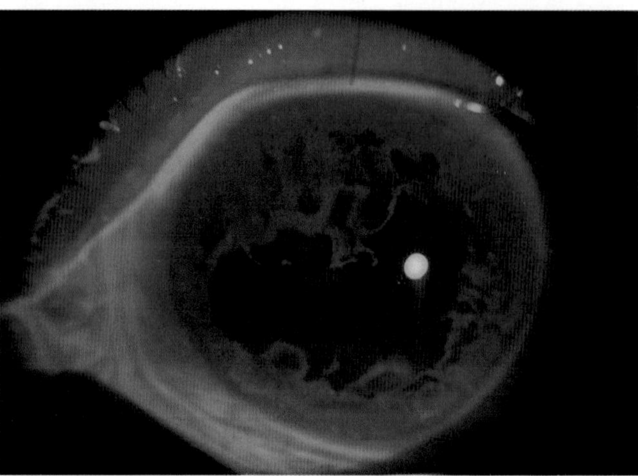

**Figure 22-4** Wave-like late fluorescein staining pattern in a patient with contact lens-wear-related limbal stem cell deficiency.

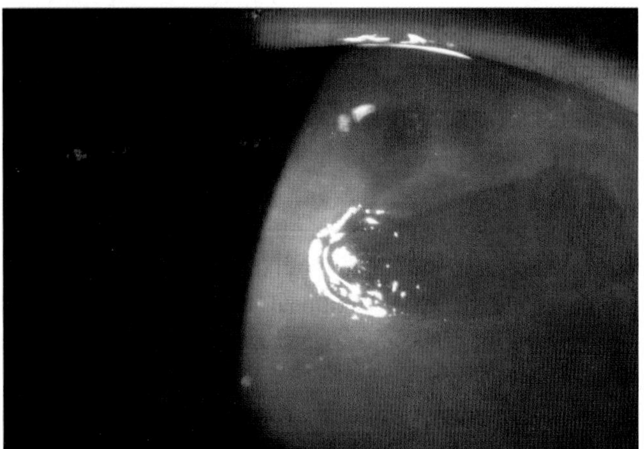

**Figure 22-5** Persistent epithelial defect in a patient with contact lens-wear-related limbal stem cell deficiency.

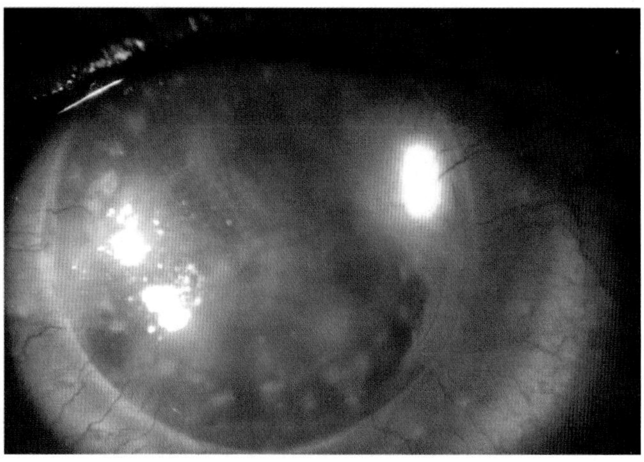

**Figure 22-6** Failed penetrating keratoplasty in a patient with congenital aniridia.

  - Wave-like late fluorescein staining pattern (Fig. 22-4)
  - Persistent or recurrent epithelial defects (Fig. 22-5)
  - Keratoplasty failure (Fig. 22-6).
- Associated conjunctival disease:
  - Symblephara formation
  - Loss of fornices
  - Surface keratinization
  - Mucin deficiency.

## PREOPERATIVE STAGING OF OCULAR SURFACE DISEASE

There are several ocular and nonocular factors that must be taken into consideration when deciding upon the optimal type and timing of surgical treatment for ocular surface reconstruction in a patient with LSCD. The most important ocular factors are laterality of disease, the extent of LSCD, and the extent of conjunctival disease (*see* Table 22-1).[1]

Additional factors include the extent of stromal scarring, mechanical eyelid problems, and other vision-limiting disease, such as glaucoma and retinal disease. Nonocular factors that should be considered include age, systemic health, and personality factors, such as ability to comply with follow-up and medications. In cases of simple focal LSCD, only limbal reconstruction is required; however, in more complicated cases, a step-by-step approach must be taken (Flowchart 22-1).

## CLASSIFICATION OF OCULAR SURFACE TRANSPLANTATION TECHNIQUES

In 2012, the Cornea Society published agreed upon nomenclature based on the following criteria: (1) anatomic source of

**TABLE 22-1** Classification of ocular surface disease based on amount of limbal stem cells and presence or absence of conjunctival inflammation

| | Normal conjunctiva (Stage a) | Previously inflamed conjunctiva (Stage b) | Inflamed conjunctiva (Stage c) |
|---|---|---|---|
| Partial limbal deficiency, < 50% (stage I) | Iatrogenic, CIN, contact lens | History of chemical or thermal injuries | Mild SJS, OCP, recent chemical injury |
| Significant total/subtotal limbal deficiency, > 50% (stage II) | Aniridia, severe contact lens, iatrogenic | History of severe chemical or thermal injuries | Severe SJS, OCP, recent chemical, or thermal injury |

(CIN:conjunctival intraepithelial neoplasia; OCP: Ocular cicatricial pemphigoid; SJS, Stevens–Johnson syndrome).

Modified with permission from Holland and Schwartz.[1]

Patients with stage IIb and IIc disease often have concomitant conjunctival scarring, decreased aqueous and tear production, potential for ocular surface keratinization, and have the poorest prognosis for surgical rehabilitation

**BOX 22-1** Tissue type, anatomic, and tissue engineered

- Type of tissue transplanted:
  - Conjunctival
  - Limbal
  - Other mucosal
- Ex vivo tissue engineered:
  - Ex vivo cultivated conjunctival transplantation
  - Ex vivo cultivated limbal transplantation
  - Other ex vivo cultivated mucosal transplantation

With permission from Daya et al.[2]

the tissue being transplanted, (2) genetic source – autologous or allogeneic and to reflect histocompatibility in the latter group, whether living-related or not, and (3) cell culture techniques.[2] The types of procedures were broadly categorized by the anatomic type, source, and whether it was tissue engineered (Box 22-1). Further categorization according to anatomic type of tissue – namely conjunctival, limbal, and other mucosal grafts – is listed in Table 22-2. Tissue engineered procedures are listed in Table 22-3 and classified according to anatomic source of tissue. These ex vivo techniques do not currently have widespread availability in North America. The most commonly performed techniques to replace absent or nonfunctional limbal stem cells include CLAU, living-related CLAL (LR-CLAL), and KLAL. Thus, the surgical techniques for these procedures will be discussed in further detail within this chapter.

**Flowchart 22-1** Schematic of a step-by-step approach that must be taken in the reconstruction of the ocular surface.

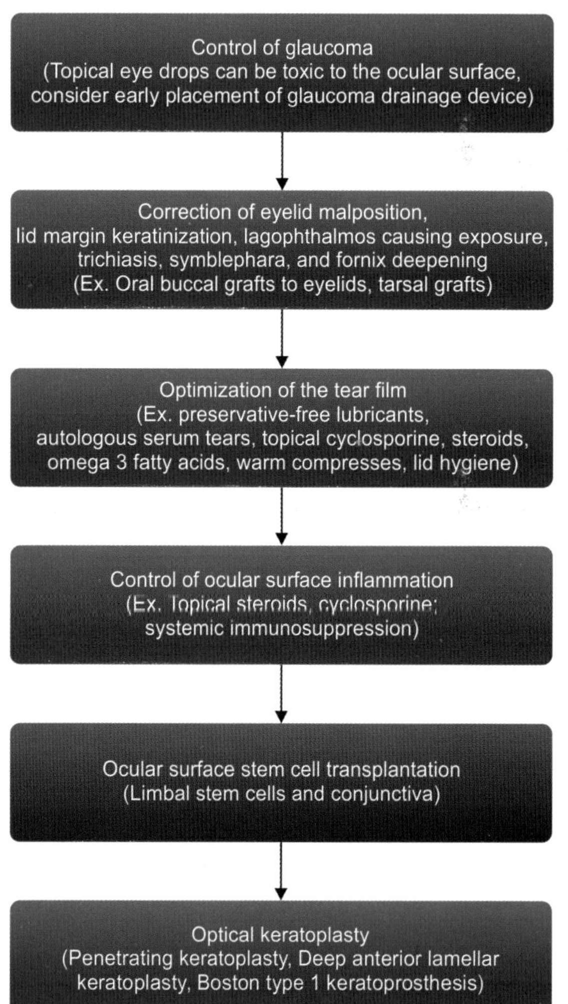


## Conjunctival Limbal Autograft

- Indications and preoperative considerations:
  - Partial (usually > 50%) or total unilateral LSCD
  - Area involved is too extensive for sequential conjunctival epitheliectomy
  - Minimal to no conjunctival inflammation
  - Normal fellow eye with no history of limbal stem cell trauma.

**TABLE 22-2** Classification of surgical procedures for ocular surface reconstruction and stem cell transplantation

| Procedure | Abbrev. | Donor | Transplanted tissue |
|---|---|---|---|
| Conjunctival transplantation | | | |
| Conjunctival autograft | CAU | Fellow eye | Conjunctiva |
| Cadaveric conjunctival allograft | c-CAL | Cadaveric | Conjunctiva |
| Living-related conjunctival allograft | LR-CAL | Living relative | Conjunctiva |
| Living nonrelated conjunctival allograft | LNR-CAL | Living nonrelative | Conjunctiva |
| Limbal transplantation | | | |
| Conjunctival limbal autograft | CLAU | Fellow eye | Limbus/conjunctiva |
| Cadaveric conjunctival limbal allograft | c-CLAL | Cadaveric | Limbus/conjunctiva |
| Living-related conjunctival limbal allograft | LR-CLAL | Living relative | Limbus/conjunctiva |
| Living nonrelated conjunctival limbal allograft | LNR-CLAL | Living nonrelative | Limbus/conjunctiva |
| Keratolimbal autograft | KLAU | Fellow eye | Limbus/cornea |
| Keratolimbal allograft | KLAL | Cadaveric | Limbus/cornea |
| Other mucosal transplantation | | | |
| Oral mucosa autograft | OMAU | Recipient | Oral mucosa |
| Nasal mucosa autograft | NMAU | Recipient | Nasal mucosa |
| Intestine mucosa autograft | IMAU | Recipient | Intestinal mucosa |
| Peritoneal mucosa autograft | PMAU | Recipient | Peritoneum |

With permission from Daya et al.[2]

**TABLE 22-3** Classification of tissue engineered surgical procedures for ocular surface reconstruction and stem cell transplantation

| Procedure | Abbrev. | Donor | Transplanted tissue |
|---|---|---|---|
| Ex vivo cultivated conjunctival transplantation | | | |
| Ex vivo cultivated conjunctival autograft | EVCAU | Recipient eye(s) | Conjunctiva |
| Ex vivo cultivated cadaveric conjunctival allograft | EVc-CAL | Cadaveric | Conjunctiva |
| Ex vivo cultivated living-related conjunctival allograft | EVLR-CAL | Living relative | Conjunctiva |
| Ex vivo cultivated living nonrelated conjunctival allograft | EVLNR-CAL | Living nonrelative | Conjunctiva |
| Ex vivo limbal transplantation | | | |
| Ex vivo cultivated limbal autograft | EVLAU | Recipient eye(s) | Limbus/cornea |
| Ex vivo cultivated cadaveric limbal allograft | EVc-LAL | Cadaveric | Limbus/cornea |
| Ex vivo cultivated living-related limbal allograft | EVLR-LAL | Living relative | Limbus/cornea |
| Ex vivo cultivated living nonrelated limbal allograft | EVLNR-LAL | Living nonrelative | Limbus/cornea |
| Other ex vivo cultivated mucosal transplantation | | | |
| Ex vivo cultivated oral mucosa autograft | EVOMAU | Recipient | Oral mucosa |

With permission from Daya et al.[2]

- Surgical technique (Figs. 22-7A to D):
  - General principles
    - Surgery can be done under local or general anesthetic
    - Both eyes prepped and draped to allow for lid speculum insertion
  - Recipient preparation
    - 360° conjunctival peritomy allowing the conjunctiva to recess posteriorly
    - Minimal resection of the conjunctiva at 12 and 6 O'clock may be performed to allow space for placement of the donor tissue, if needed

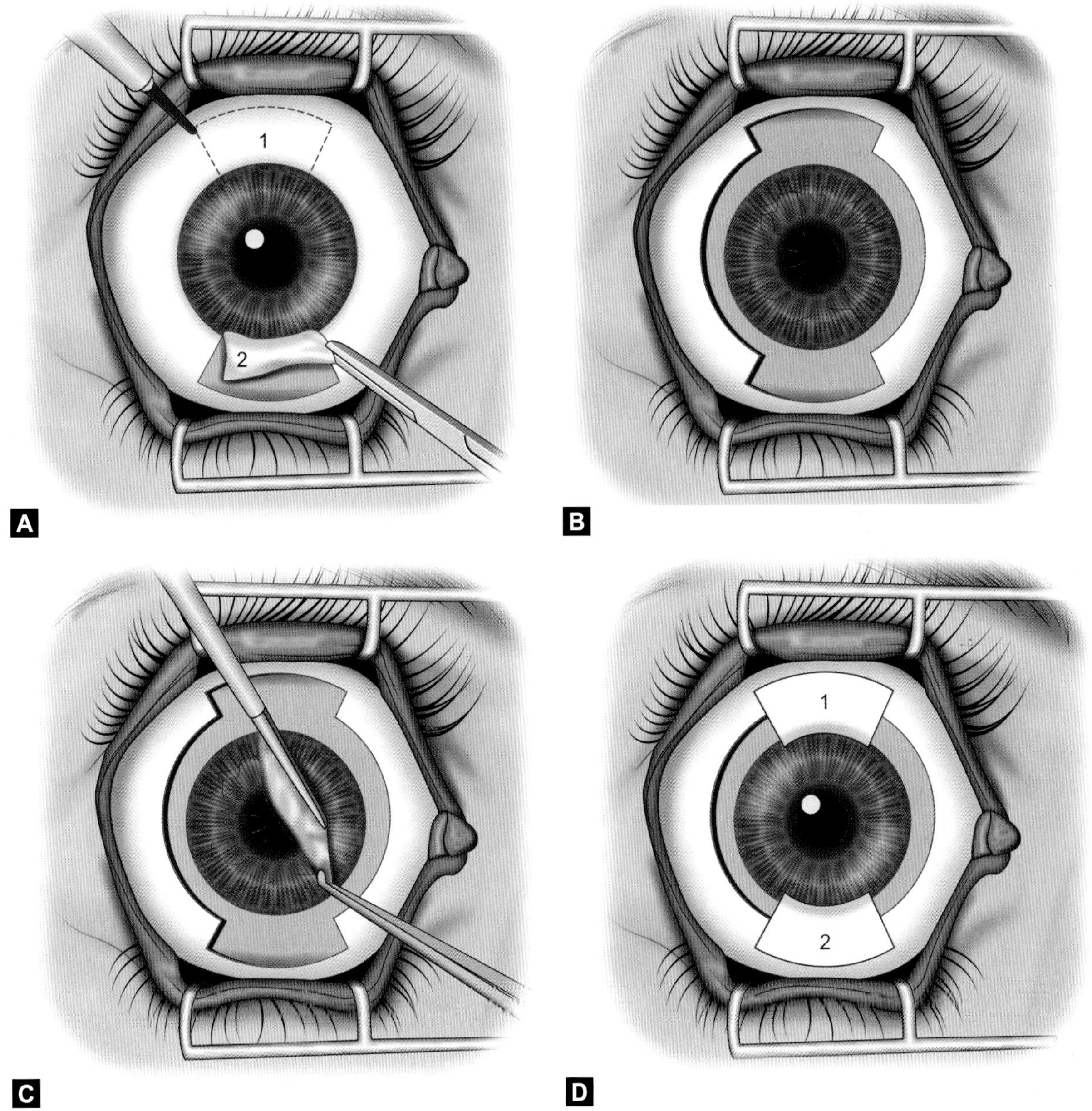


**Figures 22-7A to D** Schematic diagram of limbal autograft or living-related conjunctival limbal allograft surgery. (A) Marking and harvesting of the conjunctival and limbal grafts of the donor tissue at 12 and 6 O'clock. (B) Recipient site is prepared using a 360° peritomy and resection of the conjunctiva at 12 and 6 O'clock for placement of the donor tissue. (C) Superficial keratectomy of the recipient corneal fibrovascular pannus. (D) Securing of the grafts using tissue glue and 10-0 nylon sutures. A bandage contact lens is then placed on the eye.

- Superficial keratectomy with complete debridement of any corneal fibrovascular pannus
- Cautery may be used as needed
- The lid speculum is removed and the eye left closed, whereas the donor grafts are harvested

– Donor preparation
  - Mark the conjunctival and limbal area—2–3 O'clock hours of limbus from superior and inferior locations of the donor eye, 4–6 mm of conjunctiva (since there is more redundant conjunctiva) superiorly and 2–3 mm of conjunctiva inferiorly
  - Dissect the conjunctiva down to the adherent portion at the limbus taking care to handle with a nontoothed instrument to avoid tissue damage
  - Reflect the conjunctiva over the cornea and use a crescent blade to dissect a shallow depth about

1 mm onto the cornea prior to amputation of the graft to ensure that the limbal stem cells are harvested
    - Store the grafts in a sterile Petri dish kept wet with balanced salt solution
    - The donor sites can remain as they are, or sutured with dissolving sutures (e.g. 8-0 vicryl) or secured using tissue glue
    - Instill a drop of antibiotic and steroid, then remove the lid speculum
- Placement of donor tissue:
  - Two or more interrupted 10-0 nylon sutures may be used to ensure that each CLAU graft is secure at the limbus and tacked to the episclera. Tissue glue can alternatively be used to secure the base of the graft –taking care to ensure that it will not be dislodged
  - Subconjunctival or topical steroid and antibiotic are used, and a bandage contact lens is then placed on the eye
- Postoperative care:
  - General principles
    - No systemic immunosuppression is required, because the donor and recipient tissue are from the same patient
  - Recipient eye
    - Topical steroid and antibiotics (preservative-free if available) are given every 2–4 hours, then tapered as the cornea re-epithelializes
    - Liberal use of nonpreserved artificial tears is encouraged
    - Removal of the bandage contact lens occurs after the epithelium has stabilized
    - The 3 and 9 O'clock positions of the cornea will be the last to epithelialize
  - Donor eye
    - Topical steroid and antibiotics are given four times daily until the harvested sites are fully healed
- Variations:
  - In cases of severe unilateral conjunctival and limbal disease with significant symblepharon formation, CLAU has been combined with KLAL at the 3 and 9 o'clock meridians (modified Cincinnati procedure Figures 22-8A to E) to prevent conjunctiva invasion from the 3 and 9 o'clock meridians.[3] Systemic immunosuppression is required to prevent rejection of the KLAL tissue. The duration of immunosuppression may be less than in patients where only KLAL tissue is used.

## Living-related Conjunctival Limbal Allograft

- Indications and preoperative considerations:
  - Bilateral partial (usually > 50%) or total LSCD
  - Area involved is too extensive for sequential conjunctival epitheliectomy
  - Minimal to no conjunctival inflammation
  - Healthy conjunctiva also harvested and transplanted
  - Available and willing living-related donor (usually a sibling or parent)
  - Immunologic matching of the donor and recipient is possible (e.g. ABO blood type, human leukocyte antigens)
  - Poor candidates are patients with keratinized conjunctiva, corneal surface, and/or little to no tear production.
- Surgical technique (Fig. 22-7):
  - Recipient and donor preparation, along with placement of grafts is similar to that for CLAU.
- Postoperative care:
  - Topical and systemic immunosuppression is required for the recipient to prevent rejection of the donated allografts. Principles and protocols of topical and systemic immunosuppression are further discussed later in this chapter.
- Variations:
  - In cases of severe bilateral conjunctival and limbal disease with significant symblepharon formation, LR-CLAL has been used in combination with KLAL at the 3 and 9 O'clock meridians (Cincinnati procedure Figures 22-8A to E) to prevent conjunctiva invasion from the 3 and 9 O'clock meridians.[4]

## Keratolimbal Allograft

- Indications and preoperative considerations:
  - Unilateral severe LSCD and fellow eye has risk for limbal disease
  - Bilateral severe LSCD and no available or willing living-related donor
  - Area involved is too extensive for sequential conjunctival epitheliectomy
  - Minimal to no conjunctival inflammation
  - No healthy conjunctiva is transplanted
  - No immunologic matching of the donor and recipient
  - Poor candidates are those with keratinized conjunctiva, corneal surface, and/or little to no tear production.
- Donor tissue considerations:
  - Donor tissue selection guidelines for high quality KLAL donor tissue

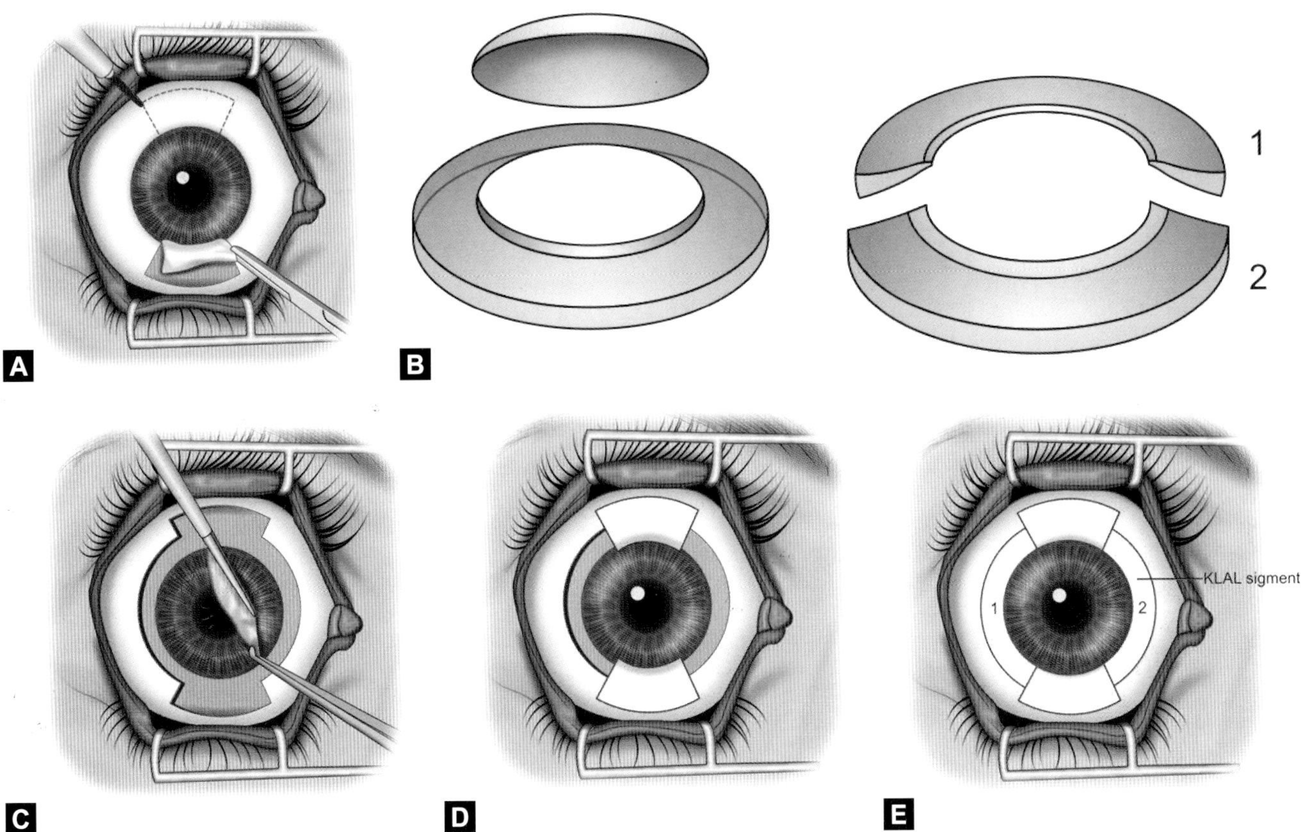


**Figures 22-8A to E** Schematic diagram of the Cincinnati or modified Cincinnati procedures where both conjunctival–limbal grafts (autografts and living-related allografts, respectively) and keratolimbal allografts (KLAL) are used. This provides enough limbal stem cells and the necessary conjunctiva for ocular surface rehabilitation in eyes with severe ocular surface disease. The conjunctival limbal autografts or living-related conjunctival limbal allografts are secured at 12 and 6 O'clock, and KLAL tissue is secured at 3 and 9 O'clock.

  - No active infection and no prior ventilator exposure to donor
    Donor age 5–70 years (ideally < 50 years)
  - Minimal time from donor death to tissue preservation
  - Use of KLAL tissue 5 to 7 days from donor time of death.
- Eye bank tissue preparation:
  - 3–4 mm skirt of peripheral conjunctiva and 4–5-mm scleral rim is left on the corneoscleral rims used for KLAL surgery
  - For KLAL transplantation, the corneoscleral rims from both eyes of 1 donor are used for 1 recipient eye
  - For the Cincinnati and modified Cincinnati procedures, just 1 corneoscleral rim is needed.
- Surgical technique (Figures 22-9A to D):
  - General principle
    - Surgery can be performed under retrobulbar or general anesthesia
  - Recipient preparation
    - 360° conjunctival peritomy releases any symblephara and the conjunctiva often will retract 2–3 mm away from the limbus
    - Tenectomy can be generously performed as tenons is often thickened and hypertrophied due to chronic inflammation
    - Topical epinephrine (1:10000 dilution) and wet-field cautery is used for hemostasis
    - Corneal fibrovascular pannus is removed by 64-beaver blade superficial keratectomy.
  - Donor tissue preparation
    - Each corneoscleral rim is trephined with a 7.5-mm blade as in routine penetrating keratoplasty (PK)
    - The rim is cut in half and trimmed, leaving 2–3 mm of sclera peripheral to the limbus
    - The posterior sclera and corneal stroma of each segment are removed using lamellar dissection

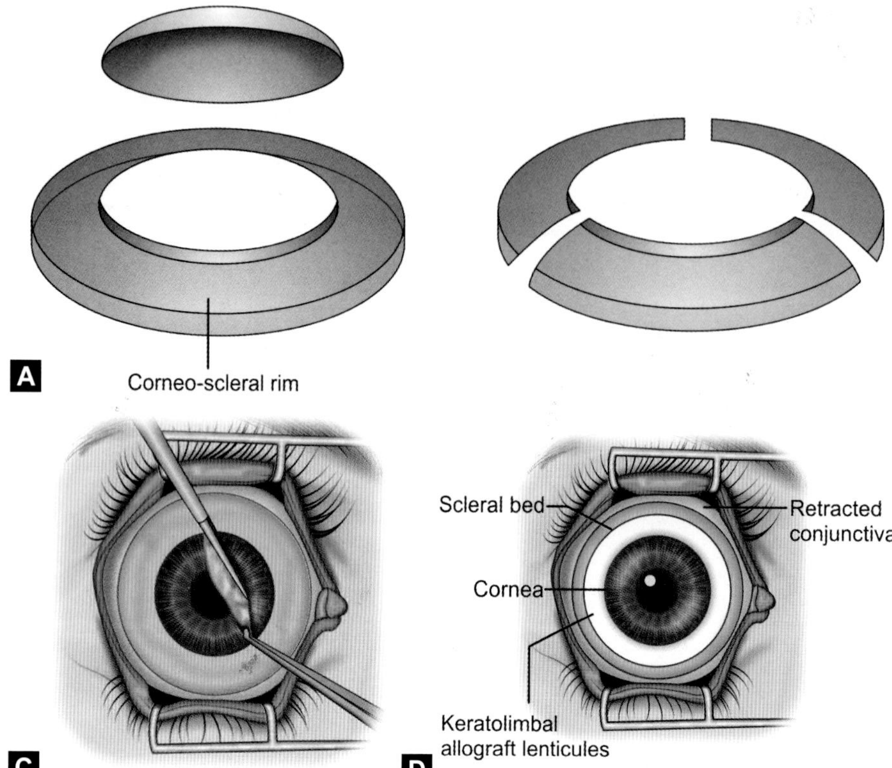


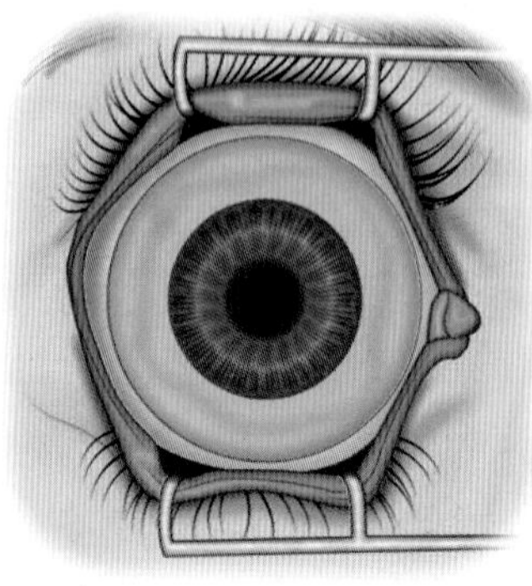


**Figures 22-9A to D** Schematic diagram of keratolimbal allograft (KLAL) surgery. (A) Donor keratolimbal allograft lenticules are fashioned from two cadaver corneoscleral rims with the central 7.5 mm of cornea removed by trephination. (B) 360° conjunctival peritomy and tenectomy is performed allowing the conjunctiva to retract. (C) Abnormal corneal epithelium and fibrovascular pannus are removed by superficial dissection using blunt and sharp techniques, such as with a 64 Beaver blade. (D) KLAL lenticules are secured to the recipient limbus using 10-0 nylon sutures and tissue glue.

techniques with a crescent blade and curved Vannas scissor. When the graft is secured, the corneal edge then sits smoothly on the plane of the cornea, avoiding a step

- The KLAL lenticules can then be stored in a Petri dish filled with storage media solution.

- Placement of donor tissue
  - Secure each KLAL segment at the limbal edge with two 10-0 nylon sutures cut very short
  - Trim the segments as needed to avoid overlap
  - Fibrin tissue glue is used to secure the base of the KLAL lenticules to recipient sclera and the posterior edge of the KLAL lenticules to the conjunctiva. The conjunctiva can even be slightly pulled over the lenticules to avoid conjunctival growth underneath the grafts, which could lead to formation of inclusion cysts
  - It is important to protect the KLAL tissue with a viscoelastic coating
  - Take care to avoid any gaps between the KLAL lenticules where conjunctival invasion could occur
  - After subconjunctival injections of antibiotic and steroid, a large diameter (18–20 mm) bandage contact lens is placed on the eye. The eye is patched for a few hours until the effects of the retrobulbar injection has worn off.

- Postoperative care:
  - Topical and systemic immunosuppression is required for the recipient to prevent rejection of the donated allografts. Principles and protocols of topical and systemic immunosuppression are further discussed later in this chapter.
- Variations:
  - KLAL lenticules used in conjunction with either CLAU or LR-CLAL tissue has been discussed previously.

## IMMUNOSUPPRESSION IN LIMBAL STEM CELL TRANSPLANTATION

Topical and systemic immunosuppression is necessary in all patients who receive any form of limbal stem cell allografts, including those who receive human leukocyte antigen (HLA)-matched tissue from a living relative.[5] Although the use of oral immunosuppression agents has been shown to have few severe adverse effects, careful monitoring and knowledge of potential side effects is important and comanagement with a solid organ transplant specialist is beneficial (*see* Table 22-4). In a patient who is elderly or with significant comorbidities

**TABLE 22-4** Adverse events reported in 136 patients (225 eyes) after ocular surface stem cell transplantation

| Severe adverse events | No. of events ($N$ = 3, 2 patients, 1.5%) |
|---|---|
| Death | 0 |
| Secondary tumors | 0 |
| Neurological events (CVA) | 0 |
| Cardiovascular events | 2 MI, 1 PE |
| **Minor adverse events** | **No. of events ($N$ = 21, 19 patients, 14.0%)** |
| Increased cardiovascular risk | 4 hypertension, 2 diabetes, 1 ↑ cholesterol |
| Bone abnormalities | 1 AVN |
| Biochemical abnormalities | 10 transient ↑ Cr, 2 transient ↑ LFT |
| Infections needing hospitalization | 1 pneumonia |

(AVN: Avascular necrosis of femoral head; CHF: Congestive heart failure; Cr: Creatinine; CVA: Cerebral vascular accident; LFT: Liver function tests; MI: Myocardial infarction; PE: Pulmonary embolus. With permission from Holland et al.[5]

and cannot tolerate systemic immunosuppression, then keratoprosthesis surgery is another option.

- Absolute contraindications:
  - History of malignancy < 5 years
  - Nonadherence with clinical or laboratory follow-up
  - History of noncompliance to medications
  - Diabetes
  - Uncontrolled hypertension
  - Renal insufficiency
  - Congestive heart failure
  - Other organ failure.
- Topical regimens:
  - Following limbal stem cell allograft transplantation, all patients begin topical immunosuppression at four times a day dosing and are maintained on a tapered dose indefinitely. Corticosteroids such as 1% prednisolone acetate and compounded 2% cyclosporine A were effective previously; however, with the advent of 0.05% difluprednate ophthalmic emulsion (Durezol, Alcon Inc., Fort Worth, TX, USA) and a more potent steroid and cyclosporine 0.05% emulsion (Restasis, Allergan, Irvine, CA, USA), these two agents now represent the mainstay of topical immunosuppression regimens after transplantation. In patients with controlled ocular surface inflammation and steroid-induced elevated intraocular pressures, topical loteprednol (Lotemax, Bausch and Lomb, Rochester, NY, USA) may be used instead
- Systemic regimens:
  - We recommend our published protocol (*see* Flowchart 22-2), which includes tacrolimus (Prograf; Astellas Pharma US, Inc, Deerfield, IL, USA), mycophenolate mofetil (MMF, CellCept; Hoffmann La Roche, Nutley, NJ, USA), and oral prednisone.[5] Once a patient and potential donor are matched in terms of their ABO blood typing (if the donor is a living relative), then the patient's immunosuppression regimen is tailored and individualized based on their immunological risk stratification (Table 22-5). Box 22-2 outlines the details of when and which pre- and post-transplant investigations are ordered to assess a patient's baseline health status and to monitor for therapeutic drug levels and adverse events.

## KERATOPLASTY AFTER LIMBAL STEM CELL TRANSPLANTATION

- Indications and preoperative considerations:
  - Central corneal scarring limiting visual acuity
  - Stable corneal epithelium
  - At least 3 months after limbal stem cell transplantation
  - Minimal to no conjunctival inflammation
  - While there is additional exposure to additional antigenic challenge, staged rather than simultaneous keratoplasty with limbal stem cell transplantation has been shown to have decreased endothelial rejection rates and better limbal graft survival.[6]
  - Keratoprosthesis surgery is an option after failed keratoplasty, in lieu of repeat keratoplasty in conditions where repeat cadaveric tissue transplantation has minimal chance of survival
  - Do not perform keratoplasty prior to limbal stem cell transplantation. The corneal graft will not survive functionally in the setting of severe LSCD.
- Surgical technique:
  - Depending on the status of the endothelium, deep anterior lamellar keratoplasty or PK may be performed using the surgeon's preferred technique
  - Larger-diameter grafts provide better apposition to the KLAL segments and decrease the risk of epithelial ingrowth.[7]
  - The recipient cornea is trephined with the same larger diameter to prevent overlap between the peripheral donor cornea and stem cell segments. An exception lies in the case of chemical injury patients where the

**Flowchart 22-2** Schematic diagram of the recommended systemic immunosuppression protocol for ocular surface stem cell transplantation. Once baseline assessment and laboratory investigations are completed, the initiation of tacrolimus, mycophenolate mofetil (MMF), prednisone, valganciclovir, and trimethoprim/sulfamethoxazole is generally started 1 week before transplantation. Basiliximab is also used on occasion for induction in higher risk patients. CMV, cytomegalovirus. With permission from Holland et al.[5]

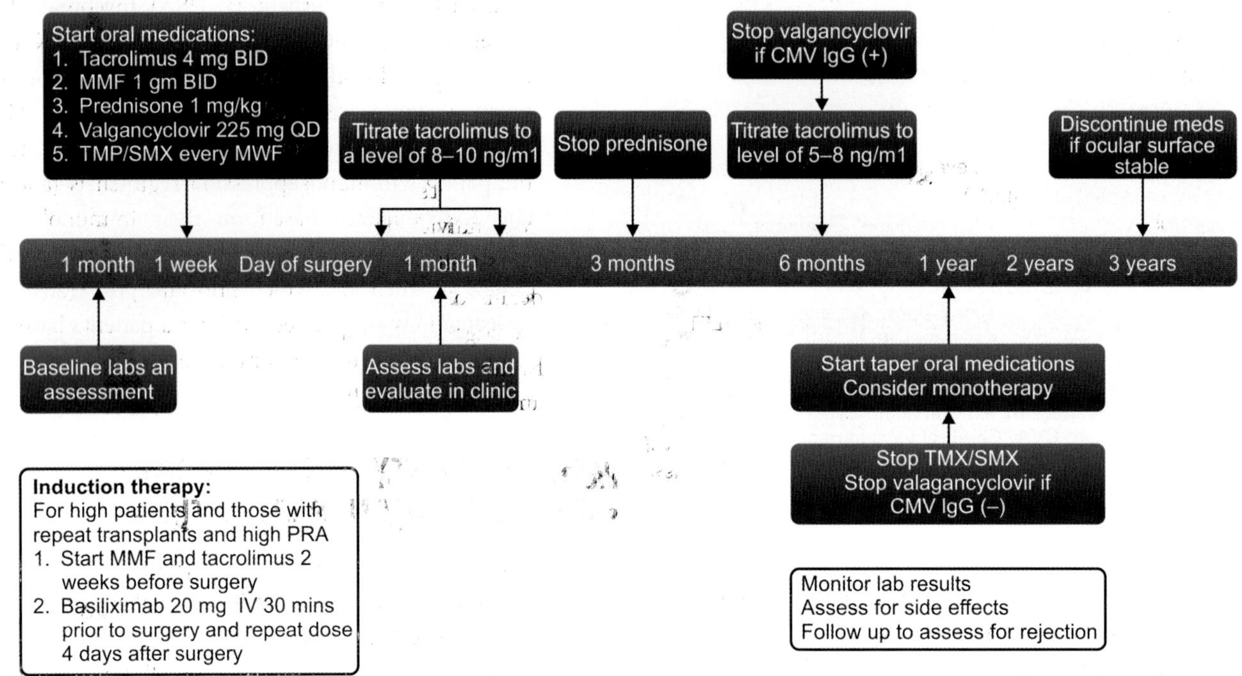


**TABLE 22-5** Tissue selection factors for the individualization of the systemic immunosuppression protocol in ocular surface stem cell transplantation once ABO-matching between a living relative donor and recipient is established

| Donor type | Living-relative donor | | | | | | Cadaveric donor | | |
|---|---|---|---|---|---|---|---|---|---|
| HLA typing | HLA identical | | | Non-HLA identical | | | Not applicable | | |
| PRA % | 0 | 0–50 | >50 | 0 | 0–50 | >50 | 0 | 0–50 | >50 |
| Induction | None | | | None | Basiliximab* | | None | Basiliximab* | |
| Maintenance[†] | Standard | | | Standard | | | Standard | | |
| Initiation of maintenance regimen | Day of surgery | 1 week before surgery | 2 weeks before surgery | 2 weeks before surgery | | | 2 weeks before surgery | | |
| Goals | Begin Prograf taper at 3 months, Cellcept monotherapy at 6 months | | | Taper Prograf at 1 year, Cellcept monotherapy at 6 months | | | Taper Prograf at 2 years, CellCept monotherapy at 2 years | | |
| Repeat transplant | OK | | | OK if DSA is negative | | | OK if PRA = 0, otherwise use living donor vs Kpro | | |

*Basiliximab (Simulect) 20 mg IV is given 30 minutes prior to transplantation with a second dose given 4 days after transplantation.
[†]Standard maintenance protocol includes oral prednisone 1 mg/kg, tacrolimus (FK-506 or Prograf) 4 mg twice daily, MMF (CellCept) 1 g twice daily, oral valganciclovir (Valcyte) 225 mg daily, and trimethoprim/sulfamethoxazole (Bactrim single strength) 1 tablet on Mondays, Wednesdays, Fridays, or dapsone 100 mg orally daily if the patient has a sulfa allergy. The higher the percentage of PRA, panel reactive antibodies, the harder it is to find a match and the patient is more likely to reject. Transplants are at higher risk of failure if DSA, donor-specific antibodies, is positive. With permission from Holland et al.[5]
(PRA: Panal Reactive Antibody; HLA: Humen Leukocyte Antigen)

donor cornea is oversized by 0.5 to 0.75 mm. After trephination, the recipient tissue tends to contract in eyes that have suffered from chemical injuries.

– Use interrupted sutures to allow for selective removal to manage astigmatism, better wound stability, and decreased risk of dehiscence.

**BOX 22-2** Schedule for standard investigations before and after ocular surface stem cell transplantation to assess a patient's baseline health status and to monitor for adverse events.

- Before transplant:
  - Medications list, previous medical history, transplant immunologist assessment
  - Physical examination completed by primary care physician within 30 days of surgery
  - Blood pressure
  - Weight
  - Lab investigations (CBC, BMP, liver function panel, UA with urinary protein, culture, and sensitivities)
  - Serology testing (Hepatitis A, B, C, HIV, EBV, CMV)
  - Tuberculosis exposure (TB skin test or chest X-ray)
  - Up-to-date mammogram, pap smear and colonoscopy
  - Pregnancy status (beta HCG)
  - Cardiac stress test if > 50 years old or history of heart problems or blood pressure
- First three visits after transplant:
  - Tacrolimus levels (target 8–10 ng/mL)
- Monthly:
  - Blood pressure
  - Lab investigations (CBC and differential, BMP, liver function panel)
  - Tacrolimus levels (target 8–10 ng/mL until 6 months, then 5–8 ng/mL for 12–18 months)
- Every 3 months:
  - Fasting lipid profile
  - $HBA_{1c}$ levels in diabetic patients
- At 6 months:
  - CMV and EBV IgG and IgM antibodies (if positive, valgancyclovir is stopped at 6 months; if negative, at 12 months)
  - UA, culture and sensitivities, random protein, and creatinine
- Every year:
  - Mammograms in patients > 40 years
  - Papsmear
- Every 2 years:
  - Mineral bone density scan if on long-term prednisone
- Other:
  - Routine colonoscopy screening in patients > 50 years, then every 5–10 years, depending on risk
  - Prostate specific antigen (PSA) levels in African Americans > 40 years and Caucasians > 50 years

(BMP: Basic metabolic panel consists of glucose, calcium, sodium, potassium, bicarbonate, chloride, blood urea nitrogen, creatinine; CBC: Complete blood count; CMV: Cytomegalovirus; EBV: Epstein–Barr virus; HCG: Human chorionic gonadotropin; HIV: Human insufficiency virus; IgG and IgM, immunoglobulin G and immunoglobulin M; UA: urinary analysis).
With permission from Holland et al.[5]

## CONCLUSIONS

Control of glaucoma and optimizing the lids (i.e. correction of lagophthalmos and trichiasis), tear film dysfunction, and conjunctival inflammation must first occur prior to any limbal stem cell transplantation surgery for successful post-operative results.

- Key considerations for deciding on surgical options in limbal stem cell transplantation:
  - Laterality of disease
  - Degree of stem cell involvement
  - Amount of baseline tear production
  - Presence of conjunctival inflammation.
- Treatment strategies are outlined in the flowcharts for unilateral and bilateral disease (Flowcharts 22-3 and 22-4):
  - Unilateral limbal disease
    - If partial (< 50%) damage, attempt sequential conjunctival epitheliectomy

**Flowchart 22-3** Ocular surface reconstruction surgical treatment options for unilateral limbal stem cell disease

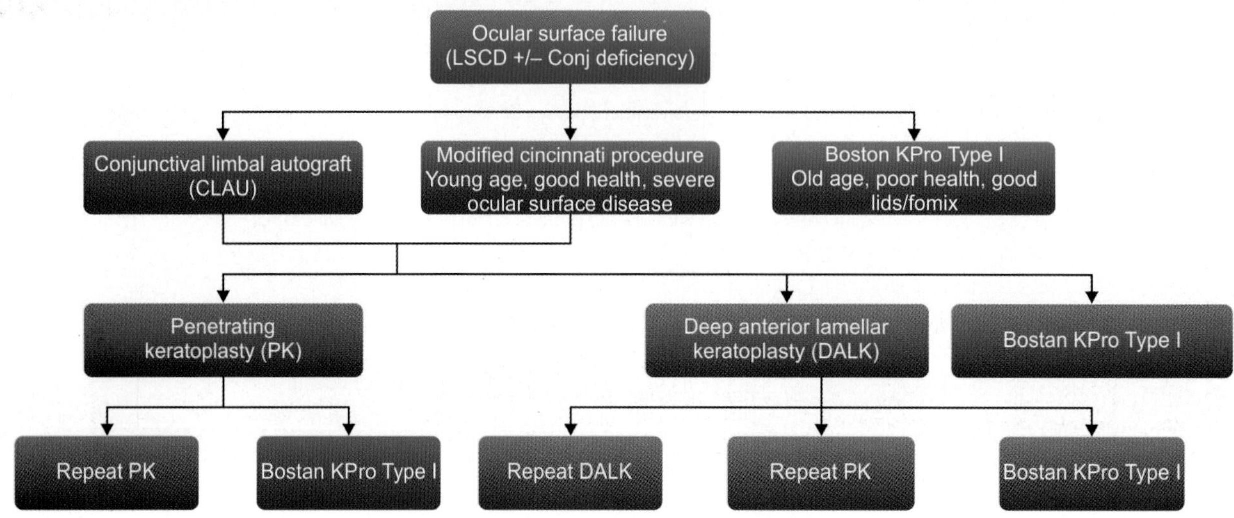


**Flowchart 22-4** Ocular surface reconstruction surgical treatment options for bilateral limbal stem cell disease

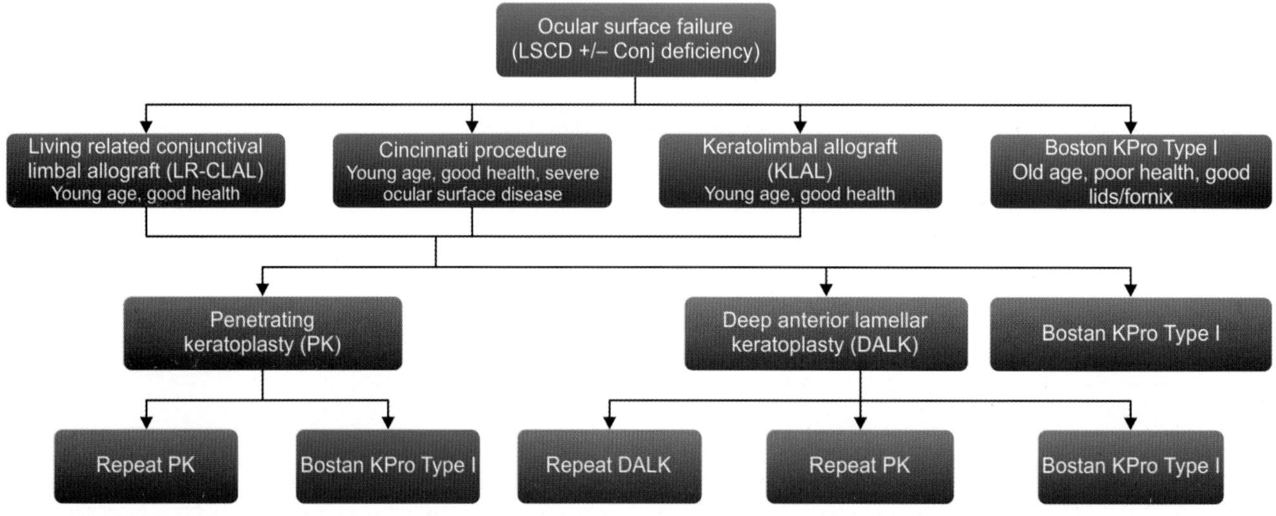


  - If > 50% limbal involvement, perform CLAU from the contralateral normal eye
- Unilateral limbal and conjunctival disease
  - Conjunctival inflammation must be controlled prior to considering any surgical techniques
  - Extensive conjunctival and limbal damage with broad symblepharon present, the "modified Cincinnati procedure" is more appropriate over CLAU alone
  - Keratoprosthesis surgery for the elderly or those with multiple systemic comorbidities who are poor candidates for systemic immunosuppression
- Bilateral limbal disease with normal conjunctiva
  - If partial (< 50%) damaged, attempt sequential conjuntival epitheliectomy
  - If > 50% limbal involvement, then consider KLAL or LR-CLAL (Figs. 22-10A to C)
  - Keratoprosthesis surgery for the elderly or those with significant systemic comorbidities who cannot tolerate systemic immunosuppression
- Bilateral limbal and conjunctival disease
  - Conjunctival inflammation must be controlled prior to considering any surgical techniques
  - If minimal conjunctival damage and/or no living-related donors, perform KLAL (Figs. 22-11A to D)

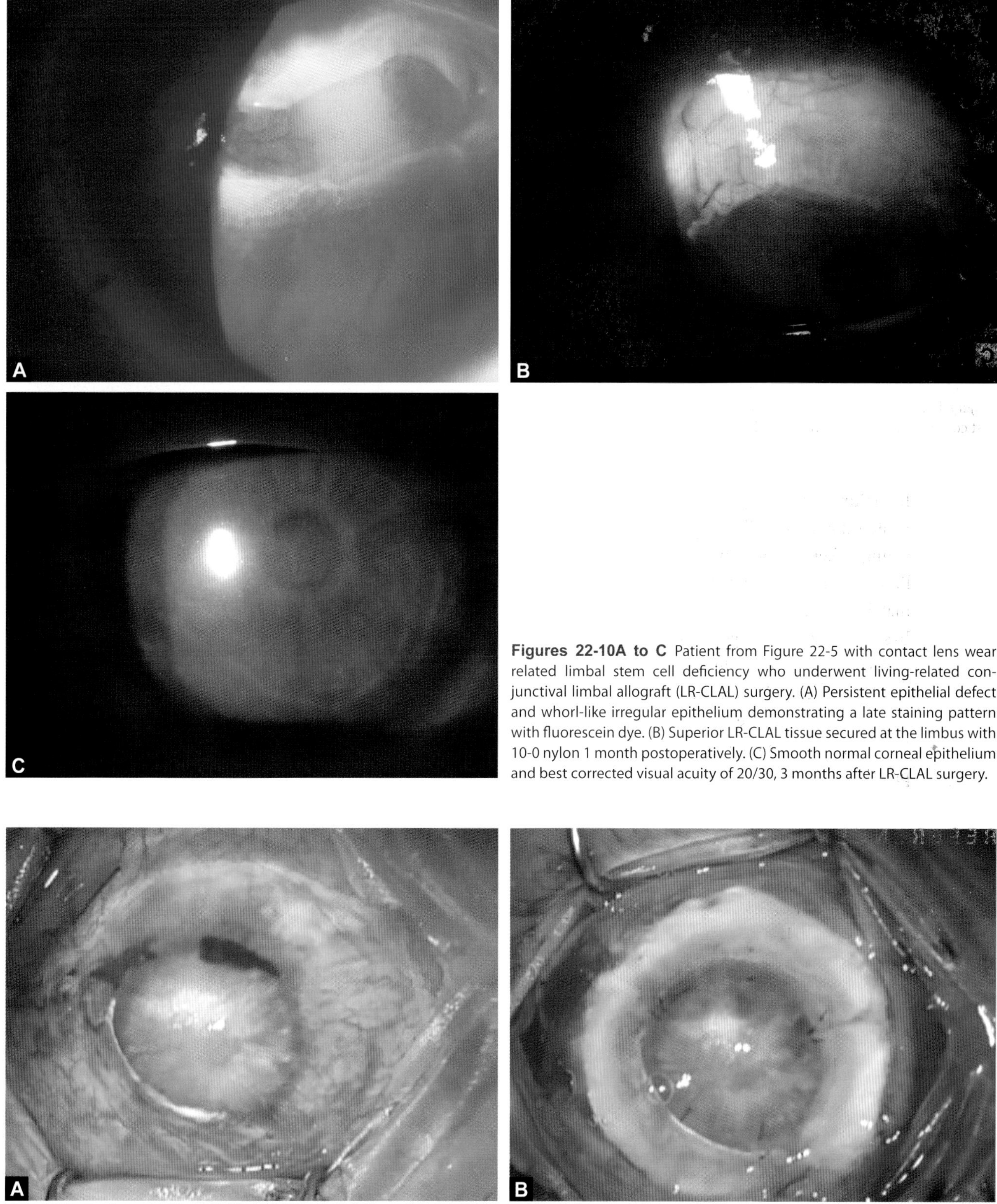

**Figures 22-10A to C** Patient from Figure 22-5 with contact lens wear related limbal stem cell deficiency who underwent living-related conjunctival limbal allograft (LR-CLAL) surgery. (A) Persistent epithelial defect and whorl-like irregular epithelium demonstrating a late staining pattern with fluorescein dye. (B) Superior LR-CLAL tissue secured at the limbus with 10-0 nylon 1 month postoperatively. (C) Smooth normal corneal epithelium and best corrected visual acuity of 20/30, 3 months after LR-CLAL surgery.

**Figures 22-11A and B** (A) Severe ocular surface disease with both limbal stem cell deficiency and conjunctival disease due to chemical and thermal injury. Visual acuity was hand motions. Glaucoma drainage device implantation was performed 3 months before ocular surface stem cell transplantation. (B) Immediately after keratolimbal allograft (KLAL) surgery.

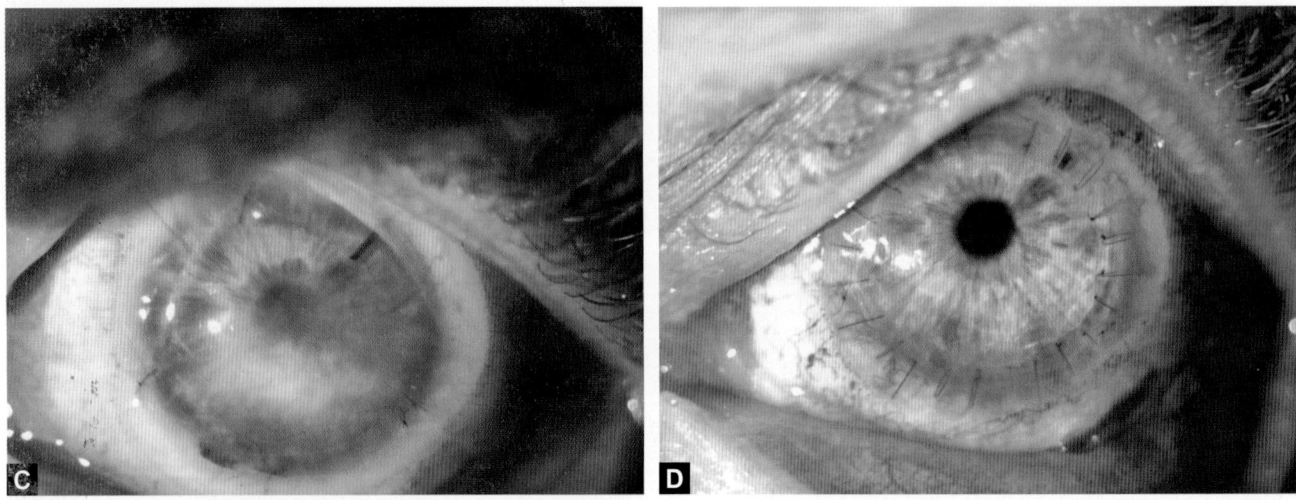


**Figures 22-11C and D** (C) Stable ocular surface, diminished conjunctival inflammation, and residual corneal stromal scarring 3 months after KLAL surgery. The glaucoma drainage device is positioned at 2 O'clock with a suture in situ. (D) Penetrating keratoplasty (PK) is performed 3 months after KLAL. Best corrected visual acuity measured 20/40 3 months after PK.

- If conjunctival damage is significant and a living-related donor is available, perform LR-CLAL in a young, otherwise healthy patient. Conjunctiva and limbal cells are provided and a tissue immunity match may be possible
- In severe cases with large amounts of symblepharon and ocular surface failure, the preferred option would be a combination of KLAL and LR-CLAL (Cincinnati procedure)
- Keratoprosthesis surgery, if systemic immunosuppression is contraindicated.

## REFERENCES

1. Holland EJ, Schwartz GS. The evolution of epithelial transplantation for severe ocular surface disease and a proposed classification system. Cornea. 1996;15:549-56.
2. Daya SM, Chan CC, Holland EJ; Members of the Cornea Society Ocular Surface Procedures Nomenclature Committee. Cornea Society nomenclature for ocular surface rehabilitative procedures. Cornea. 2011;30:1115-9.
3. Chan CC, Biber JM, Holland EJ. The modified Cincinnati procedure: combined conjunctival-limbal autografts and keratolimbal allografts for unilateral severe ocular surface failure. Cornea. 2012;31:1264-72.
4. Biber JM, Skeens HM, Neff KD, et al. The Cincinnati procedure: technique and outcomes of combined living-related conjunctival limbal allografts and keratolimbal allografts in severe ocular surface failure. Cornea. 2011;30:765-71.
5. Holland EJ, Mogilishetty G, Skeens HM, et al. Systemicimmunosuppression in ocular surface stem cell transplantation: results of a 10-year experience. Cornea. 2012;31:655-61.
6. Basu S, Mohamed A, Chaurasia S, et al. Clinical outcomes of penetrating keratoplasty after autologous cultivated limbal epithelial transplantation for ocular surface burns. Am J Ophthalmol. 2011;152:917-24.
7. Skeens HM, Holland EJ. Large-diameter penetrating keratoplasty: indications and outcomes. Cornea. 2010;29:296-301.

# Section 4

# Vitreoretinal Surgery

*Section Editors* Allen Ho, Sunir J Garg

CHAPTER 23

# Principles and Techniques of Vitreoretinal Surgery

Rajiv Shah, Omesh P Gupta

## INTRODUCTION

Machemer first introduced pars plana vitrectomy (PPV) in 1971. The original vitreous cutter was a 17-gauge (G) instrument that was 1.5 mm in diameter and was inserted through a single sclerotomy site. Early on, it became clear that smaller and more efficient instrumentation would minimize postoperative complications and improve surgical outcomes. In 1974, O'Malley and Heintz described a 20-G three-port vitrectomy system. This system used 0.9 mm incisions that were readily closed with suture. It enabled greater surgical flexibility, and was the basis of numerous innovations in retinal surgical techniques and instrumentation including evolution of cutter speeds, fluidics, surgical adjuncts, surgical instrumentation, and viewing systems through early 1980–2000s.[1]

Chen first described the idea of self-sealing sclerotomies in 1996.[2] These early tunneled incisions still required manual dissection of the conjunctiva and were associated with bleeding from sclerotomy sites and wound leakage requiring subsequent sutures. The 25-G needles used for pars plana intravitreal injections that did not require conjunctival dissection or sclerotomy suture inspired 25-G vitrectomy. De Juan and Hickingbotham designed the first 25-G instruments in 1990. In 2002, De Juanet al.[3] reported a transconjunctival vitrectomy system using 25-G instruments. The closed three-port 25-G system described by Au Eong et al.[4] is the basis for modern day 25-G PPV. Because the early 25-G systems were fairly flexible and removed the vitreous more slowly than 20-G, Eckardt introduced 23-G PPV in 2005.[5] This revised system was introduced to balance the microincision capability of 25-G surgery with the rigidity and functionality of 20-G systems. The introduction of 27-G vitrectomy system by Oshima et al. in 2010 underscores the continued evolution of smaller instrumentation.[6]

Microincision vitrectomy has been well received because of the promise of improved surgical efficacy and faster patient recovery from smaller surgical wounds. However, the transition to smaller gauge instrumentation was not without its early setbacks or controversies.[7] As with any new technology, limitations of instrumentation and new surgical techniques presented early challenges (such as instrumentation flex, poor illumination, slow rates of vitreous removal) [8-11] and complications (such as hypotony/wound leak, choroidals, breakage of instrumentation, and retinal breaks).[12-18] The most troubling complication noted was increased endophthalmitis rates following microincision surgery. Two large retrospective series from tertiary care centers reported significantly higher rates of endophthalmitis with microincision vitrectomy and caused some to question migration toward this newer technology.[19-21] Predisposing factors for endophthalmitis included wound leak, hypotony, mechanical disturbance of the wound by the patient, vitreous incarceration of the wound,[22] and the presence of fluid-filled eyes in all cases of endophthalmitis reported in the two large series.[19,20]

The majority of endophthalmitis cases seen in microincision vitrectomy patients were from nonsutured wounds with direct/straight as opposed to angled architecture.[23] The integrity of the surgical wound in microincision vitrectomy surgery, which is similar to clear cornea cataract surgery, is the presumptive mechanism through which bacteria may enter the eye and cause endophthalmitis.[24-26] Clinical reports demonstrated that direct incision versus oblique incision wounds were associated with increased postoperative hypotony and leakage (factors that would facilitate intraocular bacteria entry).[27,28] Histologic study of cadaveric human eyes demonstrated that oblique incision architecture and smaller gauge nonsutured wounds had lower migration of India ink particles, which is a reasonable surrogate for bacteria, along the scleral tunnel.[29] Noninvasive imaging with time-domain anterior segment optical coherence tomography has demonstrated adequate wound closure on the first postoperative day in 23-G-angled sclerotomies.[30] An ultrasound biomicroscope study of wound architecture in postoperative patients found that it took 15 days postoperatively for a majority (77%) of sclerotomies (straight or angled) to heal.[31] An interesting observation was that there was a higher rate of bleb formation (64% vs 25%) observed in the straight sclerotomies, suggesting a less secure wound immediately postoperatively. Furthermore, a majority of the sclerotomies (72%) were found to have vitreous incarceration, another potential risk factor for endophthalmitis.[32,33] Although initial studies raised the specter of increased endophthalmitis rates in microincision vitrectomy, other centers have found the rates of endophthalmitis were found to be similar between 20-G and 25-G vitrectomy.[34-37] A recent systematic multicenter review from Japan pooled 7 studies of 77,956 patients and did not find a statistically significant difference in endophthalmitis rates between 20-G and microincision vitrectomy.[38]

Aside instrumentation gauge, improvements in the cutter design and vitrectomy fluidics have advanced the success and adoption of vitrectomy. A significant advantage of the smaller gauge instrumentation has been the evolution of the vitrectomy cutter port design with a larger port placed more distally along the instrument shaft (Fig. 23-1). These seemingly small modifications have expanded the role of the vitrectomy cutter to function as a "multi-instrument" that may minimize the necessity of ancillary instruments such small incision forceps, pick, or horizontal scissors and facilitates more controlled segmentation/delamination of fibrovascular tissue with less risk of creating breaks in cases of complicated tractional retinal detachment cases. Early vitrectomy machines offered only low cut rates and high aspiration, which is now recognized as a scenario for increased force generation along vitreous fibers with resultant increase in iatrogenic retinal tears.[39] It is now recognized that higher cut rates decrease the force generation on vitreous and allow for a safer vitrectomy particularly when one works close to mobile retina.[39-41] Current maximum cut rates range from 2500 to 5000 cuts per minute (cpm), with newer systems touting 7500 or 8000 cpm. To achieve 5000 cpm and higher, a dual pneumatic mechanism rather than electronic or mechanical spring-loaded mechanism is necessary to drive the guillotine of the cutter. Dual pneumatic-driven cutters allow machines to control the duty cycle, which is the time a cutter port may spend opened or closed, and control of duty cycle has been a key advance toward optimizing vitrectomy fluidics toward efficiency and safety with regard to vitreous humor removal or manipulation close to the retinal surface.[42] Other studies have suggested that the use of smaller gauge instrumentation with higher cut rates creates a more precise region of fluid dynamics around the vitrector port, which is important for tissue manipulation.[43]

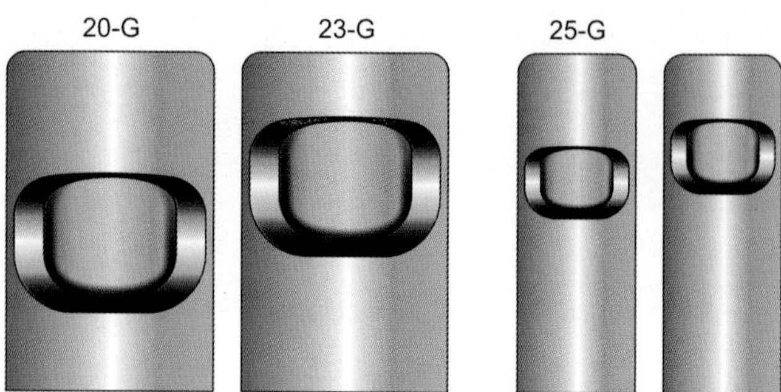


**Figure 23-1** Alterations of the port size and location between 20-gauge, 23-gauge, and 25-gauge instrumentation.

## INDICATIONS

Vitrectomy has broad applications in vitreoretinal disease or as surgical adjunct for diverse vitreoretinal surgeries. The applications include primary rhegmatogenous retinal detachment repair, recurrent retinal detachment repair, removal of visually significant vitreous opacity, vitreous or chorioretinal biopsy, aqueous misdirection/malignant glaucoma, repair of tractional retinal detachments (diabetic, retinopathy of prematurity, proliferative vitreoretinopathy), disorders of the vitreoretinal interface (vitreomacular traction, epiretinal membrane, macular hole), removal of visually significant subretinal hemorrhage, macular translocation, removal of intraocular foreign bodies, removal of subretinal choroidal neovascular membranes, posterior uveitis, placement of drug delivery reservoir, and placement of retinal bioprosthetic devices.

## CLINICAL EVALUATION

Prior to any vitrectomy surgery, a careful assessment of optical clarity (cornea and cataract) and areas of retinal pathology must be performed as these may influence surgical approaches. Meticulous biomicroscopy of the macula and careful inspection of the retinal periphery with indirect ophthalmoscopy and scleral depression are recommended prior to surgery. In scenarios where there is no view of the posterior segment (hyphema, hypopyon, corneal scar, cataract, vitreous hemorrhage, vitreous debris, vitritis, etc.), ultrasound B scan is recommended to evaluate for possible retinal tears, rhegmatogenous or tractional retinal detachment, mass lesions, or choroidal detachment. Preoperative B scan may alter surgical planning and is essential for preoperative patient counseling.

## CONTRAINDICATIONS

The main contraindications to vitrectomy are poor medical health or poor ocular media (cataract or cornea) that would impair the ability to achieve surgical goals. Consideration of cataract surgery either a week or two before vitrectomy, or in combination with vitrectomy, should be made for visually significant cataracts that would impair visualization for macular surgery. Consideration of corneal transplantation may be necessary if there is significant corneal scar impairing the macular surgical view. For the later, a temporary keratoprosthesis can be used for the vitrectomy with subsequent placement of a full thickness corneal transplant.

## SURGICAL TECHNIQUE

The first decision that requires thought is the location of port/sclerotomy placement. With the exception of two-port vitrectomy, which is utilized in some pediatric cases, the majority of vitrectomy is performed with at least three separate ports/sclerotomies (with particularly complex cases additional ports/sclerotomies may be utilized for the placement of a chandelier illumination source). Improper port/sclerotomy placement may inhibit ease of surgical manipulations such as membrane peeling or repair of a retinal detachment or may reduce surgical efficiency depending on the case. The location of sclerotomies is ultimately surgeon dependent and should be tailored to each case.

While the emphasis here is with microincision vitrectomy, one of the microincision vitrectomy incisions can be enlarged with a 20-G MVR blade to accommodate specific instruments such as a 19-gauge endoscopic probe, phacofragmatome handpiece, or for intraocular foreign body forceps. Twenty-gauge vitrectomy wounds are first constructed with conjunctival incisions (either limited peritomy or local incisions around the location of the intended sclerotomy). The same principles are applied for sclerotomy location, as noted above, and surface cautery may be necessary to achieve hemostasis prior to incision with the 20-gauge MVR blade. The MVR blade is typically inserted until the tip of the blade is readily visualized in the pupil while the blade is directed away from the crystalline lens. The infusion line in 20-gauge systems must be sutured in place. Typically this is done with a "figure of 8" suture (either 7.0 vicryl or 5.0 nylon) placed after the creation of the sclerotomy with the MVR blade. If vicryl is used, a temporary knot is placed to secure the flanges of the infusion line to the sclera, and this same suture can be released at the end of the case to close the sclerotomy without needing an additional suture pass. If nylon is used, one typically employs a permanent knot and the suture is cut, and the sclerotomy is closed with 7.0 vicryl in similar fashion to the other sclerotomies.

As noted above, proper wound construction is critical both to facilitate surgery and to reduce potential complications, particularly for microincision vitrectomy. Wound construction consists of two key elements. The first is conjunctival displacement prior to the insertion of the trocar/cannula. The displacement of conjunctiva provides surface bacteria a longer path to traverse before arriving at the sclerotomy, and it may prevent the vitreous wick phenomenon as described above. The displacement of conjunctiva can be performed with a cotton-tip applicator, 0.12 mm forceps, or specialized conjunctiva fixation device. If the conjunctiva is too scarred from either previous surgery or some alternative disease process, attempts should be made to displace the conjunctiva with hydrodissection or the wound should be sutured at the end of the case. As noted above, angled incisions are preferred as they provide improved wound closure (and less postoperative hypotony) at the end of the case and provide a longer tract for bacteria to traverse important risk factors for reducing endophthalmitis (Figs. 23-2A to C). There is no consensus regarding the angle or length of the bevel incision; some favored a bi- or triplanar wound (beveled 10–15° tunnel with completion of the tract following a straight/direct wound approach). The infusion line is inserted typically in the inferior temporal port; however, the location can be readily moved between trocars. Prior to the opening of the infusion, verify that the infusion tip is in the vitreous cavity (Fig. 23-3). Failure to verify the infusion tip position risks accidental suprachoroidal or subretinal infusion that may have catastrophic results. Should the media not allow for visualization of the infusion tip, limited vitrectomy, lensectomy, or anterior chamber infusion may be necessary to provide a safe scenario to proceed with vitrectomy. Another option is place an air bubble in the infusion line prior to opening the infusion. If the air bubble is visualized in the vitreous cavity, it is reasonable to assume the infusion tip is in the proper location for the vitrectomy to start, but verification of its location should be established once the media concerns have been alleviated.

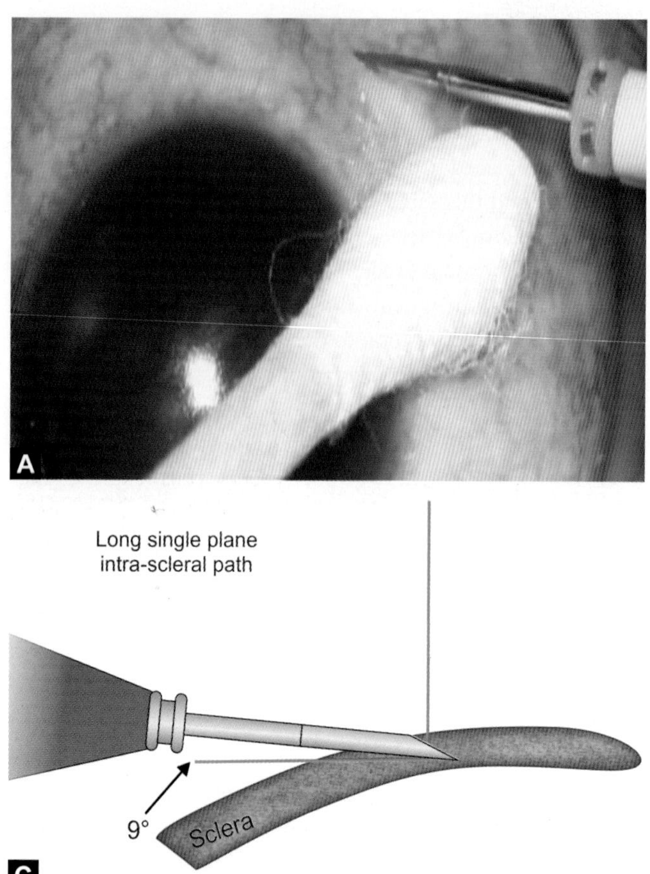

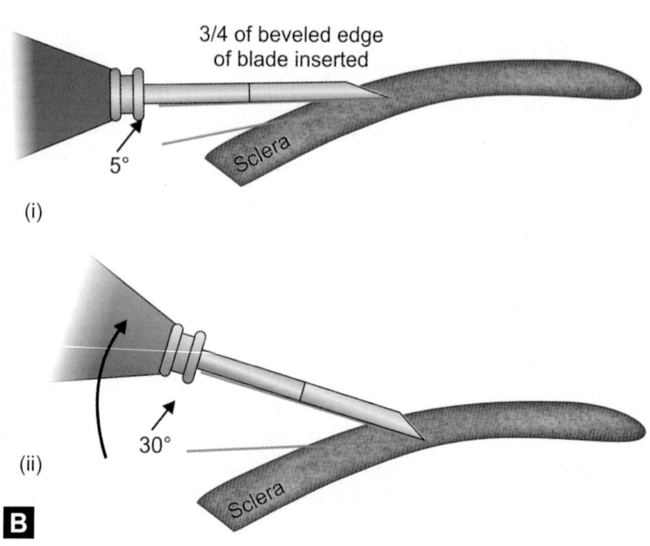


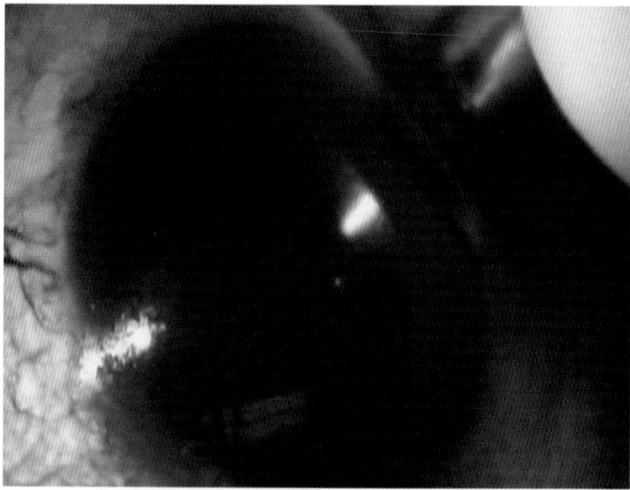


Figures 23-2A to C (A) Insertion of the trocar begins with conjunctival displacement with the cotton tip. The sclera is flattened to create a longer scleral tunnel, and the approach is flat initially prior to the elevation of the trocar thus creating a biplanar wound. (B) Creating a biplanar incision. (i) First step: Make a 5° partial thickness incision into the sclera with the trocar. The blade of the trocar is inserted with a narrow angle into the sclera until three quarters of the blade are entered. (ii) Second step: The trocar is then rotated up to 30° and the blade is inserted until it fully penetrates the sclera. Reproduced with permission from Kaiser et al.[22] (C) Alternative insertion technique with flat-angled insertion of cannula using a near-flat, narrow-angle linear incision. Care must be taken to be certain that the cannulae are not placed in the subretinal space. Reproduced with permission from Kaiser et al.[22]

Figure 23-3 The tip of the infusion line must be verified prior to infusing balanced salt solution into the eye. Light pipe is illuminated obliquely through the cornea and the tip of the infusion is found completely in the vitreous cavity.

Visualization of the posterior segment requires neutralization of the corneal converging power with some form of diverging optical lens.[44] While a complete discussion regarding all viewing systems for vitreous surgery (irrigating contact lens, direct contact viewing, etc.) is beyond the scope of this discussion, wide-field viewing has been a particular advance for vitreous surgery. Wide-field viewing applies the principle of indirect ophthalmoscopy to achieve a panoramic view of the fundus.[45] Early systems attempted to use a Rodenstock pan fundus lens to achieve a 150° optical view; a key advance was the application of a prismatic image inversion that allowed the surgeon to appreciate the panoramic view without the reversal of orientation.[46] Advances in glass manufacturing and optical engineering eventually provided for smaller, less cumbersome contact-based wide-field viewing, but eventually a noncontact system, binocular indirect operating microscope, was developed that allowed for a 130° optical view, which was independent of the pupil aperture.[44,47] Wide-field viewing systems enable a surgeon to be more independent of an assistant and improve visualization of the peripheral fundus. Macular work, however, may still require a contact lens for improved stereopsis.

A standard three-port vitrectomy is performed with an infusion line, light source, and vitrector cutter. For the beginning surgeon, the most challenging aspect of vitreous

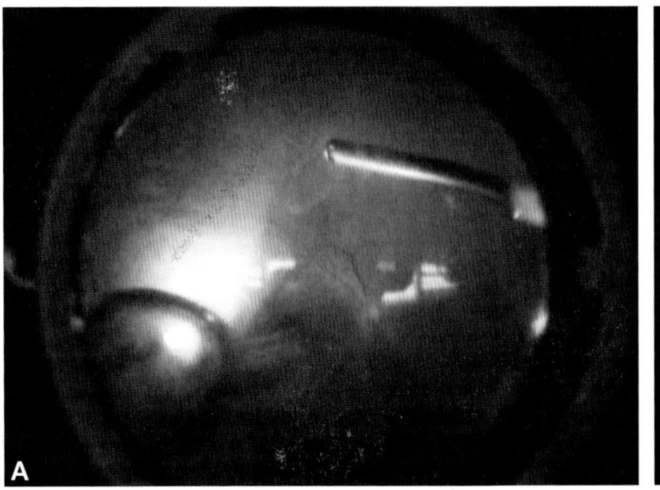
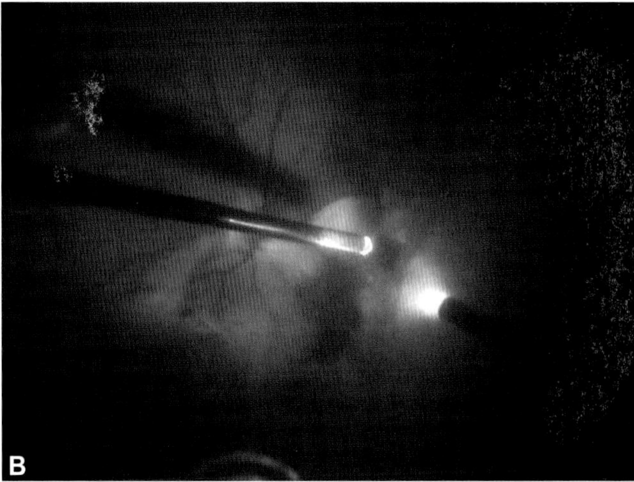

Figures 23-4A and B (A) Illumination during the vitrectomy is a challenging but important skill. Diffuse illumination helps highlight the surrounding region of retina around the vitreous being removed. This improves the safety by minimizing the chance of creating iatrogenic retinal breaks or trauma. The light pipe is typically pulled up into the trocar and directed to create broad illumination. (B) Focal illumination allows individual fibers of vitreous to be seen.

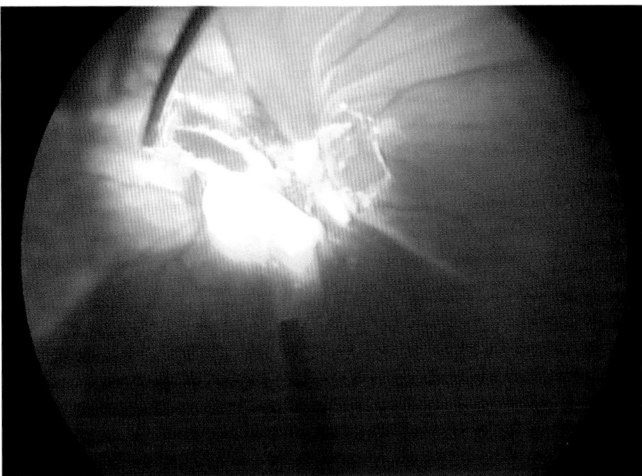

Figure 23-5 Induction of the posterior vitreous detachment with the aide of triamcinolone with the vitrectomy cutter.

removal is the orientation of the light pipe and the mechanics of instrument motion to maximize surgical efficiency and efficacy. Proper illumination is an art because it is a dynamic balance of highlighting the vitreous while illuminating the surrounding environment and minimizing iatrogenic trauma either to the retina or crystalline lens (Figs. 23-4A and B). Careful, precise, and often minute manipulations of the instruments with pivoting along the trocar/sclerotomies are necessary to achieve surgical goals.

One of the most important aspects of vitreous surgery is the induction of a posterior vitreous detachment (PVD). Meticulous technique with the vitrectomy cutter with enhanced vitreous visualization with triamcinolone in some cases usually successfully induces a PVD (Fig. 23-5).[48] To create a PVD, the mouth of the cutter should be directed to the edges of the cortical vitreous insertion at the optic nerve. Prior to attempted elevation of the posterior hyaloid, a sufficient amount of vitreous should occlude the mouth of the cutter to maximize the mechanical advantage needed to induce a complete PVD. Once the vitreous is engaged, the vitreous should be pulled anteriorly along the visual axis to disengage the vitreous while minimizing lateral tractional forces that can result in iatrogenic retinal breaks.

Following creation/confirmation of a PVD, the core vitreous is removed, followed by a peripheral vitrectomy. The goals of the peripheral vitrectomy depend on the nature of the surgery (please refer to the individual chapters regarding techniques for specific situations). In general, the goal of peripheral vitrectomy is to remove the vitreous without iatrogenic trauma to the retina or surrounding structures. Scleral depression may be necessary to access or safely remove particularly adherent vitreous, and a scleral buckle may be necessary to support the vitreous base if aggressive removal is not possible or if the retinal pathology requires it.

For tractional membranes, subretinal membranes, or foreign bodies, several types of forceps are available, including internal limiting membrane, end grasping, asymmetric, serrated, and foreign body forceps. These instruments facilitate complicated delamination, segmentation, or object removal. For particularly challenging cases, chandelier illumination or illuminated instruments may be necessary.

Regardless of the case, intraocular diathermy and careful inspection of the retinal periphery are important tools that can be used in almost any case. Intraocular diathermy is important for marking retinal breaks or for the creation of

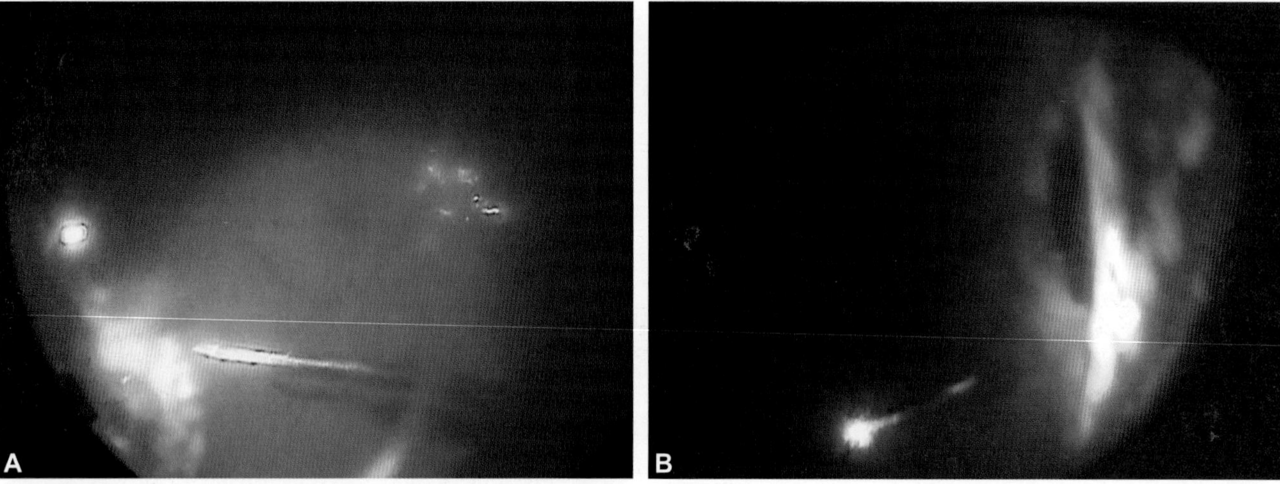


Figures 23-6A and B (A) Focal laser retinopexy with the curved illuminated probe to a retinal tear. (B) Focal laser retinopexy with the curved illuminated probe to the anterior retina with concurrent scleral depression.

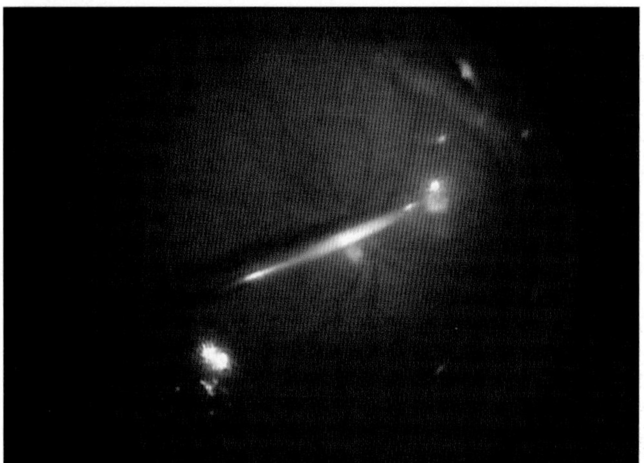

Figure 23-7 Air-fluid exchange with the drainage of subretinal fluid through the drainage retinotomy.

drainage retinotomies, and in cases when a retinal or choroidal blood vessel is broken (such as during removal of diabetic tractional membranes, relaxing retinotomies/bridging vessels, and during chorioretinal biopsies), it is vital to utilize diathermy in a meticulous fashion to maintain hemostasis. Although one may use an indirect ophthalmoscope and scleral depression to inspect the retinal periphery, the optics of wide-field lens with magnification of the operating microscope are superior and more efficient. We typically utilize a Gass muscle hook with the light pipe. The other trocar is either closed with a plug or has a sealing valve to aid in assistant independent depression and inspection of the periphery.

Creating or strengthening a chorioretinal adhesion (retinopexy) or photocoagulating areas of ischemic retina remains a common practice during vitrectomy. While cryopexy is utilized for primary scleral buckles, its role in vitrectomy has become more limited (although it may still be used for anterior retinal pathology) given the advances with lasers and particularly endolaser probes. For the majority of posterior segment surgery, a 532 nm laser is used. We prefer the use of wide-field viewing systems with the operating microscope and an endolaser probe, particularly one that is lighted with a curve to allow for access to more anterior retina (Figs. 23-6A and B). Panretinal photocoagulation of the posterior retina can be efficiently performed with the light pipe and laser probe. For the anterior/peripheral retina, we recommend scleral depression by the surgeon with one hand and use of the lighted laser curved laser probe.

Air-fluid exchange is an important and powerful tool in vitrectomy because the transition from fluid to air utilizes the large force generated by the surface tension disparity between air/fluid.[39] This force enables one to flatten retinal breaks allowing for laser treatment, to drive subretinal fluid posteriorly for drainage, displace subretinal hemorrhage peripherally, or to facilitate sclerotomy closure at the end of a microincision vitrectomy case. Although one can use passive extrusion with a soft tip needle, we recommend active extrusion with the soft tip and proportional vacuum because it offers more precision/efficiency (Fig. 35-7). For patients with a pseudophakic lens, particularly for case of an open posterior capsule or with silicone or poly-methyl-methacrylate lens implants, lens fogging is common and this may significantly limit the surgical view. Although wiping the posterior lens surface with the soft tip invariably helps, its affect is transient. For cases where continued air-fluid exchange is necessary (such as in retinal detachment repair or with the removal of perfluorocarbon liquid), we recommend the use of a dispersive viscoelastic injected via a 30-gauge needle along the posterior surface of the lens implant. Further exchange of an air-filled eye with alternate gas or silicone oil is discussed in the subsequent chapters of retinal detachment repair.

With regard to microincisional vitrectomy, after removing the cannulae inspect the wounds to detect wound leak or vitreous wicking. Any bleb formation should prompt evaluation of possible wound leak by the surgeon, and any suspicious wound or vitreous wick should prompt the surgeon to place a suture. Early studies in microincision vitrectomy had noted that air or gas-filled eyes might help close the sclerotomies and prevent postoperative hypotony.[49,50] A multicenter retrospective study of 2236 cases found only 1 case (0.04%) of endophthalmitis when a complete gas tamponade with either $SF_6$ or $C_3F_8$ was employed.[51] Gas tamponade may be beneficial because it reduces postoperative hypotony, may help close surgical wounds, and provides an additional barrier to the spread of bacteria into the vitreous cavity by the virtue of the higher surface tension.[51]

## MECHANISM OF ACTION

Removal of vitreous is safe and effective with high cut-rate vitrectomy and proper surgical technique.

### Postoperative Care

The standard antibiotic and steroid topical drop four times a day are typically sufficient for control of postoperative infection/inflammation. If gas tamponade is used, monitoring of the intraocular pressure is important for the first postoperative day.

### Complications

The most common intraoperative complication is the creation of an iatrogenic break, which occurs in approximately 5.5% of cases. Interestingly the tears are rarely found near the sclerotomies, suggesting that tear formation occurs during the PVD induction. The rate of retinal detachment was found to be 1–2%.[52] If cataract surgery is not done prior or concurrent with vitrectomy surgery, the rate of cataract progression is 81% at 2 years.[53]

## SURGICAL OUTCOMES: SCIENTIFIC EVIDENCE

Vitrectomy is a successful surgical procedure; specific outcomes and evidence depend on the particular conditions noted in other chapters.

## PLACE OF THE TECHNIQUE IN SURGICAL ARMAMENTARIUM

Vitrectomy remains the dominant vitreoretinal surgical technique.

## PEARLS AND PITFALLS

- If the infusion cannula cannot be visualized, a 6-mm cannula can be used. The light pipe can also be inserted into the cannula to confirm placement in the vitreous cavity.
- Ensure that the posterior hyaloid is separated from the retina.
- Meticulous inspection of the retinal periphery for retinal breaks is critical.
- When in doubt, suture the wounds at the end of the case. If the patient has a new IOL in place, consider suturing the wounds rather than using air/gas to prevent infection.

## REFERENCES

1. O'Malley C, Heintz RM Sr. Vitrectomy with an alternative instrument system. Ann Ophthalmol. 1975;7(4):585-8, 591-4.
2. Chen JC. Sutureless pars plana vitrectomy through self-sealing sclerotomies. Arch Ophthalmol. 1996;114(10):1273-5.
3. Fujii GY, De Juan E Jr, Humayun MS, et al. A new 25-gauge instrument system for transconjunctival sutureless vitrectomy surgery. Ophthalmology. 2002;109(10):1807-12; discussion 1813.
4. Au Eong KG , Fujii GY, de Juan E Jr, et al. A new three-port cannular system for closed pars plana vitrectomy. Retina. 2002; 22(1):130-2.
5. Eckardt C. Transconjunctival sutureless 23-gauge vitrectomy. Retina. 2005;25(2):208-11.
6. Oshima Y, Wakabayashi T, Sato T. A 27-gauge instrument system for transconjunctival sutureless microincision vitrectomy surgery. Ophthalmology. 2010;117(1):93-102 e2.
7. Thompson J. Advantages and limitations of small gauge vitrectomy. Surv Ophthalmol. 2011;56(2):162-72.
8. Ibarra MS, Hermel M, Prenner JL, et al. Longer-term outcomes of transconjunctival sutureless 25-gauge vitrectomy. Am J Ophthalmol. 2005;139(5):831-6.
9. Lakhanpal RR, Humayun MS, de Juan E Jr, et al. Outcomes of 140 consecutive cases of 25-gauge transconjunctival surgery for posterior segment disease. Ophthalmology. 2005;112(5):817-24.
10. Kellner L, Wimpissinger B, Stolba U, et al. 25-Gauge vs 20-gauge system for pars plana vitrectomy: a prospective randomized clinical trial. Br J Ophthalmol. 2007;91(7):945-8.
11. Wimpissinger B, Kellner L, Brannath W, et al. 23-Gauge versus 20-gauge system for pars plana vitrectomy: a prospective randomized clinical trial. Br J Ophthalmol. 2008;92(11):1483-7.

12. Inoue M, Noda K, Ishida S, et al. Intraoperative breakage of a 25-gauge vitreous cutter. Am J Ophthalmol. 2004;138(5):867-9.
13. Taylor SRJ, Aylward GW. Endophthalmitis following 25-gauge vitrectomy. Eye (Lond). 2005;19(11):1228-9.
14. Taban M, Ufret-Vincenty RL, Sears JE. Endophthalmitis after 25-gauge transconjunctival sutureless vitrectomy. Retina. 2006; 26(7):830-1.
15. Liu DT, Chan CK, Fan DS, et al. Choroidal folds after 25-gauge transconjunctival sutureless vitrectomy. Eye (Lond). 2005;19(7): 825-7.
16. Okuda T, Nishimura A, Kobayashi A, Sugiyama K. Postoperative retinal break after 25-gauge transconjunctival sutureless vitrectomy: report of four cases. Graefes Arch Clin Exp Ophthalmol. 2007;245:155-7.
17. Gupta OP, Weichel ED, Regillo CD, et al. Postoperative complications associated with 25-gauge pars plana vitrectomy. Ophthalmic Surg Lasers Imaging. 2007;38(4):270-5.
18. Scartozzi R, Bessa AS, Gupta OP, et al. Intraoperative sclerotomy-related retinal breaks for macular surgery, 20- vs 25-gauge vitrectomy systems. Am J Ophthalmol. 2007;143(1):155-6.
19. Kunimoto DY, Kaiser RS. Incidence of endophthalmitis after 20- and 25-gauge vitrectomy. Ophthalmology. 2007;114: 2133-7.
20. Scott IU, Flynn HW Jr, Dev S, et al. Endophthalmitis after 25-gauge and 20-gauge pars plana vitrectomy: incidence and outcomes. Retina. 2008;28(1):138-42.
21. Lewis H. Sutureless microincision vitrectomy surgery: unclear benefit, uncertain safety. Am J Ophthalmol. 2007;144(4):613-5.
22. Kaiser R, Prenner J, Scott I, et al. The microsurgical safety task force: evolving guidelines for minimizing the risk of endophthalmitis associated with microincisional vitrectomy surgery. Retina. 2010;30(4):692-9.
23. Bahrani HM, Fazelat AA, Thomas M, et al. Endophthalmitis in the era of small-gauge transconjunctival sutureless vitrectomy–meta analysis and review of literature. Semin Ophthalmol. 2010;25(5-6):275-82.
24. Thoms SS, Musch DC, Soong HK. Postoperative endophthalmitis associated with sutured versus unsutured clear corneal cataract incisions. Br J Ophthalmol. 2007;91:728-30.
25. John ME, Noblitt R. Endophthalmitis: scleral tunnel vs. clear corneal incision. In: Buzard KA, Friedlander MH, Febbraro JL (eds.), The blue line incision and refractive phacoemulsification. Thorofare, New Jersey: SLACK, 2001:53-6.
26. Nagaki Y, Hayasaka S, Kadoi C, et al. Bacterial endophthalmitis after small-incision cataract surgery: effect of incision placement and intraocular lens type. J Cataract Refract Surg. 2003;29:20-26.
27. Hsu J, Chen E, Gupta O, et al. Hypotony after 25-gauge vitrectomy using oblique versus direct cannula insertions in fluid-filled eyes. Retina. 2008;28:937-40.
28. Inoue M, Shinoda K, Shinoda H, et al. Two-step oblique incision during 25-gauge vitrectomy reduces incidence of postoperative hypotony. Clin Experiment Ophthalmol. 2007;35:693-6.
29. Gupta OP, Maguire JI, Eagle RC, et al. The Competency of Pars Plana Vitrectomy Incisions: A Comparative Histologic and Spectrophotometric Analysis. Am J Ophthalmol. 2009; 147(2):243-50.
30. Taban M, Sharma S, Ventura AA, et al. Evaluation of wound closure in oblique 23-gauge sutureless sclerotomies with visante optical coherence tomography. Am J Ophthalmol. 2009;147(1): 101-107.e1.
31. Lopez-Guajardo L, Vleming-Pinilla E, Pareja-Esteban J, et al. Ultrasound biomicroscopy study of direct and oblique 25-gauge vitrectomy sclerotomies. Am J Ophthalmol. 2007;143(5):881-3.
32. Ruiz RS, Teeters VW. The vitreous wick syndrome. Am J Ophthalmol. 1970;70(4):483-90.
33. Venkatesh P, Verma L, Tewari H. Posterior vitreous wick syndrome: a potential cause of endophthalmitis following vitreoretinal surgery. Med Hypotheses. 2002;58(6):513-5.
34. Hu AH, Bourges J-L, Shah SP, et al. Endophthalmitis after pars plana vitrectomy: a 20- and 25-guage comparison. Ophthalmology. 2009;116(7):1360-5.
35. Chen JK, Khurana RN, Nguyen QD, et al. The incidence of endophthalmitis following transconjunctival sutureless 25- vs 20-gauge vitrectomy. Eye. 2009;23(4):780-4.
36. Shimada H, Nakashizuka H, Hattori T, et al. Incidence of endophthalmitis after 20- and 25-gauge vitrectomy: Causes and prevention. Ophthalmology. 2008;115(12):2215-20.
37. Mason JO, Yunker JJ, Vail RS, et al. Incidence of endophthalmitis following 20-guage and 25-gauge vitrectomy. Retina. 2008;28(9):1352-4.
38. Oshima Y, Kadonosono K, Yamaji H. Multicenter survey with a systematic overview of acute-onset endophthalmitis after transconjunctival microincision vitrectomy surgery. Am J Ophthalmol. 2010;150(5):716-25.
39. Charles S. An engineering approach to vitreo-retinal surgery. Retina. 2004;24(3):435-44.
40. Hubschman JP, Bourges JL, Tsui I, et al. Effect of cutting phases on flow rate in 20-, 23-, and 25-gauge vitreous cutters. Retina. 2009;29(9):1289-93.
41. Teixerira A, Chong LP, Matsuoka N, et al. Vitreoretinal traction created by conventional cutters during vitrectomy. Ophthalmology. 2010;117(7):1387-92.e2.
42. Diniz B, Riberiro R, Fernandes R, et al. Fluidics in a dual pneumatic ultra high-speed vitreous cutter system. Ophthalmologica. 2013;229(1):15-20.
43. Dugel PU, Zhou J, Abulon DJ, et al. Tissue attraction associated with 20-gauge, 23-gauge, and enhanced 25-gauge dual pneumatic vitrectomy probes. Retina. 2012;32(9):1761-6.
44. Chalam K, Shah V. Optics of wide-angle panoramic viewing system-assisted vitreous surgery. Surv Ophthalmol. 2004;49(4):437-45.
45. Tolentino FI, Freeman HM, Shah VA. A new lens for closed pars plana vitrectomy. Arch Ophthalmol. 1979;97(11):2197-8.
46. Spitznas M, Reiner J. A stereoscopic diagonal inverter (SDI) for wide-angle vitreous surgery. Graefe's Arch Clin Exp Ophthalmol. 1987;225(1):9-12.
47. Spitznas M. A binocular indirect ophthalmomicroscope (BIOM) for non-contact wide-angle vitreous surgery. Graefe's Arch Clin Exp Ophthalmol. 1987;225(1):13-5.

48. Peyman GA, Cheema R, Conway MD, et al. Triamcinolone acetonide as an aid to visualization of the vitreous and the posterior hyaloid during pars plana vitrectomy. Retina. 2000; 20(5):554-5.
49. Shimada H, Nakashizuka H, Mori R, et al. Expanded indications for 25-gauge transconjunctival vitrectomy. Jpn J Ophthalmol. 2005;49(5):397-401.
50. Shaikh S, Ho S, Richmond PP, et al. Untoward outcomes in 25-gauge versus 20-gauge Vitreoretinal surgery. Retina. 2007; 27:1048-53.
51. Chiang A, Kaiser RS, Avery RL, et al. Endophthalmitis in microincision vitrectomy: outcomes of gas-filled eyes. Retina. 2011;31(8):1513-7.
52. Sjaarda RN, Flaser BM, Thompson JT, et al. Distribution of iatrogenic retinal breaks in macular hole surgery. Ophthalmology. 1995;102(9):1387-92.
53. Thompson JT, Glaser BM, Sjaarda RN, et al. Progression of nuclear sclerosis and long-term visual results of vitrectomy with transforming growth factor beta-2 for macular holes. Am J Ophthalmol. 1995;119(1):48-54.

CHAPTER

24

# Retinal Detachment Repair: Scleral Buckling Procedures

Baseer U Ahmad, Gaurav Shah, Nicholas Engelbrecht, Matthew Thomas, Bradley T Smith

## INTRODUCTION

Scleral buckling is a surgical technique for repair of rhegmatogenous retinal detachments (RRD) and as an adjunct treatment of tractional or vitreoproliferative detachments. The key principles of successful treatment of RRD are identification of all rhegmatogenous breaks, relief of traction upon the causative breaks, and closure of these breaks.[1]

## INDICATIONS

RRD repair using scleral buckling procedures (SBP) is best suited for patients who are phakic or with a formed vitreous, and any of the following:

- Uncomplicated single break
- Multiple breaks along the vitreous base
- Retinal dialysis

In particular, young, phakic patients benefit from preservation of the clear crystalline lens and normal accommodation.

## CONTRAINDICATIONS

- Posterior breaks, where proper placement of a band or element would be difficult or impossible
- Media opacities/hemorrhage that limit identification of all retinal breaks
- Scleral thinning/scleromalacia to a degree where suture placement or creation of scleral tunnels would likely result in scleral perforation

## SURGICAL TECHNIQUE

Focal indentation of the sclera to reappose retinal breaks to the underlying retinal pigment epithelium (RPE) can be done with many different buckling elements, including encircling bands, tires, and sponges. Segmental buckles, either circumferential or radial, may also be used to support a single break or multiple breaks in proximity. The most common contemporary approach involves the use of encircling silicone bands and tires.

### Preoperative Evaluation and Surgical Scheduling

Careful dilated fundus examination of both eyes is critical. A detailed preoperative drawing showing all breaks relative to the normal anatomy is necessary for surgical planning. The fellow eye should be carefully examined for any peripheral retinal pathology. After documentation, surgical scheduling should be guided as follows:

- Complete history and physical to identify contraindications to SBP, including medical instability or anticoagulation, particularly if INR > 3.0
- If the macula is attached and threatened by rapid progression, surgery should be promptly performed
- If the macula is attached and the detachment is inferior or there is known slow progression, then surgery may be performed within a few days
- Chronic extramacular detachment (evidenced by demarcation line, retinal cysts, and/or subretinal fibrosis) may be repaired on a nonemergent basis within 1–2 weeks
- If the macula has been detached for a significant period of time, surgery can be done at the convenience of the patient and surgeon within several weeks

### Setup

Instruments necessary for scleral buckling include (Fig. 24-1):

- Westcott scissors
- Needle drivers × 4 (one fine set for 8-0 suture, one large set for 5-0 suture)

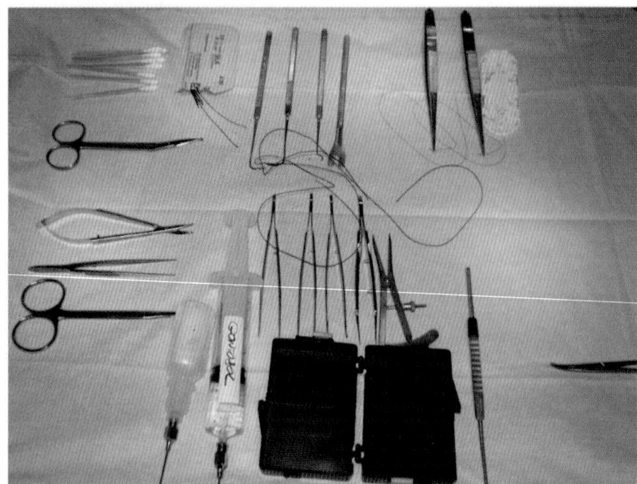
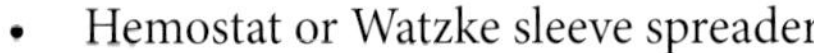

Figure 24-1 Most vitreoretinal operating rooms have standard scleral buckling surgical trays such as the one shown.

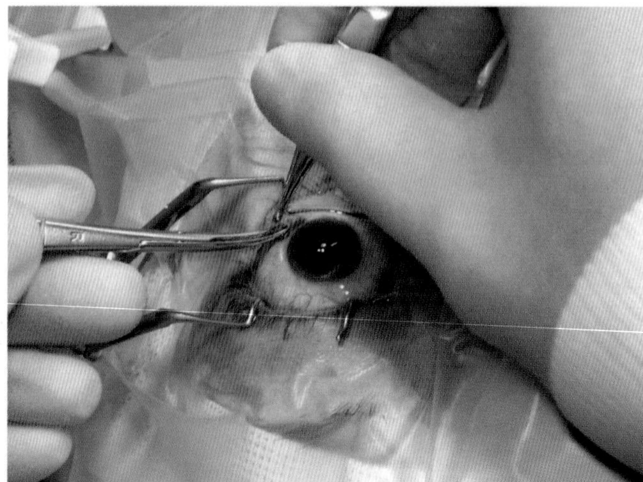

Figure 24-2 A conjunctival peritomy begins with a radial incision at 3 or 9 o'clock.

- Hemostat or Watzke sleeve spreader
- Nontoothed conjunctival forceps × 2
- Nugent forceps × 2
- Caliper
- Curved tenotomy scissors (Stephens or nurse scissors)
- Fenestrated muscle hooks × 2
- Olive tip (Jameson) muscle hook
- Schepens retractor
- Marking scleral depressor (e.g. O'connor or Urrets-Zavalia)
- Irrigating cannulae (for balanced salt solution, Goniosol, bupivacaine solutions)
- Straight tenotomy scissors ("silicone scissors")
- Toothed forceps (0.12 and/or 0.3 mm)
- Suture
  - Silk 2-0 × 1 pack (usually 12 strands)
  - Nylon 5-0 × 2 (e.g. Ethilon 18" on RD-1 spatulated needle)
  - Vicryl 8-0 × 2 (e.g. Ethilon 12" on TG140-8 spatulated needle)
- #64 or #57 blade on handle (if doing scleral cutdown or scleral tunnels)
- #66 blade on handle (if doing scleral tunnels)
- Indirect ophthalmoscope
- Condensing lenses (20 diopter and/or 28 diopter)
- Cryotherapy apparatus
  - Probe with sleeve
  - Unit
  - Nitrogen canisters
- Syringe (1 mL) and 27 or 30-gauge needle for external drainage of subretinal fluid
- Gas
  - $SF_6$ and $C_3F_8$ gas canisters
  - 3 mL and/or 1 mL syringe with 30-gauge needle
  - Millipore filter and tubing with stopcock

## Anesthesia and Preparation

Either general anesthesia or a retrobulbar block with monitored anesthesia care can be used. A retrobulbar block may be done by a transcutaneous or transconjunctival approach. If the transconjunctival approach through the inferior fornix is used, it is useful to have an idea of the axial length of the globe as the needle will pass along its contour more closely than the transcutaneous method. After anesthesia, a 5% povidine-iodine solution should be used to prep the conjunctiva, eyelids, and skin.

## Initial Dissection and Muscle Isolation

A conjunctival peritomy is done by using forceps (0.12, 0.3, or nontoothed) to lift the perilimbal conjunctiva at 3 or 9 o'clock and using a Westcott scissor to create a radial relaxing conjunctival incision (Fig. 24-2). This incision should be extended 3–4 mm in length. It is then repeated at the remaining 3 or 9 o'clock position.

Next, in a smooth continuous motion, the Westcott scissors are used to cut the conjunctiva and underlying Tenon's capsule at the limbus (Fig. 24-3). A temporal approach allows the surgeon maximal exposure to keep the blades adjacent to the corneal limbus. This helps avoid the creation of a "can-opener" peritomy with jagged edges.

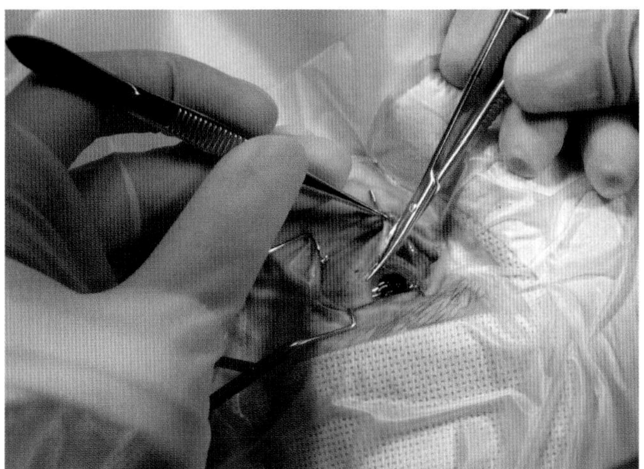

Figure 24-3 Using a Westcott scissor to cut in several smooth motions following the curve of the limbus results in conjunctival flaps with clean edges.

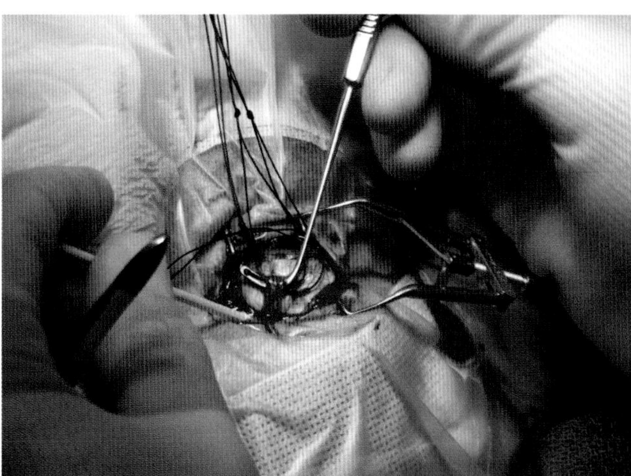

Figure 24-4 A rectus muscle is hooked, cleaned, and inspected to make sure no muscle fibers have been missed.

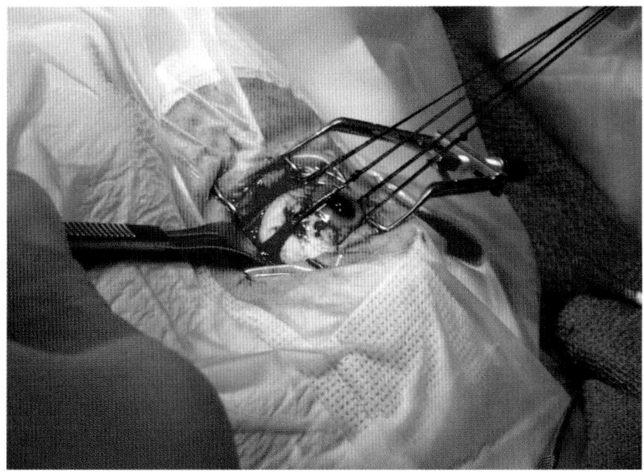

Figure 24-5 The Schepens retractor helps inspect sclera and muscle.

Curved tenotomy (Stephens or nurse) scissors are used to follow the curve of the globe underneath Tenon's capsule and to deeply enter each oblique quadrant midway between adjacent rectus muscles. They can be inserted up to the hinge of the scissor and are then opened broadly to bluntly dissect the intermuscular septum and Tenon's tissue. This allows for access to the rectus muscles.

Using a fenestrated muscle hook loaded with a 2-0 silk tie, a sweeping motion is used to pass the hook underneath and posteriorly to the medial or lateral rectus. Once the hook end is visible on the other side of the muscle, a forceps is used to grasp the tie and the hook is backed out in the same manner used for insertion. The silk tie now straddles the muscle and both ends of the tie are used to create two simple stop knots. This maneuver is repeated for the remaining horizontal muscle, followed by the inferior rectus and then the superior rectus (Fig. 24-4).

## Inspection and Identification of Breaks

Once the muscles are looped, all ties should be grasped and a Schepens retractor is then used to inspect each quadrant, look for thin/blue sclera, properly isolate the rectus muscles, and note the position of the vortex veins (Fig. 24-5). If extensive or entire quadrant(s) show scleromalacia, the scleral buckle may need to be abandoned in favor of a vitrectomy procedure. This step also enables further blunt dissection of the intermuscular septum and the Tenon's tissue back to the equator for maximal exposure. Extreme posterior dissection should be avoided as this can encourage posterior adhesion of the muscle to the scleral wall, which may increase the risk of postoperative strabismus or fat adherence syndrome.

Once scleral inspection has been performed, the surgeon should use an indirect ophthalmoscope to examine the peripheral retina with scleral depression. Since the eye has been immobilized by anesthesia, the assistant must use the silk ties to present the fundus in the appropriate direction. Usually this means turning the eye away from the surgeon's line of sight; e.g. in order for the surgeon to view the peripheral nasal fundus while standing temporally, the assistant should be positioned nasally and rotate the eye nasally.

Unlike the usual Schocket scleral depressor used in clinical exams, a marking depressor is required here, such as the Urrets-Zavalia (Fig. 24-6) or O'Connor marking depressor (Fig. 24-7). These have the feature of a sharper head on the

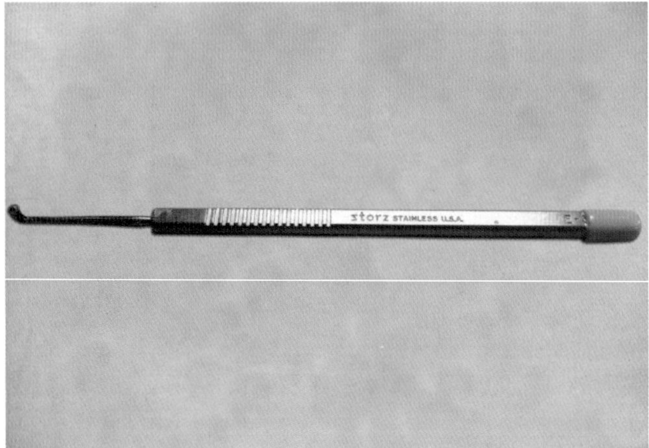


**Figure 24-6** The Urrets-Zavalia scleral depressor features a diamond-shaped tip on the marking end.

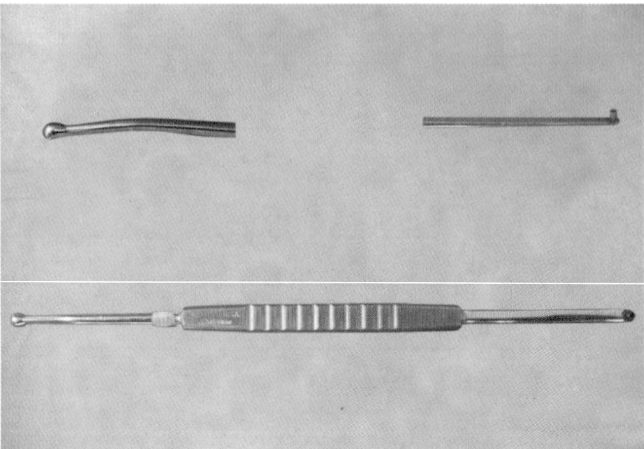

**Figure 24-7** The O'Connor scleral depressor features a ring on the marking end.

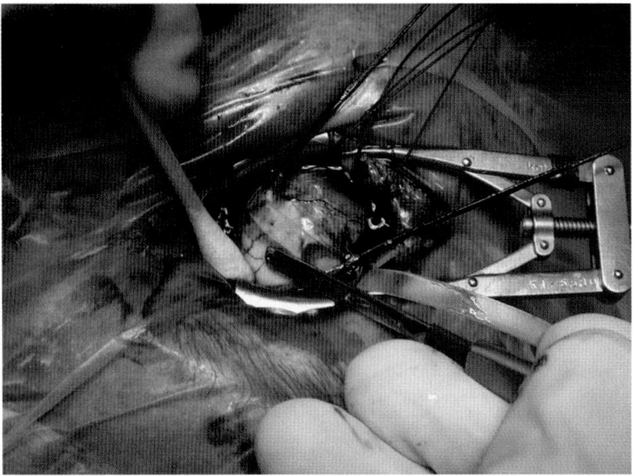

**Figure 24-8** The marking end of the O'Connor depressor is held against the sclera at the site of the break to be marked.

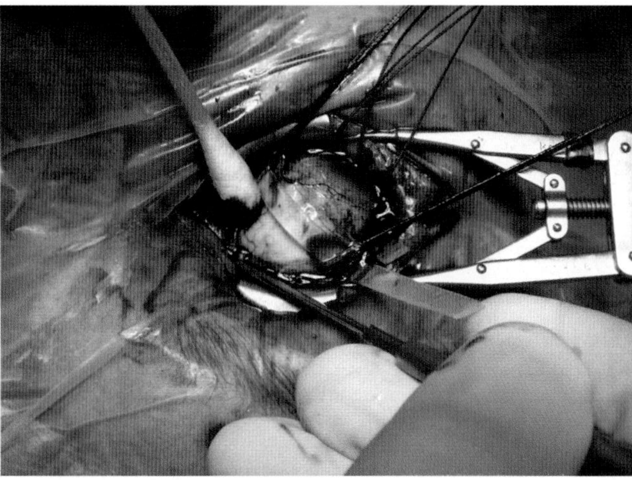

**Figure 24-9** A circular blue scleral mark results from depressing with the marking head of the O'Connor depressor.

marking side. Depression is done with the side of the depressor so that the marking tip is pointed parallel to the globe. When the causative break(s) is identified, the depressor is rotated 90° to indent the sclera with the marking head (Fig. 24-8). It is held in this position for about 5 seconds, which is sufficient to leave a blue mark caused by localized compression/scleral dehydration at this point (Fig. 24-9). For a small break, the posterior aspect should be marked. For a broad break, the horns of the break should also be marked. Marking of the lateral horns is especially important if using a segmental element. (If the sclera was noted to be thin in this region during external inspection, this should be done carefully to avoid scleral perforation.)

After the mark has been made, a cotton tip applicator should be used to dry the area and a surgical marker is used to place an indelible ink spot at the marked location. This must be done quickly as the scleral mark from depression can fade within seconds. In order to prevent smearing, a cotton tip swab should be rolled over the ink spot immediately afterward. This procedure should be repeated until all retinal breaks are identified and marked.

## Treating the Identified Breaks

Although retinal breaks can be treated postoperatively, it is preferable to treat them intraoperatively as the view through gas bubbles can be very difficult. In general, cryotherapy to the causative break is the preferred treatment method (Fig. 24-10). If the detachment is shallow, the depression of the cryoprobe is often enough to reappose the retina and RPE for treatment of the retina (either due to the mechanical indentation or by driving subretinal fluid back out through the break). During cryotherapy, the yellow glow of the circular

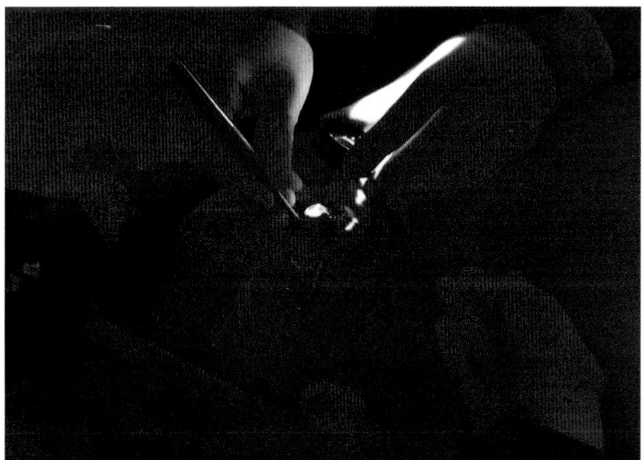

Figure 24-10 The surgeon applies cryotherapy treatment to the previously marked retinal break.

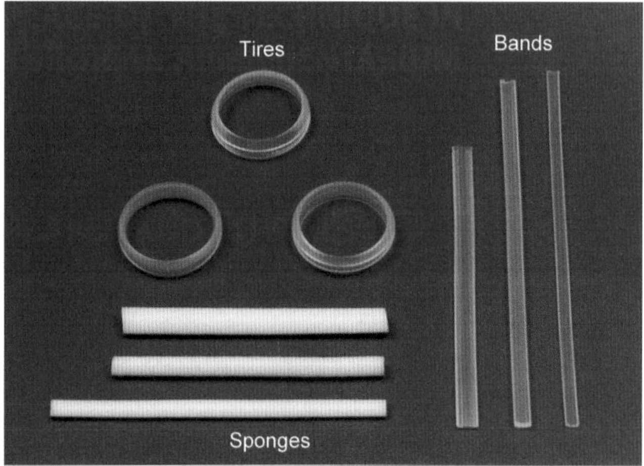


Figure 24-11 Scleral buckling can be done with an assortment of elements including bands, tires, and/or sponges. Photo courtesy of DORC Instruments, Inc.

freeze should cover the entire break for several seconds. Once completed, the treated retina should be slightly lighter in appearance than the surrounding untreated retina. For large breaks, multiple shorter contiguous applications may be used to cover the entire area of the break. If the detachment is too bullous for effective cryotherapy treatment, then external drainage may need to be done prior to this step in order to achieve adequate retinopexy (see section 'External drainage').

## Selection and Preparation of the Banding Elements

The two elements required in an encircling procedure are the band and the sleeve (Fig. 24-11). Commonly used silicone bands include the 240 (2.5 mm wide), 241 (3.5 mm wide), and 242 band (4 mm wide), which work well with the 70 or 71 sleeves. The sleeve is a long, circular silicone tube and must be cut to an appropriate width, usually about 2–3 mm.

If additional support is desired at the site of the break, a meridional element such as the 106 may be placed underneath the band. If more support or imbrication is desired around the entire circumference, a corresponding tire can be placed underneath with the band running within its groove (a 40 or 240 band will fit it a 275, 276, or 278 tire). A silicone band such as the 4050 (5 mm wide) may also be considered as an alternative for broad circumferential support.

For segmental buckling, silicone sponges or segments of silicone tires may be used. Sponges are generally preferred because they provide greater imbrication with lower risk of migration compared with other elements. In most operative rooms equipped for scleral buckling, a manufacturer's poster of available elements can be found (Figs. 24-12 to 24-15). Once the band is selected, its ends are cut with heavy/silicone scissors to create a bevel, such that the tips meet end to end or fit together like a puzzle (Fig. 24-16). Either way, it is important for the surgeon to note this orientation to help verify that it has not been twisted. The bevel also aids in passing under the rectus muscles and through any scleral tunnels.

## Localizing the Band

If placing a band in a primary SBP, the anterior edge of the band should be placed at the scleral ink marking, as the posterior aspect of the break must be supported by the anterior crest of the scleral imbrication. This distance can be measured and marked in all of the remaining quadrants so that the band is symmetrically placed (Fig. 24-17).

If doing a combined encircling band and vitrectomy procedure, the goal of band placement is often to simply support the vitreous base and this can generally be done by placing the anterior edge of the band at a distance of 11–12 mm from the limbus in each quadrant. This distance may need to be increased 1-2 mm in very long eyes where the vitreous base is likely to be more posterior.

## Placement of the Band Using Sutures

Sutures represent a common method of band fixation to the sclera. In general, it is easier to place the band before placing the sutures since placement of multiple sutures prior to the band can result in a confusing mess of suture ends. For preplaced sutures, Serrefine ("bulldog") clips can be used to keep suture ends out of the way. The band is guided with a

# SOLID SILICONE IMPLANTS

## SILICONE CIRCLING BANDS

CIRCLING BANDS ARE DESIGNED TO HOLD THE ACCESSORY IMPLANT IN PLACE, AND TO MAINTAIN OPTIMAL PRESSURE TO FORM A PERMANENT BUCKLE WITHOUT SCLERAL EROSION

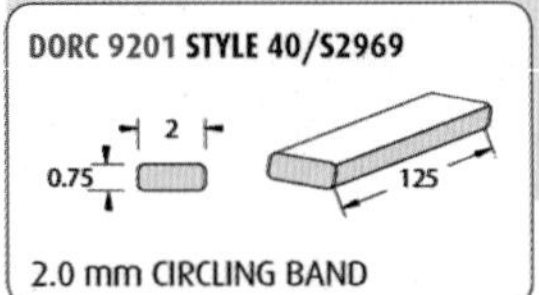


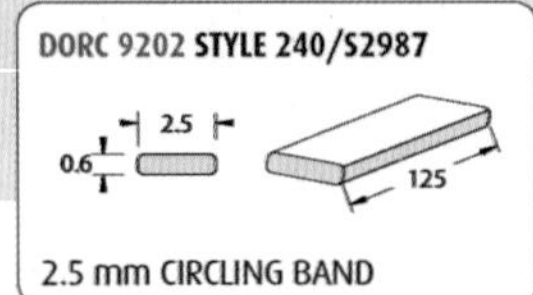


## SILICONE TIRES

TIRE-SHAPED IMPLANTS ARE DESIGNED FOR USE UNDER CIRCLING BANDS FOR WIDE SCLERAL BEDS, FOR BREAKS NEAR THE ORA SERRATA, MULTIPLE BREAKS, AND FOR HIGH SCLERAL BUCKLES

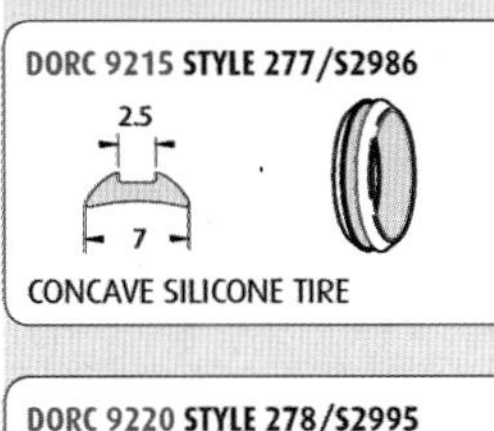


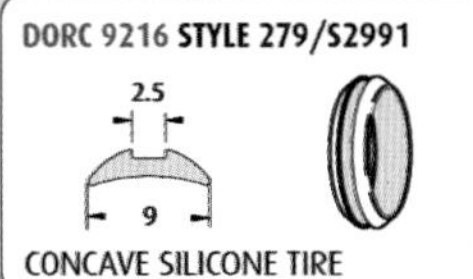


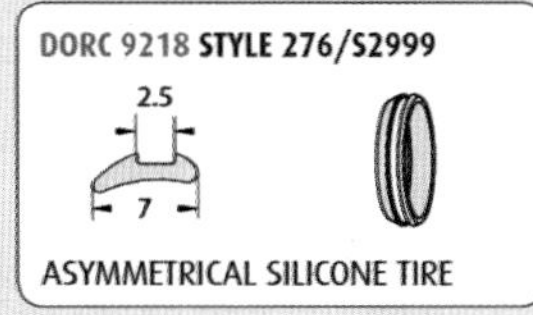


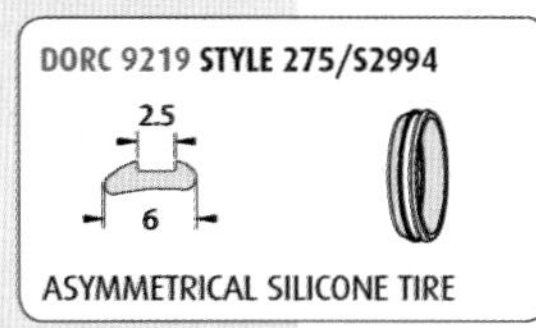


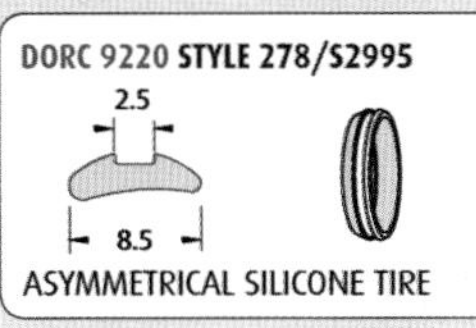


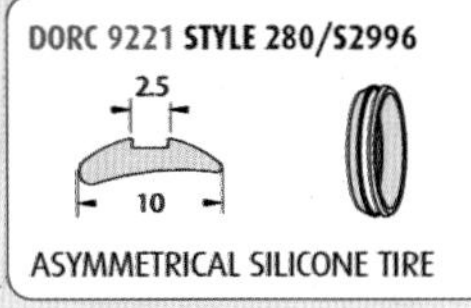


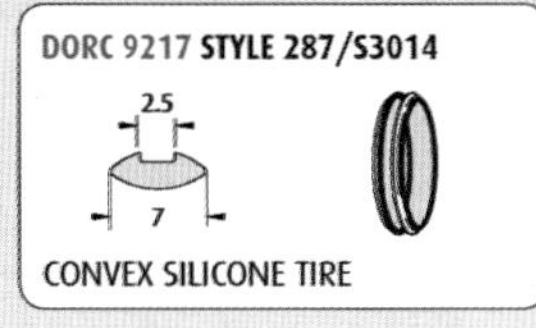


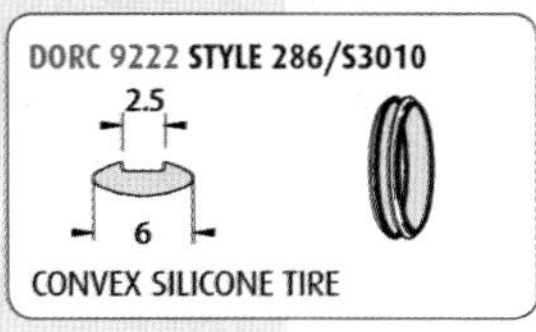


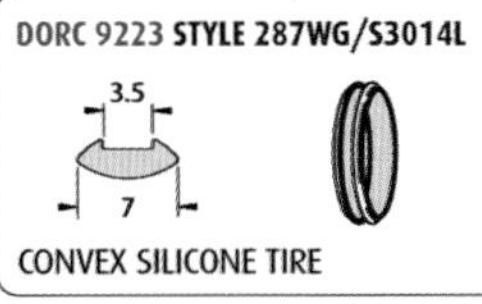


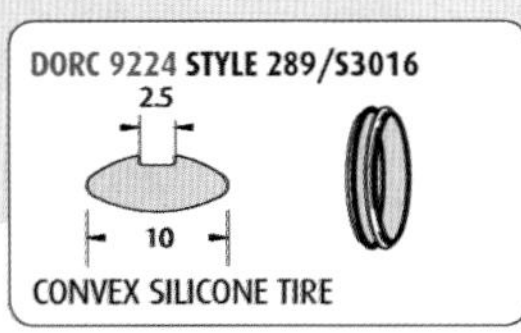


## SILICONE GROOVED STRIPS

GROOVED STRIPS ARE DESIGNED TO BE USED UNDER CIRCLING BANDS. SEVERAL DESIGNS ARE OFFERED TO FIT THE NEED FOR NARROW OR WIDE SCLERAL BEDS, AS WELL AS HIGH SCLERAL BUCKLING

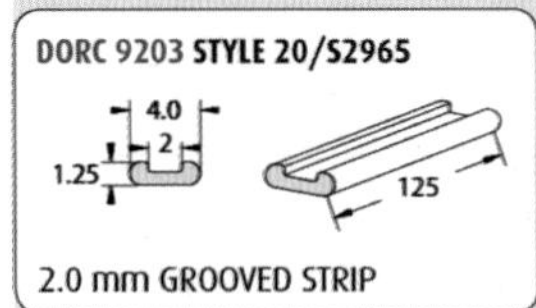


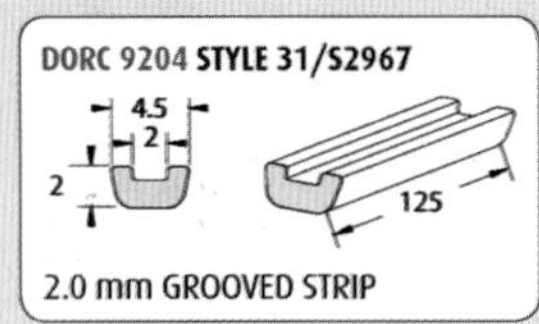


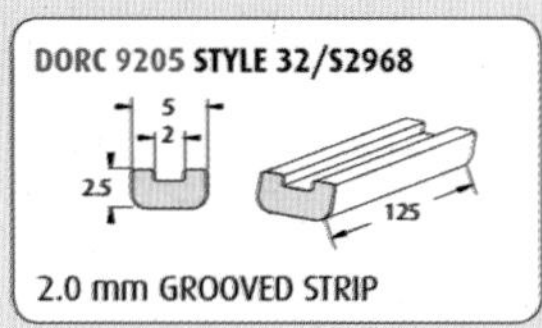


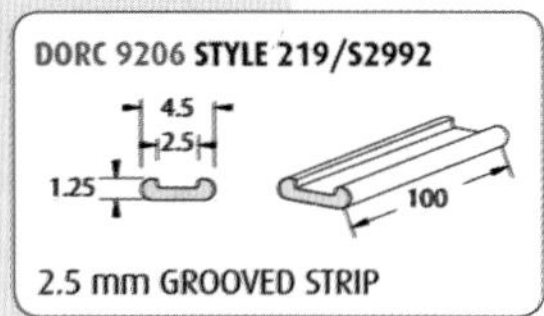


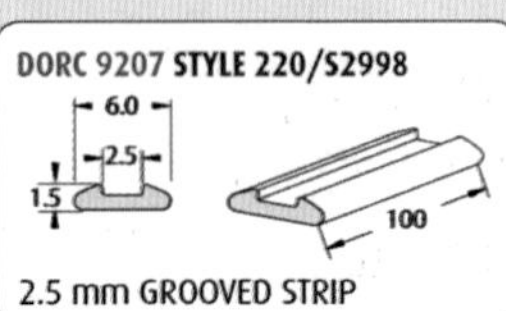


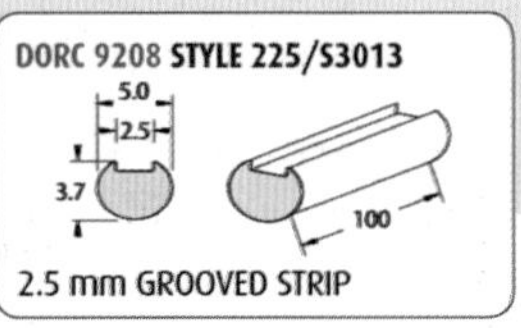


**Figure 24-12** Most operating rooms will have a standard poster of scleral buckling elements posted such as tires, grooved strips, and encircling bands shown here. Photo courtesy of DORC Instruments, Inc.

## SOLID SILICONE IMPLANTS

### SILICONE STRIPS

SILICONE STRIPS CAN BE USED ALONE, WITH WIDE GROOVED TIRES, OR WHEN 'TRAP DOOR' PROCEDURES ARE PERFORMED

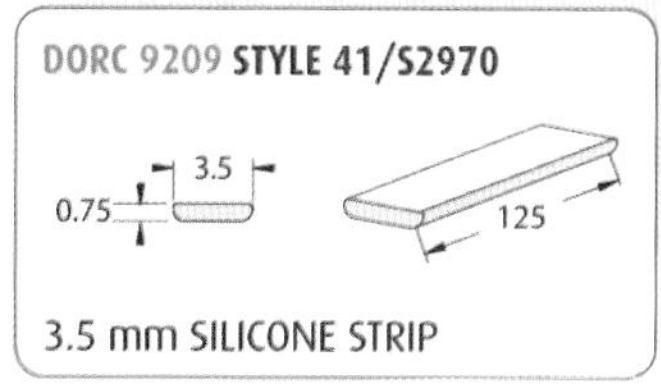


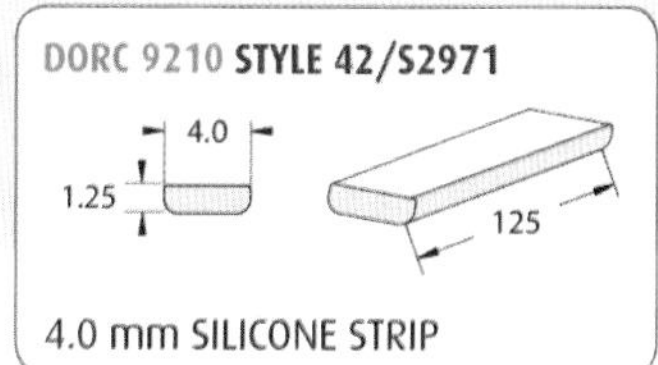


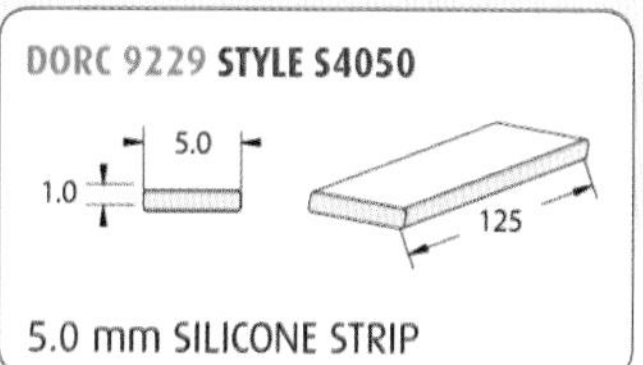


### ROUND SILICONE SLEEVES

SLEEVES ARE USED TO SECURE CIRCLING BANDS

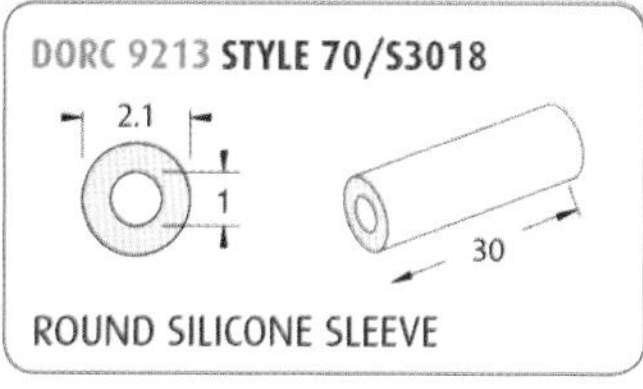


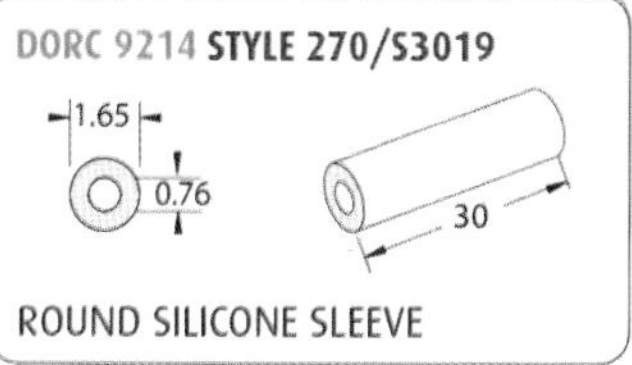


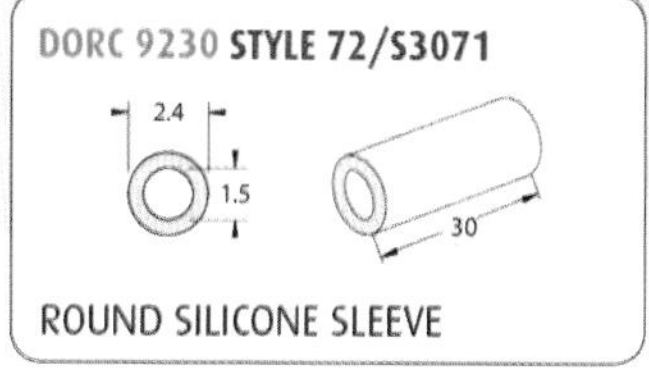


### OVAL SILICONE SLEEVES

OVAL SILICONE SLEEVES TO SECURE CIRCLING BANDS

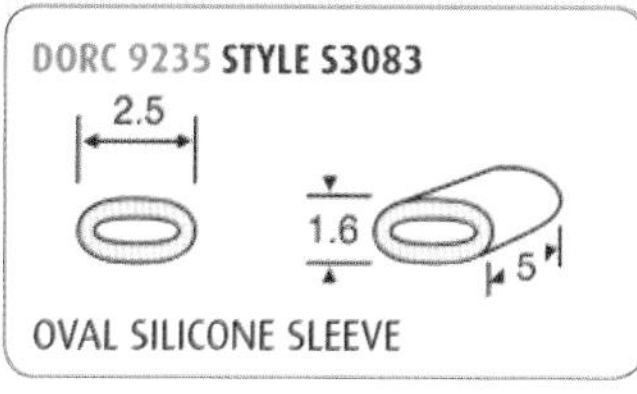


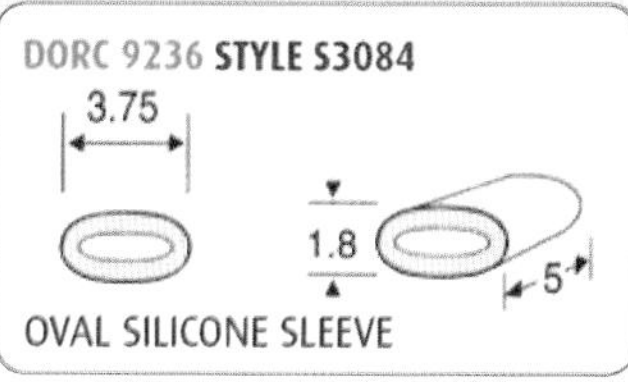


Figure 24-13 Most operating rooms will have a standard poster of scleral buckling elements posted such as encircling bands and sleeves shown here. Photo courtesy of DORC Instruments, Inc.

Nugent forceps under a muscle belly and picked up on the other side with another Nugent forceps. This is repeated until the band has been weaved under all of the rectus muscles and has encircled the globe with the beveled ends sticking out in the last quadrant.

In the quadrant of the causative or marked break, one can briefly place the band in its final desired position to get an idea of how it should rest. Then, it is slid slightly anteriorly and a partial-thickness scleral bite of is taken 1 mm posterior to the band's posterior final position using a spatulated needle with a 5-0 Prolene suture (Fig. 24-18). The band is then slid posteriorly and using the same needle and suture, another similar partial-thickness scleral bite is taken 1 mm anterior to the band's anterior final position (Fig. 24-19). The suture is tied in place with a 3-1-1 square knot (Fig. 24-20). The knot is rotated posteriorly so that it and the suture ends are not sticking out above the band (Fig. 24-21). This lessens the risk of suture erosion through the conjunctiva.

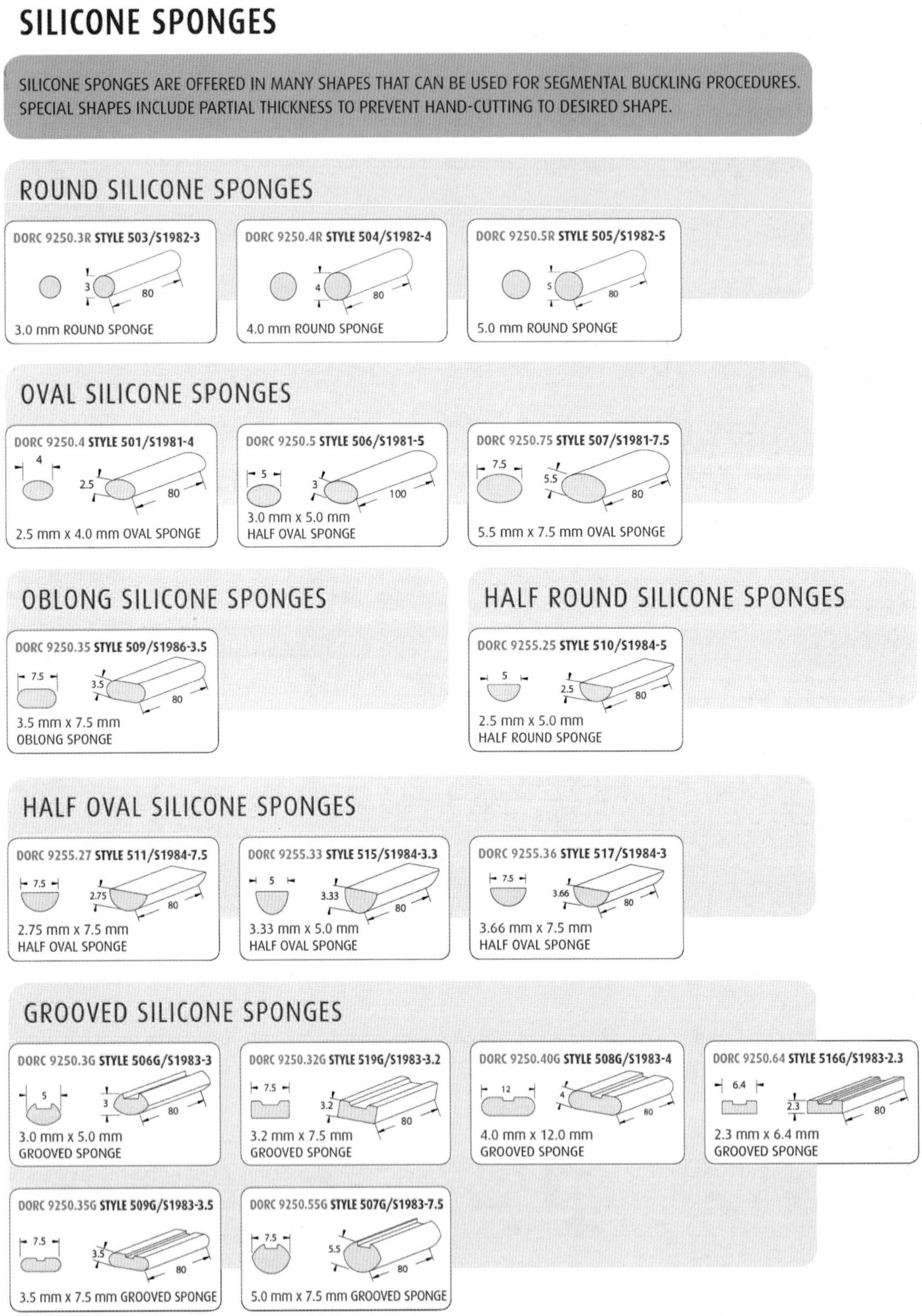

# SILICONE SPONGES

SILICONE SPONGES ARE OFFERED IN MANY SHAPES THAT CAN BE USED FOR SEGMENTAL BUCKLING PROCEDURES. SPECIAL SHAPES INCLUDE PARTIAL THICKNESS TO PREVENT HAND-CUTTING TO DESIRED SHAPE.

## ROUND SILICONE SPONGES

DORC 9250.3R **STYLE 503/S1982-3**
3.0 mm ROUND SPONGE

DORC 9250.4R **STYLE 504/S1982-4**
4.0 mm ROUND SPONGE

DORC 9250.5R **STYLE 505/S1982-5**
5.0 mm ROUND SPONGE

## OVAL SILICONE SPONGES

DORC 9250.4 **STYLE 501/S1981-4**
2.5 mm x 4.0 mm OVAL SPONGE

DORC 9250.5 **STYLE 506/S1981-5**
3.0 mm x 5.0 mm HALF OVAL SPONGE

DORC 9250.75 **STYLE 507/S1981-7.5**
5.5 mm x 7.5 mm OVAL SPONGE

## OBLONG SILICONE SPONGES

DORC 9250.35 **STYLE 509/S1986-3.5**
3.5 mm x 7.5 mm OBLONG SPONGE

## HALF ROUND SILICONE SPONGES

DORC 9255.25 **STYLE 510/S1984-5**
2.5 mm x 5.0 mm HALF ROUND SPONGE

## HALF OVAL SILICONE SPONGES

DORC 9255.27 **STYLE 511/S1984-7.5**
2.75 mm x 7.5 mm HALF OVAL SPONGE

DORC 9255.33 **STYLE 515/S1984-3.3**
3.33 mm x 5.0 mm HALF OVAL SPONGE

DORC 9255.36 **STYLE 517/S1984-3**
3.66 mm x 7.5 mm HALF OVAL SPONGE

## GROOVED SILICONE SPONGES

DORC 9250.3G **STYLE 506G/S1983-3**
3.0 mm x 5.0 mm GROOVED SPONGE

DORC 9250.32G **STYLE 519G/S1983-3.2**
3.2 mm x 7.5 mm GROOVED SPONGE

DORC 9250.40G **STYLE 508G/S1983-4**
4.0 mm x 12.0 mm GROOVED SPONGE

DORC 9250.64 **STYLE 516G/S1983-2.3**
2.3 mm x 6.4 mm GROOVED SPONGE

DORC 9250.35G **STYLE 509G/S1983-3.5**
3.5 mm x 7.5 mm GROOVED SPONGE

DORC 9250.55G **STYLE 507G/S1983-7.5**
5.0 mm x 7.5 mm GROOVED SPONGE

Figure 24-14 Most operating rooms will have a standard poster of scleral buckling elements posted such as sponges shown here. Photo courtesy of DORC Instruments, Inc.

# SILICONE SPONGES

## ROUND TUNNEL SILICONE SPONGE

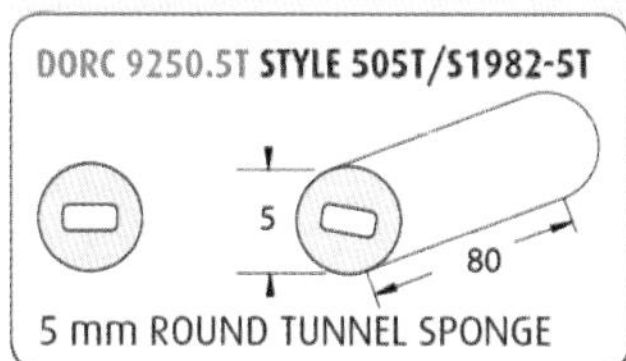


# ACCESSORIES

## MERIDIONAL IMPLANTS

THESE IMPLANTS GIVE ADDITIONAL BUCKLING IN THE MERIDIONAL DIRECTION, AND ARE USED UNDER GROOVED IMPLANTS

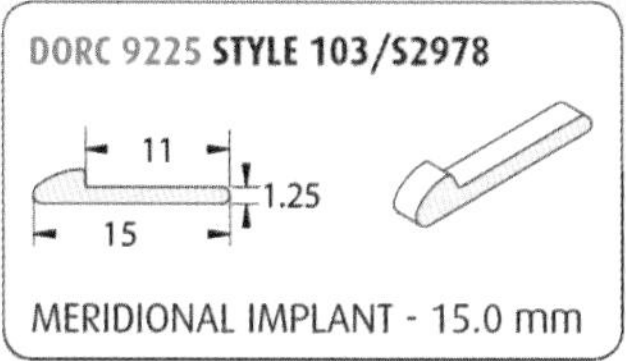


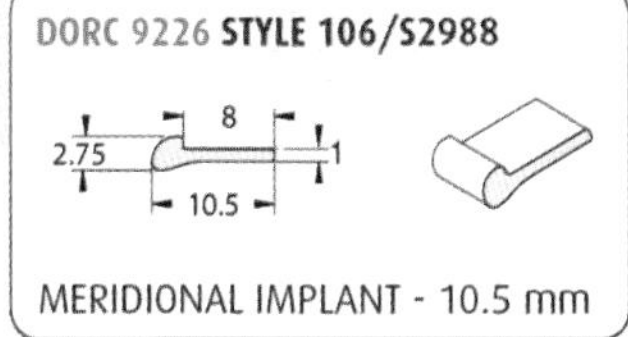


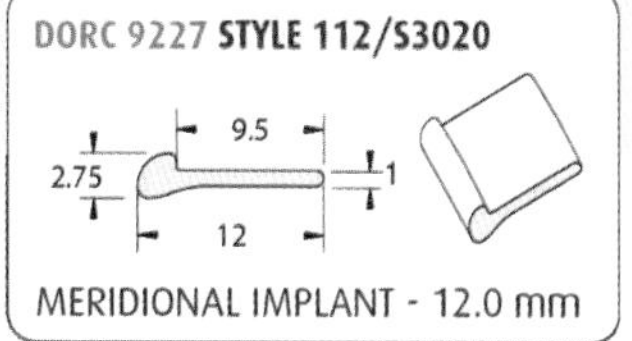


## SILICONE WEDGE

FOR HIGH SCLERAL BUCKLES. CONCAVE INNER SURFACE WITH INCREASING BUCKLE EFFECT ON TICK SIDE OF WEDGE

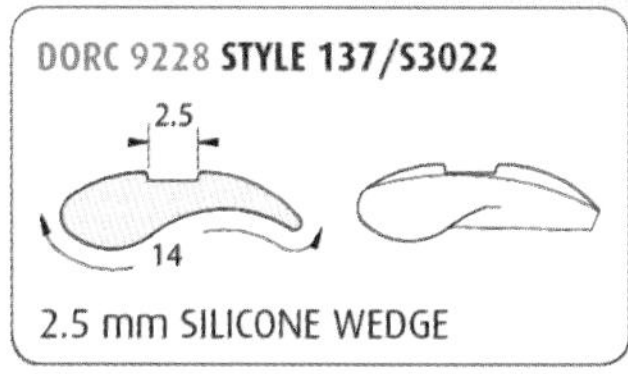


Figure 24-15 Most operating rooms will have a standard poster of scleral buckling elements posted such as wedges and meridional accessories shown here. Photo courtesy of DORC Instruments, Inc.

## Placement of the Band Using Scleral Tunnels

Another method of placing and securing a band is with the creation of partial-thickness scleral tunnels ("belt loops") in each oblique quadrant. The advantage of this method is minimization of suture-related complications such as suture migration, irritation, or infection. The primary disadvantage is a higher requirement of sclera without thinning, as the tunnel occupies a larger geographic area than a corresponding suture pass. Additional buckling materials, such as meridional elements or tire segments, must be anticipated in advanced so that the loops do not impede their placement. In some cases, sutures may be used to secure these extra elements while the encircling element is secured with scleral belt loops.

To create such a scleral tunnel, a #64 or #57 blade is used to create 2 parallel, radial, partial-thickness scleral cutdowns approximately 2–4 mm apart from each other (Fig. 24-22).

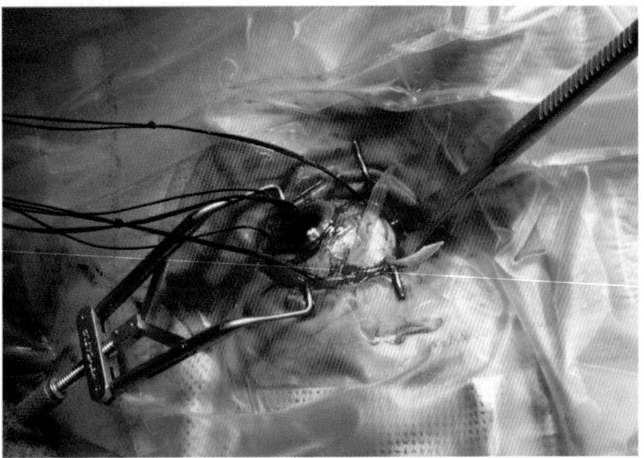

Figure 24-16 The orientation of the silicone band's beveled tips help confirm the absence of twisting.

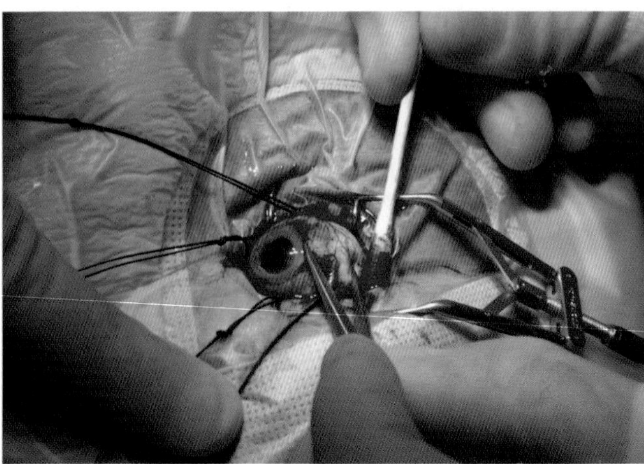

Figure 24-17 The sclera is marked with calipers to ensure proper placement of the band.

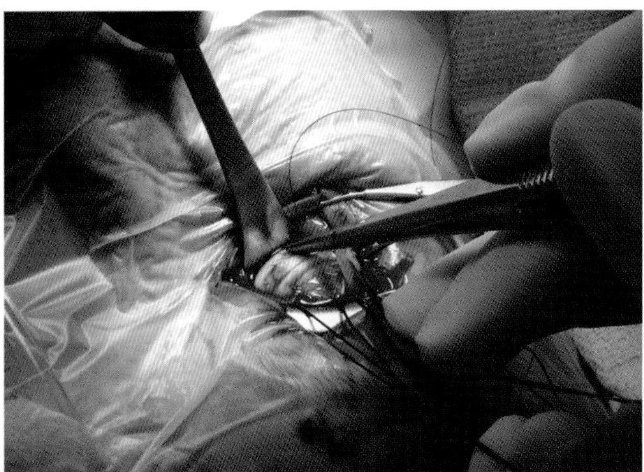

Figure 24-18 The posterior scleral bite is taken with the silicone band shifted anteriorly.

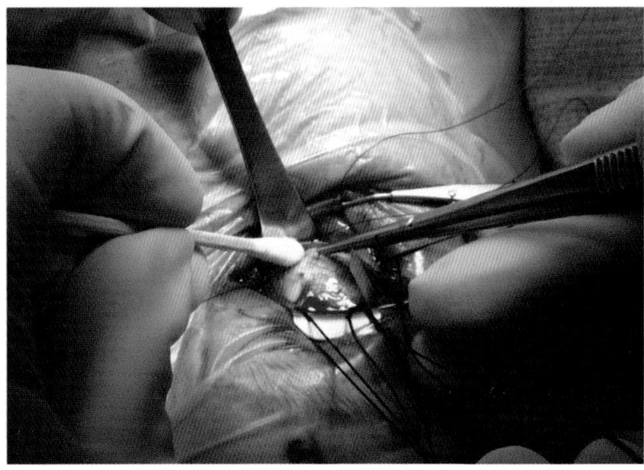

Figure 24-19 The anterior scleral bite is taken with the silicone band shifted posteriorly.

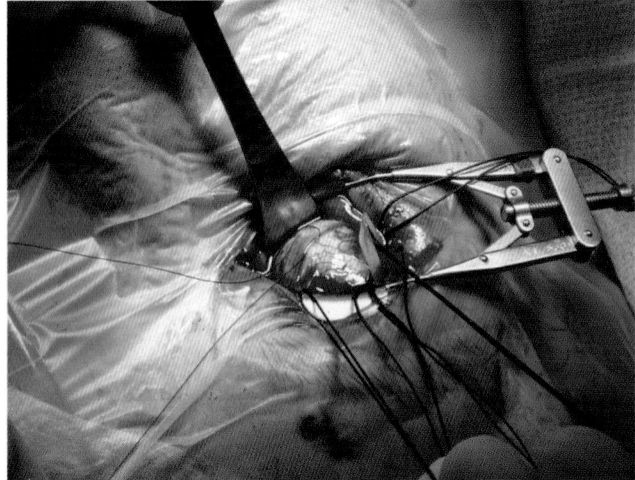

Figure 24-20 The band is moved into its resting position and the sutures are tightened.

The length of each cutdown should match the width of the selected band (e.g. 2.5 mm for a 240 band) and their orientation should be perpendicular to the limbus and parallel to each other (Fig. 24-23). A #66 (crescent-type) blade is then used to catch a lamellar plane in the sclera starting at one of the incisions. Dissection is done toward the other until the blade emerges from the second cutdown incision (Fig. 24-24). Extreme care should be taken to avoid angling in toward the eye with the blade during this step in order to avoid scleral perforation.

## Placing the Sleeve and Tightening the Band

In order to cinch the band at the correct tightness, its ends are placed through an appropriately tight silicone sleeve that

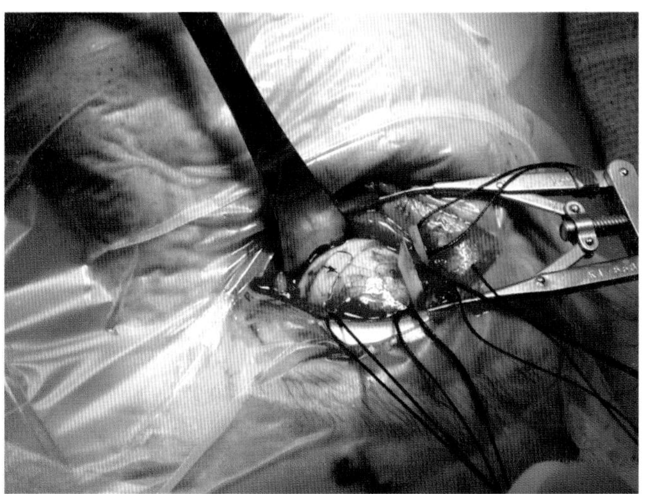

Figure 24-21 The band is finally secured in place with a square knot.

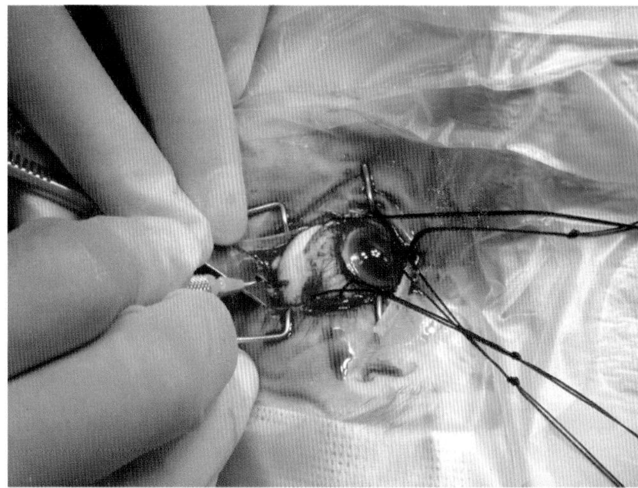

Figure 24-22 A partial-thickness scleral scratch incision for "belt-loop" can be made using a #64 blade.

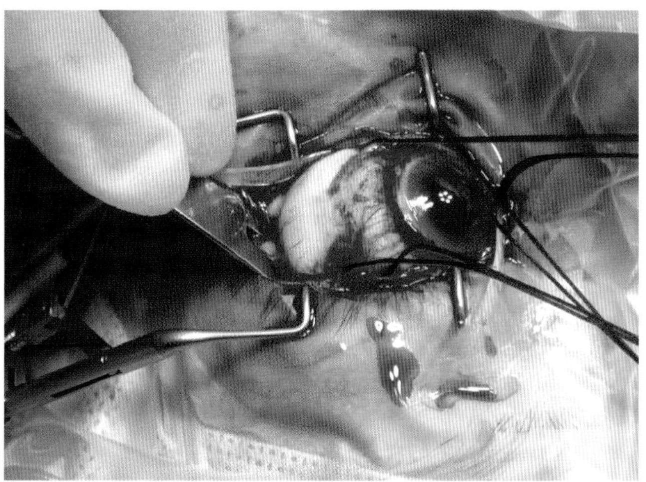

Figure 24-23 Two parallel partial-thickness scleral scratch incisions are made for the "belt-loop".

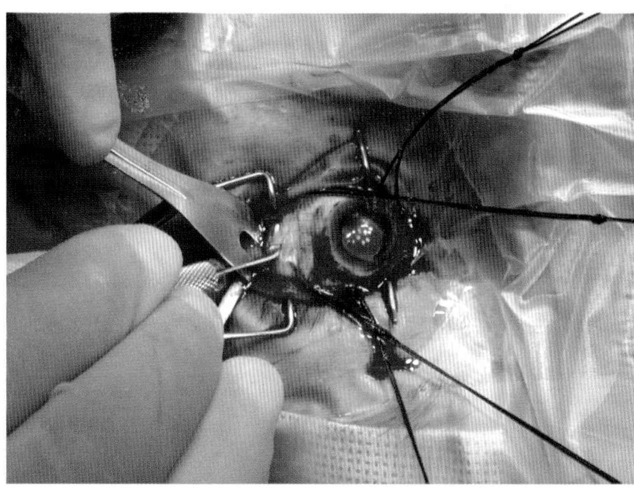

Figure 24-24 The scratch incisions are then connected with a partial-thickness scleral tunnel using a #66 blade.

will provide enough friction that the band's ends will not slide once pulled to the final desired tightness. Using a Watzke sleeve spreader or a hemostat, the previously cut silicone sleeve is spread and the band end closer to the spreading instrument's hinge is advanced through the sleeve from behind using a Nugent forceps (Fig. 24-25). The assistant will then use forceps to hold down that end while the surgeon takes the other band end and advances it through the sleeve from the front (above the previously inserted band end) using a Nugent (Fig. 24-26). Once both ends are securely through the sleeve, the Nugent is placed sideways in the open jaws of the spreading instrument between the sleeve and hinge of the instrument. The jaws are closed and the sleeve is then wiggled off the spreading instrument and the band is adjusted to its appropriate tension (Fig. 24-27).

Before tightening the band, it is good practice to again check the end-to-end points of the band tip bevels to verify that no twisting has occurred. If an external drainage procedure is to be done, it should be done now (*see* next section) prior to tightening the band. Otherwise, the band should be tightened until gently snug against the globe without increasing the intraocular pressure (IOP). It is then further tightened until gentle imbrication of the globe is noted. If a vitrectomy procedure is also to be performed, this is an appropriate time for that to be done.

## Additional Supporting Elements

If the band appears too anterior (the anterior crest of the buckle is not posterior to the causative break) or more

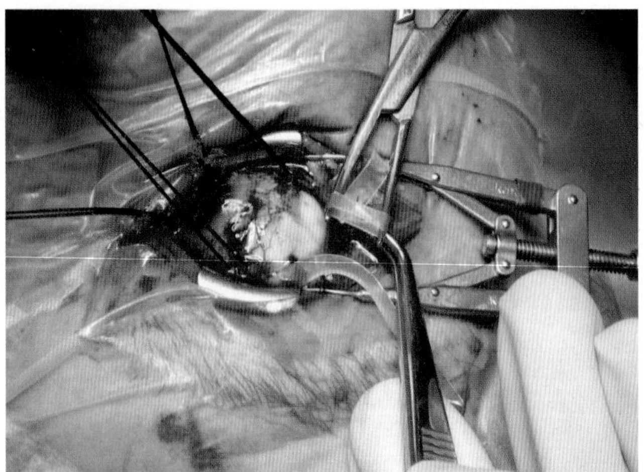
Figure 24-25 The silicone band end closer to the hemostat hinge is backed in through the silicone sleeve first.

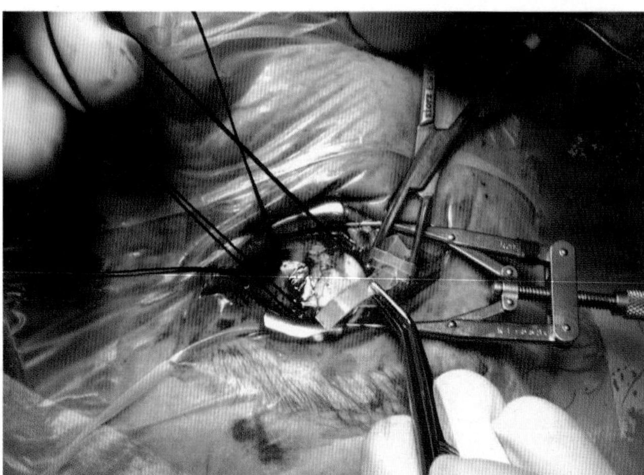
Figure 24-26 The silicone band end further from the hemostat hinge is fed through the silicone sleeve over the previously inserted band end.

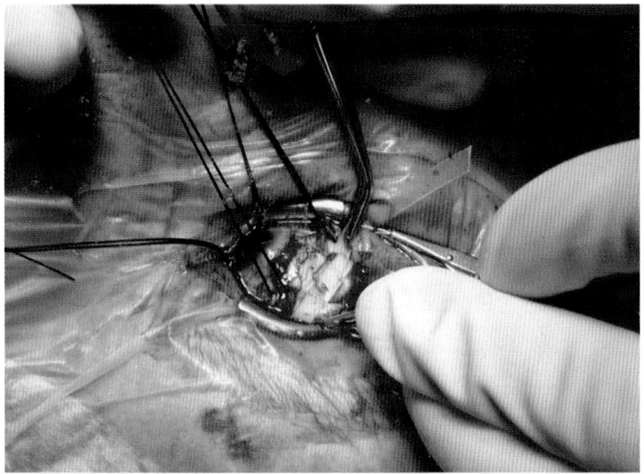
Figure 24-27 Nugent forceps are used to gently tighten the band until resting against the sclera.

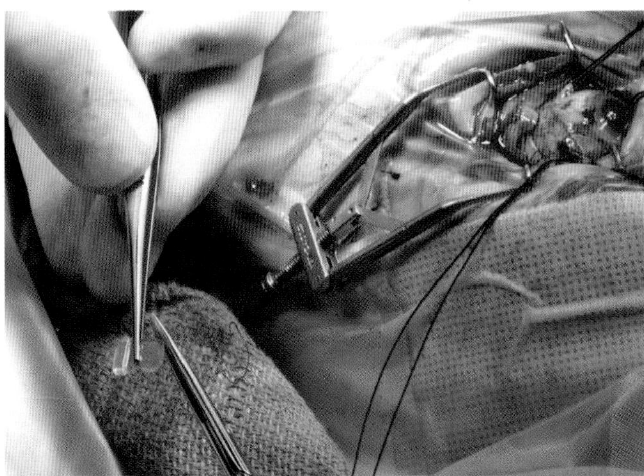
Figure 24-28 Element #106 is designed to slide under the band and offer broader support where needed.

support of the break is still required after placement of the band and tightening, meridional elements can be added. An example is the 106 meridional element (Fig. 24-28) that can be tucked under the band (Fig. 24-29) and sutured in place if desired (Fig. 24-30). Sections of various tires may also be used as alternatives.

## External Drainage

When a retinal detachment is bullous, external drainage may be necessary for the following reasons:

- To allow closure of the causative retinal break against the imbricating element
- To prevent a significant rise in IOP at the desired level of band tightening
- To prevent postoperative macular detachment from superiorly located bullous fluid
- To accommodate the volume of injected gas without causing severe rise in IOP

This step should be performed after placement of the sleeve but prior to tightening the band. The site of drainage should be such that it is as far away as possible from the causative/marked break while being near the most bullous portion of the detachment. It is often preferable to choose a site that will be covered by the band or banding elements. The band is then slid posteriorly to the selected site and the sclera is cut down to the uvea using a #64 blade (Fig. 24-31).

A fine, pointed cautery tip can be used to cauterize as the uvea is perforated. Others use a 27/30-gauge needle or a suture needle tip to perforate the uvea at the drainage site.

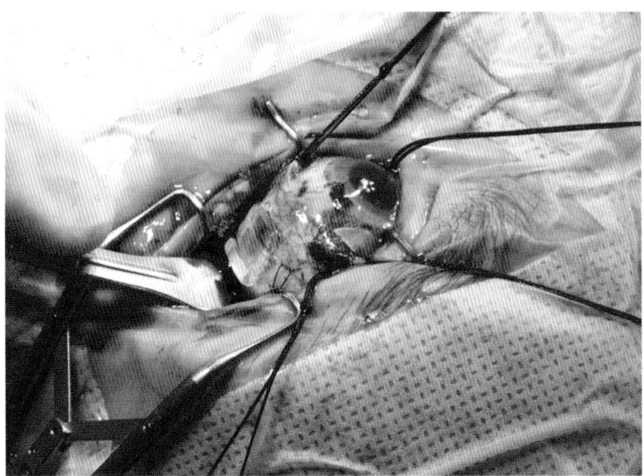

Figure 24-29 Meridional element #106 is tucked under the band and may be left in place without sutures.

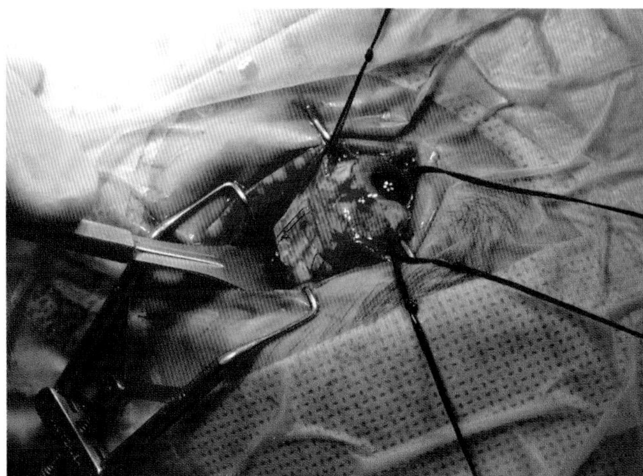

Figure 24-30 Meridional element #106 is tucked under the band and may also be sutured in place.

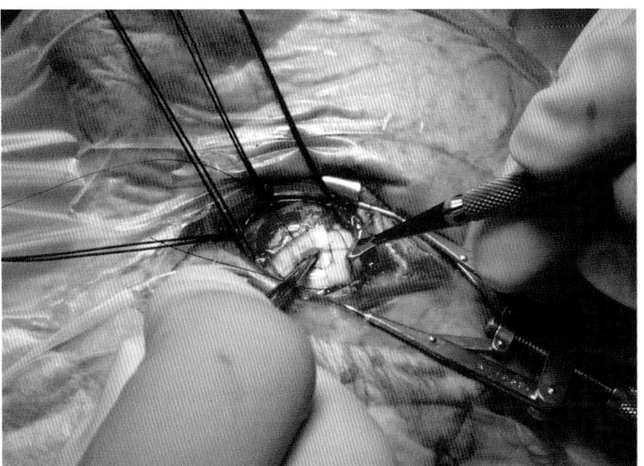

Figure 24-31 The sclera is cut down to uvea at the desired external drainage site.

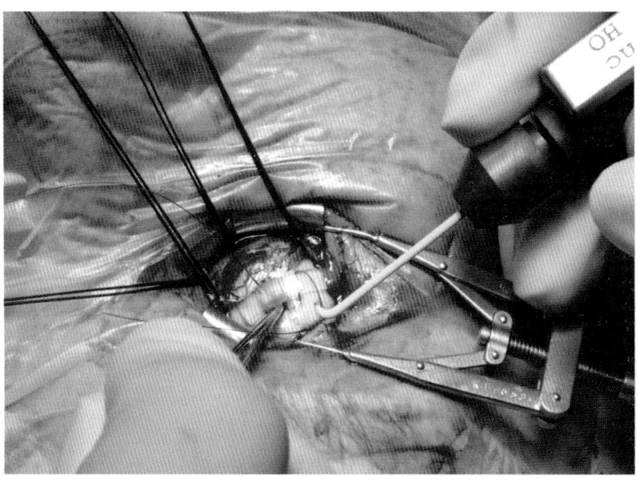

Figure 24-32 A diathermy tip used to perforate through uvea at the external drainage site.

A steady flow of subretinal fluid or thick Shlieren should ensue (Fig. 24-32). This should correlate with the surgeon's estimate of the amount of subretinal fluid during prior indirect ophthalmoscopy. Gentle depression with a cotton-tip anterior to the drainage site and sweeping toward the drain site may help initiate egress of subretinal fluid. Extreme pressure should never be applied in order to reduce the feared risk of retinal incarceration. Once spontaneous flow has stopped, adequate drainage has usually been completed. No additional pressure should be applied.

After adequate drainage has been achieved, the site may be sutured or simply covered by the band as it slid back into place. Repeat indirect ophthalmoscopy should be performed to check that no subretinal hemorrhage occurred and to confirm buckle height.

Instead of the external cutdown approach, some surgeons perform a needle drainage using a 26 or 27-gauge needle attached to a 1 mL syringe without its plunger. The surgeon dons an indirect ophthalmoscope and directly visualizes needle penetration into the subretinal space. The needle is inserted just anterior to the band with the bevel oriented posteriorly to lessen the risk of incarceration. Once the needle is inserted, the overlying detached retina begins to flutter down toward the choroid as subretinal fluid is evacuated. Any internal bleeding can quickly be addressed with pressure over the drain site.

An assistant may help with this maneuver by having previously passed a 2-0 silk tie around the band opposite the drain site. He/she then pulls on the band using the silk tie to maintain pressure and to encourage egress of the subretinal fluid through the needle into the syringe. This technique has the added advantage of directly observing the drainage procedure. However, there is a learning curve for the surgeon due to the inverted view through the indirect ophthalmoscope.

## Volume Replacement or Gas Placement

Volume replacement after external drainage can be done by injecting balanced salt solution or gas. Gas offers the added benefit of internally supporting retinal break(s) in the superior quadrants while the retinopexy scars are maturing around the treated retinal breaks.

If gas is to be placed without external drainage, anterior chamber paracentesis should be done one or more times during the preceding steps to appropriately soften the eye and prevent significant IOP elevation. Injecting into a softer eye also minimizes the risk of "fish eggs" or multiple satellite bubbles.

An injection site should be chosen remote to any breaks unsupported by the buckle or with significant traction in order to minimize the chance of subretinal gas injection. It is also helpful to rotate the eye so the injection site is the highest point of the globe. Using a 30-gauge needle on a 1 cc syringe through the pars plana (4 mm from limbus in phakic eye, 3–3.5 mm in pseudophakic eye), the needle should be advanced far into the vitreous to develop a track. It should then be retracted along the same track until just posterior to the iris. The gas should be injected in a fast, steady manner to avoid multiple small bubble formation ("fish eggs").

## Final Ophthalmoscopic Check

Indirect ophthalmoscopy is repeated to verify that the optic nerve is perfused and digital palpation is done to confirm that the eye is not unusually firm. If arterial pulsations are present or can be induced by digital pressure, it indicates that the central retinal artery (CRA) is perfused. If perfusion cannot be verified, a paracentesis should be performed or the encircling element should be loosened.

Retinal breaks, lattice degeneration, and other retinal pathology are verified to be supported by the buckle imbrication. The buckle height is also checked for appropriateness and the encircling element can be further tightened or adjusted if necessary.

## Conjunctival Closure

Once the band is trimmed and the 2-0 silk ties have all been cut away from the rectus muscles, the superior and inferior conjunctival flaps are engaged with two forceps and are walked end-over-end back to their original location near the limbus. Loosening of the lid speculum and gentle retropulsion of the globe can aid in lowering the tension of the conjunctiva.

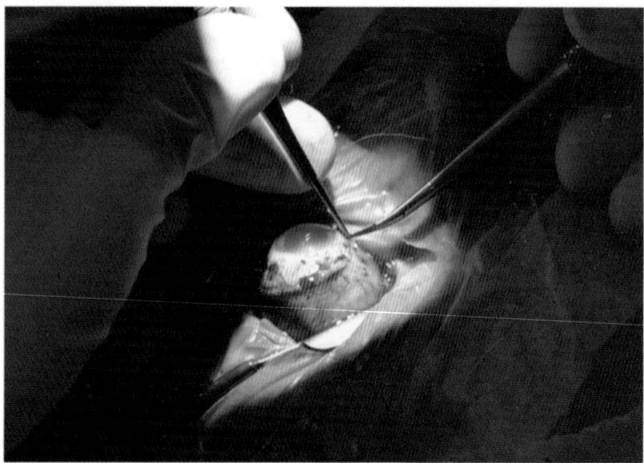

Figure 24-33 The superior and inferior conjunctival flaps are grasped with forceps and reapproximated at the horizontal aspect of limbus.

An anchoring bite is placed at the 3 or 9 o'clock site of the radial relaxing incision and the suture is guided through the conjunctival flaps such that their closure results in a buried square knot at the horizontal limbus (Fig. 24-33). Either 8-0 vicryl or 6-0 plain gut is appropriate for conjunctival closure. This is repeated for closure of the radial relaxing incision on the opposite side. Usually, a second conjunctival suture is also required for posterior closure of each of the radial relaxing peritomy incisions (Fig. 24-34). Care should be taken to avoid the caruncle during closure of the medial side. Additional retrobulbar anesthetic may be placed at this time if desired using a blunt cannula.

# MECHANISM OF ACTION

Scleral buckling results in focal indentation of the sclera to reappose retinal breaks to the underlying RPE and to relieve traction from the vitreous upon these retinal breaks. Cryotherapy (or postoperative) laser is used to create chorioretinal scars at and beyond the edges of these breaks to prevent recurrent detachment by passage of liquefied vitreous into the subretinal space.

# POSTOPERATIVE CARE

After tissue closure, a drop of IOP-lowering medication (such as timolol and dorzolamide) can be administered, particularly if a gas bubble was placed in the eye. An antibiotic drop or

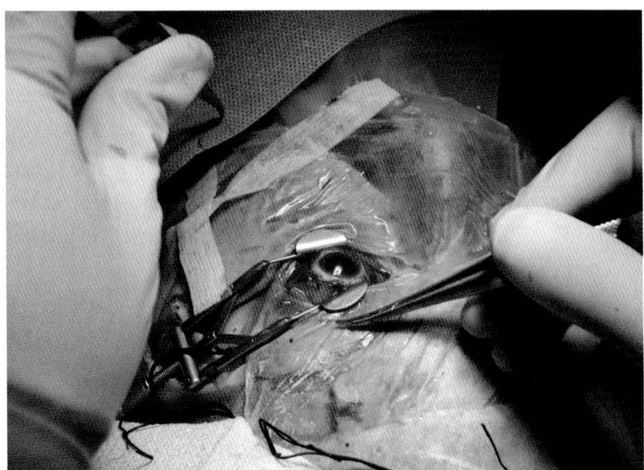

Figure 24-34 The peritomy is closed with buried sutures.

ointment should also be applied to the eye surface prior to patching. Methylprednisolone may be given intravenously at the end of the case to prevent postoperative intraorbital inflammation, swelling, and discomfort.

The five P's of postoperative care:

- *Pain*: Oral analgesics should be prescribed for postoperative pain. If worsening pain, new floaters, or decreases in vision occur (particularly if in combination), the patient should be instructed to call immediately and endophthalmitis must be ruled out.
- *Prescriptions*: Topical antibiotic should be administered for a week (e.g. moxifloxacin four times daily) and a topical steroid should be used for a month (e.g. prednisolone acetate starting four times daily and tapering after a week). Cycloplegics (e.g. homatropine twice daily) can be added for comfort and ease of postoperative examination.
- *Positioning*: If gas has been placed, the patient will need to position in a manner that the bubble supports the causative break. A general rule of thumb is to ask the patient to comply 50 minutes out of each hour with the required positioning during the first week. Drawing an arrow on the eye patch indicating which side should stay up can aid the patient and family for proper positioning.
- *Protection*: The patient should be instructed to wear glasses or the protective shield during the day and the shield at night for the first week.
- *Prohibitions*: If gas was injected into the eye, the patient must be advised that they are not to fly by air, cut off their gas armbands (often green), or undergo dental procedures. This prevents scenarios in which enlarging gas bubbles cause severe elevations in IOP. The armband is a universal flag to medical personnel that certain inhalational anesthetic agents (particularly nitrous oxide) cannot be used.

## SPECIFIC INSTRUMENTATION

Most operating rooms have standard scleral buckling trays. *See* section "Setup" for detailed description.

## POTENTIAL COMPLICATIONS

- *Scleral perforation*: This can occur from a deep pass during scleral suture placement or too deep of a cutdown during scleral tunnel creation. Evidence of perforation includes leaking of vitreous, subretinal fluid, blood, or pigment from the site especially if accompanied by softening of the eye. Pressure with a cotton tip applicator or scleral depression over the bleeding site can help raise the IOP to tamponade the wound. The retina should be carefully examined with indirect ophthalmoscopy; if retinal breaks have been created, they should be treated with laser or cryotherapy. If the wound is large, it should be sutured. If possible, the wound should be covered by the band or by adding a meridional element
- *Corneal edema*: This may occur during longer surgical cases or from increase in IOP due to tightening of the encircling element. The corneal epithelium may need to be scraped in order to complete the case
- *Miosis*: Intraoperative miosis most commonly occurs due to hypotony. Intravitreal gas in contact with the iris may also cause this. Additional cycloplegics should be given. If unsuccessful and impeding visualization, intracameral epinephrine or iris hooks may be necessary
- *Drainage complications*:
  - *Choroidal or subretinal hemorrhage*: This should be suspected if a large amount of bleeding or uveal prolapse begins to occur at the drainage site. Immediate tamponade should be done by applying pressure at the drainage site with a cotton-tip applicator. Afterward the site should be sutured as quickly as possible
  - *Retinal incarceration*: Usually occurs after perforation of the choroid and noted by a sudden cessation of drainage. Traction from silk ties should be released and ophthalmoscopy should be promptly performed to look for localized depression in the retina surrounded by radiating striae. If present, the site should be immediately sutured and covered by the encircling band or additional element. If tears have occurred, they should be treated with laser or cryotherapy
- *Gas migration*:
  - *Anterior chamber*: Adequate paracentesis and softening of the eye is critical prior to gas injection, otherwise gas may migrate around the crystalline or pseudophakic

lens into the anterior chamber. This can make the view incredibly difficult and lead to postoperative pressure issues. The gas may need to be left, as trying to tap it from the anterior chamber usually results in further gas migration into the anterior chamber. Any postoperative pressure issues should be managed as below or by tapping the anterior chamber gas at the slit lamp postoperatively

- *Subretinal gas*: If an improper injection site is chosen or large open breaks remain, it is possible for gas to end up in the subretinal space. A vitrectomy may need to be performed to evacuate it

- *'Fish-mouthing' of retinal breaks*: This results from circumferential folding of the retina at the site of a large horseshoe tear. The break may prevent reattachment if not functionally closed. It is usually due to a buckling effect that is too high and should be corrected by loosening the buckle and reducing its height. If the break is superior, intraocular gas may be injected. A radial element for added imbrication may also help

Postoperative issues can include:

- *Increased IOP*: This is most commonly due to injection of intraocular gas, but may also be related to choroidal hemorrhage. Topical IOP-lowering medications or oral acetazolamide should be given depending on the level of IOP elevation
- *Early infection*: Should be suspected if abnormal or worsening pain, chemosis, and lid edema develop. Topical and oral moxifloxacin may be used, as these achieve good intraocular and orbital penetration
- *Late infection/extrusion*: Most often due to breakdown of overlying conjunctiva and exposure. There is some evidence that bacterial biofilms may also contribute to late buckle infections. Most commonly, explantation of buckling elements becomes necessary. The retina usually remains attached after buckle removal
- *Choroidal detachments*: Usually small and self-limited. IOP should be managed as above. Uncommonly, these may be massive and if 'kissing' choroidal detachment or hemorrhage are present, these may require external drainage
- *Cystoid macular edema*: Usually occurs 4-6 weeks following successful scleral buckling. Topical steroid or NSAIDs should be used initially. Intravitreal steroid may be considered for refractory cases
- *Epimacular proliferation*: Macular puckering has been reported in 2–17% of successfully buckled cases. Observation or surgery can be pursued based on visual potential and patient motivation
- *Proliferative vitreoretinopathy*: Usually occurs within the first 3 months following surgery and is the most common cause of retinal redetachment following successful SBP. Vitrectomy with membrane stripping is most often necessary, possibly with silicone oil placement
- *Refractive error*: Myopic shift is often encountered due to an increase in axial length. This should be discussed with patients preoperatively. Studies have reported low to moderate buckle heights inducing -0.74 to -2.24 diopters of myopia
- *Diplopia*: Common in the first few weeks, but generally transient

## SURGICAL OUTCOMES: SCIENTIFIC EVIDENCE/META-ANALYSIS

Multiple, large prospective studies have demonstrated similar retinal reattachment rates between scleral buckling and vitrectomy procedures. SBP has a higher success rate for phakic patients and those with inferior pathology (Tables 24-1 and 24-2).

## PLACE OF THE TECHNIQUE IN SURGICAL ARMAMENTARIUM

SBPs were traditionally the mainstay of retinal reattachment surgery. Although they have become less common as vitrectomy procedures have become more popular, they continue to have a significant role in retinal detachment repair, particularly for children and other young phakic patients.

**TABLE 24-1** Summary of studies, phakic patients.[2-4]

| RETROSPECTIVE | SB | PPV | SB/PPV | Total eyes |
|---|---|---|---|---|
| Miki et al., 2001 | 100% | 96% | — | 225 |
| Mansouri et al., 2010 (phakic subgroup) | 86% | 78% | 84% | 168 |
| TRI recurrent RD study group, St. Louis, 2008 | 86% | 78% | 84% | 286 |
| **PROSPECTIVE** | **SB** | **PPV** | **SB/PPV** | **Total eyes** |
| Heimann et al., 2007 (phakic subgroup) | 63.6% | 61.8% | — | — |

(SB: Scleral buckling; PPV: Pars plana vitrectomy).

TABLE 24.2 Summary of studies, pseudophakic patients[3-8]

| RETROSPECTIVE | SB | PPV | SB/PPV | Total eyes |
|---|---|---|---|---|
| Mansouri et al., 2010 (pseudophakic group) | 80% | 86.5% | 80.3% | 118 |
| TRI recurrent RD study group, St. Louis, 2008 | 80% | 87% | 80% | 286 |
| **PROSPECTIVE** | **SB** | **PPV** | **SB/PPV** | **Total eyes** |
| Stangos et al., 2004 | | 98% | 92% | 71 |
| Sharma et al., 2005 | 76% | 84% | | 50 |
| Brazitikos et al., 2005 | 83% | 94% | | 150 |
| Weichel et al., 2006 | | 93% | 94% | 152 |
| Heimann et al., 2007 (pseudophakic group) | 53% | 72% | | 265 |

(SB: Scleral buckling; PPV: Para plana vitrectomy).

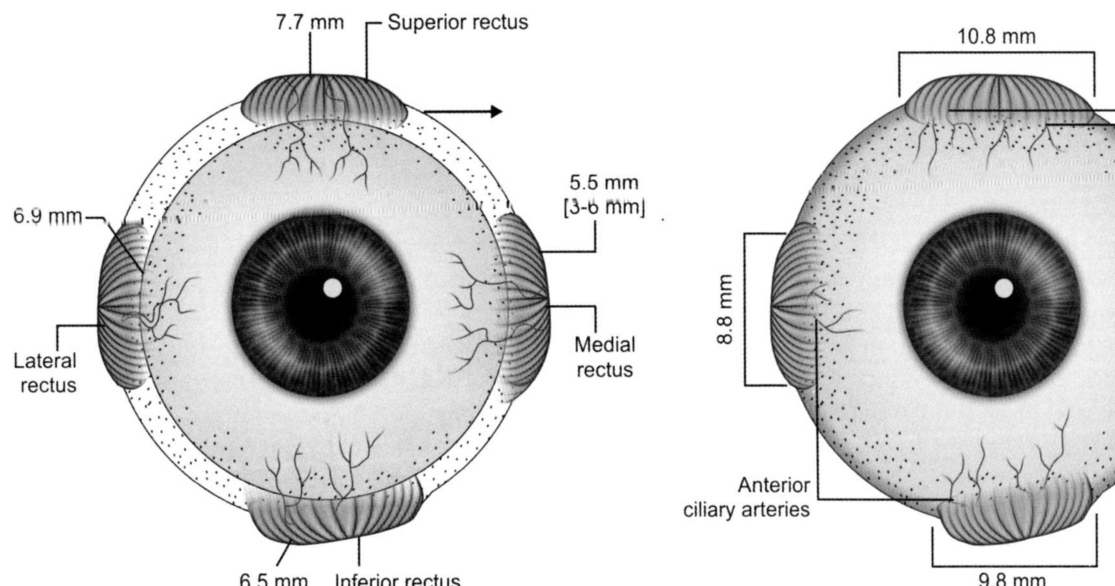


Figure 24-35 The circle of Tillaux illustrates the distance of extraocular muscles from the limbus.

Figure 24-36 Knowing the widths and anatomy of extraocular muscles aids in hooking and passing ties around them.

## PEARLS AND PITFALLS

- *Preoperative*:
  - In 50% of cases, more than one retinal break will exist in the eye with the detachment
  - In up to 20% of cases, the contralateral eye may also have retinal breaks or holes
- *Muscle anatomy*:
  - Superior and inferior rectus muscles run superiorly to their respective oblique muscles
  - Hooking the superior rectus from nasal to temporal may be less likely to incorporate or split the underlying superior oblique muscle
  - The circle of Tillaux is a guide for how far back to sweep in order to hook the muscles posterior to their insertions (Figs. 24-35 and 24-36)
- *Scleral inspection*:
  - Once the muscles have silk ties around them, it is very easy to torque the globe such that horizontal muscles end up in vertical quadrants and vice versa. It can be helpful to put three stop knots in the superior tie rather than the two for the others to help maintain orientation
  - The Schepens retractor features a broad slit that is designed to fit around the rectus muscles. In addition to visualizing the oblique quadrants, use it to inspect the muscles by placing the slit around the muscle insertion and sweeping posteriorly toward the equator. This allows further stripping of superficial Tenon's from the muscle and frees up tissue for better visualization
  - Scleral thinning is often present at the site of retinal breaks, so small areas of blue sclera may represent

areas of the fundus that deserve closer scrutiny during indirect ophthalmoscopy
  - The vortex veins are found in the middle of each oblique quadrant at the equator. These represent landmarks for orientation and areas to be avoided with sutures or scleral tunnels
- *Ciliary and vitreous anatomy*:
  - The anterior part of the ciliary body, pars plicata, extends posteriorly about 2.5 mm from the iris root. It is very vascular and can bleed heavily if traumatized. The posterior part of the ciliary body, pars plana, is relatively avascular and about 3 mm wide nasally and 4.5 mm temporally
  - The ora serrata meets the posterior aspect of the pars plana with a scalloped margin. It follows the circle of Tillaux and its most posterior extent is approximately 6.5–7.5 mm from the nasal limbus and 7.5–8.5 mm from the temporal limbus
  - The vitreous base is the place of strongest adhesion of vitreous to retina. The vitreous base is 2–4 mm wide and generally wider on the nasal side. It forms a band of 4–6 mm width (1–2 mm anterior to the ora serrata and 1–3 mm posterior to it) that overlies the posterior pars plana and the anterior peripheral retina near the ora serrata
- *Securing the band with sutures*:
  - In general, longer and shallower partial-thickness scleral passes are preferable to shorter, deep passes to reduce the risk of accidental perforation
  - The closer to the band that the sutures are placed, the more will be the imbricating effect of the band. However, they should not be closer to the height of the element or they will prevent full imbrication of the element
  - If using single-armed sutures, in order to have appropriate access to pass the scleral suture, the needle-driver handle must be pointed upward toward the ceiling while placing the suture. This means that one pass will be forehanded and the other will need to be backhanded. The more difficult posterior bite should be forehanded and the less difficult anterior bite should be backhanded
- *Securing the band with scleral tunnels ("belt loops")*:
  - Consider creating scleral tunnels slightly off-center in the quadrants to avoid risk of cutting into the vortex veins
- *Tightening the band*:
  - Once just snug against the globe, tightening the band 12 mm is often ideal, as that results in 2 mm imbrication. ($C = 2\pi r$, and a reduction in circumference of 12 mm results in 1.9 mm reduction in radius)
- *External drainage*:
  - If external drainage is done too close to the site of the causative break, you may get passage of vitreous through the break and the scleral opening, rather than or in addition to the desired subretinal fluid
  - Draining under a pre-existing subretinal vitreoproliferative band can lower the risk of retinal incarceration
  - If suturing the drainage site, an absorbable suture is adequate if covered by the band. If draining posterior to the band for maximal drainage, nonresorbable suture is preferable
- *Gas injection*:
  - A final gas volume of 0.25 mL covers 90° at the equator, and 2.5 mL covers 180° at the equator
  - Remember that pure $SF_6$ bubbles double in size over 48–72 hours and pure $C_3F_8$ bubbles quadruple in size over 72–96 hours
- *Retinal Perfusion*:
  - If arterial pulsations are spontaneously present, it indicates that the IOP exceeds the diastolic pressure but is less than the systolic pressure within the CRA
  - If arterial pulsations are not spontaneously present, it indicates that the CRA is either continuously open or closed. To determine between the two states, digital pressure is applied to the sclera, causing the IOP to increase. If pulsations are induced, it means that constant perfusion was present and the IOP had previously been lower than both the diastolic and systolic pressures in the CRA. If pulsations cannot be induced, it means that the IOP that exceeds both the systolic and diastolic pressures within the CRA

## REFERENCES

1. Brinton DA, Wilkinson CP. Retinal detachment: principles and practice, 3rd edn. Ophthalmology Monographs I. Vol. I. New York: Oxford University Press; 2009.
2. Miki D, Hida T, Hotta K, et al. Comparison of scleral buckling and vitrectomy for retinal detachment resulting from flap tears in superior quadrants. Jpn J Ophthalmol. 2001;45(2):187-91.
3. Mansouri A, Almong A, Shah GK, et al. Recurrent retinal detachment: does initial treatment matter? Br J Ophthalmol. 2010;94(10):1344-7.
4. Heimann H, Bartz-Schmidt KU, Bornfeld N, et al. Scleral buckling versus primary vitrectomy in rhegmatogenous retinal detachment: a prospective randomized multicenter clinical study. Ophthalmology 2007;114(12): 2142-54.

5. Stangos AN, Petropoulos IK, Brozou CG, et al. Pars-plana vitrectomy alone vs vitrectomy with scleral buckling for primary rhegmatogenous pseudophakic retinal detachment. Am J Ophthalmol. 2004;138(6):952-8.
6. Sharma YR, Karunanithi S, Azad RV, et al. Functional and anatomic outcome of scleral buckling versus primary vitrectomy in pseudophakic retinal detachment. Acta Ophthalmol Scand. 2005;83(3):293-7.
7. Brazitikos PD, Androudi S, Christen WG, et al. Primary pars plana vitrectomy versus scleral buckle surgery for the treatment of pseudophakic retinal detachment: a randomized clinical trial. Retina. 2005;25(8): 957-64.
8. Weichel ED, Martidis A, Fineman MS, et al. Pars plana vitrectomy versus combined pars plana vitrectomy-scleral buckle for primary repair of pseudophakic retinal detachment. Ophthalmology. 2006;113(11): 2033-40.

CHAPTER

25

# Pneumatic Retinopexy

Nikolas JS London

## INTRODUCTION

In 1986, Hilton and Grizzard popularized pneumatic retinopexy as an outpatient method to repair rhegmatogenous retinal detachments (RRD). When employed judiciously, it is an effective, minimally invasive method of retinal detachment repair. Pneumatic retinopexy offers several important advantages over other options for RRD, including significantly lower cost, better visual acuity outcomes, lack of need for systemic anesthesia, less risk of cataract induction compared to vitrectomy, no refractive change or risk of diplopia compared to scleral buckling, and the ability to intervene immediately. Despite its relatively simple appearance, pneumatic retinopexy should only be performed by experienced surgeons who understand which patients are likely to do well with the procedure and who are capable of recognizing and dealing with the potential complications.

## INDICATIONS

- Retinal break(s) within the superior 8 clock hours of the peripheral retina
- One or more retinal breaks confined to 1 clock hour

## EXPANDED INDICATIONS

- Retinal breaks up to 2.5 clock hours in length (the Pneumatic Retinopexy Clinical Trial only included retinal breaks 1 clock hour or less)
- Single or multiple breaks spanning up to 3 continuous clock hours

## CONTRAINDICATIONS

- Relative:
  - Extensive lattice degeneration (> 3 clock hours)
  - Retinal breaks or atrophic holes in attached inferior retina
  - Advanced glaucoma
  - Grade C proliferative vitreoretinopathy (PVR) not exerting traction on the break
  - Giant retinal tears
  - Moderate uveitis
- Absolute:
  - Inability to find the retinal break
  - Substantial media opacity limiting visualization
  - Poor patient cooperation
  - Grade C PVR exerting traction on the break or grade D PVR
  - Tractional or combined tractional/RRD
  - Inability to perform postoperative positioning
  - Unavoidable need to fly or travel to >4000 ft. elevation
  - Severe uveitis

Figures 25-1A to D depicts an ideal pneumatic candidate from an anatomic perspective and demonstrates the basic steps of the procedure. It is critical to accurately determine the location of all retinal breaks, not only to instruct the patient how to position postoperatively but also to predict the likelihood of success as it is directly related to the ease of maintaining the necessary position (Fig. 25-2). Tamponade with upright positioning is straightforward for breaks in the superior 2 clock hours, whereas nasal and temporal breaks are slightly more challenging to repair, as it is more difficult for patients to maintain strict side positioning. Breaks between 10 and 11 and 1 and 2 are more difficult to tamponade as these require an upright position with a head tilt. When evaluating a patient, one should consider all of the indications and contraindications for a particular case and determine how they may affect the success of the procedure. While not validated, Table 25-1 illustrates how one might approach this.

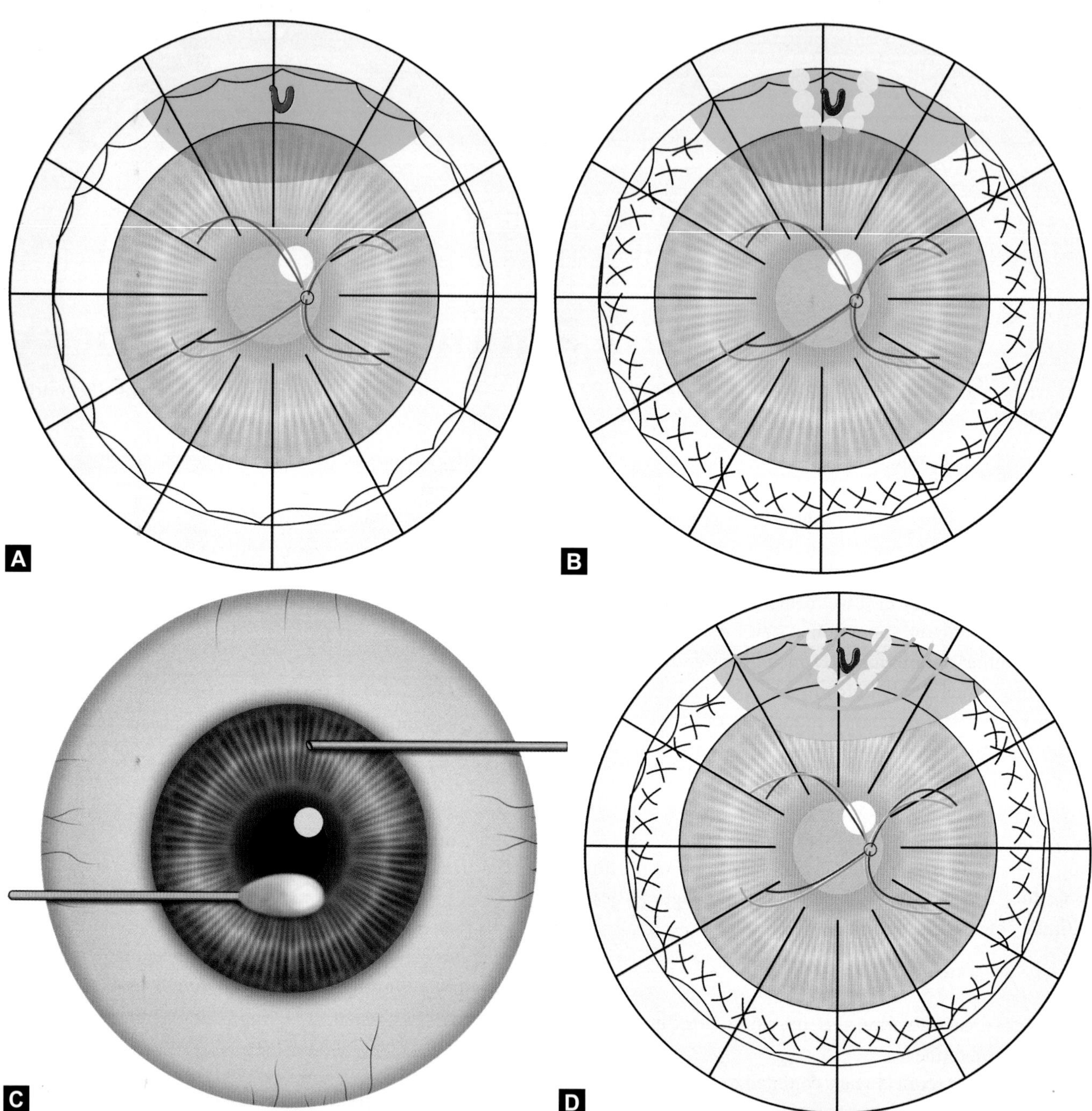


Figures 25-1A to D Ideal candidate for pneumatic retinopexy (A) and basic technique (B to D). Figure (A) depicts a patient with a single break at 12 with limited subretinal fluid. In figure (B), the patient has been treated with cryotherapy to surround the break and a band of laser in the attached periphery. Figure (C) depicts a paracentesis using a needle and syringe sans plunger and a cotton-tipped applicator for stabilization. As much aqueous as possible should be removed. Figure (D) shows the eye following injection of the gas bubble. Once the retina has completely flattened, fill-in laser should be applied for complete 360° treatment.

However, pneumatic retinopexy may still be successful in situations where it is relatively contraindicated, including eyes with multiple, separated breaks, breaks larger than 1 clock hour, grade C PVR distant from the break, and detachments associated with breaks, holes, or extensive lattice in areas of attached retina. Such "expanded indications" might be particularly necessary in situations where the patient is unable or unwilling to go to the operating room, the patient is uninsured and minimizing cost is a priority, immediate intervention is desired, and/or an operating room

TABLE 25-1 The Tornambe algorithm for single operation success rate. Start with an ideal candidate—a phakic eye with a single break in a single quadrant of detachment, which has a 97% success rate

| Question | Yes | Success rate |
|---|---|---|
| Ideal candidate: phakic eye, single break between 10 and 2, single quadrant of detachment | | 97% |
| Break in an oblique quadrant | – 10% | |
| Break in inferior 4 clock hours | – 70% | |
| Pseudophakia | – 10% | |
| ≥ 2 quadrants of detachment | – 10% | |
| Multiple breaks | – 10% | |
| Break(s) > 1 but < 2.5 clock hours | – 10% | |
| Lattice degeneration (up to 3 clock hours) | – 5% | |
| Grade A or B PVR | – 5% | |
| Grade C PVR | – 40% | |
| 360 laser retinopexy | + 10% | |

This table is largely theoretical and has not been validated, but illustrates the concept of evaluating the patient as a whole and the relative importance of various indications and contraindications.
(PVR: Proliferative vitreoretinopathy).

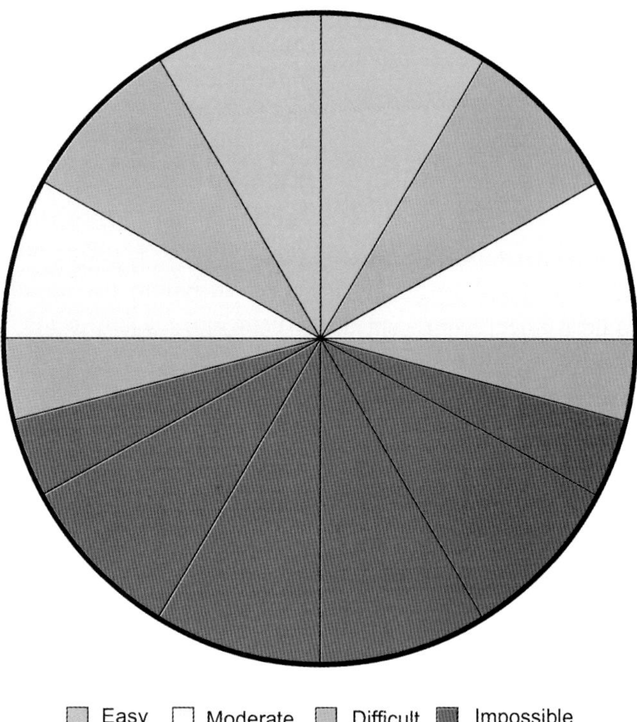


Figure 25-2 George Hilton's wheel of success. The location(s) of the causative retinal break(s) is one of the most important factors in determining the likelihood of success. This has to do with the ease of postoperative positioning. Breaks in the superior 2 clock hours are relatively easy to tamponade with upright positioning. Temporal and nasal breaks can also be tamponaded with side positioning; however, this is more difficult to maintain. Oblique breaks require a more uncomfortable position, and inferior breaks require a very awkward position in order for the gas bubble to tamponade the break.

is unavailable. It is imperative that if the pneumatic procedure fails, the subsequent rescue operation be performed within 3–5 days. Otherwise, prolonged macular detachment will affect visual recovery, and the risk of macular pucker and PVR increases. For example, Figure 25-3A illustrates the modified technique in an eye with two retinal breaks separated by several clock hours. In this scenario, both breaks are treated with cryotherapy and laser may be applied to the attached periphery. Following injection of the gas, a steamroller maneuver helps to minimize subretinal fluid and reduces the chance that the residual subretinal fluid will be displaced and elevated previously flat breaks. Postoperatively, the patient is positioned for 3 days to tamponade the suspected causative break, followed by positioning the second break for 3–4 days. Staged laser to supplement treatment around both breaks is useful once they are flat. Similarly, eyes with breaks, holes, or lattice in attached retina can be successfully treated by surrounding those areas with laser prior to gas injection and utilizing a steamroller technique (discussed below) to help prevent displaced subretinal fluid from detaching those areas. Even eyes with inferior detachments and breaks have been treated successfully with extreme positioning in limber patients. Previously vitrectomized eyes are particularly amenable to expanded indications if a fluid-gas exchange is utilized to obtain a near total gas fill. An explanation of this technique is beyond the scope of this chapter, but can be found in the reference by Landers.

## SURGICAL TECHNIQUE

Pneumatic retinopexy can be performed as a one- or two-staged procedure. In certain cases, a one-staged procedure is preferred. For example, a bullous detachment from a small, peripheral round hole close to the retinal pigment epithelium (RPE) may require minimal cryotherapy; thus, cryotherapy would be an ideal approach. One-staged procedures also may be better in cases associated with media opacity. The steps below are for a one-staged procedure. Two-staged procedures may avoid cryotherapy and associated inflammation, and may be the best option in eyes with a bullous detachment where extensive cryotherapy would be required to reach the retina. For a two-staged procedure, follow all of the steps for one-staged procedure except for the diffuse subconjunctival anesthesia and application of cryotherapy. Retinopexy, typically in the form of laser, is applied in the immediate postoperative period once the involved retina has been flattened.

The vast majority of pneumatic retinopexies in the United States are performed in an outpatient, office-based setting. The most important step is a thorough preoperative dilated fundus examination of the peripheral retina with accurate documentation of all areas of pathology, including the location and size of all retinal breaks, and the presence and extent of lattice degeneration and PVR. This enables proper patient selection and improves the ability to follow patients postoperatively, when anatomic findings may be difficult to visualize. Once pneumatic retinopexy is determined to be an appropriate option, the surgeon should have a detailed discussion of the surgical options with the patient, including the advantages and disadvantages of each procedure as well as the expected postoperative course and requirements. Patients must understand and agree to the postoperative positioning and altitude requirements. Obtain informed consent.

In preparation for the procedure, position the patient comfortably in the examination chair, reclined approximately 45°. Make sure the chair is at a good height so the surgeon is comfortable during the procedure. Confirm and then anesthetize the operative eye. Liberally apply topical anesthetic. Next, inject 2% lidocaine underneath the conjunctiva in all areas that need to be treated with transscleral cryotherapy as well as in the quadrant through which gas will be injected. Take care to avoid damage to conjunctival vessels to minimize hematoma formation. Allow the lidocaine to infiltrate the tissue and dissipate for 5–10 minutes. Although rarely necessary, peri- or retrobulbar anesthesia can be used. The ideal result is anesthesia without akinesia as it is helpful if the patient can move the eye during the procedure. During a retrobulbar block, directing 1–2 cc of anesthesia to the anterior muscle cone may help to avoid akinesia. While the anesthesia is taking effect, set up the rest of the equipment, including the appropriate gas, and verify that the cryotherapy machine is in working order and ready for use.

Retinopexy is performed with laser, cryotherapy, or a combination of the two. Consider laser retinopexy to all areas of pathology in attached retina, and consider 360° treatment in pseudophakic and high-risk eyes. Apply cryotherapy to all pathology in detached retina. For example, in a pseudophakic eye with a superior detachment associated with a break at 12 o'clock, we apply cryopexy around the break and apply peripheral scatter laser to the attached periphery (Fig. 25-3B). Once the retina reattaches a few days later, we apply fill-in laser to the untreated periphery so that the entire retina between the posterior insertion of the vitreous base and the ora is treated. The goal during cryotherapy is to surround defects with contiguous, but not overlapping, spots taken out to the ora serrata. Avoid redundant treatment as well as treatment directly to the bare RPE to minimize the liberation of RPE cells. Burns should briefly whiten

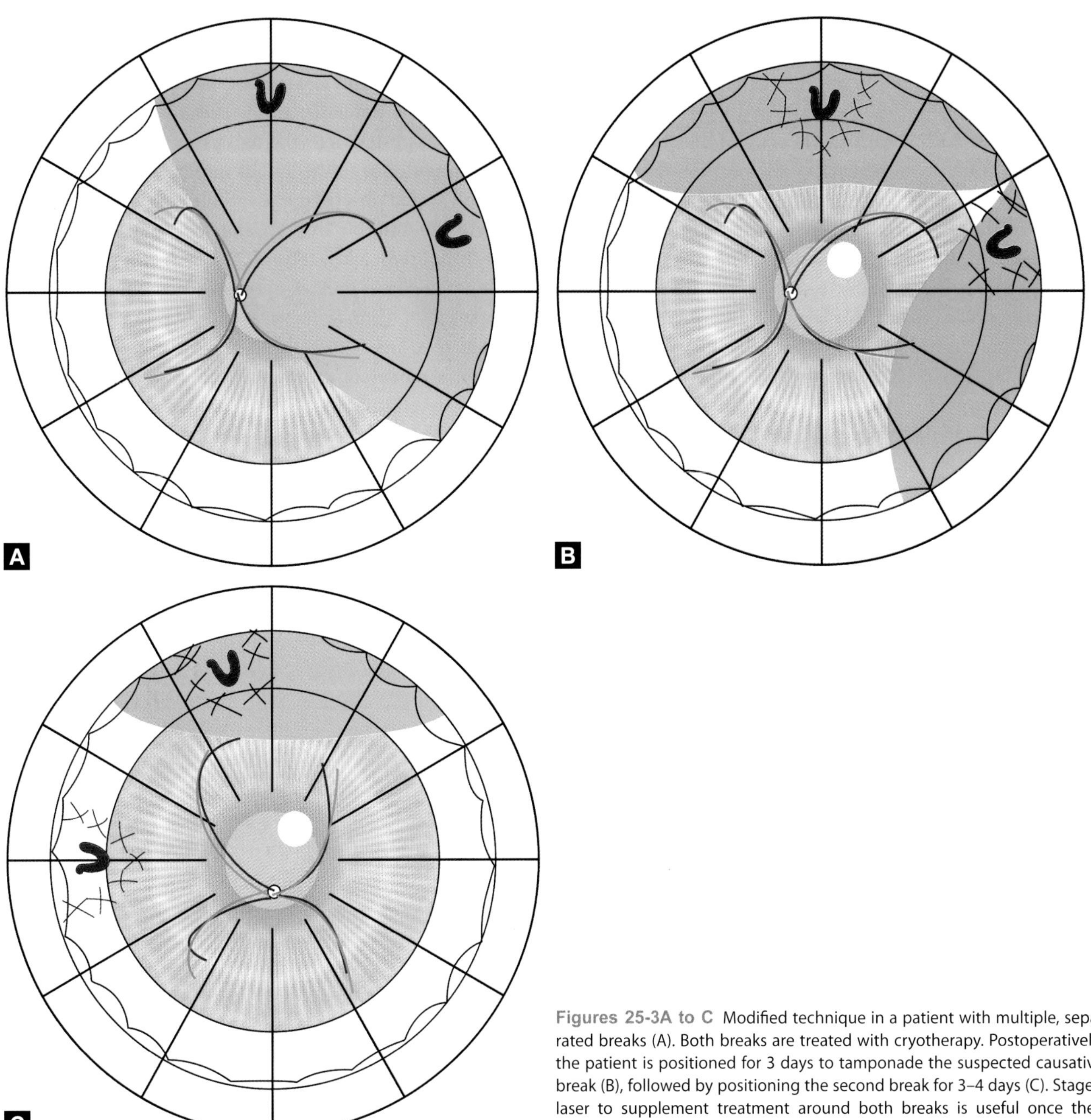


**Figures 25-3A to C** Modified technique in a patient with multiple, separated breaks (A). Both breaks are treated with cryotherapy. Postoperatively, the patient is positioned for 3 days to tamponade the suspected causative break (B), followed by positioning the second break for 3–4 days (C). Staged laser to supplement treatment around both breaks is useful once they are flat.

the retina without ice crystal formation. Excessive treatment can lead to damage and/or liberation of RPE cells and can cause exaggerated postoperative intraretinal hemorrhage and vitreous inflammation.

The next step is preparation and injection of the intraocular gas. $SF_6$, $C_2F_6$, or $C_3F_8$ may be used, depending on the clinical scenario. Only $SF_6$ and $C_3F_8$ are commonly available in the United States. Pure $SF_6$ expands two times and lasts approximately 2 weeks, whereas pure $C_3F_8$ expands four times and lasts approximately 6–8 weeks. We almost exclusively use $SF_6$, but prefer $C_3F_8$ in cases where the eye is large, and the break is large, posterior, and/or located at 4- or 8-o'clock. First, turn on the gas briefly to flush the tubing. Next, attach a 1 cc tuberculin syringe to the tubing using a Millipore filter. Fill the syringe at least two to three times with pure gas, emptying the syringe between fills. After the last fill, cap the syringe with a 30- or 32-gauge needle. Set this syringe aside in the sterile tray.

Perform an anterior chamber paracentesis. We perform this routinely on all patients and always before the gas injection in order to avoid anterior prolapse of gas and sudden intraocular pressure (IOP) elevation. This is particularly important in patients with glaucoma. Recline the patient so that the iris plane is parallel to the floor and elevate the chair to a comfortable height for you. Verify that there is no vitreous in the anterior chamber. Place a lid speculum and apply several drops of 5% povidone-iodine onto the ocular surface. Allow the povidone-iodine to work for several minutes. Approach the patient from the surgeon's view. Prepare a cotton-tipped applicator (CTA) and a tuberculin syringe with a 27- or 30-gauge needle. Remove the plunger from the syringe. Hold the CTA with the hand on the nasal side of the eye and the syringe with the hand on the temporal side of the eye. Use the CTA to apply steady pressure to the center of the cornea. This stabilizes the globe and opens the anterior chamber angle. As you are holding pressure, insert the 27- or 30-gauge needle through temporal clear cornea just anterior to the iris plane, and over the inferior mid-iris stroma to minimize the risk of injury to the anterior lens capsule (Fig. 25-3C).

A 30-gauge needle enables a slower fluid removal and is easier to insert at the limbus. If needed, you may use conjunctival forceps instead of a CTA to stabilize the globe just posterior to your entry site. As you are inserting the needle, take care to avoid contact with the lens, particularly in phakic patients. Attempt to position the syringe in such as way as it is easy to read the volume markings as well as in a way to direct the bore of the needle away from the iris to minimize incarceration. Steadily increase the pressure with the CTA as aqueous enters the syringe. Be careful not to relieve pressure suddenly or the iris will contact the needle and may result in hyphema and/or lens damage. A slight rolling maneuver of the CTA from superior to inferior on the cornea may help to maintain pressure and keep the inferior anterior chamber angle open as the volume is depleted. Remove as much aqueous as possible. Remove the needle when the anterior chamber is too shallow, while simultaneously maintaining pressure with the CTA. Note the volume of aqueous removed. Usually at least 0.25 cc of aqueous can be removed, which is appropriate if you inject 0.5 or 0.6 cc of gas. The eye is usually softer if you have already performed cryotherapy; so, ocular hypertension is not usually a problem in that situation.

Inject the gas. Choose a quadrant for injection in an area of flat retina, as far from the detachment as possible. We prefer to inject in the temporal or nasal quadrants, and almost never inject inferiorly. Have the patient look in the appropriate direction to expose the desired quadrant, and orient the injection site vertically by adjusting the height and recline of the examination chair. Apply a drop of 5% povidone-iodine. Express gas from the syringe to obtain the desired volume. Enter the eye vertically, perpendicular to the sclera 3.5 posterior to the limbus in pseudophakic eyes and 4 mm posterior to the limbus in phakic eyes. Some surgeons advocated inserting the needle 7 mm in order to penetrate the anterior hyaloid and then pull back so that only 2–3 mm remains in the eye. This may help to avoid fish eggs, but it increases the risk of the gas becoming sequestered in the space of Petit, which is a bigger cause for concern. To avoid this, inject gas in the mid-vitreous cavity. Inject the gas at a moderate, steady pace. Injection of the gas too quickly may result in multiple small bubbles or fish eggs that can potentially enter the subretinal space.

When selecting gas, consider the area that needs to be covered, phakic status, and possibility of need to travel to high altitude. For example, in an emmetropic eye, 0.5 cc of pure $SF_6$ will expand to 1cc of gas, which covers approximately 3 clock hours, whereas in the same eye 0.5 cc of pure $C_3F_8$ results in 2cc of gas, which covers approximately 4 clock hours of retina (Figs. 25-4A and B) In other words, a 0.3 cc gas bubble covers > 45° arc, but it takes at least a 1 cc bubble to cover 80–90°.

After gas injection, examine the optic nerve head for occlusion or pulsations of the central retinal artery (CRA). If pulsations are not present and it is unclear whether the CRA is perfused, apply light digital pressure to the sclera. In a normotensive eye, this should elicit pulsations of the CRA. If pulsations are not seen with digital pressure, the IOP is too high and the CRA is likely occluded. If the CRA is pulsating or closed, and the eye has no history of glaucoma, wait 10 minutes and the CRA will likely regain perfusion. Avoid the temptation to remove gas too early or aggressively, as this maneuver can be dangerous. In our experience, if you remove 0.25 cc of aqueous and inject up to 0.6 cc of gas, perfusion will generally be fine. Even with pulsations, as long as the patient has light perception vision when they leave your office they will be fine. A repeat paracentesis or controlled removal of gas can be considered, but is seldom necessary.

Consider a steamroller technique if the macula is involved or threatened, and the detachment is bullous. This technique also decreases the chances of subretinal gas, and is helpful in cases where the subretinal fluid needs to be debulked, such as those with multiple separated breaks. The purpose is to use the gas bubble to steamroll the subretinal fluid out through the retinal break and back into the vitreous cavity. Position the patient face down for approximately 10 minutes to flatten the macula, then slowly have them rotate their

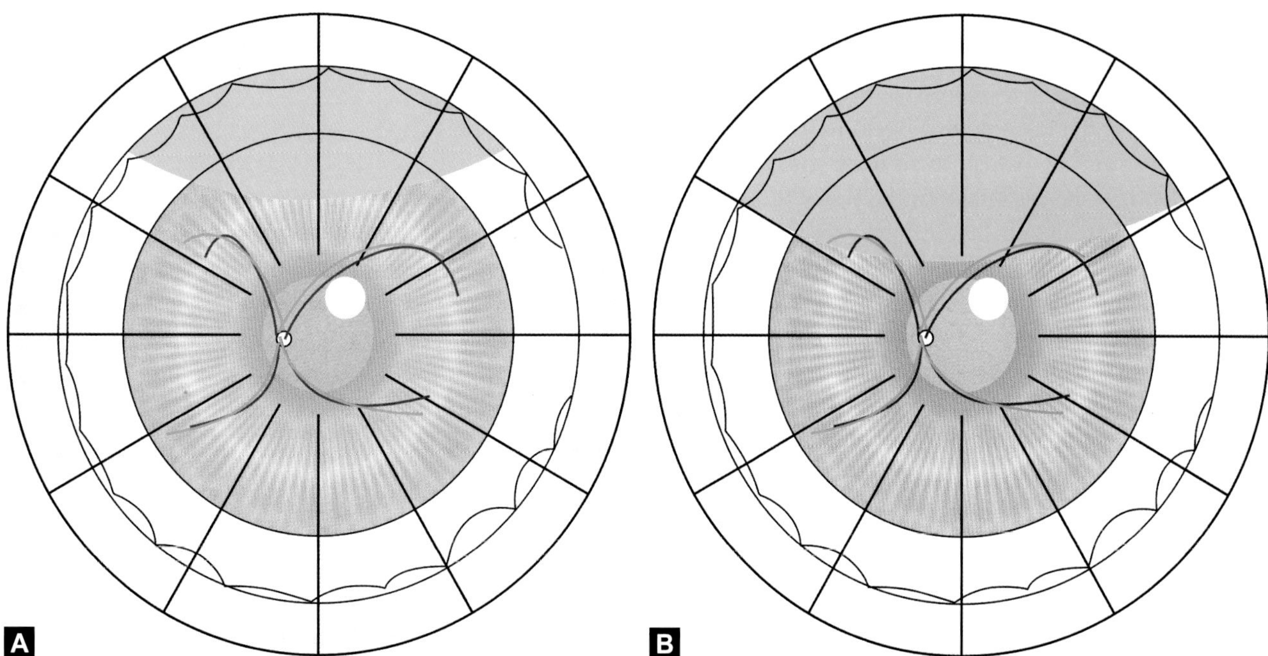


Figures 25-4A and B Bubble size versus arc of contact in emmetropic eyes. SF6 and C3F8 differ both in their expansile capacity as well as their duration. It is important to consider the desired arc of coverage when selecting a gas and the amount injected. Pure SF6 will expand to two times its volume, whereas pure C3F8 will expand four times.

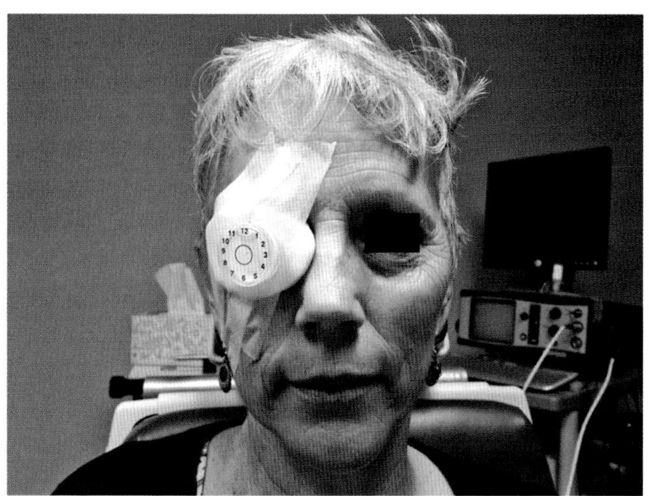

Figure 25-5 The Tornambe level (Sonomed Escalon) can help patients position correctly following pneumatic retinopexy. Patients are instructed to keep the bubble in the Pneuma level at a particular clock hour, depending on the desired location of tamponade. It may be helpful to also place a mark at the desired clock hour.

head 45° in the direction of the retinal break(s) (i.e. if the break is superior, have them sit up 45°). Position them here for another 10 minutes and then slowly have them position their head such that the bubble covers the break.

Apply an antibiotic or combined antibiotic/corticosteroid ointment and apply a patch and shield to the eye. Consider a mark or bubble device (e.g. Tornambe level, Sonomed Escalon, Lake Success, NY, Fig. 25-5) to indicate the optimal head position. Discuss postoperative care, including the optimal head position, drops, and signs/symptoms of endophthalmitis. Advise patients that they will likely have some subconjunctival hemorrhage, conjunctival and lid erythema and edema, and they may experience discomfort as the local anesthesia wears off. If cryotherapy is used, this may resemble an ice cream headache.

## MECHANISM OF ACTION

Pneumatic retinopexy works by reducing a retinal detachment to a retinal tear associated with subretinal fluid. As long as the tear is flattened, adequately surrounded with retinopexy, and allowed to remain flat during the process of wound healing, the underlying RPE should actively remove the subretinal fluid. So as long as the macula is attached and no open breaks are noted, inferior subretinal fluid is not a concern and may be allowed to last for several months. Occasionally, small pockets of subretinal fluid can develop and take several months to a year to regress. It is not necessary, nor advised, to drain these.

## POSTOPERATIVE CARE

Patients are seen on the first postoperative day, looking for signs of infection, evaluation of IOP, and examination of the retina. The subretinal fluid may not be completely resolved on the first day, and may be displaced inferiorly. Depending on the clinical scenario, patients are also seen at 1, 2, and 4 weeks. It is important to follow the eye closely until the bubble resolves and it takes up to 2 weeks for the retinopexy to mature. Instruct the patient to maintain positioning for 4–5 days to orient the gas bubble at the site of the defect(s). The patient should maintain this position as much as possible – we instruct them to position continuously with 10 minutes breaks every hour for at least the first 24 hours, followed by 16 hours per day for the next 3–4 days. Patients are advised to avoid reading for the first postoperative week to minimize saccades. An antibiotic and a corticosteroid drop are prescribed four times daily for the first postoperative week.

## SPECIFIC INSTRUMENTATION

- Cryotherapy unit or laser
- Gas ($SF_6$ or $C_3F_8$)
- 5–10% povidone-iodine (drops and/or swab)
- Topical anesthetic drops
- Injectable anesthetic (e.g. 2% lidocaine)
- Indirect ophthalmoscope and condensing lens
- 30- or 32-gauge 1/2 inch needle for injecting gas
- 27- or 30-gauge 1/2 inch needle on a 1 cc syringe for paracentesis
- 30-gauge 1/2 inch needle on a 1 cc syringe for injecting subconjunctival lidocaine
- Lid speculum
- Millipore filter × 2
- CTAs
- Mask, gloves per surgeon preference

## POTENTIAL COMPLICATIONS

- Subretinal gas
- Endophthalmitis
- Lens damage
- Subconjunctival or suprachoroidal hemorrhage
- Cryopexy to the macula
- CRA occlusion
- Missed or new retinal break
- PVR
- Recurrent retinal detachment

## SURGICAL OUTCOMES: SCIENTIFIC EVIDENCE/META-ANALYSIS

Most studies report a slightly lower single operation success rate for pneumatic retinopexy compared with scleral buckling

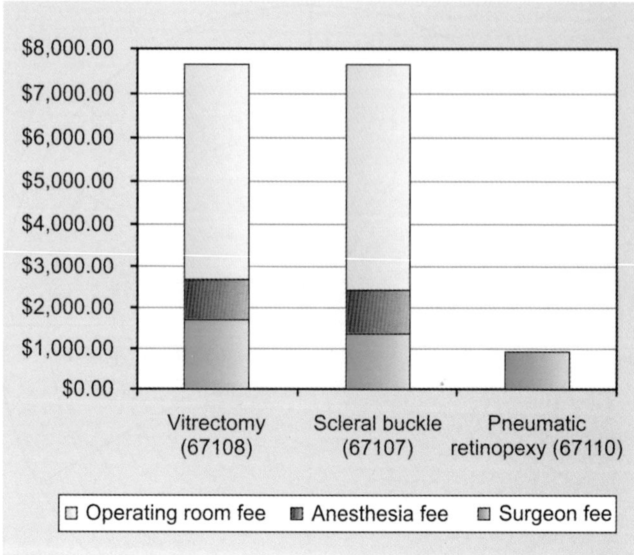


Figure 25-6 Cost comparison of retinal detachment repair procedures. These numbers are likely underestimated, particularly for hospital fees, which vary and may exceed $15,000. Data from Tornambe PE.[8]

or pars plana vitrectomy; however, it is important to note that a failed pneumatic does not damage the eye as long as excessive cryotherapy is avoided and the rescue operation, if necessary, is performed promptly. In general, successful pneumatic retinopexy cases have better postoperative visual acuity than cases repaired with vitrectomy or scleral buckle. There are reports that failed pneumatic cases have a poorer visual outcome than cases repaired with a single operation; however, careful examination of the literature reveals that many of these eyes were not repaired for several weeks. The sooner the macula is attached, the better the potential visual recovery whether one is dealing with the first, second, or third operation. Pneumatic retinopexy is often the fastest way to regain macular reattachment.

## PLACE OF THE TECHNIQUE IN SURGICAL ARMAMENTARIUM

Pneumatic retinopexy can be considered first-line treatment for selected cases and is underutilized in general. Table 25-2 compares the advantages and disadvantages of the different options for retinal detachment repair. Particularly important in our era of healthcare reform and cost reduction, the cost savings are significant compared with scleral buckling and vitrectomy, particularly when anesthesia and hospital costs are factored in (Fig. 25-6). Moreover, use of pneumatic retinopexy does no harm, and does not preclude subsequent surgical repair.

TABLE 25.2 Relative advantages and disadvantages of surgical options for retinal detachment repair

| Procedure | Advantages | Disadvantages |
|---|---|---|
| Pneumatic retinopexy | • Substantially lower cost<br>• Lowest postoperative morbidity<br>• Best postoperative visual acuity<br>• No impact on rescue surgery, if necessary<br>• Low risk of cataract induction<br>• Fewer potential complications<br>• Outpatient procedure<br>• Immediate intervention<br>• Lack of need for NPO status<br>• No change in refractive status<br>• Lowest relative difficulty<br>• Fastest visual recovery<br>• General anesthesia never necessary, retrobulbar anesthesia rarely necessary | • Lowest single operation success rate in nonideal candidates<br>• Critical importance of case selection<br>• Relatively high risk of redetachment due to new tear formation (if 360 laser not performed)<br>• Lowest reimbursement<br>• Risk of subretinal gas<br>• Risk of postoperative ocular hypertension<br>• Greatest requirements for postoperative positioning/ compliance<br>• Postoperative altitude restrictions<br>• Requires the greatest pre- and postoperative time with closer follow-up<br>• Risk of vitreous floaters with excessive cryotherapy |
| Scleral buckle | • Lowest risk of endophthalmitis<br>• 360° support of the vitreous base with encircling elements<br>• Best support of inferior pathology<br>• Slightly lower cost than vitrectomy<br>• Lowest risk of postoperative cataract | • Change in refractive status<br>• Greatest perioperative discomfort<br>• Risk of buckle extrusion/intrusion<br>• Risk of buckle infection<br>• Risk of diplopia<br>• Risk of induced myopia, anisometropia, and/or aniseikonia<br>• Risk of inadvertent globe penetration<br>• Risk of inadvertent macular treatment<br>• Risk of postoperative ocular hypertension<br>• Risk of cystoid macular edema<br>• Risk of eyelid malposition<br>• Risk of vitreous floaters<br>• Likely need for general anesthesia and associated risks (e.g. nausea, urinary retention, stroke, death)<br>• Contraindicated in eyes with glaucoma filtering blebs |
| Pars plana vitrectomy | • Only/best means of repair in certain scenarios, including giant retinal tears, advanced PVR, funnel configuration, cases with dense vitreous hemorrhage<br>• Direct repair of detachment<br>• Highest reimbursement<br>• Minimal to no change in refractive status<br>• Enables a highly detailed examination of the peripheral retinal | • Greatest risk of cataract induction<br>• Risk of traumatic optic neuropathy<br>• Risk of suprachoroidal hemorrhage<br>• Risk of subretinal perfluoron (if used)<br>• Lowest risk of post-operative ocular hypertension<br>• Postoperative altitude restrictions<br>• Risks associated with retrobulbar and/or general anesthesia |

## PEARLS AND PITFALLS

- For bullous retinal detachments, it may be helpful to have the patient lie flat in the supine position for 24 hours to allow the retinal to settle.
- While we rarely perform retrobulbar anesthesia, a retrobulbar block patient with xylocaine, just behind globe in anterior muscle cone gives prompt anesthesia with minimal akinesia.
- For staged procedures using laser retinopexy, only treat attached retina, and document all pathology well as it often becomes invisible once the retina flattens.
- 360° laser retinopexy can improve the success rate by up to 10% and is particularly useful in eyes with multiple retinal breaks (which implies abnormal vitreoretinal adhesion), eyes with lattice degeneration, and pseudophakic eyes in which breaks are easier to miss.
- Always treat detachments associated with breaks at 3- and 9-o'clock as one-stage procedures, or the breaks may reopen on the way to the office, as the patients will often end up sitting upright during transportation.
- If possible, the 3- and 9-o'clock positions should be spared from heavy cryotherapy or laser to avoid injury to the long ciliary vessels and nerves. Injury may rarely

result in permanent mydriasis and exaggerated postoperative pain.

- To avoid heavy cryotherapy, wait for the break/retina to settle onto the probe.
- During cryotherapy, be careful to allow the probe to thaw before pulling it away from the eye wall or serious injury could result.
- When injecting gas, always inject in the temporal or nasal quadrants, never inferiorly, and inject deep into the mid-vitreous cavity as occurrence of fish eggs usually do not matter and this avoids gas in the space of Petit. Also, after injecting gas hold the syringe steady for a few seconds and allow the gas in the eye to push plunger back out, if necessary, to avoid very high IOP.
- If gas becomes loculated in the anterior hyaloidal space nothing special needs to be done. It will typically break through and enter the mid-vitreous cavity within a day or two.
- If fish eggs form, have the patient position to keep the gas away from the break to prevent subretinal gas, particularly in cases with large breaks. The bubbles will usually coalesce within 24 hours. Cryotherapy remains effective for at least 5–6 days, so you lose very little with this maneuver.
- If a small bubble of subretinal gas is noted, you can try to manipulate it out through the tear through a combination of positioning and scleral depression; however, most small bubbles will resolve with no consequence, and resolve faster than the same size bubble in the vitreous cavity. However, large amounts of subretinal gas require removal with vitrectomy.
- Three important causes for poor experience with pneumatic retinopexy include poor patient selection, poor technique (particularly excessive cryotherapy), and delayed rescue operation, if needed.
- A tennis ball or sock placed in the back elastic band of a patient's pajama pants can help them position as they sleep.
- If the break is not closed on the first postoperative day there is a problem. This may be poor positioning, an insufficient gas bubble, or new break formation.
- Delayed rescue operation allows inflammatory mediators and RPE cells to fester, increasing the risk of PVR and/or ERM formation.
- While sedentary during positioning, remind patients to stretch their legs and flex their calf muscles regularly to minimize the risk of deep vein thrombosis.
- It takes up to 2 weeks for retinopexy to fully mature, so activity should be restricted for that time period, or the approximate duration of an SF6 gas bubble.
- Counsel the patient on the risk of detachment in the fellow eye, which depends on lens status and is approximately 4.5%, 16.4%, and 35.7% in phakic, pseudophakic, or aphakic eyes, respectively. Prophylactic treatment of retinal tears and lattice degeneration in fellow eyes should be considered, but treatment does not always prevent the development of a detachment.

## SUGGESTED READING


1. Hilton GF, Grizzard WS. Pneumatic retinopexy. A two-step outpatient operation without conjunctival incision. Ophthalmology. 1986;93(5):626-41.
2. Benson WE, Chan P, Sharma S, et al. Current popularity of pneumatic retinopexy. Retina. 1999;19(3):238-41.
3. Chan CK, Lin SG, Nuthi AS, et al. Pneumatic retinopexy for the repair of retinal detachments: a comprehensive review (1986-2007). Surv Ophthalmol. 2008;53(5):443-78.
4. Chan CK, Wessels IF. Delayed subretinal fluid absorption after pneumatic retinopexy. Ophthalmology. 1989;96:1691-700.
5. Grizzard WS, Hilton GF, Hammer ME, et al. Pneumatic retinopexy failures. Cause, prevention, timing, and management. Ophthalmology. 1995;102(6):929-36.
6. Hilton GF, Kelly NE, Salzano TC, et al. Pneumatic retinopexy. A collaborative report of the first 100 cases. Ophthalmology. 1987;94(4):307-14.
7. Hilton GF, Tornambe PE, Brinton DA, et al. The complication of pneumatic retinopexy. Trans Am Ophthalmol Soc. 1990;88:191-207; discussion -10.
8. Tornambe PE. Pneumatic retinopexy: the evolution of case selection and surgical technique. A twelve-year study of 302 eyes. Trans Am Ophthalmol Soc. 1997;95:551-78.
9. Tornambe PE, Hilton GF. Scleral buckling versus pneumatic retinopexy. Ophthalmology. 1992;99(11):1642-3.
10. Tornambe PE, Hilton GF, Brinton DA, et al. Pneumatic retinopexy. A two-year follow-up study of the multicenter clinical trial comparing pneumatic retinopexy with scleral buckling. Ophthalmology. 1991;98(7):1115-23.
11. Tornambe PE, Hilton GF, Kelly NF, et al. Expanded indications for pneumatic retinopexy. Ophthalmology. 1988;95(5):597-600.
12. Tornambe PE, Poliner LS, Hilton GF, et al. Comparison of pneumatic retinopexy and scleral buckling in the management of primary rhegmatogenous retinal detachment. Am J Ophthalmol. 1999;127(6):741-3.
13. Irvine AR, Lahey JM. Pneumatic retinopexy for giant retinal tears. Ophthalmology. 1994;101(3):524-8.
14. Ambler JS, Meyers SM, Zegarra H, et al. Reoperations and visual results after failed pneumatic retinopexy. Ophthalmology, 1990;97(6):786-90.
15. Landers MB, 3rd, Robinson D, Olsen KR, et al. Slit-lamp fluid-gas exchange and other office procedures following vitreoretinal surgery. Arch Ophthalmol. 1985 ;103(7):967-72.

CHAPTER

26

# Pars Plana Vitrectomy for Rhegmatogenous Retinal Detachment

Christopher J Brady, Richard S Kaiser

## INTRODUCTION

Pars plana vitrectomy (PPV), in addition to scleral buckling (SB) procedures and pneumatic retinopexy, is one of the three principal options for the repair of rhegmatogenous retinal detachment (RRD). Choosing the ideal procedure for a particular patient with their specific retinal detachment is a complex decision that varies from surgeon to surgeon. However, PPV, either alone or combined with SB, is the most common method of RRD repair for many surgeons. Instrumentation and techniques continue to evolve, making PPV safer and more effective for the treatment of RRD. Some surgeons choose vitrectomy as the first-line surgical procedure in lieu of SB, which had been the mainstay treatment of RRD for several decades.

## INDICATIONS

Indications for performing vitrectomy for RRD repair are widely debated. Some surgeons have adopted vitrectomy for virtually all retinal detachments. Others still advocate scleral buckles as the treatment of choice, reserving vitrectomy for reoperations and surgical complications such as proliferative vitreoretinopathy (PVR). A moderate approach suggests that PPV is more effective compared with SB for the treatment of RRD in pseudophakic eyes with superior retinal breaks and detachment (Figs. 26-1 and 26-2).[1-3] Other reports suggest that vitrectomy should be combined with a scleral buckle for complex detachments, or in eyes at high-risk recurrent detachment.[4]

Surgical advances have broadened the indications for primary PPV to repair RRD. Wide-field viewing systems, small-gauge vitrectomy systems, and instrumentation as well as high-quality endoillumination have improved the ability to repair these detachments. In contrast to SB during which some subretinal fluid was expected to be present at the end of the surgery, intraoperative surgical adjuvants during PPV such as perfluorocarbon liquid (PFCL) have made intraoperative reattachment of the retina possible and have increased the ability to repair complicated detachments such as those associated with a giant retinal tear. Intraocular tamponade agent such as sulfur hexafluoride ($SF_6$) and longer-acting octofluoropropane ($C_3F_8$) gas and silicone oil have also played a role in improving outcomes of vitrectomy for RD repair. In reality, almost any RD can be treated with vitrectomy but the art of repairing retinal detachments still involves considering all available treatments when assessing the particular features of a detachment.

## CONTRAINDICATIONS

Patients medically unfit for anesthesia are poor candidates for PPV. In these cases, an office-based procedure may be possible in some cases. Although other than medical health-related issues there are no contraindications for PPV, it may not always be the best option. There is no substitute for surgical experience in making this decision.

## SURGICAL TECHNIQUE

The basics of PPV and SB are covered more extensively in other chapters. Briefly, self-retaining cannulae are inserted in the pars plana, 3.5 mm posterior to the limbus for pseudophakic and aphakic patients and 4.0 mm for phakic patients, using a biplanar approach to create a wound that is more likely to be self-sealing. The technique for creating the surgical wounds is critical to prevent postoperative complications such as hypotony and theoretically to reduce

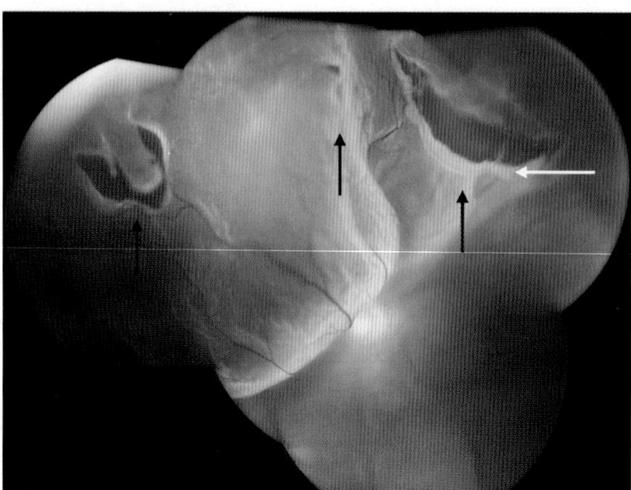

Figure 26-1 Macula-involving rhegmatogenous retinal detachment (RRD). Note the presence of three retinal tears (black arrows). The retinal tears also exhibit rolling of the edges (white arrow) consistent with Grade B proliferative vitreoretinopathy (PVR). Due to the posterior location of the tears and the presence of PVR, this RRD is a good candidate for pars plana vitrectomy.

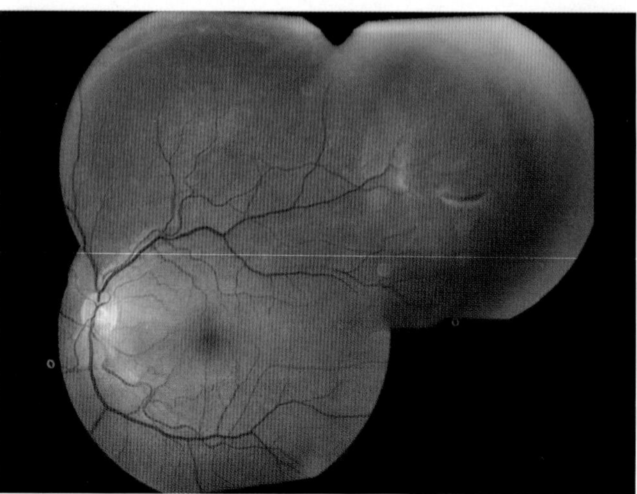

Figure 26-2 Macula-sparing rhegmatogenous retinal detachment with a single tear in the superotemporal quadrant. The posterior location of this tear makes pars plana vitrectomy a reasonable option for repair.

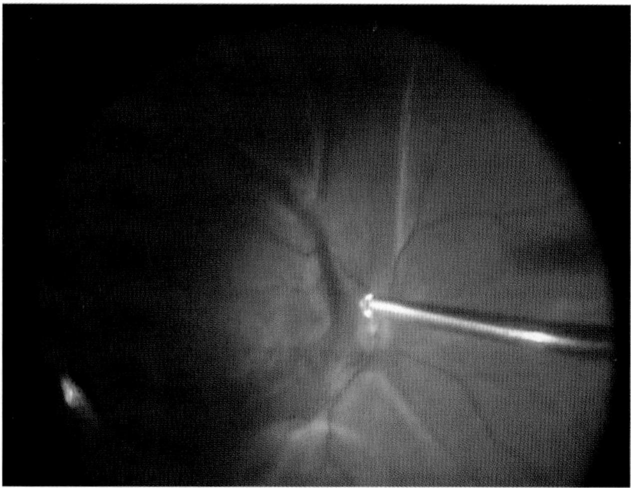

Figure 26-3 A total retinal detachment without significant proliferative vitreoretinopathy is noted in this intraoperative photograph.

the risk of endophthalmitis. An infusion cannula is placed in the inferotemporal quadrant, and placement in the vitreous cavity is confirmed by direct visualization prior to opening the infusion valve. It should be noted that cannula placement can be difficult in eyes with a bullous detachment as well as in cases of severe PVR such as a funnel detachment. The remaining two cannulae are general placed immediately superior to the horizontal meridian.

The illuminating light pipe and vitrectomy probe are inserted through the cannulae into the anterior/mid-vitreous cavity (Fig. 26-3). The retinal detachment is inspected carefully to note the configuration of the detachment, macular status, and location of retinal breaks. The vitrectomy is started peripherally on low vacuum. After clearing vitreous from around the vitrectomy port, check for the presence of a posterior vitreous detachment (PVD). If a PVD is not present, it should be created. Usually the vitrectomy probe set to suction works well, but an extrusion cannula, a pick, or a suction pick is useful when the vitreous is more adherent to the retina. Insuring complete separation of the posterior hyaloid face from the retina out to the posterior vitreous base is a crucial step in RRD repair. Visualization of the posterior hyaloid may be enhanced by instilling triamcinolone into the eye. Once a PVD is induced, the bulk of the vitreous is removed. Particular attention is paid to the anterior vitreous to ensure that all vitreous traction on retinal breaks is relieved (Fig. 26-4). This peripheral gel removal or "shaving the vitreous base" is facilitated by scleral depression, by changing the settings of the vitrectomy machine to allow for a higher cut rate and lower suction rate to minimize traction on the retina, and by the use of PFCL (Fig. 26-5). Relief of vitreous traction is the critical step for this portion of the procedure. The flaps of retinal tears may be amputated, and the breaks may be extended anteriorly to allow for more efficient drainage of subretinal fluid.

After completing the vitrectomy, the remaining subretinal fluid needs may be addressed. There are several general approaches. The first involves the injection of PFCL, a heavier than water liquid, into the eye (Fig. 26-6). The PFCL then flattens the retina in a posterior-to-anterior direction and "pushes" subretinal fluid through the peripheral break. PFCL allows stabilization of the peripheral retina, affords a good

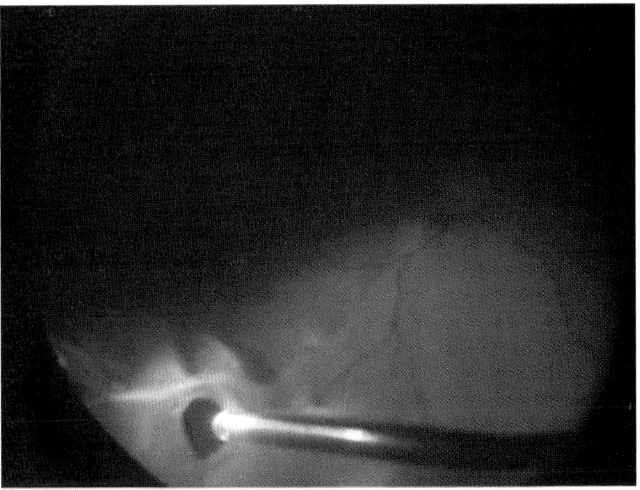

Figure 26-4 All vitreous traction must be relieved in the area of the causative retinal break. The flap of a horseshoe tear is amputated if present. Some amount of subretinal fluid may often be drained at this stage.

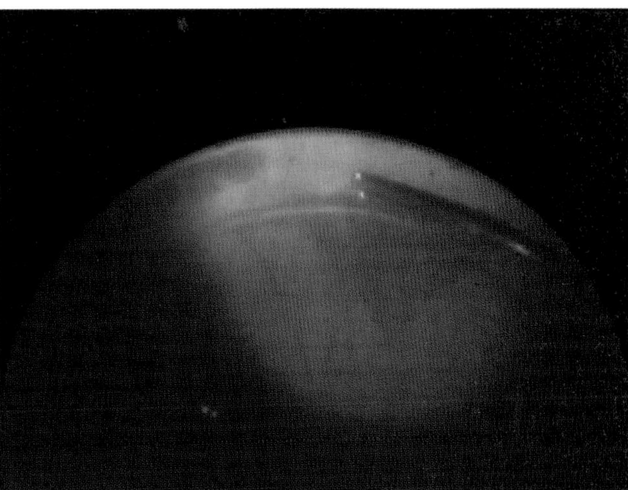

Figure 26-5 Peripheral gel removal is facilitated in this case by the instillation of perfluorocarbon liquid (PFCL) that creates an easily visualized vitreous "cushion". Additionally, the PFCL provides countertraction on the retina.

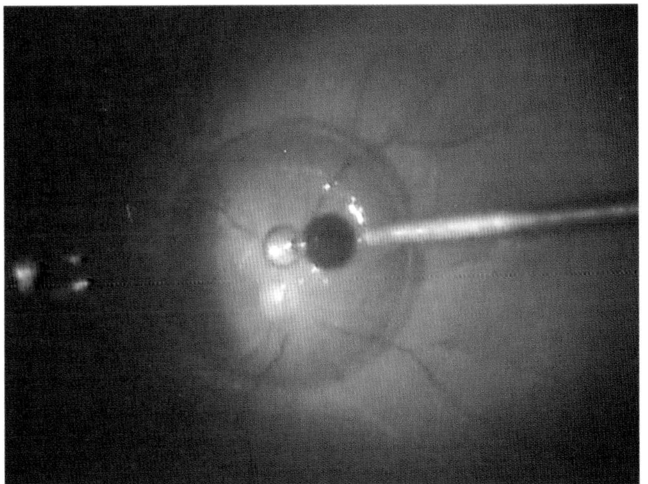

Figure 26-6 Perfluorocarbon liquid is injected over the posterior pole, over attached retina. Care is taken to ensure a single bubble is injected.

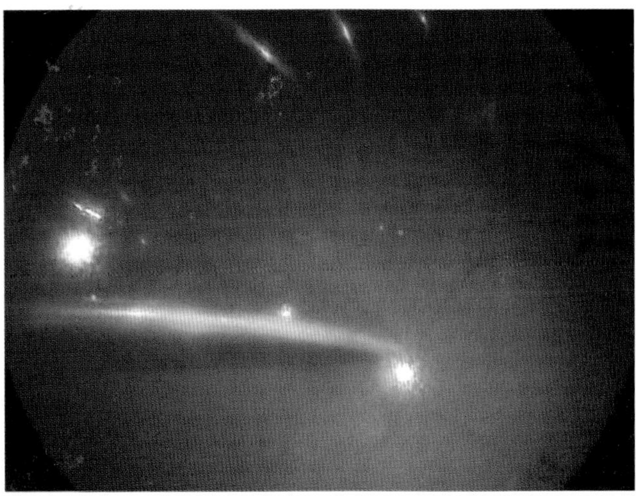

Figure 26-7 The final stages of fluid–air exchange are completed over the optic nerve head. The reflection below the soft silastic tip of the extrusion cannula is indicative of a fluid meniscus. Care must be taken to remove all perfluorocarbon liquid.

peripheral view that facilitates laser placement, and avoids making an iatrogenic hole. After performing laser, the fluid–air exchange is performed (Fig. 26-7). The second method is to create a posterior drainage retinotomy (a small hole in the retina) followed by fluid–air exchange, which flattens the retina in an anterior-to-posterior direction and permits drainage of the subretinal fluid at the dependent location at the retinotomy site. The benefit of this technique is that it avoids the expense of PFCL, and avoids complications of PFCL including retained and subretinal PFCL (*see* Figures 26-15 and 26-16). In some cases, such as with a localized superior RRD, the subretinal fluid can be left as the retinal pigment epithelium (RPE) will pump it out. Deciding which technique to utilize varies among surgeons and should be based on retinal anatomy.

Once the retina is flattened, endolaser is used to barricade the retinal breaks (Fig. 26-8). The laser energy is absorbed by the RPE, creating whitening of the retina and a focal adhesion. This adhesion becomes stronger over the following 5–10 days. There are several tamponade agents available. Air is an option. During the first 5–7 days of the postoperative period, the air will be absorbed and replaced with aqueous fluid. Air provides short-term tamponade superiorly but only fleeting tamponade for inferior retinal pathology. Other options

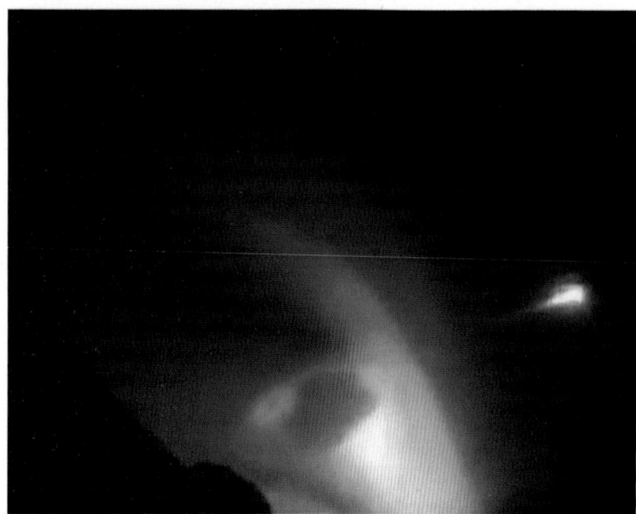

Figure 26-8 An endolaser probe is used to treat the causative break. The surgeon can perform scleral depression him or herself with an illuminated laser.

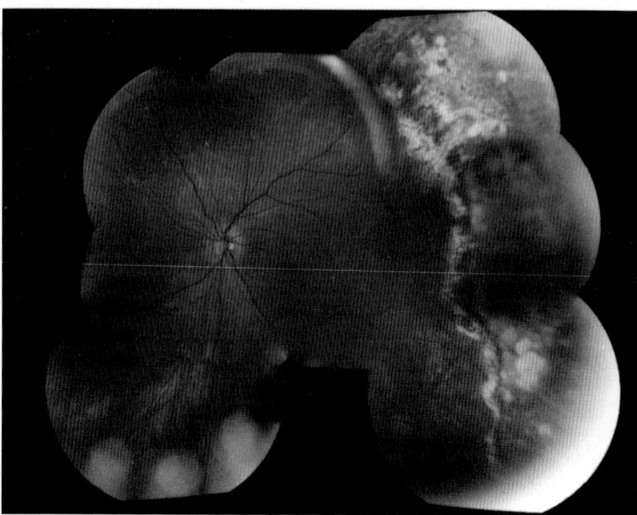

Figure 26-9 Photomontage of patient who underwent successful retinal detachment repair. Incidental note is made of slight macular translocation.

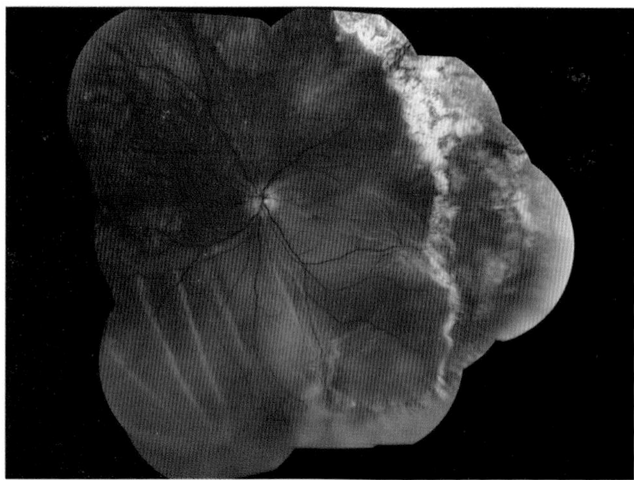

Figure 26-10 Photomontage of the patient in Figure 26-9 who presented with proliferative vitreoretinopathy redetachment.

for vitreous tamponade include inert gases that persist for longer durations. The two most commonly used gases are $SF_6$ and $C_3F_8$. $SF_6$ lasts for approximately 2 weeks, while $C_3F_8$ lasts for approximately 2 months. Each is generally used at nonexpansile concentrations (approximately 20% $SF_6$ and 14% $C_3F_8$) to minimize intraocular pressure rises. The choice of which gas to use depends on the length of desired tamponade. The gases are mixed with sterile air in the operating room to achieve the desired concentration. Silicone oil is the longest-lasting tamponade. The advantages of oil are that patients can fly with it in place, they have some vision through it, and it helps to contain a retinal redetachment. However, it remains in place until surgically removed.

The cannulae are then removed and assessed for leakage. Any leaking sclerotomies are closed with dissolvable suture. Ophthalmic ointment is instilled into the eye, which is then patched and shielded in the usual fashion.

## COMBINED SCLERAL BUCKLE PPV

If the decision to perform combined SB is made, typically the scleral buckle is placed before starting the vitrectomy. The advantage of a combined procedure is that the SB provides permanent support of the vitreous base, while the vitrectomy enables direct treatment of the specific breaks causing the retinal detachment. For RRDs with high-risk features including hemorrhage, early PVR, associated with trauma and three or more quadrants of retinal detachment, a combination of a scleral buckle with a vitrectomy has been shown to have a higher success rate than vitrectomy alone.

## PROLIFERATIVE VITREORETINOPATHY

PVR is the most common cause of recurrent RD. It has been implicated in up to 75% of redetachments, and may occur in 5–10% of all RRDs.[5] PVR is the formation of preretinal cellular membranes that subsequently contract (Figs. 26-9 to 26-12). This tractional force on the retina can cause either a rhegmatogenous or tractional retinal detachment. The formation of PVR is not completely understood, but is thought to be analogous to the anomalous wound healing that leads to skin keloid formation. The most important cell type in PVR pathogenesis are the RPE cells, which are believed

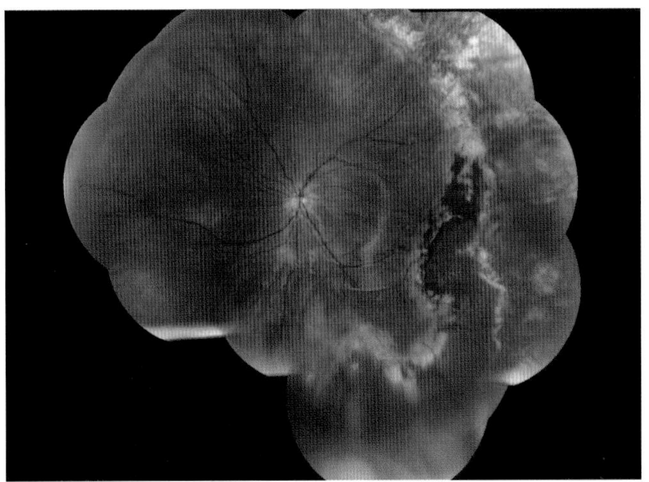

Figure 26-11 Immediate postoperative photomontage of the patient in Figure 26-9. Note the mild hemorrhage at the edge of the retinectomy.

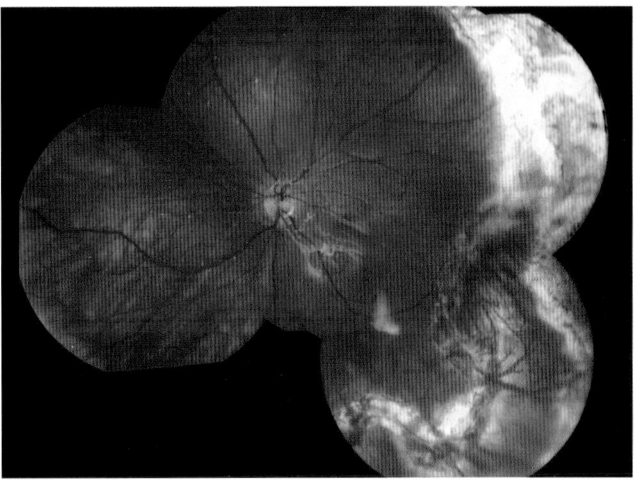

Figure 26-12 Photomontage several months after Figure 26.11 was taken. The retina is flat without recurrence of proliferative vitreoretinopathy, and silicone oil remains in the vitreous cavity.

to dedifferentiate and migrate through the retinal break and proliferate on the retinal surface. This process is driven and modulated by numerous growth factors [e.g. platelet-derived growth factor (PDGF), vascular endothelial growth factor (VEGF), tumor growth factor-beta (TGF-$\beta$), epidermal growth factor (EGF), tumor necrosis factor-alpha (TNF-$\alpha$), TNF-$\beta$, fibroblast growth factor (FGF)] and cytokines [interleukin-1 (IL-1), IL-6, IL-8, IL-10, and interferon-gamma (INF-$\gamma$)], which have been and continue to be explored as potential targets for pharmacologic prevention and treatment.[5]

The overall surgical approach for PVR is generally the same for primary retinal detachments without membranes. The principal difference is that there is significantly more retinal traction in PVR, which is caused by membranes and bands rather than vitreous gel alone. As such, additional techniques may be employed to dissect these membranes and allow the retina to flatten. Additionally, if a SB was not used at the time of the primary retinal detachment repair, it can be advantageous to place one during the PVR vitrectomy procedure. However, if an extensive inferior retinectomy is likely to be performed, a SB is likely not needed.

The primary surgical goal in PVR surgery is to remove the membranes off the retina surface and from beneath the retina (if necessary). Various forceps may be used to help remove tractional membranes. When these membranes cannot be dissected fully off the retina, the vitrectomy probe or pneumatically actuated scissors may be used to segment membranes to relieve tractional forces. If membranes are not able to be safely removed, or there is significant intrinsic thickening of the neurosensory retina itself, relaxing retinectomy may be considered. The endodiathermy instrument is used to demarcate the posterior boundary of retina to be removed, as well as to cauterize any vessels traversing the area. The retina anterior to this line is removed with the vitrectomy probe. In general if retinectomy is considered, anticipate removing 120° or more of the (usually inferior) retina. Retinectomies smaller than this size may not relieve traction sufficiently to allow the retina to flatten.

In PVR it is advantageous to use bimanual surgical techniques to manipulate the retina and associated membranes (i.e. forceps in one hand and a pick or scissors in the other hand). In order to do this, alternate forms of illumination, such as a lighted pick or chandelier, can be utilized. To use a chandelier, a fourth sclerotomy may be created inferiorly with a self-retaining illumination system. Illuminated infusion lines are also available. Lighted picks allow for semi-sharp dissection as well as endoillumination.

There are a few frequently repeated patterns of PVR. A severe form of PVR known as "anterior loop" is fairly common. With anterior loop traction, proliferation causes contraction on the vitreous that pulls the anterior retina toward the ciliary body. This can be released by relieving this traction with the vitrectomy probe or scissors, or to perform a retinectomy. In either case this anterior–posterior traction must be relieved in addition to treating the posterior disease. Thorough dissection of anterior membranes may require removal of the crystalline lens in phakic individuals.

Another common manifestation of PVR includes contracted preretinal membranes or "star-folds" that may cause stretch holes in the retina. If causing significant traction, these may be removed with forceps. Subretinal bands may also be removed with forceps, either through a pre-existing retinal break or through a small retinotomy.

After retinectomy, hemostasis is achieved with diathermy, the retina is flattened with either PFCL or air, and approximately three to four rows of near confluent laser photocoagulation is applied to the edge of the tear/retinectomy/retinotomy. For PVR cases, either $C_3F_8$ or silicone oil is instilled. Both tamponades are injected under high pressure, and another sclerotomy needs to be open to vent the eye. For all tamponades, particularly silicone oil, take care to avoid overfilling the eye. The oil may be injected under direct visualization or through a viewing system. When silicone oil is used, all sclerotomies are generally sutured.

## MECHANISM OF ACTION

*A RRD has three predisposing factors*: A retinal break, vitreous traction, and liquefied vitreous gel. Both SB and PPV address all three factors but through different mechanisms.

Laser photocoagulation is used to seal off causative retinal breaks, drainage retinotomies, and relaxing retinectomies, and works by creating an adhesion between the RPE and neurosensory retina. The laser light is absorbed by RPE and creates an inflammatory photochemical reaction that reaches peak strength within several days.

Intravitreal gas or silicone oil works through higher buoyancy and surface tension than aqueous fluid. With appropriate head positioning, as discussed below, the intravitreal bubble holds the retina in place, prevents aqueous fluid from entering the retinal breaks, and allows time for the chorioretinal adhesion to form.

## POSTOPERATIVE CARE

Postoperative head positioning plays an important role. Keeping the head in a certain position allows the intravitreal tamponade to maintain the most contact with the causative retinal break or breaks for 4–7 days allowing the laser adhesion time to strengthen. For example, a retinal detachment in the right eye caused by a temporal horseshoe tear would be best supported by maintaining the patient's left ear toward the ground. For macula involving retinal detachments, patients may be asked to maintain face-down positioning for an initial period of 24–48 hours before assuming a position to support the breaks. Customary postoperative topical therapy (steroid and antibiotic drops) is used. Cycloplegic drops and oral narcotic analgesia may be used for combined scleral buckle PPV procedures.

## SPECIFIC INSTRUMENTATION

Beyond standard instrumentation for PPV including the illuminator and vitrectomy probe, several additional instruments are needed for primary repair of RRD. These included a laser probe that may include its own illumination, endodiathermy probe, and soft-tipped extrusion cannula. PFCL may also be needed.

For the repair of PVR-RRD, an additional illumination system such as the chandelier may be needed. Retinal picks, with or without endoillumination, one or more type of small-gauge forceps, and scissors will all help in the complex dissection of retinal membranes. Such instruments permit what is known as bimanual surgery, with both hands controlling instruments capable of manipulating the retina or associated membranes. Additionally silicone oil or intravitreal gas tamponade and associated supplies for injection may be required.

## COMPLICATIONS

The main intraoperative complications seen with PPV for RRD include retinal tears, crystalline lens damage, and suprachoroidal hemorrhage. Short-term postoperative complications include intraocular pressure rise, hyphema, and vitreous hemorrhage. Late postoperative complications include retinal redetachment and PVR. The conjunctival disruption made by the vitrectomy cannulae can cause adhesions that may make glaucoma surgeries more difficult. In all phakic patients, PPV will accelerate cataract formation. Endophthalmitis is a potential rare complication of all intraocular surgery. The rates of endophthalmitis vary depending on the article referenced from the literature but for modern suture-less vitrectomy to repair a retinal detachment with a gas-filled vitreous cavity at the conclusion of the case the rate is approximately 1 in 2000.[6]

Theoretically, removal of the vitreous gel changes the pharmacokinetics of intravitreal medications by shortening the half-life of many medications. This may prove important as patients age and may need treatment of age-related macular degeneration, diabetic retinopathy, retinal vein occlusion, or other conditions.

## SURGICAL OUTCOMES: SCIENTIFIC EVIDENCE/META-ANALYSIS

There is a paucity of Level 1 evidence to guide the choice of intervention for RRD. The best-quality evidence comes from two recent systematic reviews and meta-analyses by Sun et al.[1] and by Soni et al.[7] In the study by Sun et al., three trials of phakic subjects ($n$ = 523) and four trials of pseudophakic or aphakic subjects ($n$ = 690) were analyzed. For phakic individuals, final visual success was better in the SB group (88.6%) compared with PPV (79.6). For pseudophakic and aphakic individuals, the primary anatomic success was higher with PPV (78.2%) compared with SB (68.8%), although this was not statistically significant due to heterogeneity. However, final anatomic success was significantly better in the PPV group for pseudophakic/aphakic individuals in their meta-analysis.

In contrast, the larger study by Soni et al. included seven randomized, controlled trials including 1306 eyes comparing PPV versus SB for uncomplicated RRD. There was no difference in primary reattachment rates between groups in phakic eyes (68.1% PPV; 68.1% SB). Eyes treated with SB had better best-corrected visual acuity at 6 months, perhaps attributable to cataract progression in the PPV group. There was no difference in vision between groups in pseudophakic or aphakic eyes.

A particularly large trial included in both meta-analyses was the European Scleral Buckling versus Primary Vitrectomy in Rhegmatogenous Retinal Detachment Study.[8] This individual study showed a visual acuity benefit for SB in phakic eyes.There was an anatomic benefit favoring PPV in pseudophakic and aphakic eyes, and PPV so was recommended by the authors for pseudophakic RRDs, despite the lack of a visual acuity benefit.

Two large, global, retrospective analyses explored outcomes of repair of uncomplicated (4179 patients)[2] and complicated (3499 patients)[9] RRDs. For uncomplicated RRD in phakic eyes, SB had a higher primary reattachment rate compared with PPV. In pseudophakic eyes, PPV was superior to SB alone. Combined PPV-SB had a lower primary reattachment rate than PPV alone. For complicated RRD, PPV was the procedure of choice. There was no additional benefit from combining SB with PPV in these eyes. This is in contrast to other smaller series that have shown a benefit to combining SB with PPV in high-risk eyes.[4] For eyes with RRDs with PVR the Silicone Oil Study[10] and subsequent series found tamponade with either silicone oil or $C_3F_8$ to be superior to $SF_6$.

A additional retrospective review of 152 sequential pseudophakic patients with uncomplicated RRD receiving PPV or combined PPV-SB at a single institution[11] showed no significant differences in primary reattachment rate (92.6% PPV; 94.0% PPV-SB), visual acuity, or complication rates. An interesting retrospective review of macula-off RRD comparing macular structure by spectral domain optical-coherence tomography (OCT)[12] suggested longer persistence of subretinal fluid in the macula after SB, which the authors concluded might lead to delayed recovery in this group.

## PLACE OF THE TECHNIQUE IN SURGICAL ARMAMENTARIUM

PPV is among the primary treatments of RRD, and with the parallel refinements in small-gauge sutureless instrumentation and high cut-rate vitrectomy machine engineering, is often the technique of choice for RD repair. Patient comfort has been enhanced with small-gauge instruments and surgeon efficiency has increased with modern vitrectomy machines. PFCLs have allowed surgeons to dramatically improve success rates for complex retinal detachments such as those caused by giant retinal tears (Fig. 26-13), which are outside the scope of this chapter. Many detachments are still best treated by pneumatic retinopexy or SB, but modern PPV has allowed surgeons to approach the majority of retinal detachments and has improved surgical outcomes.

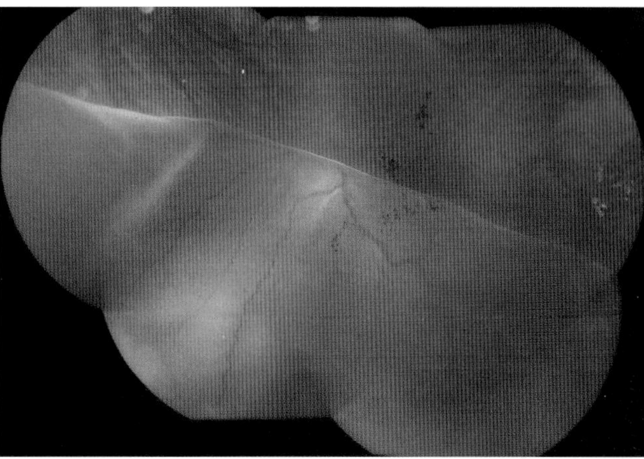

Figure 26-13 Retinal detachment caused by a giant retinal tear. Note the bare retinal pigment epithelium in the top of the photo and exposed outer retina in the bottom of the photo. This patient was treated with pars plana vitrectomy using perfluorocarbon liquid and long-term silicone oil tamponade.

## PEARLS AND PITFALLS

- Meticulous inspection of the retina preoperatively is critical to develop an operative plan.
- Proper wound construction is important to avoid patent wounds postoperatively that lead to hypotony, choroidal detachments, and possible infection.
- Visualization of the infusion cannula before turning it on is a crucial step in order to avoid choroidal or subretinal infusion.
- Care must be taken to drain all infusion fluid and subretinal fluid prior to removing the PFCL to prevent trapping and posterior migration of subretinal fluid by the air as it enters the vitreous cavity.
- Perfluorocarbon must also be removed carefully to avoid droplets from migrating under the retina—particularly under the macula/fovea (Figs. 26-14 to 26-16).
- Take care to avoid inadvertent pure (expansile) inert gas infusion.

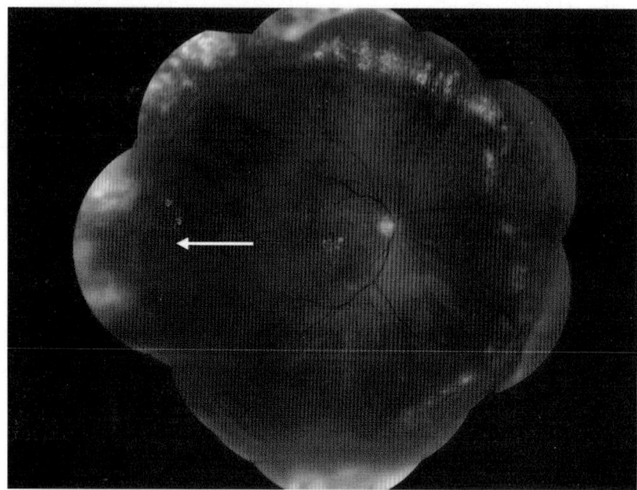

Figure 26-14 Post-operative photomontage of a patient who underwent combined pars plana vitrectomy-scleral buckling. Note the encircling band indenting the retina (white arrow) for 360°.

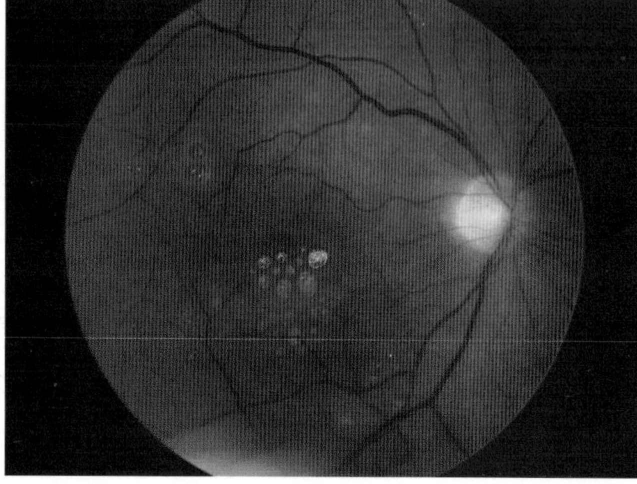

Figure 26-15 The posterior pole image of the patient in Figure 26.14 reveals several circular subretinal bubbles consistent with perfluorocarbon liquid.

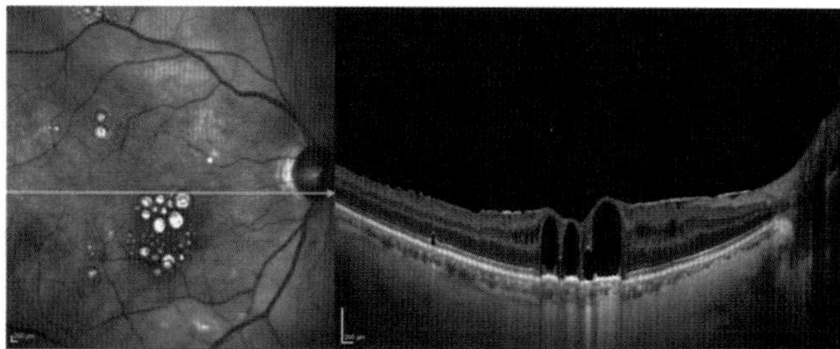

Figure 26-16 Corresponding enhanced depth optical coherence tomography of the patient in Figure 26-14 with subretinal perfluorocarbon liquid. A mild epiretinal membrane is also noted.

## REFERENCES


1. Sun Q, Sun T, Xu Y, et al. Primary vitrectomy versus scleral buckling for the treatment of rhegmatogenous retinal detachment: a meta-analysis of randomized controlled clinical trials. Curr Eye Res. 2012;37(6):492-9. .
2. Adelman RA, Parnes AJ, Ducournau D. Strategy for the management of uncomplicated retinal detachments: the European Vitreo-Retinal Society Retinal Detachment Study Report 1. Ophthalmology. 2013;120(9):1804-8.
3. Schwartz SG, Flynn HW, Jr., Mieler WF. Update on retinal detachment surgery. Curr Opin Ophthalmol. 2013;24(3):255-61.
4. Alexander P, Ang A, Poulson A, et al. Scleral buckling combined with vitrectomy for the management of rhegmatogenous retinal detachment associated with inferior retinal breaks. Eye (Lond). 2008;22:200-3.
5. Sadaka A, Giuliari GP. Proliferative vitreoretinopathy: current and emerging treatments. Clin Ophthalmol. 2012;6:1325-33.
6. Chiang A, Kaiser RS, Avery RL, et al. Endophthalmitis in microincision vitrectomy: outcomes of gas-filled eyes. Retina. 2011;31(8):1513-7.
7. Soni C, Hainsworth DP, Almony A. Surgical management of rhegmatogenous retinal detachment: a meta-analysis of randomized controlled trials. Ophthalmology 2013;120(7):1440-7.
8. Heimann H, Bartz-Schmidt KU, Bornfeld N, et al. Scleral buckling versus primary vitrectomy in rhegmatogenous retinal detachment: a prospective randomized multicenter clinical study. Ophthalmology. 2007;114(12):2142-54.
9. Adelman RA, Parnes AJ, Sipperley JO, et al. Strategy for the management of complex retinal detachments: the European Vitreo-Retinal Society Retinal Detachment Study Report 2. Ophthalmology. 2013;120(9):1809-13.
10. Abrams GW, Azen SP, McCuen BW, 2nd, et al. Vitrectomy with silicone oil or long-acting gas in eyes with severe proliferative vitreoretinopathy: results of additional and long-term follow-up. Silicone Study report 11. Arch Ophthalmol. 1997; 115(3):335-44.
11. Weichel ED, Martidis A, Fineman MS, et al. Pars plana vitrectomy versus combined pars plana vitrectomy-scleral buckle for primary repair of pseudophakic retinal detachment. Ophthalmology. 2006;113(11):2033-40.
12. Huang C, Fu T, Zhang T, et al. Scleral buckling versus vitrectomy for macula-off rhegmatogenous retinal detachment as accessed with spectral-domain optical coherence tomography: a retrospective observational case series. BMC Ophthalmol. doi: 10.1186/1471-2415-13-12.

CHAPTER

27

# Surgery for Submacular Hemorrhage due to Neovascular Age-related Macular Degeneration

Christopher J Brady, Carl D Regillo

## INTRODUCTION

Hemorrhage under the macula is one of the dreaded manifestations of neovascular age-related macular degeneration (AMD) (Fig. 27-1). Natural history studies have shown that a large submacular hemorrhage (SMH) portends a very poor prognosis, with most patients presenting with poor vision, and then worsening in up to 80% of cases without treatment.[1] Subretinal blood products cause disruption of retinal pigment epithelial (RPE) cell and photoreceptor interaction causes a dense scotoma. If not cleared, blood breakdown products, including fibrin, can be toxic to both RPE and retinal tissue.[2] In addition, formation of a fibrin clot can provide the scaffold for disciform scar formation with subsequent retraction. Despite the recent therapeutic advances of targeted therapies against vascular endothelial growth factor (VEGF), the optimal management of SMH associated with AMD is poorly defined.[3,4] This is due, in part, to the fact that patients with larger SMH were excluded from the major pivotal AMD trials testing various anti-VEGF therapeutics. The Submacular Surgery Trials (SST)[5] provide some information on the management of this condition. In one trial, surgery to remove the choroidal neovascular (CNV) complex in conjunction with evacuation of the hemorrhage prevented severe vision loss compared with observation, although it did not stabilize or improve vision. Further guidance is limited to smaller, uncontrolled published series.[6]

## INDICATIONS

The decision to manage AMD-related SMH with a hemorrhage displacement procedure (in addition to anti-VEGF therapy) is based mainly on the location, size, and thickness of hemorrhage. In the authors' opinion, patients with small, thin SMH, especially if the blood is mostly outside the foveal center, are best managed by medical therapy (anti-VEGF) alone (Figs. 27-2A and B). Patients with larger hemorrhages (> 6 disk areas) that are relatively thick and centered in the macula may be considered for a pneumatic displacement procedure, especially if the hemorrhage is < 3 weeks in duration and if the patient had reasonably good vision before the hemorrhage (Figs. 27-3 to 27-5). Displacing a SMH can be done in the office with an intravitreal injection of an expansile gas [with or without an intravitreal injection of tissue plasminogen activator (tPA)] or in the operating room with

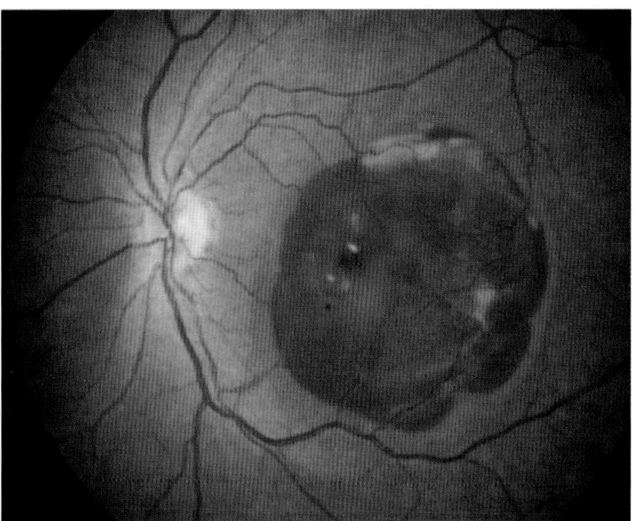

Figure 27-1 Submacular hemorrhage due to neovascular age-related macular degeneration. This patient is likely a good candidate for pars plana vitrectomy and subretinal tissue plasminogen activator.

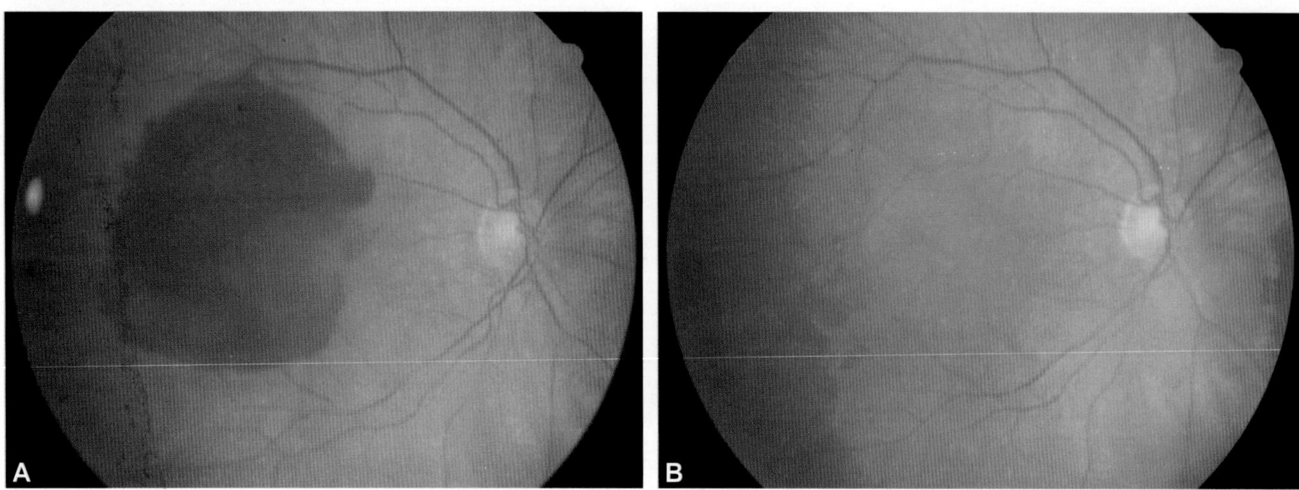


Figures 27-2A and B Due to the eccentric nature of the submacular hemorrhage, this case was managed with intravitreal antivascular endothelial growth factor (VEGF) alone. (A) At diagnosis the vision was 20/200. (B) The final vision was 20/30 after 16 months of anti-VEGF therapy without any displacement.

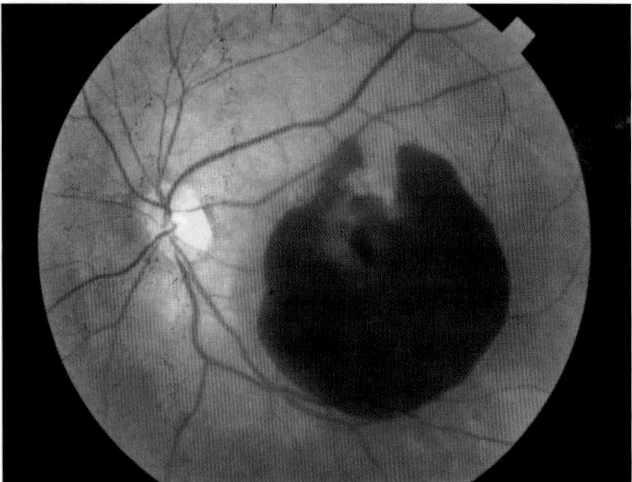

Figure 27-3 Submacular hemorrhage due to age-related macular degeneration prior to pars plana vitrectomy and subretinal tissue plasminogen activator (case A).

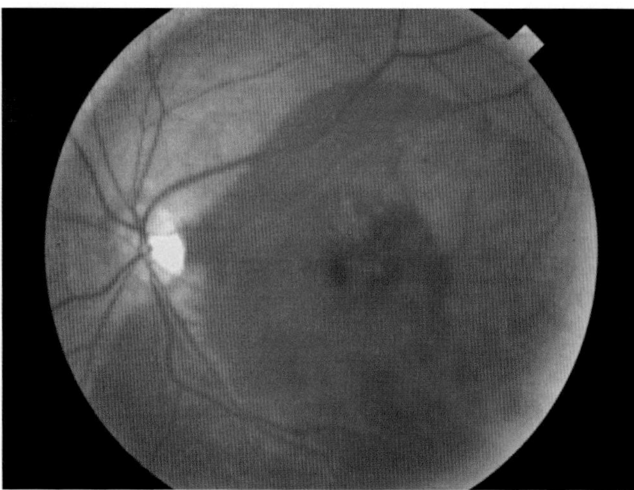

Figure 27-4 Case A shortly after vitrectomy and subretinal tissue plasminogen activator. Note the more diffuse blood extending outside the retinal arcades.

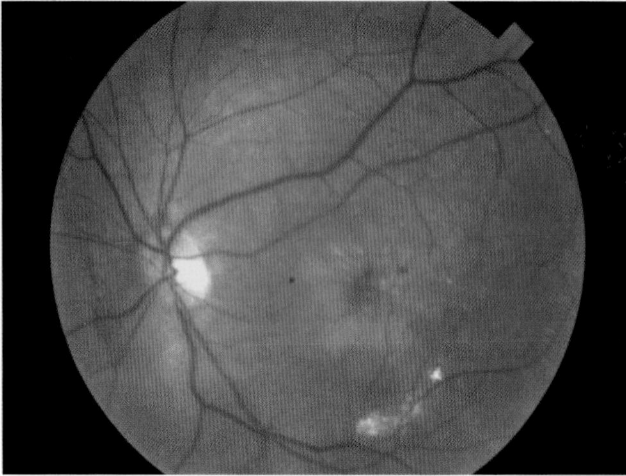

Figure 27-5 Case A several months after pars plana vitrectomy and subretinal tissue plasminogen activator. Note the neovascular complex temporal to the fovea.

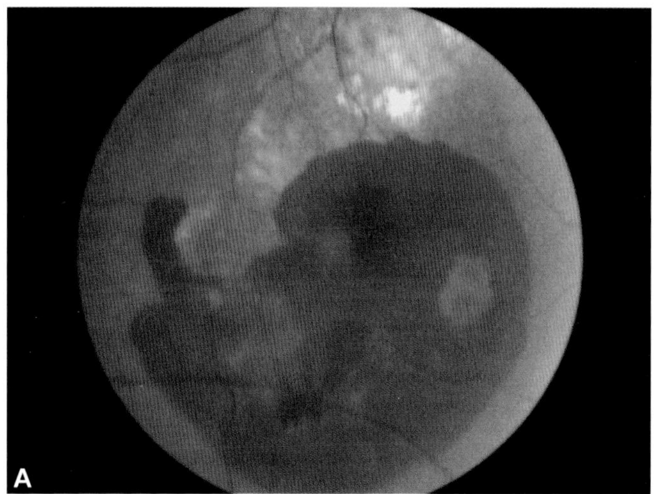


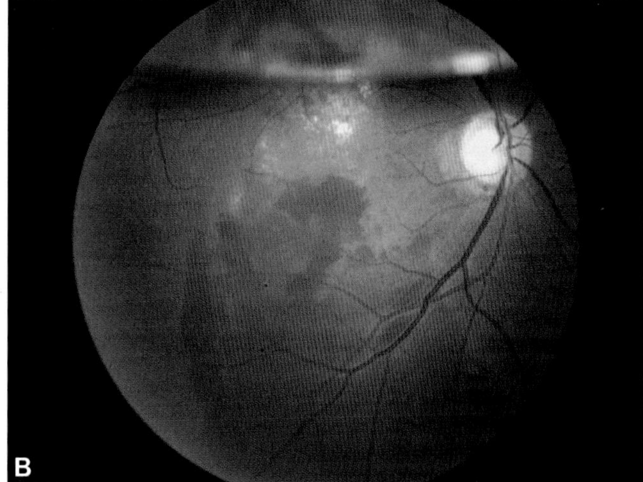


Figures 27-6A and B (A) Pre-pars plana vitrectomy (PPV), the vision was 20/300. (B) Post-PPV, the final vision was 20/50. Not the gas bubble superiorly in the frame.

a pars plana vitrectomy (PPV), subretinal tPA injection, and fluid–gas exchange.[6,7] In the authors' experience, the surgical approach produces a more reliable, complete displacement of the SMH away from the macula, and usually is the preferred technique.

## CONTRAINDICATIONS

Known poor vision prior to SMH development is a relative contraindication to surgical intervention. Patients with massive subretinal hemorrhage, such as hemorrhages that extend significantly into the peripheral retina, are not good candidates for hemorrhage displacement. Individuals with severe or uncontrolled systemic conditions may not be good surgical candidates.

## SURGICAL TECHNIQUE

If the decision is made to proceed with surgery, perioperative anti-VEGF therapy should be considered. Briefly, small-incision PPV (23- or 25-gauge) with valved cannulae is the authors' current standard procedure. Three self-retaining cannulae are placed in the pars plana 3.5 mm (4.0 mm in phakic eyes) posterior to the limbus. The infusion cannula is placed in the inferotemporal quadrant, and the two remaining cannulae are placed just superior to the horizontal meridian in beveled fashion. The endoilluminator and vitrectomy probe are then used to perform a core vitrectomy using a noncontact wide-field viewing system. The posterior hyaloid is separated from the posterior pole if there is not a pre-existing posterior vitreous detachment. Injection of triamcinolone suspension into the vitreous cavity can enhance visualization of the posterior hyaloid.

To facilitate creation of a self-sealing retinotomy, a 39- or 41- gauge needle is used to inject tPA (25 or 50 mg/0.1 mL) directly into the SMH. To ensure a good postoperative displacement, create a generous bleb of subretinal fluid that extends beyond the borders of the SMH, particularly inferiorly. (With the displacement approach, there is no attempt to evacuate the subretinal blood directly or remove the neovascular complex). The peripheral retina is inspected carefully for any retinal breaks. A 75–80% fluid–air exchange is then performed. The air may, in turn, be exchanged with 20% $SF_6$ gas if a longer lasting tamponade is desired (Figs. 27-6A and B). The cannulae are removed and assessed for leakage, and can be sutured. A subconjunctival antibiotic injection given after closure is complete. Ophthalmic antibiotic–steroid ointment is instilled into the eye, which is then patched and shielded.

### Variations in Technique

Surgeons have reported numerous variations in the technique reported above. Some are of historic interest, but are illustrative of the evolution of the management of this condition. Initially surgeons attempted mechanical drainage of the SMH/CNV complex.[5] This technique required creation of a large posterior retinotomy and aspiration of the clot. The entire choroidal neovascularization (CNV) complex was then grasped with submacular forceps and removed through the retinotomy. The complex was sometimes segmented if too large to be removed en bloc. The retinotomy was sealed with endolaser photocoagulation only if larger than 1 disk diameter. This technique was initially developed prior to the introduction of subretinal tPA, but it was permitted to be used in the SST, though interestingly its use did not improve results.[4] Other surgeons have reported preoperative intravitreal tPA 24 hours prior to PPV with heavy liquid and peripheral retinotomy to drain the SMH.[4] Surgeons in Japan have described this technique, and the majority of the included population had SMH due to polypoidal choroidal vasculopathy, so their results may not be applicable to all patients with AMD.

There are various techniques of subretinal tPA injection. Some surgeons create an initial subretinal bleb with one or more injections of BSS to dilute the SMH and fully detach the macula followed by injection of concentrated tPA into the bleb. Fluorescein dye can be added to the tPA solution. This allows for better visualization of the tPA to ensure it is injected in the proper location. Some surgeons advocate for intraoperative anti-VEGF therapy, either into the vitreous cavity or subretinally.

## MECHANISM OF ACTION

The two main ways in which the PPV displacement technique for SMH work are pharmacological and mechanical. The tPA is a 70 kDa recombinant human protein that cleaves native plasminogen into plasmin. Plasmin is an enzyme that breaks down fibrin, a principal component of clotted blood, within minutes of direct contact. The molecule is principally used as a thrombolytic in the setting of nonhemorrhagic acute stroke, but is used "off-label" for many purposes throughout medicine. After injection into the subretinal space and enzymatic lysis, the liquefied clot is then amenable to displacement. In SMH, the hemorrhage is located between photoreceptors, so this enzymatic lysis is thought to provide for a gentler reapposition of the neurosensory retina and RPE than a purely mechanical approach.[8]

Molecules that block VEGF are now the standard of care for the treatment of neovascular macular degeneration. VEGF is a cytokine that promotes angiogenesis and permeability of blood vessels. The molecule is thought to promote CNV formation and leads to subretinal and intraretinal fluid accumulation. Currently three selective pan-VEGF inhibitor drugs are available for intravitreal injection. Ranibizumab (Lucentis, Genentech, Inc., South San Francisco, CA), and aflibercept (VEGF Trap-Eye/Eylea injection; Regeneron Pharmaceuticals, Tarrytown, NY) are FDA approved for neovascular AMD. Bevacizumab (Avastin, Genentech, Inc.) is also extensively used "off-label". Pegaptanib (Macugen, Eyetech/Valeant, Mississauga, Canada) was the first anti-VEGF agent available for the treatment of exudative AMD, and is less commonly used than the above-mentioned agents. Each of these medications can lead to the stabilization or regression of the choroidal neovascular complex, and therefore reduce active bleeding into the submacular space.

Vitrectomy plays an important role in the resolution by allowing access to the subretinal space for delivery of tPA that helps dissolve the fibrin clot and the aqueous solvent that helps dilute the blood products. Removal of the vitreous gel allows for a more complex fluid–gas exchange than is possible with an office-based intravitreal gas injection. This allows for a larger and longer lasting gas bubble that, in combination with positioning, exerts direct pressure on the subretinal blood breakdown products leading to inferior displacement outside of the visual axis (Figs. 27-7 and 27-8).

## POSTOPERATIVE CARE

Patients typically are instructed to maintain face-forward positioning for 24–48 hours. Some surgeons recommend face-down positioning, while others do not feel strict positioning is necessary and recommend keeping the head upright. Postoperative topical therapy (steroid and antibiotic drops) is used per surgeon preference.

## SPECIFIC INSTRUMENTATION

Standard PPV instrumentations including the surgeon's choice of gauge of instrumentation and vitrectomy machine are needed for PPV for SMH. An endolaser probe to perform photocoagulation is only necessary if retinal breaks are found.

The principal piece of equipment not used in a standard PPV setup is a 39- or 41-gauge translocation cannula (Fig. 27-9) to inject the tPA under the retina. A small-bore needle is used in order to create a self-sealing retinotomy.

## COMPLICATIONS

Postoperative retinal tears, retinal detachment, and proliferative vitreoretinopathy are potential complications. These complications were more common with older surgical approaches that utilized larger retinotomies to directly evacuate the hemorrhage. Vitreous hemorrhage, macular hole, recurrent SMH, and RPE tear formation have all been reported following PPV with tPA for SMH displacement. PPV accelerates cataract progression, both acutely if there is inadvertent contact between the crystalline lens and the vitrectomy instruments, as well as over the long term even without lens contact. There may be an increased risk of open-angle glaucoma following PPV. Endophthalmitis is a potential rare complication of any intraocular procedure.

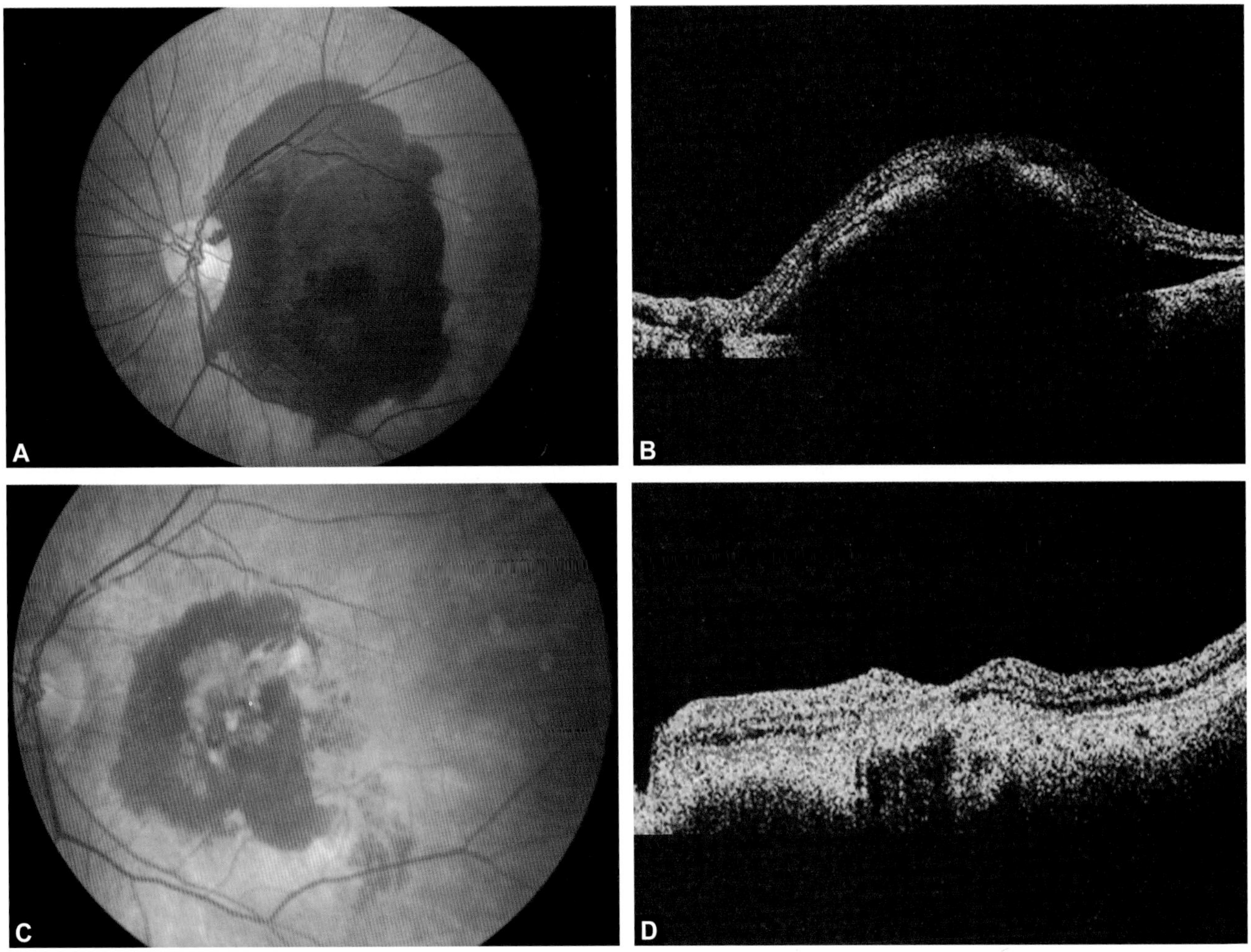

Figures 27-7A to D (A) Pre-pars plana vitrectomy (PPV), the vision was finger counting at 4 feet. (B) Preoperative optical coherence tomography (OCT) showing elevated neurosensory retina and subretinal hyperreflectivity consistent with hemorrhage. (C) The postoperative color fundus photo reveals a fibrotic choroidal neovascular membrane with decreased hemorrhage. The vision was 20/200. (D) Postoperative OCT revealing absence of subretinal blood.

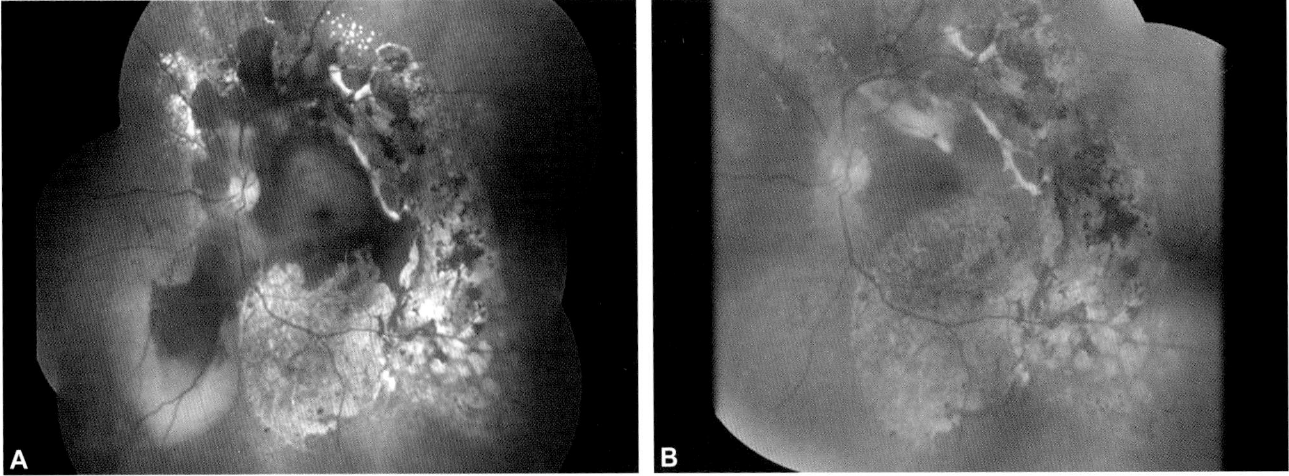


Figures 27-8A and B Submacular hemorrhage due to polypoidal choroidal vasculopathy. (A) Pre-pars plana vitrectomy (PPV), the vision was finger counting at 2 feet. (B) Post-PPV, the final vision was 20/25.

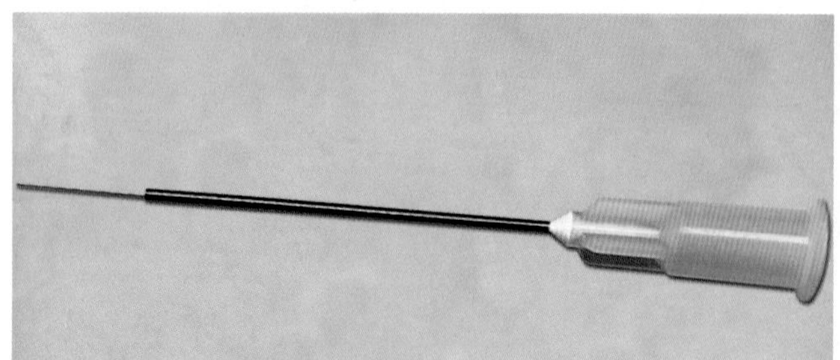

Figure 27-9 Small-gauge microcannula used to create the subretinal bleb of tissue plasminogen activator.

tPA may have theoretical retinal or RPE toxicity. All patients in one series who received 100 μg intravitreal tPA were diagnosed with inferior exudative retinal detachment following injection. None of the patients who received 50 μg experienced this.

## SURGICAL OUTCOMES: SCIENTIFIC EVIDENCE/META-ANALYSIS

Level 1 evidence supporting the efficacy of any intervention for AMD-related, large SMH is not available, but because the natural history is so poor, any evidence suggesting a favorable effect compared with the natural history is encouraging.[8] Most series that used small needles or microcannulae to create a self-sealing retinotomy have reported mean improvements in vision postoperatively, with one series reporting some visual improvement in 73% (8 of 11) eyes with a mean follow-up of 6.5 months.[9] Olivier et al. reported greater than or equal to two lines of vision gained in 68% (17 of 25) of eyes at 3 months follow-up.[10] More recently, Sandhu et al. reported 83% of patients reaching the same ≥2-line improvement end point at 6 months.[11]

## PLACE OF THE TECHNIQUE IN SURGICAL ARMAMENTARIUM

SMH in the setting of neovascular AMD can be a devastating event, and often has a poor visual outcome. High-quality evidence supporting the optimal treatment strategy is lacking, so clinicians must rely on case series to develop a management plan for each patient. Duration, location, size, and thickness of the hemorrhage determine whether or not a displacement intervention should be considered in addition to anti-VEGF therapy. PPV with subretinal tPA and gas tamponade can be a good option for patients with recent, moderate-sized, thick, central hemorrhages if there is known to be limited, pre-existing damage from AMD.

## PEARLS AND PITFALLS

- A generous amount of tPA solution injected under the retina in and around the hemorrhage helps to maximize the postoperative hemorrhage displacement success.
- Anti-VEGF therapy should continue after surgery to minimize the risk of neovascular growth and progressive exudation due to recurrent bleeding.
- After a PPV, drugs injected intravitreally are cleared faster compared with nonvitrectomized eyes and, thus, anti-VEGF therapy may need to be delivered on a regular and frequent basis to keep the neovascular process in check and maximize long-term visual outcomes.

## REFERENCES


1. Scupola A, Coscas G, Soubrane G, Balestrazzi E. Natural history of macular subretinal hemorrhage in age-related macular degeneration. Ophthalmologica. 1999;213(2):97-102.
2. Toth CA, Morse LS, Hjelmeland LM, Landers MB, 3rd. Fibrin directs early retinal damage after experimental subretinal hemorrhage. Arch Ophthalmol. 1991;109(5):723-9.
3. Tennant MT, Borrillo JL, Regillo CD. Management of submacular hemorrhage. Ophthalmol Clin North Am. 2002;15(4):445-52, vi.
4. Steel DH, Sandhu SS. Submacular haemorrhages associated with neovascular age-related macular degeneration. Br J Ophthalmol. 2011;95(8):1051-7.
5. Bressler NM, Bressler SB, Childs AL, et al. Surgery for hemorrhagic choroidal neovascular lesions of age-related macular degeneration: ophthalmic findings: SST report no. 13. Ophthalmology. 2004;111(11):1993-2006.
6. Shultz RW, Bakri SJ. Treatment for submacular hemorrhage associated with neovascular age-related macular degeneration. Semin Ophthalmol. 2011;26(6):361-71.
7. Hassan AS, Johnson MW, Schneiderman TE, et al. Management of submacular hemorrhage with intravitreous tissue plasminogen activator injection and pneumatic displacement. Ophthalmology. 1999;106(10):1900-6; discussion 1906-7.
8. van Zeeburg EJ, van Meurs JC. Literature review of recombinant tissue plasminogen activator used for recent-onset submacular hemorrhage displacement in age-related macular degeneration. Ophthalmologica. 2013;229(1):1-14.
9. Haupert CL, McCuen BW, 2nd, Jaffe GJ, et al. Pars plana vitrectomy, subretinal injection of tissue plasminogen activator, and fluid-gas exchange for displacement of thick submacular hemorrhage in age-related macular degeneration. Am J Ophthalmol. 2001;131(2):208-15.
10. Olivier S, Chow DR, Packo KH, MacCumber MW, Awh CC. Subretinal recombinant tissue plasminogen activator injection and pneumatic displacement of thick submacular hemorrhage in age-related macular degeneration. Ophthalmology. 2004;111(6):1201-8.
11. Sandhu SS, Manvikar S, Steel DH. Displacement of submacular hemorrhage associated with age-related macular degeneration using vitrectomy and submacular tPA injection followed by intravitreal ranibizumab. Clin Ophthalmol. 2010;4:637-42.

CHAPTER 28

# Macular Holes and Management

Rajiv Shah, Carl Park

## INTRODUCTION

A macular hole is a full-thickness retinal tissue defect primarily involving the fovea. Although early descriptions of macular holes focused on traumatic macular holes, 83% of macular holes are primarily idiopathic in origin while approximately 15% are related to trauma.[1,2]

Given the early reports of macular holes occurring after trauma, it was thought that a macular hole developed as a result of trauma.[3] Early histologic reports by Fuchs and Coats demonstrated cystoid intraretinal changes adjacent to the macular hole.[4,5] This led some to suggest that the coalescence of cystoid degeneration gave rise to macular holes.[6] Since many retinal vascular conditions are often associated with cystoid degeneration of the fovea, a vascular theory was also thought to play a role.[5] Lister was the first to deduce that vitreous fibrous bands distorted the macula creating cystoid spaces that eventually degenerated into macular holes.[7] There were some who believed that a combination of vitreous traction and vascular disease gave rise to cystoid degeneration and macular thinning with eventual progression to a macular hole.[8]

However, despite almost a century of work into the mechanism of onset, it was not until Gass proposed his classification scheme for idiopathic macular holes that the idea of tangential vitreous traction, the currently accepted model for pathogenesis of macular holes, became established.[9] Using only biomicroscopy, Gass recognized the four stages of macular hole formation. Optical coherence tomography (OCT) imaging studies have shown that Gass's theories and classification of macular hole formation were mostly correct.[10,11]

For almost a century, although the pathophysiology and the mechanics of macular holes were becoming better understood, there was no proven treatment for macular hole repair, and it was not known whether or not closure of the macular hole would result in visual improvement. The surgery to repair macular holes was first reported in 1991; Kelly and Wendel first described vitrectomy with removal of the cortical vitreous and epiretinal membrane (ERM) with facedown gas tamponade to help stabilize or improve vision.[12] Their approach was based on releasing tangential vitreous traction as suggested by the Gass's theory of macular hole formation. Although the surgery has been refined over the time, the principles of surgical repair are similar to what they described.

## INDICATIONS

The staging scheme proposed by Gass has been modified slightly with increasing data and OCT findings. It provides a guide as to the appropriate intervention and prognosis.[10]

### Stage 1 Impending Macular Hole

Spontaneous changes to the prefoveal cortical vitreous generate tangential and radial traction along the fovea displacing it anteriorly. This reduces the normal fovea depression. At this stage, a 100–200 micron yellow spot caused by the concentration of the xanthophyll is the characteristic finding. This is a stage 1-A macular hole (Figs. 28-1A to C).

With further vitreous contraction, as the foveola retina thins, the fovea detachment may progress. A 200–300 micron ring with radiating striae can be seen on biomicroscopy, and this is a stage 1-B macular hole (Fig. 28-1C). As the foveola thins further, a retinal break may occur and the photoreceptors, Muller cells, and xanthophyll under the internal limiting membrane (ILM) may move away form the center of the foveola. Although this configuration would represent a full-thickness hole, it is unique because the cortical vitreous bridges the hole, and reactive proliferation by Muller cells

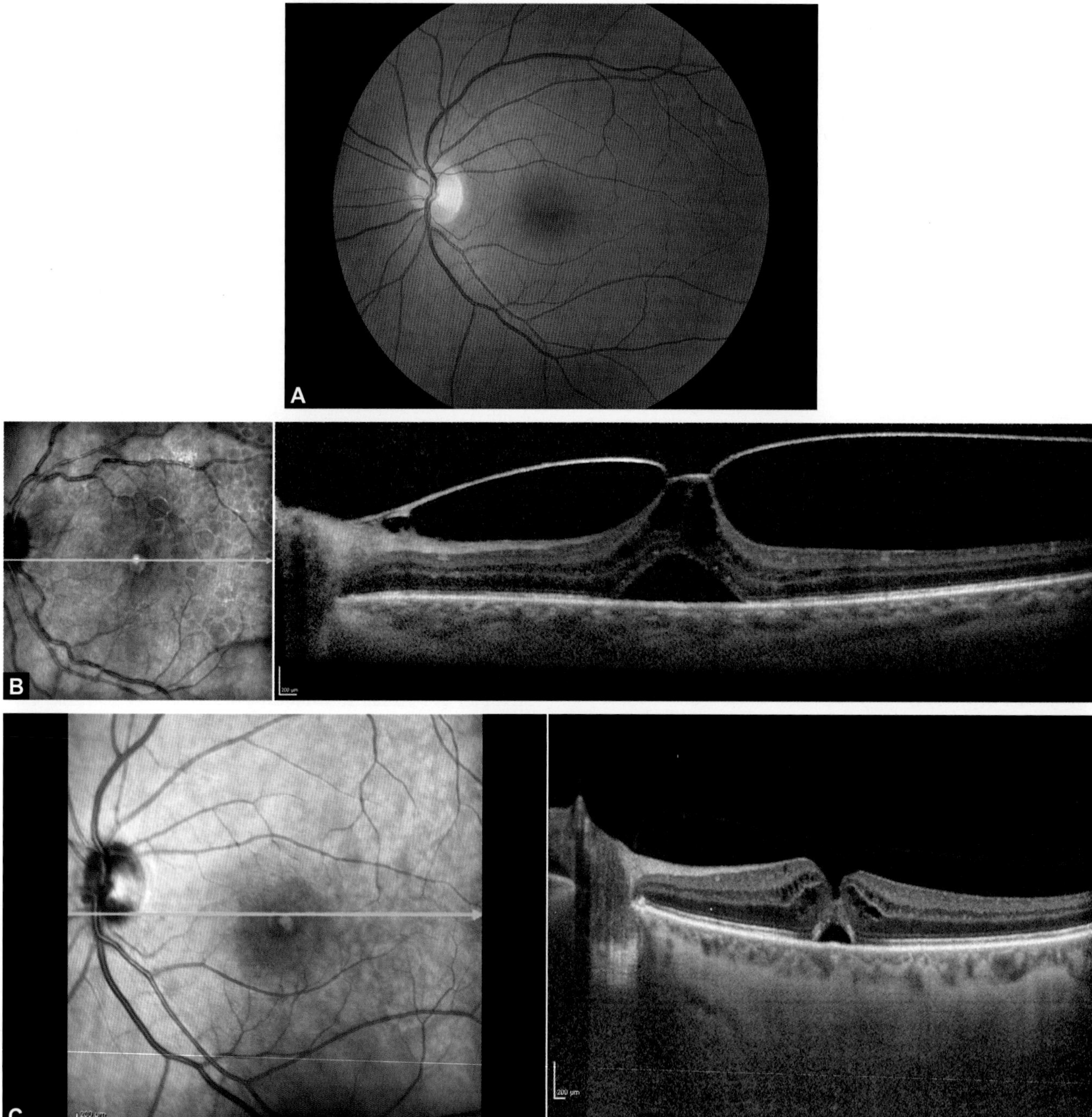

Figures 28-1A to C (A) Fundus photograph of a stage 1 macular hole. (B) Spectral domain optical coherence tomography of a stage 1-A macular hole. Note the prominent insertion of the posterior hyaloid with traction at the fovea. A pocket of subretinal fluid denotes a serous detachment of the fovea. (C) Spectral domain optical coherence tomography of a stage 1-B macular hole. Note the radial displacement of the outer retinal layer structures with beginning of a full-thickness hole (arrow).

and astrocytes creates an opacified bridging membrane across the retinal defect. This is denoted as stage 1-B occult macular hole and can only be identified with OCT.

Although patients may have symptoms and notable changes on the Amsler grid, ultimately 60% of stage 1 holes resolve spontaneously.[9] The visual acuity is usually good in the range of 20/25 to 20/40. Thus, for stage 1 holes, the typical initial management is observation. For the 40% that eventually progress to stage 2 holes, the process occurs within a few months.[13]

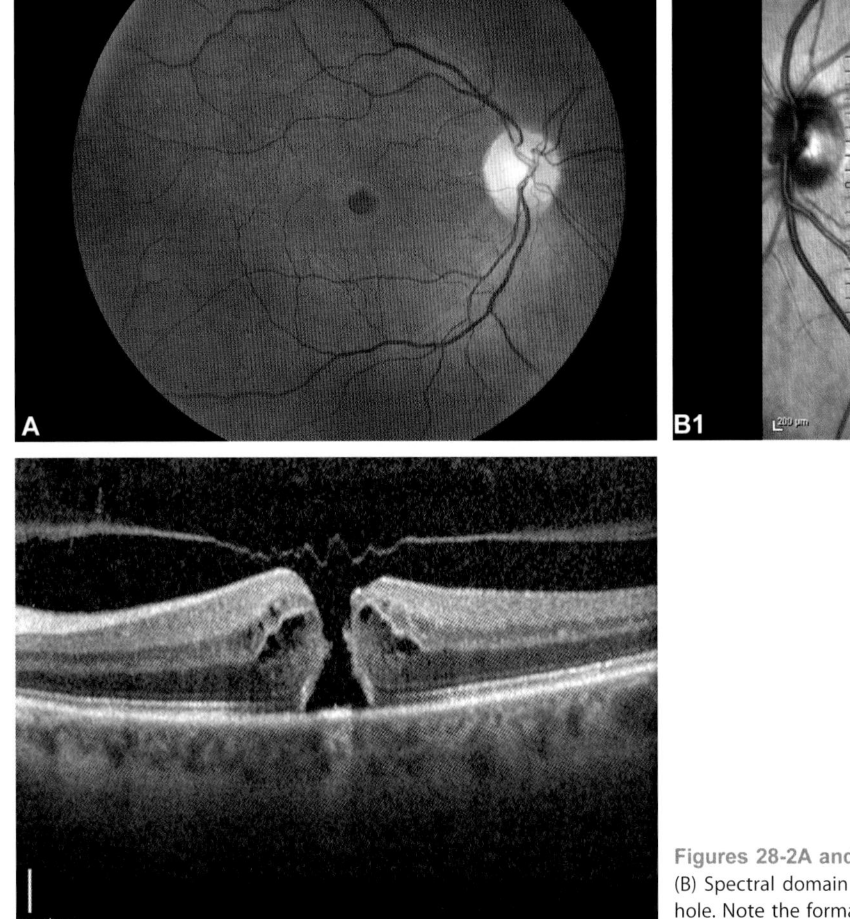


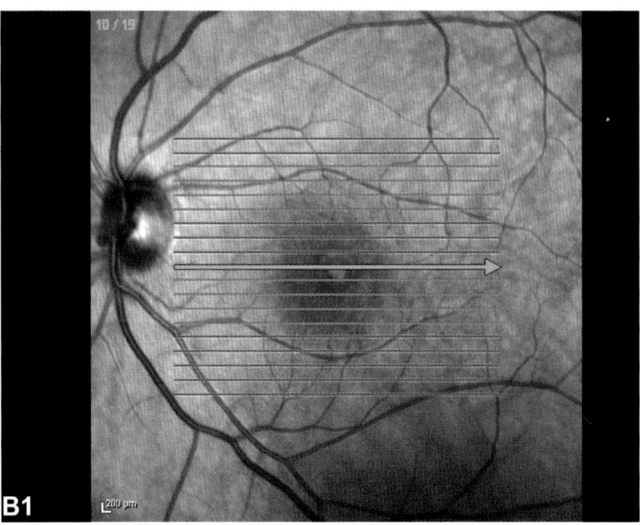


Figures 28-2A and B (A) Fundus photograph of a stage 2 macular hole. (B) Spectral domain optical coherence tomography of a stage 2 macular hole. Note the formation of the full-thickness macular hole. The posterior hyaloid is still attached but no focal vitreoretinal traction is present.

## Stage 2 Hole

With additional contraction of the cortical vitreous, the foveola continues to thin. The posterior hyaloid may be still attached to the edge of this "roof" of the macular hole (which defines a macular hole with focal vitreomacular traction) or the thin flap may become amputated forming an operculum. This full-thickness defect can be seen biomicroscopically and is the hallmark of a stage 2 hole (Figs. 28-2A and B). The size of a stage 2 hole, by definition, is less than 400 microns. Visual acuity with stage 2 holes typically range from 20/40 to 20/80.[14] Without treatment, 67–96% of stage 2 holes progress to stage 3 or 4 holes. Consequently, medical or surgical intervention is recommended for stage 2 holes.[15,16] A stage 2 macular hole with a significant component of focal vitreous traction may be a candidate for medical intervention therapy with pharmacologic vitreolysis (*see* Treatment Technique).

## Stage 3 Hole

Progressive enlargement of the macular holes to 400 microns or larger defines the stage 3 hole (Fig. 28-3). On biomicroscopy, half of stage 3 holes will demonstrate yellowish deposits at the level of the retinal pigment epithelium (RPE), and often the hole has a surrounding rim of subretinal fluid measuring 1,000–1,500 microns.[17-20] Typically, patients note metamorphopsia or a central scotoma on the Amsler grid. Average mean visual acuity is 20/200 but ranges between 20/70 and 20/400.[14] Twenty to forty percent of stage 3 holes develop a complete posterior vitreous detachment (PVD) which defines the progression to a stage 4 macular hole.[21]

## Stage 4 Hole

A stage 4 hole is a greater than 400 micron size hole (Figs. 28-4A and B) with a PVD. It should be noted that vitreous-schisis with incomplete separation of the posterior

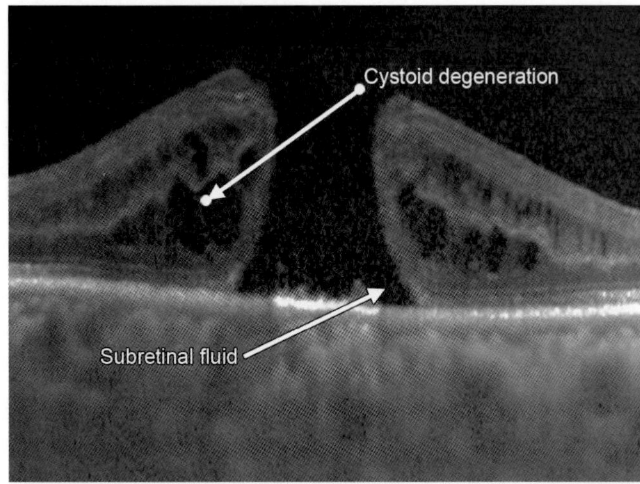


**Figure 28-3** Spectral domain optical coherence tomography of a stage 3 macular hole. Cystoid degeneration and subretinal fluid (*see* arrows) are well illustrated by the optical coherence tomography image.

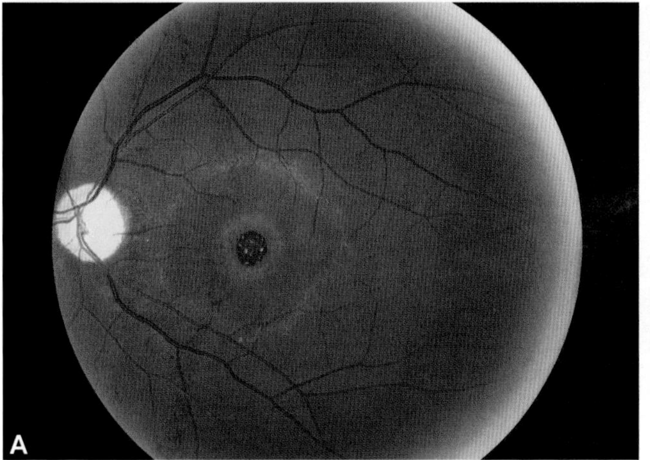


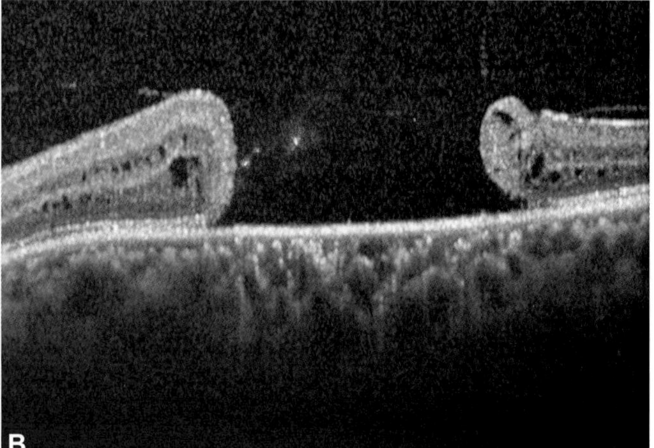


**Figures 28-4A and B** (A) Fundus photograph of a chronic stage 4 macular hole. Note the pigmentary disturbances of the retinal pigment epithelium suggested of chronicity of the hole. (B) Spectral domain optical coherence tomography of a large stage 4 macular hole.

hyaloid could mimic a PVD rendering a stage 3 hole be incorrectly classified as a stage 4 hole.[22] The clinical outcome of mistaking a stage 3 for a stage 4 hole is only relevant if the surgeon does not confirm the release of the posterior hyaloid over the optic nerve and macula during vitrectomy. Stage 1 holes that progress to full-thickness macular holes will evolve into a stage 4 hole usually within the first 6 months.[9]

Three to twenty two percent of fellow eyes develop a macular hole; however, the presence of a PVD in the contralateral eye reduces the risk to less than 1%.[20,23] The fellow eye is typically involved within 2 years of the macular hole in the first eye.[10]

## CLINICAL EVALUATION

The slit-lamp evaluation with either a noncontact lens or a contact macular lens is the most valuable tool for macular hole diagnosis. Occasionally, it can be difficult to distinguish between a full-thickness hole and a pseudohole. A useful test to differentiate between the two is the Watzke-Allen test. The Watzke-Allen test is performed by placing a narrow vertical slit beam across the fovea. If the patient notes a break in the line then this is a "positive" test that is diagnostic for a full-thickness hole. Variations on this test have utilized a 50 micron aiming beam from a laser slit-lamp delivery system. Over a full-thickness hole, the patient is unable to see the aiming beam in a "positive" test. The laser-aiming beam variant may be more sensitive than the traditional slit-beam approach.[24] As mentioned above, the Amsler grid is another means of detecting a hole prior to the biomicroscopic exam.

Despite the importance of the clinical exam, OCT imaging, particularly spectral domain OCT, offers a valuable and precise method of visualizing and staging macular holes as well as providing preoperative prognostic information.

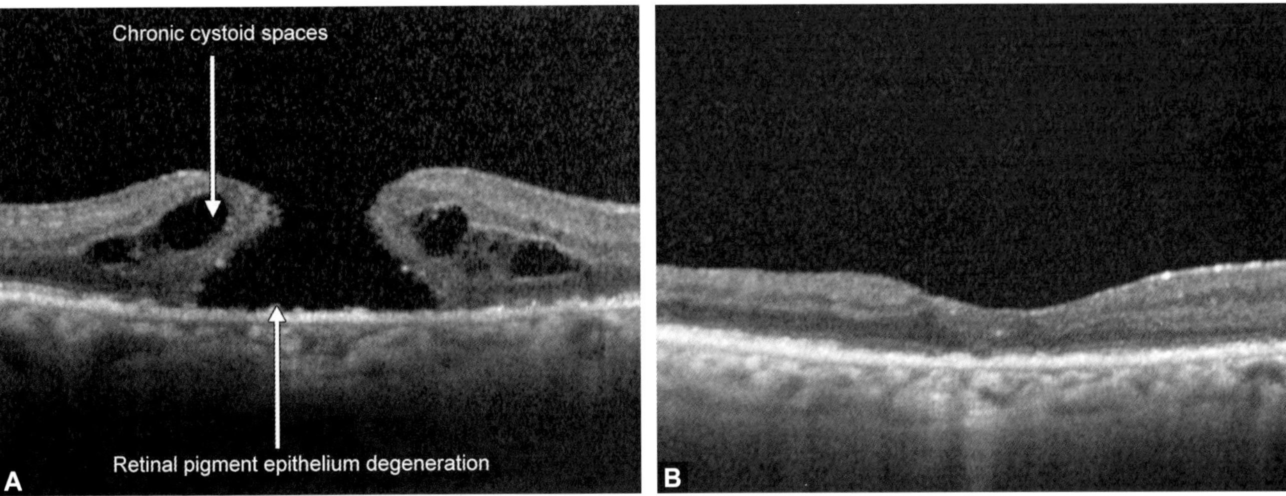


Figures 28-5A and B (A) Preoperative spectral domain optical coherence tomography of a chronic stage 4 (>1 year in duration) macular hole. Note the larger cystic spaces and the deterioration of the retinal pigment epithelium layer (arrows). (B) Postoperative spectral domain optical coherence tomography of a chronic stage 4 macular hole demonstrates hole closure. The photoreceptor layer disturbances and the retinal pigment epithelium changes suggest long-term visual limitations.

In particular, smaller macular hole size as measured by the linear distance between the two inner segment/outer segment junction tends to correlate with better visual recovery and higher macular hole closure rate.[25,26]

Chronicity of macular hole is also a consideration in the preoperative evaluation. Chronic macular holes of greater than 1 year duration have an hole closure rate comparable to macular holes less than 1 year of duration but with less visual recovery (Figs. 28-5A and B).[27] With chronic macular holes, high-resolution OCT imaging studies have shown that preoperative photoreceptor layer integrity is an important predictor of final visual recovery.[28]

In summary, the key preoperative findings with regards to prognosis of macular hole treatment outcome include macular hole staging, macular hole size, and chronicity. The presence of focal vitreomacular traction in a stage 2 macular hole may be amenable to pharmacologic treatment (discussed below). The presence or absence of a PVD or an ERM may alter the surgical approach. OCT imaging is an invaluable tool for preoperative counseling of macular hole patients and may allow for optimal planning of surgical steps.

Differential diagnosis for macular hole includes epiretinal membranes with pseudohole/lamellar holes, vitreomacular adhesion/macular cyst, atrophic age-related macular degeneration, and central serous chorioretinopathy.

## CONTRAINDICATIONS

The main contraindication to surgical vitrectomy, membrane peeling and gas tamponade for macular hole would be poor medical health or poor ocular media (cataract or cornea) to adequately perform macular surgery. Macular hole surgery is an elective surgery and can be deferred for a short term if the global medical health is not optimized or stable. Consideration of cataract surgery either a week or two before vitrectomy, or along in combination with vitrectomy, should be made for visually significant cataracts that would impair visualization for macular surgery. Coordination with a cornea surgeon may be necessary if there is significant corneal scar impairing the macular surgical view. For the later, a temporary keratoprosthesis can be used for the vitrectomy with subsequent placement of a full-thickness corneal transplant.

## TREATMENT TECHNIQUE

### Medical

Since vitreous traction plays an integral role in the pathophysiology of macular hole formation, pharmacologic vitreolysis can be considered as a nonsurgical approach to close macular holes.[29] The vitreous of the eye comprises 80% of the eye volume and it is composed of water, collagen fibers and hyaluronic acid.[30] Laminin and fibronectin, components of the extracellular matrix at the vitreomacular interface, are the key components that determine the strength of adherence of vitreous humor to the retina giving rise to macular holes and other vitreomacular pathologies.[31-33] Autologous plasmin has been studied and shown to cleave components of laminin and fibronectin,[34,35] and early work demonstrated that plasmin could induce a PVD.[36,37] Plasmin is typically collected from a patient's own serum, and the process to isolate the plasmin is

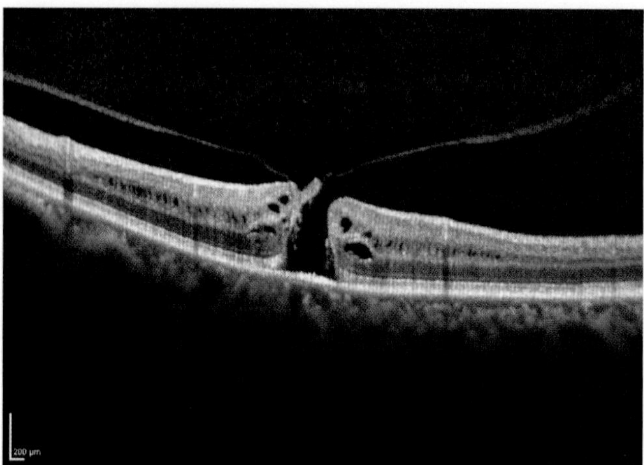


**Figure 28-6** Spectral domain optical coherence tomography for a stage 2 macular hole with focal vitreomacular traction. This configuration of a smaller macular hole (<400 micron) with focal vitreomacular traction without significant epiretinal membrane may be a candidate for nonsurgical intervention with ocriplasmin.

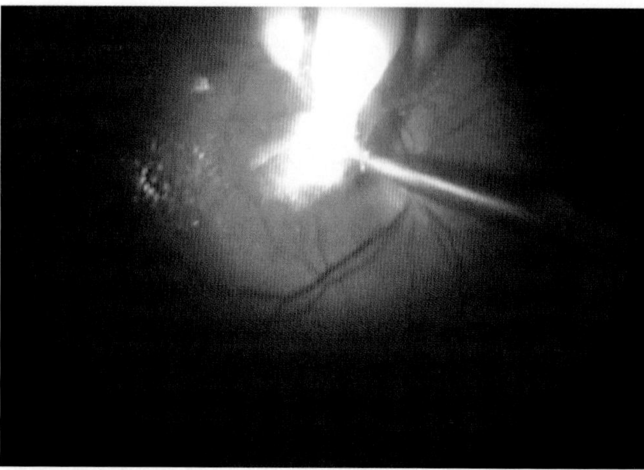

**Figure 28-7** Induction of a posterior vitreous detachment with aide of intravitreal triamcinolone visualization using a 23-gauge vitrectomy cutter in suction only mode.

expensive and intricate. Furthermore, plasmin is unstable and rapidly inactivates via autolysis.[38]

Ocriplasmin (Jetrea, Thrombogenics, Iselin, NJ) also called microplasmin is plasmin fragment created with recombinant technology that isolates only the catalytic domain of human plasmin.[39] This modification creates a smaller molecule (approximately one-fourth the size of plasmin) that more effectively penetrates the vitreous. The modification also eliminates the structural moieties of plasmin that give rise to instability. Ocriplasmin cleaves the posterior hyaloid and the ILM interface, and induces a PVD in animal and human models.[40]

In 2012, the United States (US) Food and Drug Administration (FDA) approved ocriplasmin for the treatment of symptomatic vitreomacular traction. Within their pivotal phase 3 MIVI-Trust trial, a subset of patients with macular holes was studied.[29] In this group of patients with macular holes measuring less than 400 microns in size, a single injection of ocriplasmin resulted in a 40% macular hole closure rate compared to 10.6% in the placebo injection arm. Specifically, patients with a focal macular adhesion associated with the macular hole tended to have higher closure rates (Fig. 28-6), and the presence of an ERM was found to lessen the efficacy of the ocriplasmin. The subset of macular holes less than 250 microns in size had the highest closure rate. Although the data/experience for ocriplasmin as a treatment for macular holes is limited, the MIVI-trust trial underscores the importance of careful patient selection to achieve the highest success rate of macular hole closure. As ocriplasmin does not work well in eyes that have an ERMs or for those with broad vitreomacular adhesion (>1,500 microns), it should only be considered for macular holes less than 250–400 microns in size associated with focal vitreomacular adhesion without the presence of an ERM.

## Surgical

A standard three-port vitrectomy is performed (please see the separate chapters regarding the principles of vitrectomy surgery) for vast majority of macular hole surgery. Although the size of the instrumentation probably does not affect surgical outcome, the current trend amongst surgeons is a shift toward smaller-gauge instrumentations (23-gauge, 25-gauge or 27-gauge).[41]

One of the most important aspects of macular hole surgery is the induction of a PVD. Often times the vitreoretinal adhesion can be difficult to release from around the optic nerve or premacular bursa (which obviously defines the pathophysiology of macular holes). Meticulous technique with the vitrectomy cutter with additional enhancement of vitreous visualization with triamcinolone in some cases usually results in successful PVD inducement. To engage the cortical vitreous in preparation for release, the mouth of the cutter should be directed to the edges of the cortical vitreous insertion at the optic nerve (Fig. 28-7). Prior to the attempted elevation of the posterior hyaloid, a sufficient amount of vitreous humor should be occluding the mouth of the cutter to maximize the mechanical advantage needed to induce a PVD/Weiss ring. Once the vitreous is engaged, the vitreous should be pulled anteriorly along the visual axis to disengage the vitreous while minimizing lateral tractional forces that can result in creation of iatrogenic retinal breaks. For particularly challenging cases, one can use the "fish-strike" maneuver with a soft-tip cannula attached to active extrusion to release the vitreous adhesion. During this maneuver, once the mouth of the soft tip has been occluded with vitreous humor high suction is applied. For cases that are still obstinate, consider using a membrane pick or a bent microvitreoretinal (MVR) blade to "peel" the hyaloid. A long 25-gauge needle can be bent at the tip to form a pick, and this can be attached to the extrusion to create a suction pick.[42] The sharp edges of these instruments can be used to engage the cortical vitreous at the edge of the optic nerve head to induce separation.

Following a PVD, the core vitreous is removed and this is followed by a peripheral vitrectomy. The goals of the peripheral vitrectomy are to trim the vitreous skirt to enable safe insertion of the surgical instruments and to create sufficient space within the vitreous cavity for gas tamponade at the end of the surgery.

Following the vitrectomy, often a macular contact lens is used to provide the best visualization and stereopsis for membrane peeling. The initial description of macular holes surgery advocated only ERM removal.[12] Brooks was the first to demonstrate the importance of ILM removal to improve macular hole closure rates.[43] We remove the ILM membrane in all stages of macular hole undergoing surgical repair. ILM removal ensures that the any residual overlying cortical vitreous/ERM is completely removed (partial removal would significantly reduce the closure rate) and likely aids in the symmetric mobilization of the retina surrounding the hole during closure.

There is no gold standard with regards to the style of intraocular forceps to effectively remove the ERM/ILM around the macular hole; however, we advocate an end-grasping style such as the ILM forceps because it offers a small precise gripping platform to engage and manipulate the retinal surface membranes. A further advantage of the ILM forceps design is that the skinny tip profile allows maximal visualization of the retinal surface to minimize collateral damage.

A particular advance in macular surgery over the last two decades has been the application of various membrane stains to assist in the visualization and peeling of ERM/ILM. Some have advocated peeling by direct visualization without staining; the ILM, for example, has a characteristic scrolling behavior as it is removed. The disadvantage of this approach includes the possibility of incomplete ERM/ILM removal that may result in either acute surgical failure or late failure in cases of retained traction surrounding the macular hole. Others have advocated using triamcinolone as a guide, but this does not "stain" the ERM or ILM. It settles on the surface of ERM or ILM and only provides depth perception cues for peeling.

True membrane stains include the blue stains (trypan blue and brilliant blue G, which is available in most countries) and indocyanine green (ICG). Trypan blue has been widely used for cataract surgery and has excellent intraocular safety data; the more concentrated FDA-approved version for retina surgery is also safe. Trypan blue mostly stains the ERM (and perhaps weakly the ILM), so it is mostly effective for facilitating ERM removal. Brilliant blue G staining offers an advantage as it more strongly stains the ILM and has also been found to be nontoxic. Brilliant blue approval for use in the US is pending but is more commonly available outside the US. ICG is the most commonly used ILM staining agent in the US, and is widely available throughout the world. ICG staining usually provides deep contrast of the green ILM compared to the inner retinal surface allowing for efficient peeling of the membrane around the hole. However, ICG can possibly be toxic to the RPE. Despite the concerns over possible ICG toxicity, review of the literature reports far more cases of successful ICG usage for membrane peeling rather than cases of toxicity.[44] Possible toxicity issues can be minimized by a short duration of exposure of the dye on the macular surface by rapid extrusion of the dye after introduction (direct exposure time to the macular surface prior to removal should be measured in 10–30 seconds). Longer duration of staining with ICG probably does not result in stronger staining of the ILM and may increase toxicity. In cases when a diaphanous ERM is present, one must be mindful that removal of an ERM can often mimic ILM removal. The surgeon must consider an additional peel of the ILM after the initial membrane removal. It is in these circumstances that staining dyes become an important tool aiding the complete ERM/ILM removal around the hole.

Perhaps the most challenging step in membrane (especially ILM) peeling is the creation of a free edge upon which to initiate the removal of the membrane. Options for initiating an ERM/ILM peel include a "pinch/peel" technique with the ILM forceps to generate an edge (Fig. 28-8). One can also use a Tano diamond dusted membrane scraper to generate the membrane edge or even to perform the membrane peel without the use of forceps. However, the Tano scraper can create subclinical injury to the RPE even with the proper technique and this may cause a pericentral scotoma despite successful hole closure. Another method of initiating a membrane peel is to use a MVR blade to "score" the ILM to generate a graspable edge. Although the edge of the MVR is obviously sharp and has the potential for retina trauma, with proper technique, it can be a way to engage only the most superficial membranes.

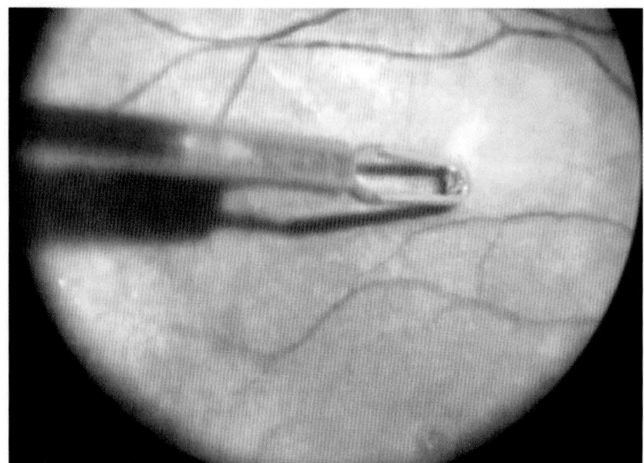

Figure 28-8 Creation of an edge in the internal limiting membrane that has been stained with indocyanine green via a "pinch/peel" technique.

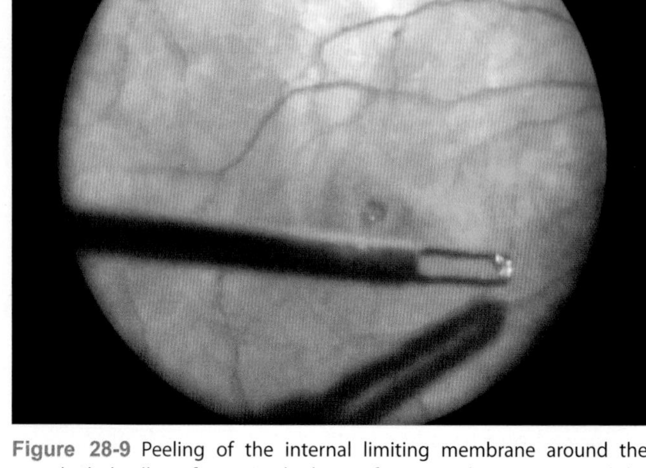

Figure 28-9 Peeling of the internal limiting membrane around the macular hole allows for optimal release of tangential traction around the hole.

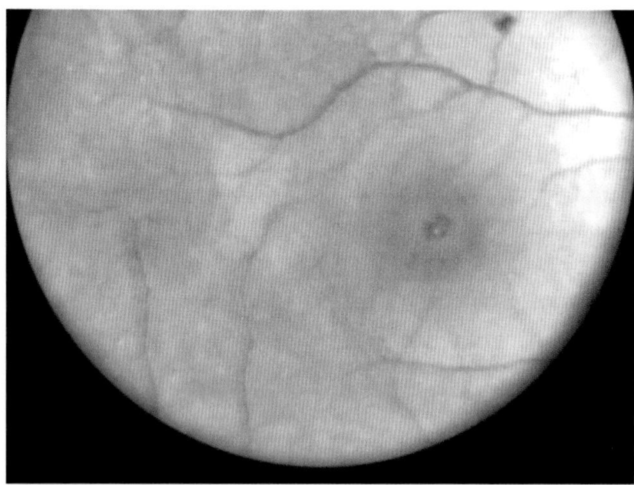

Figure 28-10 Demonstrates complete internal limiting membrane removal around the hole. The size of the internal limiting membrane removal margin should be proportional to the size of the pre-existing epiretinal membrane to ensure complete removal of the ERM/ILM complex.

Following the creation of the membrane edge, ILM forceps can be used to grasp the edge of the membrane to complete the membrane peeling (Figs. 28-9 and 28-10). During the process of membrane peeling, it may be sometimes helpful to add additional membrane stain to perform a "double stain". Staining both the anterior and posterior surface of the membrane can provide superior visualization of the membrane if the initial stain was suboptimal.

Following membrane peeling, removal of any membrane fragments from the vitreous cavity with extrusion is important as residual membrane fragments can cause highly symptomatic floaters. The peripheral retina must be inspected to identify retinal pathology such as lattice degeneration or retinal breaks. These are treated with peripheral endolaser retinopexy. Air-fluid exchange is then performed with the vitrectomy cutter or an extrusion cannula (either soft- or hard-tipped) in preparation for the gas tamponade.

With respect to tamponade agents, air or mixture gas tamponade is preferable to silicone oil because the higher surface tension aids in macular hole closure. Work from Japan has demonstrated the efficacy of air tamponade in hole closure;[45] however, we have some concern for patients who may not be able to maintain a strict facedown position for the first few days since significant air tamponade (tamponade occupying at least 60% of the vitreous cavity to cover the hole when sitting up) lasts for only 1–2 days. Between the two widely used longer-acting gas tamponade, sulfur hexafluoride ($SF_6$) and octafluoropropane ($C_3F_8$), the choice of tamponade is highly surgeon dependent, and one is not superior to the other. For patients who are less compliant with facedown positioning, a longer duration gas tamponade might be preferable to allow for significant tamponade even while the patient is sitting up. For large macular holes, chronic macular holes, or recurrent macular holes, some surgeons prefer a longer gas tamponade, but given the OCT data, which suggest that most macular holes close within the first few days, this may not be necessary.[46] Although isoexpansile concentrations of gas are often used, the surgeon may choose a slightly expansile concentration to ensure a more complete gas tamponade over the first few days.[45] For patients unable to position (such as children, those with severe mental disability, or those who have obesity or retardation), silicone oil tamponade can be utilized, although its use has become less relevant due to the efficacy of longer-acting gas tamponade without positioning.

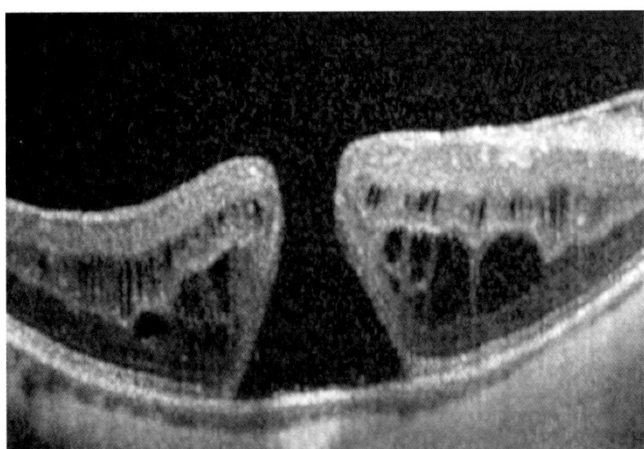

Figure 28-11 Spectral Domain optical coherence tomography for a myopic stage 4 macular hole demonstrating increased concavity of the macula. Also note prominent epiretinal membrane.

Traumatic macular holes and macular holes in high axial length myopic patients deserve separate consideration. With respect to traumatic macular holes, these typically occur in children and young adult males.[47] Traumatic macular holes are unique because the posterior vitreous is often attached (and may be difficult to induce separation) and there may be concurrent damage to the RPE, Bruch's membrane, choroid, or optic nerve that can ultimately limit visual recovery despite a successful hole closure.[48] Furthermore, some traumatic macular holes spontaneously close with in the first few weeks after the injury so the optimum timing of intervention is unknown. Early observation for traumatic macular holes especially in children and young adults is likely the best course of action.[49]

Myopic macular holes are also unusual because the cortical vitreous is often attached. Foveoschisis may play a prominent role in the pathogenesis of the disease (Fig. 28-11).[50] The axial length and posterior staphyloma also provide a technical challenge for membrane peeling, and one may need to consider extra-long forceps to comfortably reach the retina surface.

## MECHANISM OF ACTION

Surgical intervention releases the tangential traction (and in some cases oblique traction) that caused the macular hole. Release of the traction around the hole allows for "sliding closure" of the sensory retina surrounding the hole. Gas tamponade is thought to exert anterior-posterior forces and surface tension that enables hole closure. However, pharmacologic closure of certain types of macular holes suggests that gas tamponade may play a smaller role (versus release of traction) in the closure of smaller macular holes.

## POSTOPERATIVE CARE

The standard regimen of antibiotic and steroid topical eye drops four times a day for 1–4 weeks is typically sufficient to control postoperative infection/inflammation. Since gas tamponade is utilized, monitoring of the intraocular pressure is important for the first postoperative day. Expansile concentrations of gas may necessitate a more frequent evaluation of intraocular pressure.

Historically, facedown positioning following macular hole surgery has been the standard of care since the first report by Kelly and Wendel.[12] Over the years, various facedown positioning regimens from 1 week up to 1 month have been advocated. The comorbidities upon a patient's neck and back cannot be underestimated with regards to such extended positioning. Recent postoperative OCT studies have suggested that macular holes typically close in the first 1–3 days postsurgery.[44] For small macular holes (< 400 microns), we typically recommend 3 days facedown maximum, and for large macular holes (> 400 microns), we recommend 5 days facedown. Some early studies suggest that even shorter intervals of only 24 hours may be effective, and other reports suggest that no facedown positioning is required.[51]

Occasionally, postoperative development of macular edema in the setting of successful hole closure may require the use of prolonged topical or periocular steroid therapy. In cases of successful closure of chronic macular holes, a shallow pocket of subretinal fluid may persist in the fovea, and probably represents RPE dysfunction. With time and perhaps with the use of anti-inflammatory eye drops, the subretinal fluid usually resolves within 1–2 months with further visual acuity improvement. It is important to note to the patient that although most holes close within the first week, the final visual acuity recovery may take up to several months. The anatomic hole closure probably represents the initial phase of macular hole surgery recovery, with significant late healing processes that take place between the retina and the RPE.

## COMPLICATIONS

The most common intraoperative complication is an iatrogenic retinal breaks, which occurs in approximately 6% of cases.[52] Interestingly, the tears are rarely found near the sclerotomies, suggesting that tear formation occurs during PVD induction. The rate of retinal detachment following macular hole surgery is approximately 1–2%.[52] If cataract surgery is not done prior or concurrent with macular hole surgery, the rate of cataract progression is 81% at 2 years.[53]

## SURGICAL OUTCOMES: SCIENTIFIC EVIDENCE

As noted earlier, most stage 2 macular holes (other those that can be addressed with ocriplasmin) benefit from surgery and all stage 3 and 4 macular holes undergo surgery.[16] In 1998, a randomized multicenter trial was initiated for stage 3 and 4 holes but it was later abandoned because of low patient enrollment.[20] The primary surgical closure rate with ERM/ILM peeling approaches and often exceeds 90% for all stages of macular hole.[54] Smaller stage 2 holes and relatively new holes probably have even a higher closure rate. Removal of the ILM has shown to improve the closure rate of macular holes compared to just removal of the ERM and it does not affect final visual outcome when hole closure is achieved.[43] If the hole closes, nearly all patients have at least some visual improvement. Late reopening of macular holes occur 2–7% of the time.[54] Generally, reoperations of these macular holes have a high success rate as well.

## PLACE OF THE TECHNIQUE IN SURGICAL ARMAMENTARIUM

Vitrectomy with complete ERM/ILM peeling and gas tamponade is the gold standard for the repair of full-thickness macular holes.

## PEARLS AND PITFALLS

- Identification of the posterior hyaloid with assurance that it has been separated from the retinal surface is critical to the success of the surgery.
- Peripheral retinal breaks can be minimized by proper techniques during posterior hyaloid separation.
- Staining and complete removal of the ILM around the macular hole for all stages of macular hole probably increases the success rate of hole closure.
- Creation of a raised edge of ILM is often the most difficult step in membrane peeling. Regardless of which technique is used to induce an edge, one must be careful to not traumatize the retina.
- Consider removing the cataract before macular hole surgery in eyes with moderate cataracts.

## REFERENCES


1. Ho AC, Guyer DR, Fine SL. Macular Hole. Surv Ophthalmol. 1998;42(5):393-416.
2. McDonnell PJ, Fine SL, Hillis AI. Clinical Features of idiopathic macular cysts and holes. Am J Ophthalmol. 1982;93(6):777-86.
3. Alt A. Remarks of holes in the macula lutea and fovea centralis with the report of a new case. Am J Ophthalmol. 1913;30:97-106.
4. Fuchs E. Zur veranderung der macula lutea nach contusion. Ztschr Augenheilk. 1901;6:181-6.
5. Coats G. The pathology of macular holes. Roy London Hosp Rep. 1907;17:69-96.
6. Kuht H. Uber eine eigenthumliche veranderung der netzhaut ad maculam (retinitis atrophicans sive rareficans centralis). Ztschr Augenheik. 1900;3:105-12.
7. Lister W. Holes in the retina and their clinical significance. Br J Ophthalmol. 1924;8(1):14-20.
8. Morgan CM, Schatz H. Involutional macular thinning: A premacular hole condition. Ophthalmology. 1986;93(2):153-61.
9. Johnson RN, Gass JD. Idiopathic macular holes. Observations, stages of formation, and implications for surgical intervention. Ophthalmology. 1988;95(7):917-24.
10. Agarwal A. Macular dysfunction caused by vitreous and vitreoretinal interface abnormalities. Gass' Atlas of Macular Disease, 5th edition. Philadelphia: Elsevier Saunders; 2012. pp. 646-71.
11. Hee MR, Puliafito CA, Wong C, et al. Optical coherence tomography of macular holes. Ophthalmology. 1995;102(5):748-56.
12. Kelly NE, Wendel RT. Vitreous surgery for idiopathic macular holes. Results of a Pilot Study. Arch Ophthalmol. 1991;109(5):654-9.
13. De Bustros S. Vitrectomy for prevention of macular holes. Results of a randomized multicenter clinical trial. Vitrectomy for Prevention of Macular Hole Study Group. Ophthalmology. 1994;101(6):1055-9.
14. James M, Feman SS. Macular holes. Albrecht Von Graefes Arch Klin Exp Ophthalmol. 1980;215(1):59-63.
15. Hikichi T, Toshida A, Akiba J. Prognosis of stage 2 macular holes. Am J Ophthalmol. 1995;107:241-5.
16. Kim JW, Freeman WR, Azen SP. Prospective randomized trial of vitrectomy or observation for stage 2 macular holes. Vitrectomy for Macular Hole Study Group. Am J Ophthalmol. 1996;121(6):605-14.
17. Glacet-Bernard A, Zourdani A, Perrenoud F, et al. Stage 3 macular hole: role of optical coherence tomography and of B-scan ultrasonography. Am J Ophthalmol. 2005;139(5):814-9.
18. Gass JD. Reappraisal of biomicroscopic classification of stages of development of a macular hole. Am J Ophthalmol. 1995;119(6):752-9.
19. Takahashi A, Yoshida A, Nagaoka T, et al. Idiopathic full-thickness macular holes and the vitreomacular interface: a high-resolution spectral-domain optical coherence tomography study. Am J Ophthalmol. 2012;154(5):881-92.
20. Bronstein MA, Trempe CL, Freeman HM. Fellow eyes with macular holes. Am J Ophthalmol. 1981;92(6):757-61.
21. Kishi S, Takahashi H. Three-dimensional observations of developing macular holes. Am J Ophthalmol. 2000;130(1):65-75.
22. Glacet-Bernard A, Zourdani A, Perrenoud F, et al. Stage 3 macular hole: role of optical coherence tomography and of B-scan ultrasonography. Am J Ophthalmol. 2005;139(5):814-9.
23. Akiba J, Kakehashi A, Arzabe CW, et al. Fellow eyes in idiopathic macular holes cases. Ophthalmic Surg. 1992;23(9):594-7.

24. Martinez J, Smiddy WE, Kim J, et al. Differentiating macular holes from macular pseudoholes. Am J Ophthalmol. 1994; 117(6):762-7.
25. Ullrich S, Haritoglou C, Gass C, et al. Macular hole size as a prognostic factor in macular hole surgery. Br J Ophthalmol. 2002;86(4):390-3.
26. Ruiz-Moreno JM, Arias L, Araiz J, et al. Spectral-domain optical coherence tomography study of macular structures as prognostic and determining factor for macular hole surgery outcome. Retina. 2013;33(6):1117-22.
27. Roth DB, Smiddy WE, Feuer W. Vitreous surgery for chronic macular holes. Ophthalmology. 1997;104(12):2047-52.
28. Ko TH, Fujimoto JG, Duker JS, et al. Comparison of ultrahigh- and standard-resolution optical coherence tomography for imaging macular hole pathology and repair. Ophthalmology. 2004;111(11):2033-43.
29. Stalmans P, Benz MS, Gandorfer A, et al. Enzymatic vitreolysis with ocriplasmin for vitreomacular traction and macular holes. N Engl J Med. 2012;367(7):606-15.
30. Sebag J, Balazs EA. Morphology and ultrastructure of human vitreous fibers. Invest Ophthalmol Vis Sci. 1989;30(8):1867-71.
31. Kohno T, Sorgente N, Ishibashi T, et al. Immunofluorescent studies of fibronectin and laminin in the human eye. Invest Ophthalmol Vis Sci. 1987;28(3):506-14.
32. Russell SR, Shepherd JD, Hageman GS. Distribution of glycoconjugates in the human retinal internal limiting membrane. Invest Ophthalmol Vis Sci. 1991;32(7):1986-95.
33. Kohno T, Sorgente N, Goodnight R, et al. Alterations in the distribution of fibronectin and laminin in the diabetic human eye. Invest Ophthalmol Vis Sci. 1987;28(3):515-21.
34. Hermel M, Dailey W, Hartzer MK. Efficacy of plasmin, microplasmin, and streptokinase-plasmin complex for the in vitro degradation of fibronectin and laminin- implications for vitreoretinal surgery. Curr Eye Res. 2010;35(5):419-24.
35. Papp B, Kovacs T, Lerant I. Conditions of formation of the heparin-fibronectin-collagen complex and the effect of plasmin. Biochim Biophys Acta. 1987;925(3):241-7.
36. Verstraeten TC, Chapman C, Hartzer M, et al. Pharmacologic induction of posterior vitreous detachment in the rabbit. Arch Ophthalmol. 1993;111(6):849-54.
37. Kim NJ, Yu HG, Yu YS, et al. Long-term effect of plasmin on the vitreolysis in rabbit eyes. Korean J Ophthalmol. 2004;18(1): 35-40.
38. Tsui I, Pan CK, Rahimy E, et al. Ocriplasmin for vitreoretinal diseases. J Biomed Biotechnol. 2012;2012:354979.
39. Wu HL, Shi GY, Bender ML. Preparation and purification of microplasmin. Proc Natl Acad Sci U S A. 1987;84(23):8292-5.
40. Chen W, Mo W, Sun K, et al. Microplasmin degrades fibronectin and laminin at vitreoretinal interface and outer retina during enzymatic vitrectomy. Curr Eye Res. 2009;34(12):1057-64.
41. American Society of Retina Specialist. PAT Survey 2012. [Online] Available from www.asrs.org. [Accessed August, 2013].
42. Garg SJ. Use of a suction pick in small-gauge surgery facilitates induction of a posterior vitreous detachment. Retina. 2008;28(10):1536.
43. Brooks HL Jr. Macular hole surgery with and without internal limiting membrane peeling. Ophthalmology. 2000;107(10): 1939-48.
44. Thompson JT, Haritoglu C, Kampik A, et al. Should Indocyanine green should be used to facilitate removal of the internal limiting membrane in macular hole surgery. Surv Ophthalmol. 2009;54(1):135-8.
45. Hikichi T, Kosaka S, Takami K, et al. 23- and 20-gauge vitrectomy with air tamponade with combined phacoemulsification for idiopathic macular hole: a single-surgeon study. Am J Ophthalmol. 2011;152(1):114-21.
46. Shah SP, Manjunath V, Rogers AH, et al. Optical coherence tomography guided facedown positioning for macular hole surgery. Retina. 2013;33(2):356-62.
47. Atmaca LS, Yilmaz M. Changes in the fundus caused by blunt ocular trauma. Ann Ophthalmol. 1993;25(12):447-52.
48. Barreau E, Massin P, Paques M, et al. Surgical treatment of post-traumatic macular holes. J Fr Ophthalmol. 1997;20(6):423-9.
49. Kusaka S, Fujikado T, Ikeda T, et al. Spontaneous disappearance of traumatic macular holes in young patients. Am J Ophthalmol.1997;123(6):837-9.
50. Shimada N, Ohno-Matsui K, Yoshida T, et al. Progression from macular retinoschsis to retinal detachment in highly myopic eyes associated with outer lamellar hole formation. Br J Ophthalmol. 2008;92(6):762-4.
51. Forsaa VA, Raeder S, Hashemi LT, et al. Short-term postoperative non-supine positioning versus strict facedown positioning in macular hole surgery. Acta Ophthalmol. 2012.
52. Sjaarda RN, Glaser BM, Thompson JT, et al. Distribution of iatrogenic retinal breaks in macular hole surgery. Ophthalmology. 1995;102(9):1387-92.
53. Thompson JT, Glaser BM, Sjaarda RN, et al. Progression of Nuclear Sclerosis and long-term visual results of vitrectomy with transforming growth factor beta-2 for macular holes. Am J Ophthalmol. 1995;119(1):48-54.
54. Duker JS, Wendel RT, Patel AC, et al. Late re-opening of macular holes following initial successful vitreous surgery. Ophthalmology. 1994;101(8):1373-8.

CHAPTER

29

# Epiretinal Membranes

Mitchell S Fineman

## INTRODUCTION

Macular epiretinal membrane (ERM), also called macular pucker, surface wrinkling retinopathy, and cellophane retinopathy, is a semitransparent fibrocellular membrane present on the inner retinal surface, usually centered on the macula. ERM is an acquired condition that is usually idiopathic. Secondary ERMs may also occur and are usually associated with retinal breaks or detachments (Figs. 29-1A and B), uveitis and retinal vasculitis, retinal vascular disease, blunt and penetrating trauma, congenital conditions such as combined hamartoma of the retina and RPE, and previous intraocular surgery. Idiopathic ERMs are most common after 50 years of age, have no sex predilection, and are present bilaterally in up to 20% of patients.[1]

Most patients with ERM have had a previous posterior vitreous detachment (PVD), and it is thought that this separation of the posterior hyaloid from the surface of the retina may contribute to formation of ERM. During and after PVD, schisis of the vitreous may allow a portion of posterior cortical vitreous to be left behind and adherent to the macula. This residual vitreous may even be adherent to the surface of the retina in the presence of a Weiss ring. In addition, traction on the internal limiting membrane (ILM) during PVD development may alter the ILM and promote ERM development. These events set the stage for the proliferation of glial cells on the surface of the retina. Why this pathologic process occurs in certain eyes while sparing most is not well understood. It is thought that the proliferating glial cells spread and contract on the surface of the retina and develop into an ERM. Development of an ERM is more common following retinal break formation and trauma because retinal pigment epithelial (RPE) cells may escape through the retinal defect and enter the vitreous cavity. These RPE cells then undergo

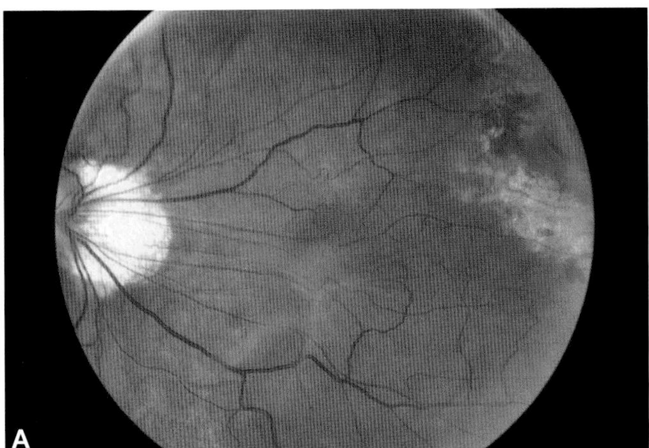


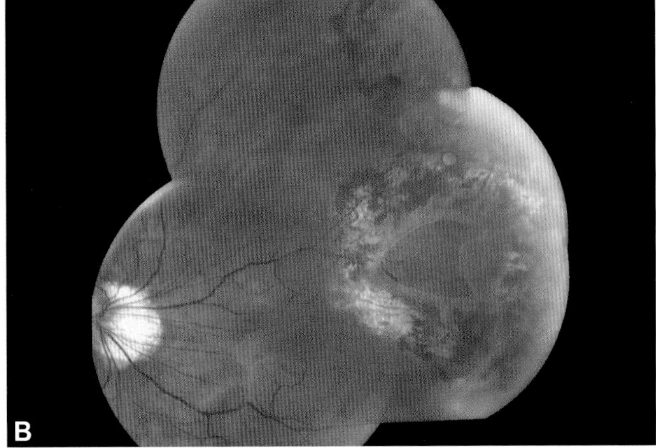


**Figures 29-1A and B** (A) An epiretinal membrane (ERM) visible in the central macula. (B) Montage fundus photograph illustrating the retinal tear previously treated with laser seen temporal to the ERM.

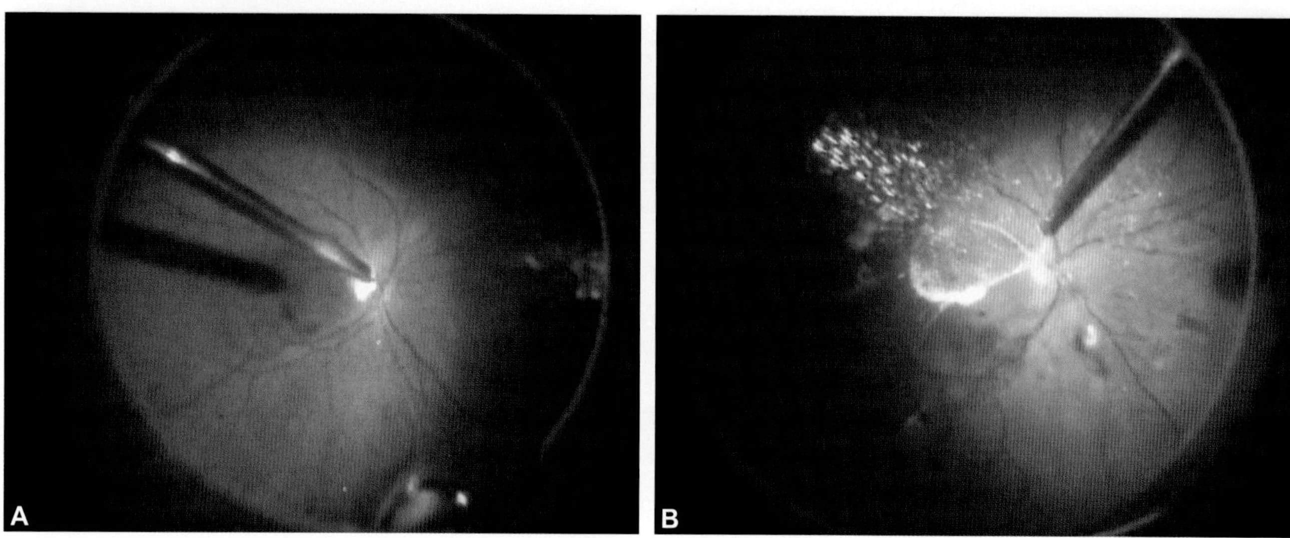

Figures 29-2A and B (A) The vitrectomy cutter applies suction over the optic nerve to engage and release the posterior hyaloid. (B) If the posterior hyaloid is very adherent, the use of triamcinolone will facilitate visualization of the posterior hyaloid and aid in its release.

transformation to glial cells, particularly in the presence of vitreous hemorrhage and inflammation, promoting the formation of ERMs.

If the macular ERM is thin and transparent and not producing distortion of the retina, then the patient is usually asymptomatic. ERMs rarely improve spontaneously and most progress slowly. With progression of the ERM, thickening and contraction of the membrane result in impaired vision, metamorphopsia, macropsia, or micropsia. If the macular traction is severe, secondary macular edema, retinal hemorrhage, and shallow tractional retinal detachment can occur.

## INDICATIONS

The following are general guidelines for patients who would benefit from surgical removal of an ERM:

- Eyes with vision of 20/60 or worse
- Patients with intolerable distortion
- Eyes with ERM and secondary macular edema recalcitrant to medical therapy
- Eyes with ERM and secondary tractional retinal detachment involving the central macula.

## CONTRAINDICATIONS

- Eyes with minimal ERM in asymptomatic patients
- Medically unstable patients
- Eyes with significant ocular comorbidities that will limit meaningful visual recovery.

## SURGICAL TECHNIQUE

### Epiretinal Membrane Removal

The removal of ERM by vitreous surgery has been performed for several decades.[2,3] While the concept remains the same, there have been significant advances in the equipment and techniques. Today, ERM peeling is now one of the most common procedures performed via a three-port pars plana vitrectomy. In recent years, small-gauge transconjunctival vitrectomy systems have largely replaced the 20-gauge vitrectomy techniques of the past. While 25 and 23-gauge systems have been used extensively, recently 27-gauge systems have been developed to perform this procedure.

Local anesthesia using either a peribulbar or retrobulbar block is required for these cases. This is necessary to achieve ocular akinesia and analgesia since even small eye movements can increase the risk of intraoperative iatrogenic retinal breaks.

A standard three-port pars plana vitrectomy is performed with removal of the core vitreous. Most patients with ERM already have a posterior vitreous separation, so the vitreous base can then be trimmed for 360°. If a posterior vitreous separation is not present, applying aspiration over the optic nerve using the vitreous cutter or silicone-tipped extrusion cannula will usually create a posterior vitreous separation that can be extended to 360°(Figs. 29-2A and B). Alternatively, the distal tip of a long 25-gauge needle can be bent to form a pick, and the needle can be attached to active extrusion. This suction pick can also help create a posterior vitreous

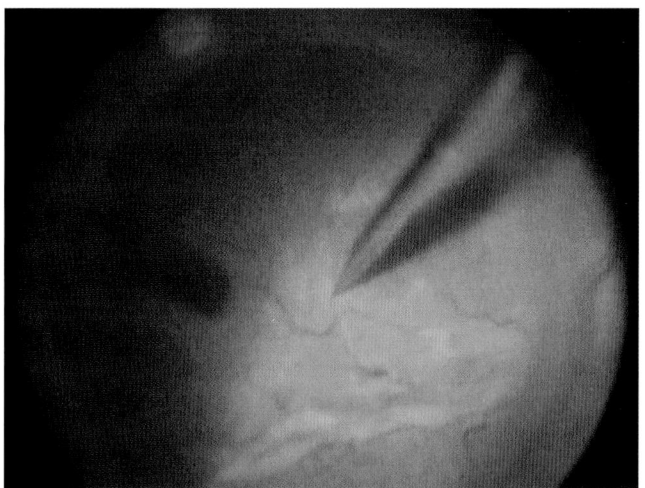

Figure 29-3 An MVR blade is used to engage and lift the edge of an epiretinal membrane.

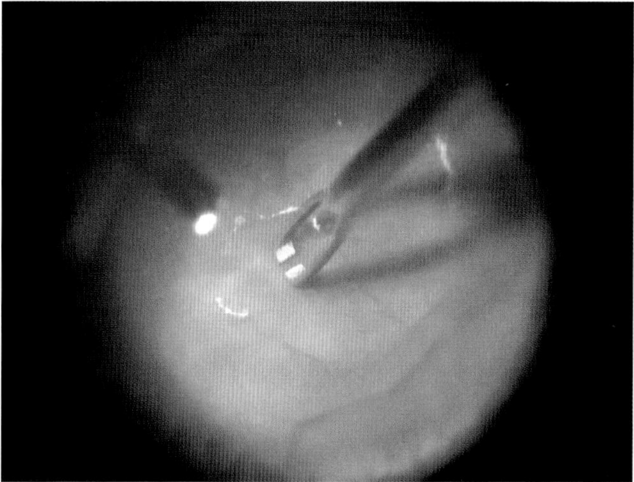

Figure 29-4 With the ILM forceps slightly opened, the epiretinal membrane is engaged.

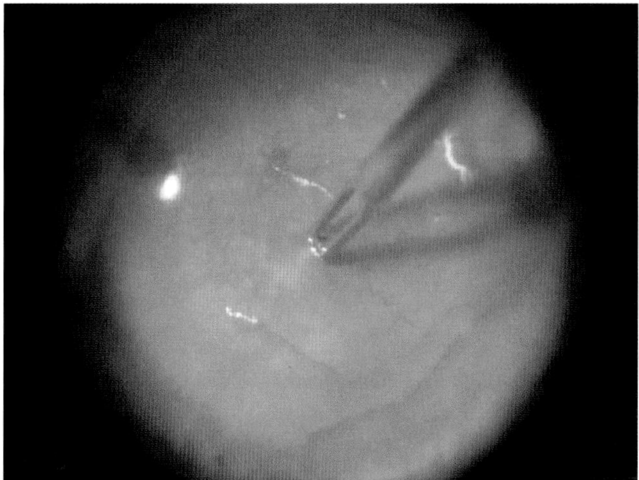

Figure 29-5 The internal limiting membrane forceps pinch and lift the epiretinal membrane to create an edge.

separation. Intravitreal instillation of triamcinolone can also help more clearly identify the vitreous.[4] Once the vitrectomy is complete, attention is turned to the macula where the extent and location of the ERM is evaluated. If an elevated edge to the ERM can be grasped with forceps, "peeling" of the ERM should commence. However, many ERMs do not have an obvious elevated edge, so an edge must be created in order to develop an appropriate plane to separate the ERM from the underlying retina.

The methods used to elevate the edge of an ERM can be generally divided into two techniques: scraping or pinching. Scraping of the ERM is performed by using one of a number of instruments designed for this purpose. These range from a Diamond Dusted Membrane Scraper, an MVR blade, a surgical needle, or even the ends of the forceps. These instruments are used to superficially "scrape" or "scratch" an approximately 3–4 mm area where the ERM meets the adjacent, unaffected retina (Fig. 29-3). This method creates an elevated edge and facilitates grasping with a forcep to begin the peel. The scraping technique can be used either before or after installation surgical adjuvants (*see* section below). To perform the pinch technique, one uses the intraocular forceps with the jaws halfway open to pinch the ERM and underlying ILM at the edge of the macula (Fig. 29-4). Special care is given not to engage the retina too deeply or one risks creating a retinal defect at the site of the pinch. After engagement of the ERM between the teeth of the forceps, the ERM is slightly pulled anteriorly to create an elevated edge (Fig. 29-5). If done correctly, an edge is created that can be used to facilitate grasping and peeling of the ERM. The following steps in ERM removal are similar, regardless of which technique is used to create an initial edge.

A forcep is used to grasp the edge of the ERM and, working in the plane between the ERM and inner retinal surface, the membrane is carefully and delicately dissected from the surface of the underlying retina. It is preferable to peel the ERM in one large sheet to ensure that the entire membrane is removed. This is accomplished by repeatedly releasing and grasping the ERM close to the surface of the retina at the outer edge of the area being peeled (Fig. 29-6). This allows for fine control of the direction of traction on the ERM while it is being separated from the surface of the retina. This also reduces the risk of retinal injury by eliminating the need to re-engage the edge of the ERM directly adjacent to the surface of the retina after the initial peel is started.

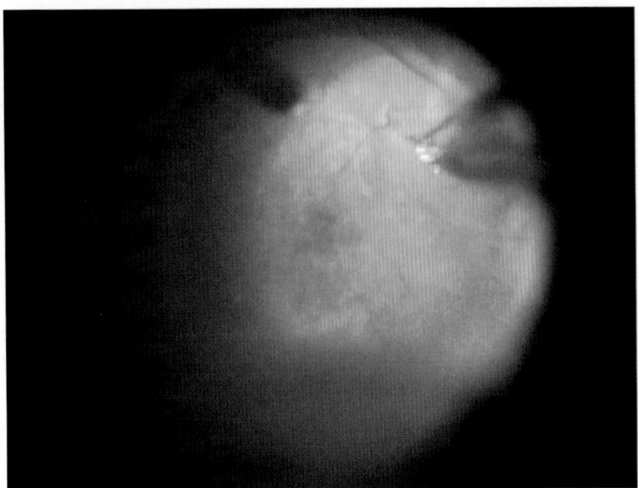

Figure 29-6 The epiretinal membrane is grasped close to the retina to allow fine control of the direction and amount of force applied.

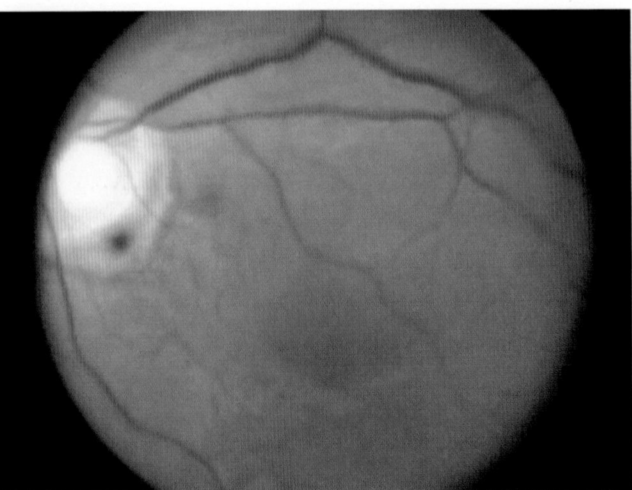

Figure 29-7 Negative staining of the epiretinal membrane is seen in the inferior macular area.

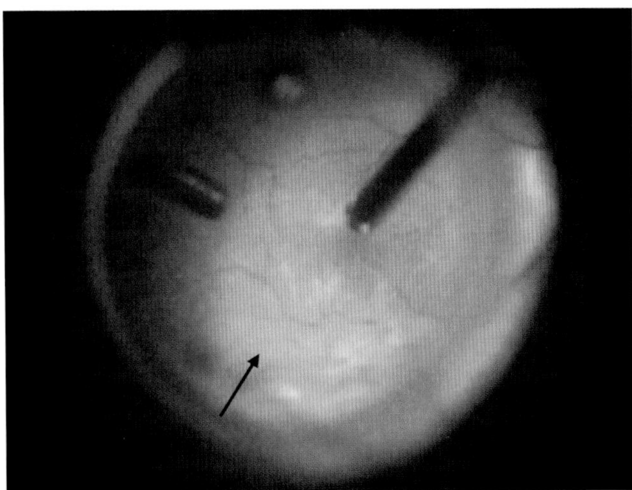

Figure 29-8 The arrow identifies the edge of residual internal limiting membrane after the epiretinal membrane has been removed.

## Internal Limiting Membrane Removal

The removal of the ILM during or following ERM removal is a commonly performed procedure.[5,6] Although whether removing the ILM following ERM removal improves postoperative visual results compare to ERM removal alone is debatable, ILM removal has been shown to significantly reduce the risk of ERM recurrence.[7,8] In more than half the cases of ERM removal, some or all of the ILM is removed along with the ERM.[9] When the ILM, or a portion thereof, is not removed completely, remaining areas of residual ILM may contract in an unbalanced fashion. This incomplete removal of the ILM is thought to contribute to what is referred to as "recurrent ERM", where, at least in some cases, contraction of the residual ILM in postvitrectomy eyes causes similar findings and symptoms as the original ERM.

## Surgical Adjuvants

The use of surgical adjuvants may aid in the visualization and therefore, the efficiency of ERM removal.[10] Although in many cases peeling of the ERM and ILM can be accomplished without the use of adjuvants, these agents decrease the risk and increase the success of this procedure by reducing the surgical time and reducing the recurrence rate. Surgical adjuvants such as indocyanine green (ICG), trypan blue, and brilliant blue G (BBG) stain the ILM very well. Intraoperative triamcinolone is also used to improve visualization of the ERM and ILM, although it achieves this by a different mechanism than that of the other adjuvants. However, none of these agents are effective in staining the ERM, giving the intraoperative appearance of "negative staining" when compared with the normal surrounding retina. This characteristic actually serves as an advantage when differentiating the normal ILM (which is effectively stained) from the area of ERM, which is devoid of stain (Fig. 29-7). This negative staining provides effective visualization of the border between the ERM and the surrounding normal retina.

Once the ERM has been removed, reapplication or "double staining" with one of the surgical adjuvants will show areas of residual ERM or ILM.[8] (Fig. 29-8) Removal of any residual ILM is facilitated by the reinstallation of surgical adjuvants, and complete removal is the only way to ensure that the risk of recurrent ERM is reduced.

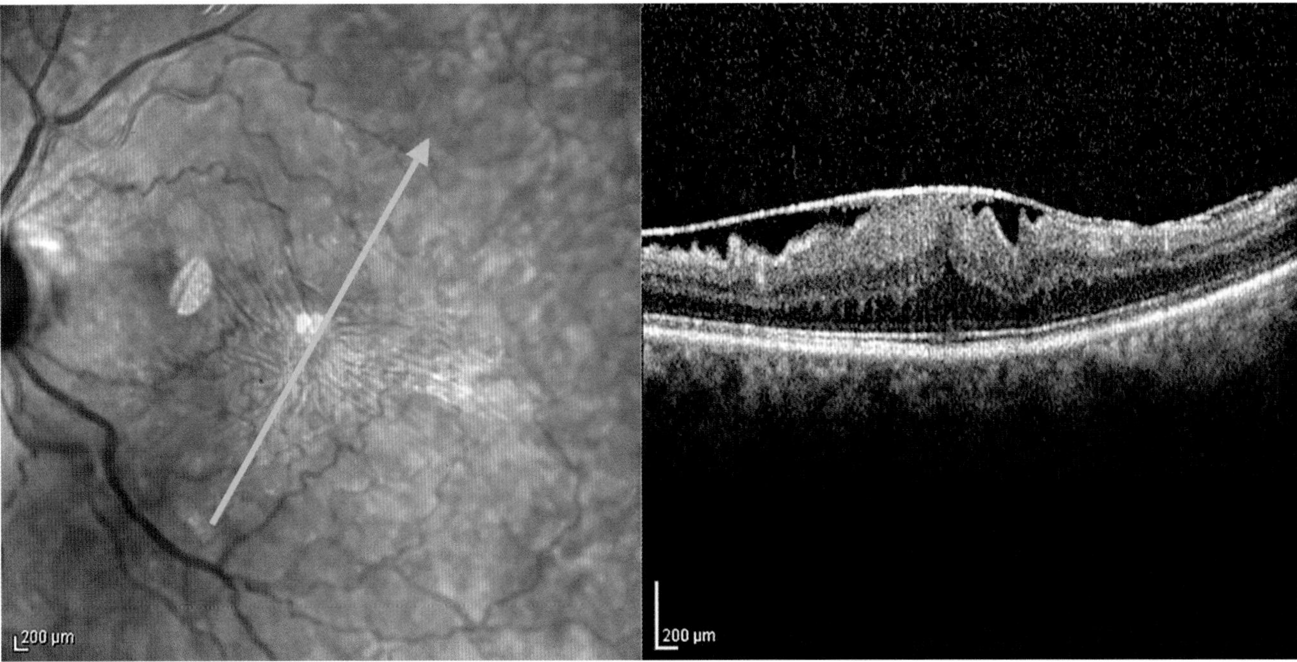


Figure 29-9 Spectral domain optical coherence tomography demonstrating retinal folds caused by a contracting epiretinal membrane.

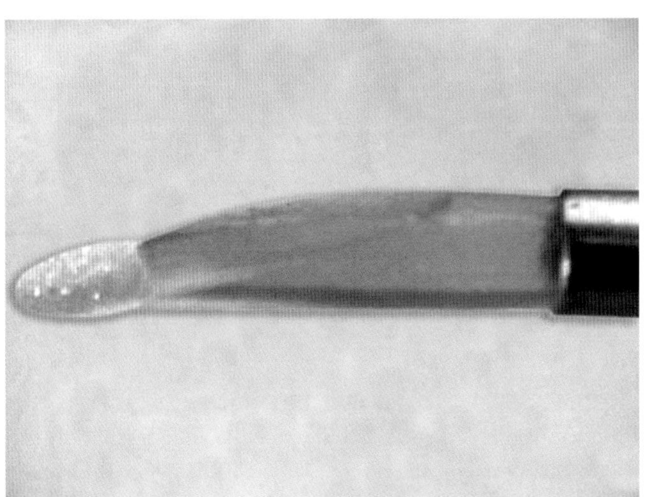

Figure 29-10 The Tano Diamond Dusted Membrane Scraper is used to engage the edge of an epiretinal membrane in an atraumatic fashion.

## MECHANISM OF ACTION

The mechanism of action for removal of ERMs involves mechanically creating a plane between the ERM and either the ILM or the inner retinal surface, and carefully separating the two layers (Fig. 29-9). The ERM is physically separated using traction by forceps to separate this membrane from the surface of the retina. Once the ERM is removed, the retina is allowed to resume its normal anatomic shape with subsequent improvement in visual acuity as well as alleviation of metamorphopsia. In most eyes, postoperative foveal thickness decreases and retinal folds smooth following removal of the ERM.

## POSTOPERATIVE CARE

After the vitrectomy procedure, the eye is patched with a combination of antibiotic/steroid ointment. The patch is usually removed approximately 6 hours following the surgery and then the patient is instructed to begin the use of topical antibiotics and steroid drops. The first postoperative examination usually occurs 24–48 hours following the procedure, specifically looking for any sign of intraocular infection and monitoring of the intraocular pressure. The antibiotic drops are used four times a day for 1 week and the steroid drops are initially used four times a day with a taper over 3–4 weeks depending on the status of the inflammation and the presence or absence of macular edema.

## SPECIFIC INSTRUMENTATION

If an edge of the ERM is not amenable to grasping, a number of devices, such as a Tano Diamond Dusted Membrane Scraper (Synergetics, O'Fallon, MO) (Fig. 29-10), a micro-vitreoretinal (MVR) blade (Fig. 29-11), a surgical needle, or even the ends of the forceps, can be used to elevate to edge of the ERM to facilitate grasping with a forcep.

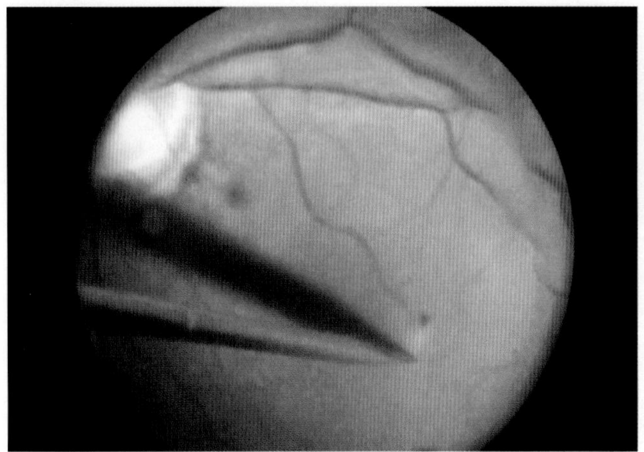

Figure 29-11 An MVR blade creates an edge in the internal limiting membrane that was previously stained with indocyanine green.

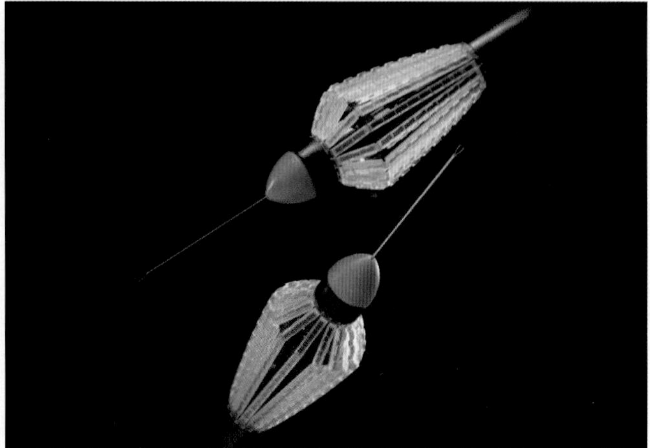

Figure 29-12 Intraocular forceps are available with different tips, sizes, and mechanisms.

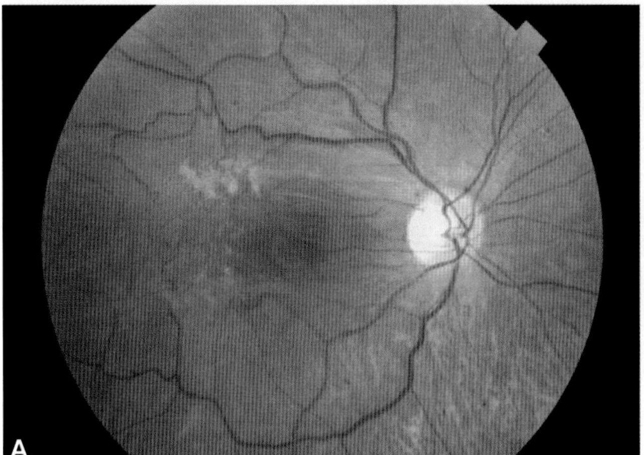

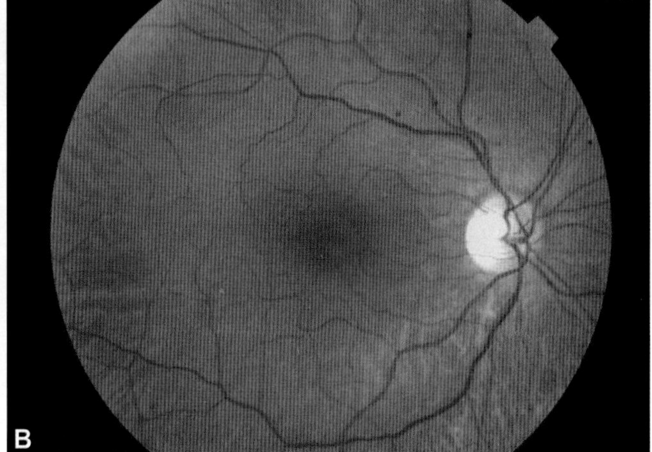

Figures 29-13A and B (A) Fundus photograph of epiretinal membrane (ERM) prior to vitrectomy with membrane peeling. (B) Postoperative appearance of same eye in Figure 29-13A. Note resolution of ERM with normalization of fundus appearance.

Once an edge of the ERM is available for grasping, there are many models and brands of forceps that are used to engage the ERM and then carefully dissect it from the underlying tissue (Fig. 29-12). The different types of forceps vary by material, size, and mechanism of action but they all share the common function of grasping the ERM and removing it from the surface of the retina.

## COMPLICATIONS

The complications related to pars plana vitrectomy surgery for ERM are similar to other types of pars plana vitrectomy surgery.[11] There are anesthesia complications related to both the intravenous sedation of the patient and complications from the periocular anesthesia such as retro-orbital hemorrhage, optic nerve, and globe perforation. The risk of infection, bleeding, retinal detachment, retinal tear, as well as iatrogenic injury to the macula can occur. Macular hole formation can occur during attempted removal of the ERM if it is abnormally adherent to the fovea. Postoperative hypotony as well as elevated intraocular pressure are also potential complications that may be seen following this type of surgery. Although considered a side effect rather than a complication, in patients with the crystalline lens, cataract progression occurs in many eyes within 6–12 months following the surgery.

## SURGICAL OUTCOMES

The vast majority of eyes undergoing surgery for ERM have a noticeable improvement in the optical coherence tomography and fundus photographic findings when compared with the preoperative testing (Figs. 29.13A and B). While anatomic improvement is the rule, the visual results can be much more variable. Most eyes undergoing surgical repair of ERM will experience some visual improvement as well as reduction in metamorphopsia.[6] The typical patient will experience two to three lines of visual improvement, although some have less and others have more improvement. The symptoms of metamorphopsia usually improve more quickly and will generally precede visual acuity improvement. One should allow at least 3–6 months to assess the final postoperative visual acuity since slow and gradual improvement is typical. Those eyes that manifested secondary macular edema due to ERM may require even more time for improvement and may require pharmacologic treatment during the postoperative period to aid in the resolution of the macular edema.

## PLACE OF THE TECHNIQUE IN SURGICAL ARMAMENTARIUM

Most patients with ERM never require surgical intervention. Many patients with mild ERM and minimal to no symptoms can be followed on a periodic basis looking for any evidence of progression. Patients with significant ERM or those associated with macular edema or those with poor vision or distorted vision are excellent candidates for this surgical technique.

## PEARLS AND PITFALLS

### Pearls

- If an edge to the ERM is present, then it should be utilized to begin the peel.
- After the ERM is removed, reinstallation of ICG, trypan blue, or BBG will help to visualize residual ILM.
- Regrasping the ERM closer to the retina as the peel is proceeding allows for greater control of the direction and force of the peel.
- Improvement in symptoms of distortion usually precedes improvement in visual acuity following ERM removal.

### Pitfalls

- Incomplete posterior vitreous separation prior to ERM removal limits enhancement by adjuvants and increases the risk of retinal tear or detachment.
- Failure to completely remove the ILM can result in "recurrent ERM" months to years later.
- All phakic patients should be informed of the side effect of cataract progression following vitrectomy for ERM.

## REFERENCES


1. Pearlstone AD. The incidence of idiopathic preretinal macular gliosis. Ann Ophthalmol. 1985;17(6):378-80.
2. de Bustros S, Thompson JT, Michels RG, et al. Vitrectomy for idiopathic epiretinal membranes causing macular pucker. Br J Ophthalmol. 1988;72(9):692-5.
3. Michels RG. Vitreous surgery for macular pucker. Am J Ophthalmol. 1981;92(5):628-39.
4. Garg SJ. Use of a suction pick in small-gauge surgery facilitates induction of a posterior vitreous detachment. Retina. 2008;28(10):1536.
5. Almony A, Nudleman E, Shah GK, et al. Techniques, rationale, and outcomes of internal limiting membrane peeling. Retina. 2012;32(5):877-91.
6. Pournaras CJ, Emarah A, Petropoulos IK. Idiopathic macular epiretinal membrane surgery and ILM peeling: anatomical and functional outcomes. Semin Ophthalmol. 2011;26(2):42-6.
7. Bovey EH, Uffer S, Achache F. Surgery for epimacular membrane: impact of retinal internal limiting membrane removal on functional outcome. Retina. 2004;24(5):728-35.
8. Shimada H, Nakashizuka H, Hattori T, et al. Double staining with brilliant blue G and double peeling for epiretinal membranes. Ophthalmology. 2009;116(7): 1370-6.
9. Kifuku K, Hata Y, Kohno RI, et al. Residual internal limiting membrane in epiretinal membrane surgery. Br J Ophthalmol. 2009; 93(8):1016-9.
10. Burk SE, Da Mata AP, Snyder ME, et al. Indocyanine green-assisted peeling of the retinal internal limiting membrane. Ophthalmology. 2000;107(11):2010-4.
11. Donati G, Kapetanios AD, Pournaras CJ. Complications of surgery for epiretinal membranes. Graefes Arch Clin Exp Ophthalmol. 1998;236(10):739-46.

CHAPTER 30

# Posteriorly Dislocated Retained Lens Material

John D Pitcher III, Marc J Spirn

## INTRODUCTION

Posteriorly dislocated lens fragments, also known as retained lens material (RLM), are a complication of cataract extraction, particularly phacoemulsification. Although improved surgical techniques have decreased the incidence of RLM, it still occurs in 0.3–1.1% of cases.[1,2] These patients are at high risk of significant intraocular inflammation, increased intraocular pressure (IOP), corneal decompensation, cystoid macular edema (CME), and rhegmatogenous retinal detachment (RRD). In many circumstances, patients require pars plana vitrectomy (PPV) and lensectomy (PPL) to restore or preserve vision, with the majority of patients ultimately achieving visual acuity of at least 20/40.[3–6] PPL may also be required for primary lens removal in settings where an anterior approach is either unsafe or impractical. In both circumstances, attention to detail and appropriate intraoperative strategy can help ensure the best possible patient outcomes.

## INDICATIONS

Postcataract extraction:

- Nuclear fragments in the vitreous
- Substantial cortical fragments in the vitreous or capsular bag.

Particularly with:

- Persistent intraocular inflammation
- Poorly controlled IOP
- Vitreous hemorrhage and/or concern for retinal tear or retinal detachment
- Unacceptably symptomatic vitreous opacities
- Need for urgent visual rehabilitation.

Primary lens removal:

- Visually significant crystalline lens subluxation or dislocation (e.g. trauma or Marfan's syndrome)
- Known or suspected prior posterior capsule violation
- Persistent fetal vasculature (some cases)
- In combination with posterior segment procedures to aid in visualization or access.

## CONTRAINDICATIONS

- Small cortical lens fragments that can be managed medically
- Corneal edema that significantly impairs visualization for PPV (consider delaying vitrectomy or using an endoscopic approach if absolutely necessary)
- Presence of moderate-to-large-sized choroidal detachments.

**Note*: Surgical planning should be accelerated in the presence of vision-threatening complications such as endophthalmitis or high IOP unresponsive to medical management, and surgery should be delayed if the patient is medically unstable or if the surgery cannot be performed safely due to ocular comorbidities.[7]

## SURGICAL TECHNIQUE

Visualization can be challenging in RLM cases due to corneal opacity and poor pupillary dilation. Wide-field, non-contact viewing systems are especially helpful in these cases. Maneuvers to deturgesce the cornea (rolling or scraping) or stretch the pupil may be necessary to improve visualization.

Standard three-port PPV involves placement of an infusion line and two other sclerotomies for bimanual surgery.

TABLE 30-1 Instrumentation in PPV/PPL is determined by the type and size of RLM

| Handpiece | Indication | Mechanism | Reference |
|---|---|---|---|
| 25-gauge vitrector | Limited cortical material | Guillotine cutting, aspiration | Kiss and Vavvas[8] |
| 23-gauge vitrector | Large soft lens<br>Dense material <50% of total lens | Guillotine cutting, aspiration | Baker et al.[6] |
| 20-gauge fragmatome | Standard PPL | Phacoemulsification, aspiration | Scott et al.[2] |
| Ozil (20-gauge) | Large, dense lens fragments | Phacoemulsification, aspiration | Chiang et al.[9] |

(PPV: Pars plana vitrectomy; PPL: Pars plana lensectomy; RLM: Retained lens material).

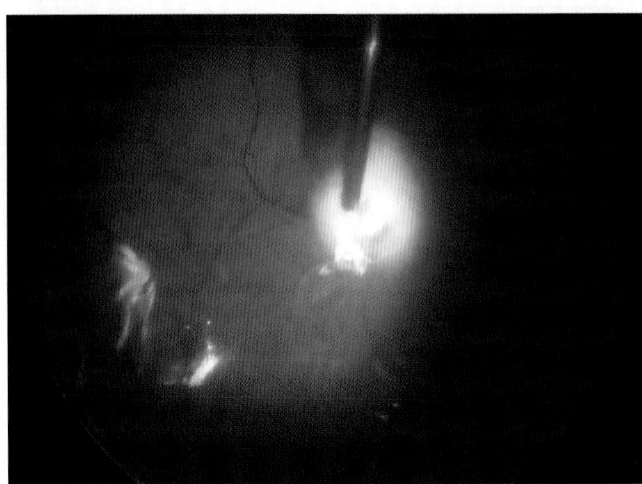

Figure 30-1 Induction of a posterior vitreous detachment. Visualization of the posterior hyaloid face is enhanced with triamcinolone particles.

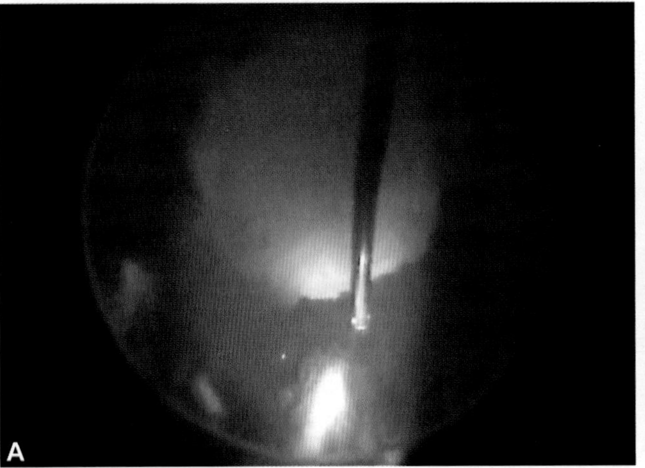


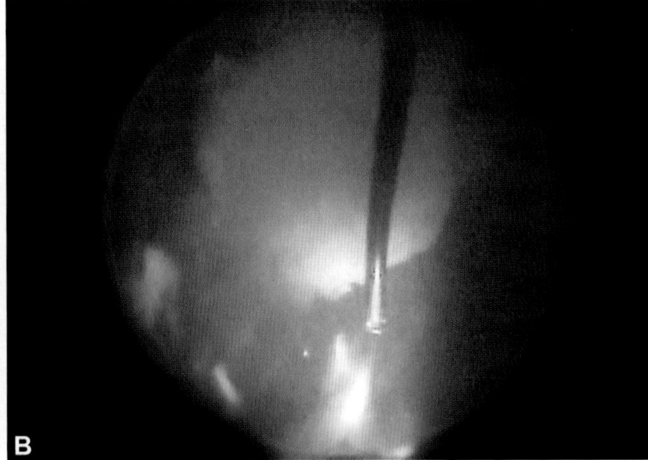


Figures 30-2A and B Peripheral vitreous removal with the aid of intravitreal triamcinolone.

Following completion of a core vitrectomy, a posterior vitreous detachment (if not already present) should be induced (Fig. 30-1). This step may be challenging if substantial RLM is acting as a counterforce. Intravitreal triamcinolone is helpful to identify residual vitreous gel (Figs. 30-2A and B). A peripheral dissection with the aid of scleral depression helps to remove small lens fragments hiding in the vitreous base, most often inferiorly. Thorough vitrectomy helps reduce the risk of retinal breaks encountered during aspiration or phacoemulsification of RLM.

The clinical scenario dictates the choice of instrumentation (Table 30-1). In settings where the vitrectomy handpiece is used for lens removal, momentary vitrectomy mode with a continuous low cut rate can help avoid clogging. It is estimated that approximately 60% of nuclear RLM cases can be managed with 23-gauge vitrectomy alone.[6] The vitreous

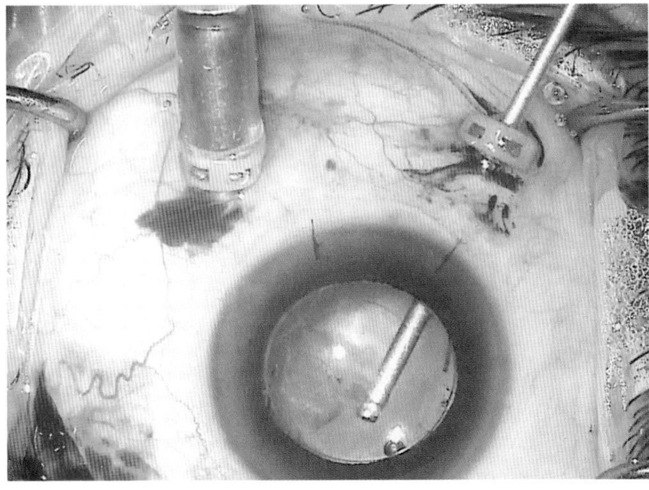

Figure 30-3 Removal of residual anterior cortical lens material just behind the intraocular lens with the vitrector. This maneuver can significantly improve visualization.

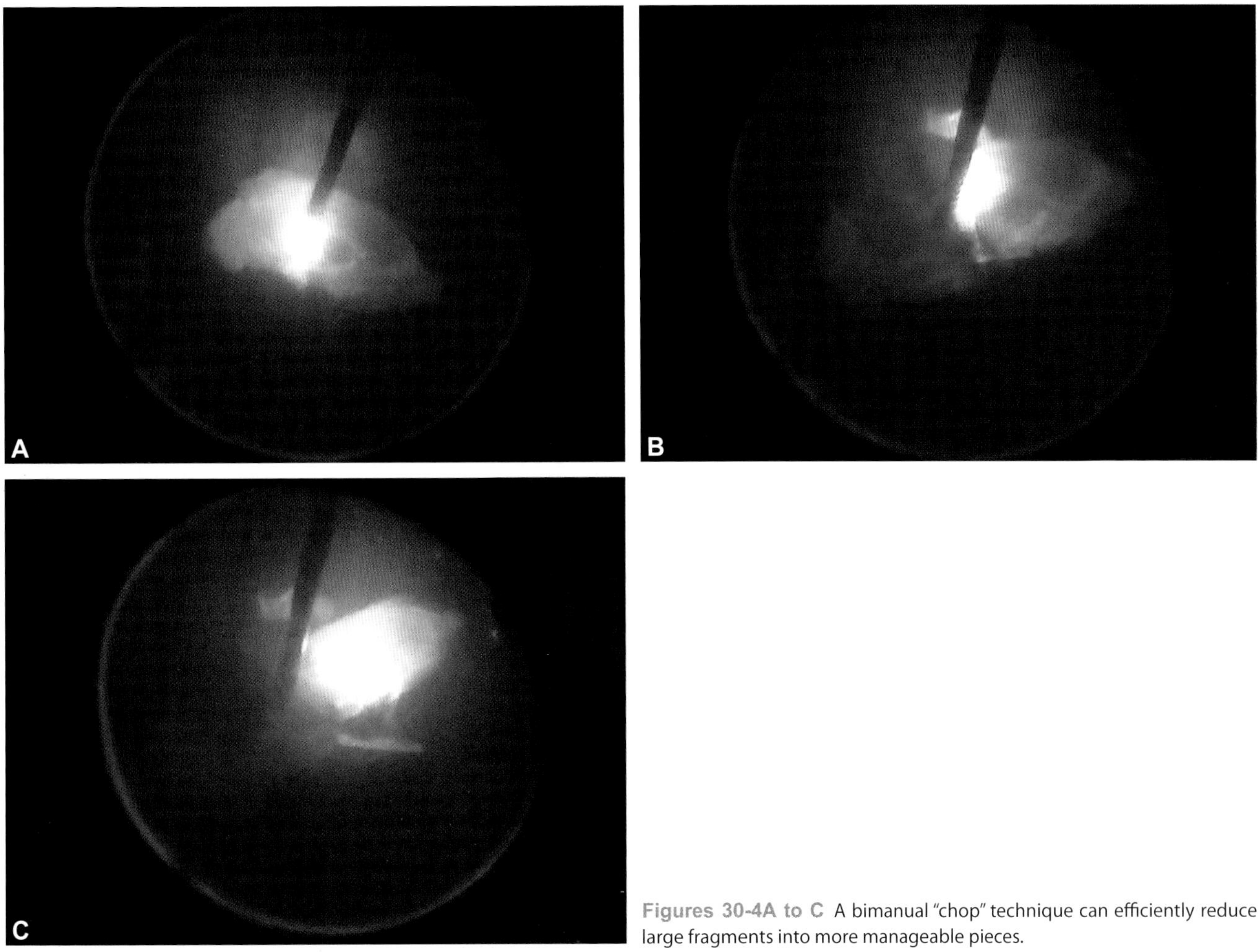

Figures 30-4A to C A bimanual "chop" technique can efficiently reduce large fragments into more manageable pieces.

cutter is optimal for removal of residual cortical fragments still adherent to the posterior capsular bag or IOL (Fig. 30-3).

In circumstances where the phacofragmatome is required, three-dimensional mode with pulse ultrasound is frequently preferable. While maintaining aspiration, the light pipe can be used in a bimanual fashion to physically chop large fragments (Figs. 30-4A to C). The second instrument is also useful to help keep the RLM at the aspiration tip. This may

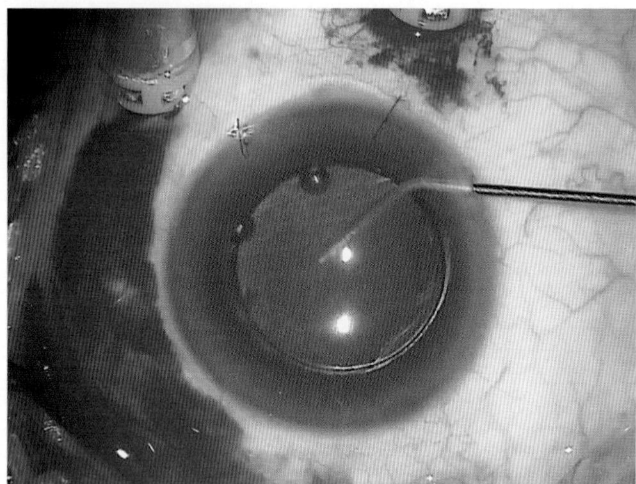

Figure 30-5 Anterior chamber irrigation can help identify any residual occult lens fragments.

also be achieved by increasing vacuum, but this should be used cautiously as high suction without occlusion can induce hypotony and choroidal detachment.

Anterior segment torsional ultrasound technology (OZil, Alcon Inc.) was recently described as a safe alternative to standard techniques and is particularly useful in cases with dense lens fragments.[9] For this method, the authors used a 20-gauge sclerotomy and removed the silicone sleeve from the phacoemulsification handpiece. Default settings included aspiration of 35 cc/min, a vacuum limit of 250 mm Hg, and bottle height of 30 cm $H_2O$. Visual acuity and anatomic outcomes were similar to the conventional fragmatome control group.

Similar principles apply when using PPL for primary lens removal. Stab incisions into the equator of the lens nucleus facilitate access while minimizing zonular injury. Placing the infusion directly into the capsule may also help. Alternatively, opening the posterior lens capsule can help facilitate lens removal. In these cases, posterior segment phacoemulsification (fragmatome) or torsional ultrasound used through the pars plana is almost always necessary since the surgeon is typically removing the whole lens. Regardless of which technique is employed, careful inspection of the retinal periphery and prompt laser retinopexy of any retinal breaks is prudent in all cases.[10]

Attention should be paid to the anterior segment, especially in the final stages of the case. Fragments that may be hiding in the angle can be identified by irrigation through a paracentesis (Fig. 30-5). Clinically significant residual anterior cortical material should be judiciously removed with the vitrector (Fig. 30-3). Injection of dilute triamcinolone into the anterior chamber can help identify vitreous anterior to the IOL. Optimally, a posterior chamber in-the-bag, sulcus, or anterior chamber lens is placed by the cataract surgeon during the initial surgery, and its stability should be confirmed. Postoperative aphakia is not ideal but may be indicated depending on the circumstances (e.g. presence of large choroidal detachments, juvenile idiopathic arthritis) and visual potential. The patient should have a peripheral iridotomy in cases with an anterior chamber lens or aphakia.

A low threshold should be maintained for prophylactic barricade photocoagulation of any suspicious lesions. Air–fluid exchange and/or gas tamponade should be performed at the discretion of the surgeon based on the presence of retinal breaks or detachment. In some eyes, 1 mg of triamcinolone can be placed in the eye at the conclusion of the case. 20-Gauge sclerotomies (if present) and any leaking smaller gauge incisions or corneal wounds should be closed with interrupted sutures. Subconjunctival antibiotic and steroid injections are often performed at the conclusion of the case.

## MECHANISM OF ACTION

PPL is the physical disassembly and aspiration of lens material. Elimination of RLM reduces the stimulus for inflammation that causes elevated IOP and CME.

### Postoperative Care

Following PPV/PPL it is critical to monitor patients for secondary complications. Intensive therapy with topical anti-inflammatory (including steroid and NSAID) eye drops can help limit persistent anterior chamber reaction. When the eye is quiet, the topical steroids can be cautiously tapered as rebound inflammation occurs in some of these eyes. If recurrence occurs, look for occult RLM. Aqueous suppressants (e.g. timolol, dorzolamide) help control elevated IOP. If medical management proves inadequate, consider consultation with a glaucoma specialist.

CME is a common cause of decreased vision in the postoperative period. Fluorescein angiography and optical coherence tomography (OCT) are essential to identify and follow this condition. If a trial of topical anti-inflammatory drops, including both a steroid and nonsteroidal medication, proves ineffective, sub-Tenon's or intravitreal steroid injections may be indicated (Figs. 30-6A to C). In those most vulnerable to elevated IOP, intravitreal antivascular endothelial growth factor (e.g. bevacizumab) injection as well as topical non-steroidal anti-inflammatory drops are alternative

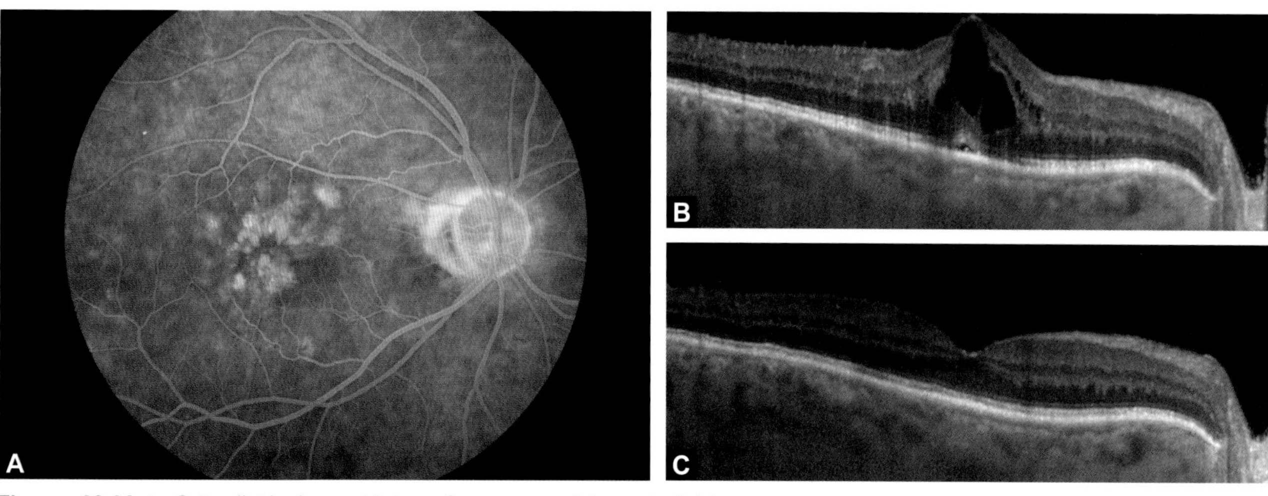


Figures 30-6A to C Petalloid edema with hyperfluorescence of the optic disk in a pin a patient who underwent pars plana vitrectomy with pars plana lensectomy for retained lens material in the right eye (A). Optical coherence tomography demonstrated significant macular edema (B). One month following sub-Tenon's triamcinolone injection, the patient's macular edema resolved (C) and her vision improved from 20/80 to 20/30.

therapeutic options. The retinal periphery should be examined with serial dilated funduscopic examinations to look for retinal tears.

### Instrumentation

- Wide-angle (preferably noncontact) viewing device
- Three-port PPV system (preferably with valved cannulae)
- Vitrector, phacofragmatome, or Ozil handpiece (Table 30-1)
- Light pipe.

As indicated:

- Paracentesis blade and BSS irrigating syringe on a blunt cannula
- Silicone soft-tip cannula (for air–fluid exchange)
- Endolaser probe
- 8-0 Vicryl, 10-0 nylon suture
- Subconjunctival antibiotics, steroid.

### Complications

Intraoperative:

- IOL instability
- Mechanical or ultrasonographic retinal damage
- Lens fragment retinal injury
- Retinal tear or detachment
- Serous or hemorrhagic choroidal detachment.

Postoperative:

- Persistent or rebound inflammation
- Elevated IOP
- Corneal decompensation
- CME
- Retinal tear or detachment
- Endophthalmitis.

## SURGICAL OUTCOMES: SCIENTIFIC EVIDENCE

Large series of patients with posteriorly dislocated lens material have concluded that most patients do quite well. Only 5% have final visual acuity of 20/200 or worse. The strongest predictors of good final vision are better vision at presentation and the presence of an IOL.[2,11] In the immediate postvitrectomy period, vision is typically limited by nonretinal pathology (corneal edema, inflammation, and elevated IOP). These issues are usually transient and can be managed medically.

The most frequent vision-limiting complication is CME, which occurs in up to 61% of patients following lensectomy.[12] Retinal detachment, while potentially more devastating, is less common. Older studies estimated the rate of postoperative RRD at 8–13%.[3,4] More recently, authors have reported lower rates of RRD (4–5%), and this is attributed to improved visualization, instrumentation, and surgical techniques.[6] Endophthalmitis and choroidal hemorrhage are even more rarely encountered. Ultimately, most patients with RLM achieve good final vision, with nearly 80% of patients seeing better than 20/40.[5]

## PLACE OF THE TECHNIQUE IN SURGICAL ARMAMENTARIUM

PPL is a common indication for PPV, and therefore represents a critical skill for any vitreoretinal surgeon.

## PEARLS AND PITFALLS

- Complete a thorough vitrectomy with careful vitreous base dissection.
- Keep lens material and instruments as far away from macula as possible to avoid mechanical trauma (perfluorocarbon liquid may be useful as a buffer in rare instances).
- Minimize turbulence by maintaining a closed system (small-incision, valved cannulae) and judiciously using vacuum.
- Caution with fragmatome will help avoid ultrasound damage to retina.
- Careful peripheral retinal inspection will help detect small retinal tears and occult lens fragments.
- Consider intravitreal triamcinolone as a tool to help identify and remove residual cortical vitreous, identify vitreous in the anterior chamber, as well as prophylaxis against postoperative CME.
- Scleral depression and anterior chamber irrigation help identify small lens fragments that can be otherwise missed.

## REFERENCES

1. Pande M, Dabbs TR. Incidence of lens matter dislocation during phacoemulsification. J Cataract Refract Surg. 1996;22: 737-42.
2. Scott IU, Flynn HW, Smiddy WE, et al. Clinical features and ouctomes of pars plana vitrectomy in patients with retained lens fragments. Ophthalmology. 2003;110:1567-72.
3. Smiddy WE, Guererro JL, Pinto R, et al. Retinal detachment rate after vitrectomy for retained lens material after phacoemulsification. Am J Ophthalmol. 2003;135(2):183-7.
4. Moore JK, Scott IU, Flynn HW Jr, et al. Retinal detachment in eyes undergoing pars plana vitrectomy for removal of retained lens fragments. Ophthalmology. 2003;110(4):709-13.
5. Merani R, Hunyor AP, Playfair TJ, et al. Pars plana vitrectomy for the management of retained lens material after cataract surgery. Am J Ophthalmol. 2007;144(3):364-70
6. Baker PS, Spirn MJ, Chiang A, et al. 23-gauge transconjunctival pars plana vitrectomy for removal of retained lens fragments. Am J Ophthalmol. 2011;152(4):624-7.
7. Colyer MH, Berinstein DM, Khan NJ, et al. Same-day versus delayed vitrectomy with lensectomy for the management of retained lens fragments. Retina. 2011;31(8):1534-40.
8. Kiss S, Vavvas D. 25-gauge transconjunctival sutureless pars plana vitrectomy for the removal of retained lens fragments and intraocular foreign bodies. Retina. 2008;28(9):1346-51.
9. Chiang A, Garg SJ, Alshareef RA, et al. Removal of posterior segment retained lens material using the OZil phacoemulsification handpiece versus Fragmatome during pars plana vitrectomy. Retina. 2012;32(10):2119-26.
10. Tan HS, Mura M, Oberstein SY, et al. Retinal breaks in vitrectomy for retained lens fragments. Retina. 2012;32(9):1756-60.
11. Ho LY, Doft BH, Wang L, et al. Clinical predictors and outcomes of pars plana vitrectomy for retained lens material after cataract extraction. Am J Ophthalmol. 2009;147:587-94.
12. Rossetti A, Doro D. Retained intravitreal lens fragments after phacoemulsification: Complications and visual outcome in vitrectomized and non-vitrectomized eyes. J Cataract Refractive Surg. 2002;28:310-5.

CHAPTER

31

# Surgical Repair of Choroidal Detachment

Andre J Witkin

## INTRODUCTION

Choroidal detachment occurs as a result of acute or chronic hypotony from inflammatory or mechanical causes, medications, and both noniatrogenic and iatrogenic trauma. Choroidal detachments are due to either choroidal vessel leak causing a serous detachment or vessel rupture causing a hemorrhagic choroidal detachment. These two types of choroidal detachment often can be differentiated with fundus biomicroscopy, but B-scan ultrasonography is frequently used to aid in the diagnosis and differentiation of these two types of fluid (hemorrhage is hyperechoic on ultrasound, while serous fluid is hypoechoic) (Fig. 31-1). Serous choroidal detachments are often asymptomatic, but hemorrhagic choroidal detachments can be extremely painful.[1]

Common causes of serous choroidal detachments include hypotony following intraocular surgery, particularly with glaucoma filtration or tube shunt surgery, extensive panretinal photocoagulation, intra- or postoperative wound leakage, certain medications, chronic retinal detachment, or chronic inflammation. Hemorrhagic detachments may occur from acute hemorrhage into a previously existing serous choroidal detachment, from ocular trauma, during or following ocular surgery, or spontaneously due to a bleeding diathesis or from abnormalities of the choroid. The visual prognosis for hemorrhagic detachment is worse than for serous choroidal detachment.[2]

Serous choroidal detachments may also occur intraoperatively during vitrectomy surgery if the infusion cannula is partially disinserted to a position where the infusion sits in the suprachoroidal space.[3] Air, gas, or silicone oil may be infused inadvertently into the suprachoroidal space during vitrectomy surgery via the same mechanism, causing a choroidal detachment from these materials.[4]

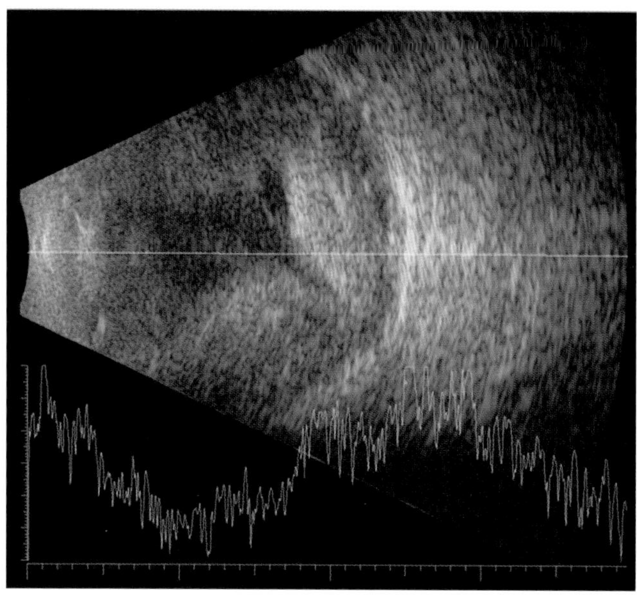

Figure 31-1 B-scan ultrasound with corresponding A-scan from a patient with an acute hemorrhagic choroidal detachment due to hypotony from a leaking glaucoma filtration bleb. Note the hyperechoic nature of acute hemorrhage. The choroidal elevation is relatively immobile on dynamic echography.

## INDICATIONS

Usually, a conservative approach using cycloplegic/mydriatic medications, and corticosteroids is advisable when a choroidal detachment is present. Surgery is reserved for cases of severe anterior chamber shallowing, concurrent rhegmatogenous retinal detachment or incarceration, retinal apposition ("kissing choroidals"), intractable pain, high intraocular pressure, or persistent decreased visual acuity due to the choroidal detachment.[5] Chronic choroidal detachment may also lead to dysfunction of the ciliary body, which eventually can lead to hypotony maculopathy and globe phthisis.

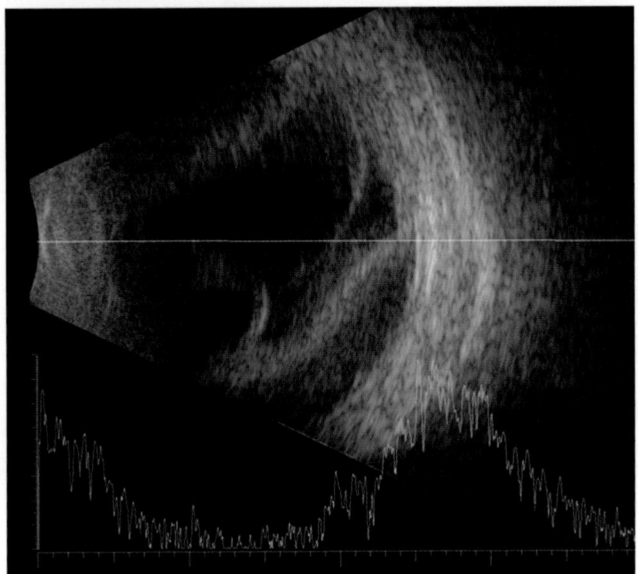

Figure 31-2 B-scan ultrasound with corresponding A-scan from the same patient, 2 weeks after presentation. Note that the choroidal detachment has become smaller, and the hemorrhage occupying the suprachoroidal space has become less hyperechoic, signifying liquefaction of the hemorrhage.

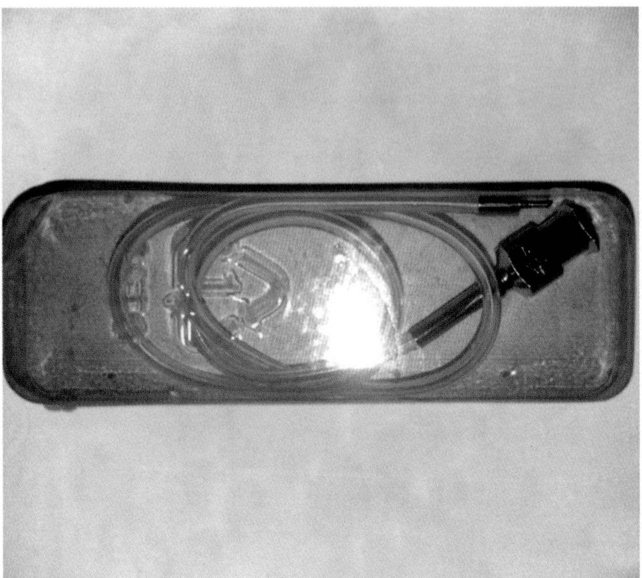

Figure 31-3 Lewicky anterior chamber maintainer.

The timing of optimal surgical intervention can be variable. For hemorrhagic choroidal detachment, if possible the surgeon should wait 7–10 days after the hemorrhagic event in order to allow the blood clot time to liquefy, as this facilitates surgical decompression of the suprachoroidal space. Ultrasonography can be helpful to decide timing of surgical intervention, as hemorrhage becomes less hyperechoic once it begins to liquefy (Figs. 31-1 and 31-2).[5,6] If the vision is no light perception or if there is a visually threatening increase in the intraocular pressure, surgical drainage can be performed earlier with more variable results.

Poor prognostic indicators are central retinal apposition ("kissing choroidals"), vitreous or retinal incarceration in surgical or traumatic wounds, and loss of intraocular contents at the time of intraoperative or traumatic choroidal hemorrhage formation. These factors also increase the urgency of performing surgical intervention.

## CONTRAINDICATIONS

As mentioned above, patients with choroidal detachments can often be managed conservatively. Surgery should be reserved for patients with higher risk characteristics as described below.

## Surgical Technique

### *Infusion of Fluid*

First, the surgeon should decide how to maintain a constant ocular pressure while the choroidal effusion or hemorrhage is drained. This can be accomplished by using an anterior chamber (limbus-based) infusion, a pars plana infusion, or repeated injections of sterile balanced salt solution or viscoelastic into the anterior chamber or posterior segment.

If an anterior chamber infusion is used, a 20- or 23-gauge anterior chamber maintainer may be inserted after the creation of an anterior chamber paracentesis, or a 23- or 25-gauge trocar may be inserted directly into the anterior chamber and the cannula may then be connected to an infusion line. After the case is finished, a 10-0 nylon suture is often necessary to close the limbal incision, as the shape of the maintainer may preclude proper wound closure without a suture (Figs. 31-3 and 31-4).

If pars plana infusion is used, the surgeon should consider using a 6 mm trocar or infusion cannula (Fig. 31-5), and/or inserting the infusion more anteriorly than normal if pseudophakic (i.e. 2.5 or 3 mm from the limbus, instead of 3.5 mm). The trocar should also be inserted more parallel to the iris plane to avoid impaling the retina/choroid. The surgeon

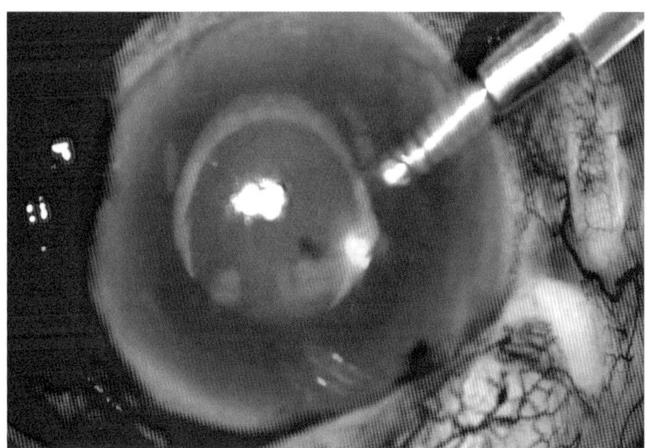

Figure 31-4 External photograph of an anterior chamber maintainer after placement into the anterior chamber through a paracentesis that was created with a 20-gauge MVR blade.

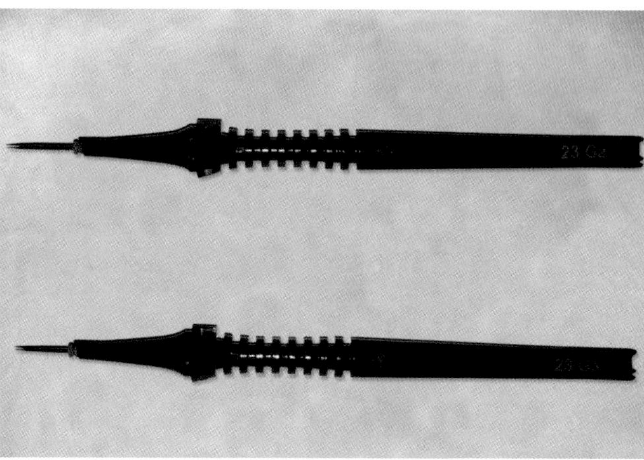

Figure 31-5 Photograph of a 6 mm 23-gauge trocar in comparison to a standard 23-gauge trocar.

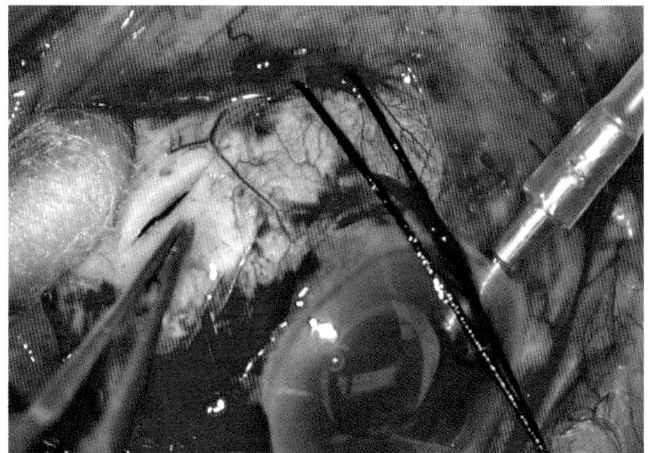

Figure 31-6 External photograph of an eye undergoing choroidal drainage. A limited peritomy has been made to isolate the extraocular muscles using 2-0 silk ties. A 2-mm-long sclerotomy has been formed parallel to and 5 mm from the limbus. A forcep and cotton-tipped swab are used to open the edge of the sclerotomy. The swab helps to express suprachoroidal fluid and to maintain constant ocular pressure. Infusion is performed with a Lewicky anterior chamber maintainer.

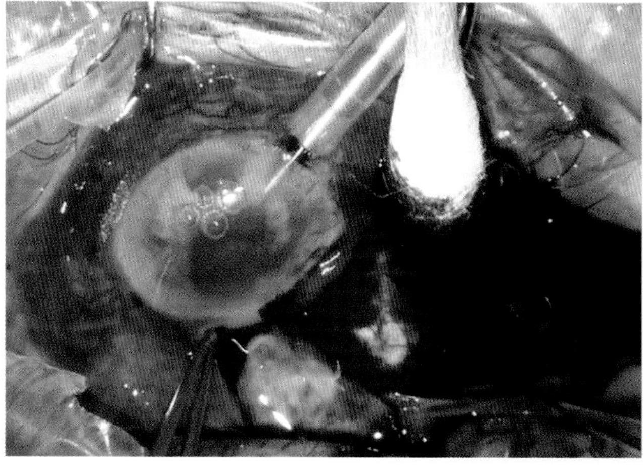

Figure 31-7 External photograph of an eye undergoing choroidal drainage. After creating a limited peritomy, a 2-mm-long radial sclerotomy has been fashioned 4–6 mm from the limbus. A cotton-tipped swab helps to express suprachoroidal fluid, and to maintain constant ocular pressure. In this case, dark liquefied hemorrhagic fluid is expressed from the suprachoroidal space. Infusion is performed with an anterior chamber maintainer.

must remember that choroidal effusions can often extend anterior to the pars plana as far as the scleral spur, which is where the ciliary body inserts. Insertion of a longer infusion cannula can run the risk of damage to the lens in phakic patients, so it might be necessary to remove the lens in phakic eyes.

## *Sclerotomy Formation*

After infusion is placed, a sclerotomy to drain suprachoroidal fluid needs to be created. A limited peritomy is performed in the quadrant of most bullous choroidal detachment. Pre- and/or intraoperative ultrasound or indirect biomicroscopy is useful to determine the ideal quadrant of choroidal drainage. Occasionally looping the extraocular muscles helps to gain exposure of the desired quadrant.

To enter the suprachoroidal space, a sharp scalpel (Microvitreoretinalblade (MVR) or #57 blade) is used to create a 2–3 mm long sclerotomy (Figs. 31-6 and 31-7). The ideal position of the sclerotomy can be debated; it should be at least 4 mm from the limbus, and some argue it should be placed as far as 9 mm from the limbus. Many surgeons prefer an incision of 6–7 mm from the limbus; however, if there is hemorrhage

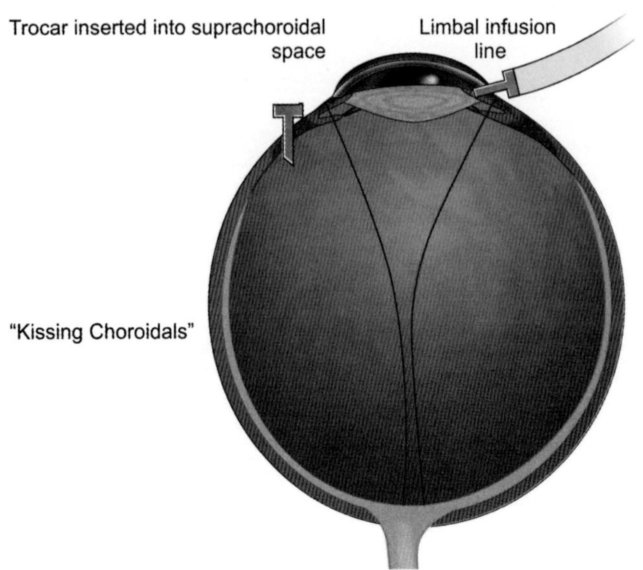


Figure 31-8 Illustration of transconjunctival choroidal fluid drainage through a 23-gauge trocar. The trocar is inserted 7 mm from the limbus, at a shallow angle to avoid damaging the choroid or retina with the sharp tip of the blade. A 23-gauge cannula can also be used as the limbus-based infusion, as shown.

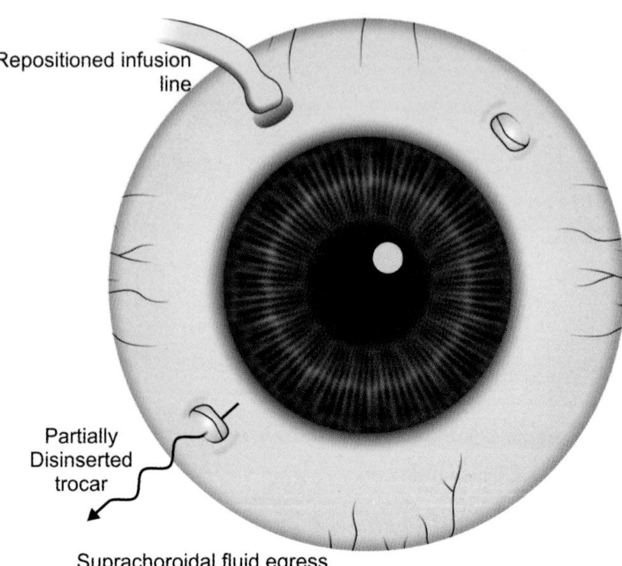


Figure 31-9 Illustration of choroidal fluid drainage via a partially disinserted trocar. The infusion line has been repositioned superotemporally, and suprachoroidal fluid is allowed to egress through the disinserted trocar, which now resides in the suprachoroidal space. The malpositioned trocar may be removed once the choroidal fluid has drained.

anterior to the ora serrata, a sclerotomy of 4 mm from the limbus may be adequate and has the advantage of potentially allowing vitrectomy to proceed from the same incision. The sclerotomy can be placed either parallel or perpendicular to the limbus depending on surgeon preference.

Once the suprachoroidal space is entered, the fluid is allowed to egress out of the sclerotomy. In hemorrhagic choroidal detachments, a sharp 25- or 30-gauge needle may be necessary to puncture through the peripheral clot to access the more liquefied area of hemorrhage. Fluid egress can be aided by gaping the edges of the wound with forceps, and a cyclodialysis spatula can be used to gently access and sweep within the suprachoroidal space (this can be helpful in hemorrhagic choroidal detachments that have not completely liquefied). Care should be taken to allow the eye to pressurize while fluid is draining from the sclerotomy. Cotton swabs may be used to depress the sclera to facilitate fluid egress and maintain adequate ocular pressure.

If inadequate drainage is attained, a second sclerotomy may be performed in an adjacent quadrant. Some surgeons argue to leave sclerotomies open to allow continued drainage of suprachoroidal fluid postoperatively, although others suggest suturing the sclerotomies at the end of the case.

An alternative technique to access the suprachoroidal space is to use a 20-, 23-, or 25-gauge trocar to drain choroidal fluid transconjunctivally. The trocar may be inserted obliquely in the area of most bullous choroidal detachment, taking care to access only the suprachoroidal space by entering at a shallow (15°) angle. Some authors suggest placing the trocar 7 mm from the limbus, although placement of the trocar 4 mm from the limbus may be sufficient to access the suprachoroidal space if the instrument is inserted at a shallow angle (Fig. 31-8).[7] Take care not to puncture the retina with the trocar.

Along the same lines, if an intraoperative choroidal detachment is caused by inadvertent infusion into the suprachoroidal space caused by partial disinsertion of the infusion cannula during pars plana vitrectomy (PPV), the infusion line may be disconnected from the partially disinserted cannula while leaving that cannula in the suprachoroidal space. Once the infusion is connected to a new properly inserted cannula, suprachoroidal fluid can be allowed to egress through the partially disinserted cannula, and choroidal detachment will often resolve (Fig. 31-9).[3]

## *Pars Plana Vitrectomy*

PPV may be indicated once choroidal fluid is drained. Indications for PPV in patients with choroidal detachment include central retinal apposition with persistent retinal adhesion after choroidal drainage, concurrent rhegmatogenous detachment, vitreous hemorrhage, or vitreous and/or retinal incarceration.[5,6] In these cases, as mentioned above, it is often helpful to use 6 mm trocars and to place them 2.5 or 3 mm from the limbus, in order to avoid entering the suprachoroidal space.

During vitrectomy, vitreous and/or retinal incarceration should be relieved. Retinal apposition requires surgical manipulation to relieve adherence. Perfluorocarbon liquid can be used to aid in flattening the retina, and help to flatten predominately serous choroidal detachments. Occasionally a relaxing retinotomy may be required to repair retinal incarceration or complex tractional retinal detachments.

At the end of vitrectomy, silicone oil may be used for tamponade, although resolution of the residual choroidal detachment postoperatively leaves the eye with a relative oil underfill. Nonexpansile or slightly expansile concentrations of gas therefore may be preferred, as they may better maintain adequate fill of the vitreous cavity during the early postoperative period.

## MECHANISM OF ACTION

The key to draining suprachoroidal fluid is to gain access to the suprachoroidal space. Preoperative planning is important to localize the area of most bullous detachment. The choroidal insertion is at the scleral spur; therefore, choroidal fluid can be drained via an incision anywhere behind the pars plana. Hemorrhagic detachments can be difficult to drain if blood is not liquefied. Liquefaction of suprachoroidal hemorrhage often occurs within 7–10 days, and is visible on serial B-scan ultrasonography.

## POSTOPERATIVE CARE

After the procedure, the eye can be patched and shielded for a few hours. Patients can then continue cycloplegic agents as well as topical anti-inflammatory medications until the residual choroidal detachment has resolved. Shallow choroidal detachments often persist after a choroidal drainage procedure, but often resolve 6–8 weeks after the procedure. Occasionally, repeat choroidal drainage procedures are necessary, particularly if there is persistent postoperative hypotony. Serous elevation of the retina initially may become more prominent as the choroidal detachment resolves; this can usually be followed without intervention as it generally spontaneously disappears.

## SPECIFIC INSTRUMENTATION

Infusion:

- Lewicky anterior chamber maintainer, and paracentesis blade OR 20-gauge MVR blade; OR 6 mm trocar/infusion cannula.

Sclerotomy:

- Westcott scissors
- Gass muscle hooks
- 20-gauge MVR blade OR #57 blade; OR, 20-gauge/23-gauge/25-gauge trocar
- Cyclodialysis spatula

Vitrectomy:

- 6 mm trocar OR infusion cannula (consider placing 2.5 to 3 mm from the limbus in pseudophakic patients)
- Perfluorocarbon liquid
- Silicone oil OR $SF_6$ gas OR $C_3F_8$ gas

## COMPLICATIONS

### Intraoperative

- New or recurrent choroidal hemorrhage
- Vitreous or subretinal hemorrhage

### Postoperative

- Cataract formation
- Recurrent or persistent choroidal detachment
- Retinal detachment
- Proliferative vitreoretinopathy
- Persistent hypotony
- Endophthalmitis
- Loss of vision
- Loss of eye

## SURGICAL OUTCOMES: SCIENTIFIC EVIDENCE/META-ANALYSIS

There have been several series of patients who have underwent surgical repair of suprachoroidal hemorrhage; all suggest a guarded visual prognosis. The evidence suggests that approximately 33% of these patients obtain a visual acuity of 20/200 or better postoperatively. Up to 25% of patients with suprachoroidal hemorrhage who require surgical intervention end up with no light perception vision. Approximately 20% of eyes have persistent hypotony. Retinal incarceration and concurrent rhegmatogenous retinal detachment portend the worst visual prognosis in this setting.[2]

Conversely, patients with a serous choroidal effusion have a better prognosis. In a large series of patients (63) who underwent surgical repair of serous choroidal detachment following glaucoma surgery, 60% of patients had complete resolution by 1 month after surgery, and 90% had complete resolution 4 months after surgery. Twenty percent of patients required more than one surgery to reattach the choroid. Seventy-seven percent of phakic eyes developed a visually significant cataract postoperatively that required phacoemulsification with intraocular lens implantation. Roughly 90% of patients attained 20/200 visual acuity or better.[5]

## PLACE OF THE TECHNIQUE IN SURGICAL ARMAMENTARIUM

Every retina surgeon and many anterior segment surgeons should understand how to repair choroidal detachment. The retina surgeon often is the specialist who has to manage the choroidal detachment, and he/she should particularly know the indications and contraindications to perform surgery in this setting. Choroidal detachment can also occur intraoperatively during vitrectomy as well as any other penetrating ocular surgery, either from hemorrhage or from infusion into the suprachoroidal space. All surgeons who perform ocular surgery should know how to recognize and manage these potentially devastating complications.

## PEARLS AND PITFALLS

- Conservative management is advisable unless there is severe anterior chamber shallowing, concurrent rhegmatogenous retinal detachment or incarceration, retinal apposition ("kissing choroidals"), intractable pain, high intraocular pressure, or persistent decreased visual acuity.
- Preoperative B-scan ultrasonography is used to detect the quadrant of most bullous detachment and to confirm liquefaction of hemorrhage.
- Maintaining constant intraocular pressure is crucial. This can be achieved with an anterior chamber infusion or a pars plana infusion.
- Pars plana infusion trocars or cannulas of 6 mm are useful in patients with choroidal detachment, particularly when performing vitrectomy.
- Suprachoroidal fluid may be drained through a sclerotomy placed 4–9 mm from the limbus.
- Conversely, a 20, 23, or 25-gauge transconjunctival trocar may be used to enter and drain the suprachoroidal space.
- Subsequent PPV may be necessary in cases of central retinal apposition with persistent retinal adhesion after choroidal drainage, concurrent rhegmatogenous detachment, vitreous hemorrhage, or vitreous and/or retinal incarceration.
- For tamponade, nonexpansile or slightly expansile gas is preferable to silicone oil as resolution of the residual choroidal detachment postoperatively leaves the eye with a relative oil underfill.

## REFERENCES

1. Bellows AR, Chylack LT Jr, Hutchinson BT. Choroidal detachment. Clinical manifestation, therapy and mechanism of formation. Ophthalmology. 1981;88(11):1107-15.
2. Wirostko WJ, Han DP, Mieler WF, et al. Suprachoroidal hemorrhage: outcome of surgical management according to hemorrhage severity. Ophthalmology. 1998;105(12):2271-5.
3. Witkin AJ, Fineman M, Ho AC, et al. A novel method of draining intraoperative choroidal detachments during 23-gauge pars plana vitrectomy. Arch Ophthalmol. 2012;130(8):1048-50.
4. Zhang ZD, Shen LJ, Zheng B, et al. Surgical management of silicone oil migrated into suprachoroidal space after vitrectomy. Int J Ophthalmol. 2011;4(4):458-60.
5. WuDunn D, Ryser D, Cantor LB. Surgical drainage of choroidal effusions following glaucoma surgery. J Glaucoma. 2005;14(2): 103-8.
6. Meier P, Wiedemann P. Massive suprachoroidal hemorrhage: secondary treatment and outcome. Graefes Arch Clin Exp Ophthalmol. 2000;238(1):28-32.
7. Rezende FA, Kickinger MC, Li G, et al. Transconjunctival drainage of serous and hemorrhagic choroidal detachment. Retina. 2012;32(2):242-9.

CHAPTER

32

# Endophthalmitis

Michael Dollin, Jason Hsu

## INTRODUCTION

Endophthalmitis, an infection of the internal ocular cavities, can be visually devastating. It can occur from exogenous sources, such as any intraocular surgery, intravitreal injection, or penetrating trauma. Endogenous endophthalmitis arises from hematogenous spread of a systemic infection. Bacteria are the most common causative organisms but fungal, parasitic, and viral cases can occur. Visual outcomes following endophthalmitis are often poor, but can be variable depending on etiology, visual acuity at presentation, and causative organism. When endophthalmitis develops, prompt diagnosis and treatment are imperative.

## THE ENDOPHTHALMITIS VITRECTOMY STUDY

Bacterial endophthalmitis following cataract surgery is the most common cause of endophthalmitis. Treatment of endophthalmitis in this clinical setting has been guided by the Endophthalmitis Vitrectomy Study (EVS), a landmark, randomized, prospective clinical trial supported by the National Eye Institute and published in 1995 (Box 32-1).[1,2]

It is important to note that the EVS results apply only to acute (within 6 weeks) postcataract surgery or postsecondary intraocular lens (IOL) implant-related endophthalmitis. It does not apply to delayed or chronic postoperative, traumatic, endogenous, bleb-related, or intravitreal injection-related endophthalmitis, although clinicians may apply the results of the EVS to these cases at their discretion.

## VITREOUS TAP AND INJECT

### Preoperative Evaluation

Any patient presenting with pain and decreased vision following ocular surgery should be examined without delay. Clinical diagnosis of endophthalmitis should be suspected based on the following slit-lamp biomicroscopic findings: lid edema, conjunctival injection, conjunctival chemosis, corneal edema, anterior chamber cell and fibrin formation, hypopyon, and vitritis (Fig. 32-1).

In the presence of significant corneal or anterior segment opacity, B-scan echography should be used to identify vitritis and rule out any posterior segment abnormalities such as choroidal or retinal detachment and retained lens material, especially in the setting of complicated cataract surgery (Fig. 32-2).

### Specific Instrumentation and Equipment (Fig. 32-3)

- *Anesthetic*: Combination of topical viscous and subconjunctival or peribulbar lidocaine (without epinephrine)
- Povidone-iodine 5%
- Bladed lid speculum
- Short 25- (preferred) or 27-gauge needle on a 3 or 5 mL Luer-lock syringe for vitreous tap
- 30-gauge needle on a 1 mL syringe should be available in the event that an anterior chamber tap is required (i.e. when a vitreous specimen is unobtainable)
- Intravitreal medications (*see* Table 32-1) each loaded in a 1 mL syringe with 30-gauge needle

**BOX 32-1 The Endophthalmitis Vitrectomy Study (EVS).[1,2]**

*Purpose*: To determine the role of immediate pars plana vitrectomy (PPV) and, separately, the role of systemic antibiotics in the management of endophthalmitis following cataract extraction or secondary intraocular lens (IOL) insertion.

*Methods*: Patients with clinical signs and symptoms of postcataract surgery or secondary IOL-related endophthalmitis, presenting within 6 weeks of surgery, and with visual acuity between 20/50 and light perception (LP) were included in the study. Patients were excluded if they had known eye disease limiting their visual acuity to 20/100 or worse before their development of cataract or if they had no LP vision at baseline. Patients were randomized to undergo either PPV or vitreous tap within 6 hours of examination, as well as receive intravenous (IV) antibiotics (ceftazidime and amikacin for 5–10 days) or no IV antibiotics. All patients, regardless of randomization, also received:

Intravitreal vancomycin 1.0 mg/0.1 mL and amikacin 0.4 mg/0.1 mL

Subconjunctival vancomycin 25 mg/0.5 mL, ceftazidime 100 mg/0.5 mL, and dexamethasone 6 mg/0.25 mL

Topical fortified vancomycin 50 mg/mL and amikacin 20 mg/mL

Topical cycloplegic and prednisolone drops

Oral prednisone 30 mg BID for 5–10 days

*Results*: Two-hundred eight patients underwent immediate (within 6 hours) PPV, 202 underwent vitreous tap, 206 received IV antibiotics, and 214 did not. The mean time from surgery to presentation was 6 days. Sixty-nine percent of microbial cultures were positive. Microbial spectrum was as follows: 70% coagulase negative *Staphylococcus* species (primarily *S. epidermidis*), 9.9% *S. aureus*, 9.0% *Streptococcus* species, 2.2% *Enterococcus*, 5.9% gram-negative organisms, and 9.3% polymicrobial. Overall visual outcomes were good, with 53% of all patients achieving 20/40 or better, and 74% 20/100 or better at 9–12 months. Only 15% had final visual acuity worse than 5/200, including 5% who had final vision of no LP. Endophthalmitis cases due to gram-positive, coagulase-negative *Staphylococci* were associated with better visual outcomes than endophthalmitis cases due to other species. Patients who were LP on initial examination and underwent immediate PPV had a three times better chance of achieving 20/40 (33% *vs* 11%), two times better chance of 20/100 (56% *vs* 30%), and less than half the risk of severe vision loss to below 5/200 (20% *vs* 47%). Immediate PPV did not confer significant benefits if patients presented with hand motions (HM) or better vision. There was no benefit of IV antibiotics.

*Conclusion*: EVS findings strongly support the use of immediate PPV in eyes with acute endophthalmitis following cataract extraction or secondary IOL implantation. Vitreous tap is equivalent to PPV in eyes with presenting vision of HM or better. Systemic IV antibiotics offer no benefit and are not necessary in the treatment of these patients.

**TABLE 32-1** Intravitreal medications used in treating endophthalmitis

| Medication | Intravitreal dose | Spectrum of coverage |
|---|---|---|
| Vancomycin | 1.0 mg in 0.1 mL | Gram-positive isolates |
| Ceftazidime | 2.25 mg in 0.1 mL | Gram-negative isolates, pseudomonas |
| Amikacin | 0.4 mg in 0.1 mL | Gram-negative isolates |
| Dexamethasone* | 0.4 mg in 0.1 mL | N/A |
| Amphotericin | 5 µg/mL (inject 0.1 mL) | *Candida, Aspergillus* |
| Voriconazole | 100 µg in 0.1 mL | *Candida, Aspergillus, Fusarium* |

*Controversy exists regarding the use of intravitreal steroid in the setting of bacterial endophthalmitis. Some believe that the majority of the damage that occurs in bacterial endophthalmitis is due to the immune response to bacterial antigen. As such, intravitreal dexamethasone or sub-Tenon's triamcinolone 40 mg/mL injection, either at the time of the tap and inject or after 24–72 hours, can be considered. In suspected fungal endophthalmitis, steroids are considered to be contraindicated.

- Syringe stopper
- Antibiotic ointment
- Patch and tape

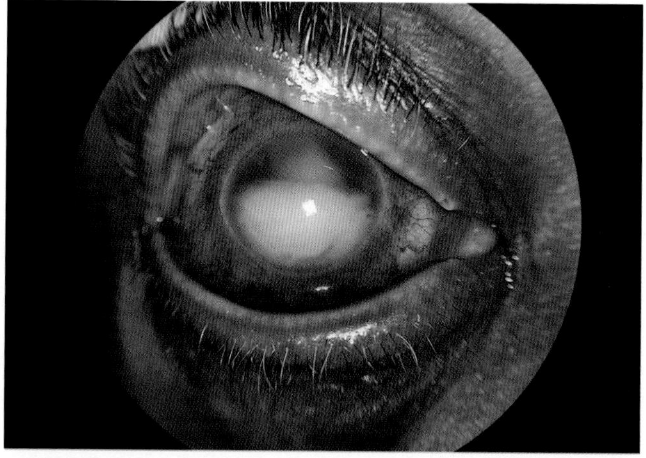

**Figure 32-1** A patient who developed endogenous endophthalmitis presented with decreased vision, redness, pain, and a hypopyon.

## Surgical Technique

- Anesthetize the patient's eye with a nonviscous topical anesthetic followed by topical povidone-iodine 5%. Viscous lidocaine may be applied at this point if desired. Subconjunctival lidocaine 2% (without epinephrine) in the quadrant of the planned tap and inject should generally

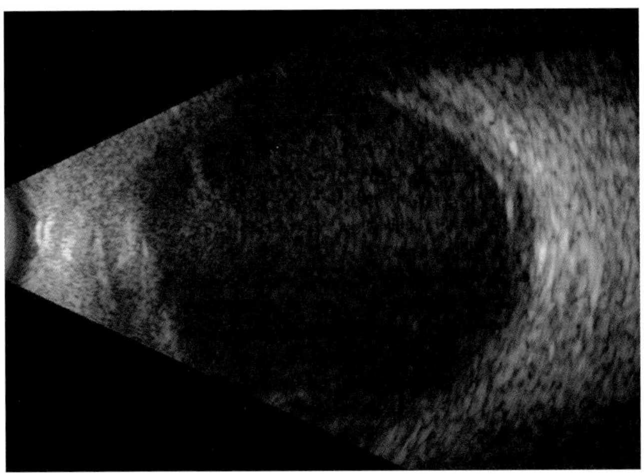

Figure 32-2 B-scan echography demonstrates vitritis in an eye with endophthalmitis.

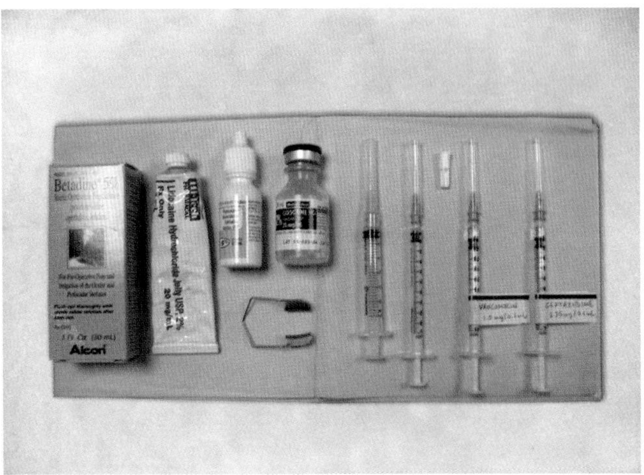

Figure 32-3 Equipment necessary for performing a tap and injection.

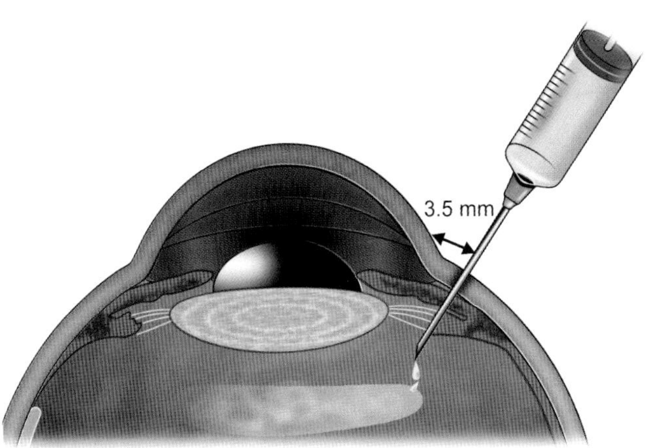


Figure 32-4 Proper location for needle insertion during a tap and inject (4 mm from the limbus in phakic eyes and 3.5 mm from the limbus in pseudophakic or aphakic eyes through the pars plana).

be performed. For patients in severe pain, peribulbar or retrobulbar injection of lidocaine 2% (without epinephrine) may be considered.

- Prep the patient's eye with povidone-iodine 5% and place a bladed lid speculum.
- Mark the site of injection using a caliper or blunt end of a tuberculin syringe (approximately 4 mm). Needles should be inserted through the pars plana 4 mm away from the surgical limbus in a phakic eye and 3.5 mm away in a pseudophakic or aphakic eye.
- Insert a short 25- or 27-gauge needle on a 3 or 5 mL syringe through the mark, aiming toward the midvitreous cavity. A 25-gauge needle is generally preferred as it may increase the chance of yielding a vitreous sample. However, a smaller gauge needle is usually sufficient in previously vitrectomized eyes. Once in the vitreous cavity, withdraw slowly on the plunger and maintain suction until egress of vitreous fluid is observed in the needle hub. In some cases, the needle may have to be repositioned within the vitreous cavity in order to obtain a sample. Release suction prior to attempting to move the needle in order to minimize the risk of traction on the vitreous and potential creation of iatrogenic retinal breaks. Withdraw between 0.1 and 0.3 mL of vitreous fluid, depending on the intended amount of medication to be injected and the preoperative intraocular pressure (IOP) (e.g. if IOP was high, consider removing additional fluid when possible). Remove the needle from the eye (Fig. 32-4).
- Inject the intravitreal medications with a 30-gauge needle on a 1 mL syringe in the same area as the tap.
- Combining the intravitreal medications into a single syringe in order to decrease the number of injections is not recommended. Combining the medications may result in dilution and/or precipitation of the medication that can reduce efficacy.
- An alternate technique involves using a single short 25-gauge needle through the pars plana, firmly grasped at the hub with a locking mosquito hemostat. The tap can be performed and the surgeon can subsequently leave the needle inserted into the eye, stabilizing it with the hemostat, and sequentially unscrewing and screwing the various syringes required, until all intravitreal medications have been administered. Only then is the needle removed from the eye.[3]
- If a vitreous sample was not forthcoming, an anterior chamber tap should be performed using a 30-gauge needle

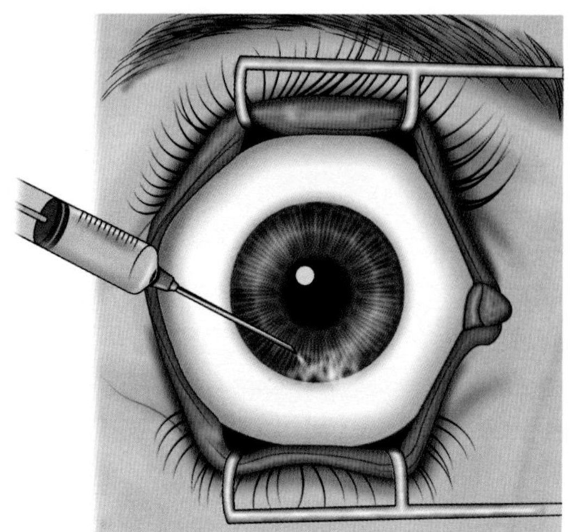

Figure 32-5 A safe position for the needle tip is over the iris when performing anterior chamber paracentesis in a phakic eye.

on a 1 mL syringe inserted through the temporal limbus into the anterior chamber. This should be performed prior to injection of intravitreal medications. In phakic eyes, be mindful to hold the tip of the needle over the iris while performing the tap, in order to avoid trauma to the anterior lens capsule. When possible, at least 0.1 mL of aqueous fluid should be removed, depending on the amount of medication to be injected and the preoperative IOP (Fig. 32-5).

- IOP should be checked after the procedure to ensure it is not elevated. If significantly elevated, an anterior chamber paracentesis may be required. Otherwise IOP-lowering drops can be prescribed.

## Postoperative Care

Following tap and inject, the authors routinely place antibiotic ointment onto the eye and patch the eye for 30–60 minutes, especially if peribulbar anesthesia was used. In addition to intravitreal antibiotics, the authors' practice is to prescribe topical fortified antibiotic drops (most commonly vancomycin 25–50 mg/mL and tobramycin 15 mg/mL) and prednisolone acetate 1% administered hourly, along with atropine 1% twice a day. In the setting of suspected fungal endophthalmitis, treatment usually consists of systemic antifungals (oral voriconazole or fluconazole), alone or in combination with intravitreal voriconazole or amphotericin.

Patients with endophthalmitis should be followed daily until there is definite sign of improvement. Often these eyes look worse the first day after the tap and inject. If patients show clinical deterioration indicated by worsening vision and/or inflammatory signs during the early postoperative course, a repeat tap and inject and/or vitrectomy should be considered. Repeat injection of intravitreal antibiotics should be tailored to the specific organism if a Gram stain or cultures are available (e.g. vancomycin alone in cases of endophthalmitis due to gram-positive cocci).

## Complications

Potential complications of tap and inject include retinal breaks and retinal detachment, intraocular hemorrhage, cataract formation due to iatrogenic lens trauma, and disruption of any pre-existing surgical wounds.

# VITRECTOMY

Performing vitrectomy surgery in endophthalmitis is analogous to draining an abscess. It allows better removal of organisms and toxins, provides a better specimen for culture, and may allow better dispersion of antibiotics. Disadvantages to treating all cases of endophthalmitis with vitrectomy as primary treatment include delay in treatment, need for operating room and equipment, surgical risks with poor visualization, and more rapid clearing of intravitreal antibiotics.

## Indications

As per the EVS, emergent vitrectomy for patients with endophthalmitis after cataract extraction or secondary IOL is indicated when they present with light perception (LP) vision. Vitrectomy is also useful to obtain a vitreous biopsy and debulk acute infectious material. Given the improvements in vitrectomy instrumentation and visualization since the EVS, however, some surgeons advocate for vitrectomy even in cases with better than LP vision, either immediately or within 24–48 hours following a tap and inject. Similarly, immediate vitrectomy may be advocated for other types of endophthalmitis (e.g. bleb-related endophthalmitis) not addressed by the EVS, or in patients showing signs of clinical deterioration despite prompt tap and inject at presentation.

Vitrectomy is also useful in managing complications or sequelae of endophthalmitis, such as traction retinal detachment, rhegmatogenous retinal detachment, nonclearing postinflammatory vitreous debris, refractory cystoid macular edema, epiretinal membrane, and hypotony. Delayed or chronic endophthalmitis, such as that caused by *Propionibacterium acnes* infection, sometimes requires IOL explantation with capsulectomy and vitrectomy.[4]

## Preoperative Evaluation

A thorough medical and ocular history and ocular examination should be performed. In cases of suspected endogenous endophthalmitis in which vitrectomy is being considered, consultation with the patient's medical team should be obtained, as a targeted systemic workup looking for the source of infection is critical (*see* section "Workup for endogenous endophthalmitis").

## Specific Instrumentation and Equipment

Standard pars plana vitrectomy equipment, preferably small (23- or 25-) gauge, is required. In cases where visualization is very poor and patients are pseudophakic or aphakic, consider using 6 mm trocar cannulae, rather than the standard 4 mm cannula to help ensure penetration through the pars plana and into the vitreous cavity. Alternatively, instead of placing the infusion cannula through the pars plana, an infusion light pipe or anterior chamber maintainer can be used instead.

## Surgical Technique

- If safe to do so from a systemic point of view, vitrectomy for endophthalmitis can generally be performed under conscious sedation with a retrobulbar, peribulbar, or sub-Tenon's block. As severe inflammation often makes local anesthesia less effective, general anesthesia can be considered.
- Prep the surface of the patient's eye along with the eyelids and eyelashes with povidone-iodine 5% and drape in a sterile fashion.
- Place a lid speculum, paying careful attention toward keeping the lashes away from the surgical field.
- Mark the sites for trocar-cannula entry. For standard three-port pars plana vitrectomy, the infusion cannula is generally inserted in the inferotemporal quadrant, while the other two instrument ports are placed superotemporally and superonasally. The cannulae should be placed 4.0 mm from the limbus in phakic eyes and 3.5 mm from the limbus in pseudophakic or aphakic eyes. When inserting the trocar-cannulae, it is important to displace conjunctiva using forceps or a cotton-tipped applicator. If the view is fairly good, enter the eye in a beveled fashion. However, in cases in which the view is not very good, entering the eye perpendicular to the sclera can help confirm that the cannula is in the vitreous cavity.
- In the presence of significant corneal edema, anterior chamber fibrin/inflammation, and vitritis, confirmation of entry of the infusion cannula through the pars plana into the vitreous cavity by direct visualization can be challenging. Options include the following:
  - 6 mm trocar cannulae (rather than the standard 4 mm cannulae)
  - Infusion light pipe
  - Anterior chamber maintainer.

  If 6 mm cannulae are not available, or if visualization is still not possible despite them, vitrectomy may have to commence without the infusion turned on, until the tip of the infusion cannula can be visualized. Alternatively, an infusion light pipe can be used or infusion can be started using an anterior chamber maintainer. In some cases, the anterior chamber maintainer can be used for the entire procedure or at least until the view clears sufficiently to allow visualization of the infusion cannula through the pars plana.
- If a tap and inject has not previously been performed in clinic, an undiluted vitreous sample should be obtained. Connect a 3 or 5 mL syringe to the aspiration line of the vitreous cutter. Without turning on the infusion, insert the vitreous cutting instrument into the middle to anterior vitreous cavity, visualizing it as best as possible. While cutting, gently aspirate vitreous into the syringe by pulling back on the plunger. Once approximately 0.3–0.5 mL has been collected, stop aspirating and open the infusion. We have found an increased yield with also sending a diluted vitreous specimen after the infusion has been opened. In this situation, we often aspirate an additional 3–5 mL. Send the vitreous sample for Gram stain and cultures and reconnect the aspiration line to the cutter. Infusing air into the eye also helps maintain pressure and can increase the volume of undiluted specimen (Fig. 32-6).

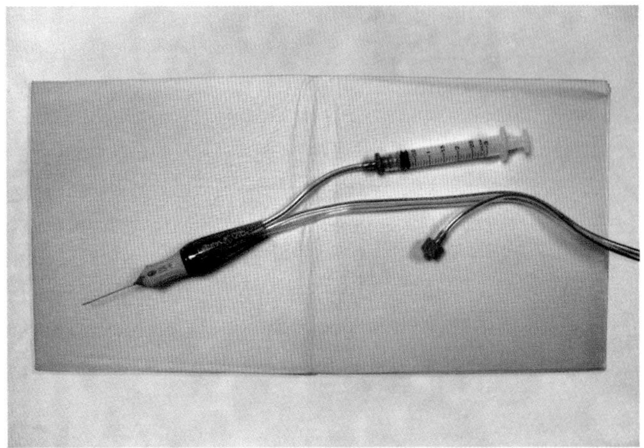

Figure 32-6 Vitreous cutter with syringe connected to aspiration line for obtaining vitreous sample during vitrectomy.

- Check that the vitreous cutting instrument is set to low suction and the highest possible cut rate (ideally, 2500–5000 cuts per minute), in order to decrease the risk of iatrogenic retinal breaks.
- If anterior chamber fibrin and a pupillary membrane significantly hinder visualization, viscoelastic can be injected into the anterior chamber to displace fibrin from the pupil. Alternatively, fibrin and membranes can be removed with the vitreous cutter and/or vitreoretinal/anterior segment forceps through a limbal paracentesis. Note that in some cases, this step may need to be performed prior to vitrectomy in order to allow for adequate visualization.
- Proceed with a core vitrectomy, removing the anterior vitreous that is visible behind the lens first. Attempt to remove core vitreous until the retina becomes visible. Keep in mind, however, that a complete vitrectomy is usually not necessary or safe in these eyes. If one is not already present, it is generally not advised to attempt to create a posterior vitreous detachment, as traction on necrotic retina can easily induce retinal breaks. Similarly, avoid using instruments, such as an extrusion cannula, which deliver only suction. Due to the difficult view in these cases, iatrogenic breaks and retinal detachments can be very difficult to repair. Moreover, given the inflammatory milieu, development of retinal tears dramatically increases the risk of proliferative vitreoretinopathy. Therefore, we cannot emphasize enough the importance of minimizing the risk of iatrogenic breaks (Fig. 32-7).
- Once as much core vitreous has been removed as is safely possible, carefully inspect the periphery under scleral depression then remove the instruments and sclerotomy cannulae. It is generally advisable to suture all sclerotomies using 8-0 polyglactin or 6-0 plain gut, and all corneal wounds using 10-0 monofilament nylon.
- Inject intravitreal medications through the pars plana as described in the previous section. With the advent of valved cannulae that prevent reflux of intraocular fluids, another option is to inject the intravitreal medications through the valved cannula prior to removal.

## Postoperative Care

Patients are placed on the same topical drops as following tap and inject (*see* section "Postoperative care"). Patients should be followed closely with peripheral fundus examination by indirect ophthalmoscopy for the presence of any retinal breaks. Serial B-scan echography may be helpful in situations where the fundus view remains obscured postoperatively in order to detect the development of retinal tears or detachment.

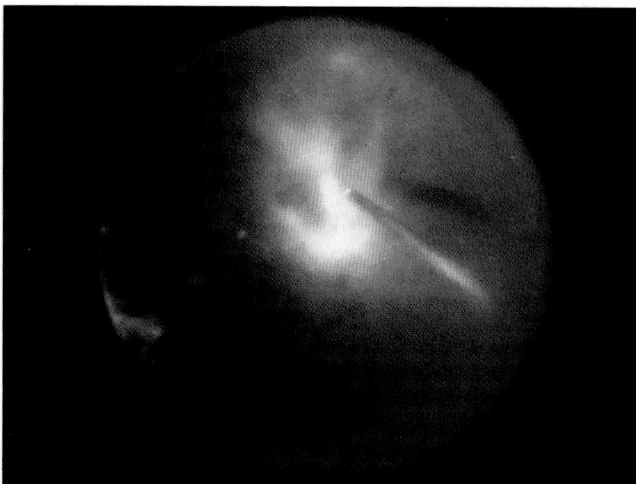

Figure 32-7 Vitrectomy in a patient with endophthalmitis. This case has a clearer view than many patients with endophthalmitis have.

## Complications

Potential complications of vitrectomy in cases of endophthalmitis include corneal decompensation, glaucoma, intraocular hemorrhage, cataract formation, choroidal hemorrhage or detachment, retinal breaks and retinal detachment.

# WORKUP FOR ENDOGENOUS ENDOPHTHALMITIS

Endogenous endophthalmitis results from hematogenous spread of a systemic infection to the eye. Workup should generally be carried out in conjunction with an internist and directed at identifying the source of the infection. History of diabetes, intravenous drug use, indwelling catheters, parenteral nutrition, nonhealing ulcers, recent surgeries, or implanted prosthetic devices should be inquired about. A complete physical examination should be performed. Investigations should include, at minimum, blood cultures and echocardiography. Further investigations may be guided by the patient's history and physical examination (e.g. culture of any indwelling catheters).[5]

# PEARLS AND PITFALLS

- Have a low threshold for treating suspected endophthalmitis.
- As these eyes are inflamed, giving subconjunctival or regional anesthesia time to work is critical.
- Visual acuity of hand motions (HM) was defined in the EVS as ability to perceive whether an examiner's hand is still, moving sideways, or moving up and down at one

motion per second 60 cm from the eye, with a lamp directed from behind the patient toward the examiner's hand. It was required in the study that patients identify the action correctly at least four out of five times.

- Using a larger (25) gauge needle for performing vitreous tap may help improve the chances of obtaining a specimen.
- Avoid combining intravitreal medications into a single syringe as precipitation of the medications may occur, which could decrease efficacy.
- Due to the severe inflammation, vitrectomy for endophthalmitis can be quite limited. Optimizing the view is critical. Performing an anterior chamber washout with removal of a fibrin clot and posterior synechiolysis may be helpful. Viscoelastic injected into the anterior chamber may also be a helpful adjunct for improving the view.
- When obtaining an undiluted specimen during vitrectomy, infusing air into the eye can help maintain pressure while at the same time not diluting the specimen.
- Retinal breaks in an eye with endophthalmitis are often difficult to identify and treat due to the limited visualization. In addition, an inflamed eye with a retinal break may increase the risk of proliferative vitreoretinopathy. Avoid placing traction on the retina and generally avoid trying to induce a posterior vitreous detachment if not already present.
- At times, getting a patient to the operating room may take longer than expected. In these cases, performing a tap and inject while waiting to go to the operating room is worthwhile.
- Cases of suspected endogenous endophthalmitis require a thorough workup for the source of systemic infection, along with empiric systemic antibiotics, not simply intravitreal antibiotics. Management should be coordinated with an internist.

## REFERENCES


1. Endophthalmitis Vitrectomy Study Group. Results of the Endophthalmitis Vitrectomy Study: a randomized trial of immediate vitrectomy and of intravenous antibiotics for the treatment of post-operative bacterial endophthalmitis. Arch Ophthalmol. 1995;113(12):1479-96.
2. The Endophthalmitis Vitrectomy Study Group. Microbiologic factors and visual outcome in the endophthalmitis vitrectomy study. Am J Ophthalmol. 1996;122(6):830-46.
3. Charles S, Calzada J, Wood B. Vitreous microsurgery, 5th edn. Philadelphia: Lippincott Williams & Wilkins; 2011. pp. 216-21.
4. Aldave AJ, Stein JD, Deramo VA, et al. Treatment strategies for postoperative Propionibacterium acnes endophthalmitis. Ophthalmology. 1999;106(12):2395-401.
5. Ryan SJ, Editor in Chief. Retina, 4th edn. Philadelphia: Elsevier Mosby; 2006. p. 2263.

CHAPTER

33

# Vitreous Implants and Intravitreal Injection

Roger A Goldberg, Chirag P Shah, Sunir J Garg

## INTRODUCTION

Over the past decade, intravitreal injections have become one of the most commonly performed procedures in the retina specialist's clinic. Intravitreal injections are an effective way to deliver therapeutic medications directly to the back of the eye and can be performed safely and comfortably in an office-based setting. New therapeutic developments will increase the number of agents available and range of diseases treated. Treating ophthalmologists require familiarity with the techniques and possible complications of the procedure.

## INDICATIONS

Intravitreal injections are performed for a range of diseases:

- Neovascular and inflammatory diseases
  - Neovascular age-related macular degeneration (AMD)
  - Retinal vein occlusion (RVO)
  - Diabetic macular edema (DME)
  - Cystoid macular edema (CME) (e.g. postsurgical or Irvine-Gass, inflammatory)
  - Retinopathy of prematurity (ROP)
  - Vitreous hemorrhage with active bleeding (e.g. due neovascularization from proliferative diabetic retinopathy or RVO)
  - Neovascular glaucoma (NVG)
  - Uveitis
  - Intraocular lymphoma.
- Infection
  - Endophthalmitis
  - Cytomegalovirus retinitis
  - Acute retinal necrosis
  - Progressive outer retinal necrosis
  - Toxoplasmosis chorioretinitis.

TABLE 33-1 Commonly used intravitreal medications

| Name | Dose | Indications |
|---|---|---|
| Ranibizumab (Lucentis) | 0.5 mg/0.05 mL<br>0.3 mg/0.05 mL | AMD, RVO<br>DME |
| Aflibercept (Eylea) | 2.0 mg/0.05 mL | AMD, CRVO |
| Bevacizumab (Avastin) | 1.25 mg/0.05 mL<br>0.625 mg/0.025 mL | AMD, RVO, DME, CNV<br>ROP |
| Triamcinolone | 4.0 mg/0.1 mL | RVO, CME, DME, uveitis |
| Dexamethasone (Ozurdex) | 0.7 mg implant | RVO, posterior uveitis |
| Ocriplasmin (Jetrea) | 0.125 mg/0.1 mL | VMT |
| Vancomycin | 1.0 mg/0.1 mL | Bacterial endophthalmitis |
| Ceftazidime | 2.5 mg/0.1 mL | Bacterial endophthalmitis |
| Voriconazole | 0.10 mg/0.1 mL | Fungal endophthalmitis, retinitis |
| Ganciclovir | 2.0 mg/0.1 mL | Viral retinitis |
| Foscarnet | 2.4 mg/0.1 mL | Viral retinitis |
| Methotrexate | 0.4 mg/0.1 mL | Noninfectious uveitis, lymphoma |

(AMD: Neovascular age-related macular degeneration; CME: Cystoid macular edema; CNV: Choroidal neovascularization; CRVO: Central retinal vein occlusion; DME: Diabetic macular edema; ROP: Retinopathy of prematurity; RVO: Retinal vein occlusion; VMT: Vitreomacular traction).

- Anatomic diseases
  - Vitreomacular traction
  - Small macular hole
  - Retinal detachment (e.g. pneumatic retinopexy)
  - Submacular hemorrhage [e.g. pneumatic displacement, tissue plasminogen activator (t-PA)].

Table 33-1 summarizes some commonly used medications, as well as their dosing and indications.

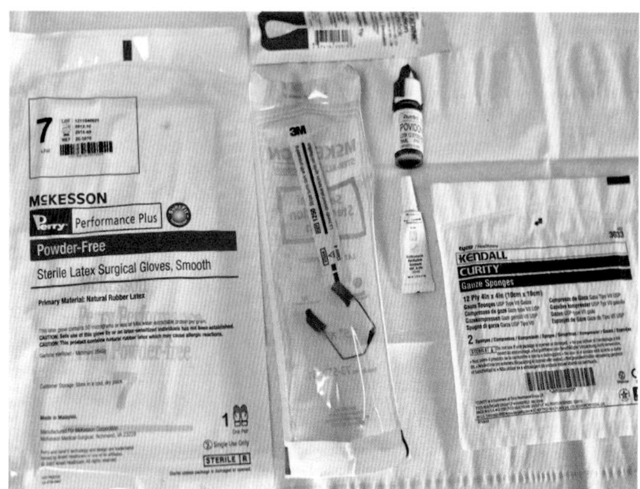


Figure 33-1 Supplies for intravitreal injections may include a sterile lid speculum, povidone–iodine topical solution and lid scrubs. Surgical gloves are used by some providers, and gauze or an eye pad can be applied to the temporal side of the face to mark the eye and prevent povidone–iodine drops from spilling into the ear or onto the patient's shirt collar.

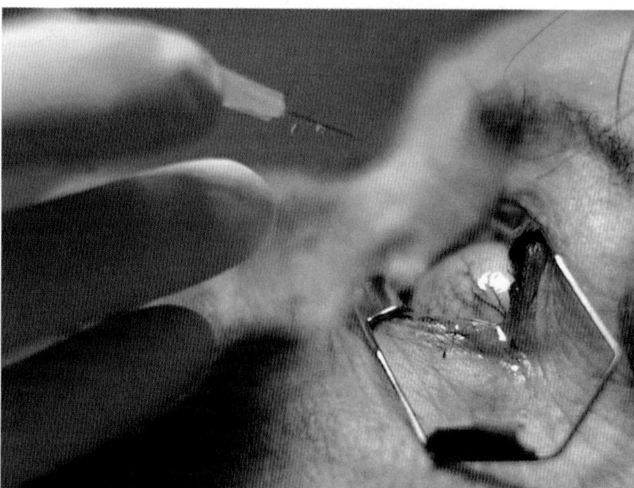

Figure 33-2 After marking the area to be injected, the syringe and needle should be brought to the eye in a controlled approach. The syringe and needle can be stabilized by balancing the ulnar aspect of the hand and fifth finger against the patient's face.

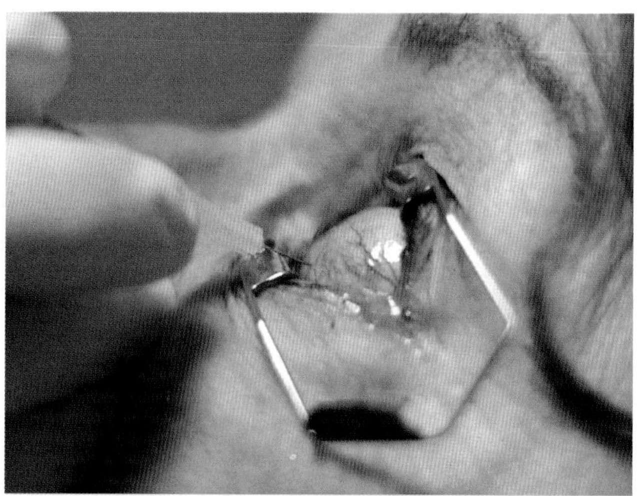

Figure 33-3 During the injection, the needle should pass perpendicular to the sclera, aiming toward the optic nerve. The needle does not need to be inserted to the hub before injecting the medicine.

## CONTRAINDICATIONS

Intravitreal injections generally should be avoided during periods of active external eye infection. In most instances, the injection can be safely postponed until after the infection is treated. An exception to this may be during the treatment of acute intraocular infections that require immediate intravitreal injection of antimicrobial agents.

Intravitreal injections are contraindicated in open globe injuries until they have undergone primary repair. Structural stability of the eye should be restored before agents are injected into the vitreous cavity, as the transient increase in pressure may lead to extrusion of intraocular contents (e.g. uveal tissue, retina, lens material, etc.).

Caution should be taken in eyes with proliferative diabetic retinopathy and retinal traction, as injection of antivascular endothelial growth factor (VEGF) agents can induce a contraction of the fibrovascular membranes. Although uncommon, tractional retinal detachment after this "crunch" has been reported, and patients should be carefully monitored.

## SURGICAL TECHNIQUE (FIGS. 33-1 TO 33-3)

Although some variation exists in specific components of intravitreal injections, the fundamental principles are generally preserved across techniques.

### Patient Positioning

In general, intravitreal injections can be safely performed in the office setting. Patients are reclined slightly in the examination chair to provide the clinician easy access to both the superior and inferior aspects of the sclera. The height of the eye should be such that the injecting physician can comfortably access the eye from a standing position without the need to bend over.

### Mark the Eye

In a busy vitreoretinal clinic, one or several other patients are often seen between when a patient is evaluated and consented for intravitreal injection, and when that injection actually occurs. Either the treating physician or the nurse or technician preparing the eye for injection should mark the eye that is to be treated. This can be performed with a surgical marking pen, a sticker, or an eye-pad/gauze taped to the side of the face the injection is to occur on (this last option also is helpful to catch any excess drops used to clean or anesthetize the ocular surface from spilling down the patient's face into the ear or onto the patient's shirt collar).

## Sterilize the Ocular Surface

Endophthalmitis is one of the most feared complications after intravitreal injection. With proper technique, however, this can be reduced to acceptably low rates (between 1 in 2000–5000 injections). Most providers use a povidone–iodine based solution to sterilize the ocular surface and eye lashes. This should be applied prior to any viscous anesthetics, which can block contact of the antiseptic with the ocular surface.

## Local Anesthetic

The quadrant to be injected should be anesthetized. Not only will this improve patient's comfort, but also will help diminish any startle reaction that may cause the patient to move their face or eye. Several options are available for local anesthesia.

Pledgetts soaked in 2–4% lidocaine can be applied directly to the sclera over the area where injection will be administered. The pledgett should be held with moderate pressure against the eye for approximately 30 seconds and can be repeated two to three times prior to injection. This technique softens the eye prior to intravitreal injection, which may limit the degree of intraocular pressure (IOP) rise after injection. Whether this has any clinical benefit (e.g. in patients with glaucoma) is unknown.

Viscous anesthetic agents can be applied to the ocular surface to provide an anesthetic effect. Examples include tetracaine 0.5% [TetraVisc; OcuSoft (Rosenberg, TX, USA)], and lidocaine 3.5% [Akten; Akorn (Lake Forest, IL, USA)]. They are typically placed on the conjunctiva 5–10 minutes prior to injection and can be repeated one to three times for pain control. These gels are generally well tolerated, although can cause conjunctival hyperemia and corneal epithelial changes. Topical povidone–iodine 5% should be placed on the eye both before and after application of the viscous anesthetic.

Subconjunctival lidocaine or xylocaine can be injected for anesthesia. A drop of proparacaine and povidone–iodine solution should be placed on the conjunctiva prior to subconjunctival injection. One typically injects 0.1–0.5 mL of lidocaine subconjunctivally to create a small bleb. The lidocaine should not contain epinephrine, as this has been rarely associated with central retinal artery occlusion.

## Lid Speculum

Many providers use a sterile lid speculum to prevent lid closure during the injection and to reflect the eyelashes away from the surgical field. Although this has not been proven to decrease the rate of infection, it should be considered a requirement for patients who are known to forcefully squeeze their eyelids. Those who do not typically use a lid speculum often use fingers to retract the eyelids.

## Injection Location

Intravitreal injections are performed through the pars plana. The pars plana extends from approximately 3–7 mm posterior to the corneoscleral limbus. To avoid hitting the crystalline lens, injections should be 3.5 mm posterior to the limbus in pseudophakic and aphakic patients, and 4.0 mm posterior to the limbus in phakic patients. The sclera can be marked using a fixed or adjustable caliper to visualize the correct distance from the limbus. Alternatively, some providers use a slip-tip 1-mL syringe placed at the limbus—the distance to the internal diameter is 3.5 mm, whereas the outer diameter measures 4.0 mm. After sufficient experience, some providers can estimate 3.5–4 mm from the limbus by visualization. An additional drop of povidone–iodine should be placed on the eye immediately prior to injection. Not only does this reduce the microbial content of the ocular surface, but also it highlights the scleral marking to ensure the correct distance from the limbus. Injections are typically performed in the temporal 6 clock hours because of better exposure, although the nasal quadrants can be used. Providers often rotate the injection location to different areas for patients receiving recurrent injections in an effort to minimize discomfort and trauma to one quadrant. Care should be taken to avoid injecting over calcific scleral plaques, as these calcified areas anterior to the rectus muscle insertions cannot be easily penetrated. In addition, the injection should not occur through an Axenfeld nerve loop, as this causes significant pain. Likewise, try to avoid the long posterior ciliary nerves along the horizontal meridian. For infants with neovascular conditions such as ROP, injections are typically 1 mm posterior to the limbus, although this varies by age.

## Needle Selection

Most intravitreal injections are performed using 27-, 30-, or 32-gauge needles. In the case of Food and Drug Administration

(FDA)-approved medications for intravitreal use, 30-gauge needles are supplied with the drug. Long-acting implants such as the dexamethasone 0.7-mg implant [Ozurdex; Allergan (Irvine, CA, USA)] come preloaded in a 22-gauge injection-needle device. Triamcinolone acetonide contains particles that should not be injected through a 32-gauge needle. Most injections use a half-inch needle to avoid penetrating the eye too deeply and injuring distal tissue.

### Injection Technique

The needle should enter the sclera nearly perpendicularly, aiming toward the optic nerve. Some providers displace the conjunctiva either with the needle tip or a sterile cotton-tip applicator. Either a one- or two-handed technique can be used. Fora two-handed technique, the thumb and first and second fingers can hold the barrel of the syringe while the pinky and ulnar aspect of the hand holding the syringe can be placed against the patient's face to stabilize the needle for injection. For a one-handed technique, the thumb and second fingers can hold the barrel of the syringe while the index finger is free to depress the plunger. The patient should be instructed to look in the opposite direction from the injection site (e.g. look superonasal for inferotemporal injections). The needle does not need to be inserted to its hub prior to depressing the plunger, as this risks unnecessary injury to distal structures. In a two-handed injection, the second hand can be used to depress the plunger. In a one-handed injection technique, the index finger can be shifted to the plunger and used to depress the plunger. In either case, the plunger should be depressed in a smooth, consistent fashion; too fast can generate excess turbulent flow, whereas too slow unnecessarily prolongs the procedure. The needle should be withdrawn quickly and discarded in a sharps container. A small amount of subconjunctival reflux after removing the needle is common. This is likely vitreous fluid and not the injected drug. Some clinicians roll a sterile cotton-tipped applicator over the injection site to limit this reflux while others keep the needle in the eye for a few seonds, giving time to let the pressure equilibrate in an attempt to reduce reflux through the puncture site.

### Postinjection Prophylaxis

Most clinicians apply an additional drop of povidone-iodine or antibiotic to the ocular surface after the injection is completed. Because povidone–iodine can irritate the ocular surface, it can be subsequently irrigated with a more mild eye drop afterward (e.g. antibiotic drops, artificial tears, sterile saline rinse). Increasing evidence suggests that short courses (1–3 days) of topical antibiotics around the time of the injection do not prevent endophthalmitis and may, in fact, increase antimicrobial resistance.

### Documentation

It is important to carefully document in the clinical chart the injection preparation technique used and the lot number of the drug injected. In addition, accurate contact information for each patient should be on file, should patients need to be contacted after their injection. Although outbreaks of infection or inflammation after intravitreal injection are rare, several have been reported, and accurate documentation can be helpful to understand and minimize the extent of these outbreaks.

## MECHANISM OF ACTION

Intravitreal injections work by delivering high concentration therapies directly to the posterior segment of the eye, to treat choroidal, retinal, and vitreoretinal diseases. The specific mechanism of action depends on the drug used. Drugs such as bevacizumab, ranibizumab, and aflibercept treat choroidal and retinal neovascularization and vascular leakage by inhibiting VEGF. Antimicrobial agents are used to treat infection and can be -cidal (direct cytotoxic effect) or -static (inhibit replication). Steroids have multiple mechanisms of action, inhibiting proinflammatory cytokine production and promoting anti-inflammatory protein production.

## POSTOPERATIVE CARE

Intravitreal injections are generally well tolerated, and postoperative care is minimal. Immediately after the injection, an antiseptic (i.e. povidone–iodine) or antibiotic drop is placed in the eye. Short-course postinjection antibiotics for 1–3 days has not been demonstrated to decrease the risk of postinjection endophthalmitis, and increasing, evidence suggests that this practice may increase antibiotic resistance. Because povidone–iodine and lid speculums are generally used during intravitreal injections, it is not uncommon for patients to experience 1–2 days of ocular surface irritation, including mild discomfort, tearing, or foreign body sensation. Artificial tears can be used up to four times per day as needed; this usually resolves the bothersome symptoms. The artificial tears can be kept chilled in the refrigerator for additional patient comfort.

Intraocular pressure measurement can be performed post-injection. An initial IOP spike occurs after the injection, and the IOP normalizes over the following 30–60 minutes. Some practitioners will check the IOP only in glaucoma patients, or, alternatively, perform indirect ophthalmoscopy to confirm optic nerve head perfusion, or ensure that the vision is finger counting or better.

Finally, patients should be given instructions regarding symptoms that should prompt a phone call to the treating ophthalmologist's office. These include retinal detachment and infection, warning signs such as new or persistent flashes of light, a curtain obscuring part of the vision, intense pain not relieved by artificial tears, or a marked decrease in vision. The patient should be provided with a phone number to call to reach the on-call provider after hours.

## SPECIFIC INSTRUMENTATION, SUBJECT TO PHYSICIAN'S PREFERENCE (FIG. 33-1)

- 1 $cm^3$ syringe
- Sterile lid speculum
- Povidone–iodine
- Anesthetic
  - Viscous lidocaine or tetracaine
  - Subconjunctival lidocaine (0.5 $cm^3$ of 2% lidocaine on a 30-gauge needle)
  - Lidocaine-soaked pledgetts
- Proparacaine drops
- Sterile cotton-tipped applicators
- Artificial tears or balanced salt solution
- Beveled needle (usually 27-, 30-, or 32-gauge)
- Sterile gloves
- Facemask

## COMPLICATIONS

- Subconjunctival hemorrhage
- Corneal abrasion
- Superficial punctate keratitis
- Endophthalmitis
- Vitreous detachment
- Vitreous hemorrhage
- Retinal tear
- Retinal detachment
- Noninfectious inflammation
- Lens trauma
- Cataract formation
- Ptosis
- Elevation in IOP (transient and persistent)
- Intravitreal silicone oil droplets

## SURGICAL OUTCOMES: SCIENTIFIC EVIDENCE

Extensive safety and efficacy data support the use of many drugs delivered by intravitreal injection. In general, agents specifically designed for intraocular use and FDA-approved for intravitreal injection are supported by randomized, controlled clinical trials. Some drugs are not FDA-approved for intravitreal injection (e.g. bevacizumab and antibiotics in endophthalmitis), but their use is often supported by data from large clinical trials. A brief summary of some of the major trials is provided below.

- *Anti-VEGF agents*: Many large, randomized, controlled clinical trials have demonstrated the efficacy of VEGF inhibition in neovascular AMD, RVO, and diabetic macular edema
  - The ANCHOR and MARINA pivotal studies demonstrated the efficacy of ranibizumab 0.5 mg [Lucentis; Genentech/Roche (South San Francisco, CA, USA)] over sham injection or photodynamic therapy for neovascular AMD. Over a 2-year period, 95% of patients receiving ranibizumab avoided severe vision loss, whereas one third of patients gained three lines of vision
  - VIEW-1 and VIEW-2 showed that aflibercept (Eylea; Regeneron/Bayer), dosed either every 4 or 8 weeks was equivalent to ranibizumab dosed every 4 weeks for patients with neovascular AMD
  - In the CATT study, which compared ranibizumab to bevacizumab (Avastin; Genentech/Roche) for the treatment of neovascular AMD, bevacizumab was demonstrated to be noninferior to ranibizumab. The head-to-head trial had two dosing regimens for each drug; all prevented vision loss and demonstrated vision gain, although greater improvements in vision were seen in the monthly dosing arms
  - BRAVO and CRUISE demonstrated the efficacy of ranibizumab in the treatment of macular edema secondary to branch and central RVOs, respectively. Among patients treated with 0.5-mg ranibizumab monthly for 6 months, 61% of patients with branch RVO improved ≥15 letters (vs 29% of sham injection patients), whereas 48% of central RVO patients improved 15 letters (vs 17% sham injection)
  - COPERNICUS and GALILEO demonstrated marked improvement in macular edema secondary to central RVO in patients treated with monthly aflibercept. After

24 weeks, 58% of patients treated with aflibercept had gained ≥15 letters of vision, compared with 17% of sham-treated patients
  - The RIDE and RISE studies led to the approval of ranibizumab for the treatment of fovea-involving diabetic macular edema. After 24 months, 34–45% of patients receiving ranibizumab 0.3 mg monthly injections had gained ≥15 letters, compared with 12–18% of sham-injected patients
  - BEAT-ROP compared bevacizumab to laser in the treatment of zone 1 or posterior zone 2 ROP and demonstrated a decreased recurrence rate of ROP with bevacizumab.
- Antimicrobials and anti-inflammatory agents:
  - The Endophthalmitis Vitrectomy Study (EVS) demonstrated in acute postcataract surgery endophthalmitis intravitreal injection of antibiotics was as effective as vitrectomy in patients with hand motion vision or better
  - The GENEVA study evaluated the safety and efficacy of a single injection of the dexamethasone implant (Ozurdex; Allergan) compared with sham in patients with macular edema secondary to RVO. Patients receiving the dexamethasone implant had more rapid resolution of macular edema, with 20–30% of subjects gaining ≥15 within 2 months of injection
  - The HURON Study evaluated the safety and efficacy of a single injection of the dexamethasone implant (Ozurdex; Allergan) for the treatment of intermediate, posterior, or panuveitis. After 26 weeks, 47% of patients versus 12% of sham patients achieved a vitreous haze score of 0 and significantly more treated patients had a three-line visual improvement compared with sham.
- Structural:
  - The MIVI-TRUST showed that a single injection of ocriplasmin [Jetrea; Thrombogenics (Leuven, Belgium)] can resolve vitreomacular adhesion in 27% of patients versus 10% of control patients at 28 days.

## PLACE OF THE TECHNIQUE IN SURGICAL ARMAMENTARIUM

Intravitreal injections are a mainstay of modern-day ophthalmology, and one of the most commonly performed procedures in a vitreoretinal clinic. As comfort with the procedure has grown, more and more drugs are being developed for delivery by intravitreal injection. Performed properly, it is a safe and effective way to deliver high concentrations of drug to the posterior aspect of the eye.

## PEARLS AND PITFALLS

- Preinjection sterilization of the ocular surface with an antiseptic agent such as povidone–iodine is key to preventing injection-related infection. Always place a drop prior to applying any viscous anesthetic to the ocular surface and consider an additional drop immediately prior to injection.
- In phakic patients, inject 4 mm posterior to the corneoscleral limbus. In pseudophakic and aphakic patients, inject 3.5 mm posterior to the limbus.
- Short courses of antibiotics after intravitreal injection do not appear necessary and may ultimately increase antibiotic resistance.
- Document the medication, dose, eye treated, and drug lot number for every injection.
- Review with patients the symptoms of retinal detachment or endophthalmitis and provide patients with an accurate phone number to call should these symptoms develop.

## SUGGESTED READING

1. Boyer D, Heier J, Brown DM, et al. Vascular endothelial growth factor trap-eye for macular edema secondary to central retinal vein occlusion: six-month results of the phase 3 COPERNICUS study. Ophthalmology. 2012;119:1024-32.
2. Brown DM, Kaiser PK, Michaels M, et al. Ranibizumab versus verteporfin for neovascular age-related macular degeneration. N Engl J Med. 2006;355(14):1432-44.
3. Haller JA, Bandello F, Belfort R, Jr, et al. Randomized, sham-controlled trial of dexamethasone intravitreal implant in patients with macular edema due to retinal vein occlusion. Ophthalmology. 2010;117:1134-46.
4. Heier JS, Brown DM, Chong V, et al. Intravitreal aflibercept (VEGF trap-eye) in wet age-related macular degeneration. Ophthalmology. 2012;119(12):2537-48.
5. Lowder C, Belfort R, Jr, Lightman S, et al. Dexamethasone intravitreal implant for noninfectious intermediate or posterior uveitis. Arch Ophthalmol. 2011;129(5):545-53.
6. Milder E, Vander J, Shah C, et al. Changes in antibiotic resistance patterns of conjunctival flora due to repeated use of topical antibiotics after intravitreal injection. Ophthalmology. 2012;119(7):1420-4.
7. Mintz-Hittner HA, Kennedy KA, Chuang AZ, et al. Efficacy of intravitreal bevacizumab for stage 3+ retinopathy of prematurity. N Engl J Med. 2011;364(7):603-15.
8. Moshfeghi AA, Rosenfeld PJ, Flynn HW, Jr, et al. Endophthalmitis after intravitreal anti-vascular endothelial growth factor antagonists: a six-year experience at a university referral center. Retina. 2011;31:662-8.

9. Nguyen QD, Brown DM, Marcus DM, et al. Ranibizumab for diabetic macular edema: results from 2 phase III randomized trials: RISE and RIDE. Ophthalmology. 2012;119(4):789-801.
10. Results of the Endophthalmitis Vitrectomy Study. A randomized trial of immediate vitrectomy and of intravenous antibiotics for the treatment of postoperative bacterial endophthalmitis. Endophthalmitis Vitrectomy Study Group. Arch Ophthalmol. 1995;113(12):1479-96.
11. Rosenfeld PJ, Brown DM, Heier JS, et al. Ranibizumab for neovascular age-related macular degeneration. N Engl J Med. 2006;355(14):1419-31.
12. Schimel AM, Scott IU, Flynn HW, Jr. Endophthalmitis after intravitreal injections: should the use of face masks be the standard of care? Arch Ophthalmol. 2011;129:1607-9.
13. Shah CP, Garg SJ, Vander JF, et al. Outcomes and risk factors associated with endophthalmitis after intravitreal injection of anti-vascular endothelial growth factor agents. Ophthalmology. 2011;118:2028-34.
14. Stalmans P, Benz MS, Gandorfer A, et al. Enzymatic vitreolysis with ocriplasmin for vitreomacular traction and macular holes. N Engl J Med. 2012;367:606-15.
15. The CATT Research Group. Ranibizumab and bevacizumab for neovascular age-related macular degeneration. N Engl J Med. 2011;364:1897-908.
16. Wykoff CC, Flynn HW, Jr, Rosenfeld PJ. Prophylaxis for endophthalmitis following intravitreal injection: antisepsis and antibiotics. Am J Ophthalmol. 2011;152:717-9.

CHAPTER

34

# Techniques of Laser Photocoagulation in Diabetic Retinopathy

Joseph I Maguire

## INTRODUCTION

The eye is an optical system whose pellucid structures allow both observation of the fundus as well as delivery of laser therapy. The retinal vasculature can be directly observed and provides measurable clues to systemic vascular disease. Laser is an acronym for light Amplification by Stimulated Emission of Radiation. Its features include coherence, both temporal and spatial, which allows a collimated, amplified and narrow wavelength light pulse to be delivered as short, focused power over brief time periods.

In retinal disease, a laser's primary function is to create a focal thermal effect. From there, the mechanisms of its impact diverge (*see* Mechanism of Action). Although retinal laser is used to treat a whole host of diseases including retinal tears and detachments, vein occlusions, macular edema from any number of causes, retinal neovascularization, macroaneurysms, central serous chorioretinopathy and age-related macular degeneration by virtue of prevalence and its multiple presentations diabetic retinopathy is the most commonly lasered retinal condition.

Diabetes is the second leading cause of visual loss in the United States and number one in working age Americans. There are currently over 25 million Americans with diabetes and that number is projected to be 39 million in 2020, a full 15% of the United States population. Currently, 28.5% of diabetics more than 40 years of age have retinopathy and 13% of that group has diabetic macular edema (DME) making it the primary form of vision threatening diabetic retinopathy.[1]

Visual dysfunction in patients with diabetes is directly related to blood vessel damage and that in turn is driven by two factors: (1) control, or lack thereof, of diabetes; and (2) time; specifically the longer one is a diabetic and the poorer the control, the greater the risk of vision loss. As a vascular disease, diabetes can affect any ocular structure, but the retina's vascular system is ground zero for the primary ocular complications leading to visual loss.[2,3]

## INDICATIONS

### High-Risk Proliferative Diabetic Retinopathy

Proliferative diabetic retinopathy (PDR) is defined by the presence of new blood vessel growth. It is divided into neovascularization of the optic nerve or disk (NVD) and neovascularization of the retina elsewhere (NVE). Patients can also develop neovascularization of the iris and trabecular meshwork. High-risk PDR is defined as NVE or NVD with vitreous hemorrhage or NVD greater than standard photograph 10a from the diabetic retinopathy study (DRS), which is roughly neovascularization one-quarter to one-third of the optic disk area.[4]

### Clinically Significant Diabetic Macular Edema

In the pre-antivascular endothelial growth factor (VEGF) era, the presence of macular thickening from DME was based on direct biomicroscopic evaluation. At the time, optical coherence tomography (OCT) did not yet exist and it has since muddied the waters in terms of exact terminology. The early treatment diabetic retinopathy study (ETDRS) defined clinically significant macular edema (CSME) as:

- Diabetic macular edema at or within 500 μm of the foveal center; or

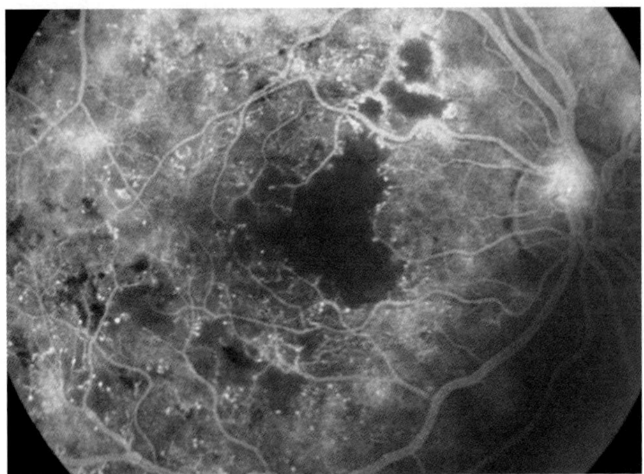

Figure 34-1 Enlargement of the foveal avascular zone due to macular ischemia.

- Diabetic macular edema with hard exudates at or within 500 μm of the foveal center and having contiguous retinal thickening; or
- Diabetic macular edema of one disk diameter (DD) any part of which is within one DD of the foveal center.[5]

### Neovascularization of the Iris and Neovascular Glaucoma

Ischemic retina causes liberation of VEGF that can diffuse into the anterior segment. Resultant neovascularization of the iris (NVI) and trabecular meshwork, if left unchallenged, can result in neovascular glaucoma (NVG).

## CONTRAINDICATIONS

Laser should be avoided in the following circumstances:
- Direct laser treatment to the foveal avascular zone (FAZ) (unless micropulse laser)
- Over areas of dense intraretinal or preretinal hemorrhage
- Near foveal telangiectasia in eyes with macular ischemia causing enlargement of the FAZ (Fig. 34-1)
- In eyes in which an adequate view cannot be obtained.

## SURGICAL TECHNIQUE

The laser can be delivered in several ways, including via:
- Slit lamp [for panretinal laser photocoagulation (PRP), direct ablation or focal]
  - Slit lamp delivery allows precise placement and modification of laser spot size
- Indirect ophthalmoscope (PRP, direct neovascular ablation)
- Endolaser probe (PRP, direct neovascular ablation, selective focal outside of fovea).

### Panretinal Photocoagulation

Panretinal photocoagulation is currently the preferred therapy for high-risk proliferative diabetic retinopathy (PDR) as well as other types of neovascularization from sickle retinopathy, branch and central retinal vein occlusion, and neovascular glaucoma. It involves applying laser burns over a wide area of extramacular retina and may be performed using a variety of delivery systems, including the slit lamp, an indirect ophthalmoscope, and intraoperatively using an endoprobe. Over time, different application methodologies have been proposed but the general principle is to treat ischemic retina.

Safe application of laser spots should start 500 μm from the disk and at least two disk diameters from the fovea proceeding peripherally; this prevents inadvertent macular laser. Moderate intensity burns of 200–500 μm (gray-white burns) are placed one spot-width apart extending to the equatorial retina for an average total of 1,200–1,600 applications (Figs. 34-2A and B). In more advanced cases, PRP can be performed more peripherally, including with scleral depression. Initial response can be judged over a 6-week period and additional laser supplementation should be added as required, including direct confluent laser treatment to small areas of persistent flat NVE (Fig. 34-3).[4] Initial DRS recommendations were to deliver laser over two to three sessions, but American Society of Retinal Subspecialists (ASRS) surveys have shown many treating physicians complete full PRP in one session if the ocular media allows. The presence of high-risk PDR is an indication for prompt treatment.

### Focal

Focal laser is placed at the slit lamp with the aid of a contact lens that allows magnified viewing facilitating precise laser placement.

Focal laser has been historically divided into two categories, direct focal or grid focal.

The strategy for treating macular edema depends on the type and extent of vessel leakage; fluorescein angiography is helpful in revealing areas of nonperfusion as well as identifying microaneurysms (MA) (Figs. 34-4A and B). If CSME is circinate or due to focal leakage, direct MA ablation is the goal. A 50–100 μm laser spot is used to achieve MA whitening. Observation of laser-whitened MA is recommended just after closure to monitor for rapid reperfusion. Focal grid laser is utilized in diffusely thickened retina and areas of

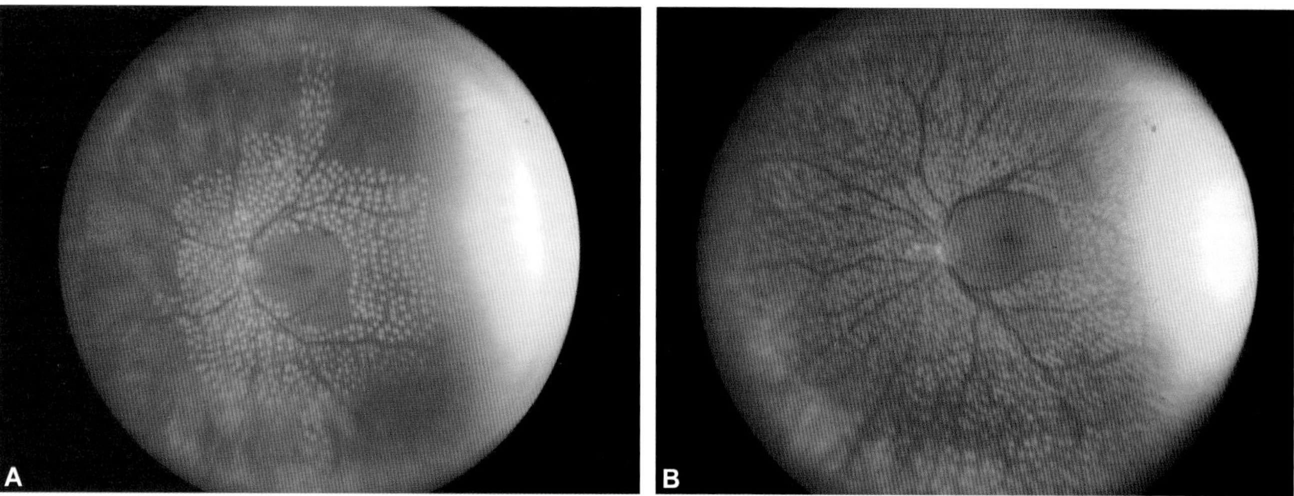

Figures 34-2A and B Equator plus photograph demonstrating (A) initial panretinal laser photocoagulation placement and (B) later completion. Currently, the initial spots would begin approximately 1–2 disk diameters away from the vascular arcades.

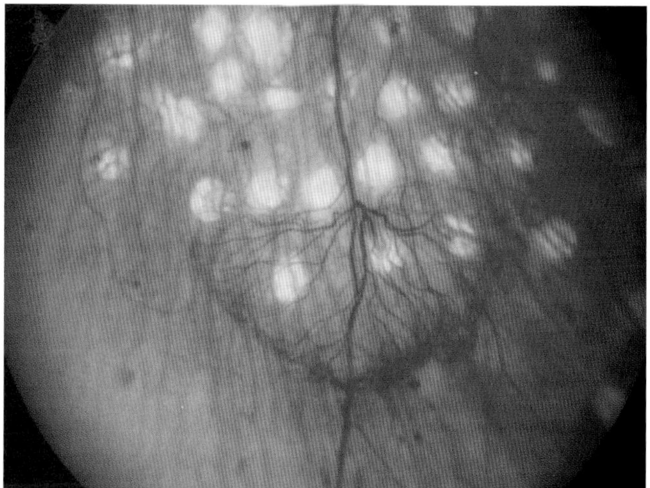

Figure 34-3 Flat neovascularization of the retina elsewhere with partial panretinal laser photocoagulation. Persistent flat neovascularization of the retina elsewhere may be ablated directly if outside the macula and no more than 2 disk areas.

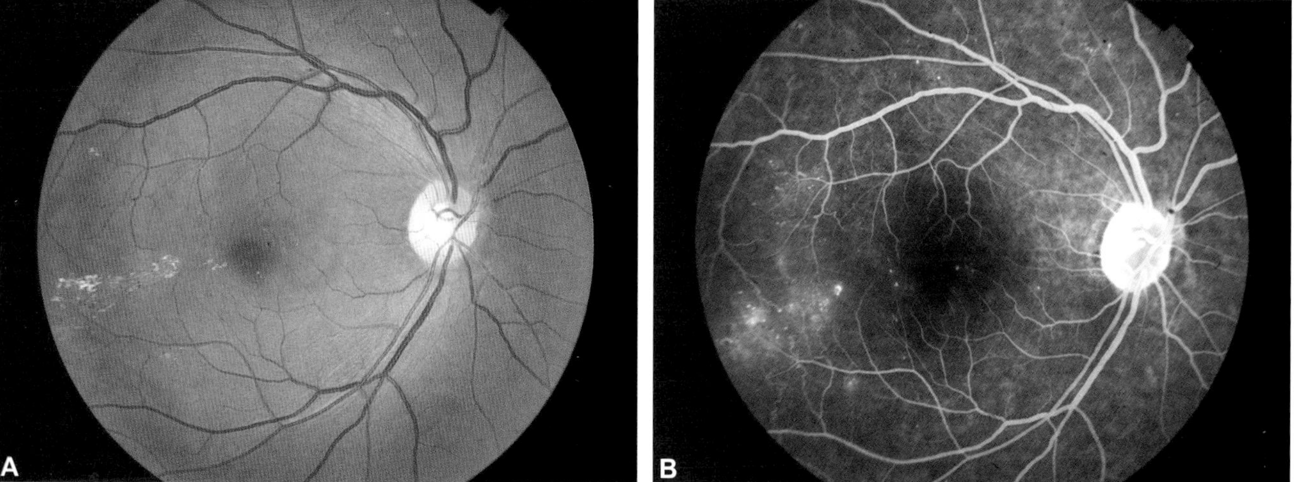

Figures 34-4A and B (A) Color and (B) fluorescein angiographic images demonstrate candidate microaneurysms for focal laser therapy.

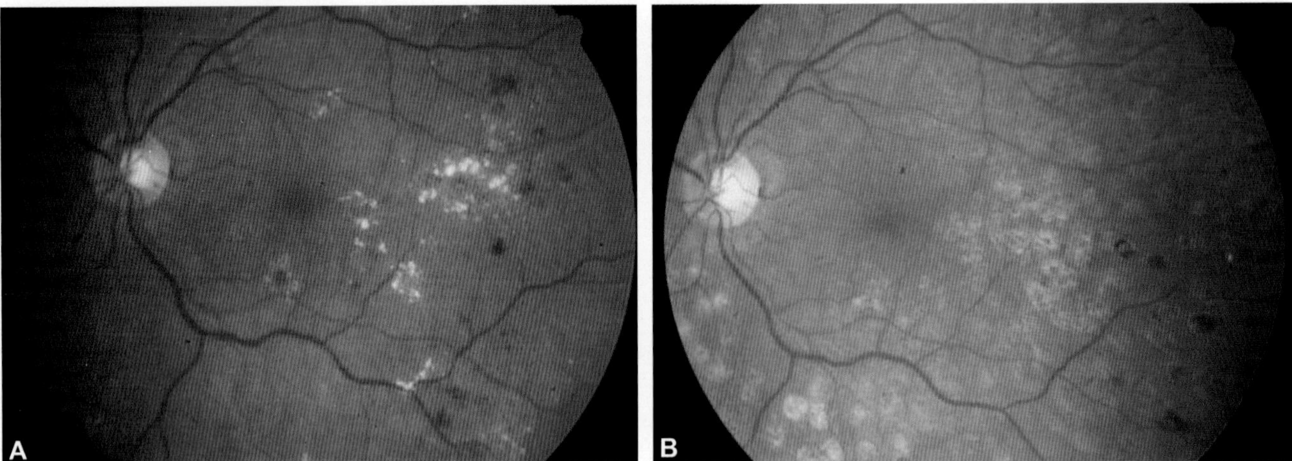


**Figures 34-5A and B** (A) Pre and (B) post-treatment fundus photos demonstrate the effective nature of focal laser in diabetic macular edema resolution with circinate clinically significant macular edema.

angiographically demonstrated nonperfusion. Light laser burns of 100–200 µm and one burn width apart are placed in a grid pattern covering the affected area.

In both grid and direct focal laser, initial therapy is placed no closer than 500 µm from the foveal center (Figs. 34-5A and B). If CSME persists three to four months after previous laser treatment, additional laser can be placed up to 300 µm from the foveal center.[5]

### Micropulse

A theoretic benefit of laser therapy is the downregulation of angiogenic growth factors such as VEGF by the retinal pigment epithelium (RPE). As such, hot, full thickness laser burns are not necessary to achieve a therapeutic effect. Micropulse laser therapy (MPLT) delivers energy in repetitive short pulses that are followed by a period of rest. Active intervals are usually 100–300 µs and the rest interval 1,700–1,900 µs encompassed within a 200–300 ms packet. MPLT produces retinal pigment epithelial thermal effects while minimizing sensory retinal and choroidal damage by using less energy. Several studies indicate subthreshold MPLT may be as effective as conventional laser therapy in DME. Sparing of the choroid and sensory retina allows confluent application to all edematous retina, including the fovea. The difficulty is determining the proper subthreshold energy required since there is no visible feedback in terms of a laser burn.[6]

### Mechanism of Action for Macular Edema

The mechanism of laser action can be subdivided into three categories:

1. Direct microaneurysmal/vasculature closure or obliteration;
2. Reduction of ischemic drive through angiogenic factor alterations, e.g. reduced VEGF production; and
3. Increased retinal oxygenation from the choroid via retinal debridement or thinning.

The exact manner by which PRP, focal and micropulse laser create an effect is not entirely understood and is most likely multifactorial. One theory suggests that destroying hypoxic retina decreases production of vasoproliferative factors, such as VEGF, that are produced in response to ischemia and are needed for both leakage as seen with DME and for growth and maintenance of neovascularization. However, the far majority of retinal oxygen is supplied by the choroid; thinning of the retina may (a) allow more free diffusion of choroidal oxygen and (b) decrease ischemic drive and secondary VEGF production.

## POSTOPERATIVE CARE

*Postoperative care includes*: (1) management of any rare post laser complications; and (2) appropriate follow-up to assess treatment effect. Comparative photos are invaluable to evaluate subtle interval changes, especially in focal laser.

With PRP, involution of neovascularization is frequently seen by six weeks after completion of full laser application. However, at least 25% of eyes with NVD treated with PRP in the Diabetic Retinopathy Study had some residual neovascular disk changes. Confluent ablation can be performed for persistent extramacular flat NVE.

Focal laser's effect is frequently more gradual than the effect of PRP. Circinate CSME not impinging on the fovea may be followed closely with follow-up in 6–12 weeks. Closer evaluation is required for near foveal exudates associated with retinal thickening to observe signs of early resolution or at least stability. Although retreatment is often carried out at

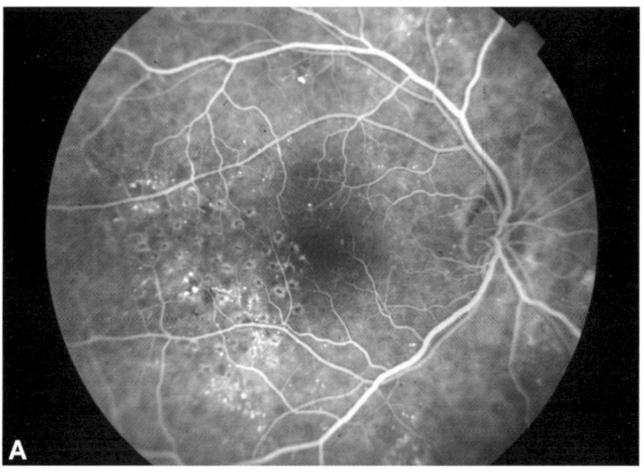


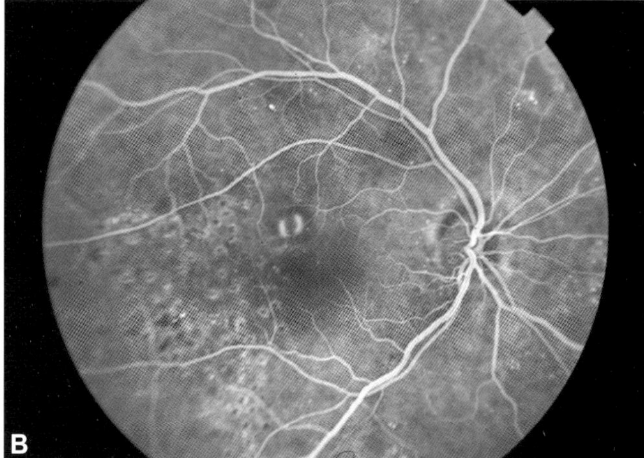


**Figures 34-6A and B** Development of choroidal neovascular membrane after focal laser treatment. (A) Demonstrates early and (B) late hyperfluorescence associated with a choroidal neovascularization. The focal laser scars are visible temporally.

4 months in cases with residual edema, if comparative photos show progressive improvement, these eyes can be followed for several additional months until improvement ceases or retinal edema resolves.

## INSTRUMENTATION

Laser technology has paralleled advances in other electronic technologies. Solid-state lasers that are both smaller in size and that have more efficient outputs are widely available. Most modern lasers use diode technology instead of glass tubes or other cumbersome laser elements, creating a dependable and portable platform that is durable and requires significantly less service.

Pattern lasers generate set multispot patterns which allow rapid delivery of multiple laser burns at shorter durations and with greater patient comfort and less time.

Micropulse modules allow reduction of collateral sensory retinal and choroidal tissues, while targeting the therapeutic effect on the RPE.

## COMPLICATIONS

Laser treatments to ocular structures involve delivery of energy to a living tissue. This necessarily results in tissue damage and localized inflammation which in turn creates risk. Laser risks include:

### PRP

- Reduced vision
- Reduced night vision
- Constriction of visual field
- Secondary macular edema
- Serous retinal detachment
- Decreased accommodation/tonic pupil (particularly if laser applied to long ciliary nerves)

### Focal Laser

- Foveal burns
- Paracentral scotomas
- Choroidal neovascular membranes (Figs. 34-6A and B)
- Reduced color vision
- Reduced contrast sensitivity
- Epiretinal membrane formation

### Contact Lens Associated Risks

- Irritation
- Corneal abrasion
- Subconjunctival hemorrhage

## SURGICAL OUTCOMES: SCIENTIFIC EVIDENCE

### Diabetic Retinopathy Study (DRS)

The diabetic retinopathy study found that adequate scatter laser PRP reduces the risk of severe visual loss (<5/200) by more than 50%.[4]

### The Early Treatment for Diabetic Retinopathy Study (ETDRS)

The early treatment for diabetic retinopathy study demonstrated that laser therapy for CSME reduces the incidence of moderate visual loss (doubling of visual angle or roughly a 2-line visual loss) from 30% to 15% over a 3-year period.[5]

### Diabetic Retinopathy Clinical Research Network

The Diabetic Retinopathy Clinical Research network (DRCR.net) randomized trial evaluating ranibizumab plus prompt or deferred laser or triamcinolone plus prompt laser for diabetic macular edema, known as the laser-ranibizumab-triamcinolone for DME study, demonstrated that ranibizumab with prompt or deferred focal/grid laser achieved superior visual acuity and OCT outcomes compared with focal/grid laser treatment alone at 2 years. In the ranibizumab groups, approximately 50% of eyes had substantial improvement (10 or more letters) and 30% gained 15 or more letters. Intravitreal triamcinolone combined with focal/grid laser did not result in superior visual acuity outcomes compared with laser alone, but did appear to have a visual acuity benefit similar to ranibizumab in pseudophakic eyes.[7]

## PLACE OF THE TECHNIQUE IN SURGICAL ARMAMENTARIUM

In the anti-VEGF era, laser photocoagulation is still a foundation therapy for diabetes-related retinopathy.

In high risk PDR, PRP is still the pre-eminent management choice.

Diffuse, center-involving macular edema with decreased vision is now initially managed with repetitive anti-VEGF injections, but supplementary grid and focal laser treatment is still the primary approach in CSME not involving fixation and as an enhancement to anti-VEGF management in center involving CSME.

Fluorescein angiography is still indicated for the diagnosis of enlarged FAZs, and areas of extrafoveal nonperfusion amenable to grid therapy.

## PEARLS AND PITFALLS

### Informed Consent

- All treatment begins with informed consent and a discussion of what therapy is designed to do, what it cannot do, and the associated risks.

### Proper Focus

- It may sound tautological, but clear visualization is imperative for proper laser therapy. This necessitates the presence of a relatively clear optical media, but also proper slit lamp technique allowing good visualization and focus with minimal reflective scatter.
- Whenever possible, whether using a contact lens at the slit lamp or an indirect ophthalmoscope as the delivery vehicle, the aiming beam should be a round circle; this ensures uniform placement of the laser pulse. Appropriate contact lens choice with maintenance of a perpendicular geometry between the contact lens optical surface and the incident laser light-resisting angling of the contact lens, allows more effective burns at a lower power.

### Comfort

- A comfortable patient is more likely to be compliant with future follow-up treatment.
- Laser power is the rate of energy delivered over time (joules or watts). Laser energy needs to be absorbed by tissue that is capable of absorption and, in the eye, this typically falls to the RPE, choroid or blood pigments.
- Manipulation of pulse duration frequently allows use of higher laser energy with comfort.
- Utilizing effective focus reduces needed power.
- Start with low power and increase it as needed.

## REFERENCES

1. Centers for Disease Control and Prevention Website. National Diabetes Fact Sheet, 2011. [Online] Available from http://www.cdc.gov/diabetes/pubs/factsheet11.htm. [Accessed July 2013].
2. Klein R. The Diabetes Control and Complications Trial. In: Kertes PJ, Conway MD (Eds). Clinical Trials in Ophthalmology: A Summary and Practice Guide. Williams & Wilkins; 1998. pp. 49-70.
3. UK Prospective Diabetes Study (UKPDS) Group. Intensive blood-glucose control with sulphonylureas or insulin compared with conventional treatment and risk of complications in patients with type 2 diabetes (UKPDS 33). Lancet. 1998;(12):352(9131):837-53.
4. Photocoagulation treatment of proliferative diabetic retinopathy. Clinical application of Diabetic Retinopathy Study (DRS) findings, DRS Report Number 8. The Diabetic Retinopathy Study Research Group. Ophthalmology. 1981;88(7):583-600.
5. Treatment techniques and clinical guidelines for photocoagulation of diabetic macular edema. Early Treatment Diabetic Retinopathy Study Report Number 2. Early Treatment Diabetic Retinopathy Study Research Group. Ophthalmology. 1987;94(7):761-74.
6. Figueira J, Khan J, Nunes S, et al. Prospective randomized controlled trial comparing sub-threshold micropulse diode laser photocoagulation and conventional green laser for clinically significant diabetic macular oedema. Br J Ophthalmol. 2009;93(10):1341-4.
7. Elman MJ, Aiello LP, Beck RW, et al. Randomized trial evaluating ranibizumab plus prompt or deferred laser or triamcinolone plus prompt laser for diabetic macular edema. Ophthalmology. 2010;117(6):1064-77.

CHAPTER

35

# Intraocular Foreign Bodies

John R Minarcik, Marcus Colyer, Eric Weichel

## INTRODUCTION

Improved vitrectomy technique and instrumentation has enabled greater success in managing difficult traumatic eye injuries. Despite the challenges of managing the complex injuries seen in intraocular foreign body (IOFB) trauma, recent data has suggested that outcomes of 20/200 or better are achievable in the majority (81%) of eyes.[1] Nevertheless, it is important that a surgeon has thorough discussion with patients regarding the uncertain visual prognosis and likely need for subsequent interventions. The ocular trauma score can be helpful. It uses individual clinical variables to predict final visual prognosis.[2]

## INDICATIONS

*The reasons to remove an IOFB are to*: (1) prevent exogenous endophthalmitis; (2) prevent the retinal toxicity of retained materials; (3) improve the clarity of the ocular media; and (4) decrease the chance of retinal detachment (RD) or other damaging sequelae to the ocular tissues. While globe closure remains the top priority after any penetrating or perforating IOFB trauma, concurrent IOFB removal is desirable to potentially decrease the risk of endophthalmitis. The decision to perform IOFB removal concurrently depends on an adequate view and the immediate availability of appropriate staff and equipment. The expected composition of the IOFB should be taken into consideration. Vegetable material or organic debris carries a considerable risk of being contaminated with virulent organisms such as Bacillus species.[3-5] Metallic IOFBs commonly contain substances known to be either acutely toxic to the retina such as copper (chalcosis) or chronically toxic to the retina such as iron (siderosis). Other metals or alloys containing zinc or lead are known to be inflammatory and arc poorly tolerated. Since the composition of a metallic IOFB is difficult to determine with certainty, they should generally be removed even if they initially appear stable.

## HISTORY AND EXAMINATION

Preoperative history should be focused to help the surgeon recreate the specifics of the trauma. Historical information helps ascertain visual prognosis, the risk of endophthalmitis, and assists surgical planning. Pertinent history includes the details of the mechanism of injury, the materials suspected as IOFBs, and the assessment of the environment for contamination risk. As an adjunct to a full eye examination, spiral computed tomography (CT) scan imaging utilizing 1 mm cuts is rapid and extremely sensitive in IOFB identification (Figs. 35-1A and B).[6] It can also approximate the composition based on radiographic density. B-scan ultrasonography can also give very valuable diagnostic information that is otherwise difficult to conclusively interpret with CT scan (Fig. 35-2). This includes the real-time dynamic movement and features of the involved tissues, which is helpful in distinguishing between choroidal detachments, RD, posterior vitreous detachment (PVD), and layered hemorrhage. B-scan can also elucidate more precise localization of metallic IOFBs, which can be shrouded in the scatter artifact of the CT. Contact ultrasonography should be used with caution. To avoid extrusion of intraocular contents, negligible globe pressure should be applied until primary globe repair is complete.

## CONTRAINDICATIONS

Nonsurgical management with close observation is sometimes warranted when the risks of IOFB removal seem to outweigh

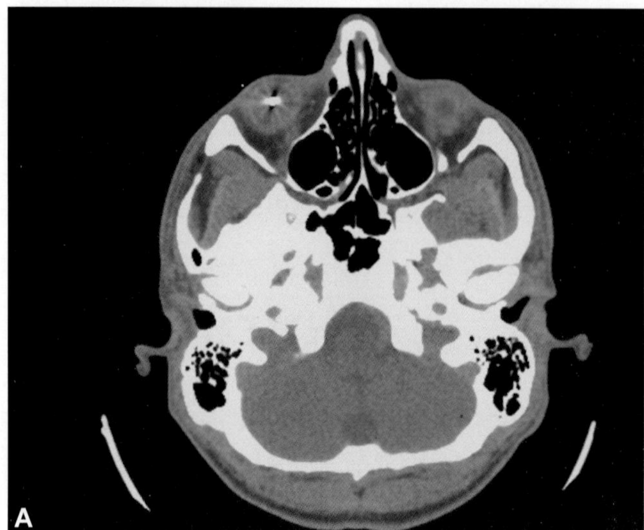


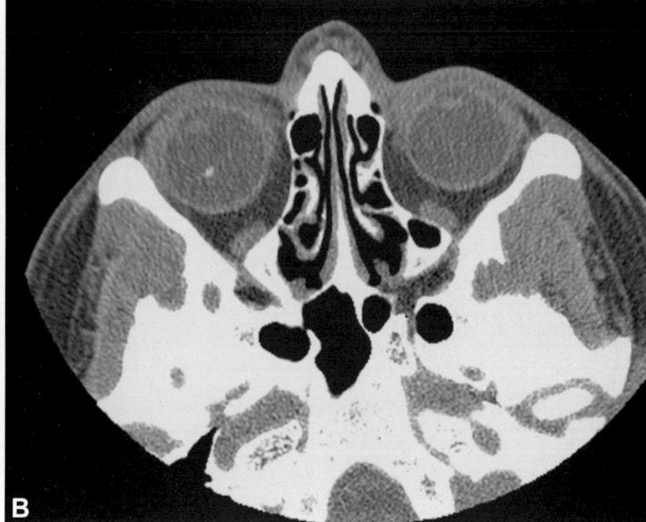


**Figures 35-1A and B** Computed tomography findings in (A) a metallic intraocular foreign body, showing scatter artifact; and (B) a lower density glass intraocular foreign body.

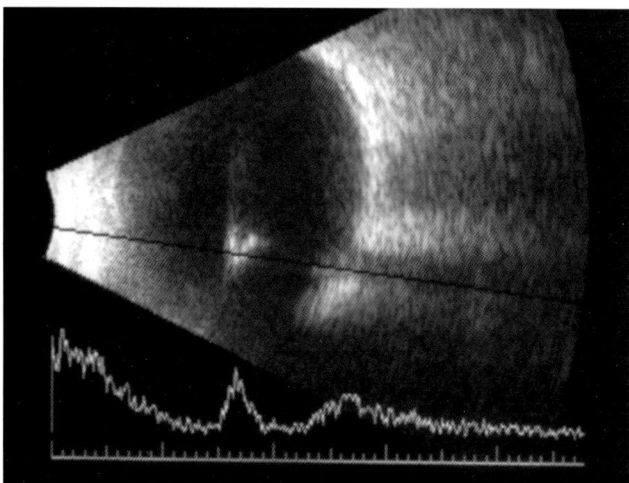

**Figure 35-2** Glass intraocular foreign body showing shadowing on B-scan ultrasonography.

the potential benefit to the patient's vision. This scenario is usually found in eyes with good vision, minimal symptoms or pathologic examination findings, and a period of demonstrated clinical stability. Some small, inert, and noninflammatory IOFBs be retained indefinitely in an encapsulated state and remain stable. Well-informed patients may also forgo IOFB removal for an eye with an otherwise poor visual prognosis, especially with no light perception (NLP) visual acuity. Occasionally, IOFBs are associated with orbital foreign bodies that transect the optic nerve. Lastly, medically unstable patients can delay IOFB removal for significant lengths of time on appropriate antibiotic prophylaxis while their other more urgent medical or surgical needs are met.

## SURGICAL TECHNIQUE

### Globe Repair

Inspection by peritomy, identification of entry and/or exit wounds, and repair of corneal and scleral lacerations or tissue defects is the first priority in any open globe traumatic injury, including cases of IOFB. Without basic globe integrity, attempts at pars plana vitrectomy (PPV) with posterior infusion can cause extrusion of intraocular contents (Figs. 35-3A to C).

### Scleral Buckling

Usually placed prior to vitrectomy, prophylactic scleral buckling is inconsistently performed in trauma. It should be a consideration for those with known RD, or judged to be at high risk for proliferative vitreoretinopathy (PVR). This decision is based on preoperative examination findings and the individual risk assessment for the case. Although somewhat more technically challenging with a softer vitrectomized eye, it can also be performed after the vitrectomy if the initial intraoperative findings suggest a benefit. It is reasonable to reserve buckling as a later secondary surgery for incarcerated folds that fail to flatten after the initial vitrectomy, or as a tool in the management of subsequent PVR related tractional retinal detachment (TRD), should it develop.

### Lens

Lens removal should be considered if a traumatic cataract precludes visualization of retina, or if there is evident capsular disruption expected to cause an inflammatory reaction.

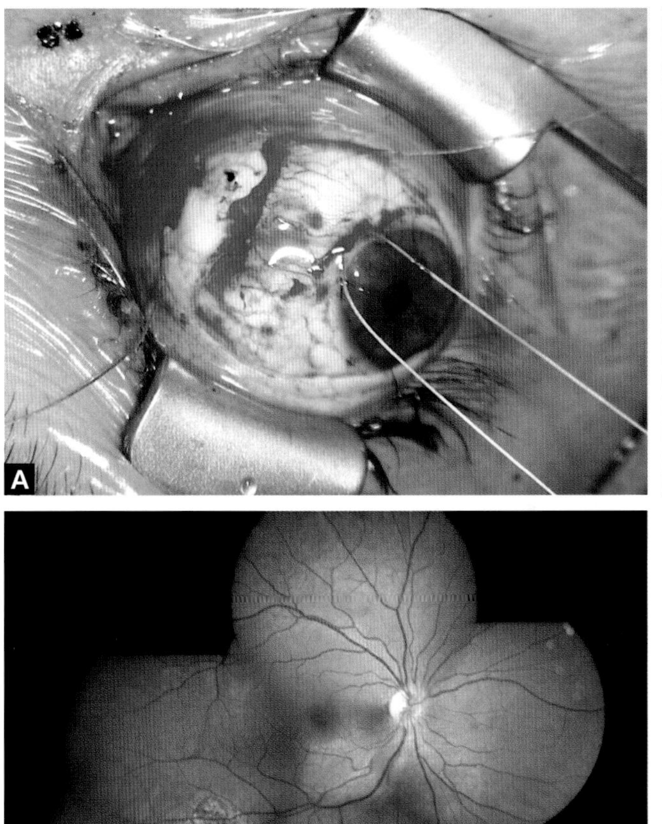

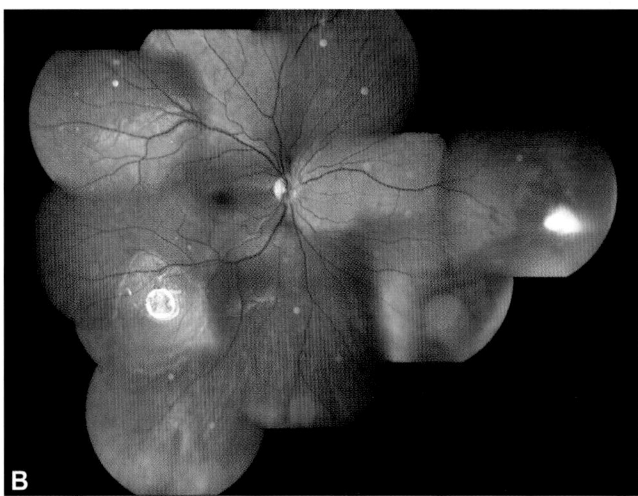

Figures 35-3A to C (A) Reflection of a rectus muscle reveals a small occult entry site. Posterior view; (B) shows reasonably clear media and a metallic intraocular foreign body embedded in the inferior retina. (C) pigmentary changes seen after removal.

Lens capsule disruption has been shown as an independent risk factor for development of endophthalmitis.[7] Lensectomy can be performed by the pars plana approach when there is trauma to the lens capsule or support structures. Alternatively, the standard phacoemulsification approach can be considered when the capsule and zonule look favorable for a future posterior chamber intraocular lens (IOL). There is some controversy regarding IOL implantation at the time of IOFB removal, particularly due to the potential risk of the implant-associated infection and inflammation.

## Culture

Prior to turning on the fluid infusion for vitrectomy, vitreous samples can be taken for culture by having an assistant manually aspirate the tubing from the cutter. This is facilitated by attachment of a syringe to a three-way stopcock. Any retrieved IOFB should also be sent for culture and analysis.

## Pars Plana Vitrectomy

Vitrectomy is performed after a traumatic eye injury for a variety of reasons, including clearing hemorrhagic media when breaks or tears are suspected, to repair RD, and to access IOFBs in the posterior segment. The most important aspect of a PPV for IOFB is the complete release of vitreous attachment prior to the mobilization of the IOFB. Any entrance wounds, exit wounds, or breaks in the retina related to the IOFB need to be completely freed of vitreous traction, therefore, elevation of the posterior hyaloid is a key step. Since the release of vitreous attachments is critical, and because patients involved in trauma tend to be younger in age, intraoperative intravitreal triamcinolone acetonide can be a useful visualization aid. Many IOFBs have irregular rough surface that require meticulous shaving and gentle manipulation to disengage from surrounding vitreous and tissues. To minimize iatrogenic RD, the successful removal of an IOFB will also

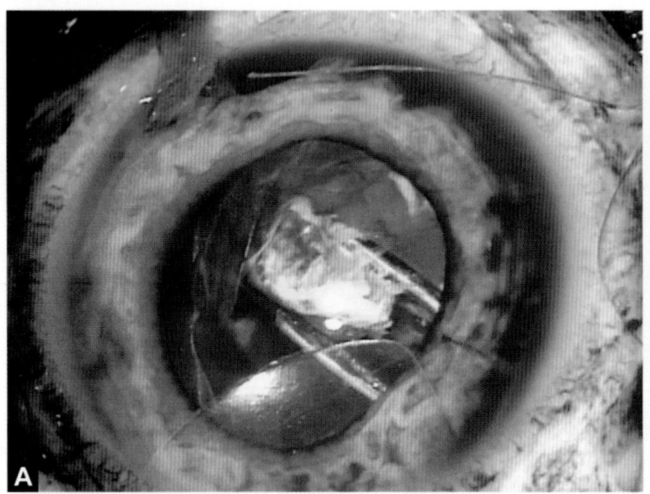

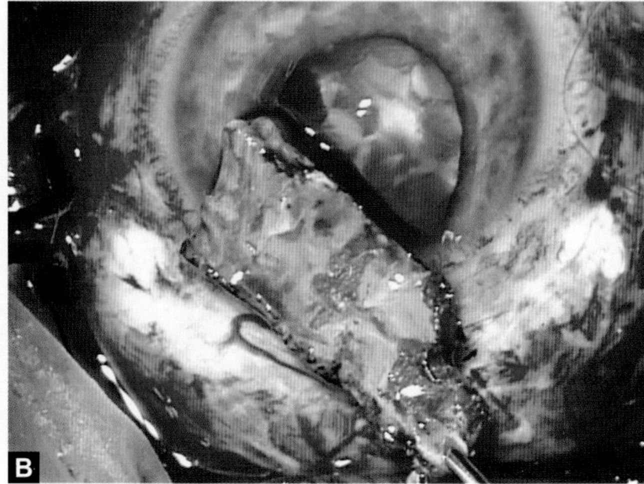

Figures 35-4A and B A diamond coated intraocular foreign body forceps is used to retrieve and extract a large irregularly shaped intraocular foreign body through a large scleral tunnel sclerotomy. Views of intraocular foreign body (A) through the anterior segment; and (B) outside of the eye.

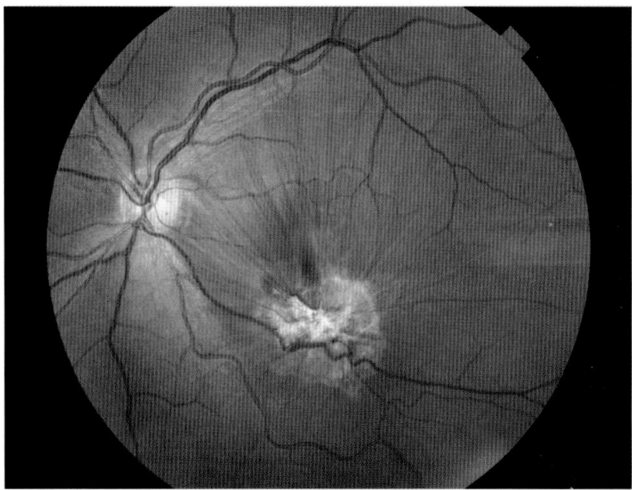

Figure 35-5 After removal of an embedded intraocular foreign body in the macula, a moderate epiretinal membrane has formed. In more severe cases, incarcerations may form. Laser was avoided in the central macula, and the patient remains 20/40, postoperatively.

depend on close vitreous base shaving so that the IOFB can be safely explanted via the pars plana. Just prior to explantation of the IOFB, pars plana sclerotomies can be enlarged to the appropriate size with a micro vitreoretinal (MVR) blade in a circumferential manner to accommodate the object. Larger IOFBs over 125 $mm^3$ or larger than 5 mm in one dimension are best removed using a scleral tunnel incision (Figs. 35-4A and B). Sclerotomies larger than 5 mm will cause globe collapse from fluid egress during IOFB removal. The surgeon has greater control of visualization and IOFB removal using a scleral tunnel removal technique.

## Retinal Tears and Detachments

Retinal breaks, tears, and dialyses are encountered relatively commonly in all traumatic eye injuries. The incidence is up to 20% in closed globe trauma,[8,9] and presumably higher in cases of penetrating or perforating open globe trauma involving the posterior segment. In all cases, meticulous removal of all traction from the breaks should be a priority during the vitrectomy, keeping in mind the high potential for later fibrocellular proliferation and contraction involving the remaining vitreous gel. Simple retinal breaks or tears without detachment are treated with endolaser and air tamponade. Retinal detachments should have treatment with $SF_6$, $C_3F_8$, or silicone oil, based on an assessment of the break location, and the anticipated compliance with optimum positioning. Strong consideration for silicone oil is recommended in cases judged to be at high PVR risk, or in perforating injuries where incarceration and folds are more likely. Retinal discontinuities in which an IOFB was impaled or embedded in the retina frequently occur in the posterior pole, and in visually significant portions of the macula. If the hyaloid can be successfully elevated with complete removal of traction, macular retinal defects do not necessarily require heavy (or even any) laser retinopexy, especially if the macular laser would be thought to decrease otherwise potentially good visual prognosis (Fig. 35-5). In this sense, they can be treated in a manner similar to that of macular holes.

## Intravitreal Antibiotics

Intravitreal injection of antibiotics is recommended at the conclusion of surgical repair in cases judged to be at significant risk for endophthalmitis. Broad spectrum coverage by

Vancomycin 1 mg in 0.1 cc and 2.25 mg Ceftazidime 0.1 cc is a standard dosing option.

### Mechanism of Action

Traumatic repairs with or without posterior vitrectomy is individually complex scenarios in which the therapeutic approach depends on the tissues involved. Some of the many goals of therapy are: preservation and reconstruction of anterior segment structures, prevention of post-traumatic endophthalmitis, prevention of toxic metallic reactions, maintaining retinal attachment, and counteraction of anticipated PVR traction. Every IOFB injury has a unique combination of intraocular injuries depending on the location and depth of IOFB penetration.

## POSTOPERATIVE CARE

Careful postoperative monitoring should be performed to watch for early signs of endophthalmitis. Special attention to intraocular pressure issues, particularly hypotony-related complications from nonpatent wounds is also warranted. Later, the risk of development of PVR and RD becomes the primary focus. Topical medications should include a long-acting mydriatic such as atropine, a steroid such as prednisolone 1%, and a broad spectrum antibiotic drop. Continuation of systemic antibiotics, such as fourth-generation fluoroquinolones, should be considered during the postoperative window of infection.

## INSTRUMENTATION

### Microincisional Vitrectomy Surgery *Vs* 20-gauge

While microincisional vitrectomy surgery has many surgical conveniences, 20-gauge instrumentation (under general anesthesia) is typically still the preferred vitrectomy approach for traumatic repairs and IOFB removal. Creating sclerotomies with an MVR blade causes less external pressure than trocars on a globe with uncertain wound integrity, and less risk of extrusion or incarceration of intraocular contents. Secondly, the forceps used in IOFB trauma are large, and significant enlargement of the pars plana sclerotomies during IOFB explantation is often anticipated (Fig. 35-6). Lastly, when younger patients are involved in trauma, the larger aperture of a 20-gauge vitrector is especially useful in getting a sound purchase on the cortical vitreous when attempting to elevate the adherent hyaloid.

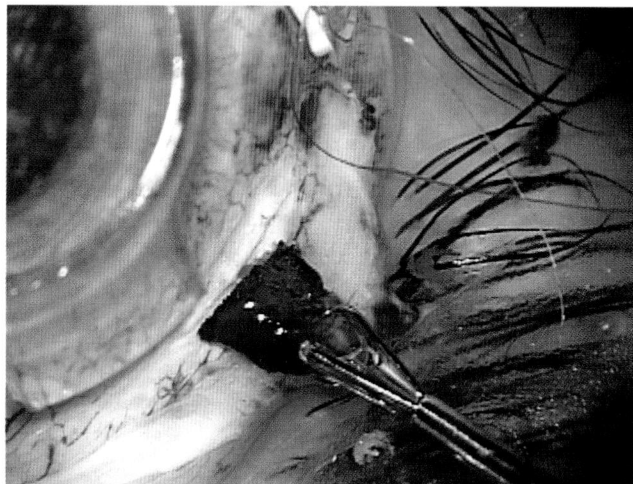

Figure 35-6 Basket forceps delivering an intraocular foreign body through an enlarged sclerotomy.

### Infusion

In the case of cataract, media opacity or choroidal thickening, the use of an extended-length (typically 6 mm) infusion cannula is advised to ensure placement within the intravitreal cavity. Limbal infusion though a needle or anterior chamber maintainer is also a cautious initial option when choroidal detachments are suspected, or visualization is too poor to confirm proper pars plana cannula placement.

### Tailoring the Forceps to the Intraocular Foreign Body

Intraocular foreign body removal forceps are chosen based on the size, shape, and magnetic characteristics of IOFB.[10] Tiny fragments can sometimes be removed by the vitrector itself. The retractable intraocular rare earth magnet is most useful in smaller (<1 mm) metallic and magnetic IOFBs that are of an appropriate size and shape to slip through a sclerotomy without a locking bite around the object. It also has the advantage of being able to engage magnetic IOFBs that are partially tissue embedded and hard to grasp with conventional forceps (Fig. 35-7). Basket forceps, on the other hand are appropriate for medium sized (1–3 mm) objects that are either non-magnetic, difficult to grasp due to a spherical shape, or having a jagged surface that will not glide easily through an enlarged sclerotomy (Figs. 35-8A and B). Reverse-action diamond-coated IOFB forceps are best suited for large (3–5 mm) or slick-surfaced IOFBs, such as glass, that have a graspable edge (Figs. 35-4A and B).With regards to external electromagnetic extraction, it is generally only recommended

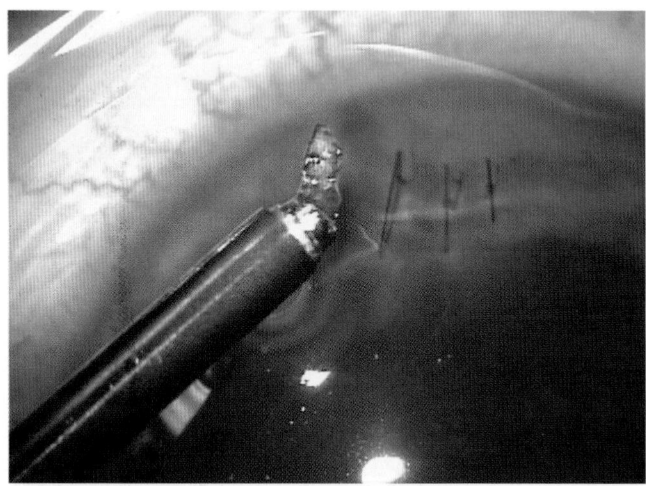

Figure 35-7 A small magnetic intraocular foreign body on a retractable rare-earth intraocular magnet.

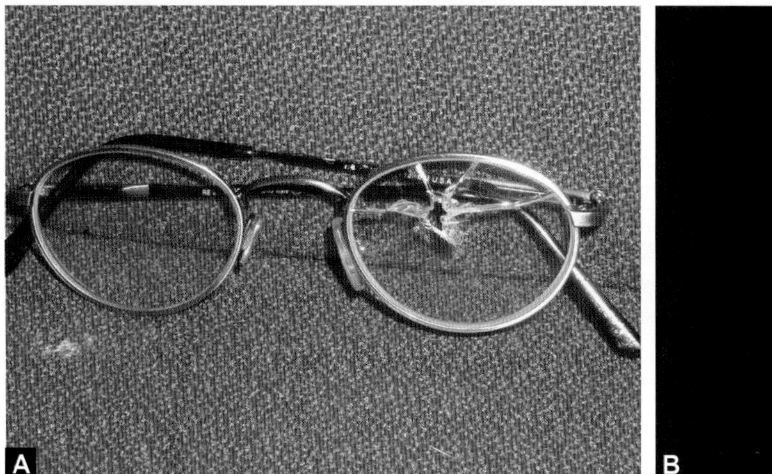

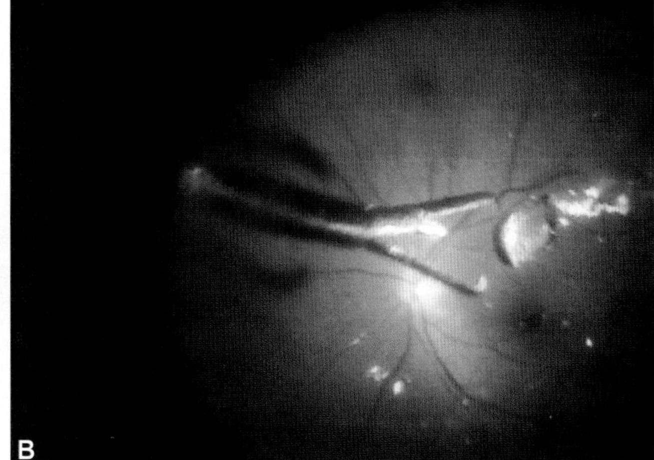

Figures 35-8A and B (A) Spectacles shattered by a projectile; and (B) a resultant Glass intraocular foreign body being approached by basket forceps.

when the IOFB is implanted in the eye wall, and is anterior enough to be immediately accessible without it traversing tissues in an uncontrolled manner (Fig. 35-9).

Intraocular foreign bodies can cause significant corneal damage obscuring the view of the retina, even when using an operating microscope with wide field viewing systems (Fig. 35-10). When significant corneal opacity is prevented, traditionally, IOFBs are removed using a temporary keratoprosthesis with penetrating keratoplasty. This procedure remains the standard of care but has high rates of graft rejection and poor visual outcomes. Endoscopic vitrectomy (Endooptiks®) is emerging as a very valuable tool in time sensitive cases, such as RD and/or IOFB, in which corneal opacity or poor media precludes safe visualization of the posterior segment structures through a wide angle viewing system. The system incorporates a 19 or 23 gauge probe with a coaxial camera, light source and laser. Its advantages over temporary keratoprosthesis include a less invasive and quicker approach, superior peripheral visualization of anterior anatomy and PVR, and it does not require coordination with a corneal specialist. It should be considered by surgeons experienced in the technique when the delay required for an adequate posterior view is expected to diminish the visual prognosis.

## COMPLICATIONS

As mentioned previously, there are multiple possible complications after IOFB removal. The most significant include endophthalmitis, intraocular pressure problems and late PVR-related RD. All patients should be made aware as early as possible that secondary, even multiple surgical interventions are common after significant traumatic ocular injuries, particularly with IOFBs.

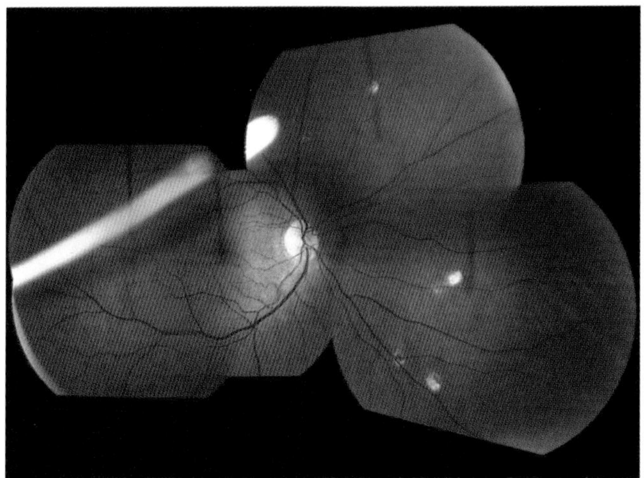

Figure 35-9 This wire from a grinding brush was retrieved atraumatically without vitrectomy by magnet, as the tail of the intraocular foreign body was still marginally accessible within the sclera. Cryotherapy was applied to the entry break.

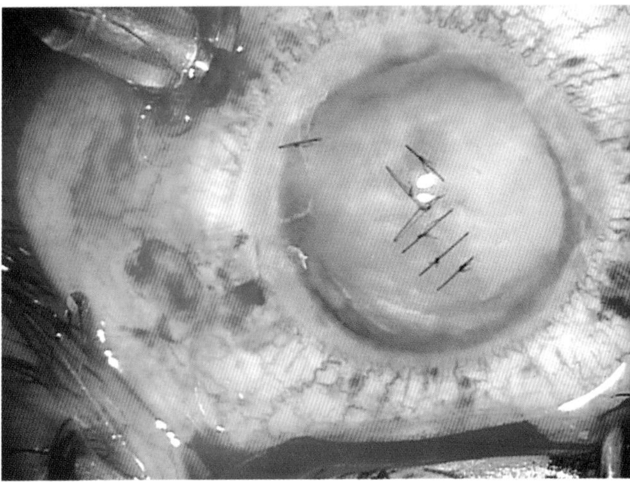

Figure 35-10 A highly opacified cornea is seen after repair of the intraocular foreign body entry site. While modern non-contact wide angle viewing systems are highly effective in obtaining a view through difficult media, endoscopic vitrectomy is an option for media that remains insufficient for surgery.

## SURGICAL OUTCOMES: SCIENTIFIC EVIDENCE

### Combat Data *Vs* Conventional Thinking

Recent data from studies involving combat ocular trauma suggest that the combination of systemic and topical fourth-generation fluoroquinolones immediately after the injury are highly effective in preventing IOFB-related endophthalmitis, even in cases of delayed IOFB removal (0% incidence).[11-13] Depending on the individual case scenario, some surgeons elect primary external globe repair first, and delaying the PPV and IOFB removal for several days. The advantages to this approach include improved anterior segment media clarity, stabilization of the patient's coexisting traumatic injuries, improved wound integrity, and optimization of the surgical resources such as securing an experienced team and a capable operating room. On the other hand, other studies which did not focus specifically on combat trauma have shown higher IOFB-related (up to 16%) endophthalmitis rates with late IOFB removal.[14] The mechanism of the injury (blast, hammering, blunt, etc.), the composition of the IOFB (metallic, vegetable, other), and the environmental contamination factors (grossly contaminated wound vs high-speed heated particle) should all be considered on a case-by-case basis in assessing the risk for post-traumatic endophthalmitis. If the patient stability, ocular media and resources allow, early IOFB removal has the advantage of a single procedure under anesthesia, a quicker opportunity to repair retinal pathology, and possibly a decreased incidence of post-traumatic eye and PVR, according to some studies. Overall, when compromising conditions are not present, it is still generally recommended to remove the IOFB as soon as possible, preferably within 24 hours at the time of the primary globe repair.

## PEARLS AND PITFALLS

- Prompt initiation of appropriate antibiotic prophylaxis and globe closure are the first most important steps in IOFB trauma.
- Preoperative assessment of associated ocular injuries, and information obtained regarding IOFB size, composition and location can assist surgical planning and choice of instrumentation.
- Delayed IOFB removal can be considered for an experienced operating room team, corneal opacity, or if the patient has other severe systemic injuries.
- Due to the significant RD and PVR risk, meticulous vitreous removal is the key. Preventative measures such as scleral buckling and silicone oil tamponade can also be considered.
- The management of the lens/IOL is a secondary objective, and should not compromise the care of the posterior segment. Patients should be made aware that periods of aphakia may be needed for adequate visualization, and subsequent operations are anticipated.
- Endoscopic vitrectomy is an emerging alternative to keratoprosthesis when corneal opacity precludes timely intervention.

## REFERENCES


1. Jonas JB, Knorr HL, Budde WM. Prognostic factors in ocular injuries caused by intraocular or retrobulbar foreign bodies. Ophthalmology. 2000;107(5):823-8.
2. Kuhn F, Morris R, Witherspoon CD, et al. Epidemiology of blinding trauma in the United States Eye Injury Registry. Ophthalmic Epidemiol. 2006;13(3):209-16.
3. Affeldt JC, Flynn HW Jr, Forster RK, et al. Microbial endophthalmitis resulting from ocular trauma. Ophthalmology. 1987;94(4):407-13.
4. Parrish CM, O'Day DM. Traumatic endophthalmitis. Int Ophthalmol Clin. 1987;27(2):112-9.
5. Al-Omran AM, Abboud EB, Abu El-Asrar AM. Microbiologic spectrum and visual outcome of posttraumatic endophthalmitis. Retina. 2007;27(2):236-42.
6. Dass AB, Ferrone PJ, Chu YR, et al. Sensitivity of spiral computed tomography scanning for detecting intraocular foreign bodies. Ophthalmology. 2001;108(12):2326-8.
7. Thompson WS, Rubsamen PE, Flynn HW Jr, et al. Endophthalmitis after penetrating trauma. Risk factors and visual acuity outcomes. Ophthalmology. 1995;102(11):1696-701.
8. Tasman W. Peripheral retinal changes following blunt trauma. Trans Am Ophthalmol Soc. 1972;70:190-8.
9. Eagling EM. Ocular damage after blunt trauma to the eye. Its relationship to the nature of the injury. Br J Ophthalmol. 1974;58(2):126-40.
10. Yeh S, Colyer MH, Weichel ED. Current trends in the management of intraocular foreign bodies. Curr Opin Ophthalmol. 2008;19(3):225-33.
11. Colyer MH, Weber ED, Weichel ED, et al. Delayed intraocular foreign body removal without endophthalmitis during operations Iraqi freedom and enduring freedom. Ophthalmology. 2007;114(8):1439-47.
12. Weichel ED, Colyer MH, Ludlow SE, et al. Combat ocular trauma visual outcomes during operations iraqi and enduring freedom. Ophthalmology. 2008;115(12):2235-45.
13. Thach AB, Ward TP, Dick JS 2nd, et al. Intraocular foreign body injuries during operation Iraqi freedom. Ophthalmology. 2005;112(10):1829-33.
14. Jonas JB, Budde WM. Early versus late removal of retained intraocular foreign bodies. Retina. 1999;19(3):193-7.

CHAPTER

36

# Diabetic Retinopathy and Its Management

Michael Dollin, James Vander

## INTRODUCTION

Diabetic retinopathy is the leading cause of blindness among adults aged 25–74 years in the United States.[1] Central to the prevention of diabetic retinopathy and its complications are optimal blood glucose and blood pressure control, population screening, and early detection. When complications do develop, treatment options include intravitreal injections of anti-vascular endothelial growth factor (VEGF) or steroid agents, focal and/or grid laser photocoagulation, and panretinal laser photocoagulation (PRP). Vitrectomy, especially with safer modern instrumentation and more efficient techniques, has become an important surgical tool through which many of the more advanced complications of diabetic retinopathy can be managed.

## LASER PHOTOCOAGULATION FOR DIABETIC MACULAR EDEMA

Laser photocoagulation has been shown in the Early Treatment of Diabetic Retinopathy Study (ETDRS) to be effective at reducing the risk of vision loss in diabetics with clinically significant macular edema (CSME).[2] CSME is defined based on the following criteria seen on biomicroscopic examination (Figs. 36-1A to C):

- Retinal thickening within 500 µ of the foveal center
- Hard exudate within 500 µ of the foveal center if associated with retinal thickening, or
- Zone of retinal thickening 1 disk diameter in size, any part of which is within 1 disk diameter of the foveal center

Intravitreal anti-VEGF agents, namely ranibizumab and off-label bevacizumab, are currently considered the standard of care for fovea-involving diabetic macular edema. Nonetheless, laser photocoagulation still plays an important role as either primary or adjunctive treatment when CSME is present.[3]

### Preoperative Evaluation

Meticulous examination of the macula using slit lamp biomicroscopy should be performed. Optical coherence tomography (OCT) scan and review of a recent fluorescein angiogram (FA) are useful (Figs. 36-2A and B).

### Instrumentation and Surgical Technique

- Instill topical anesthetic drops
- Use a macular contact lens (e.g. Goldmann 3-mirror or ocular Mainster high magnification lens)
- Set laser parameters as described in Table 36-1
- Treat with either focal or grid pattern. Focal laser consists of direct treatment of leaking microaneurysms identified on fluorescein angiography. Grid laser consists of treatment of diffuse areas of leakage with 50–200 µm burns placed 1–2 burn widths apart
- Avoid treating lesions within 500 µm of the foveal center or at the edge of the foveal avascular zone. During retreatment sessions, a cautious approach using 50–100 µm mildly white burns of 0.05–0.1 seconds in duration can be helpful

### Postoperative Care

No postoperative medications are required. Allow 3–4 months after treatment before considering retreatment for persistent or recurrent CSME.

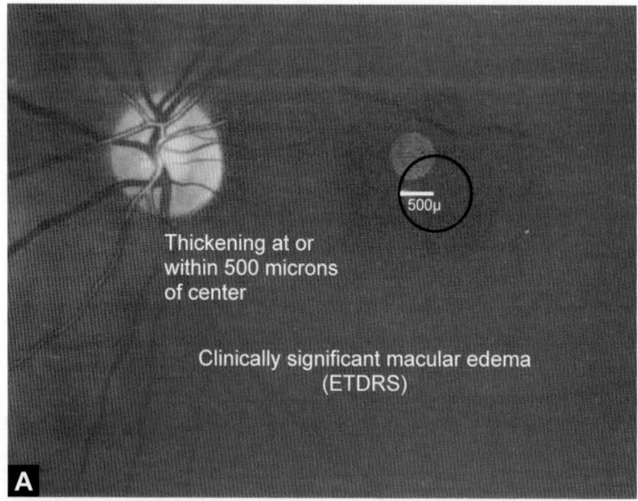


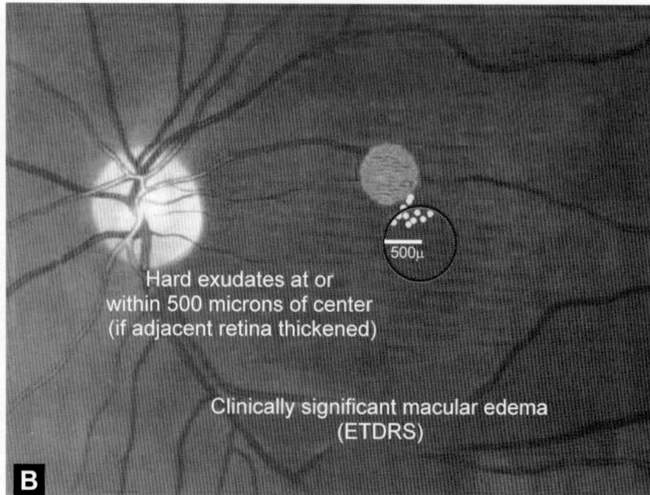


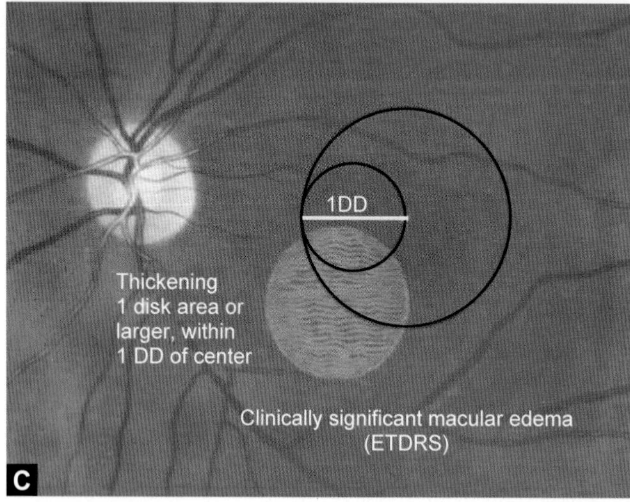


**Figures 36-1A to C** Early Treatment of Diabetic Retinopathy Study criteria for clinically significant diabetic macular edema.

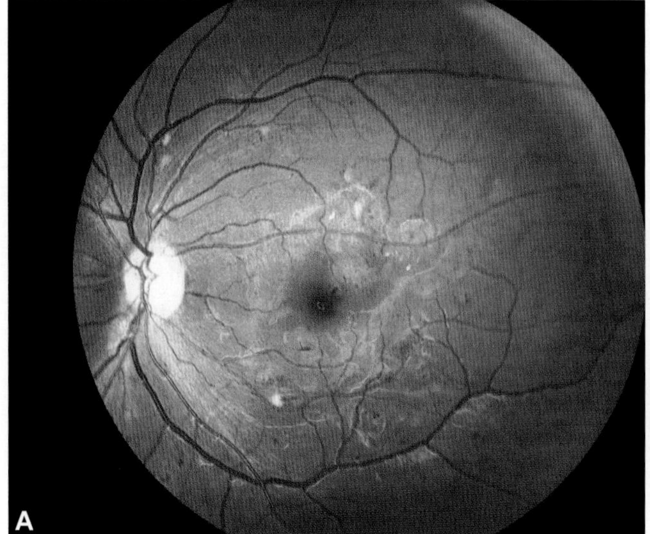


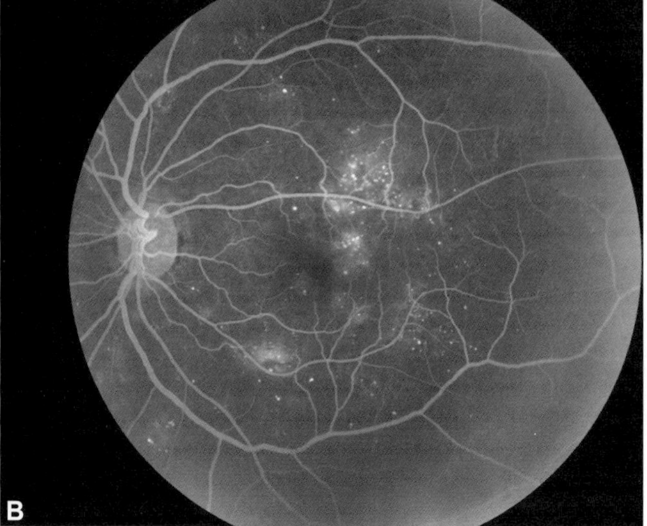


**Figures 36-2A and B** Clinical photo (A) and fluorescein angiogram (B) of a patient with clinically significant macular edema superior to the fovea.

TABLE 36-1 Parameters for laser photocoagulation in diabetic retinopathy

| Type | Lens | Spot size (μm) | Duration (seconds) | Power (mW) | Strategy |
|---|---|---|---|---|---|
| Laser for CSME | Macular contact lens<br>– Goldmann<br>– Mainster high magnification | 50–100 | 0.05–0.1 | 50–100 (begin low and titrate to create mildly white burns) | Focal: directly treat MA<br>Grid: treat zone of edema with burns placed 1–2 burn widths apart |
| PRP | Peripheral fundus contact lens<br>– Mainster 165<br>– Rodenstock | 200–500 | 0.05–0.2 | 150–200 (begin low and titrate to produce a gray-white burn) | Place burns 0.5–1 burn width apart |

(CSME: Clinically significant macular edema; MA: Microaneurysms; PRP: Panretinal photocoagulation).

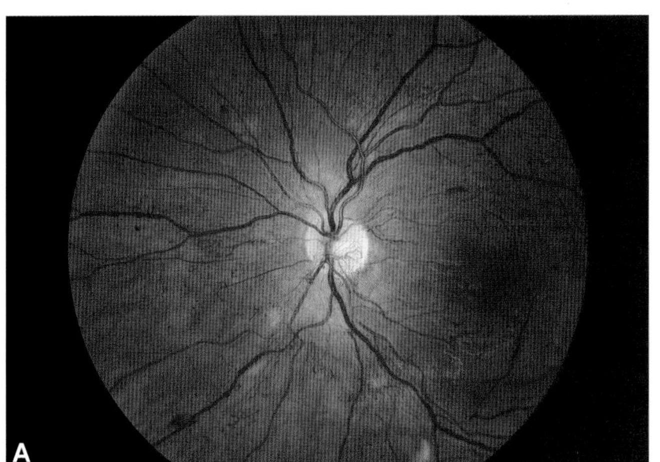


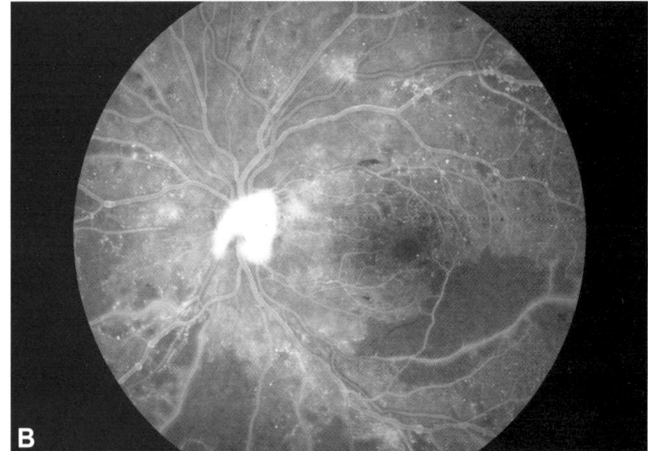


Figures 36-3A and B Clinical photo (A) and fluorescein angiogram (B) of a patient with proliferative diabetic retinopathy with high-risk characteristics.

## Complications

Potential complications of laser photocoagulation include inadvertent foveal burn, transient worsening of macular edema, subretinal hemorrhage, subretinal fibrosis, rupture of Bruch's membrane, choroidal neovascularization, scotoma, and visual loss (Table 36-1).

# PANRETINAL PHOTOCOAGULATION

The hallmark of proliferative diabetic retinopathy is neovascularization, an ischemia-driven process typically seen in advanced diabetic retinopathy. PRP was shown in the DRS to significantly reduce the rate of severe vision loss in diabetics with high-risk proliferative diabetic retinopathy,[4] defined by the presence of any of the following criteria (Figs. 36-3A and B):

- Neovascularization of the disk (NVD) greater than one-third of the disk area
- Any NVD with associated vitreous hemorrhage
- Neovascularization elsewhere in the retina (NVE) one half disk area in size or greater with associated vitreous hemorrhage

Other instances in which PRP may be considered, even in the absence of high-risk characteristics, include patients with neovascularization of the iris and/or angle, and patients with mild proliferative or severe nonproliferative diabetic retinopathy in whom regular follow-up may be questionable.

## Preoperative Evaluation

Slit lamp and dilated fundus examination to confirm neovascularization. FA is helpful for identifying subtle areas of neovascularization or capillary nonperfusion not apparent on clinical examination.

## Instrumentation and Surgical Technique

- Instill topical anesthetic drops. Peribulbar injection of anesthesia, such as lidocaine, may be considered in select patients who have difficulty tolerating the treatment, or those who require longer sessions of PRP
- Use a peripheral fundus contact lens (e.g. ocular Mainster PRP 165 or Rodenstock lens)
- Set laser parameters as indicated in Table 36-1

TABLE 36-2 Indications for vitrectomy in diabetic retinopathy

| Media opacities | Vitreoretinal traction |
|---|---|
| Nonclearing vitreous hemorrhage | Traction retinal detachment involving the macula |
| Vitreous hemorrhage with anterior segment neovascularization (especially without prior PRP) | Combined traction and rhegmatogenous retinal detachment |
| Ghost cell glaucoma | Progressive fibrovascular proliferation |
| Dense premacular hemorrhage | Diffuse diabetic macular edema associated with taut posterior hyaloid vitreomacular traction |
| | Macular heterotopias |

(PRP: Panretinal photocoagulation).

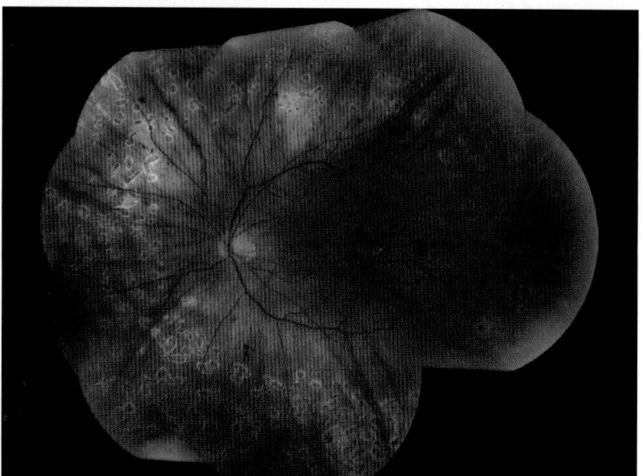

Figure 36-4 Panretinal photocoagulation in a patient with high-risk proliferative diabetic retinopathy.

- Treat in a concentric zone of retina extending from just outside the temporal arcades to just anterior to the equator. Treatment can be extended to the ora serrata in the case of persistent or recurrent neovascularization despite complete PRP or in neovascular glaucoma. PRP should extend to no closer than 0.5–1 disk diameter within the nasal aspect of the optic disk and within 2–3 disk diameters temporal to the fovea
- It is generally advisable to begin PRP in the inferior periphery, if visualization permits
- Do not treat directly over retinal vessels and avoid the long posterior ciliary arteries and nerves
- If macular edema is also present at diagnosis of PDR, consider treating macular edema first with either laser or concurrent intravitreal anti-VEGF (Fig. 36-4).

## Postoperative Care

Postoperative medications are not typically administered, unless associated conditions (e.g. neovascular glaucoma) are present. If peribulbar anesthesia was used, it is advisable to patch the eye for several hours after the procedure. Patients should be re-examined in follow-up approximately 3 weeks later to assess for regression of neovascularization. If disease is severe and sufficient PRP could not be placed at the initial session, consider re-examination of patients sooner at 1–2 weeks.

## Complications

Potential complications of PRP include cataract, iritis, tonic pupil, anterior segment ischemia, choroidal effusion with possible secondary angle-closure glaucoma, inadvertent foveal burn, macular edema, subretinal hemorrhage, subretinal fibrosis, rupture of Bruch's membrane, choroidal neovascularization, retinal tears, visual field constriction, and difficulty with night vision.

# VITRECTOMY FOR DIABETIC RETINOPATHY

Since its advent in the early 1970s, there have been remarkable advances in vitrectomy techniques and instrumentation. The earliest indication for vitrectomy in diabetic patients was nonclearing vitreous hemorrhage.[5] With refinements in surgical technique, this list of indications has expanded significantly and can generally be categorized into media opacities or vitreoretinal traction-mediated complications of diabetic retinopathy (Table 36-2).

Other indications include diffuse diabetic macular edema with and without vitreomacular traction, and postoperative complications seen in diabetics such as recurrent vitreous hemorrhage, anterior hyaloidal fibrovascular proliferation, and fibrinoid syndrome (Fig. 36-5).

## Preoperative Considerations

Both patient and ocular factors should be considered in the decision to perform surgery in patients with advanced diabetic retinopathy. Patient considerations include comorbid illness, such as hypertension, cardiovascular disease, and renal insufficiency. Prior to surgery, medical evaluation and clearance should be sought by consultation with the patient's

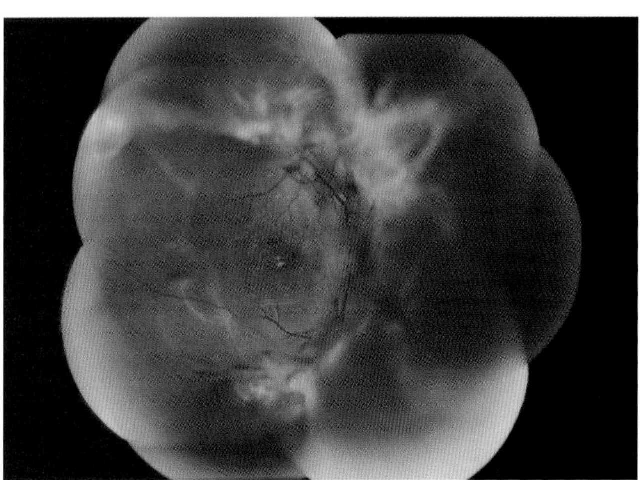

Figure 36-5 Combined traction and rhegmatogenous retinal detachment requiring vitrectomy in a patient with proliferative diabetic retinopathy.

internist. Medical status may significantly influence the risks of anesthesia, as well as the need for a hospital-based operating room where access to medical support, if needed, is readily available. Other patient considerations include status of the fellow eye, visual needs, and capacity to instill postoperative drops and return for follow-up visits.

Specific ocular considerations include the presence of cataract, as well as posterior synechiae and/or hyphema from anterior segment neovascularization. The degree of active neovascularization and amount of pre-existing PRP, if any, is also important. Wherever possible, PRP should be administered preoperatively to the extent that visualization permits. Injection of preoperative bevacizumab 2–5 days prior to surgery may also help facilitate tissue dissection and minimize bleeding intraoperatively. Another important ocular consideration is extent of macular ischemia, best evaluated by fluorescein angiography. Severe macular ischemia may significantly limit visual potential and in such cases, surgery may not be recommended. Similarly, duration of traction retinal detachment, particularly if the macula has been detached, should also be factored in to the decision for surgery versus observation. Detachments of > 6–12 months duration generally preclude the return of useful vision postoperatively. Lastly, when significant media opacity is present, preoperative echography is helpful in assessing for associated retinal detachment, which may hasten the decision towards surgery over observation.

## General Surgical Objectives in Vitrectomy for Diabetic Retinopathy

Vitrectomy is generally only considered in diabetic retinopathy when ischemia-driven neovascularization develops and complications ensue, as listed above, when vitreomacular traction is present, or when patients have persistent diabetic edema poorly responsive to other treatment.

Although surgery in these patients can range from relatively straightforward to extremely complex, the following general set of surgical objectives[6] should be kept in mind:

- Remove media opacities
- Relieve anteroposterior and tangential preretinal traction
- Achieve hemostasis
- Deliver laser treatment wherever needed (e.g. retinal breaks, flat NVE, PRP)
- Tamponade as needed.

## Instrumentation

Standard vitrectomy equipment, including infusion, fiberoptic endoilluminator, and a vitreous cutting instrument, is required. Although large-gauge vitrectomy is still utilized, small (23 and 25)-gauge microincision vitrectomy systems with transconjunctival cannula systems and high-speed vitreous cutters of 2500 to 5000 cuts per minute (CPM) are widely preferred.

Various intraocular saline infusion solutions are available. In phakic eyes, a solution containing dextrose 50% is helpful to prevent intraoperative posterior subcapsular lens changes. A helpful tool to have available when extensive dissection is anticipated is the chandelier endoilluminator, which allows for bimanual technique. Alternatively, endoilluminator probes combined with picks, cannulae, or forceps are available and help facilitate intraocular tissue dissection.

An endodiathermy probe is helpful in achieving hemostasis of bleeding fronds of NVE. It can also be utilized to create retinal whitening at the edge of retinal breaks, making them more readily identifiable and easier to treat with laser retinopexy when the eye is filled with air. The endolaser photocoagulation probe is similarly useful to achieve hemostasis from fronds of flat NVE, and greatly facilitates the delivery of intraoperative PRP and retinopexy of any retinal breaks.

Other helpful specialized instruments for surgery in diabetic retinopathy include foot-controlled vertically or horizontally oriented intraocular scissors that enable both blunt and sharp dissection for removal of fibrovascular membranes. Various other intraocular blades, picks, or forceps are also available. Wide-field viewing systems, with either contact or noncontact BIOM lenses, provide the surgeon with an overall view of the fundus. When meticulous sectioning of membranes is required, a macular contact lens helps provide both higher magnification and better depth of focus.

Particularly in the presence of iris neovascularization and small fixed pupils, iris retractors such as iris hooks, or a Malyugin ring can dramatically improve visualization of the peripheral retina. Lastly, intraocular tamponade agents should be available, especially in the management of diabetic traction and combined traction-rhegmatogenous retinal detachments. These include gases, such as sulfur hexafluoride ($SF_6$) and perfluoropropane ($C_3F_8$). Longer acting tamponade with silicone oil is available in lower (1000 centistoke) or higher (5000 centistoke) viscosities.

## Surgical Technique

- Confirm the eye to be operated on prior to surgery
- Anesthesia, either general or local, is administered
- The eye, eyelids, and periorbital skin should be prepped with povidone-iodine and draped in a sterile fashion
- Place a lid speculum, paying careful attention to keep the lashes out of the surgical field
- Mark the sites for trocar–cannula entry. For standard three-port pars plana vitrectomy, the infusion cannula is generally inserted in the inferotemporal quadrant, while the other two instrument ports are placed superotemporally and superonasally. Ports should be placed 4.0 mm from the limbus in phakic eyes and 3.5 mm from the limbus in pseudophakic or aphakic eyes. When inserting the trocar–cannulae, displace the conjunctiva using forceps or a cotton-tipped applicator, and enter in a beveled fashion
- Once the infusion port is placed, connect the infusion line. Keep the line clamped (so that no fluid is running) while connecting the infusion. Using direct visualization, confirm proper positioning of the infusion cannula with complete passage through the pars plana. Doing so is imperative to avoid suprachoroidal infusion of fluid
- If a cataract precludes adequate view of the fundus, consider performing a pars plana lensectomy prior to vitreous removal
- In small pupil cases, iris retractors may need to be inserted, both for lensectomy and subsequent vitrectomy
- Put the viewing system into position
- The endoilluminator probe should be the first instrument inserted into the eye. Subsequently turn off the microscope light and room lights. Diffusely illuminate the posterior pole by varying the probe depth within the eye. Avoid direct macular illumination until necessary
- Focus your viewing system on the posterior pole. If vitreous hemorrhage is present and view of the posterior pole is not possible, attempt to focus near the mid vitreous cavity. Refocusing may be required later in the surgery as the media is cleared
- Insert the vitreous cutting instrument and begin a core vitrectomy. Typical settings for this step would be 1500–2500 CPM and a vacuum of 400 mm Hg.
- If a posterior vitreous detachment is already present, incise the posterior hyaloid face and enlarge the opening circumferentially. Aspirate any preretinal hemorrhage overlying the posterior pole using the vitreous cutter on suction mode or a soft tipped cannula. Once sufficient hemorrhage has been cleared and visualization has improved, as much of the peripheral cortical vitreous should be removed as possible to permit more extensive laser treatment, improve peripheral fundus visualization, and reduce the chances of postoperative vitreous hemorrhage
- In eyes in which a posterior vitreous detachment is not present, broad or focal vitreoretinal adhesions often exist at foci of neovascularization. These adhesions may be associated with fibrosis, epiretinal membranes, traction detachments, or retinal breaks. General surgical techniques to approach and eliminate this vitreoretinal traction include segmentation, delamination, and "en bloc" dissection (Table 36-3, Figs. 36-6 to 36-8).
- Once vitreoretinal adhesions are eliminated using one or a combination of the above techniques, the peripheral cortical vitreous can be removed
- Remove remaining preretinal fibrovascular tissue using similar dissection techniques as used for vitreous. Removal of these tissues is generally initiated around the optic nerve and extended in a posterior to anterior direction. Blunt dissection at the retinal plane using horizontal scissors along with forceps and picks used separately or in a bimanual fashion to release pegs of neovascularization are helpful in facilitating removal of this tissue. Firm adhesions to the disk can be left in place and circumferentially trimmed using the vitreous cutter. Epiretinal membranes away from the optic nerve can be peeled toward their vascular center and then removed. Bleeding often ensues and hemostasis should be achieved promptly by transiently increasing the infusion pressure and using endocautery or endolaser (Fig. 36-9).
- In eyes in which peripheral vitreoretinal traction is present and cannot be relieved by one of the above methods, an encircling buckle or relaxing retinectomy may be required
- Apply endolaser photocoagulation to perform and/or complete pre-existing partial PRP out to the ora serrata. Any bleeding fronds of neovascularization may also be gently lasered, except at the optic nerve, to achieve hemostasis and promote regression. Full-thickness retinal breaks should be surrounded with three to four confluent rows of laser retinopexy. Note that if subretinal fluid is present,

TABLE 36-3 Techniques for eliminating vitreoretinal traction during vitrectomy

| Technique | Description | Illustration |
|---|---|---|
| Segmentation | Traction is sequentially eliminated by removing anteroposterior traction first, then removing tangential traction by severing connection between islands of vitreoretinal adhesions using the vitreous cutter or vertical scissors | Figure 36-6 Illustration of segmentation of vitreous adhesions and diabetic membranes. |
| Delamination | Anteroposterior traction is eliminated first, then preretinal fibrovascular tissue is removed in large pieces at the retinal plane using horizontal scissors, picks or forceps | 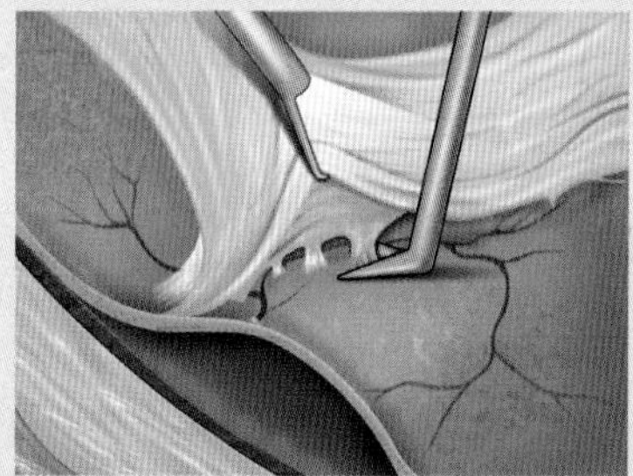 Figure 36-7 Illustration using scissors for delamination of a membrane from the retinal surface. |
| "En bloc" dissection | Tangential surface traction is removed first, leaving anteroposterior traction intact to help "assist" in elevating preretinal fibrovascular tissue and facilitating dissection. Anteroposterior traction and the bulk of the vitreous are then removed as a unit ("en bloc") | 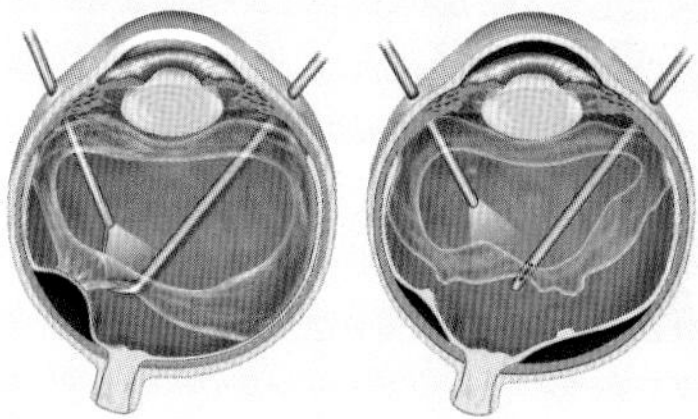 Figure 36-8 Illustration of the en bloc technique. |

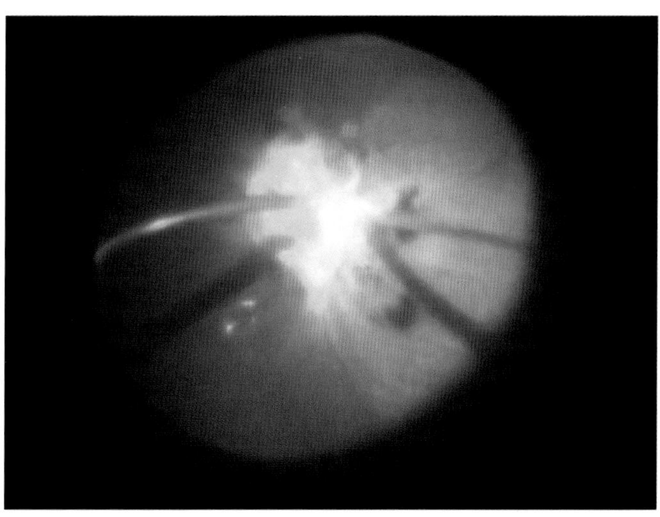

Figure 36-9 En bloc dissection can be performed using a chandelier light source and a bimanual technique.

air–fluid exchange and endodrainage will need to be performed prior to laser retinopexy to allow uptake of laser
- Inspect the peripheral retina with scleral depression to identify any peripheral retinal breaks. Any breaks should be treated completely by endolaser retinopexy
- Perform air–fluid exchange using the soft-tipped cannula if any retinal breaks are present. If no breaks are present, an air–fluid exchange can be considered to help reduce the incidence of postoperative hypotony
- If extended retinal tamponade is required, perform long-acting gas–air exchange. Nonexpansile concentrations of $SF_6$ 20% and $C_3F_8$ 14% are most commonly used. The air-filled eye should be flushed with 35–40 cc of gas through the infusion line while venting air though one of the sclerotomy ports. Valved cannulae require venting using a soft-tipped cannula or specially designed vent. If longer acting tamponade is desired, such as in reoperations, severe traction, or combined traction–rhegmatogenous retinal detachments, silicone oil can be exchanged with air. Inject silicone oil through one of the sclerotomy ports using an automated pump injection device, being careful not to introduce oil into the anterior chamber. In aphakic eyes, create an inferior peripheral iridotomy using the vitreous cutter prior to injection of oil
- Remove all sclerotomy cannulae and verify that wounds are adequately self-sealed. If any concerns for leakage become apparent, or routinely when using silicone oil, suture the sclerotomies in a transconjunctival manner using 8-0 polyglactin or 6-0 plain gut suture. A single interrupted suture will generally suffice

### Postoperative Care

Antibiotic ointment with or without steroid should be placed on the patient's eye at the conclusion of surgery. The operated eye should be patched for several hours or until the following morning. Patients are generally examined on the first post-operative day, and then subsequently at 1, 3, and 6 weeks, at the discretion of the surgeon and depending on the patient's postoperative course. Topical antibiotic drops are prescribed four times per day for 1 week following the surgery, along with topical prednisolone acetate 1% four times per day, which is tapered over 3–4 weeks as inflammation subsides. Atropine 1% twice per day may also be prescribed for cycloplegia. Patients should be instructed to position face-down and/or avoid supine positioning if phakic with gas or aphakic with oil in the eye. Heavy straining or lifting should also be avoided for the first 1–2 weeks postoperatively.

## COMPLICATIONS

Potential postoperative complications following vitrectomy for diabetic retinopathy include persistent corneal epithelial defects, cataract, vitreous hemorrhage, intraocular pressure elevation, retinal breaks or detachment, central retinal artery occlusion, optic neuropathy, cystoid macular edema, epiretinal membrane, pupillary block, neovascular glaucoma, intraocular fibrin formation (including fibrinoid syndrome), anterior hyaloidal fibrovascular proliferation, and endophthalmitis.

## PEARLS AND PITFALLS

- The effect of focal laser for CSME is not immediate. Allow 3–4 months after treatment before considering more focal laser for persistent or recurrent CSME.
- Begin PRP inferiorly. Occasionally patients may develop vitreous hemorrhage after treatment begins and this can then obscure the inferior retina and make subsequent treatment challenging.
- Even after complete PRP for proliferative diabetic retinopathy, up to 25% of patients may have persistent posterior segment neovascularization.
- When considering surgery in a patient with diabetic traction retinal detachment, the administration of as much PRP as possible preoperatively facilitates tissue dissection intraoperatively.
- Likewise, preoperative bevacizumab 2–5 days prior to surgery may help facilitate tissue dissection and minimize bleeding intraoperatively. Caution should be taken in patients whose active systemic comorbidities may postpone surgery, as bevacizumab may worsen traction retinal detachment if surgery is not imminently performed after administering it.
- Use of a chandelier endoilluminator can be very helpful in allowing bimanual tissue dissection during vitrectomy for diabetic traction retinal detachment.
- Avoid aggressive attempts to elevate the hyaloid in the presence of foci of regressed fibrovascular tissue without segmenting, cutting, or otherwise addressing the tight vitreoretinal adhesion it creates.
- If a retinal break is present, leaving any associated traction will result in failure and rhegmatogenous retinal detachment formation.

## REFERENCES

1. Klein R, Klein B. National Diabetes Data Group. Diabetes in America. Bethesda, MD: National Institutes of Health, National Institute of Diabetes and Digestive and Kidney Diseases; 1995. Vision disorders in diabetes; pp. 293-337.

2. Early Treatment Diabetic Retinopathy Study Research Group: Focal photocoagulation treatment of diabetic macular edema. ETDRS Report Number 19. Arch Ophthalmol. 1995;113:1144-55.
3. The Diabetic Retinopathy Clinical Research Network, Elman MJ, Qin H, Aiello LP, et al. Intravitreal ranibizumab for diabetic macular edema with prompt vs deferred laser treatment: 3-year randomized trial results. Ophthalmology. 2012;119:2312-8.
4. Diabetic Retinopathy Study Research Group. Preliminary report on effects of photocoagulation therapy. Am J Ophthalmol. 1976;81:383-96.
5. Machemer R, Buettner H, Norton EWD, et al. Vitrectomy: a pars plana approach. Trans Am Acad Ophthalmol Otolaryngol. 1971;75:813.
6. Scott IU, Flynn HW, Smiddy WE. Diabetes and ocular disease: past, present and future therapies, 2nd edn. New York: Oxford; 2010. pp. 207-34.

CHAPTER 37

# Endoscopic Vitrectomy

S Chien Wong, Emil Anthony T Say, Thomas C Lee

## INTRODUCTION

Most vitreoretinal surgeries are performed with good visualization using either the operating microscope or an indirect ophthalmoscope. However, in certain situations, the endoscope can be used in place of or to complement conventional contact and noncontact systems (e.g. BIOM). The endoscope has three unique attributes:

1. Posterior segment visualization is not dependent upon an optically clear anterior segment, a prerequisite of conventional viewing systems
2. It enables a distinctly different surgeon's perspective, as the intraoperative view is the image the endoscope captures looking out from one of the sclerotomy ports. Thus, the side-on perspective is approximately 90° away from the conventional top-down bird's eye view (Figs. 37-1A and B)
3. In contrast to conventional viewing systems which derive the surgeon's view from light that transmits through the patient's ocular media into the operating microscope, the endoscope both illuminates the areas of interest and captures light that reflects directly back into the endoscope. As a result, the endoscope enables better visualization of vitreous and membranes (Figs. 37-2A and B).

## INDICATIONS

- Anterior segment opacity, such as corneal scarring, hyphema or cataract, that is sufficiently dense to preclude

Conventional wide-angle
(Top-down)

A

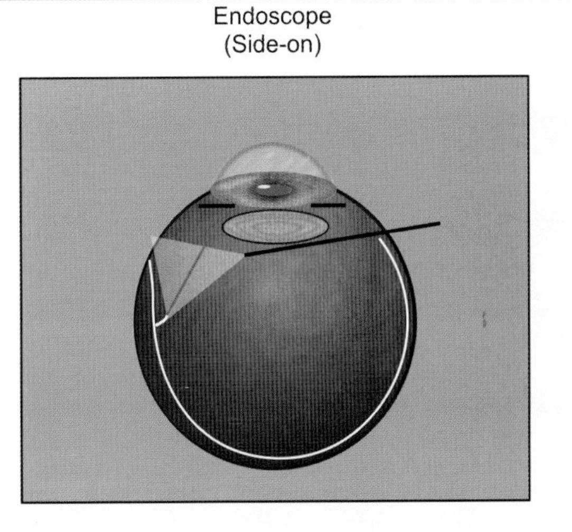


Figures 37-1A and B Illustrative comparison between (A) conventional top-down wide-angle viewing system and (B) endoscopic side-on view, i.e. 90° apart.

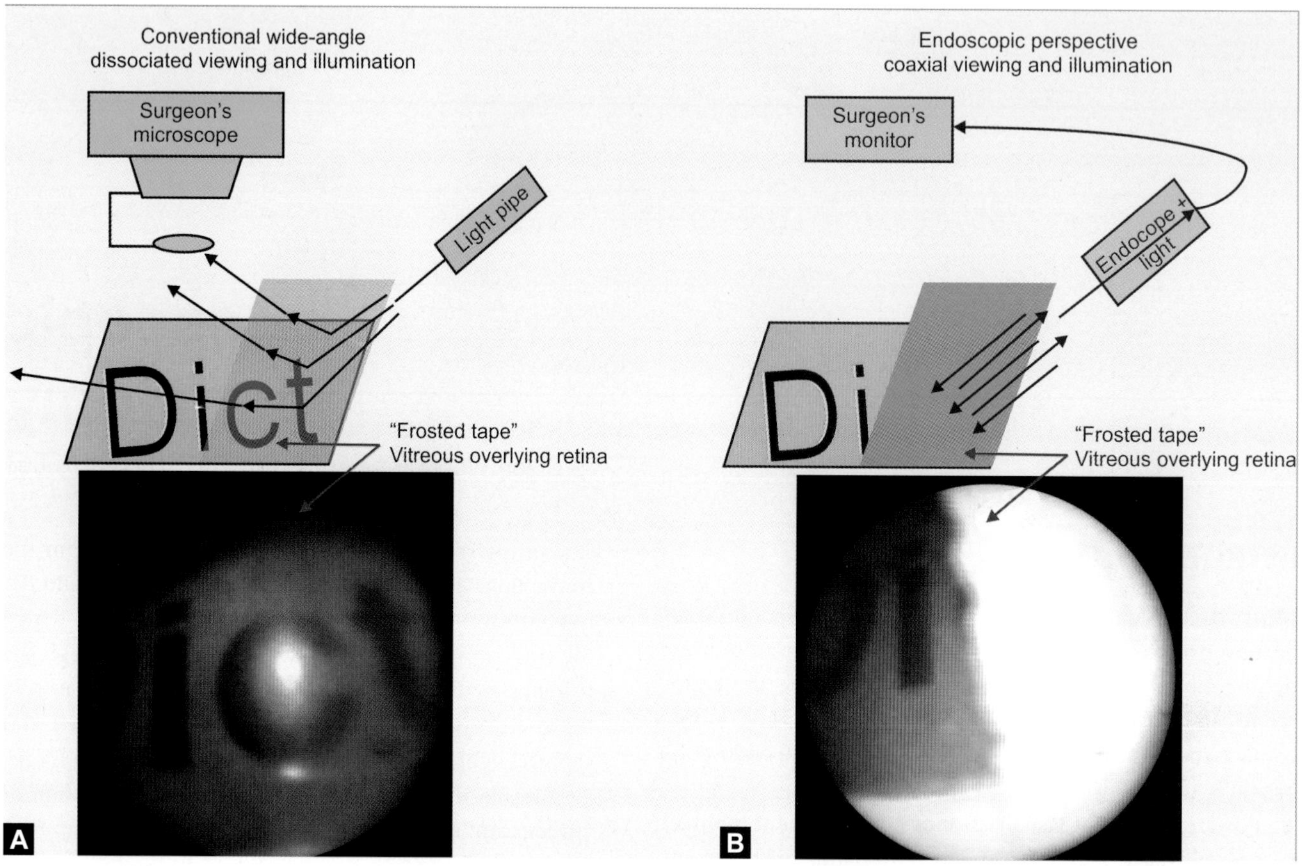

Conventional wide-angle dissociated viewing and illumination

Surgeon's microscope

Light pipe

"Frosted tape" Vitreous overlying retina

Endoscopic perspective coaxial viewing and illumination

Surgeon's monitor

Endocope + light

"Frosted tape" Vitreous overlying retina

**Figures 37-2A and B** Cellophane tape experiment differentiating transmitted (A) from reflected light (B). Conventional wide-angle viewing perspective (A) dissociates surgeon's visual axis and source of illumination, such that light is transmitted through the patient's clear vitreous and becomes difficult to visualize through the surgeon's microscope and visual axis. In comparison, an endoscopic perspective (B) combines illumination and light capture through the same endoscope probe, such that light is reflected back through the endoscope and into the surgeon's monitor for viewing.

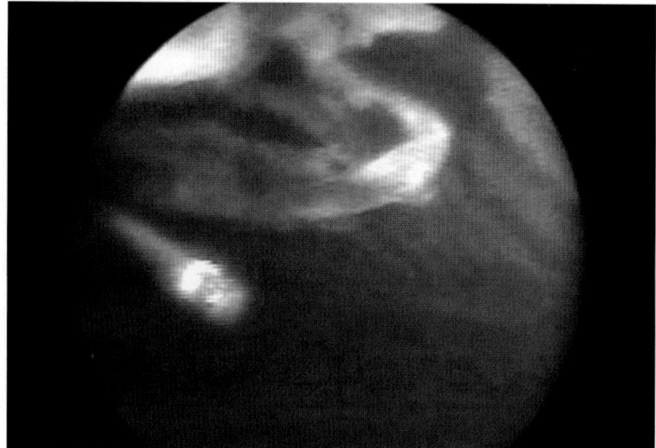

**Figure 37-3:** This patient had ectopia lentis associated with Marfan's syndrome. During endoscopic pars plana lensectomy, retained capsule remnants were carefully removed from the ciliary sulcus. Complete removal through conventional wide-angle viewing systems would have been less certain owing to the anterior location of the structures precluding direction visualization of the sulcus. This is an illustrative case—complete capsulectomy is typically more relevant in uveitis cases, particularly in children.

visualization of the vitreous cavity using conventional viewing systems.

- Any anterior vitreoretinal pathology that is difficult to access and optimally visualize using conventional systems.
- Direct visualization of the ciliary sulcus to ensure complete capsulectomy where indicated, e.g. in pediatric uveitis requiring lensectomy and vitrectomy (Fig. 37-3).
- Direct visualization and management of vitreous and/or retinal incarceration in a sclerotomy (Figs. 37-4A and B).
- Ciliary body and retroirideal pathologies (Fig. 37-5).
- Highly elevated pathologies, e.g. a traction retinal detachment (TRD) in pediatric vitreoretinopathies [retinopathy of prematurity (ROP) and familial exudative vitreoretinopathy (FEVR)] (Figs. 37-6A to C). The side-on perspective of the endoscope enables greater visualization of the entire side profile of the pathology, potentially facilitating safer tissue dissection, as compared to a conventional top-down ("bird's eye") view.

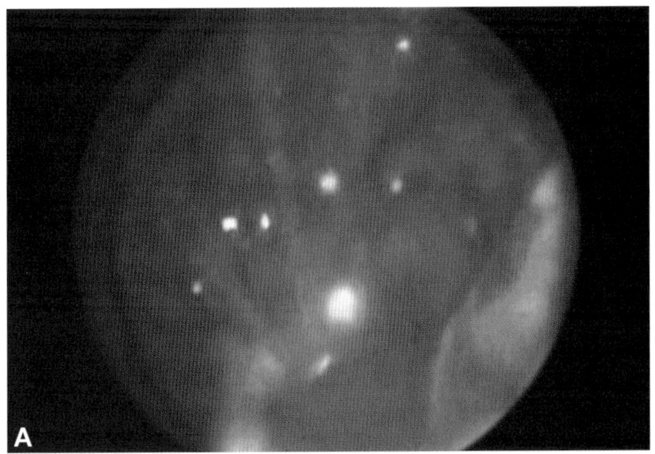


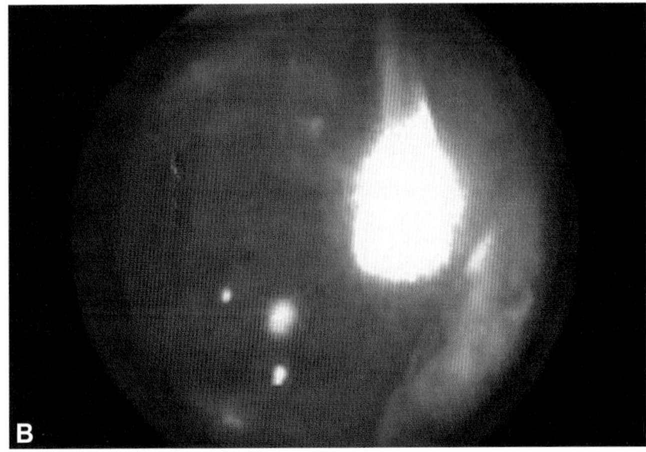


**Figures 37-4A and B** In this case of rhegmatogenous retinal detachment repair, vitreous became incarcerated into the sclerotomy port during perfluorocarbon liquid injection. (A) Vitreous can be seen as "folds" from the inside of the sclerotomy, extending toward the edge of the image circle in this figure; (B) Following release of vitreous incarceration, there was immediate relief of traction and the "folds" are no longer seen.

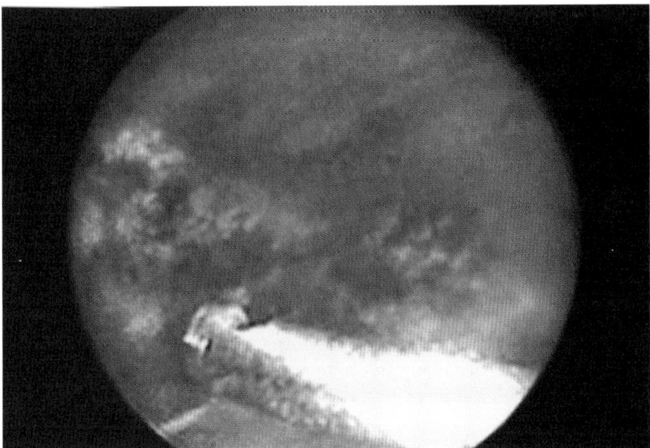

**Figure 37-5** A case of stage 4A retinopathy of prematurity with anteroposterior vitreous traction from attachment to the posterior iris surface visible only through the endoscope.

- Subretinal surgery to remove proliferative vitreoretinopathy (PVR) bands and choroidal neovascular (CNV) membranes can be easier with the endoscope (Figs. 37-7A and B).
- Any pathology that requires placement of trocars through corneal limbus rather than sclera overlying the pars plana, e.g. significant scleral thinning and total TRD in ROP or FEVR precluding safe posterior segment trocar placement.
- Enabling direct visualization of entrapped intraocular lens (IOL) haptic (Figs. 37-8A to D).
- To achieve more extensive endocyclophotocoagulation (in contrast to an anterior segment approach that glaucoma surgeons would use), also known as "ECP plus", by laser ablation of the ciliary processes and extending it into the pars plica via a posterior segment approach (Figs. 37-9A and B).

## CONTRAINDICATIONS

- Eyes that require bimanual surgery. However, endoscope instrument development is underway and may enable this.
- When 25-gauge or smaller instrumentation is required.

## SURGICAL TECHNIQUE

The setup and technique described herein refers to the Endo Optiks system (Endo Optiks Inc., Little Silver, NJ), as this is the system that the authors currently utilize.

### Setup

Endoscopic vitrectomy utilizes a standard three port setup. A 23-gauge endoscope can be inserted through a standard 23-gauge trocar (*see* section: Instrumentation). If higher resolution is required, a 19- or 20-gauge endoscope can be used. This requires creation of a sclerotomy with a 20-gauge microvitreoretinal (MVR) blade. For this, we would enlarge one sclerotomy port (usually the nondominant hand, but ultimately dependent upon site of pathology) for the 19- or 20-gauge, with the remaining ports used for a standard 23- or 25-gauge vitrectomy setup (infusion and vitreous cutter access). Alternatively, 20-gauge vitrectomy with traditional sclerotomies or 20-gauge trocars can be used for both sides for interchangeable access of the endoscope if sutureless 20-gauge vitrectomy is the technique being used.

The liquid crystal display (LCD) monitor that displays the image captured by the endoscope is placed close to the foot of the patient, in the line of sight of the surgeon. This will allow the surgeon to easily switch between viewing the LCD and operating microscope by a slight head turn.

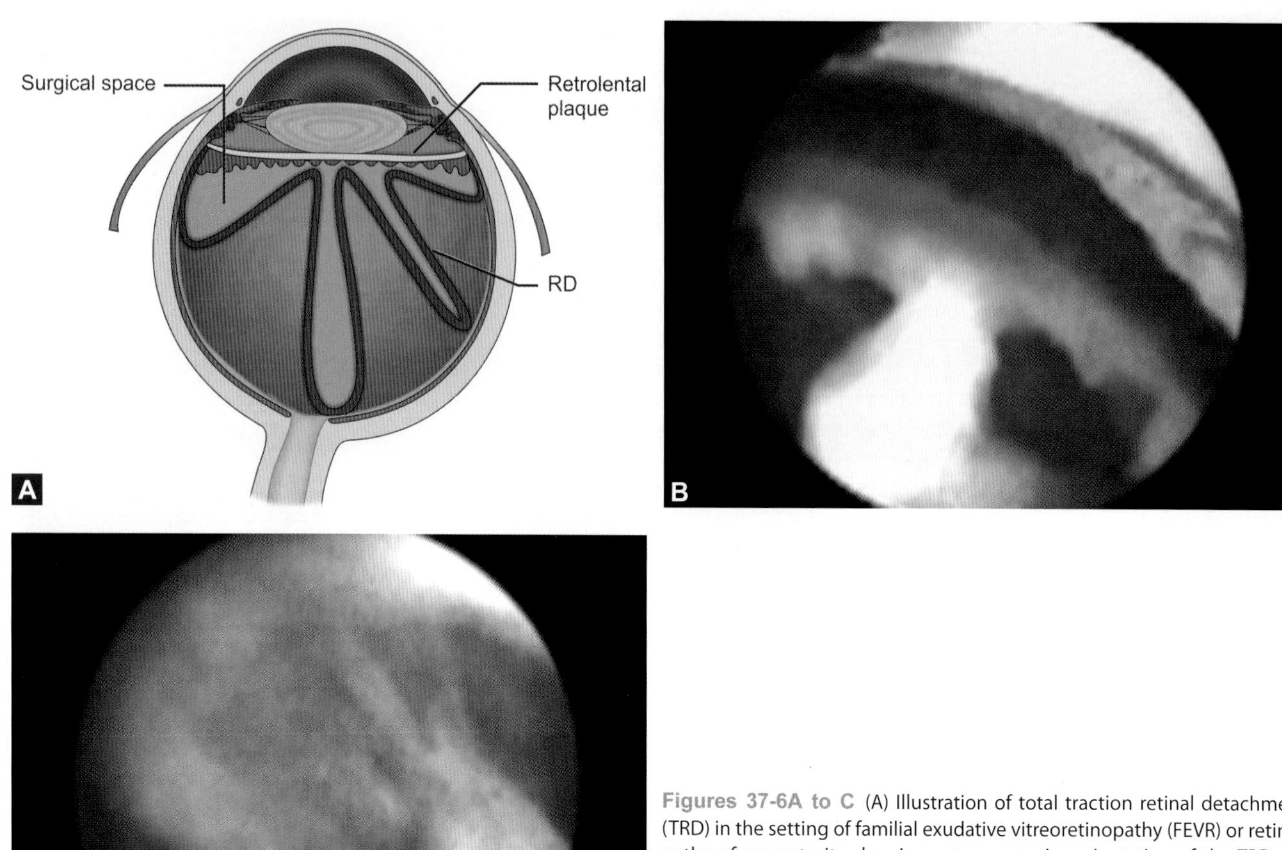


Figures 37-6A to C (A) Illustration of total traction retinal detachment (TRD) in the setting of familial exudative vitreoretinopathy (FEVR) or retinopathy of prematurity showing anteroposterior orientation of the TRD; (B) A case of total TRD from FEVR showing a top-down view of the retrolental plaque; it is difficult to visualize and address the TRD with conventional wide-angle viewing systems; (C) In the same case, a side-on view enabled by the endoscope, bypassing the retrolental plaque. The underlying fibrovascular membranes and extensive tractional retinal detachment can be appreciated.

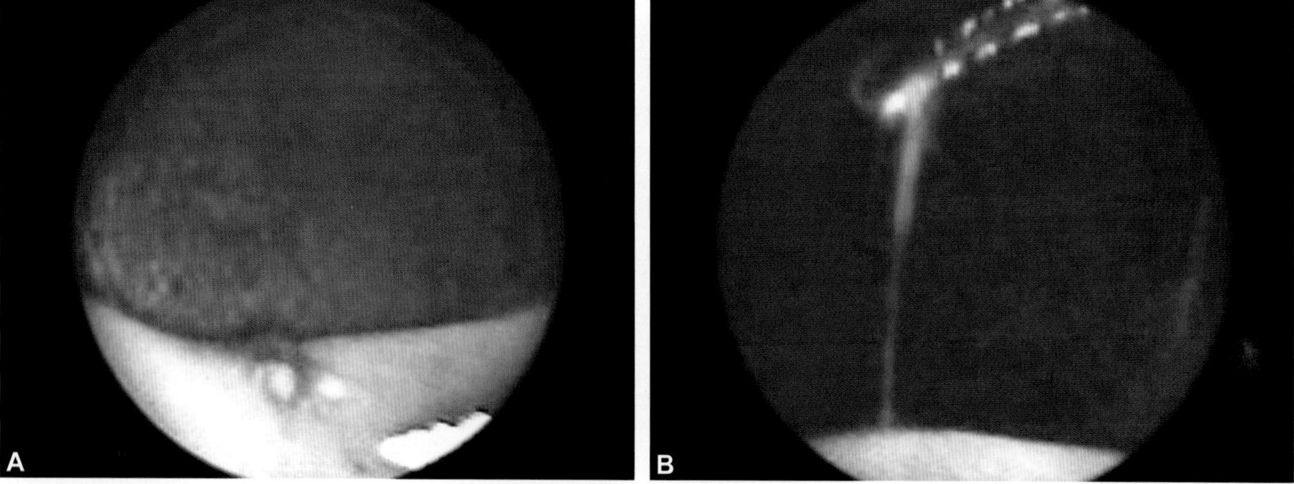


Figures 37-7A and B A case of combined traction-rhegmatogenous retinal detachment with subretinal bands. (A) An underlying subretinal band was engaged posterior to the main arcades, a reasonable distance away from the edge of the limited 3-clock-hour retinectomy. The endoscope enabled the surgeon to track posteriorly along the undersurface of the retina while avoiding the need to extend the retinectomy. Exposed retinal pigment epithelium is seen superiorly; (B) Subretinal band removed with the 23-gauge serrated forceps.

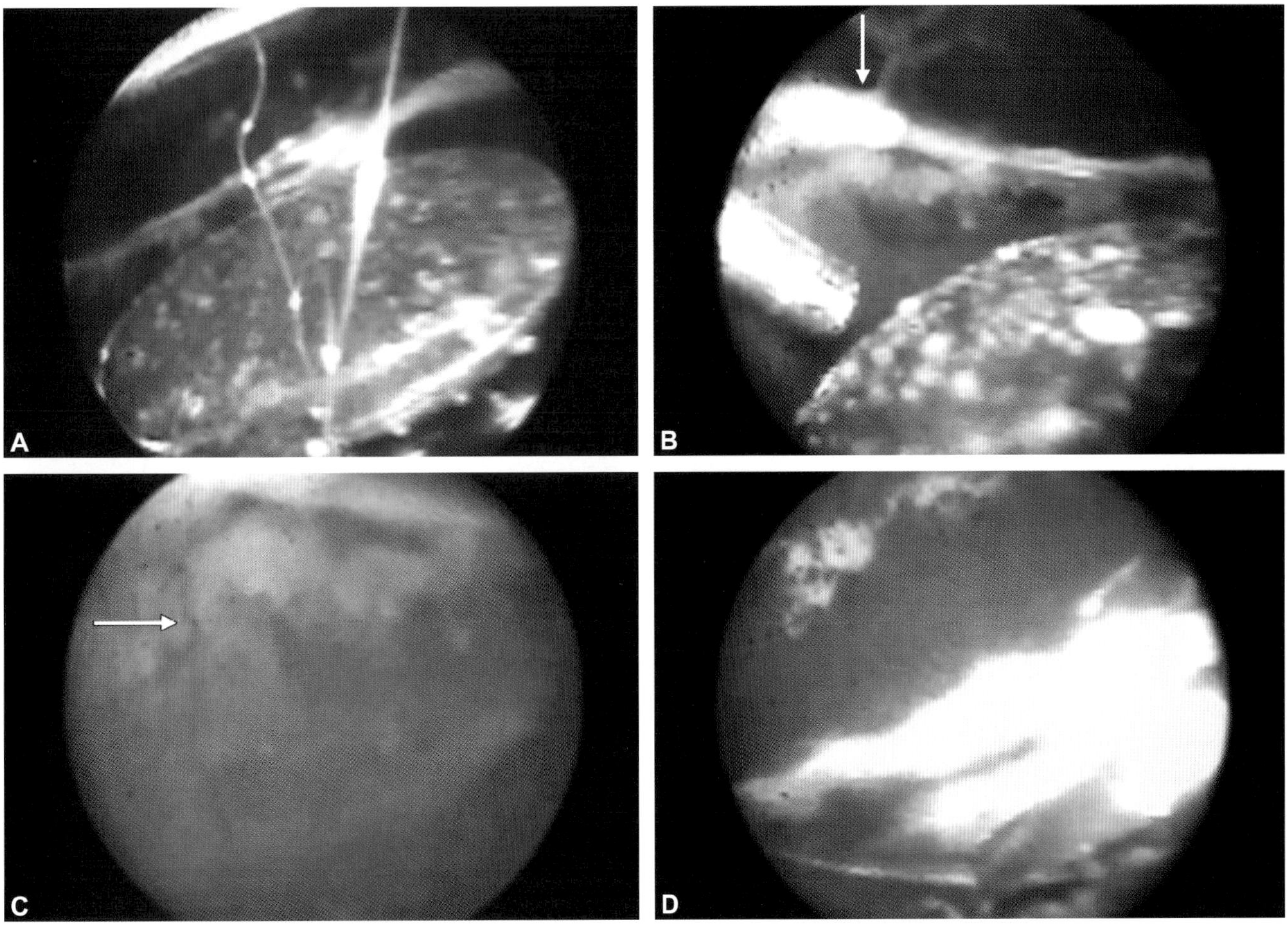

Figures 37-8A to D (A) A case of a subluxated, opacified sutured sulcus intraocular lens (IOL); (B) During IOL removal, the inferior haptic was encased in a tunnel of fibrosis (white arrow); (C) Close-up view of fibrosis with attachment to retina posteriorly as evidenced by retinal vessels (white arrow). This increases the risk for creating a retinal break. The proximity of retina to the IOL haptic could well have been missed by a conventional viewing system due to its very anterior position; (D) 23-gauge scissors were used to segment the optic-haptic junction rather than pulling it in one piece.

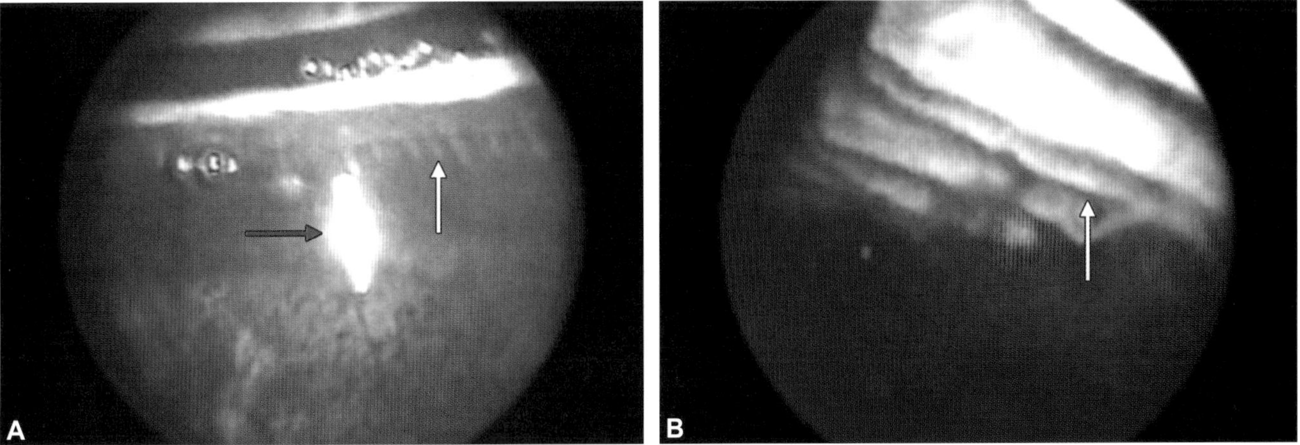


Figures 37-9A and B (A) Cyclophotocoagulation for intractable elevation of intraocular pressure can be performed more precisely and extensively with the endoscope via a posterior approach. In this aphakic patient, the previously treated ciliary processes can be visualized directly and are found to be atrophic (white arrow) surrounding the infusion cannula (red arrow); (B) Additional cyclophotocoagulation was deemed necessary because of persistently elevated intraocular pressure and laser can be performed on untreated areas under direct visualization (white arrow) across the full length of the ciliary processes into the pars plicata.

## Intraocular Use

Immediately prior to inserting the endoscope handpiece into the eye, ensure that the image on the LCD screen is oriented horizontally. This is achieved by rotating the end of the endoscope that inserts into the base unit. Following this, the image on screen is focused by rotating the black collar on the base unit where the endoscope is inserted.

After insertion of the endoscope handpiece into the eye, the following steps should be undertaken to optimize visualization:

1. *Orientation*: It is imperative to maintain orientation inside the eye at all times, both to reduce the risk of inadvertent iatrogenic ocular trauma and to optimize surgical manipulation. Start with an extraocular view of the globe in an upright position prior to entry (such that you are looking at the eye from the side with the corneal apex being the highest point on the screen). Immediately upon entering the vitreous cavity, we recommend orienting the on-screen view such that the patient's lens is at the top (12 o'clock position), with the iris on a horizontal plane. This essentially provides a sagittal view through the globe. As we approach the posterior pole, we keep the superior retina at the top of the screen.

2. *Magnification*: One can vary the size of an image by altering the distance of the endoscope from the point of interest. Due to the high magnification that can be achieved, it is possible to fill the entire LCD screen with the image of the tip of a 23-gauge vitrector, i.e. a diameter no larger than 0.9 mm. It is important to bear that in mind when manipulating vitreous and preretinal membranes (e.g. with vitreous cutter or forceps) close to the retina or uvea, as it is all too easy to get a false sense of security and distance from sensitive anatomical structures, potentially leading to iatrogenic ocular trauma.

3. *Illumination*: The amount of light that is required to illuminate and visualize an intraocular structure is heavily dependent upon its distance from the endoscope. As such, it is necessary to alter the level of illumination regularly during a case. This can be achieved either by using the dedicated foot pedal control or by having an assistant adjust the base unit controls.

4. *Safe surgical zone*: The image projected on screen has a circular border due to the shape at the tip of the endoscope handpiece. The center of the image is the safest area for surgical manipulation, as one can fully visualize the surrounding structures along the circumference of the image circle. It is important to maintain the area of interest in the center by making small adjustments to the endoscope position (Fig. 37-10). Manipulation at the edge of the image circle significantly increases the risk of inadvertent iatrogenic trauma that may go unrecognized as it is outside the field of view.

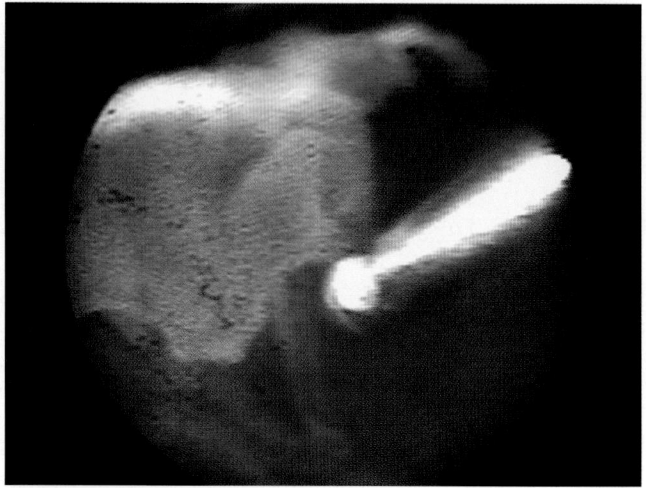

**Figure 37-10** Vitreous cutter centered on endoscope field during retinectomy in a case of complex rhegmatogenous retinal detachment repair.

5. *Overcoming the learning curve*: The learning curve relates to three principal factors: (1) a lack of stereopsis; (2) dissociation between the surgeon's hand movement and the intraoperative view, as the surgeon is looking at an LCD screen rather than down an operating microscope and directly at the surgical instruments and (3) maintaining intraocular orientation (see above). In our experience, early in adoption of endoscopy, it is useful to have both the endoscope and a conventional wide-angle viewing system setup, to enable one to quickly switch to the microscope to regain orientation. Thus, it is preferable that the initial cases have clear optical media to enable this. It may also be useful to practice in a wet-lab type setup with an artificial eye (to avoid cross species issues with animal eyes).

## MECHANISM OF ACTION

Endoscopes generally function as an optical conduit that transfer light captured through an objective lens from otherwise inaccessible areas in the human body at its distal end and then transfers the images obtained through a relay system to the operator for viewing. A basic endoscope has a source of illumination, an objective lens at its distal end, an image relay system and either an eyepiece or a sensor at its proximal end to allow direct or indirect viewing of the captured images. Major differences in endoscope design arise from the image relay system.

In ophthalmology, there are two major types of endoscopes available: ones that use a series of refractive relay lenses called gradient index (GRIN) lens system or those that use fiberoptics. GRIN lens systems offer higher image quality because of less light loss during image transmission from the distal to the proximal end for viewing. An eyepiece rather than a camera can also be used at its proximal end to expand the depth of field by taking advantage of the viewer's own accommodative amplitude. Disadvantages are its limited field of view and the need for rigid housing for the individual lenses. This causes limited instrument flexibility that is critical for maneuvering through tight spaces during vitreoretinal surgery.

Most ophthalmic endoscopes currently available use fiberoptic cables to transmit images to the viewer. The main advantage for using fiberoptics is the ability to create smaller diameter instruments that are easier to manipulate, and offer a significantly increased field of view. Although image quality is relatively better with GRIN lens endoscopes, today's fiberoptic endoscopes allow sufficient image quality sufficient for use in vitreoretinal surgery.

## POSTOPERATIVE CARE

Generally, patient care after endoscopic vitreoretinal surgery is no different from conventional pars plana vitrectomy. As such, in addition to anti-inflammatory, antibiotic and pain medications, postoperative positioning may also be required if a gas tamponade is used. Further, eye patch and clear instructions to minimize manipulation of the postoperative eye are recommended.

## INSTRUMENTATION

Today's fiberoptic endoscopes are available in 19-, 20- and 23-gauge sizes. The systems used by the authors offer 19- and 20-gauge endoscopes that produce 17,000 pixel images with a 140° field of view, while 23-gauge systems are capable of 6,000 pixels and a smaller 90° field of view. There are also variations in the endoscope handpiece, with either a curve or straight probe. In our experience, the additional axis of rotation provided by a curved probe can be quite disorientating even for more experienced endoscopic surgeons and may increase the risk of inadvertent trauma to ocular structures.

The Endo Optiks E2 endoscopic system has an 810 nm diode laser, combined with a camera and either a 175 W or 300 W xenon light source. Although the laser settings and illumination can be manipulated by a footswitch, camera focusing requires manual adjustment outside the sterile surgical field. Alternatively, the Endo Optiks E4 system incorporates both a illumination with a 175 W xenon light source and a camera but requires a separate stand alone laser console. Both systems can provide video outputs using video graphics array (VGA) or S-video signals. The probes come in sterile packs that are recommended for single-use but are sterilizable. Other manufacturers produce endoscopes such as those produced by FiberTech Co., Ltd. (Tokyo, Japan) but these are not commonly available in the United States.

## COMPLICATIONS

The complication profile is similar to traditional pars plana vitrectomy using a top-down wide-field viewing systems. However, the learning curve is steep. This is primarily related to a lack of stereopsis, a closer working distance, a smaller field of view compared to wide-field systems, and a completely different surgeon's perspective (side view) compared to a traditional top-down view through an operating microscope. There is also an additional challenge to the surgeon's dissociated hand-eye coordination when viewing the surgical field from a monitor farther away rather than the operating microscope most are accustomed too (see Surgical Techniques). These challenges are difficult in the beginning but when overcome, complication rates are similar compared to traditional pars plana vitrectomy.

## SURGICAL OUTCOMES: SCIENTIFIC EVIDENCE

Since its inception and acceptance as part of a vitreoretinal surgeon's armamentarium, there have been several publications on outcomes following endoscopic vitrectomy that are mostly small case series or case reports. The most obvious benefits are for cases with a cloudy cornea. Although a keratoprosthesis allows arguably a better image quality and a stereoscopic view compared to the endoscope, it requires additional procedures, surgical time and adds complexity to a case that is usually already difficult. In one series comparing outcomes of vitrectomy for severe ocular trauma with media opacities, Chun et al. concluded that "endoscopy allows earlier diagnosis and treatment of occult pathology and requires less time and fewer procedures to implement than the temporary keratoprosthesis".

Comparatively, anatomic and visual outcomes are similar using either conventional wide-angle and endoscopic vitrectomies for rhegmatogenous retinal detachment, globe trauma, proliferative diabetic retinopathy, placement of pars plana tube shunts and transcleral sutured IOLs, ciliary body dissection or endophthalmitis. Although the endoscope was previously used to visualize the ciliary processes and peripheral retina during fluorescein angiography, today's wide-field cameras have largely supplanted its use in this regard. Table 37-1 lists a summary of some published outcomes of vitreoretinal surgery through an endoscopic approach for various indications.

TABLE 37-1 Summary of studies on endoscopic vitrectomy for various indications

| Study (year) | Indication (number of eyes) | Endoscopic procedure | Result/s | Follow-up (months) | Complications (number of eyes) |
|---|---|---|---|---|---|
| Uram (1992) | Neovascular glaucoma (10) | Ciliary body photocoagulation | 90% with IOP < 21 mm Hg | 9 | None |
| Uram (1994) | RRD with anterior PVR (10) | PPV | 60% retinal reattachment | 9 | None |
| Boscher et al. (1998) | Retained lens fragments and/or posterior IOL dislocation (30) | PPV | 63% final visual acuity ≥ 20/40 | 21 | Retinal tear (2); CME (2); retinal detachment (2) |
| Ciardella et al. (2001) | Complicated proliferative diabetic retinopathy (9) | PPV | 75% visual improvement | 11 | Retinal tear (1) |
| Hammer and Grizzard (2003)‡ | Chronic hypotony (9) | PPV + Ciliary body dissection | 67% postoperative IOP > 5 mm Hg | Not available | None |
| Sasahara et al. (2005) | IOL dislocation (26) | PPV + Transscleral IOL sulcus suture fixation | 96% stable or improved visual acuity<br>0% postoperative IOL dislocation<br>0% CME | ≥ 3 | IOP elevation (1) |
| De Smet and Carlborg (2005) | Endophthalmitis with coexistent corneal opacities (15) | PPV | 100% final retinal reattachment<br>100% stable or improved vision | ≥ 6 | Retinal detachment (2) |
| Sonoda et al. (2006) | Subretinal fluid drainage during PPV for RRD (10) | Subretinal fluid drainage | 100% retinal reattachment | 6 | Transient retinal hemorrhage (2) |
| De Smet and Mura (2008) | RRD with media opacities (9) | PPV | 89% retinal reattachment<br>100% stable or improved visual acuity | 11 | Retinal detachment (1) |
| Olsen and Pribila (2011) | Sutured posterior chamber IOL implantation (74) | Transscleral sulcus suture fixation | 4% IOL decentration<br>0.7 logMAR (children) and 0.6 logMAR (adult) average postoperative visual acuity improvement | 29 | IOP elevation (11); corneal decompensation (6); transient vitreous hemorrhage (2) |
| Tarantola et al. (2011) | Uncontrolled chronic angle closure glaucoma (19) | PPV + Pars plana tube shunt placement | Significant reduction in IOP from 31.3 mm Hg to 11.4 mm Hg ($p < 0.001$) at final follow-up visit | 62 | Phthisis (2); shunt retraction (1); shunt blockage (3); suprachoroidal hemorrhage (1) |
| Kita and Yoshimura (2011) | RRD with undetected breaks (20) | PPV | Breaks found in 19/20 (95%) eyes<br>100% retinal reattachment<br>100% stable or improved vision | 24 | None |
| Sabti and Raizada (2012) | Ocular trauma (50) | PPV | 82% visual acuity improvement<br>90% retinal reattachment | 14 | Not available |
| Ren et al. (2013) | Endophthalmitis and RD (21) | PPV | 62% visual acuity better than LP | ≥ 18 | Recurrent infection (2) |

‡This series used a GRIN type endoscope; all other series were performed with fiberoptic endoscopes

(PPV: Pars plana vitrectomy; RRD: Rhegmatogenous retinal detachment; PVR: Proliferative vitreoretinopathy; CME: Cystoid macular edema; IOL: Intraocular lens; IOP: Intraocular pressure; LP: Light perception; RD: Retinal detachment).

## PLACE OF THE TECHNIQUE IN SURGICAL ARMAMENTARIUM

Endoscopy is highly complementary to conventional viewing systems, and can be used in conjunction with, or sometimes in place of the latter. The disadvantage of a lack of stereopsis is, in our opinion, outweighed by a number of significant advantages, making it a valuable addition to our surgical armamentarium.

In summary, endoscopy is the system of choice for viewing posterior segment structures in the presence of significant anterior segment media opacity. Secondly, the endoscope offers distinct advantages with pathology that is anteriorly positioned and/or orientated anteroposteriorly, due to the angle from which the image is captured as well as the surgeon's perspective that is conferred (*see* Indications). Finally, the ability to better visualize vitreous should not be underestimated, making it very useful for a wide range of vitreoretinal conditions where vitreous and membrane removal is important for an optimal outcome.

## PEARLS AND PITFALLS

- Maintaining intraocular orientation is essential. Start with an extraocular view of the globe in an upright position prior to entry. Maintain orientation by keeping the patient's lens (if looking anteriorly) or superior retina (if looking posteriorly) at the 12 o'clock position on-screen.
- Only perform surgical manipulation in the center of the image circle to maintain a safe peripheral zone that is constantly in view.
- There is a potential increased risk of iatrogenic trauma due to the high magnification that is possible. For example, the tip of the vitrector could be within 200–300 μm of the retina, retinal pigment epithelium (RPE)-choroid complex or ciliary body, but the surgeon could be lulled into a false sense of distance and security due to the on-screen magnification.
- Always have the manipulating instrument, for example the vitreous cutter or forceps in full view.
- Constantly adjust illumination, particularly to avoid image white-out when very close to an area of interest.

## SUGGESTED READING


1. Boscher C, Lebuisson DA, Lean JS, et al. Vitrectomy with endoscopy for management of retained lens fragments and/or posteriorly dislocated intraocular lens. Graefes Arch Clin Exp Ophthalmol. 1998;236:115-21.
2. Chun DW, Colyer MH, Wroblewski KJ. Visual and anatomic outcomes of vitrectomy with temporary keratoprosthesis or endoscopy in ocular trauma with opaque cornea. Ophthalmic Surg Lasers Imaging. 2012;43:302-10.
3. Ciardella AP, Fisher YL, Carvalho C, et al. Endoscopic vitreoretinal surgery for complicated proliferative diabetic retinopathy. Retina. 2001;21:20-7.
4. De Smet MD, Carlborg EA. Managing severe endophthalmitis with the use of an endoscope. Retina. 2005;25:976-80.
5. De Smet MD, Mura M. Minimally invasive surgery—endoscopic retinal detachment in patients with media opacities. Eye (Lond). 2008;22:662-5.
6. Hammer ME, Grizzard WS. Endoscopy for evaluation and treatment of the ciliary body in hypotony. Retina. 2003;23:30-6.
7. Kita M, Yoshimura N. Endoscope-assisted vitrectomy in the management of pseudophakic and aphakic retinal detachments with undetected retinal breaks. Retina. 2011;31:1347-51.
8. Olsen TW, Pribila JT. Pars plana vitrectomy with endoscope-guided sutured posterior chamber intraocular lens implantation in children and adults. Am J Ophthalmol. 2011;151:287-96.
9. Ren H, Jiang R, Xu G, et al. Endoscopy-assisted vitrectomy for treatment of severe endophthalmitis with retinal detachment. Graefes Arch Clin Exp Ophthalmol. 2013;251:1797-800.
10. Sabti KA, Raizada S. Endoscope-assisted pars plana vitrectomy in severe ocular trauma. Br J Ophthalmol. 2012;96:1399-403.
11. Sasahara M, Kiryu J, Yoshimura N. Endoscope-assisted transscleral suture fixation to reduce the incidence of intraocular lens dislocation. J Cataract Refract Surg. 2005;31:1777-80.
12. Sonoda Y, Yamakiri K, Sonoda S, et al. Endoscopy-guided subretinal fluid drainage in vitrectomy for retinal detachment. Ophthalmologica. 2006;220:83-6.
13. Tarantola RM, Agarwal A, Lu P, et al. Long-term results of combined endoscope-assisted pars plana vitrectomy and glaucoma tube shunt surgery. Retina. 2011;31:275-83.
14. Uram M. Laser endoscope in the management of proliferative vitreoretinopathy. Ophthalmology. 1994;101:1404-8.
15. Uram M. Ophthalmic laser microendoscope ciliary process ablation in the management of neovascular glaucoma. Ophthalmology. 1992;99:1823-8.
16. Wong SC, Lee TC. Endoscopic vitrectomy. In: Hartnett ME, Trese M, Capone A, Keats BJB, Caputo G (Eds). Pediatric Retina, 2nd edition. Philadelphia: Lippincott Williams & Wilkins; 2013.

# CHAPTER 38

# Surgical Uveitis

Sal Porbandarwalla, G Atma Vemulakonda

## INTRODUCTION

For patients with uveitis, surgical procedures may be necessary when either the diagnosis or adequate therapeutic response remains elusive despite medical diagnostics such as imaging and blood labs, or when the patients have not responded as expected to medical therapy. More invasive procedures should be considered under the following circumstances: all other appropriate diagnostic testing fails to confirm a diagnosis, and the patient is progressing despite appropriate therapy; or the fellow eye is threatened despite appropriate therapy; or a malignancy is suspected; and if the results of the biopsy will alter the treatment plan.

There are several diagnostic and therapeutic surgical interventions available for patients with uveitis. As these differ from one another, they are discussed individually.

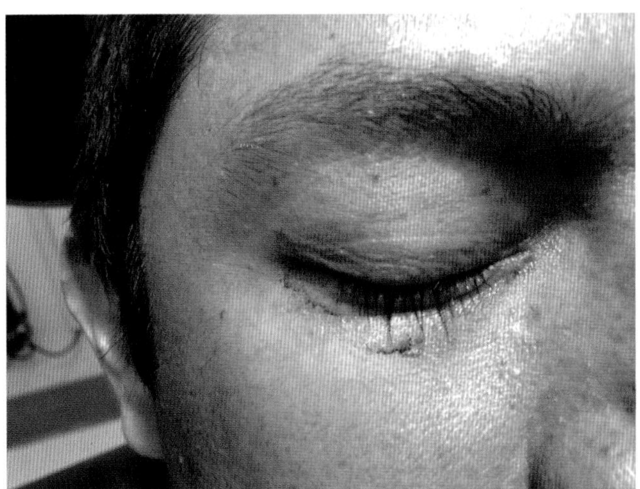

Figure 38-1 Prep the eyelids and lashes with povidone-iodine.

## SURGICAL OPTIONS/INDICATIONS/TECHNIQUES

### Aqueous Tap for Molecular Diagnostics/Culture

*Indications:* An anterior chamber tap is particularly useful for suspected viral, bacterial, and fungal etiologies. These indications include viral retinitis, endophthalmitis, and presumed viral anterior uveitis among others. It has the advantage of being straightforward and minimally invasive and can be performed even on very ill patients.

*Technique:* After applying a topical anesthetic such as proparacaine/tetracaine, prep the eyelids and eyelashes with povidone-iodine 5% (Fig. 38-1) and apply 1–3 drops of povidone-iodine 5% to the conjunctival surface and allow at least 30 seconds of contact time (Fig. 38-2). After placing the lid speculum, use a 30-gauge needle on a 1 cc syringe to enter the anterior chamber through the temporal peripheral cornea and slowly withdraw 0.1–0.2 cc of fluid. Take care to avoid the central anterior chamber, corneal endothelium, or iris (Fig. 38-3). Slowly remove the needle from the eye and place a sterile or povidone-iodine-soaked cotton swab over the paracentesis site. After removing the speculum, the eye can be rinsed with sterile balanced salt solutions (BSS). Remove the needle from the syringe, place a cap over the syringe (Fig. 38-4), and send the specimen to the lab for appropriate diagnostics including viral/fungal/bacterial/mycobacterial polymerase chain reaction (PCR), culture, and cytology.[1] Postoperatively, some providers use topical antibiotics, although this can be left to the physician's preference. Patients may benefit from post-procedural artificial tears.

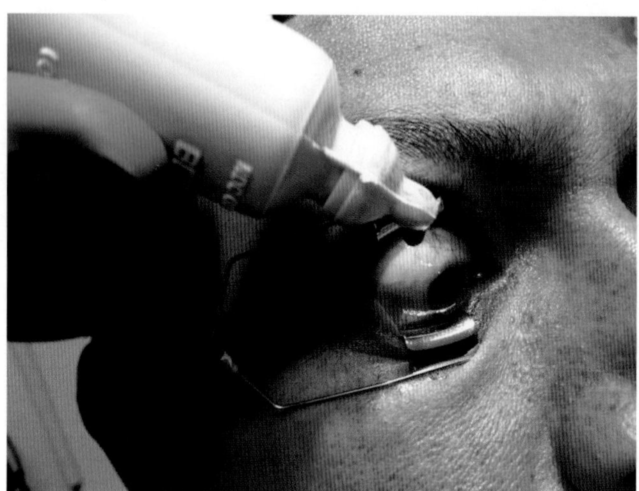

Figure 38-2 After placing a lid speculum, apply povidone-iodine to the ocular surface for at least 30 seconds of exposure.

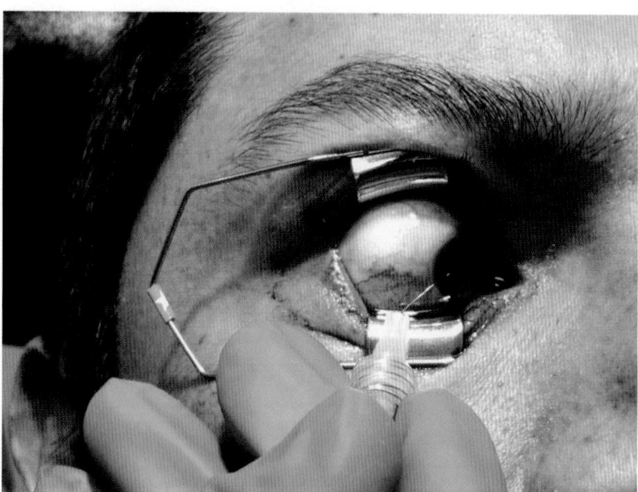

Figure 38-3 Enter the anterior chamber through the temporal peripheral cornea and slowly, but actively, withdraw 0.1–0.2 cc of fluid using a bent needle. Take care to avoid the central anterior chamber, corneal endothelium, or iris.

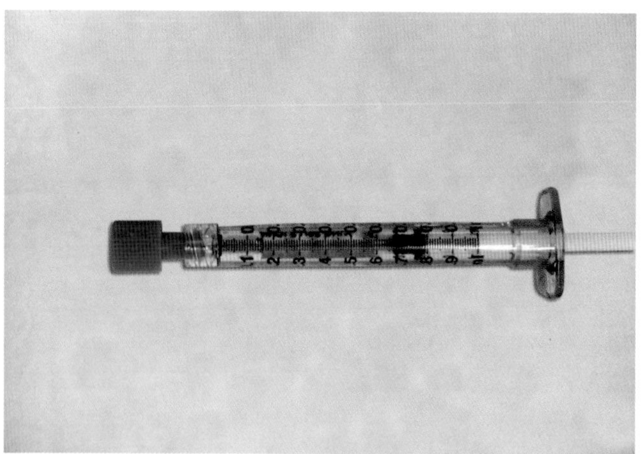

Figure 38-4 Remove the needle and cap the syringe for transport to the laboratory.

*Complications:* Although uncommon, these include infection, bleeding, hypotony, choroidal effusion, damage to the crystalline lens, and in pseudophakic patients dislocation of intraocular lens (IOL).

## Vitreous Tap for Molecular Diagnostics/Culture

*Indications:* A vitreous tap is useful in patients suspected of having endophthalmitis, chorioretinitis, panuveitis, or retinitis from viral, bacterial, parasitic, or fungal etiologies.[2] This procedure is less invasive than surgery and can be performed at bedside and is especially useful in patients with severe comorbidities.

*Techniques:* Topical anesthetic medications including proparacaine, tetracaine, or lidocaine can be applied directly to the conjunctiva or can be placed via a pledget held against the site of injection. In more inflamed eyes, a subconjunctival injection can be performed after prepping the eye with a topical anesthetic and povidone-iodine. Sometimes a retrobulbar block can be used, and this is particularly useful in cases of endophthalmitis where the patient is in pain and cannot otherwise tolerate the procedure. In the authors' experience, the need for a retrobulbar block for vitreous tap is uncommon. After applying povidone-iodine 5% to prep the lids and lashes, place a lid speculum. Apply another drop of povidone-iodine 5% over the site of injection and let it sit for approximately 30 seconds. Using a sterile or povidone-iodine-soaked sterile cotton-tipped applicator, displace the conjunctiva. Use a 25-gauge 27-gauge needle on a 3 cc syringe to enter the vitreous cavity 3–4 mm posterior to the limbus. A 23-gauge can be used if the initial tap is dry. Once in the vitreous cavity, slowly withdraw plunger to aspirate 0.2–0.4 cc. Prior to withdrawing the needle, its helpful to push a tiny amount of fluid back into the eye to ensure that all suction on the vitreous has been released. Remove the needle from the eye and use a sterile/povidone-iodine-soaked cotton swab to reposition the conjunctiva over the vitreous aspiration site. Remove the speculum and rinse the eye with sterile BSS. Remove the needle from the syringe, place a cap over the syringe, and send the specimen to the lab for molecular diagnostics (cultures, as well as viral/fungal/bacterial/mycobacterial PCR, cytology, etc.).[3] Some providers use topical antibiotics after the procedure, although this is unnecessary. Artificial tears may reduce patient discomfort.

*Complications:* These are typical of any vitreoretinal procedure and include infection, bleeding, retinal tear/detachment, choroidals, hypotony, and cataract.

## Sub-Tenon's Injection of Steroid for Local Therapy

*Indications:* A sub-Tenon's injection of steroid effectively treats many patients with noninfectious uveitis including those with cystoid macular edema (CME) due to either uveitis or cataract extraction (Irvine Gass syndrome). In addition, patients with CME who have partially responded to topical steroids without history of steroid responsive glaucoma may benefit from this procedure.[4]

*Technique:* Topical anesthetic medications including proparacaine, tetracaine, or lidocaine can be applied directly to the conjunctiva or can be placed via a pledget held against the site of injection. Prep the eyelids and eyelashes with povidone-iodine 5% and place a lid speculum. Some physicians prefer a 0.1–0.5 cc subconjunctival lidocaine injection using a 27- or 30-gauge needle. The steroid, typically triamcinolone or dexamethasone, should be injected into the desired quadrant. In eyes with macular edema, some physicians recommend a superotemporal injection with an attempt made to inject the steroid as close to the macula as possible, but this likely does not affect success of the procedure. While avoiding the conjunctival vessels, it is useful to move the needle side to side in the sub-Tenon's space to ensure the sclera is not engaged. Remove the speculum and rinse the eye with sterile BSS. Postoperative care includes monitoring of intraocular pressure (IOP) beginning a few weeks after the procedure.

*Complications:* These include inadvertent globe perforation, elevated postinjection IOP, cataract, infection, and conjunctival/sub-Tenon's scarring.

## Intravitreous Injection for Local Therapy: Antibiotics, Antifungals, Antivirals, Steroids, Anti-VEGF Agents, and Chemotherapeutics

*Indications:* Intravitreal injections of various therapeutic agents are indicated for patient with both infectious and noninfectious etiologies. Infectious etiologies include infectious chorioretinitis/retinitis, endophthalmitis, and select cases of anterior segment infection such as blebitis. Other indications for treatment of noninfectious etiologies include but are not limited to primary intraocular/vitreoretinal lymphoma (PIOL), CME, and inflammatory choroidal neovascularization.

*Technique:* Topical anesthetic medications including proparacaine, tetracaine, or lidocaine can be applied directly to the conjunctiva or can be placed via a pledget held against the site of injection. Prep the eyelids and eyelashes with povidone-iodine 5% and place a lid speculum. Apply povidone-iodine 5% to prep the lids and lashes, and retract the lashes using a lid speculum. Place a drop of povidone-iodine 5% to site of the injection 3–4 mm posterior to the limbus. Then using a sterile or a povidone-iodine-soaked sterile cotton-tipped applicator, displace the conjunctiva.[5] Use a 27-gauge to 32-gauge needle on a 1 cc syringe and enter the vitreous cavity 3–4 mm posterior to the limbus and perform the injection. Once completed, slowly remove the needle from the eye to allow time for the IOP to equilibrate and apply pressure to the injection site using a cotton swab over the vitreous injection site. Remove the speculum and rinse the eye with sterile BSS. For postop care some providers use topical antibiotics, although this is unnecessary. Patients may benefit from postprocedural artificial tears.

*Complications:* These include endophthalmitis, bleeding, retinal detachment, elevated IOP, and cataract.

## Cryo/Laser for Local Therapy

*Indications:* Five percent of patients with pars planitis can develop anterior or posterior segment neovascularization. Cryotherapy/laser therapy not only helps decrease neovascularization of the vitreous base but also reduces vitritis. Cryo/laser therapy is indicated for the treatment of pars planitis, viral retinitis, and neovascular complications of inflammatory eye diseases.

*Technique:* Cryo: For patients with noninfectious intermediate uveitis/pars planitis and media opacity/haze that precludes laser, treatment should be applied immediately anterior and posterior to the snow bank as well as to areas of peripheral nonperfusion. If patients have obvious vitreoretinal traction, cryotherapy should be avoided. Patients should also receive concurrent local and/or systemic steroids.

*Laser (532 nm) for pars planitis:* This is appropriate for noninfectious intermediate uveitis/pars planitis with relatively clear media. Treatment should surround the snow bank with three or four rows of nearly confluent laser. Patients should be treated with concurrent topical and/or systemic steroids during the periprocedural period.

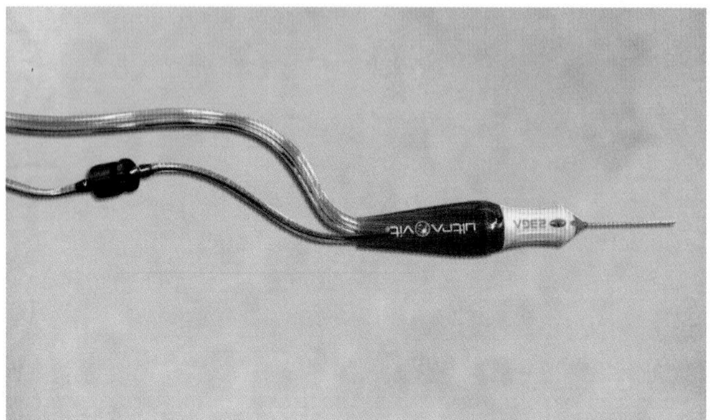

Figure 38-5 Standard vitrectomy hand piece setup.

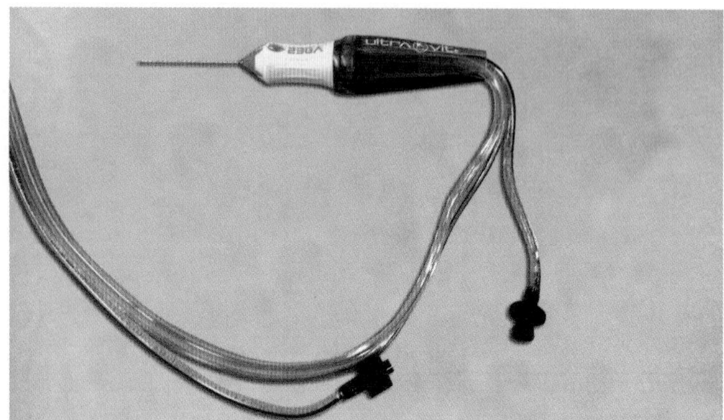

Figure 38-6 Disconnect the aspiration line from the hand piece.

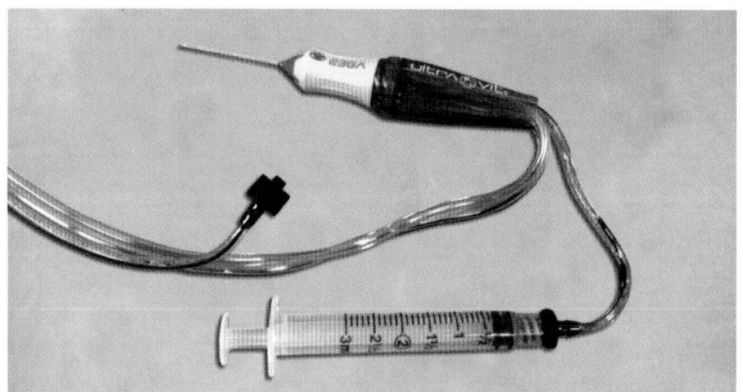

Figure 38-7 Attach a syringe to the hand piece aspiration line to allow for manual aspiration of sample.

*Laser for retinitis:* Same as above. Placing laser barricade around inactive areas of cytomegalovirus retinitis decreases the risk of subsequent retinal detachment. The use of laser barricade around areas of acute retinal necrosis remains controversial as complete treatment is challenging.[6]

*Complications:* These include inflammation, epiretinal membrane, retinal detachment (seen more with cryoablation), and tonically dilated pupil (may improve in some cases).

## Diagnostic Vitrectomy/Vitreous Biopsy

*Indications:* Since the etiology of many of the cases of intermediate uveitis remains unclear, a diagnostic vitrectomy/vitreous biopsy can be helpful to establish a diagnosis and help guide therapy. Noninfectious causes include intraocular lymphoma, while infectious causes of uveitis can include bacterial, parasites, fungi, and viruses.

*Techniques:* Any gauge vitrectomy system can be used for this procedure. Preoperative treatment with topical, peribulbar, and sometimes systemic corticosteroids may be indicated to decrease inflammation prior to vitrectomy. Preoperative cycloplegia may also be used to maximize pupillary dilation, increase comfort, and limit posterior synechiae. It is best to obtain undiluted as well as semidiluted or diluted samples. To obtain an undiluted sample, place the infusion and trocars or create sclerotomies (*see* sections on vitrectomy as well as principles and techniques). The infusion cannula must be directly visualized and confirmed to be in the vitreous cavity; however, it should NOT be turned on. The aspiration line of the vitrectomy hand piece should be disconnected from the machine (Fig. 38-5) and attached to a 3–5 cc syringe (Figs. 38-6 and 38-7). The vitrectomy hand piece then is placed in the vitreous using high cut rate. An assistant then slowly manually aspirates until the vitreous sample enters the syringe. A larger sample may be obtained, but the fluid in the tubing alone often can provide a reasonable sample. This author usually obtains approximately 0.6–1 cc depending on the patient's bleeding risk and overall ocular health. Once the vitrector is out of the eye and the cannula or sclerotomy is occluded, the posterior infusion can be turned on. If the eye hypotonous after obtaining a sample, the infusion may be turned prior to removing the hand piece from the eye on as long as the assistant does not aspirate further. Once the infusion is on and the instruments are out of the eye, the sample is prepared depending on the testing required.

- *Cytology*: The sample should be mixed 50:50 with RPMI (tissue culture) medium
- Samples for PCR should either be frozen as soon as possible or immediately sent to the lab
- *Culture*: The vitrectomy can then be continued as usual and the dilute vitreous and the vitrectomy cassette can be directly sent for culture. This dilute vitreous should be further diluted in RPMI (tissue culture) medium for flow cytometry in cases of presumed lymphoma[7]

Postoperative care includes local, periocular, and occasionally systemic anti-inflammatory treatment, topical antibiotics, and cycloplegia.

*Complications:* These include endophthalmitis, bleeding, retinal detachment, elevated eye pressure, and cataract.

## Chorioretinal Biopsy

*Indications:* Although chorioretinal biopsy and other more invasive procedures carry the potential for serious complications, these results may assist in the proper diagnosis and guide management in difficult cases, especially when other less invasive testing proves inconclusive or unhelpful. Examples include a patient with poor vision in an affected eye who is getting worse despite treatment, a case in which a malignancy is suspected, or a patient who is getting worse in the better seeing eye despite presumed appropriate treatment.[8]

*Techniques:* Perform a complete vitrectomy and ensure that the posterior hyaloid is separated from the retina. Next, raise the infusion pressure above the ocular perfusion pressure (somewhere between 60 and 80 mm Hg) and use endodiathermy to demarcate the area of the biopsy down to bare sclera. The biopsy specimen should include both normal and involved retina. If the chorioretinal biopsy is not freed from the surrounding tissue with the diathermy, then intraocular scissors may be used. The retina often separates from the underlying choroid, so use all efforts to maintain apposition of the tissues when sending them to pathology. Once the specimen is created, it can be removed either at this stage or after the infusion pressure normalizes. The infusion pressure should be lowered slowly to allow careful use of diathermy to address any bleeding that arises. Once hemostasis has been achieved at a physiologic infusion pressure, create a pars plana incision large enough to remove the biopsy without a great deal of tissue manipulation (which can damage this delicate tissue). Laser the edges of the biopsy site (as long as there is no retinal detachment–if there is a detachment then reattach the retina first). After closing the pars plana incision, perform 360° scleral depression to ensure there are no retinal tears. After performing an air-fluid exchange, place a short-acting or long-acting gas, or silicone oil.

*Complications:* These include endophthalmitis, bleeding, retinal detachment, elevated eye pressure, and cataract.

## Fluocinolone Acetonide 0.59 mg Implant

*Indications:* The fluocinolone acetonide implant (Retisert, Bausch and Lomb, Rochester, New York) is FDA approved for the treatment of chronic non-infectious posterior uveitis.

*Techniques:* This is placed in the operating room. After creating a conjunctival peritomy using 0.3 forceps and Westcott scissors in a quadrant (usually inferotemporal), obtain hemostasis with cautery. A 4-mm long sclerotomy is created 3–4 mm posterior to the limbus using an MVR or v-lance blade. Place the double-armed 8-0 prolene that is included in the pack through the suture strut of the implant followed by three simple interrupted throws. The edges of the sclerotomy are grasped with fine forceps and the implant is placed though the incision. Use direct visualization to ensure that the implant is in the vitreous and not in the subretinal or choroidal space. There are two ways to close the wound. In the first way, each arm of the 8-0 prolene suture placed through the wound in 90% depth and suture to the sclera in a 3-1-1 manner. The tails are left long and are laid along the wound. The rest of the wound is closed using 9-0 prolene suture. Rotate the 9-0 prolene suture to bury the knots. The tails of the 8-0 prolene are held against the sclera by the interrupted 9-0 prolene sutures. In the second approach, place the 8-0 prolene needles with sutures through the apices of the wound in order to bury the sutures. The rest of the wound can then be closed with either the 8-0 prolene or 9-0 prolene (both included with the implant).[9] A concomitant vitrectomy may or may not need to be performed.

The fluocinolone acetonide 0.59 mg implant allows for long-term (30 months) high-dose intravitreal steroid administration. Postoperative care includes monitoring for IOP, cataract, and infection. Continue topical steroid, antibiotic, and cycloplegia for the immediate postoperative course (similar to other intraocular retinal surgery). Systemic anti-inflammatory treatment should be continued in patients with bilateral disease until the second eye is also implanted.[10] A number of patients can then have the systemic immunosuppression reduced or eliminated.

*Complications:* These include high risk of elevation in IOP requiring medication and sometimes surgery, high risk of cataract formation, endophthalmitis, and hypotony (especially if the wound is not properly closed).

## PEARLS

- When aspirating fluid from the anterior chamber with a syringe, it is useful to actively withdraw aqueous (with the plunger) as it allows more reliable transfer to the laboratory.
- The hub of a 1 cc syringe can be used to mark 3–4 mm from the limbus.
- When performing sub-Tenon's steroid injection, care should be taken to ensure that the sclera and hence the globe has not been penetrated with the needle, so the needle should be bevel down (the opening of the needle should face the ocular surface). Infectious etiologies should be ruled out before administration of periocular steroids.

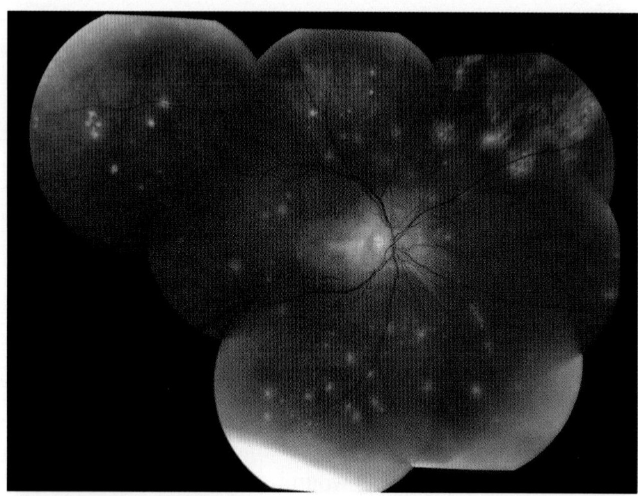

Figure 38-8 Patient with diffuse chorioretinitis.

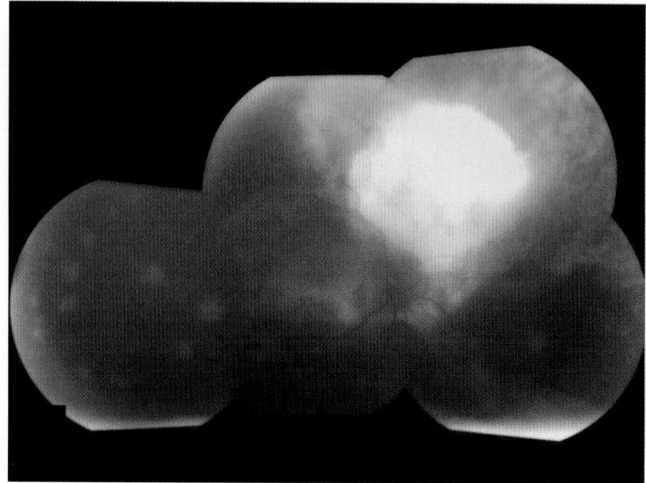

Figure 38-9 Postoperative appearance of chorioretinal biopsy site with surrounding laser barricade.

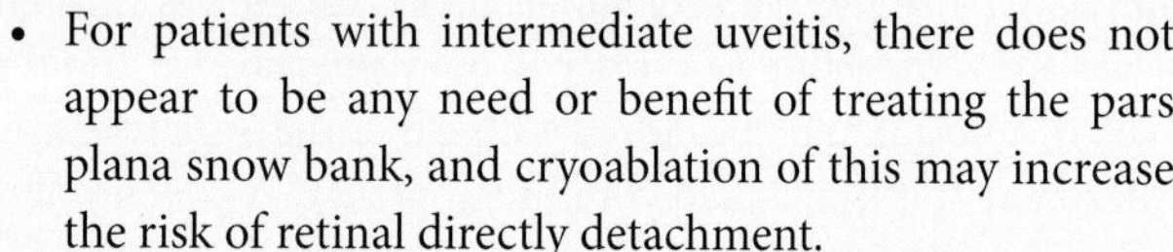

- For patients with intermediate uveitis, there does not appear to be any need or benefit of treating the pars plana snow bank, and cryoablation of this may increase the risk of retinal directly detachment.
- If the eye becomes hypotonous during the vitreous biopsy, air rather than BSS can be infused to maintain a physiologic pressure. Care should be taken at the end of the surgery to examine the retinal periphery to treat any retinal tears, breaks, or detachment.
- During a chorioretinal biopsy, excellent hemostasis is critical, otherwise the risks of subretinal hemorrhage, choroidal hemorrhage, retinal detachment, and other complications are high.
- A superior and nasal location is an ideal site of a chorioretinal biopsy as it can be supported with gas tamponade and easy positioning (Figs. 38-8 and 38-9).
- Given the high risk of cataract, it can be useful to perform cataract extraction with lens implantation at the same time as Retisert implantation. If the patient is known to have steroid responsive glaucoma, then it can be useful to perform glaucoma surgery (often with tube shunt placement) at time of Retisert implantation.

## REFERENCES


1. Anwar Z, Galor A, Albini TA, et al. The diagnostic utility of anterior chamber paracentesis with polymerase chain reaction in anterior uveitis. Am J Ophthalmol. 2013;155(5):781–6. doi: 10.1016/j.ajo.2012.12.008. Epub 2013 Feb 12.
2. Endophthalmitis Vitrectomy Study Group. Results of the Endophthalmitis Vitrectomy Study: a randomized trial of immediate vitrectomy and of intravenous antibiotics for the treatment of postoperative bacterial endophthalmitis. Arch Ophthalmol. 1995;113:1479-96.
3. Nandi K, Ranjan P, Therese L, et al. Polymerase chain reaction in intraocular inflammation. Open Ophthalmol J. 2008;2:141-5.
4. Choudhry S, Ghosh S. Intravitreal and posterior subtenon triamcinolone acetonide in idiopathic bilateral uveitic macular oedema. Clin Experiment Ophthalmol. 2007;35:713.
5. Bhavsar AR Googe JM, Jr, Stockdale CR, et al., for the Diabetic Retinopathy Clinical Research Network. The risk of endophthalmitis following intravitreal injection in the DRCR.net laser-ranibizumab-triamcinolone clinical trials. Arch Ophthalmol. 2009;127(12):1581-3.
6. Pulido JS, Mieler WF, Walton D, et al. Results of peripheral laser photocoagulation in pars planitis. Trans Am Ophthalmol Soc. 1998;96:127-41.
7. Yeh S, Weichel ED, Faia LJ, et al. 25-Gauge transconjunctival sutureless vitrectomy for the diagnosis of intraocular lymphoma. Br J Ophthalmol. 2010;94(5):633-8. doi: 10.1136/bjo.2009. 167940.
8. Martin DF, Chan CC, de Smet MD, et al. The role of chorioretinal biopsy in the management of posterior uveitis. Ophthalmology. 1993;100(5):705-14.
9. Berger BB, Mendoza WBS. Sclerotomy closure for Retisert implant. Retina. 2013;33(2):436-8.
10. Pavesio C, Zierhut M, Bairi K, et al. Evaluation of an intravitreal fluocinolone acetonide implant versus standard systemic therapy in noninfectious posterior uveitis. Ophthalmology. 2010;117(3):567-75, 575.e1. doi: 10.1016/j.ophtha.2009.11.027. Epub 2010 Jan 15.

# *Section* 5

# Glaucoma Surgery

*Section Editors* Ronald Leigh Fellman, Davinder S Grover

CHAPTER 39

# Indications for Glaucoma Surgery

George L Spaeth

## INTRODUCTION

The surgeon contemplating treatment of a patient with glaucoma must take into account the present state of the affected individual and the projected future state. The approach to an individual who is asymptomatic, which is the case for many patients with glaucoma, is totally different from that in a person who has virtually no vision left and is already, or rapidly becoming, totally incapacitated. Furthermore, the risks to the patient vary dramatically depending on the stage and the type of glaucoma. It is not possible to make an asymptomatic person better. Thus, surgery on an individual who has no awareness that he or she even has a disease called glaucoma is not likely to be well received if following the surgery the best the surgeon can say is, "Well I know you don't see as well as you used to, and your eye is uncomfortable, but at least you are going to keep your sight now". Nor is the patient happy who has a tiny island of vision, but is able to read with great difficulty, who after glaucoma surgery the surgeon says is successful because of a controlled intraocular pressure, can no longer read at all.

The first principle with regard to glaucoma surgery, is to keep in mind clearly the purpose of the surgery, the risks, and the benefits, and to make absolutely certain that the patient is fully aware of the purpose, the risks, and the benefits.

Physicians tend to forget that what matters to the patient is how the patient feels and functions. Patients are not always interested in their intraocular pressure, their corneal thickness, or even their visual field unless they have been brainwashed by the doctor to think those things are of primary importance. They know better, and they know that what counts is quality of life and their ability to act.

Glaucoma is an imperfect word because it suggests a homogeneity that does not exist. Some patients with glaucoma (i.e. optic nerve damage of a characteristic type, related to pressure higher than the optic nerve can tolerate) do not need any treatment at all, because they are asymptomatic and will probably remain asymptomatic for the rest of their lives. In contrast, some patients who have normal vision, but who develop glaucoma, can lose their vision within hours. Clearly, preventive care in such cases is warranted. Patients who are functioning quite well despite far-advanced glaucoma can become nonfunctional within several weeks as their advanced glaucoma progresses rapidly. Patients with mild angle-closure glaucoma can be cured by a 5-minute, almost totally asymptomatic Nd:YAG laser iridotomy, whereas even a superbly performed tube-shunt procedure on a patient with neovascular glaucoma may be ineffective in saving any sight. It is wise, then, not to think in general terms about "indications for surgery in patients with glaucoma", but rather to be highly specific, recognizing that each person is different, each person's needs and wants are different, and that glaucoma comes in many forms from benign to malignant.

A helpful principle is to think that no treatment of any kind is necessary unless without treatment the individual will develop a decrease in quality of life or a troublesome disability. Every treatment of every kind carries risks; more accurately, every treatment of every kind makes the treated person worse in some way: indeed just telling a person that he or she has glaucoma immediately reduces the person's quality of life. Consequently, there must be a certainty, especially when considering surgery, that the person will become significantly worse and, when considering surgery, that the person's life will become worse in the absence of surgery. The

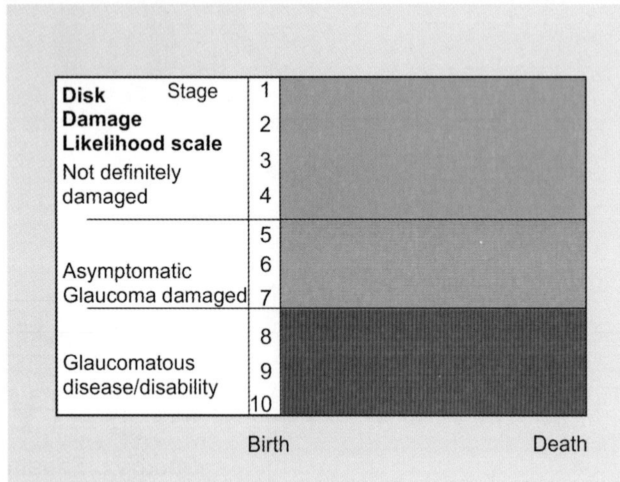


**Figure 39-1** The Colored Glaucoma Graph.

most important word in that last sentence is "significantly". Gradual deterioration is not always an indication for surgery. Deterioration has to be enough that it has some harmful effect on the person, i.e. on how the person feels or functions. The fact that the optic nerve has become more cupped or the visual field damaged is not always a sufficient indication for surgery. However, surgery may well be indicated in individuals in whom documented deterioration is minimal or even absent, because the certainty that they will develop disability in the future is so great that the risk of the surgery is warranted. This certainly applies to most individuals in early chronic angle closure glaucoma in whom laser iridotomy is virtually always indicated.

A helpful way for both the patient and physician to consider whether or not surgery is appropriate is to plot their course graphically on the Glaucoma Graph (Fig. 39-1). The Glaucoma Graph illustrates (in green) the fact that nobody starts with glaucoma damage (excludes infantile glaucoma) and that even those with moderate field loss are largely asymptomatic (yellow). It also shows, in red, that those with glaucoma which has progressed toward its end stages become disabled and have a decreased quality of life. The goal of treatment, then, is not to keep people from getting into the yellow zone, that is to say having some mild field loss, but rather to keep them out of the red zone, or if already in the red zone to prevent any further worsening whatsoever. When an individual already has disability related to glaucoma, any deterioration will result in a worsening of how they feel and how they function. The four critical considerations are (1) the stage of glaucoma, (2) the rate of change (either documented or anticipated), (3) the number of years the disease is likely to continue to be present, and (4) socioeconomic factors.

The stage of glaucoma is relatively easy to establish, the disk damage likelihood scale (DDLS) is useful in that regard.[1-5] The DDLS is based on the amount of damage in terms of rim/disk ratio, and the size of the optic disk. A nomogram calculating the DDLS is shown in (Fig. 39-2). The method of calculating the DDLS is to estimate the disk size by any of a variety of ways, and then determine the extent of rim narrowing in terms of rim/disk ratios, or the circumferential amount of rim absence. The largest possible rim/disk ratio would be .5. In an average-sized disk (disk diameter between 1.5 and 1.75 mm) when there is almost no rim left, i.e. <0.1 rim/disk ratio, the DDLS would be 5. In a small disk (disk diameter <1.25 mm) with the same very narrow rim, the DDLS score would be 6, and in a large disk (disk diameter greater than 1.75 mm), the DDLS grade would be a 4.

Patients are rarely symptomatic in terms of noticing visual loss until their nerves are severely damaged, usually around a DDLS of 7. Of course, this relates to whether one or both eyes are involved. Determining the rate of change is probably best done by estimating the structural changes in the optic nerve. Visual field changes do not usually occur until the patients develop enough damage, so they are at about a DDLS of 4, or perhaps even 5. In some patients surgery should have been done long before they get to that stage. For example, a 20-year-old woman in excellent health who has juvenile-onset open-angle glaucoma, intraocular pressures in the 40s and 50s on treatment, and has gone from a DDLS of 2–4 in a period of 2 years will be blind before she dies. It is unwise to wait until field loss develops in such an individual to decide that surgery is necessary. It is not wise to try to compare the rate of deterioration of the disk or of the field to a normative rate of change. The issue is the rate of change for the particular person being considered. That rate of change will cause him or her to have a worsening of function or feeling.

Socioeconomic factors are often key to determine whether surgery should or should not be performed. The individual who has limited understanding of how to care for himself or herself, poor access to care, and severe, rapidly progressing disease is often best treated surgically, whereas an individual with the same amount of disease that is progressing as rapidly, but who has a good comprehension of what glaucoma entails, and how to care for himself, and has the finances to care for himself or herself well, may well not need surgery.

A factor that often influences whether surgery is done or not is the nature of the surgeon. Some ophthalmologists and

**THE DISK DAMAGE LIKELIHOOD SCALE**

| | Narrowest width of rim (rim/disk ratio) | | | | | Examples | |
|---|---|---|---|---|---|---|---|
| DDLS Stage | For Small Disk < 1.50 mm | For Average Size Disk 1.50-2.00 mm | For Large Disk > 2.00 mm | Orignal DDLS stage | 1.25 mm optic nerve | 1.75 mm optic nerve | 2.25 mm optic nerve |
| 1 | 0.5 or more | 0.4 or more | 0.3 or more | 0a | | | |
| 2 | 0.4 to .49 | 0.3 to 0.39 | 0.2 to 0.29 | 0b | | | |
| 3 | 0.3 to 0.39 | 0.2 to 0.29 | 0.1 to 0.19 | 1 | | | |
| 4 | 0.2 to 0.29 | 0.1 to 0.19 | less than 0.1 | 2 | | | |
| 5 | 0.1 to 0.19 | less than 0.1 | 0 for less than 45° | 3 | | | |
| 6 | less than 0.1 | 0 for less than 45° | 0 for 46° to 90° | 4 | | | |
| 7 | 0 for less than 45° | 0 for 46° to 90° | 0 for 91° to 180° | 5 | | | |
| 8 | 0 for 46° to 90° | 0 for 91° to 180° | 0 for 181° to 270° | 6 | | | |
| 9 | 0 for 91° to 180° | 0 for 181° to 270° | 0 for more than 270° | 7a | | | |
| 10 | 0 for more than 180° | 0 for more than 270° | | 7b | | | |

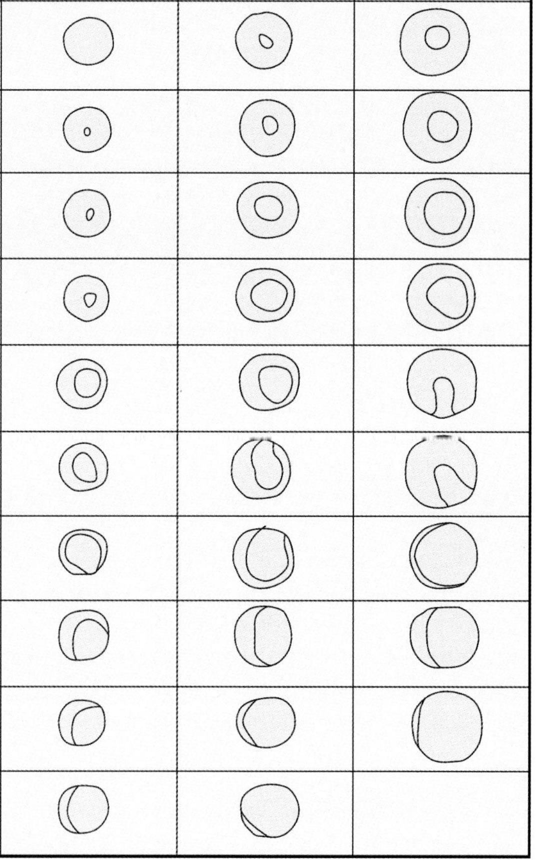

**Figure 39-2** The disk damage likelihood scale. The current method of assigning a Disk Damage Likelihood Scale score is shown in the lefthand most column in this figure. The stages in the fifth column represent the original scoring system, when the system was first published. "0A" and "0B" seemed awkward and difficult to manage. Consequently, the rim system was changed resulting in the figures shown in the lefthand most column".

other physicians are in the "when in doubt, cut it out" category, whereas others are extremely risk adverse and see surgery as something to be avoided if at all possible. The former camp is dangerous, so also is the latter camp. Risk cannot be avoided in people who have glaucoma. Determining the severity of the risk is highly important. Where there is little risk of blindness, there is little justification for taking risk. But, where the patient is at great risk for going blind, not to take needed risks (including surgery) is unethical.

It is also important to recall that medicinal treatment is not without risks itself. Long-term treatment with preservative-containing eye drops may cause significant ocular surface disease (OSD). OSD is frequently far more troublesome to the patient than is mild or even severe field loss. The cost of medications is a factor for all except the very wealthy, and even these individuals frequently are concerned by the cost associated with expensive, long-term use of glaucoma medications. Cataract is frequently cited as a reason not to perform glaucoma surgery, but properly performed glaucoma surgery with judicious use of postoperative corticosteroids, in my opinion, is not likely to lead to an increased incidence of cataract. It is complicated glaucoma surgery that leads to cataract. With modern techniques, including trabeculectomy, it should be possible to avoid most of those complications in almost all cases. The Ocular Hypertension Treatment Trial and other studies have demonstrated conclusively that cataract is a consequence of long-term therapy with ocular medications. Additionally, there are some physicians who believe that the trabecular meshwork is damaged by glaucoma medications; these individuals also feel strongly that mild

**TABLE 39-1** Factors influencing whether treatment of an individual with or suspected of glaucoma have incisional surgery, laser surgery, or medicinal therapy.

| FACTOR | FAVORS | | |
|---|---|---|---|
| **Patient** | **Incisional surgery** | **Laser surgery** | **Medicinal therapy** |
| Inability to care for himself/herself | X | | |
| Able to access care easily | | | X |
| Need to lower IOP below 10 mm Hg | X | | |
| Urgent need to lower intraocular pressure | X | | |
| Field loss cuts into fixation and vision still better than 20/200 | | | X |
| Visual acuity poor due to glaucoma (between 20/40 and 20/200) | | | X |
| Need to lower IOP and demonstrated non-adherence | X | | |
| **Disease** | | | |
| Narrow angle with peripheral anterior synechia, IOP < 35 mm Hg, and no optic nerve damage | | X | |
| Chronic angle-closure glaucoma with minimal field loss and IOP < 30 mm Hg | | X | |
| Chronic angle-closure glaucoma with poorly controlled IOP | X (usually with cataract extraction) | | |
| Open-angle glaucoma with DDLS < 5 and IOP < 35 mm Hg | | | X |
| Open-angle glaucoma with DDLS < 5 and IOP > 35 mm Hg and EYR > 10 | X or | X | |
| Open-angle glaucoma with DDLS > 5 and rate of change likely to lead to DDLS > 7 prior to death | X | | |
| Open-angle glaucoma with questionable control of IOP and DDLS > 7 | | X | |
| Open-angle glaucoma with IOP in range expected to cause further damage and DDLS > 7 and no predisposition to wipe out | X | | |
| Open-angle glaucoma with documented worsening despite maximum tolerated medical therapy and DDLS > 7 | X | | |
| Glaucoma secondary to intraocular malignancy | No | CPC | X |

(IOP: Intraocular pressure; DDLS: Disk damage likelihood scale; EYR: Estimated years remaining).

glaucoma can be turned into severe glaucoma as a result of using glaucoma medications. The default position frequently taken that "medicines are safer", then, may not be the case. It all depends on duration of treatment, the type of medication, and the response of the eye, and the nature of the person.

Aggressive surgeons are not automatically competent surgeons. As with everything else in life, the single most important principle is to "know oneself". Surgeons with lack of insight into their abilities and limitations are not likely to make wise decisions as to when surgery is to be performed.

## CONCLUSION

Knowledgeable, honest, appropriate individualization is the key to deciding whether or not glaucoma surgery is appropriate. Many of the points made in this chapter are summarized in Table 39-1 that provides rough guidelines. This table should be used in conjunction with the Glaucoma Graph; this combination provides guidance helpful in almost all cases.

## REFERENCES

1. Bayer A, Harasymowycz P, Henderer JD, et al. Validity of a new disc grading scale for estimating glaucomatous damage: correlation with visual field damage. Am J Ophthalmol. 2002; 133(6):758-63.
2. Henderer JD, Liu C, Kesen M, et al. Reliability of the disk damage likelihood scale. Am J Ophthalmol. 2003;135(1):44-8.
2a. Spaeth GL, Henderer J, Steinmann W. The Disk Damage Likelihood Scale (DDLS): its use in the diagnosis and management of glaucoma. Highlights of Ophthalmology. 2003;31(4):4-19.
3. Danesh-Meyer HV, Ku JYF, Papchenko TL, et al. Regional correlation of structure and function in glaucoma, using the disc damage likelihood scale, Heidelberg retina tomograph, and visual fields. Ophthalmology 2006;113(4):603-11.
4. Spaeth GL, Henderer J, Liu C, et al. The disc damage likelihood scale: reproducibility of a new method of estimating the amount of optic nerve damage caused by glaucoma. Trans Am Ophthalmol Soc. 2002;100:181-86.
5. Read RM, Spaeth GL. The practical clinical appraisal of the optic disc in glaucoma: the natural history of cup progression and some specific disc-field correlations. Trans Am Acad Ophthalmol Otolaryngol. 1974;78:OP255-74.

CHAPTER 40

# Guarded Filtration Surgery

Marlene R Moster, Augusto Azuara-Blanco

## INTRODUCTION

Lowering intraocular pressure (IOP) was established as a treatment of glaucoma more than 100 years ago. Guarded filtration surgery, commonly named trabeculectomy, is currently the most commonly used operation for glaucoma. Cairns reported the first series in 1968.[1]

## INDICATIONS

Guarded filtration surgery is generally indicated when medicine or laser therapy is insufficient to control the disease, and can be considered in selected cases as initial therapy. Treatment of glaucoma aims to prevent visual disability and maintain the quality of life of the patient. IOP is the only risk factor that can be treated and lowering IOP has been shown to be beneficial at reducing progression of visual field loss in glaucoma. Two fundamental questions arise every time glaucoma therapy is initiated: (1) the degree to which the IOP should be lowered and (2) how to reach that level, with medical or surgical interventions.

- Setting a target pressure is part science and part of the art of medicine. The decision must take into account the characteristics of each individual patient, including the severity and natural course of the disease, and the life expectancy. The target IOP can be adjusted depending on the response to therapy and the anticipated iatrogenic risk of the next treatment or intervention.
- There remains uncertainty as to whether the initial treatment should be medical or surgical as their relative effectiveness in terms of IOP reduction and its relationship to long-term visual outcomes and quality of life are not well understood. Should the treatment choice be different for individuals identified at high risk of blindness, i.e. black race and/or severe disease at presentation? Generally, medications are started when glaucoma is first diagnosed. If initial medical management fails should the further management be surgical or additional medical treatments?

In general, glaucoma surgery is indicated when neither medical nor laser therapy is sufficient to control the glaucoma and when the progression of the disease is likely to diminish the patient's quality of life. Medical therapy may be considered insufficient if it cannot maintain the IOP within a range believed low enough to prevent further damage, if it is not tolerated, or if compliance is a problem. This general principle of the indication for glaucoma surgery allows room for individual interpretation, as the decision must take into account the characteristics of each individual patient. Patients' visual needs and the vision-related quality of life differ greatly and should be assessed individually. Another factor to consider in determining whether surgery is appropriate is the likelihood of success and risk of complications (*see* below). Glaucoma filtration surgery may also be considered as an initial treatment of newly diagnosed glaucoma patients. Evidence from the CIGTS trial supports this possibility, which may be particularly helpful for those patients with severe disease at presentation.[2,3]

## CONTRAINDICATIONS

Contraindications include (1) eyes with extensive superior scarring of the conjunctiva when it would be technically very difficult to dissect the conjunctiva and sclera, and it would have very little chances of success; (2) eyes with very disorganized anterior segment, such as extensive peripheral anterior synechiae, active neovascularization, or vitreous in the anterior chamber; (3) patients with very high risk of failure and complications, such as those with active inflammation, aphakic, nanophthalmos, elevated episcleral venous pressure, epithelial downgrowth; (4) in situations where postoperative visits and care cannot be conducted.

## MECHANISM OF ACTION

Filtration surgery lowers the IOP by creating a fistula between the inner compartments of the eye and the subconjunctival space (i.e. filtering bleb). This alternative path allows aqueous humor to accumulate under the conjunctiva and form a blister-like dome, or filtering bleb. The fistula is covered by a scleral flap that provides some resistance to the outflow, thus preventing profound hypotony.

## SURGICAL TECHNIQUE (FIGS. 40-1 TO 40-10)

Any type of regional anesthesia (retrobulbar, peribulbar, and sub-Tenon's) can be used. Topical anesthesia is also possible, with topical 2% lidocaine gel, 0.1 mL of intracameral 1% nonpreserved lidocaine, and 0.5 mL of subconjunctival 1% lidocaine injected from the superior–temporal quadrant to balloon the conjunctiva over the superior rectus muscle.

Filtration surgery should be done at the superior limbus, because inferiorly located blebs are associated with a much higher risk of bleb-associated infections. A fixation or traction suture is used to keep the eye in downward position giving a good area of exposure. A corneal traction suture in the quadrant of the planned surgery (7-0 or 8-0 black silk or nylon, or 8-0 Vicryl on a spatulated needle) is ideal for this purpose. The needle is passed through clear, midstromal cornea approximately 2 mm from the limbus for approximately 3–4 mm. Alternatively a superior rectus traction suture (4-0 or 5-0 black silk on a tapered needle) can be used to rotate the globe inferiorly and bring the superior bulbar conjunctival into view. Using a muscle hook to rotate the globe downward, the conjunctiva and superior rectus are grasped with toothed forceps and the threaded needle is passed through the tissue bundle.

A limbus- or fornix-based conjunctival flap is made with Westcott-type scissors and nontoothed forceps. When forming limbus-based flaps, the conjunctival incision is placed 8–10 mm posterior to the limbus. The conjunctival and Tenon's wound should be lengthened to approximately 8–12 mm cord length. The flap is then extended anteriorly to expose the corneoscleral sulcus. When making fornix-based flaps, the conjunctiva and Tenon's are disinserted. Approximately a 2–3 clock hour limbal peritomy (6–8 mm) is sufficient. Blunt dissection is carried posteriorly. A fornix-based flap is more likely to be associated with diffuse blebs.

After gently cauterizing the bleeding vessels a sclera flap is dissected. Differences in the shape or size of the scleral flap probably have little effect on surgical outcome. The flap thickness should be between one half and two thirds. It is important to dissect the flap anteriorly (approximately 1 mm into clear cornea) to ensure that the fistula is created anterior to the scleral spur and ciliary body.

A corneal paracentesis is made before opening the globe with either a 30- or a 27-gauge needle or a sharp point blade. A block of tissue at the corneoscleral junction is then excised.

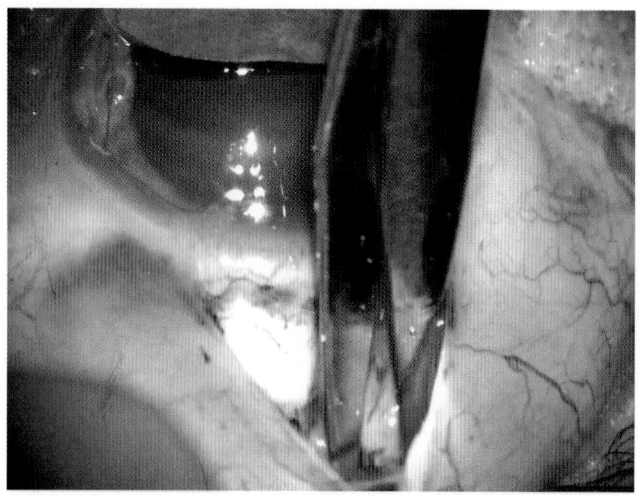

**Figure 40-1** Fornix-based conjunctival dissection, extended posteriorly with Westcott scissors.

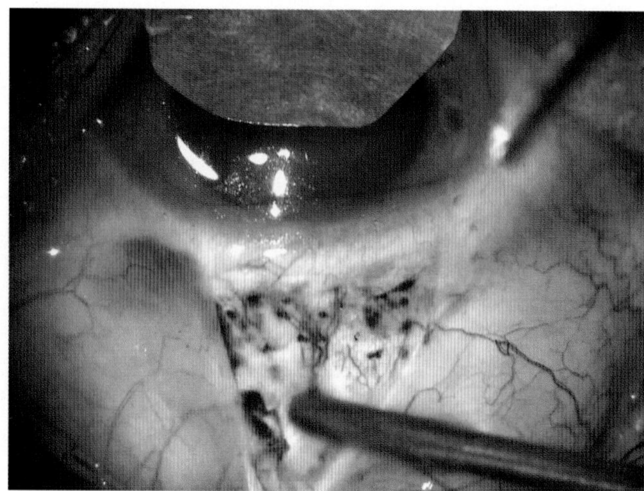

**Figure 40-2** Gentle use of cautery on the scleral surface.

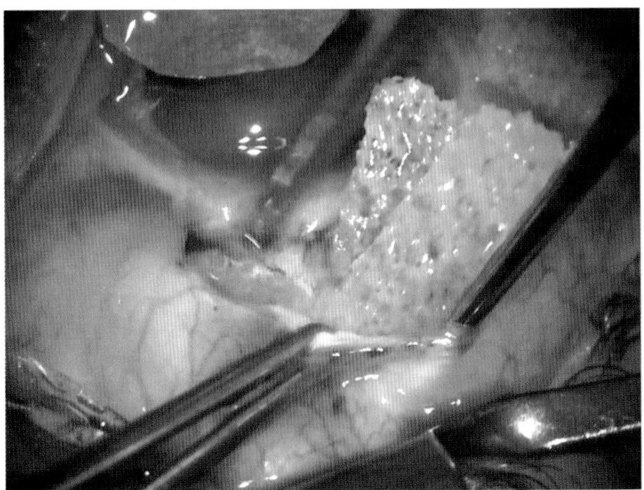

**Figure 40-3** Insertion of sponges soaked in mitomycin C, with the aim of treating a large area.

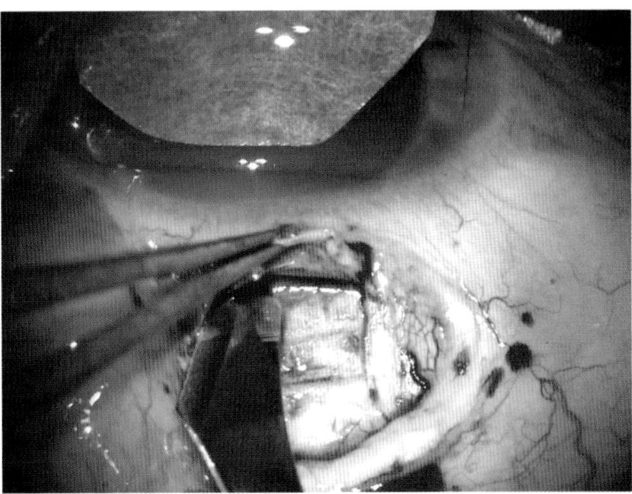

**Figure 40-4** The scleral flap is dissected well into the cornea.

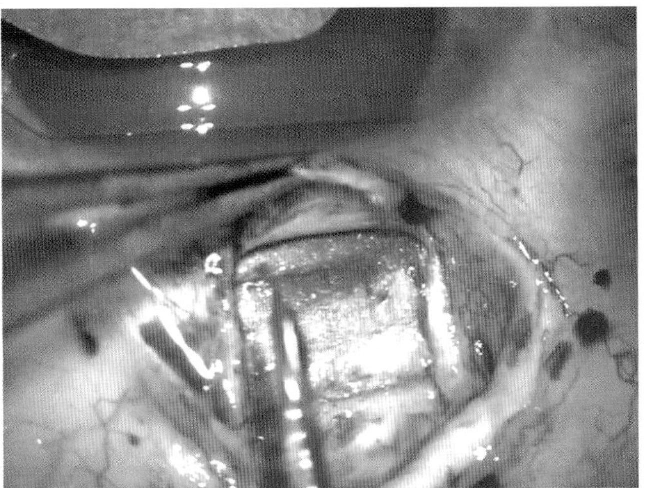

**Figure 40-5** The scleral flap is fully dissected and ready for the creation of the fistula.

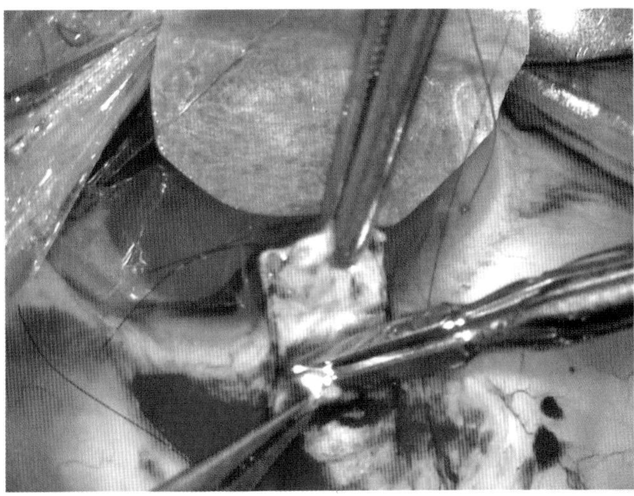

**Figure 40-6** A fistula is created by excising corneolimbal tissue. In this case, a sharp point blade and Vannas scissors were used. Note the preplaced scleral flap sutures.

Two radial incisions are made first with a sharp blade or knife starting in clear cornea, and extending posteriorly approximately 1–1.5 mm. The radial incisions are made approximately 2 mm apart. The blade or Vannas scissors are used to connect the incisions; thereby a rectangular piece of tissue is removed. Alternatively, an anterior corneal incision, parallel to the limbus and perpendicular to the eye, is made to enter into the anterior chamber and a Kelly or Gass punch is used to excise the tissue. The scleral flap should completely cover the fistula to provide resistance to the aqueous outflow.

A peripheral iridectomy may then be performed. Iridectomy is not necessary in many cases (e.g. pseudophakic eyes with deep anterior chamber and open angle), but recommended in patients with shallow anterior chamber and angle-closure glaucoma. The iris is grasped near its root with toothed forceps. The iris is retracted through the sclerostomy, and an iridectomy is performed with Vannas or DeWecker scissors. The iridectomy should avoid damage to the iris root and ciliary body or bleeding.

The scleral flap is sutured initially with two interrupted 10-0 nylon sutures (in case of rectangular flap) or with one suture (in a triangular flap). Slipknots are useful to adjust the tightness of the scleral flap and the rate of aqueous outflow. Additional sutures can be used to better control the outflow. During the suturing of the scleral flap, the anterior chamber is filled through the paracentesis, and the flow around the scleral flap is observed. If flow seems excessive, or the anterior chamber shallows, the slipknots are tightened

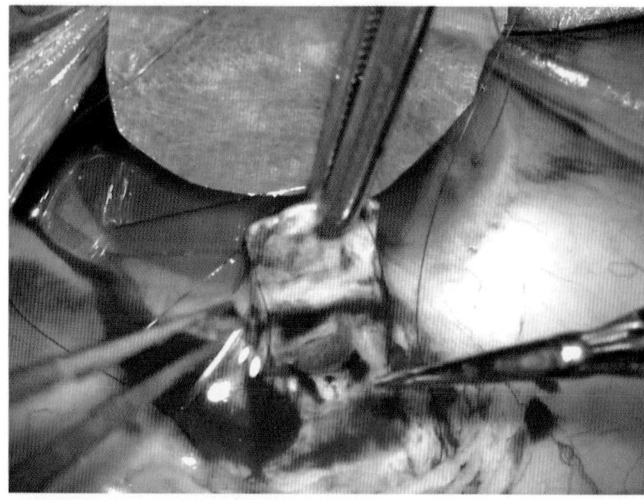

**Figure 40-7** Peripheral iris is protruding through the fistula, and thus should be excised (i.e. peripheral iridectomy).

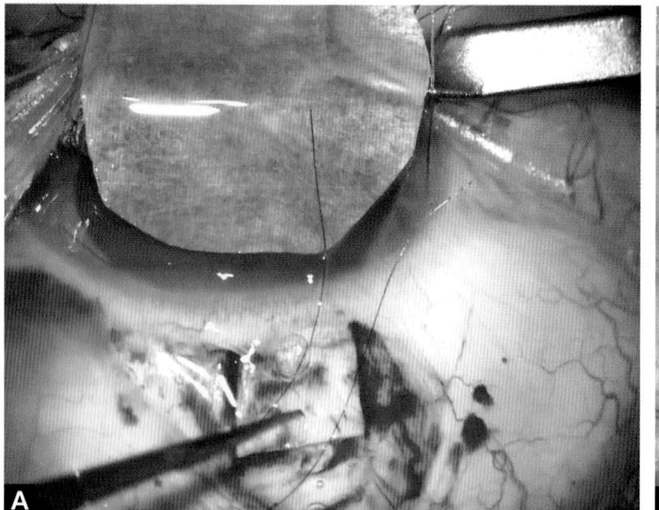

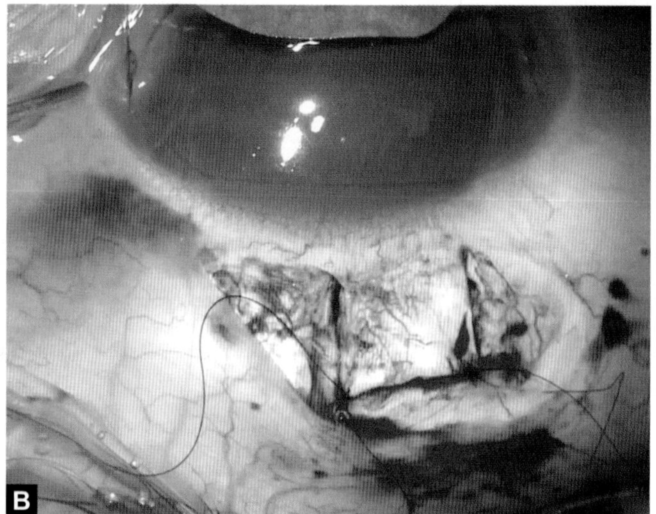

**Figures 40-8A and B** Suturing the scleral flap with two 10-0 nylon corner sutures. (A) The sutures are tied with a slipknot to allow for evaluation of aqueous flow around the scleral flap. (B) The corner sutures are tied and trimmed.

or additional sutures are placed. If aqueous does not flow through the flap, the surgeon may loosen the slipknots, or replace tight sutures with looser ones. In some situations the scleral flap is tightly closed to avoid hypotony, e.g. angle-closure glaucoma and high preoperative IOP. Releasable sutures can be used instead of interrupted ones. Externalized releasable sutures are easily removed and are effective in cases of inflamed or hemorrhagic conjunctiva or thickened Tenon's capsule.

Conjunctival closure in limbus-based flaps is done with a double or single running suture with an 8-0 or 9-0 absorbable suture, or with 10-0 nylon. Many surgeons favor a rounded-body needle. In fornix-based flaps, a tight conjunctival-corneal apposition is needed. Sutures (e.g. mattress 10-0 nylon suture) at the edges of the incision can be used to anchor the conjunctiva to the cornea.

After the wound is closed, a 30-gauge cannula is used to fill the anterior chamber with balanced salt solution through the paracentesis track to elevate the conjunctival bleb and test for leaks (Figs. 40-11A and B) Intracameral or subconjunctival antibiotics can be used, as well as subconjunctival corticosteroids. Patching the eye can be individualized depending on the patient's vision and the anesthesia used.

## Technique of Intraoperative Application of Antimetabolites

To reduce postoperative subconjunctival fibrosis, especially important in cases at high risk of failure, mitomycin C (MMC)

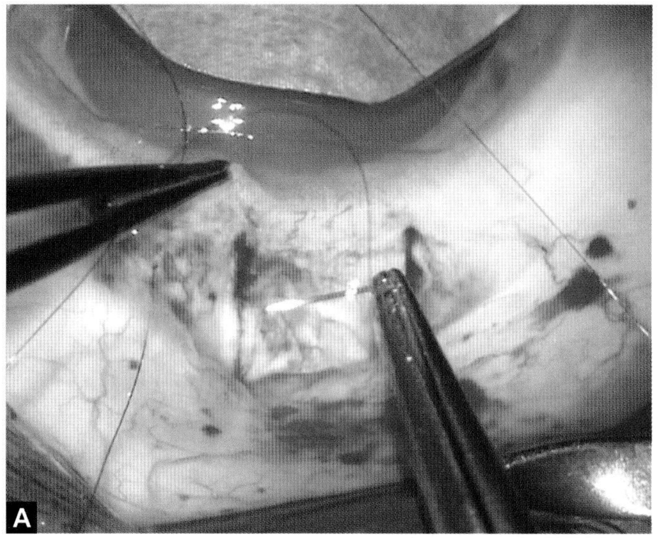


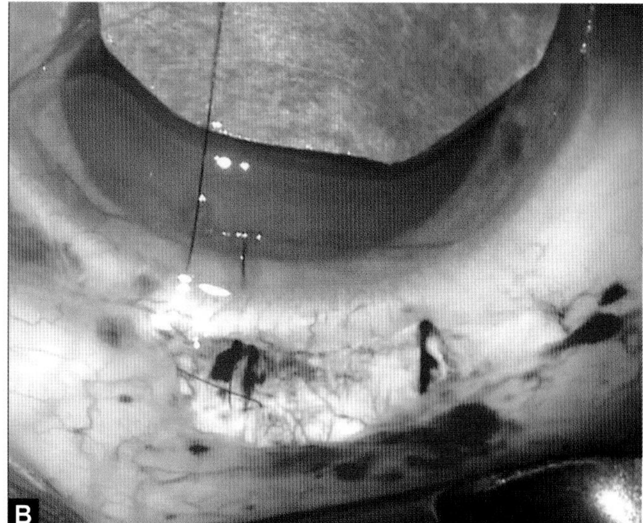


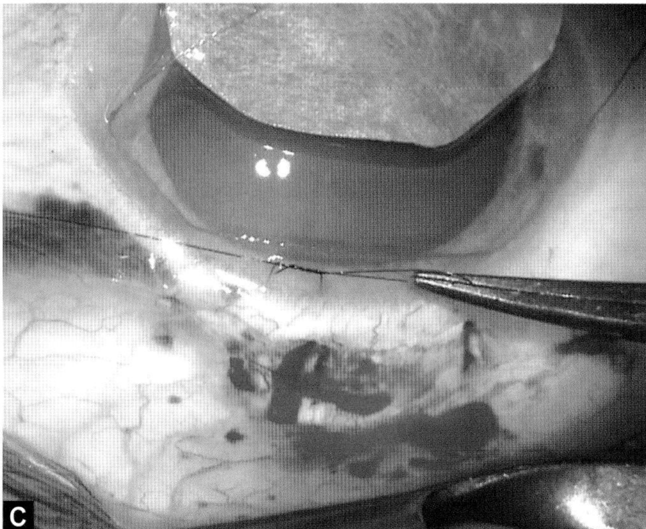


**Figures 40-9A to C** Releasable suture. The use of a releasable suture allows for tighter closure of the scleral flap to restrict the aqueous outflow during the immediate postoperative period. First, A 10-0 nylon releasable suture is placed at the side of the scleral flap. Second, the needle goes through the scleral flap (A) and then is led from the adjacent sclera to the cornea (B). The suture is tied and trimmed at the cornea (C).

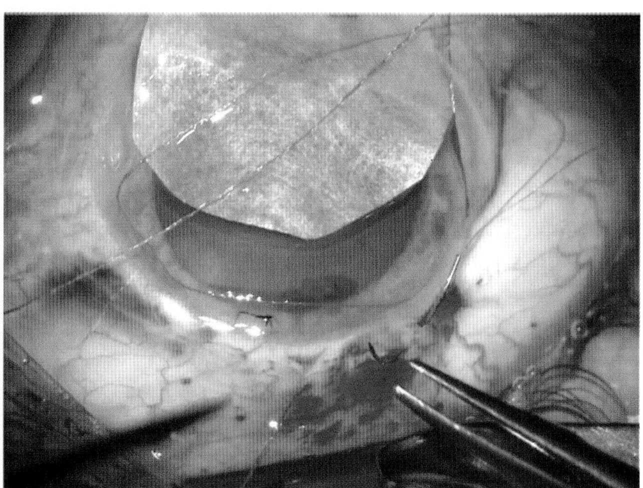

**Figure 40-10** Conjunctival suturing with 8-0 polyglactin.

and 5-fluorouracil (5-FU) are used. The use of antifibrotic agents is associated with a higher success rate, although the risk of complications may also increase. An individualized consideration of the risk/benefit ratio is recommended.

MMC (0.2–0.5 mg/mL solution) or 5-FU (50 mg/mL solution) is applied for 1–5 minutes using soaked cellulose sponges placed over the episclera. Application under the scleral flap is also possible. The conjunctival–Tenon's layer is draped over the sponge, avoiding contact of the MMC with the wound edge. After the application, the sponge is removed and the entire area is irrigated thoroughly with balanced salt solution. The plastic devices that collect the liquid runoff are changed and disposed of according to toxic waste regulations. Alternatively it can be injected subconjunctivally (0.1–0.2 mL) at the beginning of the surgery.

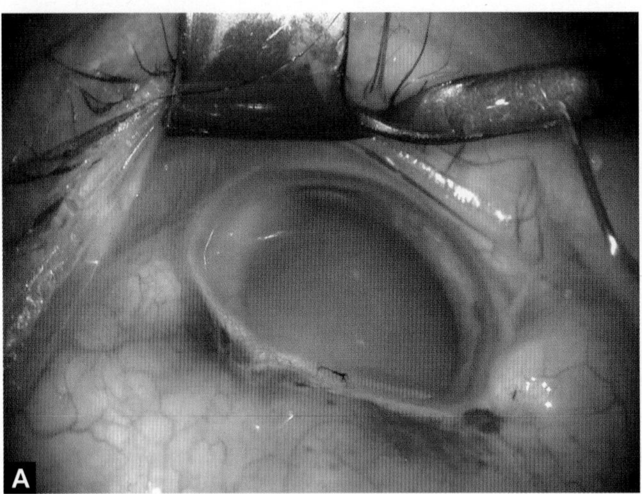


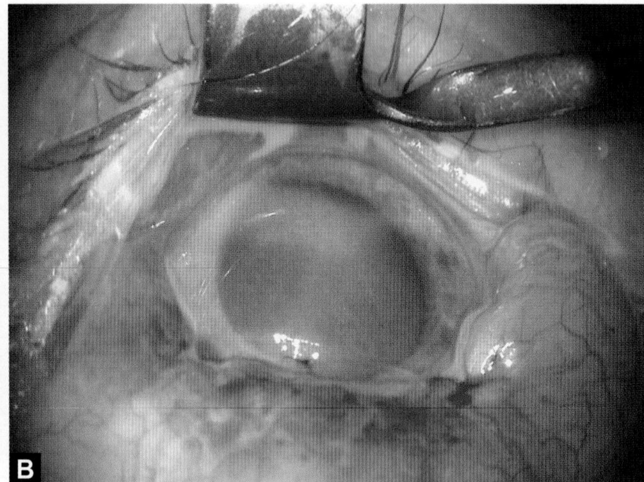


**Figures 40-11A and B** Raising the filtering bleb. (A) The bleb is raised to confirm that the closure is watertight. (B) Fluorescein drops can be used to confirm absence of leakage.

## POSTOPERATIVE CARE

Patients can resume daily activities promptly, but those with postoperative hypotony should avoid Valsalva maneuvers and brisk physical activities. Topical steroids (e.g. difluprednate or prednisolone acetate 1%, four times daily) are tapered over 6–8 weeks. In addition some clinicians use topical nonsteroidal anti-inflammatory agents (e.g. one times a day for 1 month or longer to control inflammation.). Antibiotics are required for 1–2 weeks after surgery. Postoperative cycloplegics are utilized on an individual basis, particularly in patients with shallow anterior chambers or intense inflammation.

During postoperative visits, digital ocular compression applied to the inferior sclera or cornea through the inferior eyelid, and focal compression with a moistened cotton tip at the posterior edge of the scleral flap, can be useful to elevate the bleb and reduce the IOP in the early postoperative period, especially after laser suture lysis. Suture lysis and cutting releasable sutures are necessary when there is a high IOP, a flat filtration bleb, and a deep anterior chamber. Gonioscopy must be performed prior to the laser treatment to confirm an open sclerostomy with no tissue or clot occluding its entrance. Suture lysis and removal of releasable sutures should be done within the first few weeks after surgery, although it may be successful even months after surgery in patients in whom MMC had been used. In cases prone to early failure (e.g. vascularized and thickened blebs), repeated subconjunctival applications of 5-FU (5 mg in 0.1 mL solution) and anti-VEFG therapy (see below) over the first few weeks are recommended.

### Anti-VEGF Therapy

The use of anti-vascular endothelial growth factor (VEGF) agents (bevacizumab and ranibizumab) as an adjunct to filtration surgery has recently been proposed. The wound healing process is potentiated through both fibroblast activity and angiogenesis. Therefore, an anti-VEGF agent should decrease new vascular growth and potentially lead to a healthier bleb with less scarring and better long-term IOP control. Anti-VEGF agents may have a synergistic effect with MMC and 5-FU in those patients whose trabeculectomies may fail with the use of MMC or 5-FU alone.

### Bleb Needling

In cases of subconjunctival–episcleral fibrosis, an external revision or bleb needling can be tried. A 27- or 25-gauge needle is used to cut the edge of the scleral flap and restore aqueous outflow. Entry of the needle tip into the anterior chamber beneath the flap may be required but should be undertaken with extreme caution in phakic eyes. The outcome may be more favorable if there was a previously well-established filtration bleb before the fistula became occluded. Repeated subconjunctival injections of 5-FU after revision increase the probability of success. MMC before or after needling has been also proposed in conjunction with needling of blebs. We are currently using 0.1 cc of nonpreserved 1% lidocaine mixed with 0.1 mL of 0.4 mg/mL MMC at the time of the needling.

## SPECIFIC INSTRUMENTATION

No specific instrumentation is required for glaucoma surgery, and there is large variability in the type of instruments used among surgeons. As a general principle, blunt dissection of the conjunctiva is better done with blunt-tipped scissors (e.g. Westcott). Forceps to handle the conjunctiva and sclera should have no teeth. Scleral flap dissection can be done with any sharp knife. A Kelly or Gass punch may be useful to create the fistula; otherwise Vannas or DeWecker scissors are helpful. Suturing material can also vary, but 10-0 nylon is the preferred suture material by the authors.

## COMPLICATIONS OF FILTRATION SURGERY

Transient hypotony is very common after glaucoma surgery, and often well tolerated, but occasionally it may lead to other possible complications including flat anterior chamber, Descemet's membrane folds, choroidal effusions, or suprachoroidal haemorrhage. Persistent hypotony can lead to macular and optic disk edema, and chorioretinal folds (predominantly in young myopic patients). Hyphema and early bleb leak are not rare, but often resolve with conservative management.

Late bleb-related infection can be a very severe complication, potentially leading to endophthalmitis. It is more common in surgeries supplemented with MMC and in leaking, avascular, thin, localized filtering blebs. Cataract is a very common development after filtration surgery. Cataract surgery may impair the function of the filtering bleb, especially if it is done within the first year after the glaucoma operation.

## SURGICAL OUTCOMES: SCIENTIFIC EVIDENCE/META-ANALYSIS

The use of intraoperative MMC or postoperative 5-FU reduces the risk of surgical failure both in eyes at high risk of surgical failure and in eyes that have not undergone previous surgery.[4,5] The use of an antifibrotic agent carries with it an increased likelihood of complications such as hypotony, hypotony maculopathy, late-onset bleb leak, and bleb-related infections.

Filtration surgery has been compared with topical medical treatment as primary treatment of newly diagnosed open-angle glaucoma (OAG).[2,3] The most recent trial included participants with average mild OAG.[2] At 5 years, the risk of progressive visual field loss, based on a three-unit change of a composite visual field score, was not significantly different according to initial medication or initial filtration surgery. In an analysis based on mean difference (MD) as a single index of visual field loss, the between treatment group difference in MD was -0.20 decibel (dB) (95% CI -1.31 to 0.91). For a subgroup with more severe glaucoma (MD -10 dB), findings from an exploratory analysis suggest that initial filtration surgery was associated with marginally less visual field loss at 5 years than initial medication, (MD 0.74 dB (95% CI -0.00 to 1.48). Initial filtration surgery was associated with lower average IOP (MD 2.20 mm Hg (95% CI 1.63–2.77) but more eye symptoms than medication. Beyond 5 years, visual acuity did not differ according to initial treatment.[2]

In patients with advanced glaucoma on maximum medical treatment, the Advanced Glaucoma Intervention Study (AGIS) suggested that an IOP of 12 was the optimum to avoid further loss of visual field with an acceptable risk of side effects.[6] However, there was a racial difference in the relative efficacy of laser trabeculoplasty and filtration surgery. In whites, filtration surgery was the best option after failure of medical treatment, while in blacks argon laser trabeculoplasty was the best initial choice (AGIS).

In patients with high risk of failure (e.g. with a history of previous ocular surgery) trabeculectomy has been compared with glaucoma drainage device in a relatively small-randomized trial. The results did not show a clear superiority of IOP control or complications with either technique.[7] An ongoing trial with a similar study design is comparing the results of filtration surgery and glaucoma drainage device in eyes with low risk of failure, i.e. as an initial surgical intervention for glaucoma.

## PEARLS AND PITFALLS

- Consider early surgery in patients with advanced glaucoma, high IOP, and fast rate of progression.
- Intensive postoperative care is as important as proper surgical technique to optimize surgical outcomes. Consider increasing topical steroids, 5-FU injections, and perhaps subconjunctival anti-VEGF if the bleb becomes vascularized and thickened in the early postoperative period. Timing of suture lysis and release of scleral flap sutures is critical.
- *Manage patients expectations*: Visual acuity may be impaired after trabeculectomy, commonly due to cataract, and failure or need for glaucoma medications is not uncommon.
- Create the fistula as anterior as possible, e.g. into the cornea. A large fistula (excision of tissue) is not required.
- Peripheral iridectomy is not required in patients with open angle, especially if they are pseudophakic. However, if the iris protrudes into the fistula it would be best then to perform the peripheral iridectomy.
- After placing the scleral flap sutures confirm there is flow under the flap by raising the IOP injecting BSS through the paracentesis. Try to estimate how high is the IOP for the aqueous humor to start flowing under the

flap, and how low is the IOP for the aqueous humor to stop flowing. The amount of flow can be controlled: to decrease flow, add further tighten sutures. To increase flow, loosen a suture(s). It may preferable to have a low filtration and relatively high IOP in the first postoperative visit than excessive filtration and low IOP.

- Confirm there is no bleb leak after closing the conjunctiva.

## REFERENCES


1. Cairns JE. Trabeculectomy. Preliminary report of a new method. Am J Ophthalmol. 1968;66:673-9.
2. Musch DC, Gillespie BW, Lichter PR, etal. CIGTS Study Investigators. Visual field progression in the Collaborative Initial Glaucoma Treatment Study the impact of treatment and other baseline factors. Ophthalmology. 2009;116:200-7
3. Burr J, Azuara-Blanco A, Avenell A, et al. Medical versus surgical interventions for open angle glaucoma. Cochrane Database Syst Rev. 2012(9). Art. No.: CD004399. DOI: 10.1002/14651858.CD004399.pub3
4. Wilkins M, Indar A, Wormald R. Intraoperative mitomycin C for glaucoma surgery. Cochrane Database Syst Rev. 2005(4). Art. No.: CD002897. DOI: 10.1002/14651858.CD002897.pub2.
5. Wormald R, Wilkins M, Bunce C. Postoperative 5-fluorouracil for glaucoma surgery. Cochrane Database Syst Rev. 2001(3). Art. No.: CD001132. DOI: 10.1002/14651858.CD001132.
6. Anonymous. The Advanced Glaucoma Intervention Study (AGIS): 7. The relationship between control of intraocular pressure and visual field deterioration. The AGIS Investigators. Am J Ophthalmol. 2000;130:429-40.
7. Gedde SJ, Schiffman JC, Feuer WJ, et al. Tube versus Trabeculectomy Study Group. Treatment outcomes in the Tube Versus Trabeculectomy (TVT) study after five years of follow-up. Am J Ophthalmol. 2012;153:789-803.

CHAPTER

41

# Microincisional Glaucoma Surgery

Steven D Vold, Mary Anne Ahluwalia

## INTRODUCTION

With the marketing advantages potentially associated with this new class of glaucoma procedures, utilization of the term minimally invasive glaucoma surgery (MIGS) became widespread when discussing any procedure other than filtration or tube shunt surgery. Consequently, Ahmed and his colleague Hady Saheb, MD, further clarified the intent of the term MIGS. MIGS was defined as microinvasive glaucoma surgery and described as having the following characteristics: (1) ab interno surgical approach, (2) minimal tissue trauma, (3) superior safety and low complication profile, (4) at least modest intraocular pressure (IOP) lowering efficacy, and (5) rapid patient recovery (Table 41-1).[1] In an attempt to further decrease confusion regarding these procedures, Vold published a surgical classification system of currently available glaucoma procedures (Flowchart 41-1).[2]

Incisional glaucoma surgical techniques are in a period of remarkable evolution. With recent advances in glaucoma microincisional surgical techniques and innovative microstent technologies, a complete transformation of the glaucoma treatment paradigm appears to be underway. The intent of this chapter is to provide a useful framework for thinking about this promising new class of glaucoma surgical techniques.

### Indications

The advent of MIGS procedures opens the door to earlier surgical intervention in patients with less advanced glaucomatous disease. Previous conventional wisdom relegated incisional glaucoma surgery to patients with more advanced glaucomatous disease or disease refractory to both medical and laser therapies.[3] Furthermore, MIGS potentially offers a more palatable option than filtration surgery in patients who struggle with medical compliance issues. Although the indications for MIGS have yet to be fully elucidated, clinicians are now beginning to approach glaucoma as a surgical disease.

**TABLE 41-1** Microinvasive surgery characteristics

| |
|---|
| • Ab interno surgical approach |
| • Minimal tissue trauma |
| • Superior safety and low complication profile |
| • At least modest intraocular pressure lowering |
| • Rapid patient recovery |

### Trabecular Bypass Procedures

#### *Trabectome*

Ab interno trabeculotomy utilizing the Trabectome (NeoMedix Corporation, Tustin, CA) (Fig. 41-1) is indicated for patients with open-angle glaucomas. Surgeons frequently combine Trabectome surgery with phacoemulsification in the setting of both visually significant cataract and mild-to-moderate open-angle glaucomas, but may also perform this surgery as a stand-alone procedure. Some surgeons advocate its utilization in both congenital and advanced open-angle glaucomas.[4,5]

#### *iStent, iStent Inject trabecular bypass microstents and Hydrus*

iStent and iStent Inject trabecular bypass microstents (Glaukos Corporation, Laguna Hills, CA) (Figs. 41-2 and 41-3) and Hydrus ((Ivantis, Inc., Irvine, CA) (Fig. 41-4) are novel ab interno MIGS devices. The iStent procedure is FDA approved in the United States for use in eyes with mild-to-moderate primary open-angle glaucoma at the time of cataract surgery.[6-8] FDA-approved clinical trials for both the iStent Inject and Hydrus procedures are currently evaluating the efficacy and safety of these devices in this setting as well.

**Flowchart 41.1** Proposed Classication of Surgical Procedures for Glaucoma

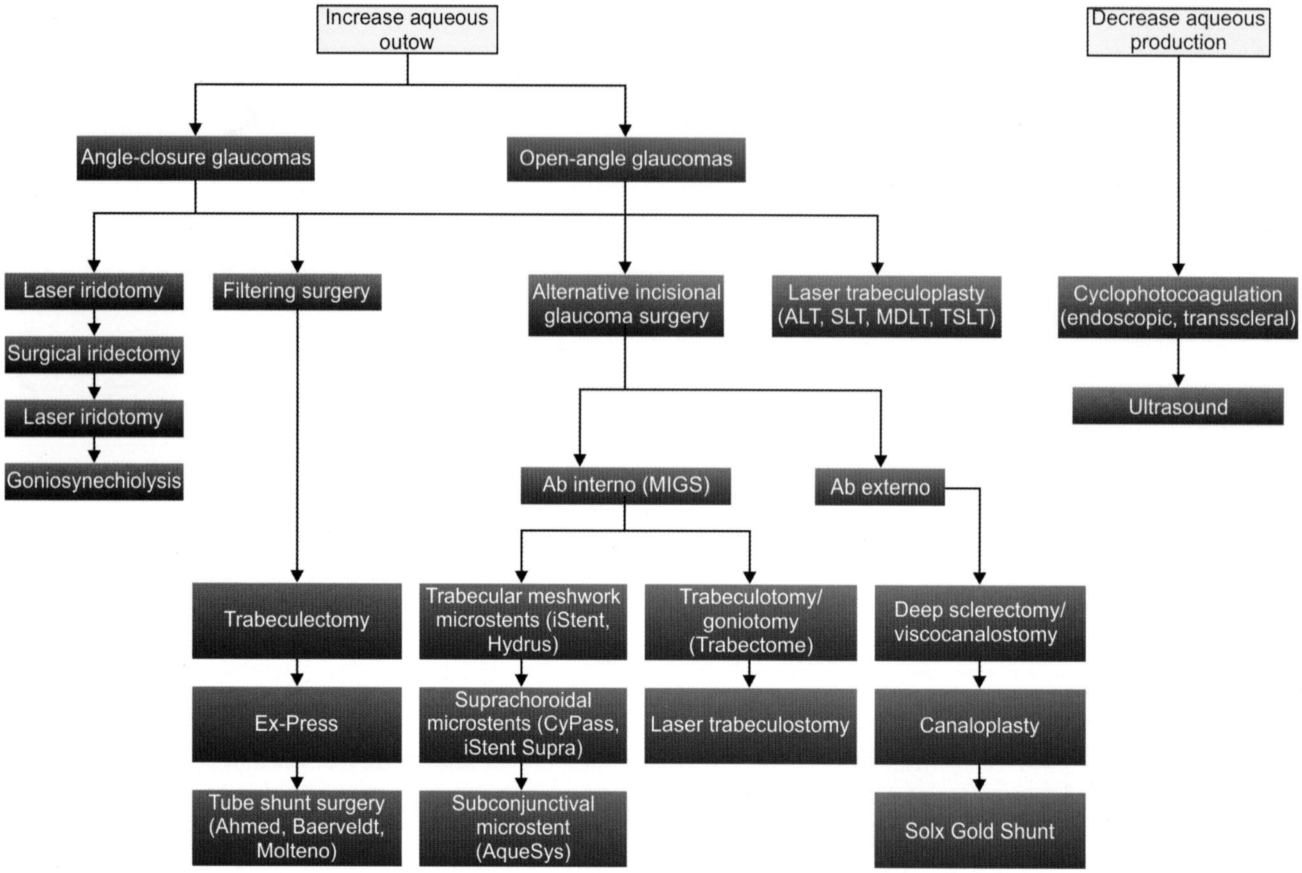

- Increase aqueous outow
  - Angle-closure glaucomas
  - Open-angle glaucomas
    - Laser iridotomy → Surgical iridectomy → Laser iridotomy → Goniosynechiolysis
    - Filtering surgery
      - Trabeculectomy → Ex-Press → Tube shunt surgery (Ahmed, Baerveldt, Molteno)
    - Alternative incisional glaucoma surgery
      - Ab interno (MIGS)
        - Trabecular meshwork microstents (iStent, Hydrus) → Suprachoroidal microstents (CyPass, iStent Supra) → Subconjunctival microstent (AqueSys)
        - Trabeculotomy/ goniotomy (Trabectome) → Laser trabeculostomy
      - Ab externo
        - Deep sclerectomy/ viscocanalostomy → Canaloplasty → Solx Gold Shunt
    - Laser trabeculoplasty (ALT, SLT, MDLT, TSLT)
- Decrease aqueous production
  - Cyclophotocoagulation (endoscopic, transscleral) → Ultrasound

(ALT: Argon laser trabeculoplasty; SLT: Selective laser trabeculoplasty; MDLT: Micropulse diode laser trabeculoplasty; TSLT: Titanium:sapphire laser trabeculoplasty: MIGS: Microinvasive glaucoma surgery. Manufacturing information: Express Glaucoma Filtration Device (Alcon Laboratories, Inc.), AqueSys device (AqueSys), Ahmed Glaucoma Valve (New World Medical, Inc.), Baerveldt glaucoma implant (Abbott Medical Optics Inc.), Molteno Implant (Molteno Ophthalmic Limited), iStent and iStent Supra (Glaukos Corporation), Hydrus (Ivantis Inc.), CyPass Micro-Stent (Transcend Medical), Trabectome (NeoMedix Corporation), Solx Gold Shunt (Solx, Inc.).

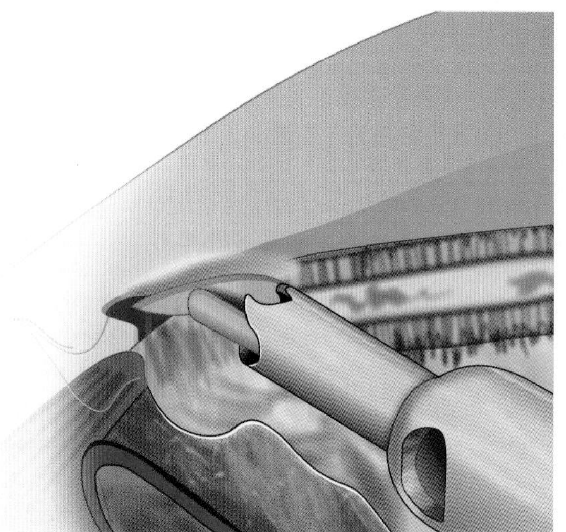

**Figure 41-1** Ab interno trabeculotomy using the Trabectome.

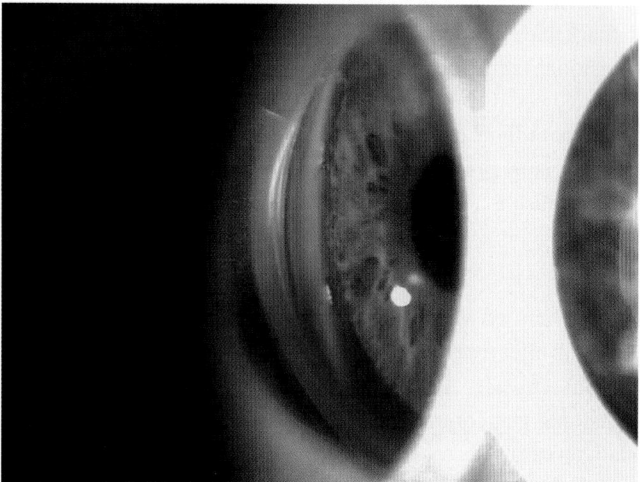

**Figure 41-2** Proper placement of two trabecular bypass iStents within Schlemm's canal.

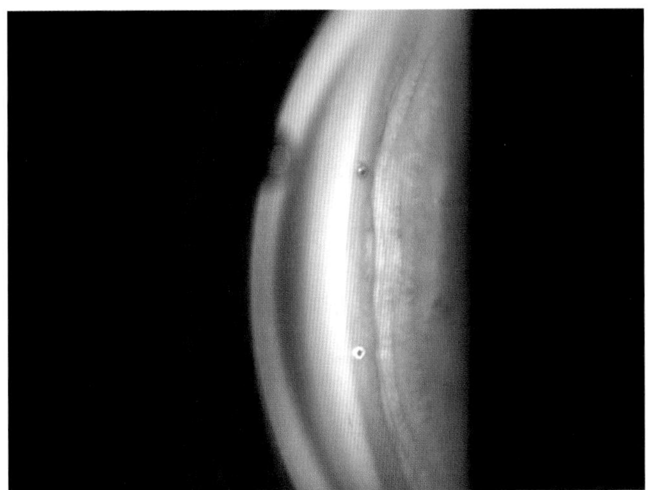

**Figure 41-3** Two iStent Inject devices.

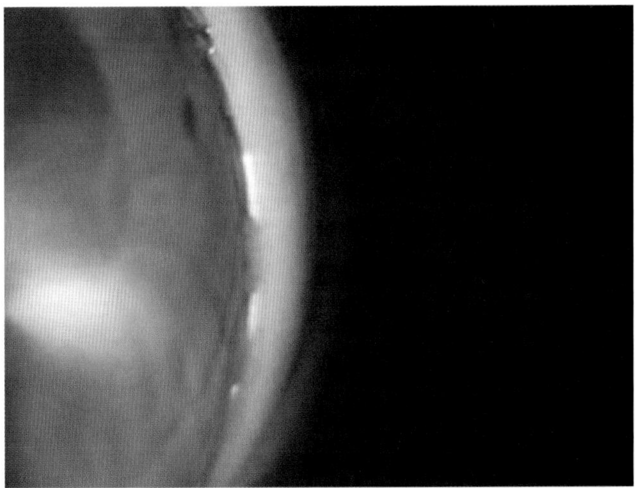

**Figure 41-4** Hydrus trabecular scaffold.

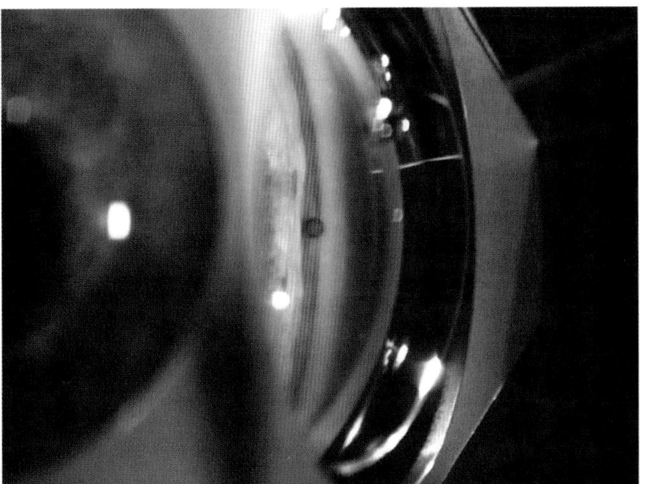

**Figure 41-5** CyPass supraciliary microstent.

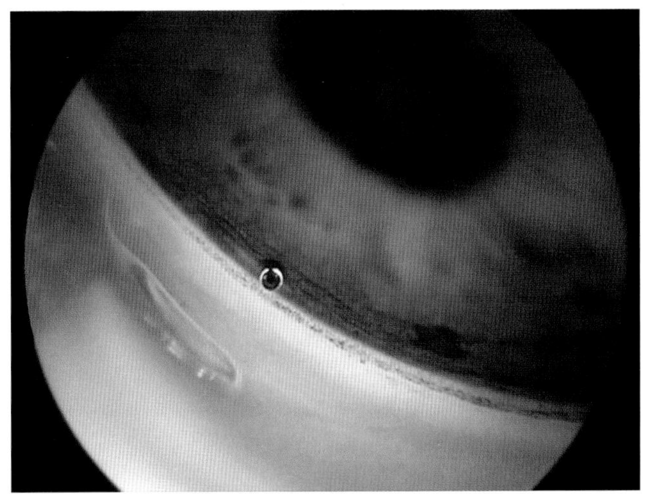

**Figure 41-6** iStent Supra microstent.

### Suprachoroidal Microstents

CyPass supraciliary microstent (Transcend Medical, Menlo Park, CA) (Fig. 41-5) and iStent Supra (Glaukos Corporation, Laguna Hills, CA) (Fig. 41-6), are ab interno supraciliary microstents currently under investigation in the United States for use in eyes with mild-to-moderate primary open-angle glaucoma at the time of cataract surgery. These devices potentially offer benefit in more advanced glaucomatous disease and may eventually play a role in angle-closure glaucomas.

## SUBCONJUNCTIVAL MICROSTENT

The XEN implant (AqueSys, Inc., Irvine, CA) is another MIGS device currently being investigated in select refractory glaucoma patients in an FDA-approved clinical trial in the United States (Figs. 41-7A and B). The hope of investigators is that this procedure will ultimately replace standard filtration surgery and potentially be indicated in earlier stages of glaucomatous disease as well.

## CONTRAINDICATIONS

MIGS contraindications have yet to be fully elucidated. However, trabecular bypass procedures are generally avoided in advanced open-angle glaucomas in eyes where the collector system has been significantly compromised. In addition, eyes with secondary glaucomas and angle closure are generally believed to be less than ideal MIGS cases. Further study is required to better define the relative and absolute contraindications of these procedures.

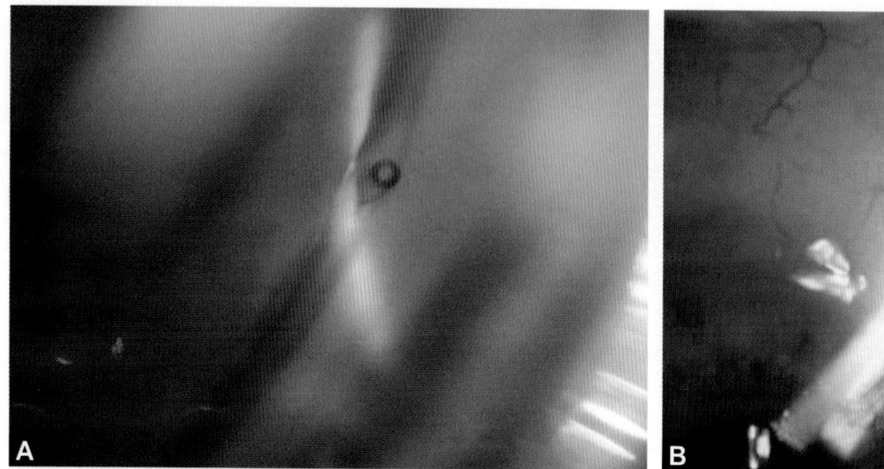


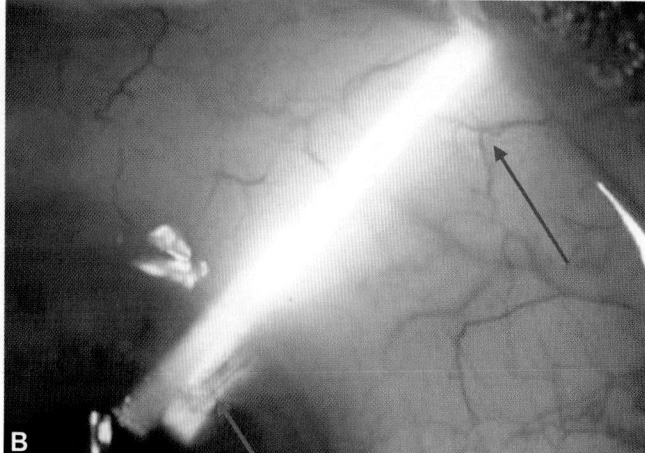


**Figures 41-7A and B** AqueSys XEN implant. (A) Gonioscopic view of AqueSys. (B) Slit lamp view of device.

## MECHANISM OF ACTION

Trabecular bypass procedures restore normal physiologic aqueous outflow by connecting the anterior chamber to Schlemm's canal bypassing the trabecular meshwork. Supraciliary microstents enhance uveoscleral aqueous outflow by connecting the anterior chamber to the suprachoroidal space. Subconjunctival microstents connect the anterior chamber to the subconjunctival space creating filtering blebs. Interestingly, the blebs associated with the use of AqueSys XEN Implant appear to actually restore lymphatic drainage as well.

## SURGICAL TECHNIQUE

### Ab Interno Trabeculotomy Using the Trabectome

When combining Trabectome and cataract surgery, ab interno trabeculotomy may be performed either before or after phacoemulsification. When inserting the Trabectome handpiece into the eye, the insulator footplate should be held parallel to the iris, its tip placed against the posterior lip of the wound, and gentle posterior pressure applied to allow the device to move into the eye easily. This technique maintains a watertight seal around the infusion sleeve as the handpiece is guided into the anterior chamber. Placing viscoelastic in the wound may facilitate the instrument's insertion. The footplate can then be advanced across the eye while using continuous irrigation to maintain the anterior chamber. The tip of the footplate should be pointed into the canal under direct visualization and the handpiece gently wiggled to ensure that the unit is properly seated. Once in position, the footswitch can be used to activate the handpiece's aspiration and electrosurgical functions and the instrument tip can be slowly rotated along Schlemm's canal. To maximize the treated area, 90–120° of the inner wall of the canal should be ablated before rotating the footplate 180° within the anterior chamber to remove tissue from the opposite direction.[4-5,9]

### iStent

The iStent is the first FDA-approved trabecular bypass microstent. This titanium microstent is 1.0 mm in length, 0.33 mm in height with a snorkel size of 0.25 mm × 120 um. The iStent is preloaded in a single-use inserter. After completing small incision cataract surgery and filling the anterior chamber of the eye with an ophthalmic viscoelastic device, remove the apparatus from the packaging and carefully avoid dislodging the iStent on the corneal wound. Gently depressing the corneal wound causes blood reflux into the canal allowing for easier identification of Schlemm's canal. Left-directed iStents require a forehand motion for proper device placement with a right-handed surgeon. A forehand maneuver may be easier for novice MIGS surgeons. Approach the upper one-third of the trabecular meshwork at an approximately 15° angle with the iStent. Once the microstent is in Schlemm's canal, surgeons must flatten their approach to allow the device to slide into the canal. Push the button on the inserter to release the iStent. Blood reflux after iStent placement confirms proper device placement. The iStent should be seated securely along the outer wall of Schlemm's canal. Regrasping the iStent to ensure the device is in proper position occasionally may be required. The iStent placement near larger collector channels in the nasal quadrants is recommended. Conscientious viscoelastic removal following device placement helps prevent postoperative pressure spikes. Although only one iStent placement per procedure is FDA approved, placement of two or three iStents may ultimately prove to maximize IOP lowering.[10]

### iStent Inject

In an effort to simplify and automate implantation of iStent devices, the iStent Inject system was developed to allow for deployment of multiple iStents with a single injector. These modified titanium microstents have a rivet-shaped appearance. Under direct gonioscopic visualization, the needle of the injector is placed on the anterior aspect of the trabecular meshwork, and the button on the injector gently depressed deploying the device into position within Schlemm's canal. Placement of the microstents near large collector channels in the two nasal quadrants is recommended.[11]

### Hydrus

The Hydrus is a 6-mm, flexible "scaffold" of Schlemm's canal. It is composed of nitinol and is designed to re-establish aqueous flow to the collector channels. The Hydrus dilates and supports Schlemm's canal and targets approximately 3 clock hours of the collector system. Its unique design may permit later enhancements to aqueous outflow through the application of YAG laser energy to three trabecular meshwork windows in the device.[12]

### Ab Interno Canaloplasty

In an effort to increase surgeons' intraoperative efficiency, iScience Interventional is making a significant effort to allow them to place a 360° trabecular-suture microstent from an ab interno approach. The overall impact of this surgical approach on IOP lowering and surgeons' technique has yet to be fully determined.

### CyPass Microstent

The CyPass microstent is a supraciliary device composed of a polyimide material. It has a 300-μm lumen and is 6 mm long. The device is implanted via a curved insertion device through an approximately 2.0 mm clear corneal incision. Anterior chamber deepening using a viscoelastic facilitates a proper insertion angle for the CyPass microstent.[13]

### iStent Supra

The design of the iStent Supra is similar to that of the CyPass microstent. It is also implanted via an ab interno approach into the supraciliary space.

### XEN Implant

The XEN implant is a porcine 6.0 mm collagen-derived, gelatin implant that is soft and flexible when hydrated. It is noninflammatory and may mitigate the problem of implant migration. The porcine tube is injected into the subconjunctival space 3.0 mm posterior to the limbus utilizing a specially designed inserter that allows device implantation to occur without utilizing a direct gonioscope. Ideally, 1.0–2.0 mm of the implant should reside in the anterior chamber.[14]

## POSTOPERATIVE CARE

Recommended follow-up for these patients is similar to that of cataract surgery alone. Patients generally are examined 1 day, 1 week, and 1 month postoperatively. Topical antibiotics are currently administered perioperatively to prevent infection. Patients should also use a topical anti-inflammatory medication such as prednisolone acetate 1% or loteprednol 0.5% (Lotemax, Bausch & Lomb, Rochester, New York) for approximately 1 month postoperatively. Patients undergoing trabecular bypass procedures are prone to developing steroid-induced IOP spikes. Consequently, loteprednol or a nonsteroidal anti-inflammatory medications are sometimes advocated in these patients rather than difluprednate or prednisolone acetate. As an alternative, prednisolone acetate 1% can be tapered relatively rapidly to avoid steroid-induced IOP spikes. For XEN implant surgeries, more aggressive steroid therapy utilizing difluprednate may be considered. Following Trabectome surgery, topical pilocarpine is sometimes utilized for several weeks postoperatively to prevent peripheral anterior synechiae formation. Topical nonsteroidal anti-inflammatory medication may help prevent cystoid macular edema formation following combined MIGS and cataract extraction procedures.

### Instrumentation

At the present time, MIGS is generally combined with cataract surgery in the United States. However, these procedures are commonly performed as stand-alone procedures in other countries. The frequent use of intraoperative gonioscopy under an operating microscope is a common component of all these procedures. For many ophthalmic surgeons, intraoperative gonioscopy represents the single most challenging acquired skill in the performance of MIGS. It is important for the novice MIGS surgeon to perform gonioscopy in the clinic prior to surgery in order to most easily identify angle anatomy. Most direct intraoperative goniolenses used to perform ab interno angle surgery require tilting of the operating microscope approximately 30° toward the surgeon and tilting of the patient's head 30° away from the surgeon as well as significant dexterity from the surgeon to obtain clear visualization of the anterior chamber angle (Fig. 41-8). With use of these gonioprisms, it may be preferred to use topical anesthesia, because this permits the patient to gaze nasally for an optimal view of the structures in the anterior chamber. Care must be taken not to compress the cornea during gonioscopy, potentially compromising visualization of the angle and shallowing the anterior chamber during surgery.[15]

Each MIGS procedure also has its own insertion device. All of these inserters have their own particular characteristics to facilitate ab interno deployment through as small a corneal incision as possible, and are in rapid evolution. Recent iterations appear to be moving toward more automated insertion technologies.

## COMPLICATIONS

In addition to complications associated with cataract surgery, potential complications of trabecular bypass procedures include hyphema, microstent malpositioning, corneal endothelial damage, iris touch/incarceration, anterior synechiae, chronic uveitis, postoperative IOP elevation, and failure to lower IOP.[16] In addition to these potential complications, suprachoroidal microstents have been occasionally associated with chronic inflammation, device occlusion, device extrusion, and hypotony. The subconjunctival XEN implant potentially may result in complications observed with conventional filtration surgery. Published studies evaluating the iStent technology demonstrated that the iStent did not significantly increase the risk of intraoperative complications when compared with cataract surgery alone.[6-8]

## SURGICAL OUTCOMES: SCIENTIFIC EVIDENCE/META-ANALYSIS

At this time, the amount of long-term published data regarding the majority of MIGS procedures is quite sparse. As expected, the Trabectome currently has the most long-term data of MIGS procedures. Published studies demonstrate IOP lowering and reduction in medication use in the majority of glaucoma patients with this procedure. Complications were minimal and comparable with those in an earlier series of Trabectome-only procedures. Phacoemulsification appears to be additive to the Trabectome in achieving improved glaucoma control. With combined surgery, clinicians commonly expect IOP lowering of at least 20% from preoperative levels with a reduction in the need for 1–2 glaucoma medications following surgery.[4-5,9]

Similarly, at 12 months, Samuelson et al. demonstrated that 72% of iStent subjects maintained IOPs ≤21 mm Hg without medication in contrast to only 50% with cataract surgery alone. IOP in both treatment groups was statistically significantly lower from baseline values. In addition, at 1 year, 66% of treatment eyes versus 48% of control eyes achieved ≥20% IOP reduction without medication ($P$ = 0.003). The overall incidence of adverse events was similar between groups with no unanticipated adverse device effects. The incidence of adverse events was low in both groups through 24-month follow-up. Furthermore, the mean IOP remained stable between 12 months and 24 months [17.0 mm Hg ± 2.8 (SD) and 17.1 ± 2.9 mm Hg, respectively] in the stent group but increased (17.0 ± 3.1 mm Hg to 17.8 ± 3.3 mm Hg, respectively) in the control group. Ocular hypotensive medication was statistically significantly lower in the stent group at 12 months; it was also lower at 24 months, although the difference was no longer statistically significant.

The other microstent technologies still undergoing further FDA evaluation appear to be quite effective in lower IOPs into the mid-teens as well. However, peer-reviewed publication of key FDA pivotal trials will be helpful in assisting surgeon as to the role of each procedure in the treatment of glaucoma.

## PEARLS AND PITFALLS

- Several critical factors play a significant role in determining patient visual outcomes. First, proper patient selection is mandatory. If surgeons select patients with poor collector systems or significant scarring in the area of the trabecular meshwork and Schlemm's canal, trabecular bypass procedures are doomed for failure. Consequently, surgeons are generally advised to select patients with more mild-to-moderate open-angle glaucomas for early cases. Furthermore, eyes with inflammatory or vascular components to their glaucoma etiology likely will do poorly with MIGS procedures.
- Second, surgical success is heavily dependent on knowing the internal-angle anatomy. Understandably, the importance of precise placement of these microstents cannot be underestimated. Placing of trabecular bypass microstents near large collector channels appears to be critical to optimizing postoperative IOP lowering for these patients. Suprachoroidal and subconjunctival devices need to be placed precisely and with care to avoid damaging the corneal endothelium.
- In summary, MIGS procedures offer promising new technologies that potentially may significantly enhance patient glaucoma care. However, much study remains to determine exactly when and where to utilize these procedures.

## REFERENCES

1. Saheb H, Ahmed II. Micro-invasive glaucoma surgery: current perspectives and future directions. Curr Opin Ophthalmol. 2012;23(2):96-104.
2. Vold S. What's in a name? Glaucoma Today [Internet]. 2012 Apr [cited 2013 June 1]. Available from: http://bmctoday.net/glaucomatoday/pdfs/gt0312_meded.pdf.
3. Francis BA, Singh K, Lin SC, et al. Novel glaucoma procedures: a report by the American Academy of Ophthalmology. Ophthalmology. 2011;118(7):1466-80.
4. Minckler DS, Baerveldt G, Alfaro MR, et al. Clinical results with the Trabectome for treatment of open-angle glaucoma. Ophthalmology. 2005;112(6):962-7.
5. Francis BA, Minckler D, Dustin L, et al. Combined cataract extraction and trabeculotomy by the internal approach for coexisting cataract and open-angle glaucoma: initial results. J Cataract Refract Surg. 2008;34(7):1096-103.
6. Samuelson TW, Katz LJ, Wells JM, et al. Randomized evaluation of the trabecular micro-bypass stent with phacoemulsification in patients with glaucoma and cataract. Ophthalmology. 2011;118(3);459-67.
7. Craven ER, Katz JK, Wells JM, et al. Cataract surgery with trabecular micro-bypass stent implantation in patients with mild-to-moderate open-angle glaucoma and cataract: two-year follow-up. J Cataract Refract Surg. 2012;38(8):1339-45.
8. Fea A. Phacoemulsification versus phacoemulsification with micro-bypass stent implantation in primary open-angle glaucoma: randomized double-masked clinical trial. J Cataract Refract Surg. 2010;36(3):407-12.
9. Vold SD. Int Ophthalmol Clin. 2011;51(3):65-81.
10. Belovay GW, Naqi A, Chan BJ, et al. Using multiple trabecular micro-bypass stents in cataract patients to treat open-angle glaucoma. J Cataract Refract Surg. 2012; 38 (11):1911-7.
11. Bahler CK, Hann CR, Fjield T, et al. Second-generation trabecular meshwork bypass stent (iStent inject) increases outflow facility in cultured human anterior segments. Am J Ophthalmol. 2012;153(6):1206-13.
12. Camras LJ, Yuan F, Fan S, et al. A novel Schlemm's Canal scaffold increases outflow facility in a human anterior segment perfusion model. Invest Ophthalmol Vis Sci. 2012;53(10):6115-21.
13. Hoeh H, Ahmed II, Grisanti S, et al. Early postoperative safety and surgical outcomes after implantation of a suprachoroidal micro-stent for the treatment of open-angle glaucoma concomitant with cataract surgery. J Cataract Refract Surg. 2013; 39(3):431-7.
14. Xen Glaucoma Implant [Internet]. Aliso Viejo: AqueSys; c2012. http://aquesys.com/xen.aspx [accessed 1 June 2013].
15. Vold SD, Ahmed IK. Intraoperative gonioscopy: past, present, and future. Glaucoma Today [Internet]. 2010 Sep 9cited 2013 June 1]. Available from: http://bmctoday.net/glaucomatoday/pdfs/gt0810_techtoday_vold.pdf.
16. Ahuja Y, Malihi M, Sit AJ. Delayed-onset symptomatic hyphema after ab interno trabeculotomy surgery. Am J Ophthalmol. 2012;154(3):476-80.

CHAPTER

42

# Glaucoma Drainage Devices

Joseph F Panarelli, Steven J Gedde

## INTRODUCTION

A recent shift in practice patterns is apparent among glaucoma surgeons. Sequential surveys of the American Glaucoma Society membership demonstrated that selection of glaucoma drainage device (GDDs) as the preferred surgical approach in various clinical settings increased from 17% in 1996 to 51% in 2008.[1] A study based on Medicare claims data found that the number of trabeculectomies performed between 1995 and 2004 decreased by 51%, and the number of tube shunts implanted increased by 184% during the same time period.[2]

### Indications

GDDs have traditionally been reserved for patients at high risk of failure with standard filtering surgery. This includes eyes with extensive conjunctival scarring from prior ocular surgery, trauma, or cicatrizing diseases (e.g. ocular cicatricial pemphigoid, Stevens–Johnson syndrome). Several secondary glaucomas are best managed with GDDs, such as neovascular glaucoma, uveitic glaucoma, epithelial or fibrous downgrowth, and iridocorneal endothelial (ICE) syndrome. GDDs are favored over trabeculectomy in eyes requiring long-term contact lens use (e.g. aphakia, high myopia) because of concerns about the risk of infection with a perilimbal filtering bleb. The Tube Versus Trabeculectomy (TVT) Study found that GDDs may be effectively used to surgically manage glaucoma in eyes with previous cataract and/or glaucoma surgery without significant conjunctival scarring (a population at lower risk of failure than the one that has historically undergone GDD surgery).[3] Eyes that may need additional ocular surgery in the future are good candidates for GDD, as they appear less prone to failure relative to trabeculectomy. The safety and efficacy of these devices suggest that they may be appropriate as a primary incisional procedure, even in eyes at low risk of surgical failure.

## CONTRAINDICATIONS

GDDs may have a complicated postoperative course and should be avoided in patients who are unable to comply with postoperative follow-up. An anatomically narrow angle and reduced corneal endothelial function are relative contraindications for anterior chamber placement of a tube. Caution should also be taken in patients with extensive conjunctival scarring, as conjunctival closure could extremely challenging.

## MECHANISM OF ACTION

All modern GDDs consist of a silicone tube that shunts aqueous humor from the anterior chamber or posterior chamber to an end plate located in the equatorial region of the globe. A fibrous capsule forms around the end plate over a period of several weeks after implantation. Aqueous humor pools in the potential space between the end plate and surrounding capsule. It then passively diffuses through the capsule wall into periocular capillaries and lymphatics. The fibrous capsule provides the primary resistance to aqueous outflow with GDDs.

## SURGICAL TECHNIQUE

Adequate anesthesia for GDD surgery may be achieved with a retrobulbar or peribulbar block, although general anesthesia may be required in select patients. The patient is then prepped and draped in a sterile manner, and a lid speculum is placed.

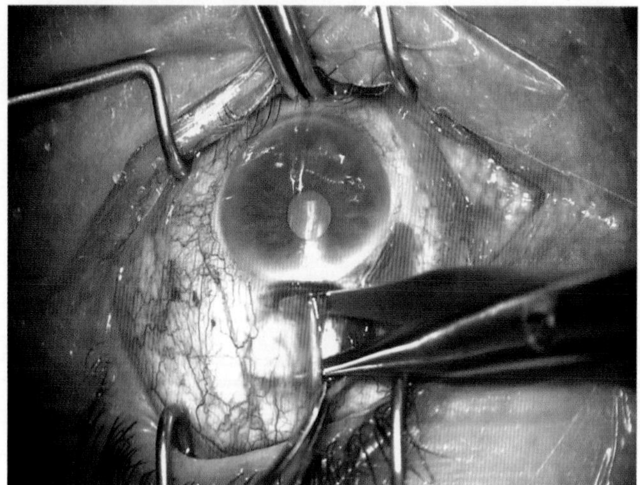

**Figure 42-1** The conjunctiva and Tenon's capsule are dissected from sclera to create space for the implant.

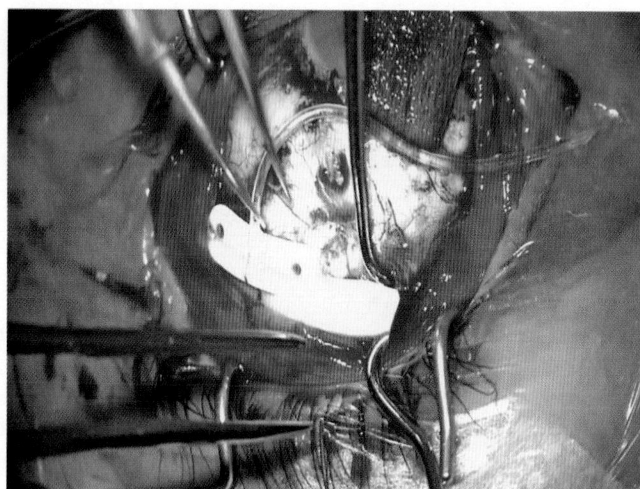

**Figure 42-2** The end plate is positioned between the rectus muscles.

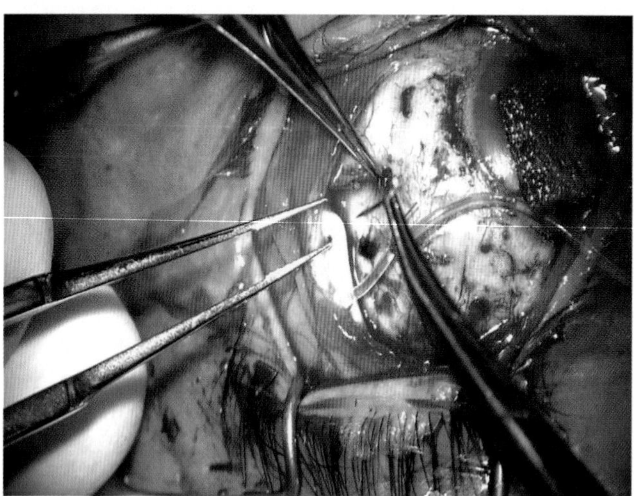

**Figure 42-3** The end plate is attached to sclera approximately 8–10 mm posterior to the limbus with nonabsorbable sutures (nylon or polypropylene) on a spatulated needle.

## Conjunctival Incision

A limbus-based or fornix-based conjunctival flap is dissected in the quadrant for GDD implantation. The superotemporal quadrant is generally selected as the site for placement of the initial implant because surgical exposure is better and postoperative strabismus is less frequent. The superonasal quadrant is generally avoided, as it is associated with a higher incidence of diplopia. Additionally, posteriorly positioned implants in this quadrant can encroach on the optic nerve.[4-6] The presence of the inferior oblique muscle fibers as well as cosmetic issues with the lower eyelid makes the inferotemporal quadrant a less satisfactory choice as well. For eyes that cannot undergo superotemporal implant placement, the inferonasal quadrant is a safe and effective alternative option.

## Quadrant Dissection

The conjunctiva and Tenon's capsule are dissected from sclera to create space for the implant (Fig. 42-1). Cautery is applied to bleeding episcleral vessels. A corneal traction suture may be used to enhance exposure.

## Attachment of the End Plate

The implant is placed in antibiotic solution before insertion. Adjacent rectus muscles are identified with muscle hooks. The end plate is positioned between the rectus muscles (Fig. 42-2). The lateral wings of the 350 mm$^2$ Baerveldt glaucoma implant are designed for positioning under the adjacent rectus muscles. The end plate is attached to sclera approximately 8–10 mm posterior to the limbus with nonabsorbable sutures (nylon or polypropylene) on a spatulated needle (Fig. 42-3). The knots are rotated into the fixation holes to prevent erosion through the conjunctiva. When using double-plate implants, one plate is positioned in each of two quadrants and the tube connecting them may be positioned under or over the rectus muscle.

## Preparation of the Implant

### *Restriction of Aqueous Flow in Non-valved Implants*

When using non-valved implants, temporary occlusion of the tube is required until fibrous encapsulation of the plate

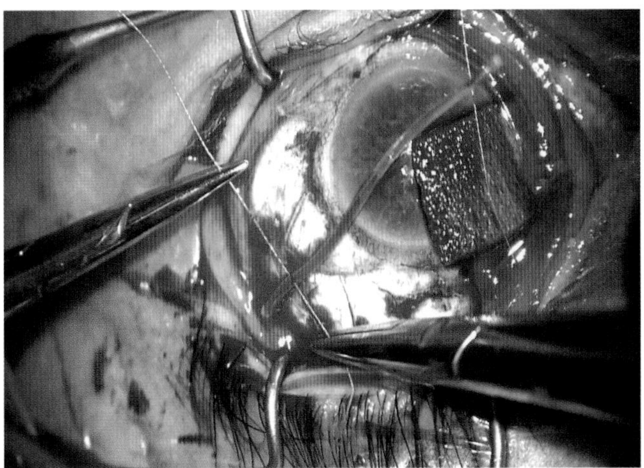

**Figure 42-4** Ligating the tube with a 7-0 polyglactin suture near the tube-plate junction restricts aqueous flow for the first 4–6 weeks after surgery.

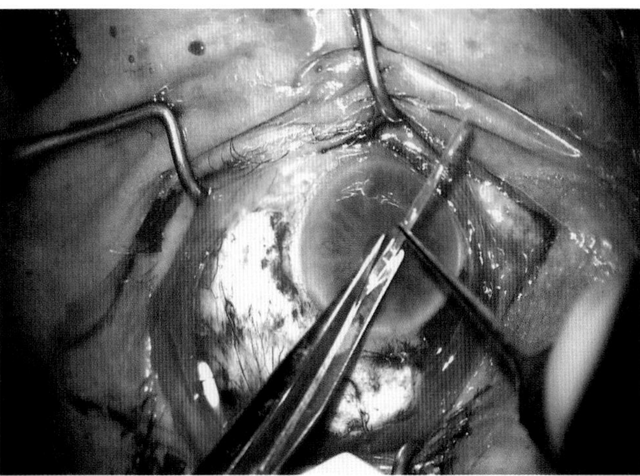

**Figure 42-5** The tube is draped across the cornea and cut with an anterior bevel so that a 2–3 mm segment of tube extends into the anterior chamber from the site of entry.

occurs. Ligating the tube with a 7-0 polyglactin suture near the tube-plate junction restricts aqueous flow for the first 4–6 weeks after surgery (Fig. 42-4). Complete closure is confirmed by attempting to irrigate balanced salt solution (on a 30-gauge cannula) through the tube. The polyglactin suture lyses 4–6 weeks postoperatively, causing spontaneous opening of the tube. If needed, the surgeon can perform laser suture lysis in the clinic prior to the suture releasing on its own. Other techniques for temporarily occluding the tube involve the use of a 4-0 chromic or polypropylene intraluminal suture, or placement of a 4-0 or 5-0 nylon or polypropylene suture alongside the tube and incorporating it within the ligating suture. These "ripcord" sutures are positioned subconjunctivally in a different quadrant from the implant and can be removed easily after several weeks with Vannas scissors and forceps. The final option is to use an intracameral 9-0 polypropylene suture to ligate the tube. An argon laser is subsequently applied to melt the stitch and open the tube.

After occluding the tube, fenestrations can be made anterior to the tube ligature to provide pressure control during the early postoperative period. The surgeon may place one or multiple fenestrations using the needle on a 7-0 polyglactin suture (TG-140). Alternatively, a 9-0 or 10-0 monofilament polyglactin suture may be left in a tube fenestration to serve as a wick promoting continued aqueous egress. No general consensus exists for which method is best, as results with each technique can vary greatly.

### *Priming Valved Implants*

Valved implants must be "primed" by injecting balanced salt solution through the tube using a cannula. This breaks the surface tension between the two silicone sheets of the Ahmed implant and allows the valve mechanism to function. The same procedure is done with the Krupin valve to ensure that the valve slits are functional.

## Insertion of the Tube

A paracentesis may be placed at this time to allow for better control of the anterior chamber. The tube is draped across the cornea and cut with an anterior bevel so that a 2–3 mm segment of tube extends into the anterior chamber from the site of entry (Fig. 42-5). An anterior bevel should be made if the tube is to be positioned in the anterior chamber or the pars plana, while a posterior bevel is indicated when the tube is placed in the ciliary sulcus. A 23-gauge needle is used to make an entry incision as this size needle creates a tight entry wound for the tube (Fig. 42-6). The tube is inserted through the needle track with nontoothed forceps. The tube can be secured to the sclera with either an 8-0 or 9-0 nylon suture.

## Tube Coverage with a Patch Graft

The limbal portion of the tube is covered with a patch graft to decrease the risk of tube exposure postoperatively. Donor sclera, cornea, pericardium, or amniotic membrane grafts can all be used as patch graft material. The graft is secured in place with absorbable sutures (Fig. 42-7).

## Conjunctival Closure

Conjunctiva is then reapproximated and closed using an interrupted and/or continuous suturing technique, depending on if a fornix- or limbus-based approach was used (Fig. 42-8).

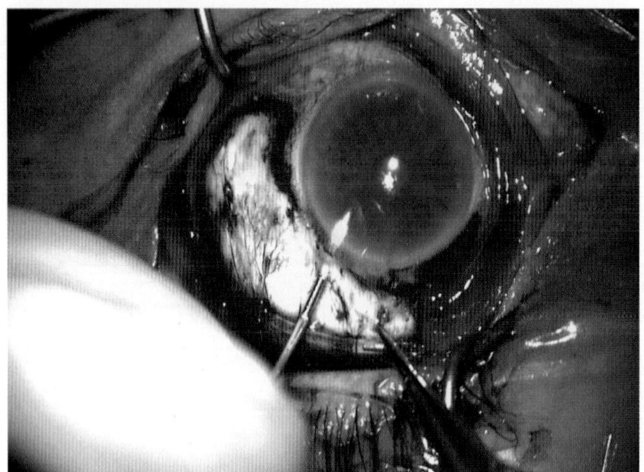

**Figure 42-6** A 23-ga needle is used to make an entry incision as this size needle creates a tight entry wound for the tube.

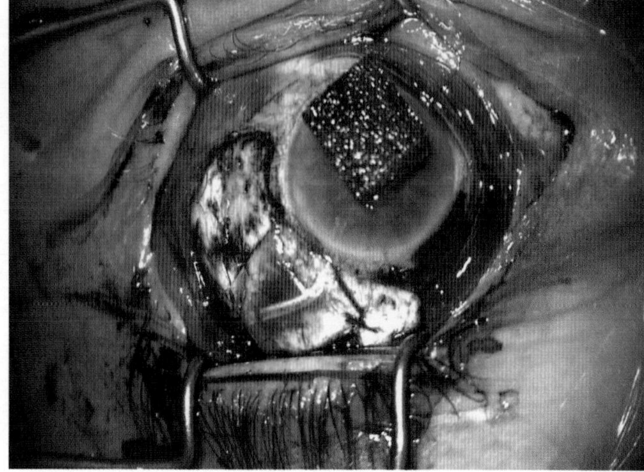

**Figure 42-7** The graft is secured in place with absorbable sutures.

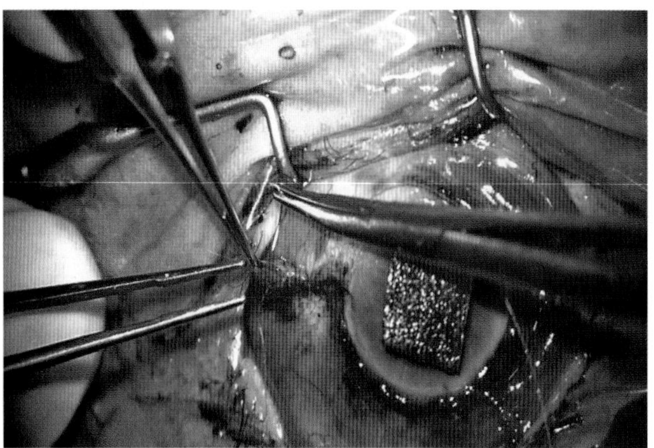

**Figure 42-8** Conjunctiva is then reapproximated and closed using an interrupted and/or continuous suturing technique, depending on if a fornix- or limbus-based approach was used.

At the conclusion of the case, a subconjunctival injection of an antibiotic and corticosteroid can be given.

## POSTOPERATIVE CARE

Patients are evaluated on the first postoperative day and started on topical antibiotic and steroid drops. If the intraocular pressure (IOP) is elevated, prior glaucoma medications can be resumed. Patients then follow up at 1 week, and every 1–2 weeks thereafter until the tube has opened when using non-valved implants. Steroid drops can be reduced during the early postoperative period. However, an increase in topical steroid therapy is generally required when a non-valved implant opens, as this event is usually associated with increased inflammation. Once the inflammation is controlled, the steroid medication can be tapered off over the course of a few weeks. Occasionally, the IOP may become elevated due to a "hypertensive phase" after tube placement. This occurs as a result of reduced permeability of the bleb. Aqueous suppression can be used to support the IOP during the hypertensive phase, and the condition typically improves with gradual remodeling of the bleb capsule.

## SPECIFIC INSTRUMENTATION

### Non-valved Implants

#### *Baerveldt Glaucoma Implant*

The Baerveldt glaucoma implant (Abbott Medical Optics Inc, Santa Ana, CA) has a silicone end plate with a surface area of 250 mm$^2$ (103–250) or 350 mm$^2$ (101–350). The increased surface area of the end plate produces a larger surface area of encapsulation around the plate and greater IOP reduction. Both models have fenestrations in the plate that allow for the growth of fibrous bands, thereby reducing bleb height. The pars plana version (102–350) has a 90° elbow that aides in the placement of the tube in the pars plana.

#### *Molteno Implant*

The Molteno 3 implant (Molteno Ophthalmic Limited, Dunedin, New Zealand) has a larger, thinner, more flexible end plate when compared with previous models, and it is shaped to fit the curvature of the globe. Single-plate implants are available with a surface area of 185 mm$^2$ or 245 mm$^2$. These devices have a lower profile and more anteriorly positioned suture holes, which allow for easier implantation of the device. The double-plate Molteno implants (R2/L2 and DR2/DL2) are connected by a 10 mm silicone tube, which may be positioned over or under the superior rectus muscle and have a maximum surface area of 530 mm$^2$. The Molteno3 and the DR2/DL double-plate Molteno implant have a pressure ridge on the upper surface of the end plate that was designed to reduce postoperative hypotony.

## Valved Implants

### *Ahmed Glaucoma Valve*

The Ahmed glaucoma valve (New World Medical, Rancho Cucamonga, CA) has a scarab-shaped end plate made of silicone (models FP7, FP8, FX1, FX4, PC7, and PC8) or polypropylene (models S2, S3, B1, B4, PS2, and PS3). Single-plate versions of the Ahmed implant are available with a surface area of 96 mm$^2$ (S3 and FP8) or 184 mm$^2$ (S2 and FP7). The major differences between the FP7 and the S2 are the presence of plate fenestrations and a thinner profile in the former. The smaller S3 and FP8 implants are designed for use in the pediatric population. The double-plate implants have a surface area of 364 mm$^2$ (FX1 and B1). Four of these models (PC7, PC8, PS2, and PS3) are fitted with a Pars Plana Clip designed for insertion into the posterior segment. The newest implant that was recently introduced is the M4. This implant has a surface area of 191 mm$^2$ and its end plate is composed of a biocompatible, porous polyethylene shell. The Ahmed glaucoma valve utilizes a tapered trapezoidal chamber to create a Venturi effect to aid in the flow of fluid through the device. IOP is regulated by a valve mechanism consisting of elastic membranes that consistently change their shape to control flow and reduce the risk of hypotony.

### *Krupin Valve with Disk*

The Krupin valve (Benson Hood Laboratories, Pembroke, MA) with disk has an oval silastic endplate with a surface area of 183 mm$^2$. The distal end of the tube contains horizontal and vertical slits that function as a valve.

# COMPLICATIONS

## Intraoperative Complications

Complications that may develop during implantation of a GDD include hyphema, scleral perforation, suprachoroidal hemorrhage, and vitreous prolapse.

## Early Postoperative Complications

Hypotony, suprachoroidal hemorrhage, diplopia, tube obstruction, and aqueous misdirection are complications that typically arise within the first few months after placement of a GDD.

## Late Postoperative Complications

Late complications of GDD surgery include erosion of the tube or plate, migration of the tube, endophthalmitis, diplopia, and corneal decompensation.

# SURGICAL OUTCOMES: SCIENTIFIC EVIDENCE

## Comparison with Trabeculectomy

Wilson et al. conducted the first prospective, randomized trial comparing a GDD to trabeculectomy. A total of 123 patients were randomized to receive an Ahmed glaucoma valve or trabeculectomy as a primary surgical procedure for glaucoma. With an average follow-up of 31 months, the mean IOPs and adjunctive medications were comparable in the two groups. No statistically significant differences between groups were found in visual acuity, visual field, and short- or long-term complications. The cumulative probabilities of success were similar between both procedures at final follow-up (68.1% trabeculectomy group versus 69.8% Ahmed group).[7,8]

The TVT Study is a multicenter randomized clinical trial that evaluated the safety and efficacy of the 350-mm$^2$ Baerveldt glaucoma implant to trabeculectomy with mitomycin C in patients who had undergone previous cataract extraction with intraocular lens implantation and/or failed filtering surgery. Tube shunt surgery had a higher success rate than trabeculectomy throughout 5 years of follow-up (70.2% tube group vs 53.1% trabeculectomy group). No significant differences in IOP and glaucoma medical therapy were observed between the two procedures at 5 years. Early postoperative complications were more frequently seen after trabeculectomy compared with tube shunt placement, although most were transient and self-limited. The rates of late postoperative complications, serious complications, and vision loss were similar with both procedures. A higher rate of reoperation for glaucoma was seen after trabeculectomy relative to tube shunt surgery.[3,9]

## Comparison of Different Aqueous Shunt Types

There have been numerous retrospective case series comparing different aqueous shunts. Several studies found significant differences with regard to surgical success, but average follow-up in these studies was under 2 years.[10-12] Tsai et al. conducted one of the larger studies with an average follow-up of 4 years and found similar success with the Ahmed valve and Baerveldt implants.[13,14] Several other case series also found similar outcomes between different aqueous shunt types.[15-18] Patient selection bias and surgeon shunt preference may have affected results in these retrospective studies.

Two ongoing randomized clinical trials are comparing the safety and efficacy of the Ahmed glaucoma valve implant (model FP7) and Baerveldt glaucoma implant (model 101-350). The Ahmed Baerveldt Comparison (ABC) study enrolled 276 patients with refractory glaucoma and found that there was no significant difference in the cumulative probability of failure between treatment groups at 1 year (16.4% Ahmed group vs 14.0% Baerveldt group). More patients experienced early postoperative complications and serious complications associated with reoperation and vision loss following Baerveldt implantation.[19] The Ahmed Versus Baerveldt (AVB) study compared these implants in 238 patients, but a higher cumulative probability of failure was observed with the Ahmed implant compared with the Baerveldt implant (43% Ahmed group vs 28% Baerveldt group). The overall rate of complications was similar in both treatment groups, although there was a higher incidence of corneal edema in the Baerveldt group and a higher incidence of bleb encapsulation in the Ahmed group.[20,21] The Baerveldt implant produced lower IOPs and a lesser need for adjunctive glaucoma medications when compared with the Ahmed implant in both the ABC and AVB study, but this difference did not reach statistical significance in the ABC study.

### Comparison of Similar Aqueous Shunts with Different End Plate Size or Composition

Several retrospective case series have compared similar aqueous shunts with different endplate size or composition. No significant differences in the rates of surgical success were detected in any of the studies comparing various Baerveldt, Molteno, or Ahmed implants. Siegner et al. did a find a lower mean IOP when evaluating the 350 mm$^2$ Baerveldt implant compared with the 200 mm$^2$ and 250 mm$^2$ Baerveldt implants, while Hinkle et al. reported lower IOP in patients with the silicone plate (model FP7) Ahmed implant compared with the polypropylene plate (model S2) implant.[22,23] Law et al. performed a similar study looking at the silicone and polypropylene implants and did not observe a difference in IOP reduction.[24]

There have been three randomized clinical trials comparing similar aqueous shunts with different end plate size or composition. Heuer et al. compared the single-plate and double-plate Molteno implants in 132 patients with non-neovascular glaucoma. The double-plate group had a higher rate of success, although there was also a higher incidence of choroidal hemorrhages, flat anterior chambers, phthisis bulbi, and serous choroidal effusions requiring surgical drainage.[25] Lloyd et al. enrolled 73 patients with uncontrolled non-neovascular glaucoma with aphakia, pseudophakia, or failed filters and randomized them to placement of a 350 mm$^2$ or 500 mm$^2$ Baerveldt implant. At 18 months, similar rates of surgical success were found.[26] Britt et al. recruited an additional 34 patients and provided long-term follow-up on all 107 patients. At 5 years, there was a higher rate of success in the 350 mm$^2$ Baerveldt group with no significant difference in the rate of vision loss or complications.[27] Ishida et al. performed a multicenter trial comparing the silicone plate (model FP7) Ahmed implant to the polypropylene plate (model S2) implant. A higher rate of success and lower mean IOP was observed in the silicone plate group. There was no significant difference with regard to vision loss, but there was a higher incidence of surgical complications in the polypropylene plate group.[28]

## PLACE OF THE TECHNIQUE IN SURGICAL ARMAMENTARIUM

GDDs are now being used more frequently in the management of glaucoma. These devices are no longer solely indicated for patients with refractory glaucoma. GDDs are an acceptable treatment option for patients with medically uncontrolled glaucoma who are at lower risk of filtration failure, such as those with prior cataract extraction and/or failed filtering surgery. There are numerous types of GDDs that are commercially available, and they differ in the composition and size of the end plate. Results from the aforementioned studies provide valuable information to guide surgical decision making. Ultimately, the choice of surgical procedure depends not only on evidence from the literature and specific patient characteristics but also on the surgeon's comfort and experience with each implant.

## REFERENCES

1. Desai MA, Gedde SJ, Feuer WJ, et al. Practice preferences for glaucoma surgery: a survey of the American Glaucoma Society in 2008. Ophthalmic Surg Lasers Imaging. 2011;42(3):202-8.
2. Ramulu PY, Corcoran KJ, Corcoran SL, et al. Utilization of various glaucoma surgeries and procedures in Medicare beneficiaries from 1995 to 2004. Ophthalmology. 2007;114(12):2265-70.
3. Gedde SJ, Schiffman JC, Feuer WJ, et al. Treatment outcomes in the Tube Versus Trabeculectomy (TVT) study after five years of follow-up. Am J Ophthalmol. 2012;153(5):789-803.
4. Prata JA Jr., Minckler DS, Green RL. Pseudo-Brown's syndrome as a complication of glaucoma drainage implant surgery. Ophthalmic Surg. 1993;24(9):608-11.

5. Ball SF, Ellis GS Jr., Herrington RG, et al. Brown's superior oblique tendon syndrome after Baerveldt glaucoma implant. Arch Ophthalmol. 1992;110(10):1368.
6. Smith SL, Starita RJ, Fellman RL, et al. Early clinical experience with the Baerveldt 350-mm$^2$ glaucoma implant and associated extraocular muscle imbalance. Ophthalmology. 1993;100(6): 914-8.
7. Wilson M, Mendis U, Smith S, et al. Ahmed glaucoma valve implant vs. trabeculectomy in the surgical treatment of glaucoma: A randomized clinical trial. Am J Ophthalmol. 2000;130:267-73.
8. Wilson M, Mendis U, Paliwal A, et al. Long-term follow-up of primary glaucoma surgery with Ahmed glaucoma valve implant versus trabeculectomy. Am J Ophthalmol. 2003;136: 464-70.
9. Gedde SJ, Herndon LW, Brandt JD, et al. Postoperative complications in the Tube Versus Trabeculectomy (TVT) study during five years of follow-up. Am J Ophthalmol. 2012;153(5):804-14.
10. Aung T, Seah SK. Glaucoma drainage implants in Asian eyes. Ophthalmology. 1998;105(11):2117-22.
11. Goulet RJ, 3rd, Phan AD, Cantor LB, et al. Efficacy of the Ahmed S2 glaucoma valve compared with the Baerveldt 250-mm$^2$ glaucoma implant. Ophthalmology. 2008;115(7):1141-7.
12. Taglia DP, Perkins TW, Gangnon R, et al. Comparison of the Ahmed Glaucoma Valve, the Krupin Eye Valve with Disk, and the double-plate Molteno implant. J Glaucoma. 2002;11(4):347-53.
13. Tsai JC, Johnson CC, Dietrich MS. The Ahmed shunt versus the Baerveldt shunt for refractory glaucoma: a single-surgeon comparison of outcome. Ophthalmology. 2003;110(9):1814-21.
14. Tsai JC, Johnson CC, Kammer JA, et al. The Ahmed shunt versus the Baerveldt shunt for refractory glaucoma II: longer-term outcomes from a single surgeon. Ophthalmology. 2006;113(6): 913-7.
15. Smith MF, Doyle JW, Sherwood MB. Comparison of the Baerveldt glaucoma implant with the double-plate Molteno drainage implant. Arch Ophthalmol. 1995;113(4):444-7.
16. Syed HM, Law SK, Nam SH, et al. Baerveldt-350 implant versus Ahmed valve for refractory glaucoma: a case-controlled comparison. J Glaucoma. 2004;13(1):38-45.
17. Wang JC, See JL, Chew PT. Experience with the use of Baerveldt and Ahmed glaucoma drainage implants in an Asian population. Ophthalmology. 2004;111(7):1383-8.
18. Yalvac IS, Eksioglu U, Satana B, et al. Long-term results of Ahmed glaucoma valve and Molteno implant in neovascular glaucoma. Eye. 2007;21(1):65-70.
19. Budenz DL, Barton K, Feuer WJ, et al. Treatment outcomes in the Ahmed Baerveldt Comparison Study after 1 year of follow-up. Ophthalmology. 2011;118(3):443-2.
20. Christakis PG, Tsai JC, Zurakowski D, et al. The Ahmed Versus Baerveldt study: design, baseline patient characteristics, and intraoperative complications. Ophthalmology. 2011;118(11): 2172-9.
21. Christakis PG, Kalenak JW, Zurakowski D, et al. The Ahmed Versus Baerveldt study: one-year treatment outcomes. Ophthalmology. 2011;118(11):2180-9.
22. Siegner SW, Netland PA, Urban RC Jr., et al. Clinical experience with the Baerveldt glaucoma drainage implant. Ophthalmology. 1995;102(9):1298-307.
23. Hinkle DM, Zurakowski D, Ayyala RS. A comparison of the polypropylene plate Ahmed glaucoma valve to the silicone plate Ahmed glaucoma flexible valve. Eur J Ophthalmol. 2007; 17(5):696-701.
24. Law SK, Nguyen A, Coleman AL, et al. Comparison of safety and efficacy between silicone and polypropylene Ahmed glaucoma valves in refractory glaucoma. Ophthalmology. 2005; 112(9):1514-20.
25. Heuer DK, Lloyd MA, Abrams DA, et al. Which is better? One or two? A randomized clinical trial of single-plate versus double-plate Molteno implantation for glaucomas in aphakia and pseudophakia. Ophthalmology. 1992;99(10):1512-9.
26. Lloyd MA, Baerveldt G, Fellenbaum PS, et al. Intermediate-term results of a randomized clinical trial of the 350- versus the 500-mm$^2$ Baerveldt implant. Ophthalmology. 1994;101(8): 1456-63.
27. Britt MT, LaBree LD, Lloyd MA, et al. Randomized clinical trial of the 350-mm$^2$ versus the 500-mm$^2$ Baerveldt implant: longer term results: is bigger better? Ophthalmology. 1999;106(12): 2312-8.
28. Ishida K, Netland PA. Ahmed Glaucoma Valve implantation in African American and white patients. Arch Ophthalmol. 2006; 124(6):800-6.

CHAPTER

# 43

# Angle Surgery: Trabeculotomy and Goniotomy

Ronald Leigh Fellman, Davinder S Grover

## INTRODUCTION

The conventional outflow pathway is the pressure-dependent trabecular route (trabecular-juxtacanalicular-canal-collectors-aqueous veins) compared with the pressure-independent uveo-scleral pathway (Fig. 43-1). Both trabeculotomy and goniotomy remain dependable angle procedures for congenital glaucoma; in addition, the indications for modern-day trabeculotomy continue to expand for adult glaucomas. This is because circumnavigation of the canal improves outcomes for congenital and juvenile glaucomas and has broadened the indications for adult primary and secondary glaucomas. The impetus to expand trabeculotomy continues due to the intense desire to improve flow into the natural drainage channels and thereby avoid bleb formation. Improved methods of cleaving the canal open along with the use of an illuminated microcatheter (iTrack, Ellex, Minneapolis, MN) to explore the canal have made this possible. The ability to cleave open the canal for 360° has enhanced success rates compared with the more antiquated trabeculotomy methods of 50 years ago. Most recently, gonioscopy-assisted conjunctival sparing sutureless ab interno trabeculotomy alternatives have become available. Trabectome surgery, a form of ab interno trabeculotomy, is reviewed in another chapter.

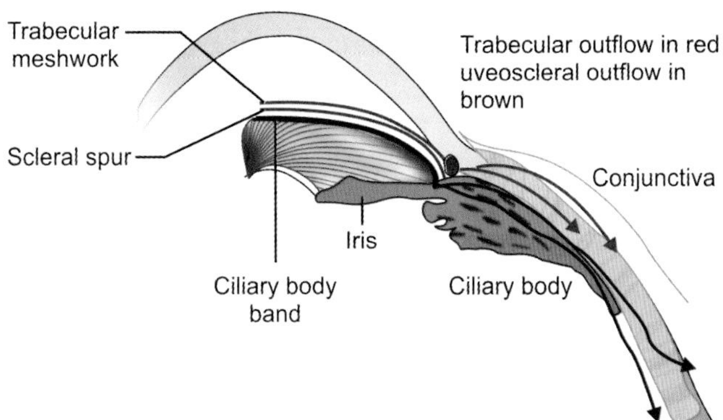


**Figure 43-1** Aqueous outflow pathways. There are two known major outflow pathways in the human eye: (1) the pressure-dependent trabecular, collector channels, aqueous veins pathway comprises approximately 75% of outflow and (2) the pressure-independent uveoscleral path comprises approximately 25%.

Goniotomy surgery remains similar to the original description by Barkan[1] but with improvements in goniolenses to view the angle along with viscoelastics to maintain chamber. One disadvantage for goniotomy is a cloudy cornea that limits visualization of the angle. Some authors have tried endoscopic goniotomy,[2] which eliminates this problem; however, this needs further study. The lack of a three-dimensional view makes this approach very challenging. Only a segment of the circumference of the canal system is opened at one sitting with goniotomy, but both trabeculotomy and goniotomy remain steadfast angle procedures for congenital glaucomas.

## INDICATIONS

### Congenital Glaucoma

Trabeculotomy and goniotomy are both highly effective in primary congenital glaucoma, but they are less effective in secondary forms of congenital and developmental glaucomas such as aniridia, Axenfeld–Reigers syndrome, and many other syndromes related to various chromosomal abnormalities where severe anterior segment dysgenesis may exist.

### Juvenile Glaucoma

Glaucoma diagnosed between the ages of 4 and 35, namely juvenile glaucoma, is usually associated with a less severe component of trabeculodysgenesis and both angle procedures may be highly effective.

### Adult Glaucoma

Worldwide, trabeculotomy is a primary procedure for many forms of open angle glaucoma as well as some forms of secondary glaucoma such as pseudoexfoliation and pigmentary glaucoma. Goniotomy sometimes termed goniotrabeculotomy is used to a lesser extent for adult glaucoma.

### Steroid-Induced Glaucoma

Trabeculotomy may be effective in steroid-induced glaucoma[3] because the procedure cleaves open the trabecular meshwork, the site thought to be most responsible for the elevated intraocular pressure (IOP) in the setting of steroids.

### Failed Filtration and Shunt Surgery

Filtration and shunt surgery both abandon the patient's natural drainage system; however, when these procedures fail, trabeculotomy may still lower IOP by improving flow into the natural collector system, rejuvenating this abandoned pathway.

## CONTRAINDICATIONS

- Newborn glaucoma, glaucoma discovered during the first month of life, typically carries a poorer prognosis for angle surgery; this is not an absolute contraindication but an established fact. The family should be informed that the success of the angle procedure is much lower when glaucoma is discovered within the first month of life
- A cloudy cornea may prevent an adequate view of the angle during goniotomy, even after denuding the epithelium. The surgeon should have a backup procedure in mind prior to surgery
- Extensive peripheral anterior synechiae (PAS) due to NVG or uveitis prevent adequate cleavage of the angle with trabeculotomy or goniotomy, and reformation of PAS is common
- Aniridic patients usually have a severely malformed canal preventing external cannulation during a trabeculotomy ab externo and may be better initial candidates for goniotomy or drainage implant surgery
- Adult patients with far advanced glaucoma may not tolerate the IOP spike associated with transient hyphema from an angle procedure and may require additional urgent filtration or shunt surgery.

## SURGICAL TECHNIQUES

### Goniotomy

Goniotomy is most commonly performed in congenital and juvenile glaucomas, and is rarely used today in adult glaucoma. An examination under anesthesia (EUA) is imperative for several reasons: to verify IOP measurement (measured immediately upon induction), to evaluate the disk, to describe the iridocorneal angle and ultimately decipher the mechanism of IOP elevation, and to formulate the surgical plan. A relatively clear cornea greatly facilitates the ease of goniotomy. Under general anesthesia, the chamber angle is visualized through a Swan–Jacob goniolens, or similar goniolens. If the cornea is cloudy, the epithelium may be removed with a Q-tip to improve visualization. Typically, the surgeon is seated temporally, the microscope is tilted toward the surgeon for approximately 30°, and the head of the patient tilted away from the surgeon to view the angle. A temporal paracentesis is made followed by an intracameral miotic to protect the lens as well as a viscoelastic to keep the chamber formed. The goniotomy blade is inserted into the chamber followed by application of the goniolens to view the blade tip near the angle. The angle is incised just under Schwalbe's line and advanced clockwise and counterclockwise to open several clock hours of the malformed angle. Avoid excessive pressure with the goniotomy blade, as the tissue is typically delicate. During the goniotomy, the peripheral angle tissues are seen to fall posteriorly as the canal is visualized. Upon completion of the goniotomy, one should remove the vast majority of the viscoelastic. One can leave a small amount of viscoelastic in the anterior chamber (10–20% fill) in an attempt to minimize postoperative hypotony and protect against blood reflux from the canal.

### Trabeculotomy Ab Externo

Ab externo technique implies using an external approach to identify and open Schlemm's canal, which usually involves a conjunctival dissection and a scleral flap. There are three major advancements regarding ab externo surgery: the first involves instrumentation and technology, the second is extent of angle opened at one sitting, and the third is innovative techniques. Regarding instrumentation to open the canal, the procedure has evolved from using a metal trabeculotome, to a filamentary suture, and lastly to an illuminated microcatheter to cannulate and cleave the canal.

### Description of Technique

*Identification of Schlemm's canal*: Following adequate anesthesia, a superior corneal traction suture is placed and the eye rotated inferiorly. Some surgeons, however, prefer the opposite and place the traction suture inferiorly to expose the inferior tissues for surgery. This spares the superior tissues for future filtration surgery. For simplicity, the superior site approach will be described. After the globe is rotated inferiorly, a fornix-based conjunctival peritomy is created dissecting the Tenon's and conjunctiva posteriorly in order to undermine both layers. Minimal wet-field cautery is used for hemostasis in the intended area of scleral dissection. A two-third thickness limbal-based scleral flap is outlined in the sclera and dissected evenly into clear cornea. As the limbus is approached, one can identify the scleral spur as the circumlinear white area of condensation of scleral fibers. Schlemm's canal is usually located directly anterior to the scleral spur. Make a 1–2 mm long scratch incision with a microsurgical blade directly perpendicular to the scleral spur, equidistant across the spur. If the location is correct, the canal is identified. Clues that one has correctly identified Schlemm's canal are the presence of a darker zone or visualizing blood or aqueous leak out once the canal is unroofed. At this juncture, slightly extend the incision laterally, perpendicular to the initial scratch incision (parallel to the spur). The canal zone appears darker than surrounding tissue. Once the canal is identified, there are three methods to cleave it open: (a) metal trabeculotomy with a trabeculotome, (b) suture trabeculotomy with 6-0 prolene suture, and (c) iTrack microcatheter.

## Metal Trabeculotomy

After identifying the canal, a viscoelastic is injected into the anterior chamber to tamponade the bleeding that refluxes through the collector system once the trabecular meshwork is incised. A metal trabeculotome, either a Harms, McPherson, or similar probed instrument, is carefully inserted into the canal in one direction, using the designated right- or left-handed curvature of the instrument. An overlying guide is usually present on the instrument to aide in tracking the extent and location of the trabeculotome in the canal. Once fully inserted to the hilt, the instrument is gently rotated into the anterior chamber, staying parallel to the iris during the rotation, cleaving open the corresponding segment of the canal. After opening approximately 5 clock hours of the angle with right and left approaches, the majority of the viscoelastic is removed, the scleral flap sutured in a watertight fashion, and the fornix-based conjunctival incision closed according to surgeon preference. A miotic is instilled along with topical and/or subconjunctival antibiotic and corticosteroid and the eye is patched and shielded. In adults, it is common to administer an oral carbonic anhydrase inhibitor, CAI, in the recovery room for an IOP spike is common on postoperative day one.

## Circumferential Trabeculotomy

After the external identification of Schlemm's canal (as described above), a 5-0 or 6-0 prolene suture is prepared for entry and cleavage of the canal. When the suture is removed from its casing, it typically has an inherent curvature. This curved portion of the suture is useful for it serves as a guide to follow the natural contour of the canal as the suture is advanced. Thermally blunt one end of the suture with a high temperature fine tip cautery to create a small bulb on the end of the suture. Insertion of this thermally blunted end is less likely to tear or hang up in the canal. Prepare a length of suture that will easily circumnavigate the canal for 360° along with an additional 10 mm in order to pull the suture ends after canal circumnavigation. Once the prolene suture is prepared, rest the suture with its curvature aligned over the limbus with the blunted end parallel to the limbus ready for insertion into the canal. Thus, the suture rests with its natural curvature aligned over the limbus. Carefully insert the blunted end of the suture into the canal, without tearing through into the anterior chamber. Slowly, methodically, advance the suture until it traverses 360° and emerges form the other side of the cutdown site.

Once the suture has circumnavigated the canal for 360°, grasp each end and pull tangentially along the limbus to cleave open the entire canal. Pre-place viscoelastic in the anterior chamber to tamponade the bleeding, maintain the anterior chamber, and protect the lens. The suture can be seen through the cornea as it cleaves the canal and appears in the anterior chamber. After opening the canal, the suture or catheter is removed and the anterior chamber washed out. If the iris presents through the initial scleral cutdown site, a small iridotomy is necessary. Typically some viscoelastic remains in the eye to reduce bleeding. The scleral flap is closed in a watertight fashion along with the conjunctiva. Great care is exercised to make sure the flap closure is watertight in order to avoid bleb formation. Antibiotic and corticosteroid are used per surgeon's preference. The technique is similar for the microcatheter (which is currently our preferred ab externo procedure, *see* Figs. 43-2A to W).

## Options for Failure to Circumnavigate the Canal

Occasionally, the suture or microcatheter will not advance the entire length of the canal and will stop around 180°. There are numerous methods to troubleshoot this situation. The most common approaches are (in order of complexity) as follows: (1) Retract the probe 2 clock hours, apply external limbal pressure with the tip of a muscle hook (or similar instrument) slightly before the point of obstruction, and advance the suture again. Oftentimes, the suture or catheter will pass the point of prior obstruction because external pressure closes off

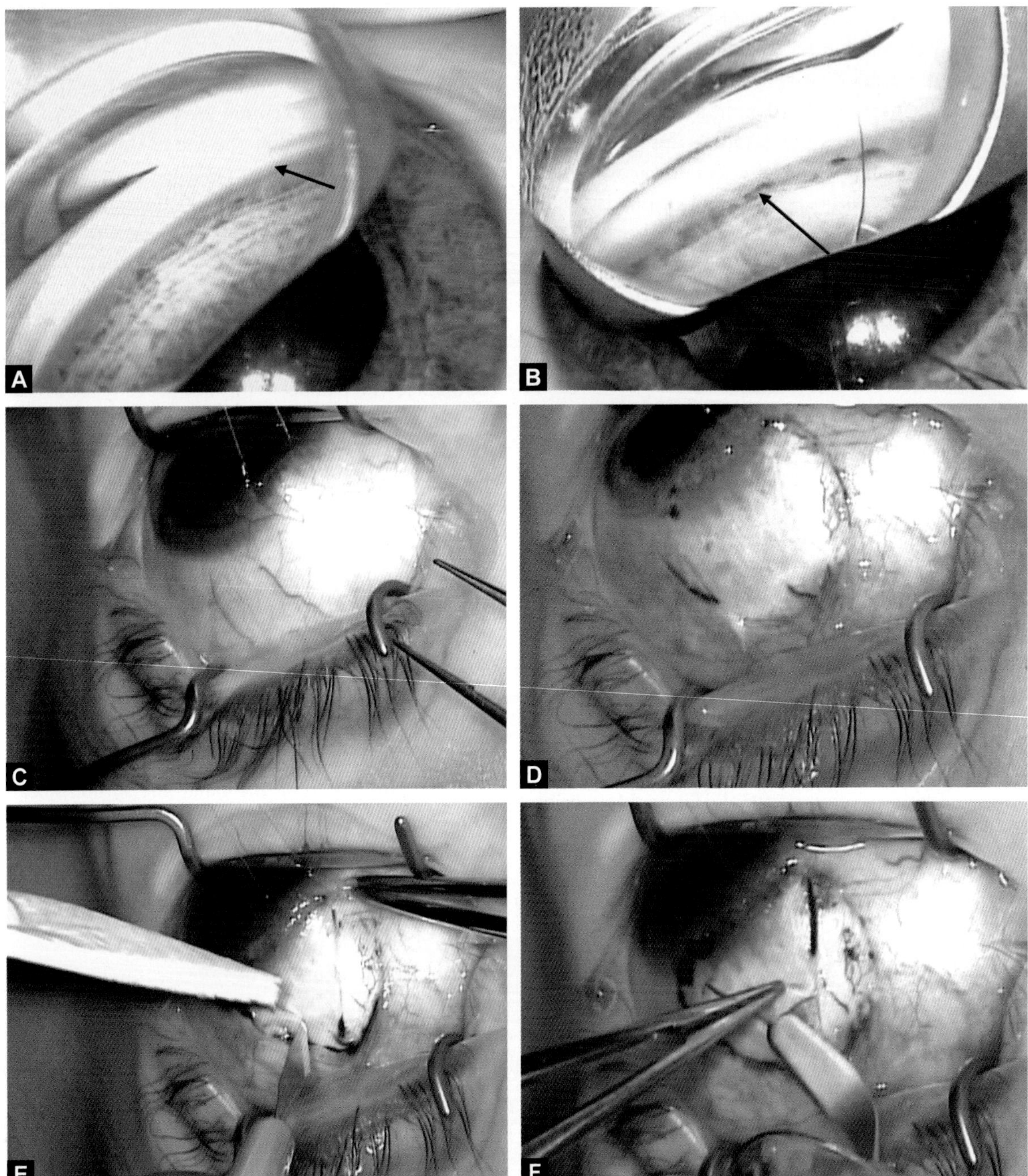


**Figures 43-2A to F** Trabeculotomy ab externo with iTrack microcatheter. (A) Age-appropriate angle of right eye. Relatively normal-appearing angle of the unaffected right eye of 6-month-old infant. The intraocular pressure (IOP) was 15 mm Hg, cornea clear, disk normal, and angle appeared immature with a difficult to visualize scleral spur, but overall relatively normal compared with OS. The arrow points to the ground glass appearance of the lightly pigmented trabecular meshwork region. (B) Dysgenic angle of fellow left eye. The arrow indicates peripheral iris atrophy. These darker areas occur due to show through of the posterior iris neuroepithelium, a common finding in congenital glaucoma. The outflow structures above the arrow appear poorly developed, with poor identification of normal angle structures, a form of trabeculodysgenesis. The IOP was 34 mm Hg, Haab striae were noted and the disk revealed glaucomatous damage, requiring surgery that follows in the following figures. (C) Corneal traction suture. Pass a 7-0 or 8-0 vicryl suture through the superior cornea and rotate the globe inferiorly. This provides excellent exposure of the superior tissues. (D) Fornix-based conjunctival flap. Prepare a fornix-based conjunctival flap followed by light wet-field cautery. Avoid excessive cautery that causes scleral shrinkage and potential unwanted filtration through the flap. (E) Outline the scleral flap. This large 5 × 5 mm scleral flap provides an adequate scleral bed area to allow for exploration of the canal. Sometimes the canal is more anterior or posterior to the scleral spur and a large flap allows adequate area to search for the flap with more than one radial incision if necessary, and adequate coverage of the entry site to allow for a watertight closure. (F) Initiate the scleral flap. The tendency is to make the flap too thin for oftentimes the scleral tissue is stretched from glaucoma. Persist to create a thick two-third thickness even scleral flap.

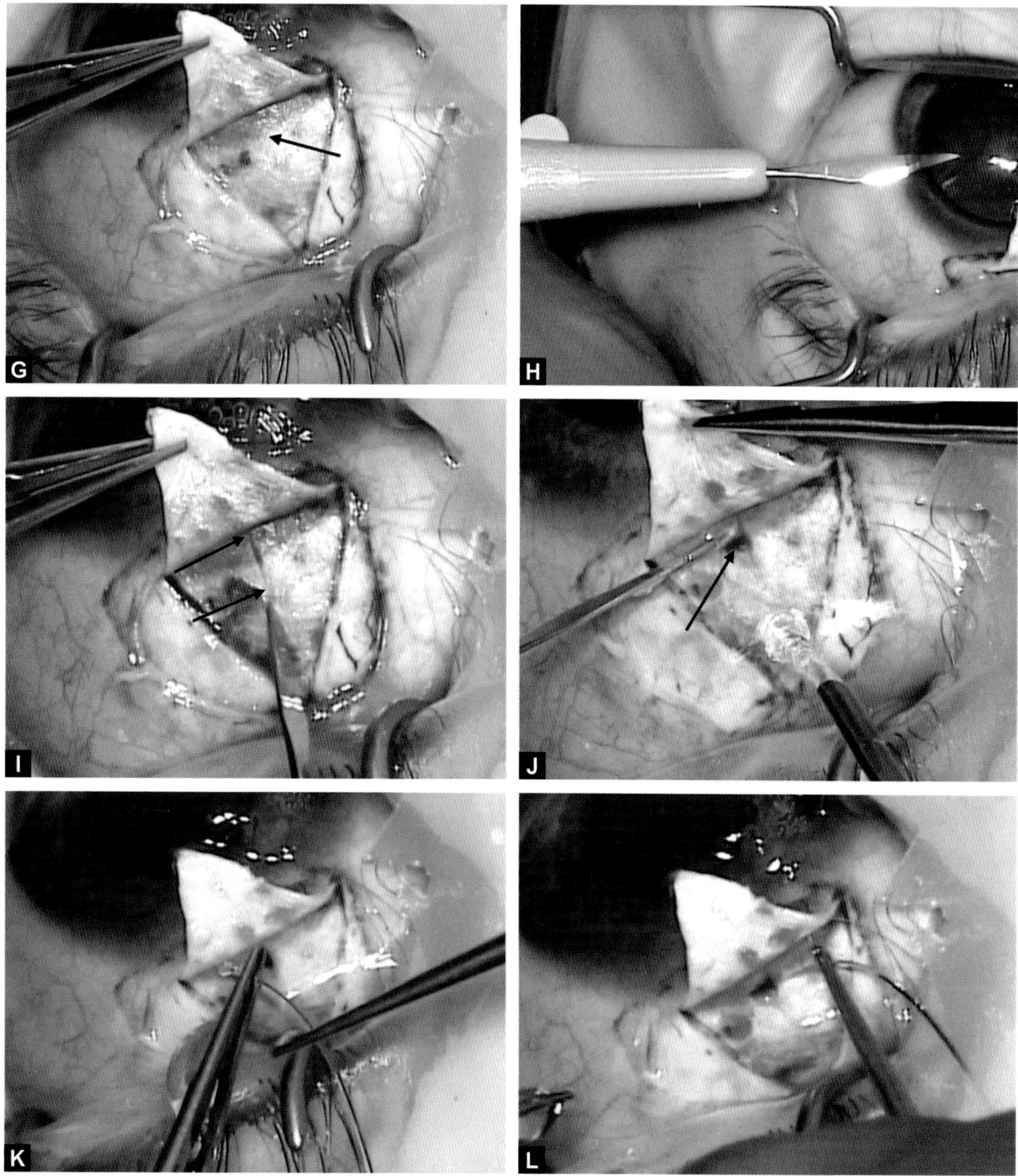


**Figures 43-2G to L** (G) Fashion scleral flap. The flap is fashioned into clear cornea to allow for anterior access to the canal. This flap is uniform and exceptionally well prepared, the first step for successful trabeculotomy. The arrow points to the scleral spur for the canal anticipated to be directly anterior to this vital landmark, but not always. (H) Temporal paracentesis. The paracentesis allows for administration of intracameral acetylcholine and viscoelastic along with washout of blood and viscoelastic as needed. (I) Radial incision traversing scleral spur. Use a super sharp blade to cut down, fiber by fiber over the spur. The black arrows indicate the extent of the incision, approximately 1–2 mm on each side of the spur. This is necessary for the canal could be anterior or posterior to the spur. Once the roof of the canal is pierced, a darker color is seen, sometimes pigment and oftentimes blood. (J) T-cut to expose floor of canal. Upon suspecting the canal, enlarge the incision in a tangential direction in order to expose the canal. Typically, the canal appears darker than the surrounding tissue and aqueous may ooze from it. If the canal is not easily seen with the first T-cut, prepare a second one on the opposite side. (K) Flexible iTrack microcatheter. The 250 μ tip of the microcatheter is illuminated allowing the surgeon to know its location at all times, an excellent safety feature. Line the tip up tangential to the uncovered canal, making it easier to insert. (L) Insertion of iTrack into Schlemm's canal. The canal access site should be large enough from the T-cut to accommodate the microcatheter. If insertion is difficult, try and enlarge the incision site. Do not force the microcatheter for if it is in the proper location, the catheter is easy to insert and advance.

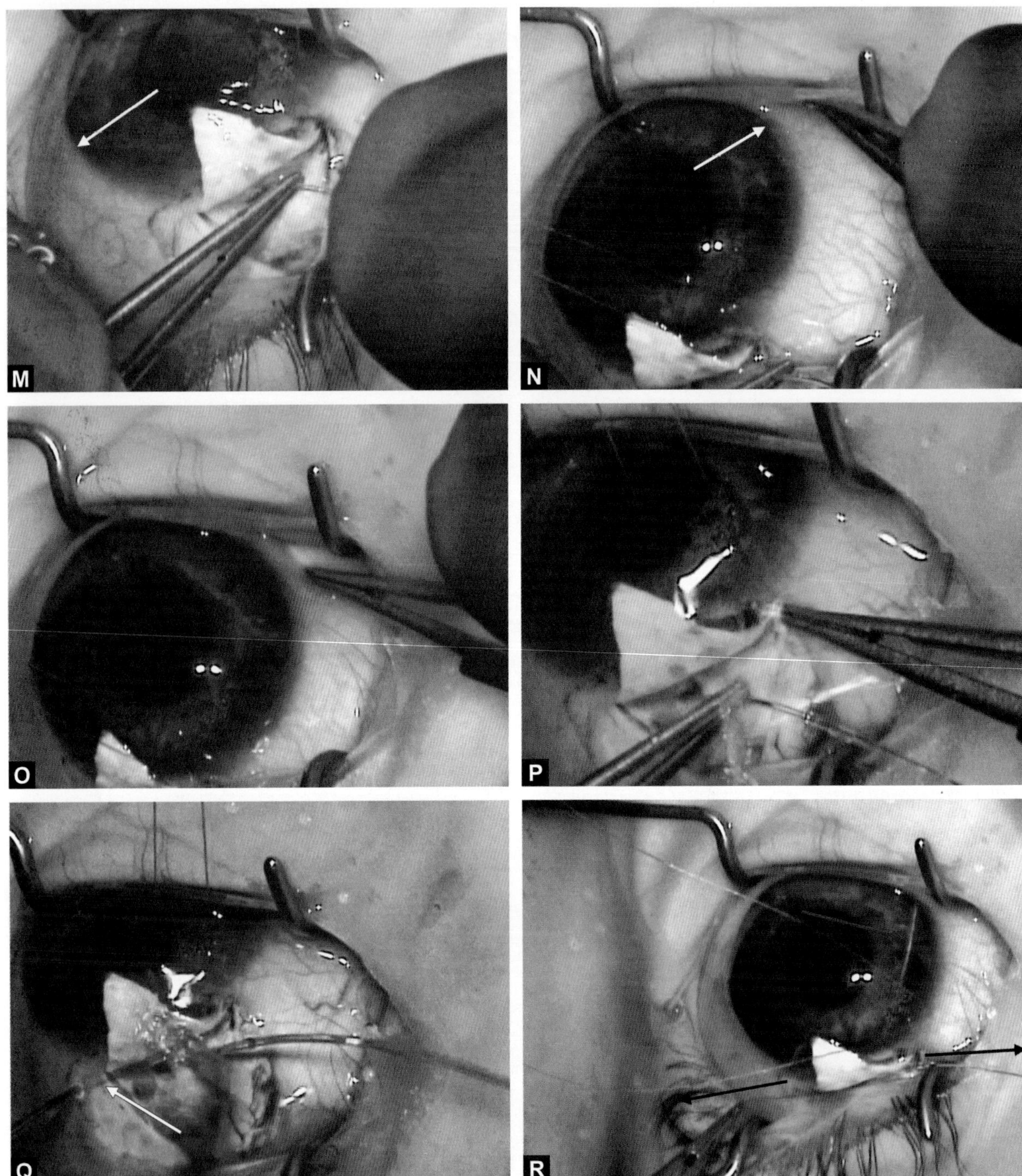


**Figures 43-2M to R** (M) Advance ITrack microcatheter. Initially, a minimal amount of force is necessary to advance the catheter in the canal. Dim the microscope light and track the location of the probe by observing its circumferential progress. The white arrow indicates the illuminated tip seen through the canal at the limbus. (N) Difficulty advancing iTrack. Occasionally the iTrack becomes difficult to advance. This usually occurs because the tip slides into a collector channel. See chapter text for solutions to this dilemma. (O) Focal limbal pressure to advance iTrack. Simultaneously retract the probe 1 clock hour, apply focal pressure slightly before the stopping point and then advance the probe again. It usually will stay in the main canal and advance for the side channel is compressed and closed. (P) Near complete iTrack circumnavigation. The illuminated tip indicates the catheter probe has nearly completed its journey. None of these illuminated advantages are seen with a prolene or nylon suture. (Q) Isolate and grasp the distal catheter tip from the canal. Gently use jewelers or a similar instrument to secure the distal tip of the catheter probe from the canal and pull tangentially to prepare for the drawstring maneuver. (R) Drawstring 360° trabeculotomy maneuver. Grasp both ends of the catheter, black arrows, and pull in a tangential manner in order to cleave the canal for 360°. The red arrow indicates the position of the catheter in the anterior chamber after it first penetrates through the nasal angle. The circumferential process is completed and catheter removed.

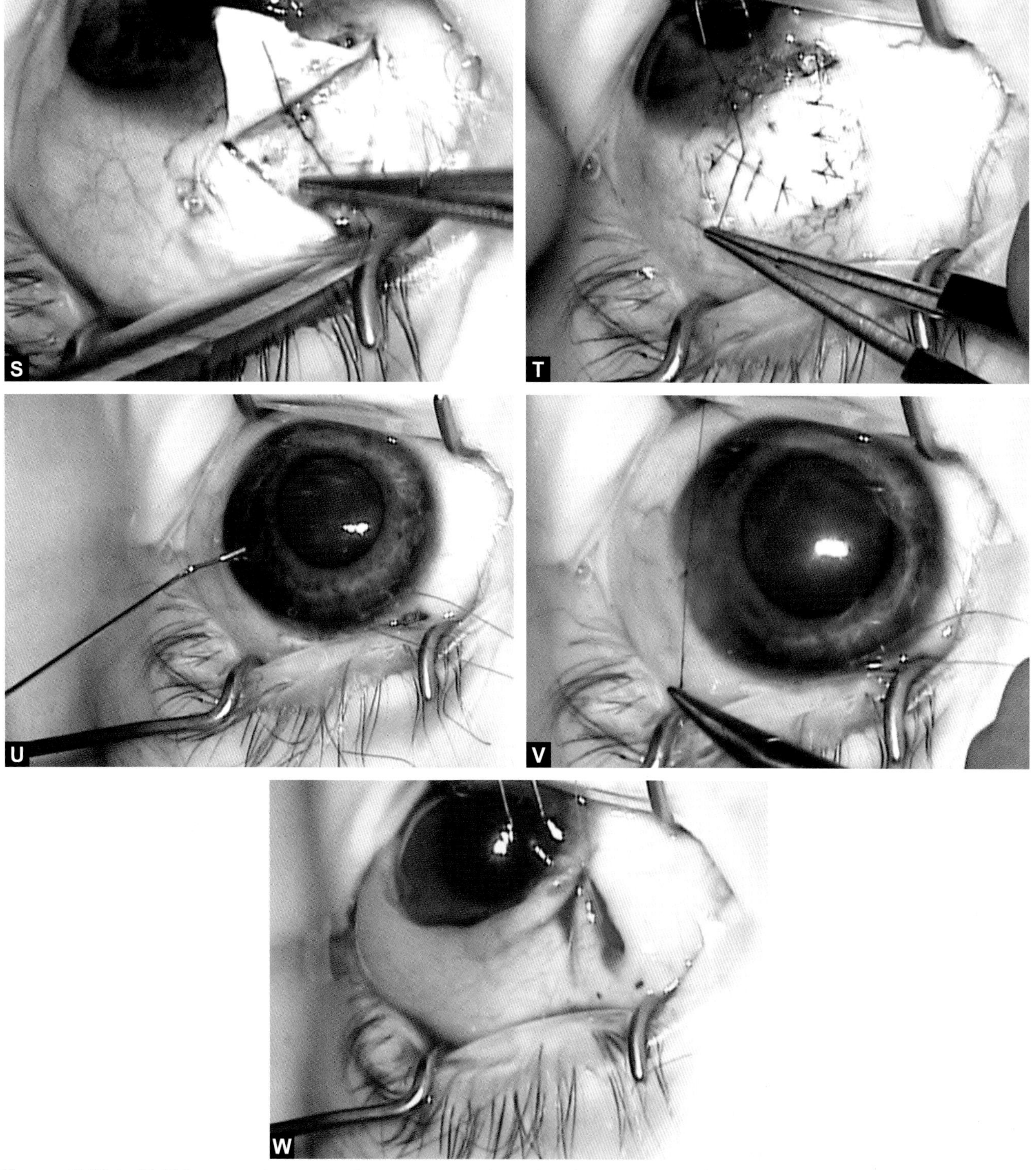

**Figures 43-2S to W** (S) Suture canal access site. Some surgeons prefer to close this site, especially if it enlarges during the procedure. Oftentimes, a small basal iridotomy is necessary if the iris prolapses. (T) Close scleral flap. Close the scleral flap in a watertight fashion with several nylon sutures. Check repeatedly for leaks and add sutures as necessary. (U) Irrigation of anterior chamber. Hyphema is common with trabeculotomy. Once the wound is watertight, repeatedly irrigate blood from the anterior chamber, firm the globe by adding BSS, and then hydrate the wound. Recheck the scleral flap for leakage. (V) Suture paracentesis site. Endophthalmitis is a grave consequence of any intraocular surgery. Unquestionably secure the paracentesis site, especially in infant eyes where the tissue is very elastic. Invariably, this suture may be removed during an examination under anesthesia or at the slit lamp in adults. (W) Closure of conjunctiva. Secure the conjunctiva much like a trabeculectomy closure. This is necessary because no matter how well the scleral flap is closed, a small percentage will leak. A transient bleb may form, but usually disappears within a few weeks.

the side collector channel that the probe initially went down, thus allowing it to continue in the main canal. (2) If this fails, completely retract the probe and reinsert into the canal in the opposite direction. Oftentimes, the probe will go around 360° with ease. (3) If the above two maneuvers fail, consider changing to a microcatheter if a suture was utilized. It is easier to circumnavigate the canal with the microcatheter.

If the suture will not advance past 180°, try and observe the angle with the aide of a gonioprism and visualize the blue prolene suture in the canal or the illuminated catheter tip. Mark the corresponding limbal position where the tip stops, as seen gonioscopically. Open the conjunctiva at this area and fashion a scleral flap over the anticipated spot. Use the same technique to identify the canal and unearth the tip of the suture. Pulling both ends of the suture will cleave half the angle and create a 180° trabeculotomy, which is typically sufficient to control IOP. Depending on the clinical scenario, one may wish to open the other half of the canal by passing the suture in the opposite direct. Remove the suture and close both scleral sites in a watertight fashion. The methodology for using the iTrack microcatheter is very similar to the suture. However, there are numerous advantages to using the microcatheter. The illuminated tip acts as a beacon and immediately shows the surgeon if the tip is following the path of Schlemm's canal. The catheter aids in identification of the canal, enhances safety for the procedure, and minimizes the chance of unknowingly passing the suture into the suprachoroidal space. Moreover, it is easier to circumferentially cannulate the canal with the microcatheter, which decreases surgical and anesthetic times.

## Circumferential Trabeculotomy ab Interno

The ab interno approach is a sutureless, conjunctival sparing two-handed technique and is an exercise in hand–eye coordination. This method involves viewing the canal through a gonioprism, much like goniotomy, but in addition to incising the trabecular meshwork, the canal is subsequently cannulated internally with the iTrack microcatheter. Using microsurgical instruments within the anterior chamber, the catheter is passed 360° around the canal. Thus, a complete circumferential trabeculotomy is performed without violating the conjunctiva or sclera (Figs. 43-3A to M).

## Mechanism of Action

The general concept is that both goniotomy and trabeculotomy improve outflow facility by cleaving open the site of greatest resistance to conventional outflow, the trabecular, and juxtacanalicular tissue. It is likely that the mechanism of action may be different between adults and infants for the healing processes, and etiology of the glaucoma is not the same. A recent histopathology report in adult glaucomas suggests that the enhancement of conventional routes may not be the sole reason for IOP lowering, but that newly created unconventional routes may also play a significant role.[4]

## Postoperative Care

Postoperative care after a trabeculotomy or goniotomy is much simpler than a filtering procedure. The care is very

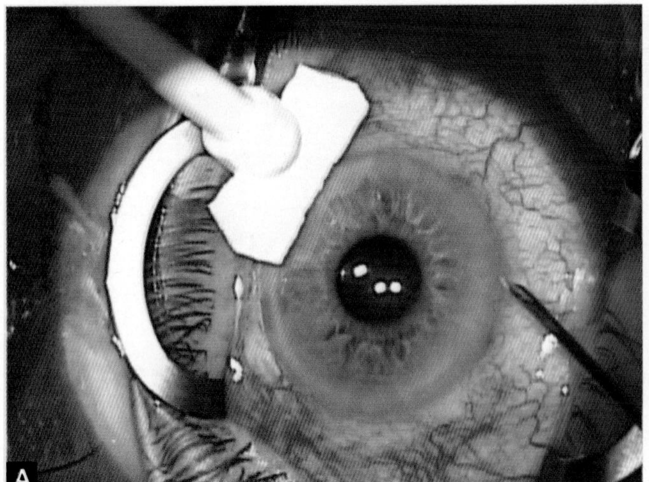


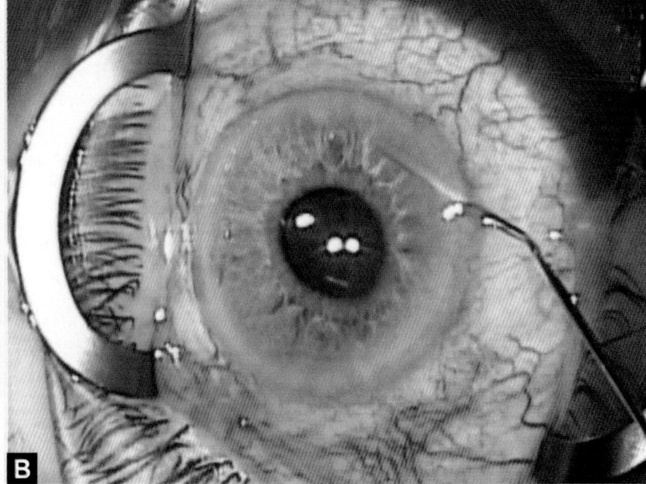


**Figures 43-3A and B** Trabeculotomy ab interno (gonioscopy-assisted transluminal trabeculotomy). (A) Paracentesis track for iTrack microcatheter. Use a 23-gauge needle to create a paracentesis track in this right eye of an 80-year-old with POAG and an open-angle, post failed trabeculectomy. The needle tract should not be radial but more tangential and serves as the insertion site for the microcatheter probe. (B) Inject viscoelastic. Inject Healon GV to maintain anterior chamber depth.

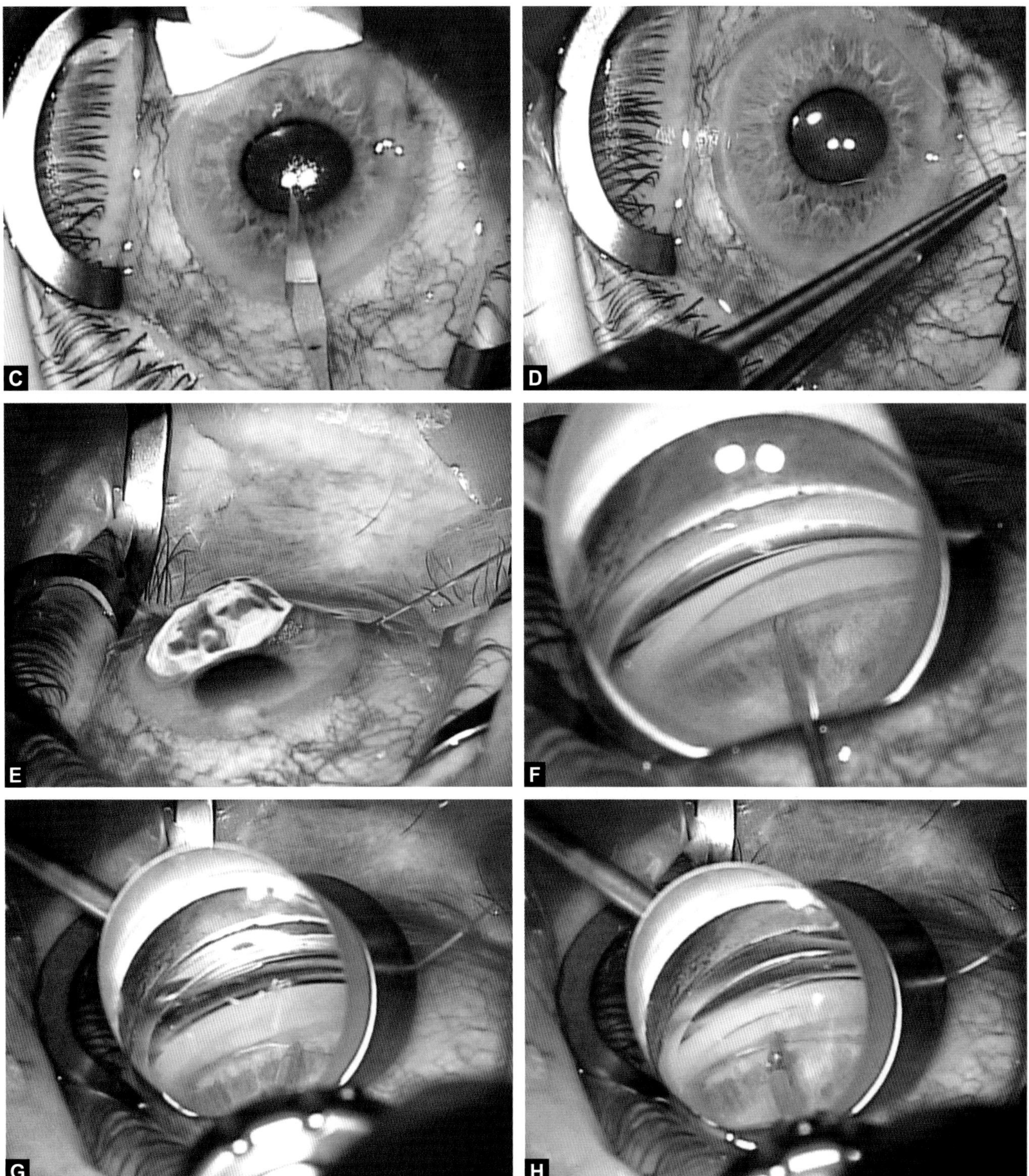


**Figures 43-3C to H** (C) Temporal paracentesis. The temporal paracentesis serves as the access site for the microsurgical instruments. (D) iTrack microcatheter insertion. The microcatheter is inserted at approximately the 5 o'clock hour aiming for the nasal angle. (E) Microscope and head tilted for temporal approach. The eye is positioned to gain visualization of the nasal angle and a viscoelastic coupling agent applied to the cornea. (F) Goniotomy canal entry site. Use a gonitomy blade visualized through a Swann–Jacob goniolens in order to incise the trabecular meshwork. (G) iTrack insertion into Schlemm's canal. Inside the anterior chamber, gently grasp the iTrack with a microsurgical instrument and guide it through the incision created by the goniotomy knife. (H) Advance iTrack catheter. Continue to advance the iTrack until it circumnavigates the canal.

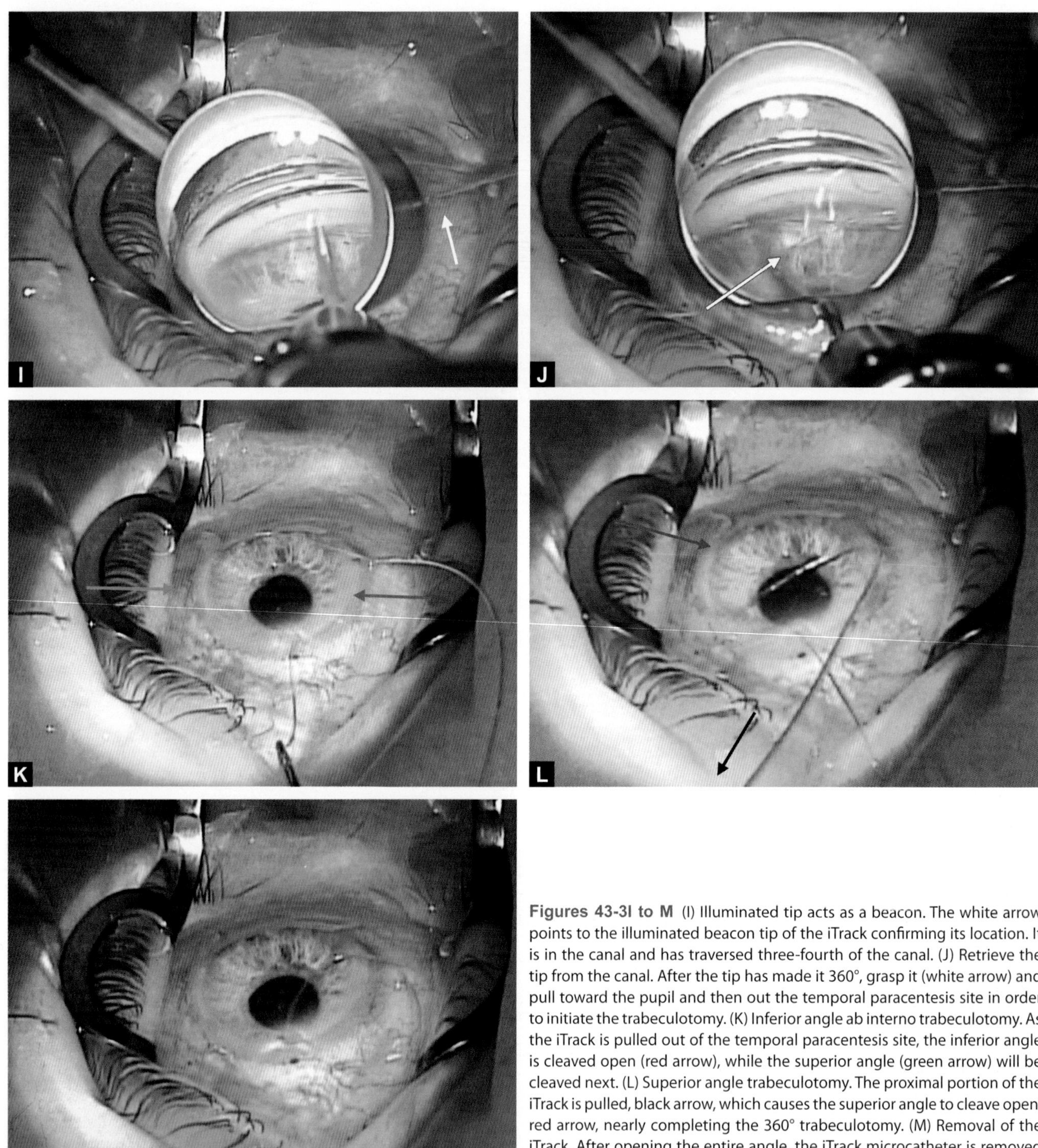


**Figures 43-3I to M** (I) Illuminated tip acts as a beacon. The white arrow points to the illuminated beacon tip of the iTrack confirming its location. It is in the canal and has traversed three-fourth of the canal. (J) Retrieve the tip from the canal. After the tip has made it 360°, grasp it (white arrow) and pull toward the pupil and then out the temporal paracentesis site in order to initiate the trabeculotomy. (K) Inferior angle ab interno trabeculotomy. As the iTrack is pulled out of the temporal paracentesis site, the inferior angle is cleaved open (red arrow), while the superior angle (green arrow) will be cleaved next. (L) Superior angle trabeculotomy. The proximal portion of the iTrack is pulled, black arrow, which causes the superior angle to cleave open, red arrow, nearly completing the 360° trabeculotomy. (M) Removal of the iTrack. After opening the entire angle, the iTrack microcatheter is removed and viscoelastic irrigated from the anterior chamber and paracentesis sites hydrated. The procedure is completed.

similar to that of a cataract procedure with the use of a topical antibiotic for one week and a tapering dose of topical corticosteroid. The IOP may rise due to hyphema during the first week or later due to steroid responsiveness necessitating glaucoma therapy. The judicious use of a weak miotic at bedtime may help reduce PAS formation. Additionally, until the blood clears, standard hyphema precautions are given, such as limited activity and head of bed elevation.

## Specific Instrumentation

Overall, the instrumentation for trabeculotomy and goniotomy are relatively simple and straightforward.

### Goniotomy

- Koeppe goniolens to evaluate the angle preoperatively
- Handheld biomicroscope to view the angle and understand the landmarks stereoscopically prior to surgery through the Koeppe lens
- Barkan or similar goniolens to view the angle during surgery
- Goniotomy knife.

### Trabeculotomy Ab Externo

- For suture trabeculotomy, 5-0 or 6-0 prolene suture or 4-0 or 5-0 nylon suture
- Intraoperative sterile gonioprism handy to view angle if necessary
- For microcatheter trabeculotomy, iTrack catheter.

### Trabeculotomy Ab Interno

- Swann–Jacob or similar goniolens, both right- and left-handed versions
- iTrack microcatheter
- 23-gauge needle for paracentesis track for iTrack
- Irrigation/aspiration setup.

## COMPLICATIONS

### Management of Hyphema

Postoperative care largely centers on managing early IOP spikes from hyphema formation, especially with full circumference canal opening. The majority of the blood comes from Schlemm's canal. In most cases, this is a limited problem for the blood clears from the anterior chamber and IOP drops. The IOP spike may be significant. Glaucoma medications are restarted during this time, typically aqueous suppressants. A weak dose of a miotic, typically 1% pilocarpine, may be instituted at bedtime to try and reduce PAS formation due to blood in the angle.

### Steroid Response

Theoretically, IOP elevation from topical corticosteroids should not occur because the resistance in the trabecular meshwork has been drastically reduced. However, steroid response is a significant problem post-trabeculotomy in some patients. The weakest steroid along with least frequency necessary to reduce inflammation to acceptable levels is the best option. Corticosteroids should be discontinued as soon as feasible for the IOP typically falls 1–2 weeks after topical steroids are discontinued. Topical nonsteroidal anti-inflammatory medications can also be used. Unfortunately, our knowledge of wound healing in and around Schlemm's canal is limited at this time.

### Gonioscopy, the Canal and PAS

Serial postoperative gonioscopy is critical to visualize the canal. It often takes 7–10 days for blood to completely clear from the canal. If IOP is elevated, yet the canal appears open; it may be due to a steroid response. Topical corticosteroids should be tapered as soon as possible. If PAS are seen obstructing the angle, this would obviously explain an elevated IOP.

## SURGICAL OUTCOMES

### Adult Glaucomas

The concept of modern-day circumferential trabeculotomy in adults is still a new one; for prior results with older metal trabeculotomes opening segments of the canal were not as favorable, ultimately leading to its demise decades ago. However, the ability to circumnavigate the canal with a suture or a flexible microcatheter has improved outcomes and success rates for congenital, juvenile, and adult cases. Trabeculotomy is performed in the United States and globally for congenital glaucomas but infrequently in the United States for adult glaucomas. However, with the advent of newer techniques and devices, trabeculotomy, especially in Europe and Japan, continues to gain leverage as a primary procedure for adult glaucomas. A recent report concerning outcomes for circumferential trabeculotomy in adults found that 360° suture trabeculotomy ab externo was significantly more effective in lowering IOP in adult primary and secondary glaucomas than metal trabeculotomy.[6] The success rate was higher with the circumferential trabeculotomy, 84% versus 31%. The IOP was lower with fewer medications in the circumferential group versus metal trabeculotomy, with a mean postoperative IOP of 13.1 mm Hg on 0.5 medications versus 15.2 mm Hg on 1.4 medications at 12 months, respectively. Goniotomy for adult open-angle glaucoma is not as popular as trabeculotomy but Quaranta found success in 87.5% of eyes undergoing goniotomy, termed ab interno goniotrabeculotomy, using a Swann goniotome as visualized through a Barkan lens.[7]

### Congenital and Juvenile Glaucomas

The overall success rate for goniotomy in juvenile glaucoma, with a mean age of 16 years, was 77% with a mean follow-up of 8 years as reported by Yeung and Walton.[8] These cases are almost always bilateral with a fairly normal appearing angle. Tamcelik[9] reported excellent results in congenital glaucoma with viscotrabeculotomy, using a viscoelastic in conjunction with a standard angled Harms trabeculotome, while others have found excellent results with standard metal trabeculotomy.[10] However, a movement continues for many surgeons who use either a suture or microcatheter to circumnavigate the canal. Beck and Lynch[11] reported excellent results using a suture to open the canal for 360°, while more recent studies support the use of catheter-assisted circumferential trabeculotomy[12,13] for congenital and juvenile glaucomas with success rates of up to 90%. A recent study, although small, demonstrates better outcomes with circumferential trabeculotomy compared with goniotomy for congenital glaucoma.[14]

## PLACE OF THE TECHNIQUE IN SURGICAL ARMAMENTARIUM

### Congenital Glaucoma

Both goniotomy and trabeculotomy are well-accepted procedures for congenital and developmental glaucomas. However, if the cornea is cloudy, the view for goniotomy is suboptimal. The authors prefer circumferential trabeculotomy over goniotomy for the childhood glaucomas because a cloudy cornea is not a problem and the entire angle can usually be cleaved open at one sitting. This may significantly decrease the number of surgical procedures.

From an adult glaucoma viewpoint, many patients with mild-to-moderate glaucoma may not need a complex filtering or drainage implant procedure. The ability to lower IOP by increasing flow into the patients natural drainage system and avoid a bleb is an excellent alternative for many of these patients. In addition, trabeculotomy may be combined with phacoemulsification with excellent results. The IOP reduction with successful trabeculotomy is not as substantial as a filter, but many glaucoma patients will do well with an IOP in the midteens on one glaucoma medication. It is likely (though unproven), that in the adult glaucomas, an angle procedure may work better and last longer when performed earlier rather than later in the disease before the distal collector channels atrophy from years of disuse and the tissue aggravated by years of topical glaucoma therapy.

## PEARLS AND PITFALLS

### Failure to Identify Schlemm's Canal

If the surgeon is completely unable to identify Schlemm's canal during a trabeculotomy, the procedure is typically converted to a filtration procedure or the site is closed and a tube inserted. This should be discussed preoperatively and consented appropriately.

### Additional Maneuvers to Identify Schlemm's Canal

Considerable effort should be expended on identifying the canal. It may be necessary to make a second adjacent cutdown in the scleral bed in order to search for the canal. In addition, inserting a segment of 4-0 clear nylon suture with a blunted tip partly into the canal may be helpful in trying to identify the canal. With the 4-0 nylon suture in position within the suspected canal, flex the proximal end of the suture posteriorly over the sclera. If the suture is actually nestled in the angle, not in the canal, the distal tip will present into the anterior chamber. In addition, if the distal tip is over the suprachoroidal space, when the proximal end is flexed anteriorly, upon release, it will not spring back into its original position. Also, if the illuminated microcatheter is not available, the tip of a light pipe may be placed onto the proximal end of a clear 4-0 nylon suture and the blunted end may light up revealing its subscleral location.

### Lack of a Visible Outcome Marker for Canal Surgery

The success of canal-based procedures is based on improving flow into the episcleral venous collector system; however, at this time, we do not have a reliable method of measuring flow in the episcleral and collector veins.[15] This makes it difficult to study our newer procedures and determine their outcomes. For example, bleb formation is associated with successful filtration surgery and correlates with the clinical course, an excellent visible outcome marker. We can study the aqueous veins of Ascher, but this is laborious and very difficult, but possible in the operating room.[16] We await episcleral venous flow technology to better understand outcomes of canal-based surgeries.

## REFERENCES

1. Barkan O. A new operation for chronic glaucoma. Restoration of physiological function by opening Schlemm's canal under direct magnified vision. Am J Ophthalmol. 1936;19:951-66.

2. Kulkarni SV, Damji KF, Fournier AV, et al. Endoscopic goniotomy early clinical experience in congenital glaucoma. J Glaucoma. 2010;19:264-9.
3. Honjo M, Tanihara H, Inatani M, et al. Trabeculotomy for the treatment of steroid-induced glaucoma. J Glaucoma. 2000;9: 483-5.
4. Amari Y, Hamanaka T, Futa R. Histologic investigation failure of trabeculotomy. J Glaucoma. 2013 DOI: 10.1097/IJG.0b013e31829e1d6e.
5. Grover DS, Godfrey DG, Smith O, et al. Gonioscopy-assisted transluminal trabeculotomy, ab interno trabeculotomy: Technique report and preliminary results. Ophthalmol 2014;121: 855-61.
6. Chin S, Nitta T, Shinmei Y, et al. Reduction of intraocular pressure using a modified 360-degree suture trabeculotomy technique in primary and secondary open-angle glaucoma: a pilot study. J Glaucoma. 2012;21(6):401-7.
7. Quaranta L, Hitchings RA, Quaranta CA. Ab-interno goniotrabeculotomy versus MMC trabeculectomy for open angle glaucoma. Ophthalmology. 1999;106:1357-62.
8. Yeung HH, Walton DS. Goniotomy for juvenile open-angle glaucoma. J Glaucoma. 2010;19:1-4.
9. Tamcelik N, Ozkiris A. Long-term results of viscotrabeculotomy in congenital glaucoma: comparison to classic trabeculotomy. Br J Ophthalmology. 2008;92:36-9.
10. Ikeda H, Ishigooka H, Muto T, et al. Long-term outcome of trabeculotomy for the treatment of developmental glaucoma. Arch Ophthalmol. 2004;122:1122-8.
11. Beck AD, Lynch MG. 360 degrees trabeculotomy for primary congenital glaucoma. Arch Ophthalmol. 1995;113:1200-02.
12. Sarkisian SR Jr. An illuminated microcatheter for 360-degree trabeculectomy in congenital glaucoma: a retrospective case series. J AAPOS. 2010;14:412-6.
13. Girkin CA, Marchase N, Cogen MS. Circumferential trabeculotomy with an illuminated microcatheter in congenital glaucomas. J Glaucoma. 2012;21:160-63.
14. Girkin CA, Rhodes L, McGwin G, et al. Goniotomy versus circumferential trabeculotomy with an illuminated microcatheter in congenital glaucoma. J AAPOS. 2012;16:424-7.
15. Fellman RL. Lack of a visible outcome marker fuels the perfect storm of Dr Singh's editorial. Ophthalmol. 2014:121;2,e12
16. Fellman RL, Grover DS. Episcleral venous fluid wave: evidence for patency of the conventional collector system. J Glaucoma. 2014;23:347-50.

CHAPTER 44

# Complications of Glaucoma Surgery and their Management

Sunita Radhakrishnan, Andrew G Iwach

## COMPLICATIONS OF TRABECULECTOMY

### Intraoperative Complications

Most intraoperative complications can be avoided with meticulous surgical technique. Conjunctival buttonholes can ultimately result in bleb failure and are managed best by prevention. Poor visualization and use of inappropriate instruments are common causes of conjunctival tears and should be avoided. Inflating the bleb at the end of surgery by instillation of fluid in the anterior chamber (AC) can detect small conjunctival buttonholes, which should then be sutured closed. Scleral flap complications are minimized by dissecting a flap of adequate thickness and gentle handling of the flap. Partial flap tears may be dealt with by modifying the flap suture placement or using a new flap at a deeper plane or a new site altogether. Total flap amputations may be repaired with a scleral patch graft. Intraoperative bleeding should be controlled with cautery as needed. Suprachoroidal hemorrhage during surgery is fortunately rare, and if it does occur, the primary goal is to immediately close all wounds. In high-risk cases [e.g. aphakia, prior vitrectomy, pathological myopia, high preoperative intraocular pressure (IOP), Sturge–Weber syndrome] preventive measures include use of preplaced scleral flap sutures, gradual reduction in IOP with a controlled paracentesis and maintenance of blood pressure control during surgery.

## POSTOPERATIVE COMPLICATIONS

### Early Postoperative Complications

#### *Hypotony*

Transient hypotony is common after filtering surgery and usually requires no intervention. Hypotony is generally defined as an IOP <5 mm Hg, but in many eyes, this IOP is compatible with normal visual acuity and does not lead to structural changes in the anterior or posterior segment. "Nonphysiological" hypotony is usually accompanied by decreased visual acuity and varying combinations of anatomical changes such as shallow or flat AC, corneal folds and/or edema, cataract, ciliochoroidal effusions, hypotony maculopathy and optic disk edema.

The first step in managing hypotony after filtering surgery is to identify the cause. In the following list of possible factors, overfiltration and wound leak are the most common culprits. Careful slit lamp examination with particular attention to the bleb is important to identify the cause of hypotony; gonioscopy and anterior segment imaging should be utilized as appropriate. An elevated bleb is present in overfiltration, whereas hypotony in the presence of a flat or low bleb raises the suspicion of an aqueous leak. In some cases, examination with a fluorescein strip and/or application of gentle pressure on the eye may be necessary to identify the site of aqueous leak.

- Hypotony due to increased outflow:
  - Overfiltration
  - Wound leak
  - Unrecognized intraoperative conjunctival buttonhole
  - Inadvertent cyclodialysis cleft.
- Hypotony due to reduced aqueous production:
  - Uveitis
  - Extensive prior cyclophotocoagulation
  - Annular ciliary detachment
  - Use of aqueous suppressants—inadvertent or intentional to treat the fellow eye.

*Hypotony and shallow or flat AC*: The Spaeth classification of a shallow AC in the presence of hypotony is useful for

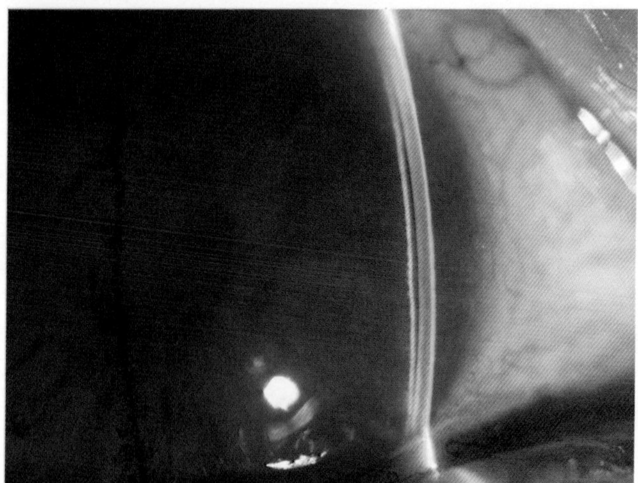

**Figure 44-1** Shallow anterior chamber.

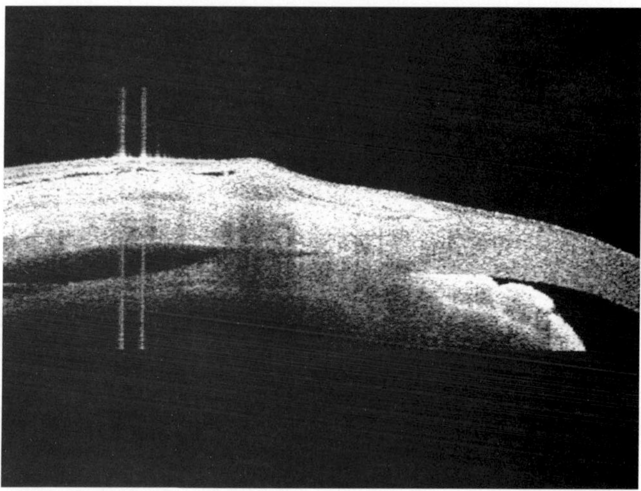

**Figure 44-2** Anterior segment optical coherence tomography image showing supraciliary effusion.
*Source* Sunita Radhakrishnan

postoperative management. A Grade 1 shallow AC has peripheral iridocorneal contact (Fig. 44-1), a Grade 2 shallow AC has more iridocorneal contact extending from the peripheral iris to the pupillary margin, and a Grade 3 AC is flat with total iris apposition and contact between the corneal endothelium and the lens (or vitreous). For monitoring of Grade 1 and 2 shallow AC, it is useful to also semiquantify the AC depth in terms of the number of "corneal thicknesses" between the corneal endothelium and the pupillary plane. The management of Grade 1 and 2 shallow AC is conservative with steroids and cycloplegics, closer follow-up is usually performed for eyes with Grade 2 AC. When the AC is flat, immediate intervention is indicated to prevent complications such as corneal decompensation and cataract formation. Management options in this situation include AC reformation with viscoelastic, closure of site of aqueous leak (suture line or conjunctival buttonhole) or tightening of scleral flap as appropriate and drainage of choroidal effusion. One or more of these approaches may be used depending on the clinical situation.

The management of wound leak depends on the size and position of the leak, the AC depth and the bleb appearance. Small leaks along the suture line in the presence of a formed AC will often resolve spontaneously, whereas a large dehiscence of the conjunctival closure will require resuturing.

*Hypotony and choroidal effusion:* Hypotony is often accompanied by choroidal effusion of varying degrees ranging from annular supraciliary fluid accumulations that can only be detected by imaging studies (*see* Fig. 44-2) to appositional "kissing" choroidals. The incidence of choroidal effusion reported in the Collaborative Initial Glaucoma Treatment Study (CIGTS) was 11%[1] and in the National Survey of Trabeculectomy performed in the United Kingdom, choroidal detachment was reported in 14% of 1240 cases.[2] Certain ocular conditions such as Sturge–Weber syndrome and nanophthalmos are associated with a higher risk of postoperative choroidal detachment. Choroidal effusion in the setting of overfiltration usually resolves with conservative management. Inflammation is a contributory factor and aggressive treatment with topical steroids is warranted, in this setting the more potent steroid difluprednate is often helpful. Surgical intervention is indicated only if there is appositional choroidal detachment or if other clinical findings such as a large conjunctival buttonhole or flat AC require surgery at which time a large nonappositional choroidal effusion may also be drained. Choroidal effusions due to overfiltration will often reaccumulate if the scleral flap is not tightened at the time of drainage.

*Hypotony maculopathy:* This complication is characterized by decrease in vision due to chorioretinal folds in the macula, with or without accompanying macular and optic disk edema (*see* Fig. 44-3). Not all patients with hypotony will develop maculopathy and the classic demographic associated with this complication is the young, male, myope. Tighter suturing of the scleral flap in this group of patients is advisable to minimize this complication. Identifying the underlying cause of hypotony is the first step in management and initial conservative treatment is typical. Surgical intervention consisting of tightening the scleral flap or bleb compression sutures may be required when conservative measures are ineffective. A transconjunctival method of suturing the scleral flap is especially useful.[3] There is no agreement on the timing of intervention for hypotony maculopathy. Although permanent

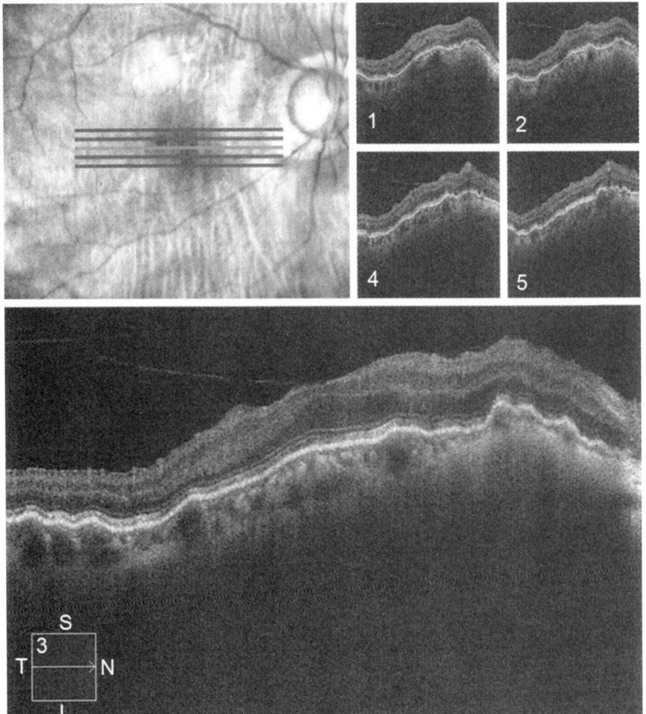


Figure 44-3 Spectral domain optical coherence tomography image of the macula showing chorioretinal folds in a patient with hypotony maculopathy.
*Source* Sunita Radhakrishnan

retinal changes are more likely with longer duration of hypotony, visual recovery has been reported after correction of hypotony in eyes that had maculopathy for several years.[4,5]

## *Intraocular Pressure too High*

Very early elevation of IOP usually indicates a technical problem with the surgery. Of the following list, tight sutures and retained viscoelastic are the most common causes of higher than desired IOP after filtering surgery.

1. Plugged sclerostomy—by iris, blood clot, or vitreous
2. Retained viscoelastic material
3. Scleral flap sutured too tightly
4. Ciliary block glaucoma
5. Suprachoroidal hemorrhage
6. Encapsulation of the bleb may occur in the first 2–4 weeks.

Management of elevated IOP after filtering surgery depends on the cause; this is usually evident by careful clinical examination including gonioscopy and ultrasound imaging as needed. Iris plugging the sclerostomy usually occurs after a shallow/flat AC or if the peripheral iridectomy is too small. Pilocarpine and/or laser iridoplasty are helpful in this situation. Plugging of the sclerostomy with vitreous strands usually occurs in eyes with prior cataract surgery and is a more difficult complication to resolve with nonsurgical measures. Retained viscoelastic material can be managed conservatively if the eye can tolerate temporary IOP elevation. If not, digital massage of the bleb site or release of viscoelastic through the paracentesis may be performed with the caveat that the viscoelastic may leave the eye in a sudden bolus resulting in a flat AC. Although not ideal, temporary use of aqueous suppressants may be necessary in some cases. Tight scleral flap sutures are easily addressed by laser suturelysis or removal of releasable sutures; however, it is best to avoid this in the first few days after surgery—digital pressure to separate the edges of the scleral incision will usually lower the IOP until sutures can be loosened. It is also advisable to release sutures one at a time to prevent hypotony and its resultant effects. Encapsulated blebs (Fig. 44-4) are reported to be more common in trabeculectomies with limbus-based conjunctival flaps[6] and in eyes with prior beta-blocker treatment.[7] Medical management with aqueous suppressants is recommended, and this may be tapered or discontinued eventually. Bleb needling and/or surgical revision is necessary in some cases.

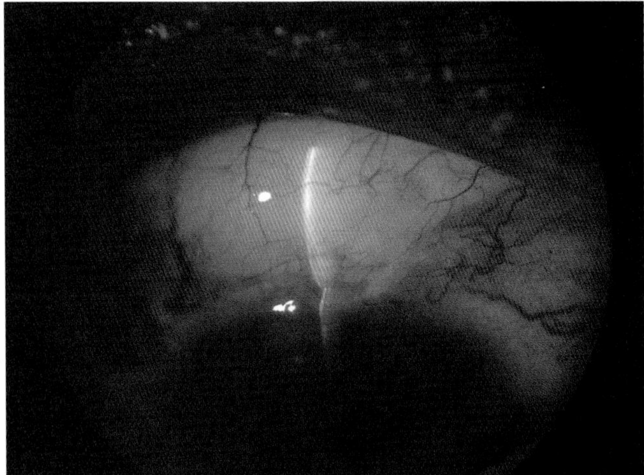

Figure 44-4 Encapsulated bleb.

*Ciliary block or malignant glaucoma:* This complication is more common in eyes with primary angle closure and is characterized by elevated IOP and a uniformly shallow or flat AC in the presence of a patent iridectomy. When occurring after filtering surgery, the IOP may only be modestly elevated and the diagnosis may be missed until several interventions have failed to resolve the problem. The absence of pupillary block or a posterior pushing mechanism such as suprachoroidal hemorrhage must be established before diagnosing ciliary block glaucoma.

Initial management consists of cycloplegia with a long-acting agent like atropine and IOP lowering medications including oral carbonic anhydrase inhibitors and hyperosmotic

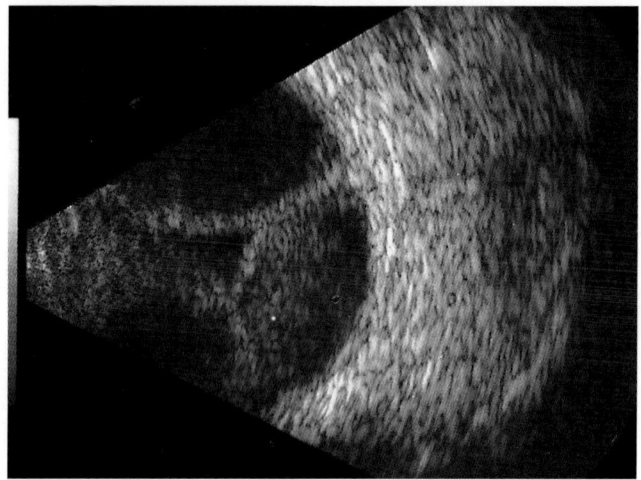

**Figure 44-5** Suprachoroidal hemorrhage.
*Source* Bradley F Jost, MD, Dallas, Texas.

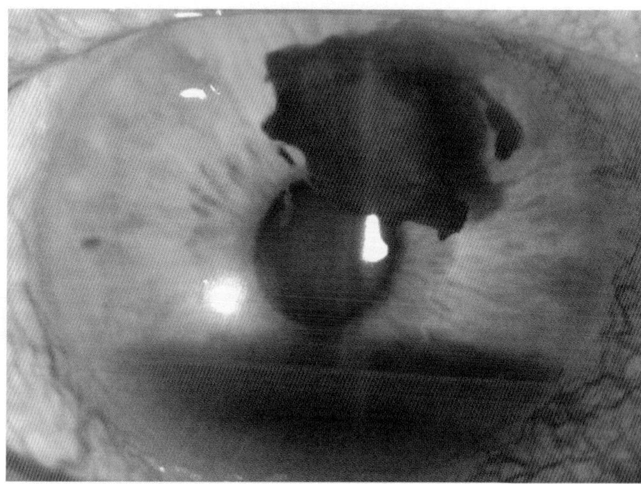

**Figure 44-6** Hyphema.

agents when feasible. In pseudophakic eyes, an Nd-YAG laser hyaloidotomy may resolve the situation. The goal is to create an opening from the AC through the iris, posterior capsule, and anterior hyaloid face into the vitreous to facilitate free passage for aqueous. This can be achieved either through an existing peripheral iridectomy or within the dilated pupil at the edge of the IOL optic. A new iridectomy site should be created if there is any doubt about the patency of a preexisting iridectomy or iridotomy. If these measures fail, surgical intervention is required; several management techniques have been described, including irido-zonulo-hyaloido-vitrectomy through an anterior segment approach,[8] pars plana vitrectomy (PPV) alone, complete PPV with iridectomy and zonulectomy, PPV with pars plana aqueous drainage device (ADD) and cyclophotocoagulation. A recent retrospective review of management options in 24 eyes with malignant glaucoma showed the highest relapse rate with medical therapy (100%) and the best outcome (0% relapse rate) with complete PPV combined with iridectomy, zonulectomy, and phacoemulsification if phakic. The mean follow-up time in this study was relatively short at 2 months (range 13 days to 7.5 months).[9] Another retrospective review of 28 eyes with malignant glaucoma showed successful resolution in 27 eyes; a single intervention was sufficient in 63% of these. Resolution was achieved in four eyes (15%) with medical treatment, seven eyes (26%) with laser hyaloidotomy, four eyes with vitrectomy-hyaloidotomy-iridectomy (15%), and 12 eyes with trans-scleral cyclophotocoagulation (44%). The median duration of follow-up was longer in this study at 6.4 months.[10]

*Suprachoroidal hemorrhage:* This is a rare but potentially devastating complication after filtering surgery. Ocular risk factors include myopia, previous vitrectomy, aphakia, and postoperative hypotony. Systemic risk factors include anticoagulant therapy, bleeding disorders, hypertension, and arteriosclerosis. Postoperative hemorrhage usually occurs within the first week after surgery in a hypotonous eye. The typical history is sudden onset of severe pain and loss of vision after exertion with a Valsalva maneuver. Examination shows a shallow or flat AC with variable IOP depending on the extent of the hemorrhage. Fundus examination usually reveals the pathology and an ultrasound is helpful if the posterior segment cannot be visualized (Fig. 44-5). Initial management consists of pain control, cycloplegia, and IOP lowering medications. Surgical intervention is warranted when there is a flat AC, large or kissing choroidal detachments, uncontrolled pain, or uncontrolled IOP. Drainage of a hemorrhagic choroidal is best performed 5–10 days after the onset so that the clot has lysed and can be easily drained through one or more posterior sclerotomies.

## *Hyphema*

Hyphema (Fig. 44-6) in the early postoperative period is usually small and self-limiting. Common sources of bleeding are the ciliary body, iris, corneoscleral incision and cut ends of the Schlemm's canal. Most cases require no intervention, and the hyphema resolves within a few days. Restriction of activity and elevation of the head of the bed are usually recommended. A blood clot blocking the sclerostomy site may result in temporary IOP elevation and can usually be managed medically until the clot lyses in a few days and aqueous flow is re-established through the scleral flap. The need for surgery is rare, and the decision to operate largely depends on the extent of hyphema, the level of IOP, and the presence of sickle cell

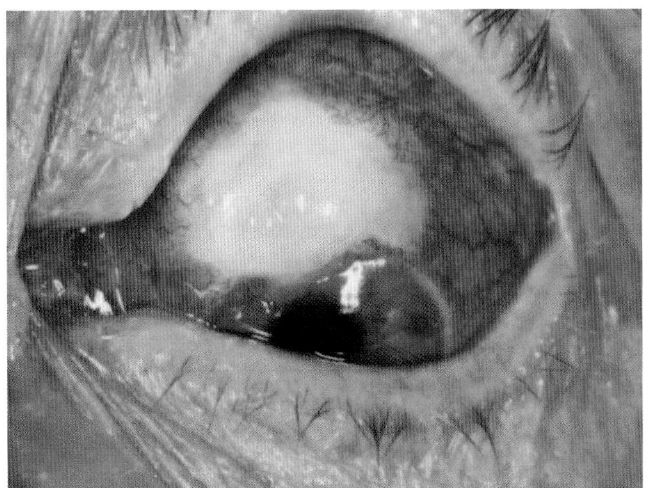

Figure 44-7 Bleb-related infection.

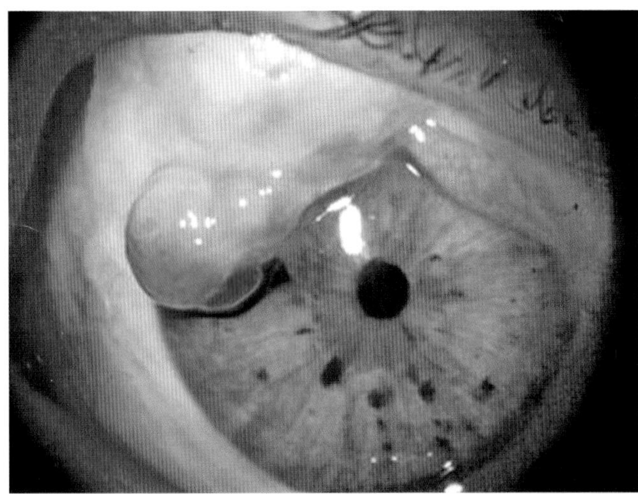

Figure 44-8 Avascular, thin bleb with corneal extension.

trait or disease. If the hyphema has liquefied, simple irrigation and aspiration is sufficient to clear the AC. A large blood clot requires expression via a corneal incision or removal with the aid of a vitrectomy instrument.

## Late Postoperative Complications

*Bleb-related infections*: Blebitis and bleb-related endophthalmitis (BRE) (Fig. 44-7) are potentially devastating complications that can occur months to years after surgery. Because even a superficial infection has the potential to quickly spread into the eye and result in permanent visual impairment and because patients may not always associate symptoms of infection with a surgery perhaps performed many years ago, it is imperative that patients who have undergone filtering surgery be regularly reminded about the symptoms of bleb-related infections and instructed to start topical antibiotics while also immediately contacting their ophthalmologist.

The incidence of BRE after filtering surgery with mitomycin has been reported as 1.3% per patient-year in two retrospective studies.[11,12] In the study by DeBry et al.,[12] the 5-year probability of developing blebitis or BRE was estimated to be 6.3% and 7.5%, respectively. A recent retrospective study from the United Kingdom reported a decrease in cumulative incidence of bleb-related infections (blebitis and endophthalmitis) from 5.7% during the period 1993–1997 to 1.2% during the period 1999–2005.[13] Although the retrospective nature of this study precluded conclusions regarding causality, the most significant change in surgical technique between the two periods was a transition from limbus-based to fornix-based conjunctival flaps.

The common causative organisms in bleb-related infections are Staphylococcus and Streptococcus. Presenting symptoms include redness, pain, tearing or discharge, photophobia, and decreased vision. Examination shows conjunctival injection, which is usually most intense around the bleb. The bleb itself has a milky-white appearance and a bleb leak is often present. A mild AC reaction is often seen. The presence of hypopyon or vitritis is indicative of endophthalmitis. If the diagnosis is in doubt, it is prudent to err on the side of caution and aggressively treat with antibiotics.

Initial management of blebitis is with frequent topical broad spectrum antibiotics and very close supervision—daily follow-up is recommended until an improvement is noted. If an AC reaction is also present, oral moxifloxacin may be used. Aqueous suppressants may be added in the presence of a bleb leak. BRE warrants immediate referral to a vitreoretinal specialist and is treated with intravitreal antibiotic injections and/or vitrectomy. Referral to a vitreoretinal specialist should also be considered in cases of blebitis, which does not improve with initial management. The prognosis is good in most cases of blebitis, whereas BRE usually results in a poor visual outcome.

Prevention of bleb-related infections may be aided by treatment of blepharitis and conjunctivitis, timely diagnosis and management of bleb leaks, avoiding mechanical bleb microtrauma such as from contact lenses and the use of eye protection in situations such as swimming where the bleb may be exposed to potential contaminants.

*Late bleb leak:* Avascular, thin blebs are more prone to develop spontaneous late bleb leaks (Fig. 44-8). Bleb leak may be asymptomatic or may present as decreased vision and tearing. Associated findings include varying combinations of low IOP, shallow/flat AC, choroidal detachment, and bleb infection. Many bleb leaks heal spontaneously and initial conservative management with topical antibiotics and aqueous suppressants

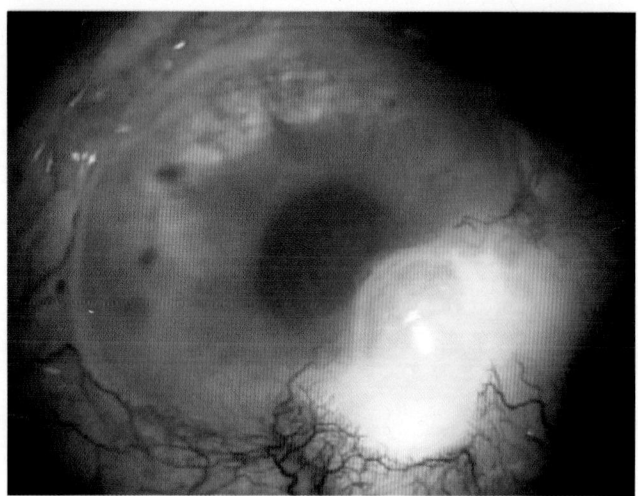

Figure 44-9 Bleb extension onto cornea.
*Source*: Andrew G Iwach

is recommended. The decision to perform bleb repair and its timing is highly variable among surgeons and is based on the level of IOP, the AC depth, level of visual impairment, prior history of bleb-related infections, and the risk of bleb failure. Numerous techniques to treat bleb leaks have been described with varying degrees of success–these include autologous blood injection, bandage contact lens, bleb compression sutures, bleb needling, and cautery of the bleb. The definitive method to repair a bleb leak is by surgical revision, most commonly consisting of bleb excision or denudation followed by conjunctival advancement. Further IOP lowering surgery after a surgical bleb repair is necessary in approximately 10% of cases.[14,15]

*Bleb dysesthesia:* Large, cystic blebs that encroach onto the cornea may cause discomfort and tear film abnormalities with dellen formation (Figs. 44-8 and 44-9). Artificial tears and lubricant ointments are helpful for initial management and various chemical and thermal methods to shrink the bleb have been described. Other interventions include bleb compression sutures, bleb needling to increase the bleb surface area while decreasing its height, "bleb-window" pexy (creation of a conjunctival window in the palpebral fissure and anchoring the free edges to bare sclera) and simple excision of the portion extending onto the cornea. As with repair of bleb leaks, surgical revision by bleb excision and conjunctival advancement has a high success rate.

*Bleb failure:* Late bleb failure is usually due to scarring in the subconjunctival and episcleral plane, and common risk factors for this type of bleb failure are young age, black race, and inflammation. Failure due to internal closure of the sclerostomy is rare and is classically seen in patients with the iridocorneal endothelial syndrome. Signs of a failing filtering bleb include increased vascularization and thickening. Bleb needling can prolong the survival of a bleb and is best performed on a failing as opposed to a failed bleb. Various techniques have been described, and adjunctive use of intraoperative and postoperative antimetabolites is typical. The authors' preferred bleb needling technique is performed in the operating room with a relatively large, 25-gauge, needle, transconjunctival application of mitomycin and suturing of the needle entry site.[16] Bleb elevation by aqueous is easily visualized with this technique since the subconjunctival space is not already inflated with antimetabolite or anesthetic (Figs. 44-10A and B).

### Complications of Filtering Surgery with the ExPress Shunt

The ExPress shunt is a modified trabeculectomy procedure in which aqueous outflow occurs via a small stainless device inserted under a partial thickness scleral flap. Complications are similar to trabeculectomy with additional considerations relating to the presence of an implant. An adequate scleral bed and scleral flap are important for good positioning of the device. In eyes with postoperative shallowing of the AC, iris tissue may occlude the ExPress shunt tip as well as side ports resulting in elevated IOP (Fig. 44-11); this can usually be managed with Nd-YAG laser iridoplasty. Bleb needling after an ExPress shunt has to be modified since there is no fistulous connection between the AC and the episcleral plane. After elevation of the scleral flap, the needle may be advanced into the AC taking care that the entry site is not adjacent to the ExPress shunt.

## COMPLICATIONS OF AQUEOUS DRAINAGE DEVICES

Aqueous drainage devices are associated with similar complications as occurs with trabeculectomy with additional unique device-related adverse events.[17]

### Tube Exposure

Conjunctival erosion over the tube (Figs. 44-12A to C) can occur years after surgery and should be surgically repaired to reduce the risk of endophthalmitis. The incidence of tube exposure in the Tube versus Trabeculectomy (TVT) study was 5% after 5 years of follow-up[18] and in a recent meta-analysis of 3255 eyes with a mean follow-up of 26 months, the overall

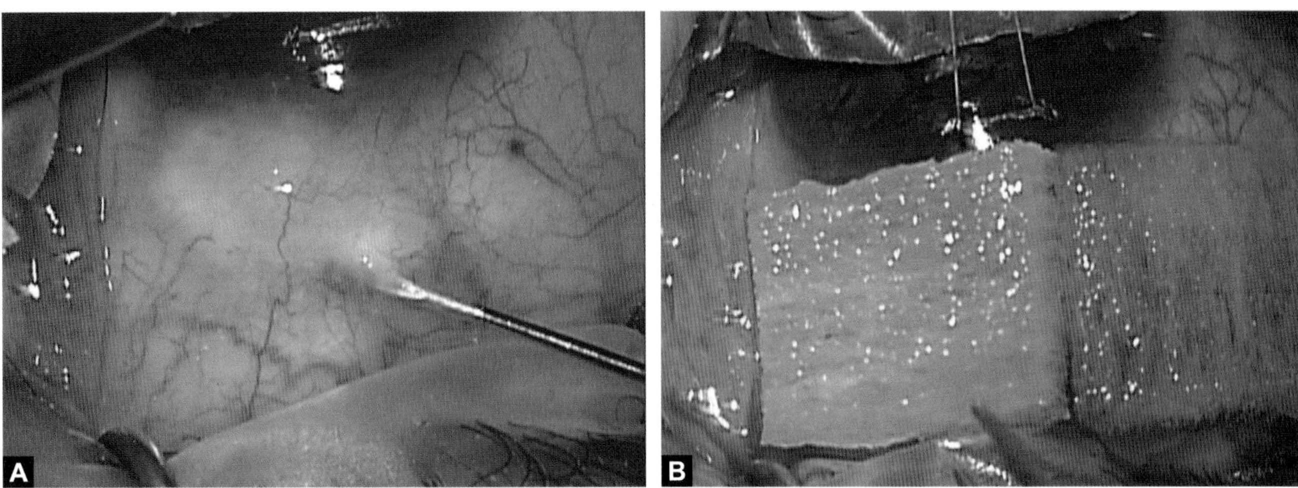

**Figures 44-10A and B** (A) Bleb needling. (B) Transconjunctival application of mitomycin.
*Source* Sunita Radhakrishnan, Andrew G Iwach

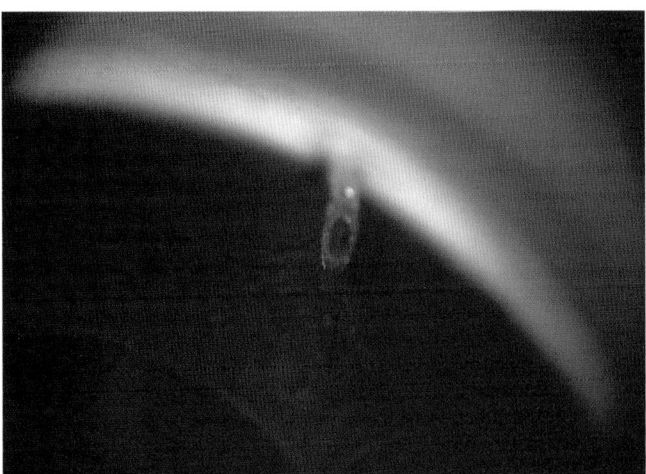

**Figure 44-11** Iris occluding ExPress shunt tip.
*Source* Sunita Radhakrishnan, Terri-Diann Pickering, San Francisco

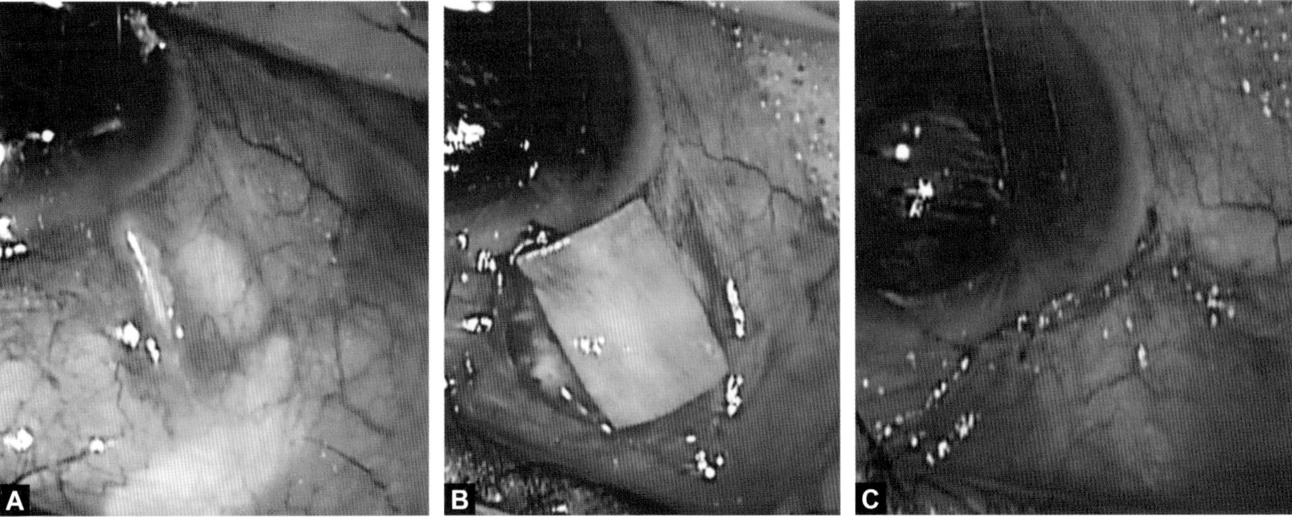

**Figures 44-12A to C** (A) Conjunctival erosion over tube. (B) Tube revision with patch graft placement. (C) Conjunctival closure.
*Source* Sunita Radhakrishnan, Andrew G Iwach

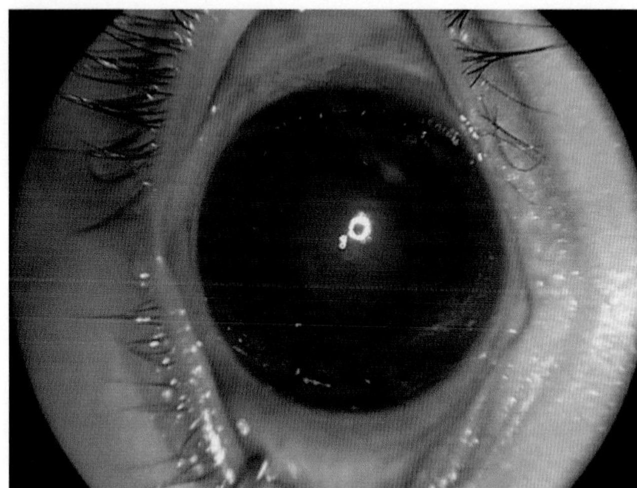

**Figure 44-13** Tube corneal touch.
*Source* Ta Chen Peter Chang, MD, Bascom Palmer Eye Institute, Miami, Florida.

incidence of tube exposure was 2%.[19] Revision of the tube is performed with placement of a new patch graft and conjunctival closure (*see* Figs. 44-12A to C). This may be combined with redirecting the tube either more posteriorly in the same quadrant or creating a new entry site in a different quadrant. In contrast to tube exposure, exposure of the implant plate almost always necessitates removal of the device.

## Diplopia

Motility disturbances associated with ADDs are attributed to mechanical extraocular muscle (EOM) restriction by the plate, stretching of EOM due to a large bleb, scarring involving the EOM adjacent to the implant or mass effect from a large bleb over the plate. In the TVT study, new onset persistent diplopia was reported in 6% patients at 5 years follow-up after implantation of a Baerveldt implant.[18] The one-year results of two randomized controlled trials comparing the Ahmed and Baerveldt implants showed diplopia or motility disturbances in 3–7% with no statistically significant difference between the two devices.[20,21] Strabismus associated with ADDs can be managed with spectacle prisms, EOM surgery or device explantation.

## Persistent Corneal Edema

The pathogenesis of corneal edema after ADD placement is multifactorial with mechanical tube-corneal touch (Fig. 44-13), and progressive endothelial loss from multiple prior surgeries being important factors. Persistent corneal edema was reported in 16% at 5 years in the Baerveldt arm of the TVT study.[18] In the one-year outcomes reported in two randomized controlled trials, persistent corneal edema was more common in the Baerveldt group (12–22%) than in the Ahmed group (2–12%) and the difference was statistically significant.[20,21] The risk of corneal edema may be minimized by placing the tube far from the corneal endothelium in the iris plane. In eyes at high risk for endothelial cell damage and those with corneal transplants, sulcus or pars plana placement of the tube should be considered.

# CONCLUSION

Glaucoma surgery can be associated with a number of complications. A combination of prevention, immediate identification, and timely management of problems usually results in a good outcome. Bleb-related infections are a dreaded long-term complication of filtering surgery, and patients must be periodically reminded about the symptoms of infection and instructed regarding immediate measures such as topical antibiotics and contacting their glaucoma specialist.

# REFERENCES


1. Jampel HD, Musch DC, Gillespie BW, et al. Perioperative complications of trabeculectomy in the Collaborative Initial Glaucoma Treatment Study (CIGTS). Am J Ophthalmol. 2005;140:16-22.
2. Edmunds B, Thompson JR, Salmon JF, et al. The National Survey of Trabeculectomy. III. Early and late complications. Eye. 2002;16:297-303.
3. Shirato S, Maruyama K, Haneda M. Resuturing the scleral flap through conjunctiva for excess filtration. Am J Ophthalmol. 2004;137:173-4.
4. Delgado MF, Daniels S, Pascal S, et al. Hypotony maculopathy: improvement of visual acuity after 7 years. Am J Ophthalmol. 2001;132:931-3.
5. Oyakhire JO, Moroi SE. Clinical and anatomical reversal of long-term hypotony maculopathy. Am J Ophthalmol. 2004;137:953-5.
6. Scott DR, Quigley HA. Medical management of a high bleb phase after trabeculectomies. Ophthalmology. 1988;95:1169-73.
7. Yarangumeli A, Koz OG, Kural G. Encapsulated blebs following primary standard trabeculectomy: course and treatment. J Glaucoma. 2004;13:251-5.
8. Lois N, Wong D, Groenewald C. New surgical approach in the management of pseudophakic malignant glaucoma. Ophthalmology. 2001;108:780-3.
9. Debrouwere V, Stalmans P, Van Calster J, et al. Outcomes of different management options for malignant glaucoma: a retrospective study. Graefes Arch Clin Exp Ophthalmol. 2012;250:131-41.
10. Dave P, Senthil S, Rao HL, et al. Treatment outcomesin malignant glaucoma. Ophthalmology. 2013;120(5):984-90.
11. Greenfield DS, Suner IJ, Miller MP, et al. Endophthalmitis after filtering surgery with mitomycin. Arch Ophthalmol. 1996;114:943-9.

12. DeBry PW, Perkins TW, Heatley G, et al. Incidence of late-onset bleb-related complications following trabeculectomy with mitomycin. Arch Ophthalmol. 2002;120:297-300.
13. Rai P, Kotecha A, Kaltsos K, et al. Changing trends in the incidence of bleb-related infection in trabeculectomy. Br J Ophthalmol. 2012;96:971-5.
14. Radhakrishnan S, Quigley HA, Jampel HD, et al. Outcomes of surgical bleb revision for complications of trabeculectomy. Ophthalmology. 2009;116:1713-8.
15. Lin AP, Chung JE, Zhang KS, et al. Outcomes of surgical bleb revision for late onset bleb leaks after trabeculectomy. J Glaucoma. 2013;22:21-5.
16. Iwach AG, Delgado MF, Novack GD, et al. Transconjunctival mitomycin-C in needle revisions of failing filtering blebs. Ophthalmology. 2003;110:734-42.
17. Gedde SJ, Parrish RK, Budenz DL, et al. Update on aqueous shunts. Exp Eye Res. 2011;93:284-90.
18. Gedde SJ, Herndon LW, Brandt JD, et al. Postoperative complications in the Tube versus Trabeculectomy study during five years of follow-up. Am J Ophthalmol. 2012;153:804-14.
19. Stewart WC, Kristoffersen CJ, Demos CM, et al. Incidence of conjunctival exposure following drainage device implantation in patients with glaucoma. Eur J Ophthalmol. 2010;20:24-30.
20. Budenz DL, Barton K, Feuer WJ, et al. Treatment outcomes in the Ahmed Baerveldt Comparison study after one year of follow-up. Ophthalmology. 2011;118:443-52.
21. Christakis PG, Kalenak JW, Zurakowski D, et al. The Ahmed versus Baerveldt Study. One-year treatment outcomes. Ophthalmology. 2011;118:2180-9.

CHAPTER

# 45

# Laser Trabeculoplasty

Fabiana Q Silva, Scott D Smith

## INTRODUCTION

The application of light energy to the anterior chamber angle for glaucoma treatment was first described by Zweng and Flocks in 1961. They used the xenon-arc photocoagulator of Meyer-Schwickerath and selectively coagulated the anterior chamber angles of animal models resulting in ciliary body and trabecular burn.[1]

In the 1970s, studies by Krasnov et al. were not encouraging due to transient intraocular pressure (IOP) reduction and complications.[2-6] However, in 1979, Wise and Witter reported a high rate of success in treating phakic open-angle glaucoma (POAG) with low-energy, non-penetrating argon laser burns applied to the trabecular meshwork (TM). This was considered to be the first successful laser trabeculoplasty protocol, and despite some modifications, remains the technique used at present.[7]

In 1995, Latina and Park designed a new laser procedure to treat patients with primary open-angle glaucoma (POAG) using a Q-switched 532-nm neodymium: yttrium-aluminum-garnet (Nd:YAG) laser called selective laser trabeculoplasty (SLT). This technique selectively targets pigmented cells in the TM without producing collateral thermal damage to non-pigmented cells or structures.[8]

## INDICATIONS

Laser trabeculoplasty may be indicated in the treatment of any phakic, aphakic, or pseudophakic eye in which the angle is at least 180° open.[9] The procedure has been found to be effective in POAG, normal tension glaucoma, ocular hypertension, juvenile open-angle glaucoma and is particularly effective in patients with pseudoexfoliation glaucoma, and pigmentary glaucoma.[9-15] It is also indicated in eyes in which conventional glaucoma surgery has failed, and when noncompliance to medical therapy results in uncontrolled glaucoma.

Recently, the effectiveness of SLT in steroid-induced glaucoma was evaluated by Tokuda et al. This study demonstrated significant decreases in IOP after laser treatment.[16] In addition, several investigators suggested that SLT should be considered in patients with elevated IOP after intravitreal triamcinolone–acetonide injection as a temporizing treatment and prophylactic procedure.[17-19]

Initial treatment with laser trabeculoplasty can also be considered in particular cases. The Glaucoma Laser Trial (GLT) randomly assigned patients to receive argon laser treatment (ALT) in one eye and standard topical medication in the other eye to determine whether ALT was effective in patients with newly diagnosed POAG. Over the course of this trial and of the Glaucoma Laser Trial Follow-Up Study, the eyes treated initially with ALT had lower IOP and better visual field and optic disk status than their fellow eyes treated initially with topical medication.[20,21] However, medical therapy is still more commonly used than laser trabeculoplasty as initial therapy, especially with the advent of more effective IOP-lowering topical medications since those studies were performed.

## CONTRAINDICATIONS

Trabeculoplasty is probably not beneficial in the treatment of:

- Angle-closure glaucoma
- Congenital glaucoma
- Glaucoma secondary to uveitis
- Glaucoma secondary to trauma
- Iridocorneal endothelial (ICE) syndrome
- Axenfeld–Rieger syndrome
- Glaucoma with elevated episcleral venous pressure

## MECHANISM OF ACTION

The mechanism of action of laser trabeculoplasty remains uncertain. A mechanical theory was proposed by Wise who suggested that coagulation caused by the laser burns results in a contracture of adjacent tissue, tightening the trabecular ring and perhaps widening the adjacent trabecular pores.[22] Histopathological evidence supporting this theory has been provided, with demonstration of widening of the intratrabecular spaces in the adjacent untreated regions of a series of nonglaucomatous monkey eyes 4 weeks after ALT.[23]

Additional theories of the mechanism of action of laser trabeculoplasty have been proposed based upon cellular and biochemical changes presumed to be induced by this procedure. Laser application to the TM has been proposed to dislodge some trabecular cells, stimulating the remaining cells to renew more active synthesis and/or turnover of the trabecular extracellular matrix.[24,25] It also may generate the renewal of matrix metalloproteinases on the beams and may stimulate the macrophage-like capacity of the trabecular-lining cells.[26] Of course, these concepts of the mechanism of action of ALT are not mutually exclusive.

Furthermore, different lasers can lead to different types of response. Kramer and Noecker performed a study comparing the histopathological appearance of the TM after ALT and SLT. It showed that SLT seemed to cause no coagulative damage and less structural damage to the human TM when compared with ALT supporting the evidence that the mechanism of action of SLT is biological rather than mechanical. The short pulse duration of SLT is below the thermal relaxation time of the tissue and thus causes no thermal damage. In addition, the laser energy is more uniformly distributed to the TM, suggesting that SLT may be a safer and more repeatable procedure than the ALT.[27,28]

## SURGICAL TECHNIQUE

After instilling a drop of topical anesthetic and an alpha-agonist, a goniolens is filled with gonioscopic solution and placed on the cornea. A standard Goldmann three-mirror lens or a single-mirror gonioscopy lens can be used. Specific gonioscopy lenses have been designed for ALT and SLT that incorporate an antireflective coating matched to the corresponding laser wavelength. With the lens in place, the surgeon identifies the anterior chamber angle structures and their variations regarding pigmentation and width of the angle.

### ALT

Argon laser treatment is performed with an argon green laser with wavelength of 514 nm. The settings most commonly used are a spot size of 50 µm and a pulse duration of 0.1 seconds. The energy level used varies between 600 and 1200 mW based on a clinical endpoint of mild blanching of the TM. The amount of energy is adjusted until a bubble is formed on the TM. It is, then, decreased until there is blanching with minimal bubble formation. Laser applications are spaced two to three spot diameters apart. The laser burns should be placed along the border of the pigmented and nonpigmented anterior TM, which may reduce the occurrence of peripheral anterior synechiae. Studies have shown that the application of 50 burns to either 180° or 360° have a similar effect on IOP reduction as a treatment of 100 burns to 360° of the TM.[29-31]

### SLT

Selective laser trabeculoplasty is performed with a 532-nm frequency-doubled, Q-switched Nd:YAG laser with a pulse duration of 3 ns and spot size of 400 µm coupled to a slit lamp delivery system and a Helium–Neon aiming laser. The spot size and pulse duration are fixed and cannot be adjusted by the surgeon. The pulse energy is initially set between 0.5 and 0.8 mJ and increased in 0.1 mJ increments until fine bubbles are noted on the TM. The energy is then decreased by 0.1 mJ for the rest of the applications. A total of approximately 100 adjacent, nonoverlapping spots are placed over 270° to 360° of the TM.

The parameters of ALT and SLT are summarized in Table 45-1.

## POSTOPERATIVE CARE

Postoperatively, another drop of an alpha-agonist is instilled and topical steroid, or non-steroidal anti-inflammatory drops are prescribed for 3–7 days. The IOP should be checked approximately 1 hour after the procedure to determine whether a short-term increase in IOP has occurred. The patient's glaucoma medications should be continued as usual. Tapering of glaucoma medications can be considered several weeks after laser trabeculoplasty if a substantial reduction of IOP has been achieved.

**TABLE 45-1** Typical parameters for ALT and SLT

| Type | Power/energy × no. of spots | Circumference treated |
|---|---|---|
| ALT | 600–1200 mW for 0.1 second × 50–100 | 180°–360° |
| SLT | 0.5–1.2 mJ × 100 | 270°–360° |

(ALT: Argon laser trabeculoplasty; SLT: Selective laser trabeculoplasty).

## COMPLICATIONS

The most serious early complication of laser trabeculoplasty is a transient elevation of the IOP. In most cases, these spikes are transitory and do not exceed 10 mmHg. Normally, such events respond well to medical therapy and resolve within the first 24 hours.[32-34] Some patients are at higher risk of IOP spikes than others. Pseudoexfoliation and pigmentation of the TM are the main patient characteristics associated with transient pressure rise. In addition, eyes that had an IOP rise after the first laser session are more likely to have a rise after a second session.[35] Theoretically, modifying the laser settings with lower energy, fewer applications and/or treating a lesser amount of TM may decrease this risk.

Iritis is another common early complication after laser trabeculoplasty. In most of cases, the inflammation is transitory and may be more frequent in eyes with pigmentary glaucoma and exfoliation syndrome. It can be treated with prednisolone 1% or equivalent, four times daily for 5–7 days.[36]

Another complication of ALT is peripheral anterior synechiae, which is related to the location of the laser applications. This complication does not generally occur after SLT when performed correctly.

## SURGICAL OUTCOMES: SCIENTIFIC EVIDENCE

Studies have shown that ALT provides useful IOP reduction in up to 90% of eyes.[20] SLT has been reported to induce an effect on IOP, with a mean reduction of 30% after 18 months of follow-up as a primary treatment in patients with POAG.[33]

Many factors influence the IOP response to laser trabeculoplasty. Higher initial IOP is associated with a greater fall in pressure.[9] Glaucoma subtype also influences the results, with a better response in pseudoexfoliation glaucoma and pigmentary glaucoma.[9,13] The higher success rate with these conditions is related to the favorable influence of increased TM pigmentation.[37]

Although the IOP reduction may last for several years after this procedure, a considerable number of patients show an increase in IOP over the time. Failure is most common during the first year after treatment, with a reported rate of 23%, and a subsequent failure rate of 5–9% per year. As a result, up to one-half of eyes within 5 years of trabeculoplasty and two thirds of eyes within 10 years may require additional treatment.[38]

In cases of failure, trabeculoplasty can be repeated with a wide range of reported results. Repeat ALT after an initially successful treatment has had reported success rates of 21–73% at 1 year.[39,40] However, eyes that demonstrate a poor response to initial treatment with failure in <12 months are unlikely to respond to a second treatment.[39] ALT should not be performed more than two times in the same area of TM, as photocoagulative damage may make additional treatments ineffective, or may actually lead to an increase in IOP.

The absence of structural damage to the TM after SLT suggests that this treatment may be amenable to multiple retreatments. Hong et al. reported no difference in efficacy between eyes that received SLT 6–12 months after the first treatment compared with those that received a second treatment at >12 months, concluding that this procedure can be repeated as early as 6 months.[41]

Treatment with SLT can be effective following previous ALT. In a prospective randomized trial study, patients with previously failed ALT were shown to have a significantly greater drop in IOP when treated with SLT when compared with repeat ALT.[42]

## PLACE OF THE TECHNIQUE IN SURGICAL ARMAMENTARIUM

Laser trabeculoplasty is a good option to consider in treating patients with POAG whose IOP is about 30% or less above the desired target and in patients with pseudoexfoliation or pigmentary glaucoma whose IOP is 40–50% above the desired target. Patients with higher IOP are unlikely to achieve a successful result, as the procedure does not often lower the IOP more than this amount.

Laser trabeculoplasty may be used as initial therapy, or early in the course of treatment in patients where medical therapy is undesirable or impractical. For example, when barriers to reliable ongoing medical treatment exist due to patient aversion to the use of medications, the cost of treatment, side effects, or poor patient reliability in the use of eyedrops, laser trabeculoplasty can be an attractive alternative.

## REFERENCES


1. Zweng HC, Flocks M. Experimental photocoagulation of the anterior chamber angle. A preliminary report. Am J Ophthalmol. 1961;52:163-5.
2. Krasnov MM. Laseropuncture of anterior chamber angle in glaucoma. Am J Ophthalmol. 1973;75(4):674-8.
3. Krasnov MM. Q-switched laser goniopuncture. Arch Ophthalmol. 1974;92(1):37-41.
4. Worthen DM, Wickham MG. Argon laser trabeculotomy. Trans Am Acad Ophthalmol Otolaryngol. 1974;78(2):OP371-5.
5. Ticho U, Zauberman H. Argon laser application to the angle structures in the glaucomas. Arch Ophthalmol. 1976;94(1):61-4.

6. Wickham MG, Worthen DM. Argon laser trabeculotomy: long-term follow-up. Ophthalmology. 1979;86(3):495-503.
7. Wise JB, Witter SL. Argon laser therapy for open-angle glaucoma. A pilot study. Arch Ophthalmol. 1979;97(2):319-22.
8. Latina M, Park C. Selective targeting of trabecular meshwork cells: in vitro studies of pulsed and CW laser interactions. Exp Eye Res. 1995;60:359-72.
9. Brooks AM, Gillies WE. Do any factors predict a favourable response to laser trabeculoplasty? Aust J Ophthalmol. 1984; 12(2): 149-53.
10. Latina MA, Tumbocon JA. Selective laser trabeculoplasty: a new treatment option for open angle glaucoma. Curr Opin Ophthalmol. 2002;13(2):94-6.
11. Mao AJ, Pan XJ, McIlraith I, et al. Development of a prediction rule to estimate the probability of acceptable intraocular pressure reduction after selective laser trabeculoplasty in open-angle glaucoma and ocular hypertension. J Glaucoma. 2008;17(6): 449-54.
12. Popiela G, Muzyka M, Szelepin L, et al. Use of YAG-Selecta laser and argon laser in the treatment of open angle glaucoma. Klin Oczna. 2000;102(2):129-33.
13. Ritch R, Liebmann J, Robin A, et al. Argon laser trabeculoplasty in pigmentary glaucoma. Ophthalmology. 1993;100(6):909-13.
14. Lieberman MF, Hoskins HD, Jr, Hetherington J, Jr. Laser trabeculoplasty and the glaucomas. Ophthalmology. 1983;90(7): 790-5.
15. Lunde MW. Argon laser trabeculoplasty in pigmentary dispersion syndrome with glaucoma. Am J Ophthalmol. 1983;96(6): 721-5.
16. Tokuda N, Inoue J, Yamazaki I, et al. Effects of selective laser trabeculoplasty treatment in steroid-induced glaucoma. Nihon Ganka Gakkai Zasshi. 2012;116(8):751-7.
17. Bozkurt E, Kara N, Yazici AT, et al. Prophylactic selective laser trabeculoplasty in the prevention of intraocular pressure elevation after intravitreal triamcinolone acetonide injection. Am J Ophthalmol. 2011;152(6):976-81.
18. Rubin B, Taglienti A, Rothman RF, et al. The effect of selective laser trabeculoplasty on intraocular pressure in patients with intravitreal steroid-induced elevated intraocular pressure. J Glaucoma. 2008;17(4):287-92.
19. Aktas Z, Deniz G, Hasanreisoglu M. Prophylactic selective laser trabeculoplasty in the prevention of intraocular pressure elevation after intravitreal triamcinolone acetonide injection. Am J Ophthalmol. 2012;153(5):1008-9.
20. The Glaucoma Laser Trial (GLT). 2. Results of argon laser trabeculoplasty versus topical medicines. The Glaucoma Laser Trial Research Group. Ophthalmology. 1990;97(11):1403-13.
21. The Glaucoma Laser Trial (GLT) and glaucoma laser trial follow-up study: 7. Results. Glaucoma Laser Trial Research Group. Am J Ophthalmol. 1995;120(6):718-31.
22. Wise JB. Glaucoma treatment by trabecular tightening with the argon laser. Int Ophthalmol Clin. 1981;21(1):69-78.
23. Melamed S, Pei J, Epstein DL, et al. Delayed response to argon laser trabeculoplasty in monkeys. Morphological and morphometric analysis. Arch Ophthalmol. 1986;104(7):1078-83.
24. Van Buskirk EM, Pond V, Rosenquist RC, et al. Argon laser trabeculoplasty. Studies of mechanism of action. Ophthalmology. 1984;91(9):1005-10.
25. Bylsma SS, Samples JR, Acott TS, et al. Trabecular cell division after argon laser trabeculoplasty. Arch Ophthalmol. 1988; 106(4):544-7.
26. Johnson DH, Richardson TM, Epstein DL, et al. Trabecular meshwork recovery after phagocytic challenge. Curr Eye Res. 1989;8(11):1121-30.
27. Kramer TR, Noecker RJ. Comparison of the morphologic changes after selective laser trabeculoplasty and argon laser trabeculoplasty in human eye bank eyes. Ophthalmology. 2001; 108(4):773-9.
28. Cvenkel B, Hvala A, Drnovsek-Olup B, et al. Acute ultrastructural changes of the trabecular meshwork after selective laser trabeculoplasty and low power argon laser trabeculoplasty. Lasers Surg Med. 2003;33(3):204-8.
29. Schwartz LW, Spaeth GL, Traverso C, et al. Variation of techniques on the results of argon laser trabeculoplasty. Ophthalmology. 1983;90(7):781-4.
30. Weinreb RN, Ruderman J, Juster R, et al. Influence of the number of laser burns administered on the early results of argon laser trabeculoplasty. Am J Ophthalmol. 1983;95(3):287-92.
31. Lustgarten J, Podos SM, Ritch R, et al. Laser trabeculoplasty. A prospective study of treatment variables. Arch Ophthalmol. 1984;102(4):517-9.
32. Weinreb RN, Wilensky JT. Clinical aspects of argon laser trabeculoplasty. Int Ophthalmol Clin. 1984;24(3):79-95.
33. Melamed S, Ben Simon GJ, Levkovitch-Verbin H. Selective laser trabeculoplasty as primary treatment for open-angle glaucoma: a prospective, nonrandomized pilot study. Arch Ophthalmol. 2003;121(7):957-60.
34. Lanzetta P, Menchini U, Virgili G. Immediate intraocular pressure response to selective laser trabeculoplasty. Br J Ophthalmol. 1999;83(1):29-32.
35. Glaucoma Laser Trial Research Group. The Glaucoma Laser Trial. I. Acute effects of argon laser trabeculoplasty on intraocular pressure. Arch Ophthalmol. 1989;107(8):1135-42.
36. Hoskins HD, Jr, Hetherington J, Jr, Minckler DS, et al. Complications of laser trabeculoplasty. Ophthalmology. 1983;90(7): 796-9.
37. Rouhiainen H, Leino M, Teräsvirta M. The effect of some treatment variables on long-term results of argon laser trabeculoplasty. Ophthalmologica. 1995;209(1):21-4.
38. Shingleton BJ, Richter CU, Dharma SK, et al. Long-term efficacy of argon laser trabeculoplasty. A 10-year follow-up study. Ophthalmology. 1993;100(9):1324-9.
39. Feldman RM, Katz LJ, Spaeth GL, et al. Long-term efficacy of repeat argon laser trabeculoplasty. Ophthalmology. 1991;98:1061-5.
40. Grayson DK, Camras CB, Podos SM, et al. Long-term reduction of intraocular pressure after repeat argon laser trabeculoplasty. Am J Ophthalmol. 1988;106:312-21.
41. Hong BK, Winwe JC, Martone JF, et al. Repeat selective laser trabeculoplasty. J Glaucoma. 2009;18:180-3.
42. Damji KF, Shah KC, Rock WJ, et al. Selective laser trabeculoplasty v argon laser trabeculoplasty: a prospective randomized clinical trial. Br J Ophthalmol. 1999;83(6):718-22.

CHAPTER

# 46

# Laser Peripheral Iridotomy and Iridoplasty

Jocelyn L Chua, Monisha E Nongpiur, Andrew Tsai, Tin Aung

## LASER PERIPHERAL IRIDOTOMY

### INTRODUCTION

Laser peripheral iridotomy (LPI) is the first-line treatment option in the management of angle closure caused by pupil block (Fig. 46-1). Considered to be the main mechanism for angle closure pathogenesis, pupil block is characterized by the presence of a resistance to the flow of aqueous from the posterior to anterior chamber (AC) at the level of the pupil. An LPI alleviates this pressure differential.[1-3]

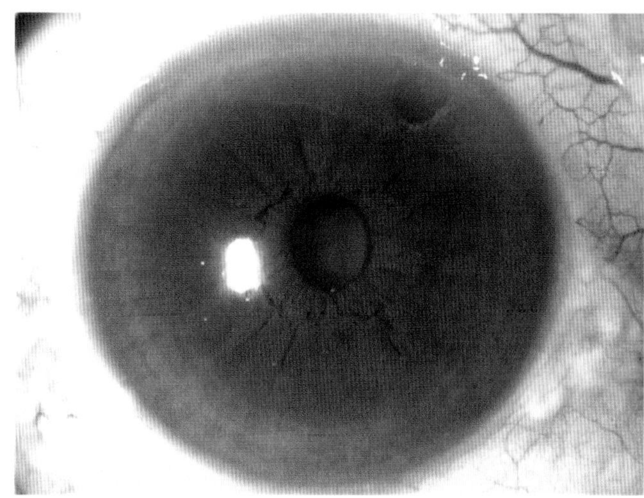

**Figure 46-1** Laser peripheral iridotomy visible at the superonasal quadrant of the iris.

### INDICATIONS

- The most definitive indication for an LPI is acute primary angle closure (APAC).[4] An acute presentation of PAC is characterized by headache, nausea, blurred vision, redness, mid-dilated pupils, and considerable elevations of intraocular pressure (IOP). Performing an LPI in an APAC eye is often difficult due to the presence of corneal edema. Initial efforts to reduce the IOP with medications may improve the corneal clarity. Other alternatives for IOP reduction include corneal indentation, AC paracentesis, and iridoplasty, all of which may be necessary to facilitate the laser procedure.
- Prophylactic LPI in the fellow eye of unilateral APAC has been shown to be effective in preventing the development of an acute attack in that eye.[5]
- Several studies have reported lowering of IOP after an LPI in eyes with PAC glaucoma and PAC.[1,6] While an LPI may not be the definitive treatment in eyes with glaucomatous optic neuropathy, it still remains the initial treatment in such eyes, but patients should be followed and monitored regularly for a rise in IOP.
- It is also common practice to perform a prophylactic LPI in eyes with anatomically narrow angles or PAC suspects (PACS). However, there is currently insufficient evidence to show that a prophylactic LPI is beneficial in preventing disease progression in all PACS. The Zhongshan angle closure prevention trial is designed to further evaluate the indications of an LPI in PACS and help determine who is at greatest risk for progression.[7]

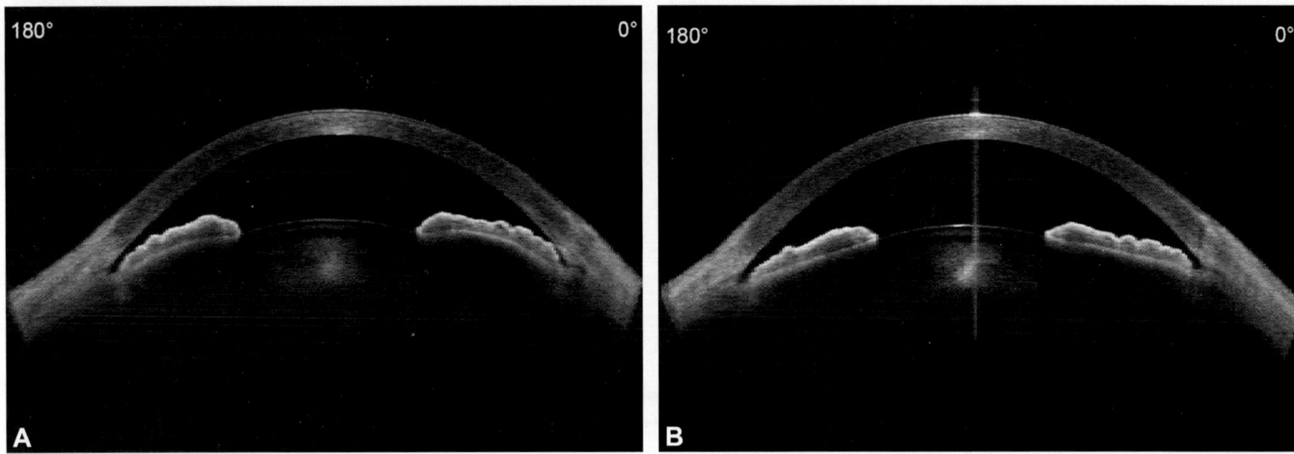


**Figures 46-2A and B** (A) Anterior segment optical coherence tomography image prelaser peripheral iridotomy. (B) Anterior segment optical coherence tomography image after laser peripheral iridotomy showing widening of the angles.

- The other indications for an LPI include the relief of pupil block resulting from other causes such as aphakic and pseudophakic pupillary block, and uveitic glaucoma producing 360° of posterior synechiae and iris bombe.

## Surgical Technique

The LPI is performed using either sequential argon-neodymium: yttrium-aluminum-garnet (Nd:YAG) laser or Nd:YAG laser alone. The former technique is usually performed in darker pigmented irides as the argon laser is helpful to obtain a partial-thickness focal thinning of the iris while minimizing surrounding iris tissue damage. The Nd:YAG laser causes a photodisruptive effect and is responsible for creating a wider iridotomy site. An Nd:YAG laser alone is often sufficient to complete an LPI in lighter pigmented irides.

### *Preoperative*

- Topical pilocarpine (1–4%) to induce miosis and stretch the iris stroma.
- Topical brimonidine is used to blunt any postprocedure IOP spike.

### *Intraoperative*

- The procedure is performed under topical anesthesia, using either the Abrahams or Weiss contact lens. The contact lens has a lenticule, which concentrates the laser energy to a focal point on the iris.
- The authors' preferred placement of the iridotomy site is the superior or superonasal quadrant of the peripheral one third of the iris. However, some surgeons treat at the 3 or 9 o' clock positions as they feel it reduces the chance of a prismatic interaction with the upper eyelid tear film.
- The argon laser energy is delivered using a 50-µm spot size, at 500–1000 mW energy per shot over a duration of 50 ms. Full-thickness penetration of the iris is identified with the presence of a pigment plume.
- The Nd:YAG laser (2.0–3.0 mJ) is then used to enlarge the iridotomy. Patency of the iridotomy is confirmed with the presence of positive retroillumination and deepening of the AC.

### *Postoperative care*

- IOP measurement is usually taken 30 minutes after the procedure.
- Topical steroids are used four to six times a day for a week to control inflammation.
- IOP lowering medications may be necessary in the presence of laser-induced IOP spike.

## Anatomical Changes After LPI

In addition to relieving the underlying pupil block and lowering IOP, an LPI also results in deepening of the AC and widening of the AC angles (Figs. 46-2A and B).[3,8-10] The predictive factors for the amount of angle opening after LPI include a greater lens vault, thicker iris, and higher baseline IOP.[10]

Deepening of the AC is demonstrated by an increase in the AC depth, AC area, and AC volume. AC angle widening has been documented qualitatively by gonioscopy and quantitatively by an increase in the angle opening distance, trabecular-iris space area, and angle recess area as obtained from ultrasound biomicroscopy and anterior segment optical coherence tomography (ASOCT) imaging. Likewise, imaging studies also revealed flattening of the iris following LPI as assessed both qualitatively and quantitatively by a reduction of the iris curvature.[3,8-10]

## Complications

The common complications associated with LPI include postlaser IOP spike,[11,12] inflammation and hyphema. These side effects are often self-limiting and resolve without sequelae. Other less common but more adverse complications include monocular visual disturbances, cataract formation, corneal decompensation, and malignant glaucoma.[13]

Pretreatment with IOP lowering medications have been shown to be efficacious in preventing postlaser IOP spikes, and treatment with argon prior to Nd:YAG iridotomy has also been found to minimize the occurrence of bleeding.[14]

Visual disturbances such as ghost images, bright horizontal lines, and glare have been described after an LPI. These symptoms can be visually debilitating; patients therefore need to be counseled appropriately prior to the laser procedure. Although the etiology of these visual disturbances has not been fully elucidated, the visual disturbances are often (but not always) transient. While the symptoms were initially attributed to a poorly sited iridotomy that was not fully covered by the upper eyelid,[15] one study showed that neither the size nor site of iridotomy were associated with these post-laser visual symptoms.[16] Alternatively, it is speculated that a worsening of cortical cataract severity may be a contributor to this complication. Cataract progression in the form of nuclear, cortical, and/or posterior-subcapsular opacity has been demonstrated to occur during the first 12 months after LPI.[17] When a patient experiences a visual disturbance after an LPI, they should be reassured that it is normal to experience these symptoms and that they are likely transient. If their symptoms have not resolved over a month or two and are debilitating, there are various strategies to fix the problem, such as a colored contact lens, enlarging the iridotomy, corneal tattoo overlying the LPI, or cataract surgery. Open communication with the patient when this situation occurs is essential to maintain a healthy patient–doctor relationship.

The prevalence of post-LPI corneal decompensation ranges between 1.8% and 20%,[18] and the related risk factors include pre-existing corneal endothelial pathology such as Fuchs' endothelial dystrophy, a previous history of acute angle closure, and direct laser damage to the endothelium either as a result of high laser energy and/or extensive number of laser shots. Studies have also demonstrated a reduction of the cornea endothelial cell count over the treated area in these eyes.[19]

## PEARLS AND PITFALLS

- Pretreatment with pilocarpine to achieve miosis and thinning of the iris; use topical glaucoma medications such as brimonidine and dorzolamide to prevent post-laser IOP spikes.
- Pretreatment with argon laser (i.e. sequential Argon-Nd:YAG) at the intended iridotomy site to reduce the risk of hyphema.
- Avoid placement of iridotomy at the 12 o'clock position as the air bubble created by the laser procedure may obscure further laser application.
- In eyes with APAC, the IOP should be adequately lowered to ensure a clear cornea through which the LPI can be performed.
- Laser should be applied through a focusing lens to minimize damage to the cornea.
- When possible, place the LPI over an iris crypt or thin area of iris stroma.
- In the setting of inflammation (associated with either uveitis or APAC), it is occasionally difficult to complete a full-thickness LPI in one session. After a first attempt, one can treat with topical corticosteroid and IOP lowering medications and complete the LPI a few days later.
- If a patient presents with angle closure in one eye, perform gonioscopy on the fellow eye as this will provide insight into the underlying mechanism.
- If a patient presents with bilateral angle closure, one must rule out anterior rotation of the ciliary body, which can be seen with topiramate use or certain drugs with sulfa-based moieties.

# LASER IRIDOPLASTY

## INTRODUCTION

Argon laser peripheral iridoplasty (ALPI, Fig. 46-3) is a non-invasive, simple and effective procedure to open an appositionally closed AC angle (ACA).

## INDICATIONS

Argon laser peripheral iridoplasty can be performed in various angle closure situations or can be used as an adjunctive procedure.

- In eyes with plateau iris configuration, in which a patent iridotomy fails to open the ACA, ALPI is indicated to pull the iris root away from the trabecular meshwork.
- In eyes with APAC, ALPI may be indicated as initial therapy or when there are factors that preclude a successful iridotomy. This includes corneal edema, shallow AC, severe inflammation or extreme mydriasis. An ALPI may be indicated to relieve angle closure and lower the IOP before definitive management in the form of LPI is carried out.[20]
- In chronic angle closure, appositionally closed angles may be treated with ALPI.
- Iridoplasty can be used when there are other causes of secondary angle closure such as in a microphthalmic or nanophthalmic eye, iris cyst or where there is forward rotation of the ciliary body, e.g. postscleral buckle surgery. In these situations, the angles are often closed in the absence of a pupil block mechanism.
- In eyes with phacomorphic glaucoma or if the lens is anteriorly subluxed, ALPI may be used as a temporizing measure to relieve angle closure.
- Iridoplasty may be used as an adjunctive procedure to deepen the ACA so as to facilitate subsequent laser trabeculoplasty.
- The success of ALPI in eyes with peripheral anterior synechiae (PAS) is usually limited. However, some authors have described the use of ALPI in eyes with a short duration of PAS. The laser is performed with a gonioscopy lens and should then be applied to the base of the synechiae. This is also known as gonioplasty. It should be noted that ALPI is generally more successful for appositional angle closure.[21]
- After incisional goniosynechialysis, ALPI can be used as an adjunctive procedure to open areas of persistent or recurrent synechial closure.[22]

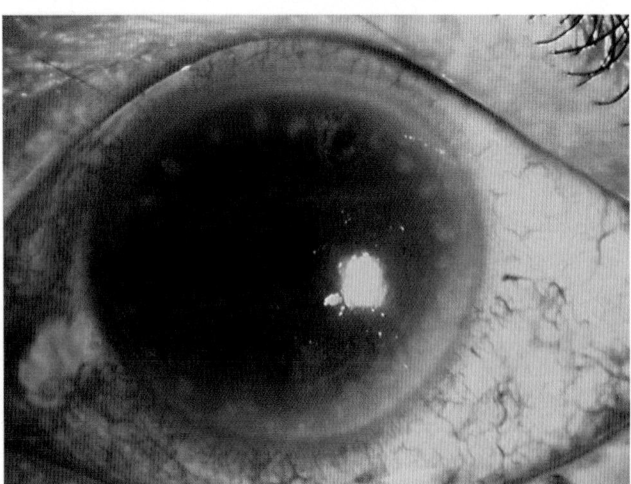

**Figure 46-3** An eye with acute angle closure that underwent laser iridoplasty (as well as laser peripheral iridotomy).

### Contraindications

There are few contraindications to ALPI. In eyes with a flat or very shallow AC, there is a risk of inadvertent damage to the corneal endothelium, and ALPI should not be performed.

In cases where there is extensive corneal edema or opacification, this obscures the surgeon's view and results in poor focusing of the laser. Iridoplasty is contraindicated due to the risk of damage to contiguous ocular structures. Synechial angle closure secondary to uveitis, neovascular glaucoma, or iridocorneal endothelial syndrome is also a contraindication to ALPI.[20]

A relative contraindication is light colored irides, as ALPI can cause a type of traumatic mydriasis, which can sometimes be asymmetric when performed bilaterally.

### Surgical Technique

The ALPI is performed in an outpatient under topical anesthesia.

#### *Preoperative*

- Topical pilocarpine 2% or 4% is used 1 hour before the procedure to stretch the iris stroma.
- Topical brimonidine is used to blunt any post procedure IOP spike.

- Lowering the IOP will also aid in decreasing corneal edema and improving visualization of the iris. Options include topical and systemic hypotensive agents such as acetazolamide or mannitol, performing AC paracentesis or use of topical glycerin.

### *Intraoperative*

Argon laser is most commonly used. The laser settings should be of low power, large area, and long duration. The Abraham iridotomy contact lens is recommended.

The initial laser setting is usually 100–400 mW, 300–500 µm, and 300–500 ms. Others have reported laser settings of 50–500 µm, 500 ms, and 150–1000 mW.

The subsequent power and duration of the laser is then titrated accordingly. It is increased if no iris contraction is observed. If pigments are liberated, a pop sound is heard or gas bubble seen, the power should be reduced. Lighter irides require more power due to reduced absorption of laser.

*Treatment zone:* 5–6 burns per quadrant are placed on the peripheral iris. A total of 20–24 spots (2 spot size apart) are applied 360°. In APAC eyes, if ALPI is used as initial treatment, treatment of 180° of the peripheral iris may be sufficient to abort the attack.

The laser is applied perpendicular to the iris surface for uniform contraction. If required, an additional row can be applied more peripherally to the first row of burns.[20] Care should be taken to avoid PAS, radial iris vessels, iris defects, or abnormalities.

Some authors have described the use of diode laser or double frequency Nd:YAG with good results.[23,24]

### Mechanism of Action

Iridoplasty tightens the peripheral iris to physically pull it posteriorly from the trabecular meshwork. Consequently, the ACA is opened.

Histopathological studies show that there is contraction furrow formation, proliferation of fibroblast like cells, collagen deposition on iris surface, denaturation of stromal collagen, and coagulative necrosis of blood vessels in anterior two thirds of the iris stroma.[25] The short-term effect is achieved via heat shrinkage, and in the long term, there is contraction of a fibroblastic membrane in the region of laser application.

### Postoperative Care

Topical brimonidine is given to prevent IOP elevation. Topical steroids four to six times a day can be given for 5 days to reduced inflammation.

### Complications

The most common complication of ALPI is a mild transient iritis, which is usually amenable to topical steroids. IOP can be elevated due to pigment dispersion, protein leakage, or inflammation. This is usually managed using topical hypotensive agents.

Corneal endothelial burns can occur especially in eyes with shallow AC and extensive corneal edema. Mild endothelial burns resolve spontaneously within a few days, but rarely there is a long-term risk of corneal decompensation, especially in patients with pre-existing Fuchs' endothelial corneal dystrophy. To prevent corneal endothelial burns, some authors have described placing the initial contraction burn more centrally to deepen the AC before placing the peripheral burns.[20]

Other complications include pupil distortion, focal iris atrophy, and iris perforation. Rarely, over treatment may also lead to iris necrosis.

## SURGICAL OUTCOMES

### Acute Angle Closure

The definitive procedure for acute angle closure is an LPI. Iridoplasty can be used as an initial treatment modality. It has been shown to reduce IOP more rapidly than systemic medications in the first 2 hours.[26] Lai et al. compared the use of ALPI versus systemic hypotensive agents such as acetazolamide and/or mannitol. At a mean follow-up of 15 months, there were no differences in mean IOP and requirement for glaucoma medications between eyes treated with ALPI and systemic hypotensive agents.[27]

### Plateau Iris Syndrome

Iridoplasty is the definitive treatment in plateau iris syndrome. It relieves appositional angle closure in plateau iris after LPI. A study found that after >6 years, 87% of treated eyes had ACA which remained open after only one session of treatment.[28]

### Phacomorphic Glaucoma

The definitive treatment in phacomorphic glaucoma is cataract extraction. Tham et al. assessed the efficacy of ALPI as an initial treatment in 10 consecutive patients who received topical atropine and timolol. After ALPI, the mean IOP reduced from 56.1 ± 12.5 to 45.3 ± 14.5 mm Hg at 15 minutes, 37.6 ± 7.5 mm Hg at 30 minutes, 34.2 ± 9.7 mm Hg at 60 minutes, 25.5 ± 8.7 mm Hg at 120 minutes, and 13.6 ± 4.2 mm Hg at 1 day. There were no ALPI-related complications.[29]

## PLACE OF THE TECHNIQUE IN SURGICAL ARMAMENTARIUM

The ALPI is useful in treating appositionally closed ACA. In other angle closure situations where mechanism other than pupil block is present, ALPI can be a temporizing measure. However, definitive treatment to eliminate the underlying mechanism will be needed.

## PEARLS AND PITFALLS

- A prerequisite for the success of ALPI is appositionally closed angles. Ideally, preoperative indentation gonioscopy should be performed by an experienced examiner.
- Good visualization is essential to prevent contiguous damage to the cornea. Ideally, preoperative IOP should be well control, although this may not be possible in some cases of APAC attack.
- To achieve a peripheral iris burn, it is useful to allow a thin crescent of aiming beam to overlap the sclera at the limbus. The patient may be instructed to look in the direction of the beam.[20]
- Careful titration of the power and duration is also important so as to prevent excessive inflammation and elevated IOP.
- The peripheral iris should be targeted for maximum efficacy of iris contraction.

## REFERENCES


1. Nolan WP, Foster PJ, Devereux JG, et al. YAG laser iridotomy treatment for primary angle closure in East Asian eyes. Br J Ophthalmol. 2000;84:1255-9.
2. Snow JT. Value of prophylactic peripheral iridectomy on the second eye in angle closure glaucoma. Trans Ophthalmol Soc U K. 1977;97:189-91.
3. Gazzard G, Friedman DS, Devereux JG, et al. A prospective ultrasound biomicroscopy evaluation of changes in anterior segment morphology after laser iridotomy in Asian eyes. Ophthalmology. 2003;110:630-8.
4. Saw SM, Gazzard G, Friedman DS. Interventions for angle-closure glaucoma: an evidence-based update. Ophthalmology. 2003;110(10):1869-78.
5. Friedman DS, Chew PT, Gazzard G, et al. Long-term outcomes in fellow eyes after acute primary angle closure in the contralateral eye. Ophthalmology. 2006;113:1087-91.
6. Salmon JF. Long-term intraocular pressure control after Nd-YAG laser iridotomy in chronic angle-closure glaucoma. J Glaucoma. 1993;2:291-6.
7. Jiang Y, Friedman DS, He M, et al. Design and methodology of a randomized controlled trial of laser iridotomy for the prevention of angle closure in southern China: the Zhongshan angle Closure Prevention trial. Ophthalmic Epidemiol. 2010;17:321-32.
8. Ang GS, Wells AP. Changes in Caucasian eyes after laser peripheral iridotomy: an anterior segment optical coherence tomography study. Clin Experiment Ophthalmol. 2010;38:778-85.
9. Lei K, Wang N, Wang L, et al. Morphological changes of the anterior segment after laser peripheral iridotomy in primary angle closure. Eye (Lond). 2009;23:345-50.
10. How AC, Baskaran M, Kumar RS, et al. Changes in anterior segment morphology after laser peripheral iridotomy: an anterior segment optical coherence tomography study. Ophthalmology. 2012;119:1383-7.
11. Jiang Y, Chang DS, Foster PJ, et al. Immediate changes in intraocular pressure after laser peripheral iridotomy in primary angle-closure suspects. Ophthalmology. 2012;119:283-8.
12. Lee TL, Yuxin Ng J, Nongpiur ME, et al. Intraocular pressure spikes after a sequential laser peripheral iridotomy for angle closure [published online ahead of print Feb 19, 2013]. J Glaucoma.
13. Cashwell LF, Martin TJ. Malignant glaucoma after laser iridotomy. Ophthalmology. 1992;99:651-8.
14. Goins K, Schmeisser E, Smith T. Argon laser pretreatment in Nd: YAG iridotomy. Ophthalmic Surg. 1990;21:497-500.
15. Spaeth GL, Idowu O, Seligsohn A, et al. The effects of iridotomy size and position on symptoms following laser peripheral iridotomy. J Glaucoma. 2005;14:364-7.
16. Congdon N, Yan X, Friedman DS, et al. Visual symptoms and retinal straylight after laser peripheral iridotomy: the Zhongshan Angle-Closure Prevention Trial. Ophthalmology. 2012;119:1375-82.
17. Yip JL, Nolan WP, Gilbert CE, et al. Prophylactic laser peripheral iridotomy and cataract progression. Eye (Lond). 2010;24:1127-34.
18. Ang LP, Higashihara H, Sotozono C, et al. Argon laser iridotomy-induced bullous keratopathy a growing problem in Japan. Br J Ophthalmol. 2007;91:1613-5.
19. Park HY, Lee NY, Park CK, et al. Long-term changes in endothelial cell counts after early phacoemulsification versus laser peripheral iridotomy using sequential argon:YAG laser technique in acute primary angle closure. Graefes Arch Clin Exp Ophthalmol. 2012;250:1673-80.
20. Ritch R, Tham CC, Lam DS. Argon laser peripheral iridoplasty (ALPI): an update. Surv Ophthalmol. 2007;52:279-88.
21. Wand M. Argon laser gonioplasty for synechial angle closure. Arch Ophthalmol. 1992;110:363-7.
22. Tanihara H, Nagata M. Argon-laser gonioplasty following goniosynechialysis. Graefes Arch Clin Exp Ophthalmol. 1991;229:505-7.
23. Chew PT, Wong JS, Chee CK, et al. Corneal transmissibility of diode versus argon lasers and their photothermal effects on the cornea and iris. Clin Experiment Ophthalmol. 2000;28:53-7.
24. Lai JS, Tham CC, Chua JK, et al. Immediate diode laser peripheral iridoplasty as treatment of acute attack of primary angle closure glaucoma: a preliminary study. J Glaucoma. 2001;10:89-94.

25. Sassani JW, Ritch R, McCormick S, et al. Histopathology of argon laser peripheral iridoplasty. Ophthalmic Surg. 1993;24: 740-5.
26. Lam DSC, Lai JSM, Tham CCY, et al. Argon laser peripheral iridoplasty versus conventional systemic medical therapy in treatment of acute primary angle-closure glaucoma: a prospective, randomized, controlled trial. Ophthalmology. 2002;109: 1591-6.
27. Lai JSM, Tham CCY, Chua JKH, et al. To compare argon laser peripheral iridoplasty (ALPI) against systemic medications in treatment of acute primary angle-closure: mid-term results. Eye. 2006;20:309-14.
28. Ritch R, Tham CCY, Lam DSC. Long-term success of argon laser peripheral iridoplasty in the management of plateau iris syndrome. Ophthalmology. 2004;111:104-8.
29. Tham CCY, Lai JSM, Poon ASY, et al. Immediate argon laser peripheral iridoplasty (ALPI) as initial treatment for acute phacomorphic angle-closure (phacomorphic glaucoma) before cataract extraction: a preliminary study. Eye. 2005;19:778-83.

CHAPTER

47

# Cyclophotocoagulation

Donna Nguyen, Kimberly A Mankiewicz, Nicholas P Bell

## INTRODUCTION

Cyclodestructive procedures were first introduced in the 1930's using diathermy to produce selective destruction of ciliary processes to reduce the rate of aqueous production.[1,2] Several other modalities have since evolved, including β-irradiation,[3] electrolysis,[4] cryotherapy,[5] ultrasound,[6] and surgical excision.[7] Cryotherapy was thought to be less destructive and more predictable in inducing ciliary process necrosis and atrophy; however, there was a high incidence of intense postoperative pain and inflammation, as well as high rates of phthisis and vision loss.[8,9]

The concept of using light energy to photocoagulate the ciliary body led to today's current method for performing cyclophotocoagulation (CPC).[10] Initially, a ruby laser (693 nm)[11] was used, but the neodymium:yttrium-aluminum-garnet (Nd:YAG) laser (1064 nm) was found to be more effective in penetrating the sclera and optimizing energy absorption by the ciliary epithelium.[12] Now, the semiconductor diode laser (750-850 nm)[13,14] has become the laser of choice for transscleral cyclophotocoagulation (TSCPC), even though there is less scleral transmission than with Nd:YAG CPC. The diode laser results in greater absorption of energy by the melanin in the ciliary epithelium[15] and thus more focused treatment with less collateral damage. Endoscopic cyclophotocoagulation (ECP) uses an 810 nm diode laser to directly treat the ciliary processes under endoscopic guidance with a Xenon light source and video camera. This chapter will focus on TSCPC and ECP.

## INDICATIONS

### Transscleral Cyclophotocoagulation (TSCPC)

- Glaucoma insufficiently controlled after filtering or tube shunt surgery where scarring of conjunctiva limits success with additional incisional glaucoma surgery.
- Refractory glaucoma in eyes with poor visual acuity/potential where risks associated with incisional surgery (endophthalmitis, significant hemorrhage, sympathetic ophthalmia) exceed potential benefits. These often include neovascular, traumatic, aphakic, pediatric, developmental, inflammatory, and silicone oil-induced glaucomas, as well as glaucoma associated with corneal transplantation or in eyes with scarred conjunctiva.
- Patients in poor health where general anesthesia would be unsafe.
- To control intractable pain associated with elevated intraocular pressure (IOP) in eyes with severe vision loss or no light perception.
- As a primary surgical treatment for glaucoma when access to medical care is limited.
- Patients with loss of IOP control due to failure of previous TSCPC.
- Patients who are at high risk of intraoperative suprachoroidal hemorrhage especially due to inability to discontinue anticoagulants, bleeding diathesis, blood dyscrasias, or high risk anatomy (extreme myopia) may be reasonable candidates for TSCPC.

### Endoscopic Cyclophotocoagulation (ECP)

- Refractory and pediatric glaucoma in pseudophakic eyes.
- Primary glaucoma surgery in conjunction with cataract surgery.

Indications for TSCPC and ECP have both evolved over the last decade, and the procedures are performed in situations that traditionally would have been treated by filtration procedures. CPC is typically reserved to treat refractory glaucoma. However, studies on CPC as primary surgical treatment in eyes with good vision have shown positive results. In a prospective randomized study in Ghana, of primary open-angle glaucoma (POAG) patients who underwent TSCPC, 47% of eyes (37 of 79), had an IOP reduction of 20% or more. There were no serious complications such as hypotony, phthisis bulbi, or sympathetic ophthalmia; however, 28% developed an atonic pupil. In 76% of eyes (60 of 79 eyes), the vision remained the same or was better after the laser.[16] A retrospective study of eyes with POAG and mean pretreatment visual acuity in the range 20/20 to 20/120 underwent a single application of diode TSCPC between 60 and 160 Joules. Mean visual acuity did not deteriorate, although the final visual acuity was worse in three cases (13% of 23 eyes), two of which were due to cataract progression.[17] Other studies evaluating TSCPC as primary surgical treatment have shown good success with few, if any, serious complications.[18-20]

## CONTRAINDICATIONS

Because of the significant risk of vision loss, TSCPC is typically not performed as first-line therapy in eyes of young patients with good vision. However, as mentioned, TSCPC has been evaluated as a primary surgical treatment, especially in developing countries where conventional glaucoma therapy is unavailable or adequate surgical follow-up to ensure good outcomes is not feasible. Elderly pseudophakic patients who are unable to undergo incisional glaucoma surgery are good candidates for TSCPC with the slow coagulation settings (*see* Table 47-2). Caution should be taken with TSCPC on eyes with thinned sclera from pre-existing inflammatory connective tissue disease, such as rheumatoid arthritis and Wegner's granulomatosis, and prior large scleral incision cataract surgery.

With lower risks of hypotony, phthisis, and severe vision loss, ECP is being combined with intraocular procedures, such as cataract surgery,[21,22] in an effort to reduce the need for IOP-lowering medications. However, because the extent of IOP-lowering with ECP seems modest,[22] eyes with very high pressures may benefit more from TSCPC, particularly if visual potential is limited. In the setting of excessively high IOP with good vision in a healthy patient with minimal intraoperative surgical risk, filtering procedures or drainage devices provide better results.

## MECHANISM OF ACTION

CPC reduces IOP by coagulation and destruction of the ciliary body to reduce aqueous production. The mechanism is thought to involve both destruction of the ciliary epithelial tissue and reduced blood flow to the ciliary body. Studies in rabbits following TSCPC with the Nd:YAG laser showed coagulative necrosis of the ciliary epithelium and destruction of ciliary vessels in the overlying area[23] with similar findings in human eyes.[24,25] In another study, tissues treated with diode TSCPC showed pronounced disruption of the ciliary body muscle and stroma, ciliary processes, and ciliary epithelium. In contrast, tissues treated with ECP showed sparing of the ciliary body muscle with less architectural disorganization.[26] Another study also demonstrated immediate and severely reduced or nonexistent blood flow in the areas of treatment with both TSCPC and ECP; however, transscleral-treated processes remained nonperfused, whereas endoscopic-treated processes showed some reperfusion that increased over time.[27] Thus, the conclusion that chronic poor perfusion of the ciliary body after diode TSCPC may partly account for its efficacy and the significant complications, including hypotony and phthisis. Additionally, the resulting inflammatory response from the procedure has been hypothesized to reduce IOP by increasing aqueous outflow via the uveoscleral outflow pathway.[28]

## SPECIFIC INSTRUMENTATION

The most widely used semiconductor for contact TSCPC is the Oculight SLx (Iridex, Mountain View, CA: Figs. 47-1 and 47-2). The G-probe handpiece can be reused several times without loss of power, even if cleaned by alcohol each time.[34]

The ECP laser unit (Endo Optiks, Little Silver, NJ) consists of the laser endoscope and the equipment console. The laser endoscope contains fiber optics for an 810 nm diode laser, xenon light source, a helium-neon laser aiming beam, and a video imaging camera connected to the console. The console contains features to adjust laser power and duration and light and aiming beam intensity. A foot pedal controlled by the surgeon is used to control the progress of surgery by viewing the video monitor, rather than viewing through the operating microscope.[22]

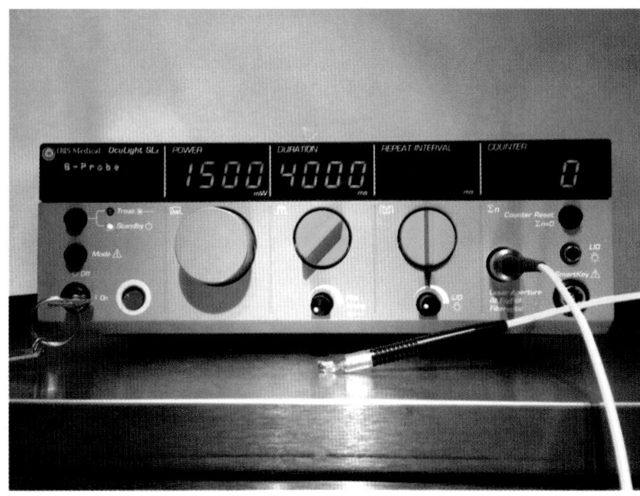

**Figure 47-1** Oculight SLx (Iridex, Mountain View, CA) diode laser system for transscleral cyclophotocoagulation.

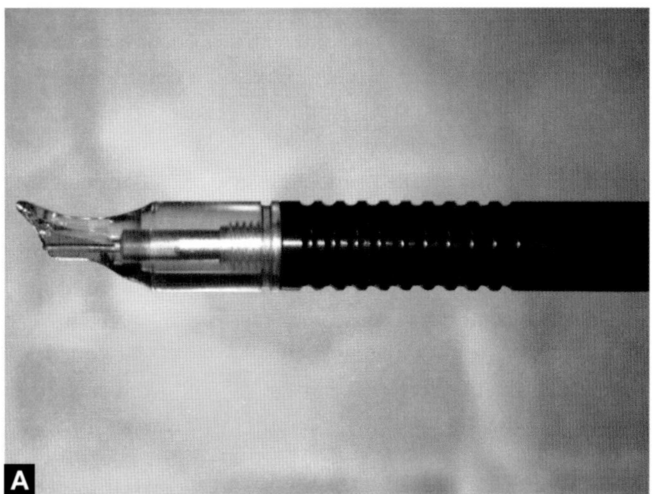

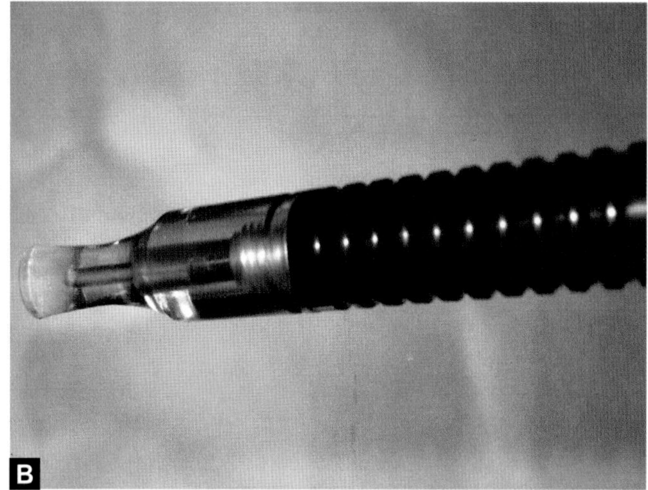

**Figures 47-2A and B** G-probe (Iridex, Mountain View, CA) fiber optic handpiece for Oculight SLx viewed from the side (A) and from the top (B).

## SURGICAL TECHNIQUE

### Transscleral Cyclophotocoagulation

If performed in a minor procedure or laser suite, a retrobulbar or peribulbar injection is necessary for the awake patient due to significant intraoperative pain with TSCPC. We recommend a 1:1 mixture of 2% lidocaine and 0.75% bupivacaine, as it also provides a few hours of postoperative pain control. Treatment should not be initiated until the eye is adequately anesthetized. Diode TSCPC is usually performed with the patient in the supine or reclined position. If the patient is unable to tolerate the procedure with a local anesthetic block (young or anxious patients), general anesthesia (endotracheal or laryngeal mask) can be induced in an operative suite. Even for the patient under general anesthesia, a retrobulbar injection is recommended when feasible to limit postoperative discomfort for the first few hours. An eyelid speculum is typically placed for optimal exposure.

**TABLE 47-1** Diode transscleral cyclophotocoagulation settings*

| | |
|---|---|
| Power | 1500–2500 mW |
| Duration | 2.0 s |

*Applications are spaced one-half of the probe tip apart.

Contact TSCPC was initially performed with the Nd:YAG laser[15] using a round sapphire probe tip but was replaced by the more portable, compact, and relatively inexpensive semiconductor solid-state diode laser system. The diode laser utilizes an 810 nm wavelength that exhibits less scleral transmission than the Nd:YAG laser but considerably greater

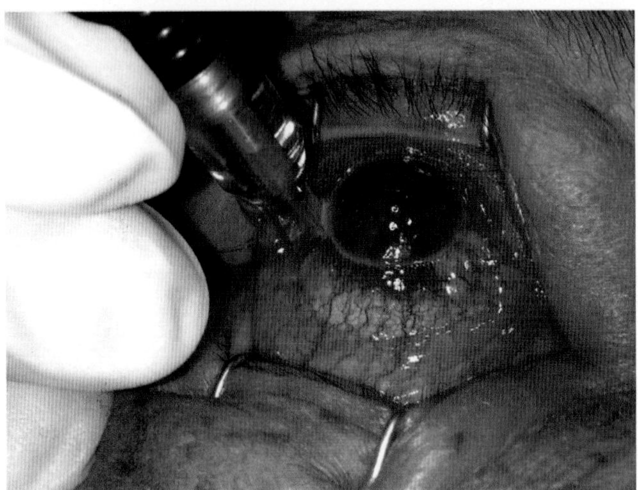

**Figure 47-3** Application of transscleral cyclophotocoagulation.

absorption by melanin. One commonly used commercially available diode laser is the Oculight SLx (Fig. 47-1). The laser energy is transmitted by a fiber optic handpiece called the G-probe (Iridex, Mountain View, CA). The G-probe footplate is curved spherically to match the perilimbal curvature of the eye. The heel of the probe is placed on the conjunctiva adjacent to the limbus so the fiber optic tip is 1.2 mm behind the limbus and thus over the ciliary body (Figs. 47-2A and B). The probe is held firmly against the conjunctiva and sclera for the entire duration of each laser application (Fig. 47-3). Traditional initial power settings are 1500–1750 mW and duration set at 2000 ms (2 seconds) (Table 47-1).[13] The power is increased in 250 mW increments until an audible popping sound is heard, then reduced in smaller increments until no pop is heard. The rest of the treatment is completed at this power. The audible pop is caused by excessive tissue explosion; therefore; it is believed that a power setting one increment below this level is preferred to limit the inflammatory response.[29] The laser is applied circumferentially with each application spaced one-half the width of the probe tip apart by aligning the lateral edge of the plastic probe on the indentation mark created by the fiber optic point of conjunctival indentation from the previous laser placement. Approximately 17–19 applications can be placed over 270°, sparing a temporal quadrant to minimize risk of anterior segment ischemia.[13] However, an alternative is to treat with 20–24 applications for 360° sparing only the 3- and 9-o'clock positions.

Lower energy levels with longer duration have also been used with success.[8,30] This 'slow coagulation technique' is the authors' preferred treatment (Table 47-2).[31] The duration is doubled to 4000 ms, and the initial power settings are lower

**TABLE 47-2** Slow Coagulation Technique Settings*[30,31]

| Iris color | Power | Duration |
|---|---|---|
| Dark and light brown | 1200–1250 mW | 4–4.5 s |
| Others | 1500 mW | 4.0 s |

*Applications are spaced one full width of the probe tip apart.

(1250 mW). As with traditional treatment settings, the power is titrated to just lower than is needed to achieve audible pops. Because the longer time duration results in a larger area of ciliary body destruction, fewer applications are spaced one probe tip apart (instead of one-half).

If repeat treatments are needed to titrate IOP control, laser may be applied over 180° to lower the risk of over treating and causing phthisis. Additional TSCPC (3rd or greater procedure) can be administered in 180° increments as well, overlapping 90° with the previous 180° treatment.

Although not common currently, noncontact TSCPC can be performed with a Nd:YAG laser, a continuous-wave thermal mode laser at 1064 nm in wavelength. With the patient seated at the laser slit lamp, the beam is aimed onto the conjunctiva over the proposed ciliary body but defocused approximately 1.0–1.5 mm posteriorly (sub-scleral), thus coagulating the ciliary body processes. A contact lens with 1.0 mm markings parallel to the limbus can be used to hold the lids open and blanch the conjunctiva or a lid speculum can also be used. Approximately 8–10 applications per quadrant are placed from 270° to 360° but can be adjusted to 180° in patients at risk of hypotony.

## Endoscopic Cyclophotocoagulation

Retrobulbar, peribulbar, topical, or intracameral anesthesia is appropriate for ECP treatments. General anesthesia can be considered in certain cases. There are two main approaches to access the ciliary processes with ECP: limbal or pars plana.

In the limbal approach, after dilation, a temporal incision 1.5–2.0 mm in length is created. Both clear cornea and scleral tunnel incisions commonly used in cataract surgery provide adequate access for the ECP probe. The anterior chamber is filled with a cohesive viscoelastic between the iris and lens to deepen the ciliary sulcus space and allow for easier approach to the pars plicata with the ECP probe. The 18-gauge or 20-gauge probe is then inserted through the incision and into the posterior sulcus. The ciliary processes are viewed on the ECP unit monitor and treatment can begin. The laser is set on continuous wave, and the energy setting is titrated to between 300 and 900 mW.[22] The ECP probe is placed 1.0–3.0 mm from the tissue, and laser energy is applied to each ciliary process until shrinkage and whitening occur. The ciliary processes are treated individually or in a "painting" fashion across multiple processes. If excessive energy is used, the ciliary process will explode (or "pop") with bubble formation, possibly resulting in excessive inflammation. Approximately 180° of ciliary processes can be treated with one incision site but more can be treated with the curved probe. After the nasal 180° of ciliary processes are treated, a second incision nasally is created to treat the tissue underneath the initial incision. It is recommended to treat at least 270–360° through two incision sites to lower IOP to a greater degree and for a longer period.[32] Before closure of the wounds, the viscoelastic is thoroughly removed from the anterior chamber with irrigation and aspiration to prevent a postoperative IOP spike.

A pars plana approach is preferred if there is an anterior chamber IOL, disrupted anterior segment, or difficult view. A pars plana incision can be easily placed in a vitrectomized eye that is either pseudophakic or aphakic, allowing for complete visualization of the ciliary processes. In phakic eyes or those that are not vitrectomized, unless simultaneous vitrectomy can be done, this is often more difficult. An infusion port is inserted through the inferior pars plana or the anterior chamber. Two superior entries are created for the ECP probe (and vitrector, if being performed) and illumination. The ECP probe is inserted through each of the superior entries, and the opposite 180° processes are treated.

## POSTOPERATIVE CARE

- Postoperative inflammation can be significant following diode TSCPC and should be addressed prophylactically. Subconjunctival injection of a short-acting steroid at the end of the procedure is recommended.[33] Immediately after the procedure, atropine and steroid ointment should be applied prior to patching the eye. The patch may be removed later in the evening when the anesthetic block has worn off, and glaucoma medications should be resumed
- Prostaglandins or cholinergics may be temporarily discontinued if worried about exacerbating cystoid macular edema or inflammation. Preoperative glaucoma medications are restarted as necessary to control IOP.
- Postoperative topical steroids should be used at least four times daily but may be needed as frequently as every 1–2 hours. Topical steroids should be tapered slowly over 1–2 months as the inflammation recedes.
- Atropine 1% applied 1–2 times daily should be used to relax the ciliary muscle. Atropine dosing can be titrated to the level of ocular throbbing and pain.
- Postoperative pain is typically mild to moderate, and a weak analgesic is usually sufficient for a few days following the procedure. However, if the pain is more severe, oral narcotic medications may be necessary.
- We recommend re-examining the patient within 7–14 days to assess the IOP, the level of inflammation, and the degree of patient discomfort. If only a modest IOP lowering is achieved, we prefer to wait until the eye is quiet before repeating the procedure.

Postoperative management of both ECP alone and ECP combined with cataract surgery is similar to that with cataract surgery alone, except that anti-inflammatory medications should be tapered slowly over 1–2 months. Subconjunctival or sub-Tenon's injection of a short-acting steroid at the end of the procedure and topical cycloplegics can also be utilized.

## COMPLICATIONS

After TSCPC, pain and conjunctival hyperemia are common but typically lessen over the first few days to weeks. Hyphema is also common, especially in patients with neovascular glaucoma. Anterior chamber inflammation ranges from mild to moderate, although some patients rarely may develop fibrin clots or hypopyon, which resolve with postoperative steroids. A transient IOP rise may occur. Other reported complications include hypotony,[35] malignant glaucoma from possible ciliary body edema,[36,37] necrotizing scleritis,[38] and sympathetic ophthalmia.[39,40] Although rare, phthisis bulbi is a possible condition that can develop following prolonged hypotony after CPC.

The most significant complication is loss of visual acuity. In many cases, the visual loss is partially related to the underlying disease process and not entirely a direct result of the laser treatment.[41] CPC has historically been used in those with poor visual potential but is also being used successfully as primary surgical treatment in eyes with good vision as previously discussed.

Reported complications for ECP include fibrin exudates, hyphema, cystoid macular edema, vision loss, and choroidal detachment.[42] There have been no reported cases of endophthalmitis, choroidal hemorrhage, or sympathetic ophthalmia with ECP, but these are always potential risks due to the intraocular nature of the procedure. Early postoperative IOP spikes can occur from retained viscoelastics[32] and iris trauma from an improperly placed ECP probe.[43] With the limited literature on ECP, potential and late complications may not yet have been encountered or reported.

## SURGICAL OUTCOMES

TSCPC is a well-established treatment of intractable glaucoma and is widely used in advanced cases with minimal visual potential.[44] A case series of 27 eyes with recalcitrant, severe glaucoma consisting of phakic, pseudophakic, and aphakic patients with POAG and various secondary open-angle and closed-angle glaucomas underwent TSCPC with a cumulative probability of success of 72% at 1 year and 52% at 2 years, with failure defined as <20% IOP reduction from baseline or IOP >22 mm Hg.[30] A retrospective study with an extended follow-up of up to 10 years (mean of 5.85 years) reviewed 68 eyes treated with Nd:YAG TSCPC. The preoperative IOP was 36.3 mm Hg and dropped to 22.6 mm Hg at 1 year, 18.9 mm Hg at 5 years, and 18.9 mm Hg at 10 years. The overall success rate (IOP 3–25 mm Hg and no secondary intervention) by 10 years was 48%.[45] In a randomized trial comparing diode TSCPC with the Ahmed Glaucoma Valve (New World Medical, Inc.) in neovascular glaucoma patients, the diode TSCPC group had a 57% IOP reduction, whereas the Ahmed group had 47% decrease in IOP. Visual acuity decreased in 6 eyes that had TSCPC (24% of 33 eyes) and in 9 eyes (27% of 33 eyes) in the Ahmed group.[46]

ECP is becoming more widely used in the treatment of glaucoma within the past decade. In a study of 68 eyes with refractory glaucoma, with the exception of those undergoing combined cataract extraction and ECP, all patients had failed maximal medical therapy and most had undergone one or more prior glaucoma surgeries. Eyes were treated between 180° and 360° of the ciliary body via a limbal or pars plana approach. The preoperative mean IOP was 27.7 mm Hg. Mean IOP reduction was 34%, and glaucoma medications were reduced from an average of 3.0 preoperatively to 2.0 postoperatively over a mean follow-up period of 12.9 months. Success in controlling IOP <22 mm Hg was 90% at last follow-up.[42]

A randomized trial of 68 eyes comparing ECP and the Ahmed Glaucoma Valve for refractory glaucoma found both procedures to be equally effective in reducing IOP. Success rates of IOP 6–20 mm Hg with or without topical medications were 73.6% and 70.6% for the ECP and Ahmed groups, respectively. Overall, there was lower frequency of complications in the ECP group than the Ahmed group.[47]

Combined phacoemulsification cataract extraction with ECP was compared with phacotrabeculectomy in a randomized prospective study involving 58 eyes of 58 patients. Reports showed 30% of participants treated with ECP achieved IOP control (below 19 mm Hg) without medication, and 65% achieved IOP control with medication. In the trabeculectomy group, 40% and 52% achieved IOP control without and with medication, respectively.[43]

## PEARLS AND PITFALLS

### Transscleral Cyclophotocoagulation

- The original study on diode TSCPC with the G-probe used a 2000 ms (2s) duration to place laser applications circumferentially along the limbus one-half width of the G-probe apart.[13] With the longer duration of 4000 ms (4s), especially for heavily pigmented eyes, the authors suggest laser applications placed one entire width of the G-probe apart to prevent excessive conjunctival and scleral burns due to longer treatment duration.
- Transscleral illumination with a light pipe or similar probe is extremely useful to delineate the location and extent of the ciliary body, especially in eyes with altered anatomy, prior cyclodestruction, staphylomatous areas, or intraocular surgery. This may be performed preoperatively or intraoperatively by placing the light pipe on the sclera in a dimly lit room and observing for limbal areas of irregular transillumination (prior cyclodestruction or trauma) or lack of transillumination that typically indicates the location of the ciliary body.
- Eyes that are acutely inflamed and with highly elevated IOP, especially in cases of neovascular glaucoma, may be difficult to achieve good anesthesia due to low tissue pH and thus poor penetration of anesthetic agents into the tissues. Thus, multiple retrobulbar injections and allowing sufficient time for infiltration of anesthetic agents to the tissues may be necessary. Supplementing the retrobulbar block with an injection into the superior orbit may be helpful.
- Laser energy dose should be titrated. To minimize the risk of ciliary body shutdown with resultant chronic hypotony and eventual phthisis, do not be overly aggressive with initial settings.
- In our experience, the ciliary body of younger people with healthier eyes seems to recover more rapidly and often requires more treatment sessions to achieve the desired IOP. Older people with recalcitrant neovascular glaucoma due to proliferative diabetic retinopathy or central retinal vein occlusion (or even end stage POAG) tend to respond better to CPC, possibly due to pre-existing vascular compromise of the ciliary body.

### Endoscopic Cyclophotocoagulation

- Although ECP can be performed with topical or intracameral anesthesia, for the novice ECP surgeon, lasting pain control and akinesia may be advantageous with retrobulbar injection.[48]

- For a pars plana approach, if the anterior segment surgeon has not had extensive experience in posterior segment surgery, assistance from a retinal surgeon should be sought for the establishment of the pars plana entry ports and the limited anterior vitrectomy.[22]
- During ECP, it is best to hold the probe within 2 mm of the ciliary processes. This distance can be judged by counting the ciliary processes in view on the monitor as the probe tissue distance of 2 mm corresponds to six processes in view.[32]
- During treatment of the ciliary processes, it is important to treat the entire process that is visible, not just the tip to obtain optimal results.[49]
- Iris hooks may provide a safe alternative for the elevation of the iris during ECP treatment in aphakic eyes, or those with posterior capsule compromise in which viscoelastic removal is more difficult, to prevent a postoperative IOP spike.[32]
- When combined with cataract surgery, performing ECP after extracting the cataract but before implanting the IOL may improve the visibility of the ciliary processes.[32]

## CONCLUSION

In summary, both TSCPC and ECP have a role in the surgical treatment of glaucoma. The mechanism of action is to decrease aqueous production by photocoagulation and subsequent destruction of ciliary processes. Postoperative inflammation is common with both but more pronounced following TSCPC. Good IOP reduction has been reported with both TSCPC and ECP, although the effect appears more modest in the latter. TSCPC has been historically performed in endstage, refractory glaucoma with poor visual acuity due to risk of vision loss. However, TSCPC as primary surgical treatment and in those with good visual acuity has recently shown good success. ECP is commonly performed in patients with mild-to-moderate glaucoma with good visual potential, especially in the setting of cataract surgery. Further, studies are required to better assess the long-term efficacy of ECP, but it appears to be a relatively safe surgical treatment. Both TSCPC and ECP will continue to evolve and remain important tools in the surgical treatment of glaucoma.

## REFERENCES


1. Vogt A. Versuche zur intraokularen Druckherabsetzung mittels Diatermieschadigung des Corpus ciliare (Zyklodiatermiestichelung). Klin Monastbl Augenheilkd. 1936;97:672-7.
2. Weve H. Die Zyklodiatermie das Corpus ciliare bei Glaukom. Zentralbl Ophthalmol. 1933;29:562-9.
3. Haik GM, Breffeilh LA, Barber A. Beta irradiation as a possible therapeutic agent in glaucoma. Am J Ophthalmol. 1958;31(8):945-52.
4. Berens C, Sheppard LB, Duel AB. Cycloelectrolysis for glaucoma. Trans Am Ophthalmol Soc. 1949;47:364-82.
5. Bietti G. Surgical intervention on the ciliary body; new trends for the relief of glaucoma. J Am Med Assoc. 1950;142(12):889-97.
6. Coleman DJ, Lizzi FL, Driller J, et al. Therapeutic ultrasound in the treatment of glaucoma. II. Clinical applications. Ophthalmology. 1985;92(3):347-53.
7. Freyler H and Scheimbauer I. [Excision of the ciliary body (Sautter procedure) as a last resort in secondary glaucoma (author's transl)]. Klin Monbl Augenheilkd 1981;179(6):473-7.
8. Pastor SA, Singh K, Lee DA, et al. Cyclophotocoagulation: a report by the American Academy of Ophthalmology. Ophthalmology. 2001;108(11):2130-38.
9. Shields MB. Cyclodestructive surgery for glaucoma: past, present, and future. Trans Am Ophthalmol Soc. 1985;83:285-303.
10. Vucicevic ZM, Tsou KC, Nazarian IH, et al. A cytochemical approach to the laser coagulation of the ciliary body. Bibl Ophthalmol. 1969;79:467-78.
11. Beckman H, Kinoshita A, Rota AN, et al. Transscleral ruby laser irradiation of the ciliary body in the treatment of intractable glaucoma. Trans Am Acad Ophthalmol Otolaryngol. 1972;76(2):423-36.
12. Beckman H, Sugar HS. Neodymium laser cyclocoagulation. Arch Ophthalmol. 1973;90(1):27-28.
13. Gaasterland DE, Pollack IP. Initial experience with a new method of laser transscleral cyclophotocoagulation for ciliary ablation in severe glaucoma. Trans Am Ophthalmol Soc. 1992; 90:225-43; discussion 226-243.
14. Peyman GA, Naguib KS, Gaasterland D. Trans-scleral application of a semiconductor diode laser. Lasers Surg Med. 1990; 10(6):569-75.
15. Schuman JS, Puliafito CA, Allingham RR, et al. Contact transscleral continuous wave neodymium:YAG laser cyclophotocoagulation. Ophthalmology. 1990;97(5):571-80.
16. Egbert PR, Fiadoyor S, Budenz DL, et al. Diode laser transscleral cyclophotocoagulation as a primary surgical treatment for primary open-angle glaucoma. Arch Ophthalmol. 2001;119(3):345-50.
17. Ansari E and Gandhewar J. Long-term efficacy and visual acuity following transscleral diode laser photocoagulation in cases of refractory and non-refractory glaucoma. Eye (Lond). 2007;21(7):936-40.
18. Kramp K, Vick HP, Guthoff R. Transscleral diode laser contact cyclophotocoagulation in the treatment of different glaucomas, also as primary surgery. Graefes Arch Clin Exp Ophthalmol. 2002;240(9):698-703.
19. Lai JS, Tham CC, Chan JC, et al. Diode laser transscleral cyclophotocoagulation as primary surgical treatment for medically uncontrolled chronic angle closure glaucoma: long-term clinical outcomes. J Glaucoma. 2005;14(2):114-9.
20. Rotchford AP, Jayasawal R, Madhusudhan S, et al. Transscleral diode laser cycloablation in patients with good vision. Br J Ophthalmol. 2010;94(9):1180-83.

21. Lin S. Endoscopic cyclophotocoagulation. Br J Ophthalmol 2002;86(12):1434-8.
22. Lin SC. Endoscopic and transscleral cyclophotocoagulation for the treatment of refractory glaucoma. J Glaucoma. 2008;17(3): 238-47.
23. Devenyi RG, Trope GE, Hunter WS. Neodymium-YAG transscleral cyclocoagulation in rabbit eyes. Br J Ophthalmol. 1987; 71(6):441-4.
24. Marsh P, Wilson DJ, Samples JR, et al. A clinicopathologic correlative study of noncontact transscleral Nd:YAG cyclophotocoagulation. Am J Ophthalmol. 1993;115(5):597-602.
25. Feldman RM, el-Harazi SM, LoRusso FJ, et al. Histopathologic findings following contact transscleral semiconductor diode laser cyclophotocoagulation in a human eye. J Glaucoma. 1997; 6(2):139-40.
26. Pantcheva MB, Kahook MY, Schuman JS, et al. Comparison of acute structural and histopathological changes in human autopsy eyes after endoscopic cyclophotocoagulation and trans-scleral cyclophotocoagulation. Br J Ophthalmol. 2007; 91(2):248-52.
27. Lin SC, Chen MJ, Lin MS, et al. Vascular effects on ciliary tissue from endoscopic versus trans-scleral cyclophotocoagulation. Br J Ophthalmol. 2006;90(4):496-500.
28. Liu GJ, Mizukawa A, Okisaka S. Mechanism of intraocular pressure decrease after contact transscleral continuous-wave Nd:YAG laser cyclophotocoagulation. Ophthalmic Res. 1994; 26(2):65-79.
29. Simmons RB, Prum BE, Jr., Shields SR, et al. Videographic and histologic comparison of Nd:YAG and diode laser contact transscleral cyclophotocoagulation. Am J Ophthalmol. 1994; 117(3):337-41.
30. Kosoko O, Gaasterland DE, Pollack IP, et al. Long-term outcome of initial ciliary ablation with contact diode laser transscleral cyclophotocoagulation for severe glaucoma. The Diode Laser Ciliary Ablation Study Group. Ophthalmology. 1996; 103(8):1294-1302.
31. Oculight SLx [manufacturer's instructions]. Mountain View, CA: Iridex; 2009.
32. Kahook MY, Lathrop KL, Noecker RJ. One-site versus two-site endoscopic cyclophotocoagulation. J Glaucoma. 2007;16(6): 527-30.
33. Hampton C, Shields MB, Miller KN, et al. Evaluation of a protocol for transscleral neodymium: YAG cyclophotocoagulation in one hundred patients. Ophthalmology. 1990;97(7):910-17.
34. Carrillo MM, Trope GE, Chipman ML, et al. Repeated use of transscleral cyclophotocoagulation laser G-probes. J Glaucoma. 2004;13(1):51-4.
35. Maus M and Katz LJ. Choroidal detachment, flat anterior chamber, and hypotony as complications of neodymium: YAG laser cyclophotocoagulation. Ophthalmology. 1990;97(1):69-72.
36. Hardten DR, Brown JD. Malignant glaucoma after Nd:YAG cyclophotocoagulation. Am J Ophthalmol. 1991;111(2):245-7.
37. Wand M, Schuman JS, Puliafito CA. Malignant glaucoma after contact transscleral Nd: YAG laser cyclophotocoagulation. J Glaucoma. 1993;2(2):110-11.
38. Ganesh SK, Rishi K. Necrotizing scleritis following diode laser trans-scleral cyclophotocoagulation. Indian J Ophthalmol. 2006; 54(3):199-200.
39. Bechrakis NE, Muller-Stolzenburg NW, Helbig H, et al. Sympathetic ophthalmia following laser cyclocoagulation. Arch Ophthalmol. 1994;112(1):80-84.
40. Pastor SA, Iwach A, Nozik RA, et al. Presumed sympathetic ophthalmia following Nd: YAG transscleral cyclophotocoagulation. J Glaucoma. 1993;2(1):30-31.
41. Shields MB, Shields SE. Noncontact transscleral Nd:YAG cyclophotocoagulation: a long-term follow-up of 500 patients. Trans Am Ophthalmol Soc. 1994;92:271-83; discussion 277-83.
42. Chen J, Cohn RA, Lin SC, et al. Endoscopic photocoagulation of the ciliary body for treatment of refractory glaucomas. Am J Ophthalmol. 1997;124(6):787-96.
43. Gayton JL. Traumatic aniridia during endoscopic laser cycloablation. J Cataract Refract Surg. 1998;24(1):134-5.
44. Vernon SA, Koppens JM, Menon GJ, et al. Diode laser cycloablation in adult glaucoma: long-term results of a standard protocol and review of current literature. Clin Experiment Ophthalmol. 2006;34(5):411-20.
45. Lin P, Wollstein G, Glavas IP, et al. Contact transscleral neodymium:yttrium-aluminum-garnet laser cyclophotocoagulation Long-term outcome. Ophthalmology. 2004;111(11): 2137-43.
46 Yildirim N, Yalvac IS, Sahin A, et al. A comparative study between diode laser cyclophotocoagulation and the Ahmed glaucoma valve implant in neovascular glaucoma: a long-term follow-up. J Glaucoma. 2009;18(3):192-6.
47. Lima FE, Magacho L, Carvalho DM, et al. A prospective, comparative study between endoscopic cyclophotocoagulation and the Ahmed drainage implant in refractory glaucoma. J Glaucoma. 2004;13(3):233-7.
48. Kahook MY and Noecker RJ. Endoscopic cyclophotocoagulation. Glaucoma Today 2005;November:24-9.
49. Allingham RR, Damji KF, Freedman SF, et al. Cyclodestructive Surgery. In: Shields' Textbook of Glaucoma, 6th edn. Philadelphia: Lippincott Williams & Wilkins; 2011.

CHAPTER

# 48

# Endoscopic Cyclophotocoagulation: Limbal and Pars Plana Approaches

Brian A Francis, Alexander K Nugent

## INTRODUCTION

The endoscopically guided limbal or pars plana approach delivers laser energy in an accurate and effective manner for a wide variety of glaucoma scenarios and severities. For the following patient selections, endoscopic cyclophotocoagulation (ECP) is best performed in combination with cataract surgery or in an aphakic or pseudophakic eye.

## PATIENT SELECTION

- *Glaucoma and visually significant cataract*: Combined ECP with phacoemulsification has a synergistic effect on intraocular pressure (IOP) lowering and can be performed through the same incision. Additionally, ECP spares the sclera and conjunctiva so that traditional transconjunctival filtration procedures such as aqueous tube shunt or trabeculectomy may be performed in the future[1,2]
- *Uncontrolled glaucoma after traditional filtration surgery*: Eyes after failed drainage implant or filtration surgery often have badly scarred conjunctiva and therefore are good candidates for ECP.[3,4] The reduction in aqueous can augment the aqueous drainage with a prior tube shunt and help to control IOP in these patients without the need for multiple tube shunts
- *Eyes at high risk of decompression complications following filtration surgery*: For a select group of patients who are at high risk of complications after filtration surgery such as aphakia, high myopia, patients with very long or short axial length, prior vitrectomy, natural bleeding diatheses, and/or anticoagulants, eyes prone to aqueous misdirection, and severe conjunctival scarring after scleral buckling, ECP offers a possible alternative.[4]
- ECP can even be used in patients who have had prior failed transscleral cyclophotocoagulation (TCP).[4,5] In these cases, the endoscopic approach is more directed, and mayreveal that the external ablation approach missed the target tissue
- Pediatric glaucomas are typically difficult to treat, and may require multiple surgical approaches to control long-term IOP. ECP has been employed with some limited success in these cases and is generally used as an adjunct to angle based or external filtration surgeries.[6-7]

## INDICATIONS

- Primary or secondary, open or closed angle glaucoma
- Mild-to-moderate glaucoma on multiple medications with preoperative IOP in the 18–30 mm Hg range
- Advanced glaucomatous damage on maximal medical therapy and having failed trabeculectomy as well as having one or more tube shunts implanted. In these cases, the pars plana approach (ECP plus) can be employed
- Patients having newer angle-based glaucoma surgeries such as canaloplasty (iScience, Menlo Park, CA), Trabectome (trabeculotomy internal approach, Neomedix, Tustin, CA), or iStent (canalicular bypass stent, Glaukos, Laguna Hills, CA) can have ECP concurrently or if the primary surgery fails to control IOP. In cases where a target IOP is in the low teens and external filtration surgery is to be avoided, combining an internal filtering procedure and aqueous reduction procedure may achieve this goal.

## CONTRAINDICATIONS/CAUTIONS

- Patients with advanced pseudoexfoliation with dense white fibrillar material coating the ciliary processes will have limited laser uptake secondary to lack of pigment

- Patients with a compromized blood aqueous barrier, such as neovascular glaucoma or uveitic glaucoma, should be approached with caution due to the possibility of severe inflammatory response and hypotony with formation of a cyclitic membrane
- Patients with advanced disk damage with high IOP on maximal medical therapy who undergo phaco-ECP may have a damaging IOP spike within the first few hours after surgery and should be monitored and treated accordingly.

## SURGICAL TECHNIQUE

### Basic Considerations

The ciliary processes are sensitive to manipulation therefore topical anesthesia is not adequate. Intracameral injection of preservative-free lidocaine is normally adequate and can also be used with phacoemulsification cataract extraction. Peribulbar, sub-Tenon's or retrobulbar anesthesia with lidocaine, and bupivacaine can be used for more aggressive treatments.

The surgeon will typically sit at the superior or temporal position. The settings on the console should be a power of 0.25–0.4 Watts, with a continuous (surgeon controlled) ablation time, and an aiming beam setting of 20–40. The intensity of the light source is varied depending on how far away the endoscope is from the target tissue.

### Anterior Approach

The anterior chamber is partially filled with viscoelastic and the ciliary sulcus is expanded with viscoelastic to create space between the lens and the iris. A 2 mm clear corneal incision is made adjacent to the limbus. The wound should be large enough to allow entry of the probe without much resistance. Due to certain viscoelastic products producing bubbles, the authors recommend a cohesive viscoelastic such as sodium hyaluronate (Healon, Abbott Medical Optics, Santa Ana, CA). Thicker forms of hyaluronate (Healon GV, Abbott Medical Optics, Santa Ana, CA) can also be used. For eyes that are aphakic or have had prior vitrectomy, an anterior chamber maintainer with BSS is used to keep the eye pressurized.

The endoscope tip is advanced in the anterior chamber to the pupillary margin, and then the surgeon changes gaze from the microscope to the monitor. The probe is then advanced toward the ciliary sulcus until 6–8 ciliary processes are visualized. This view gives the optimal distance for laser energy for tissue absorption. The aiming beam is centered over a process and depressing the foot pedal activates the laser. The ciliary process will shrink and whiten, signifying that it has been properly treated. It is important to treat the entire visible ciliary process (Fig. 48-1). Adjacent processes are treated until 180° has been treated. Going back over the same area is recommended to ensure adequate energy absorption and also to treat the areas in between ciliary processes that are now more accessible. A second incision is made to allow treatment of the remaining processes. At the end of treatment, irrigation and aspiration are necessary to fully remove viscoelastic in order to avoid damaging postoperative IOP spikes.

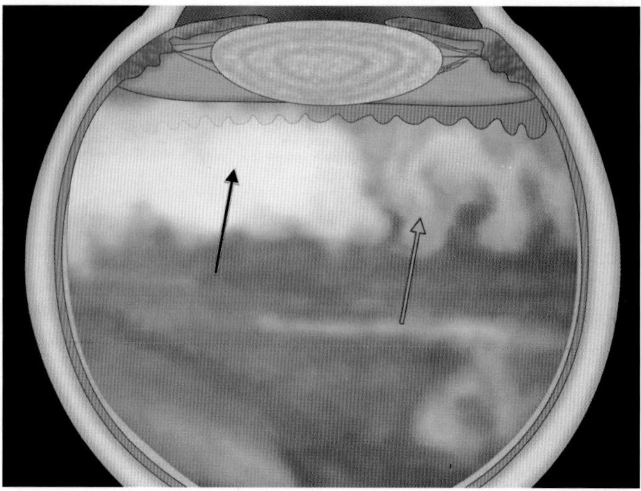

**Figure 48-1** Endocyclophotocoagulation of the ciliary body processes. The black arrow indicates the typical whitish appearance of the ciliary body processes immediately after treatment with laser energy. The green arrow represents the adjacent untreated tissue. The white appearance is the typical treatment endpoint associated with shrinkage of the tissue.

### Phaco-ECP

ECP combined with phacoemulsification cataract surgery is one of the most common indications for the procedure.[8-10] The procedure can be used in open-angle glaucoma patients with cataract in order to lower IOP and reduce their medication use. In addition, Phaco-ECP can be used in patients with chronic synechial angle closure, in whom angle-based procedures or aqueous tube shunts may be difficult.

An interesting indication is in the population of refractory plateau iris syndrome, where it is used to shrink the ciliary processes away from the posterior iris and angle structures.[11-12] Removal of the cataract is completed first, followed by removal of viscoelastic after intraocular lens implantation. Then the anterior chamber is refilled with viscoelastic with the ciliary sulcus also expanded and the procedure conducted as mentioned above. A single temporal incision will allow for treatment of 270° of ciliary processes. If 360° treatment is desired, a second incision made 90° from the temporal incision (enlarging the paracentesis) facilitates the treatment of the remaining processes.

## Pars Plana Approach and "ECP-Plus"

The pars plana approach provides the best view of the ciliary processes and can be used in cases where pathology in the anterior chamber precludes a clear pathway for the endoscope probe. It cannot be performed in eyes that are phakic. A conjunctival peritomy is made nasally and temporally followed by a sclerotomy made 3 mm posterior to the limbus with a 20-gauge MVR blade. Using either a three-port or two-port technique, a full or limited posterior vitrectomy is performed prior to ECP. In the two-port setup, the infusion is used as the anterior chamber maintainer or in one sclerotomy (while the ECP probe is placed in the other). In the three-port approach, the infusion is left in the inferior sclerotomy and one port is plugged or used to hold the vitrector. The ECP probe is placed through one of the sclerotomies and positioned so that the ciliary processes are visible. Treatment is conducted in the same fashion as the anterior approach. However, the posterior approach allows for the entire ciliary process to be treated so extra care should be taken not to overtreat in eyes with neovascular and uveitic glaucoma to avoid hypotony. Lastly, for eyes with recalcitrant glaucoma, the entire ciliary process can be treated leading to profound IOP reductions but again care must be taken to avoid hypotony.

*ECP plus:* In eyes with glaucoma refractory to other treatments, additional treatment of the pars plana can be added to the usual ciliary process treatment performed via a pars plana approach.[13] This can result in greater IOP reduction due to two possible reasons. The first is that the ciliary epithelium may extend onto the pars plana from the adjacent pars plicata, and treatment of the pars plana results in more complete aqueous suppression. The second is that treatment of the pars plana may result in an increase in uveoscleral outflow of aqueous.

## MECHANISM OF ACTION

The diode laser emits a beam of light with a wavelength of 810 nm that is well absorbed by melanin chromophores in the CB tissues generating sufficient thermal energy to coagulate them.[14]

Histopathologic analysis of ECP shows preservation of the normal architecture of the ciliary processes with changes in the ciliary epithelium such as a decrease in pigment granules and loss of smaller blood vessels.[15-17] This is in contrast to TCP and other cyclodestructive procedures that exhibit the permanent loss of both ciliary epithelial layers, and extensive coagulative necrosis with permanent damage of some or all of the ciliary body structures. There is substantially less disruption of the ciliary body stroma or adjacent tissues with evidence of regeneration of the epithelial bilayer and partial reperfusion of the vasculature over time.

## POSTOPERATIVE CARE

The two most common postoperative complications are inflammation and IOP spike. The first can be avoided with aggressive anti-inflammatory medication. In the perioperative period, intravenous steroids can be given (prednisone or dexamethasone 10 mg), and intracameral preservative-free dexamethasone (500–800 μg), as well as subconjunctival steroids. Longer acting steroids are generally avoided to prevent steroid response. Topical nonsteroidal anti-inflammatory drugs are used to prevent cystoid macular edema. A tapering dose of oral steroids is helpful if needed postoperatively.

For IOP control, it is imperative to remove all viscoelastic from the anterior chamber and ciliary sulcus space. Patients are kept on all topical glaucoma medications and sometimes intravenous or oral carbonic anhydrase inhibitors are added to prevent IOP spike in the early postoperative period. As time progresses, the medications can be reduced. The extent of steroid and antiglaucoma medication treatment generally depends on the severity of glaucoma damage and the degree of treatment. Pars plana ECP and ECP plus require the most aggressive postoperative care.

## SPECIFIC INSTRUMENTATION

The only systems currently approved by the FDA for use in the United States are the E2 and E4 by Endooptiks, Inc (Little Silver, NJ). The E2 combines a diode laser, aiming beam, and fiberoptic camera for viewing, while the E4 is an endoscope only. ECP in the treatment of glaucoma is the most common indication for their uses. ECP employs a diode laser with a wavelength of 810 nm, a 175-Watt xenon light source, a helium-neon aiming beam, and video imaging integrated into a fiberoptic system delivered through an 19–20-gauge probe. There is also a 23-gauge probe that has a viewing system only (no diode laser) and can be used to assist in anterior or posterior segment surgery.

## COMPLICATIONS

Inflammation has been discussed, will vary by severity, and is likely dependent on the amount of energy used as well as type of glaucoma diagnosis and ocular comorbidities. This is most common in patients with uveitis or neovascular glaucoma. Inflammation can cause ciliary body shut down and lead to hypotony post operatively, cystoid macular edema, or corneal transplant graft rejection in patients with a prior penetrating keratoplasty.

It is possible to treat phakic patients with a deep anterior chamber, but this clearly carries a risk of anterior capsule trauma and cataract formation. When there is significant anterior segment scarring such as posterior or anterior synechiae, this makes the view more difficult and increases the risk of bleeding, corneal trauma, intraocular lens implant dislocation, and postoperative inflammation.

The pars plana approach carries an increased risk of retinal detachment and vitreous hemorrhage and care should be taken to examine the retina with the endoscope at the end of the surgery. The diode laser can be used to create a laser retinopexy if needed. Other rare complications of ocular surgery such as endophthalmitis and hemorrhage are comparable with other anterior and posterior segment procedures.

## SURGICAL OUTCOMES/SCIENTIFIC EVIDENCE AND META-ANALYSIS

Chen et al. described a retrospective case series of 68 limbal or pars plana ECP procedures in refractory glaucoma cases with or without combined phacoemulsification surgery. All patients had failed maximal medical therapy and prior filtration surgery and some had failed prior TCP. After a mean follow-up of over 1 year, IOP decreased from 27.7 ± 10.3 mm Hg to 17.0 ± 6.7 mm Hg, with a reduction in glaucoma medications from 3.0 ± 1.3 to 2.0 ± 1.3. At 1 year, 94% of patients achieved IOP ≤21 mm Hg, with 82% at 2 years, without any incidences of hypotony or phthisis bulbi.

Uram[18] reported his success with the pars plana approach in 10 patients with neovascular glaucoma, showing IOP <21 mm Hg at 9 months after surgery, despite a mean preoperative IOP of 43.6 mm Hg. More recently, Uram also reported ECP through a limbal incision and combined with phacoemulsification showed in 10 patients with preoperative IOP of 31.4 mm Hg and a mean IOP of 13.5 mm Hg 19.2 months after surgery.

Kahook et al.[19] retrospectively compared the results between 15 patients treated with one-site corneal incision ECP (240–300°) and 25 patients treated with two-site corneal incision ECP (360°) both combined with phacoemulsification. After 6 months of follow-up, postoperative mean IOP was significantly lower in the group treated with two-site ECP (mean 13 mm Hg) versus the group treated with one-site ECP (mean 16 mm Hg), without any higher incidence of complications related to the procedure.

Gayton et al. compared combined limbal-based cataract surgery with ECP to cataract surgery with trabeculectomy in a randomized trial. Cataract surgery with ECP produced significantly less postoperative inflammation than cataract surgery combined with trabeculectomy. In patients followed for at least 6 months after treatment, 32% of patients treated with ECP had IOP controlled (≥21 mm Hg) without medication and 45% with medications, as compared with 54% of patients treated with trabeculectomy without medications and 18% with medications. The IOP reduction was similar between the two groups.

Lima et al.[20] studied the success of ECP when compared with the Ahmed drainage implant in refractory glaucoma patients. Sixty-eight pseudophakic patients who had failed trabeculectomy with antimetabolite underwent either ECP or Ahmed drainage implant in alternating allocation. The mean preoperative IOP was high in both groups (41.2 mm Hg Ahmed, 41.6 ECP), and was similar at the 2-year follow-up (14.7 and 14.1, respectively). The group that underwent Ahmed drainage implant surgery had a higher rate of decrease in visual acuity and early postoperative hypotony, requiring additional postoperative visits.

Neely and Plager reported a study of 36 pediatric patients' eyes treated with single-incision limbal ECP over 6 years, with a minimum of 6 months of follow-up. Thirty-four percent were successfully controlled after the procedure with a mean follow-up of 10 months. Sixty percent were not successfully controlled after ECP and went on to require further treatment. An advantage of ECP in the pediatric population where anatomy is likely to be abnormal was demonstrated by Barkana et al.[5] In this case report, prior TCP was unsuccessful, and at the time of ECP it was discovered that the laser burns had been placed in the pars plana.

ECP can also be performed after outflow procedures. Francis et al.[3] reported a prospective case series of 25 patients with uncontrolled IOP after prior Baerveldt Glaucoma Implant 350 (AMO, Santa Ana, CA) aqueous tube shunt. At 1 year, the mean IOP decreased from 24.0 to 15.4 mm Hg, and medications from 3.2 to 1.5, with 88% achieving a reduction in IOP of 3 mm Hg or greater.

In summary, ECP is a useful tool for glaucoma surgeons. It can be combined with a standard phacoemulsification and intraocular lens implant surgery. It has been shown to be comparable with other filtering or shunting procedures in control of intraocular pressure. It can be used to effectively treat refractory glaucomas that have failed other forms of treatment. In pediatric patients, outcomes have been less favorable. This may be due to the degree of abnormality of the eye structures often present in congenital glaucomas, especially those associated with other anterior segment pathologies, or the increased ability for tissue regeneration in children.

## PLACE OF THE TECHNIQUE IN SURGICAL ARMAMENTARIUM

Ciliary body ablation procedures remain an effective tool in glaucoma management. Evidence suggests that ECP is an effective procedure with a favorable side effect profile that can be used earlier in the surgical management of glaucoma as in medically controlled mild glaucoma (in conjunction with cataract extraction) to ultrarefractory glaucoma with multiple failed filtration surgeries. It can also be used as a combination procedure with any outflow surgery from newer angle-based, minimally invasive glaucoma surgery to trabeculectomy or aqueous tube shunt. Further research evaluating the long-term complications and outcomes of ECP beyond the traditionally studied 1- to 2-year postoperative period is needed.

## PEARLS AND PITFALLS

- Generally, as much of the ciliary processes as possible should be treated to achieve the maximum IOP reduction.[19] This usually means 270–360° of treatment, including the entire visible process and the areas of ciliary epithelium in between the processes. An area that is already treated can be treated again as the probe sweeps in the other direction to ensure that adequate energy has been absorbed. Care should be taken not to overtreat in a specific spot, as this will result in explosion of the process. Do not treat the posterior surface of the iris, as this will only result in more inflammation and pupillary irregularities
- *Inflammation*: Intensive topical steroids, subconjunctival injection, intracameral injection of preservative free steroid, postoperative oral steroids, or perioperative intravenous steroids can be used to prevent the most common complication of ECP. In eyes with uveitis or neovascular glaucoma, a less aggressive approach is recommended for these patients, treating for 180–270° instead of 360° and reducing the energy applied.[20] Steroid use can sometimes mask IOP lowering due to steroid response. Therefore, once inflammation is controlled, we recommend tapering of the steroid and reevaluation of IOP if the desired lowering has not yet been achieved
- Scleral depression can be used to facilitate treatment of the ciliary processes via an anterior or posterior approach. This maneuver will splay out the processes and allow more complete treatment of the processes and the areas in between. It will also allow more of the posterior aspect of the processes to be visible and treated from an anterior approach
- If there is significant anterior segment pathology, consider a pars plana approach
- Anterior and posterior synechiae can be broken to access the ciliary sulcus. Residual lens material or posterior iris synechiae can be removed if necessary, but often can be circumvented by manipulation of the probe. This generally results in the probe tip being in close proximity to the ciliary processes, and thus requires lowering of the power
- Patients with an anterior chamber intraocular lens implant can still be treated via an anterior approach, with the probe entering the pupil posterior to the lens
- In postvitrectomized eyes, an anterior chamber maintainer is critical, as viscoelastic will not keep the eye sufficiently inflated. This can also be used for infusion for a pars plana approach
- The amount of power and duration of treatment should be titrated depending on how close the probe tip is to the ciliary processes. If too much energy is absorbed by the process, it may explode, causing a severe inflammatory reaction
- The endoscope may be used as a stand-alone device to better visualize altered anterior segment anatomy including but not limited to capsular bag problems, dislocated intraocular lens, cyclodialysis clefts, foreign bodies, and drainage device tube malpositions.

## REFERENCES

1. Lin SC. Endoscopic and transscleral cyclophotocoagulation for the treatment of refractory glaucoma. J Glaucoma. 2008;17(3): 238-47.
2. Uram M. Endoscopic cyclophotocoagulation in glaucoma management. Curr Opin Ophthalmol. 1995;6(2):19-29.
3. Francis BA, Kawji AS, Vo NT, et al. Endoscopic cyclophotocoagulation for glaucoma after tube shunt surgery. J Glaucoma. 2011;20(8);523-7.
4. Chen J, Cohn RA, Lin SC, et al. Endoscopic photocoagulation of the ciliary body for treatment of refractory glaucomas. Am J Ophthalmol. 1997;124(6):787-96.
5. Barkana Y, Morad Y, Ben-nun J. Endoscopic photocoagulation of the ciliary body after repeated failure of trans-scleral diode-laser cyclophotocoagulation. Am J Ophthalmol. 2002;133(3): 405-7.

6. Neely DE, Plager DA. Endocyclophotocoagulation for management of difficult pediatric glaucomas. J AAPOS. 2001;5(4):221-9.
7. Plager DA, Neely DE. Intermediate-term results of endoscopic diode laser cyclophotocoagulation for pediatric glaucoma. J AAPOS. 1999;3(3):131-7.
8. Friedman DS, Jampel HD, Lubomski LH, et al. Surgical strategies for coexisting glaucoma and cataract: an evidence-based update. Ophthalmology. 2002;109(10):1902-13.
9. Gayton JL, Van Der Karr M, Sanders V. Combined cataract and glaucoma surgery: trabeculectomy versus endoscopic laser cycloablation. J Cataract Refract Surg. 1999;25(9):1214-9.
10. Uram M. Combined phacoemulsification, endoscopic ciliary process photocoagulation, and intraocular lens implantation in glaucoma management. Ophthalmic Surg. 1995;26(4):346-52.
11. Ahmed IK, Podbielski DW, Naqi A, et al. Endoscopic cycloplasty in angle-closure glaucoma secondary to plateau iris. Poster presented at: American Glaucoma Society Annual Meeting; March, 2009, San Diego, CA.
12. Francis BA, Tan J, Chopra V, et al. Endoscopic cilioplasty and lens extraction in the treatment of severe plateau Iris syndrome. Poster presented at: American Glaucoma Society annual meeting: February, 2012, New York, NY.
13. Tan J, Vakili G, Noecker R, et al. "ECP-plus" to treat refractory glaucoma. Poster presented at: American Glaucoma Society annual meeting, March, 2011, Dana Point, CA.
14. Vogel A, Dlugos C, Nuffer R, et al. Optical properties of human sclera, and their consequences for transscleral laser applications. Lasers Surg Med. 1991;11(4):331-40.
15. Lin SC, Chen MJ, Lin MS, et al. Vascular effects on ciliary tissue from endoscopic versus trans-scleral cyclophotocoagulation. Br J Ophthalmol. 2006;90(4):496-500.
16. Pantcheva MB, Kahook MY, Schuman JS, et al. Comparison of acute structural and histopathological changes in human autopsy eyes after endoscopic cyclophotocoagulation and trans-scleral cyclophotocoagulation. Br J Ophthalmol. 2007; 91(2):248-52.
17. Alvarado J, Francis B. Characteristics of ciliary body lesions after endoscopic and transscleral laser cyclophotocoagulation. Poster presented at the American Academy of Ophthalmology Annual Meeting; November, 1998, New Orleans, LA.
18. Uram M. Ophthalmic laser microendoscope ciliary process ablation in the management of neovascular glaucoma. Ophthalmology. 1992;99(12):1823-8.
19. Kahook MY, Lathrop KL, Noecker RJ. One-site versus two-site endoscopic cyclophotocoagulation. J Glaucoma. 2007;16(6):527-30.
20. Lima FE, Magacho L, Carvalho DM, et al. A prospective, comparative study between endoscopic cyclophotocoagulation and the Ahmed drainage implant in refractory glaucoma. J Glaucoma. 2004;13(3):233-7.

CHAPTER

# 49

# Nonpenetrating Glaucoma Surgery

Richard A Lehrer

## INTRODUCTION AND HISTORY

The distinguishing feature of nonpenetrating glaucoma surgery (NPGS) is the development of two scleral flaps with the subsequent removal of the deep flap (deep sclerectomy) forming an intrascleral lake. The remaining TDM, or trabeculodescemetic membrane, serves as a protective tissue barrier to excessive outflow in the early postoperative period (Fig. 49-1A). The intraocular pressure (IOP) is lowered by three potential methods. There is no fistula because the anterior chamber is not entered, making this a safer procedure with less likelihood of blebitis, endophthalmitis, or hypotony. Canaloplasty, the latest addition to NPGS, adds 360 degree viscodilation of Schlemm's canal (SC) and suture tensioning (Fig. 49-1B) of SC along with the typical NPGS features.

The first NPGS was performed by Epstein[1] in South Africa in 1959. He suggested that a "deep lamellar sclerectomy overlying Schlemm'scanal" would be a means of forming new aqueous canals. Walker and Kanagasundaram[2] in 1964 felt that by leaving a layer of trabecular tissue between the anterior chamber and the subconjunctival space, many complications of filtration procedures could be avoided. Their procedure was called EFSC (external fistulization of SC). In EFSC, a trephination was made over forceps placed into SC, and then

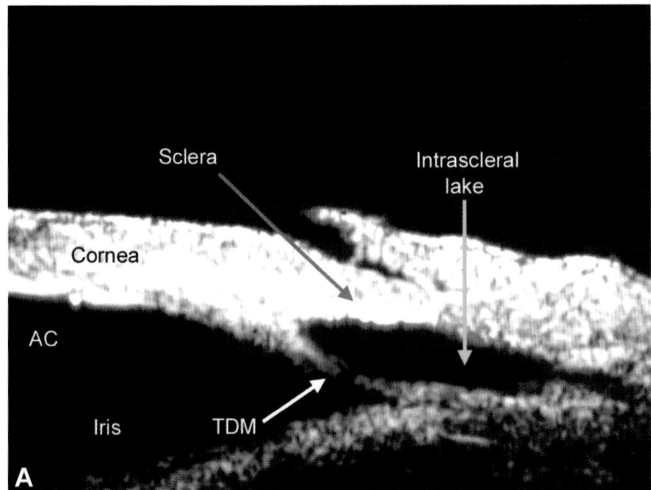


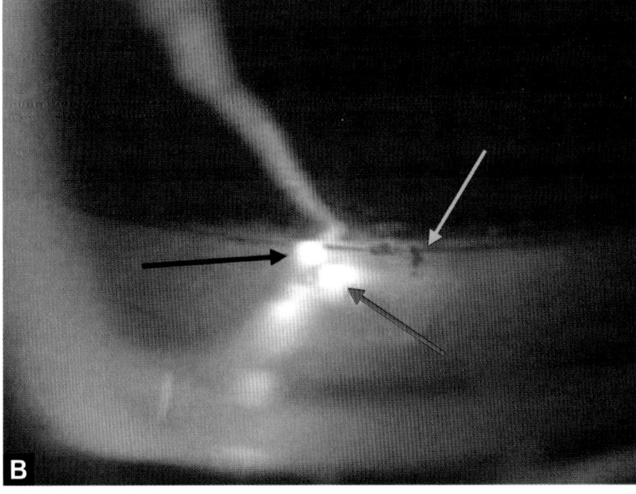


**Figures 49-1A and B** Nonpenetrating glaucoma surgery (NPGS). (A) Intrascleral lake. Both the intrascleral lake (green arrow) and TDM (trabeculodescemetic membrane, white arrow) are created by removal of the deep scleral flap (deep sclerectomy), the hallmark of all NPGS. Aqueous must pass through the TDM to enter the lake, which serves as the intrascleral (no bleb) conduit for the exit of aqueous. (B) Goniophotograph of canaloplasty site. The blue polypropylene suture (green arrow) is inside the canal for 360°. The black arrow indicates the amount of suture tension, pulling the canal and trabecular meshwork inward, an important feature for success of the procedure. Suture tension is best seen by examining the bend in the slit beam as it traverses the suture. The red arrow indicates a goniopuncture site, which was necessary to improve flow to the lake at 1 year.

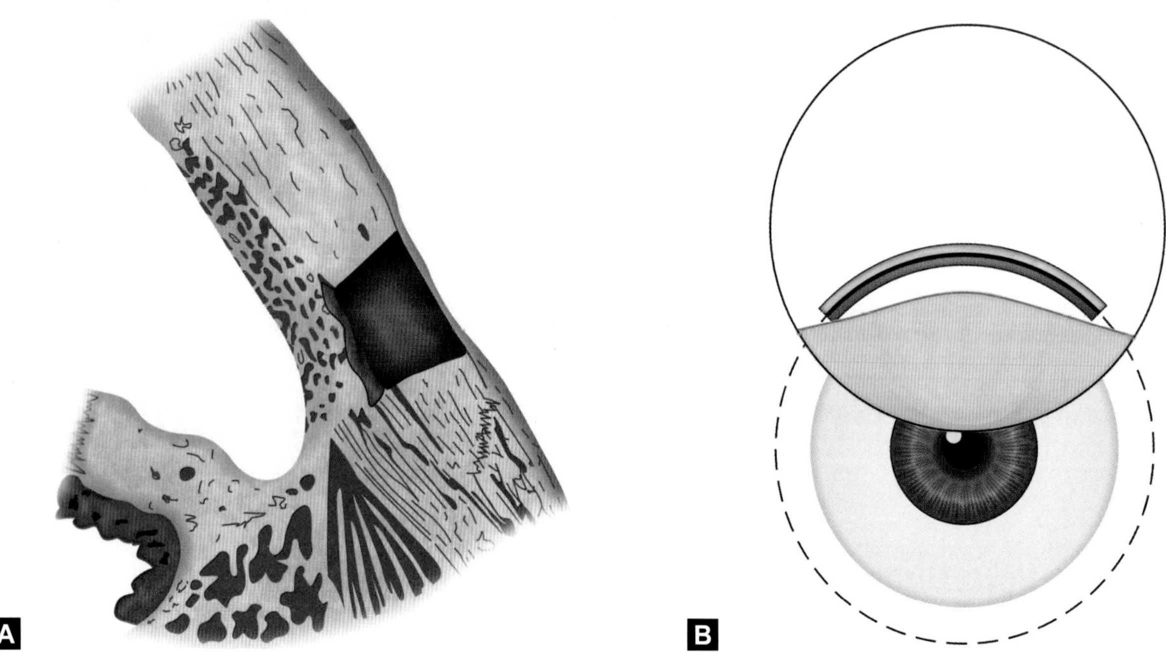


**Figures 49-2A and B** Sinusostomy. (A) Krasnov[3] sinusostomy diagram showing externalization of Schlemm's canal (SC) (side view). (B) Krasnov[3] sinusostomy diagram showing externalization of SC (top view) extending 4 clock hours or approximately 120°.

covered by conjunctiva and Tenon's capsule. Krasnov[3] published on sinusostomy (SOS) in 1968. He wrote that the majority of glaucomas were the "intrascleral" type as opposed to the "trabecular" type, and SOS was specifically targeting the outflow system distal to SC. If he opened the canal and found little flow, then he felt the glaucoma was "trabecular" in mechanism. In SOS (Figs. 49-2A and B), dissection was carried down to SC and extended circumferentially for 120°. The authors noted that this was a somewhat difficult dissection, and that it was possible to damage the internal portion of SC. The conjunctiva also tended to scar over the canal leading to poor long-term results and was abandoned, especially with the rise in popularity of the guarded trabeculectomy of Sugar and Cairns in the late 1960s to present.

In the 1980s, Zimmerman[4] et al. in the United States proposed that in aphakic glaucomas, the complications of vitreous prolapse could be avoided by nonpenetrating trabeculectomy (NPT) (Fig. 49-3). By performing the procedure under a scleral flap (Figs 49-3A to C), they would avoid conjunctival fibrosis and have improved success and lower complications compared with trabeculectomy[5] in phakic eyes. Fyodorov et al.[6] and Koslov et al.[7] in Russia also published results with nonpenetrating deep sclerectomy (NPDS). The NPDS was further modified by others with the addition of a spacer device after the deep scleral flap was excised to improve long-term success. Many different spacers have been used including collagen[6,7,9] (Aqua-Flow, STAAR surgical, Monrovia, CA, USA), reticulated hyaluronic acid[10] (SK-Gel, Corneal, Paris, France), autologous sclera,[11] PMMA[12] (T-Flux, IOLTECH, La Rochelle, France), ceramic,[13] and several others. The antimetabolite mitomycin-C[14] (MMC) has also been added to improve success. Modifications of these are still in use at this time.

Stegmann et al.[8] in the 1990s was concerned with complications of bleb-forming glaucoma surgeries and modified the NPT by dilating SC with high-viscosity sodium hyaluronate (HVSH) and leaving it in the resultant intrascleral "lake" to promote success (Figs. 49-4A and B). They also found that by tight closure of the superficial scleral flap, the formation of a bleb could be avoided in most cases. To improve success, a catheter and light source, iTrack and iLumin (Figs. 49-5A and B), was developed in conjunction with John Kearney in the United States and Ellex/iScience (Menlo Park, CA, USA) and called the procedure canaloplasty.[15] This involved threading a catheter 360° around the canal and dilating it with HVSH. This was later modified by placing a stent consisting of one or two 9-0 or 10-0 polypropylene sutures.[16] By adding tension to the sutures (CPST), additional outflow was observed. Barnebey added MMC[17] to the procedure to try to further improve success.

In addition, all of these procedures have been combined with modern small incision cataract surgery for even greater success.

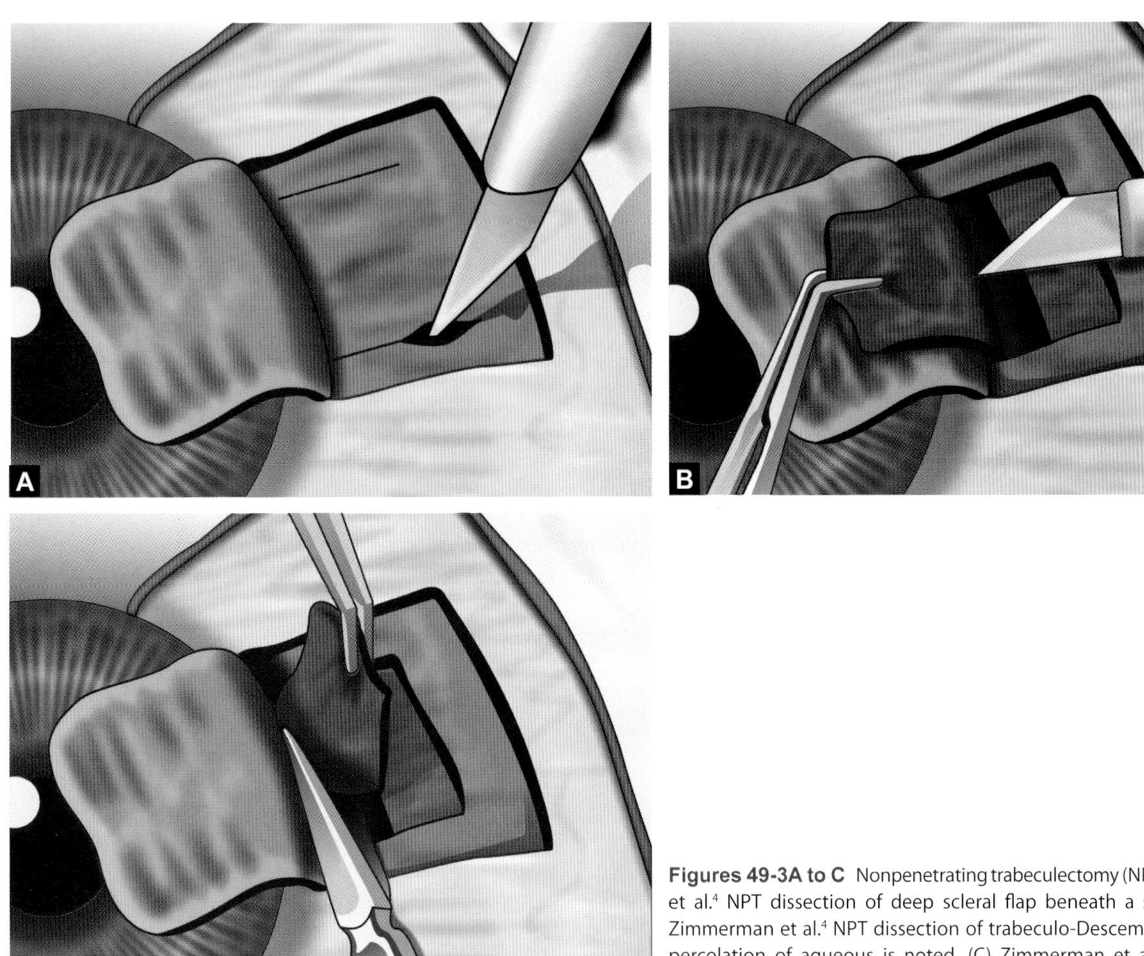


**Figures 49-3A to C** Nonpenetrating trabeculectomy (NPT). (A) Zimmerman et al.[4] NPT dissection of deep scleral flap beneath a superficial flap. (B) Zimmerman et al.[4] NPT dissection of trabeculo-Descemet's window where percolation of aqueous is noted. (C) Zimmerman et al.[4] NPT excision of deep scleral flap (deep sclerectomy) prior to closure of the superficial flap.

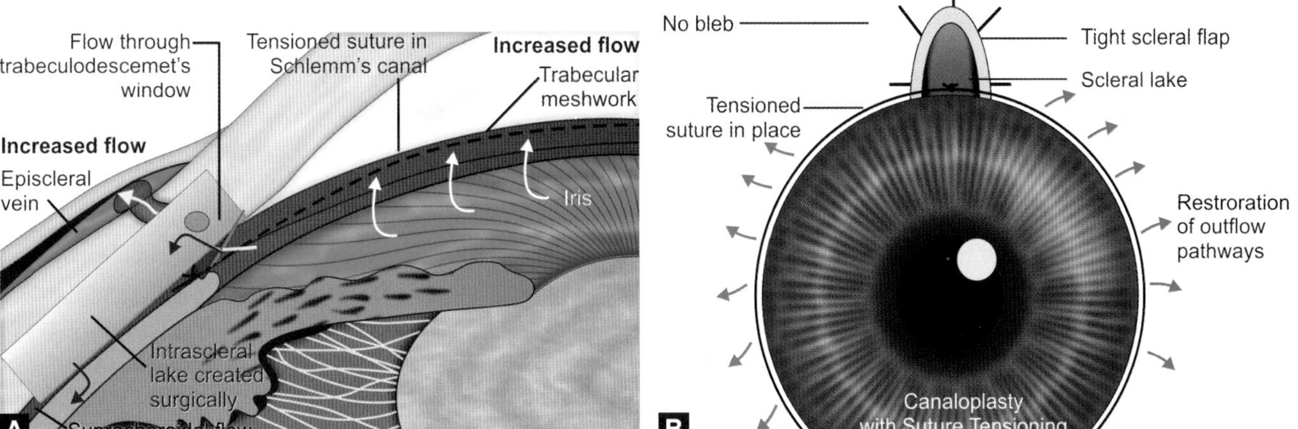


**Figures 49-4A and B** (A) Schematic drawing of canaloplasty with suture tensioning (CPST) side view. (B) Schematic drawing of CPST top view. All mechanisms of CPST are not entirely understood. Several things are occurring simultaneously: 1) Viscodilation and catheterization of the canal has been shown to create microtears in it along with the juxtacanalicular meshwork, increasing its permeability and thereby decreasing the resistance to outflow. 2) The suture or stent, which is tensioned, has also been shown to facilitate this outflow and flow is tension dependent. 3) Viscodilation may improve the distal collector channel system, opening previously poor functioning channels and allowing for increased outflow via this system. 4) There is egress of aqueous from the TDW into the intrascleral lake. It may then go into Schlemm's canal or may drain to some extent by the suprachoroidal route.

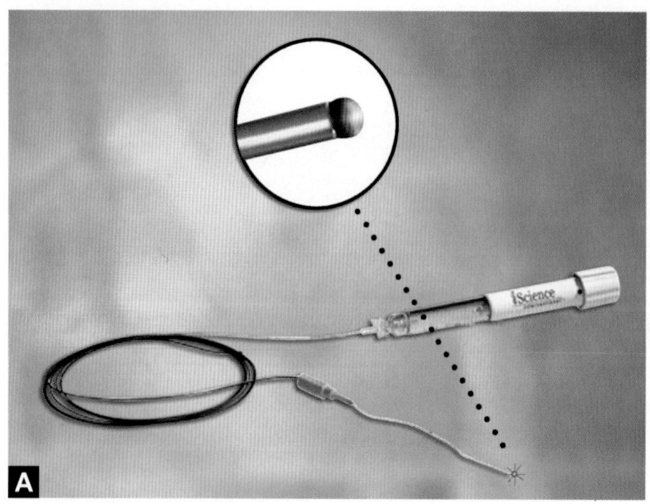


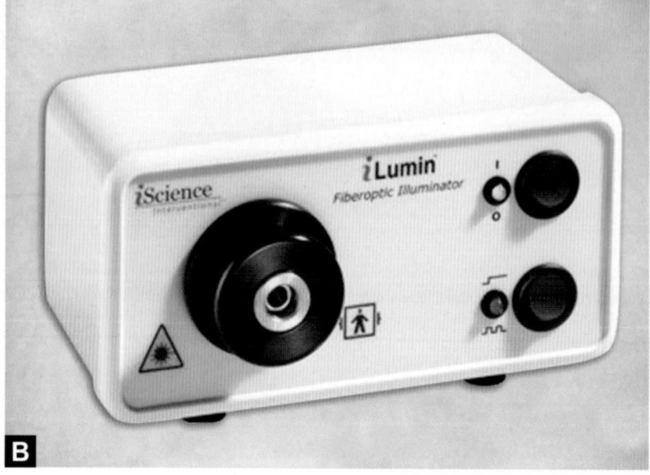


**Figures 49-5A and B** (A) iTrack catheter (B) iLumin light source.

## INDICATIONS

- Open angle glaucoma (OAG) and ocular hypertension (OHT).
- Other secondary OAGs can be considered including pseudo-exfoliation, pigmentary, traumatic, and uveitic glaucomas
- NPDS may be considered for eyes where a filtering bleb is not contraindicated and target IOP ≥12 mm Hg.
- CPST may be considered especially when an eye is at risk for bleb-related complications such as ocular surface disease, s/p corneal transplantation, bleb-related complications in the fellow eye and target IOP ≥15 mm Hg.
- Also consider CPST for eyes at high risk for hypotony such as high myopia, young patients, prior hypotony in the fellow eye.
- Easy to combine with phacoemulsification and intraocular lens (IOL) surgery.

## CONTRAINDICATIONS

- Narrow angle glaucoma (NAG)
- Neovascular glaucoma (NVG)
- Developmental glaucomas
- Prior incisional surgery that disrupts SC may preclude CPST and make catheterization of SC impossible. This may include SC stents and trabeculotomy/goniotomy type procedures
- Significant conjunctival scarring from injury or prior surgery
- Prior heavy argon laser trabeculoplasty (ALT) may make some canal surgeries more difficult.

## TECHNIQUE

Currently, NPDS and CPST are most widely used. There are common elements to both procedures. They involve conjunctival and Tenon's dissection, creation of a superficial scleral flap, creation and removal of a deep scleral flap (deep sclerectomy), unroofing SC, and creating a trabeculo-Descemet's window (TDW).

### Common Elements

Anesthesia is achieved in the usual manner for glaucoma filtration. The author prefers topical tetracaine 1%, followed by subconjunctival/sub-Tenon's 1% lidocaine with epinephrine 1:100,000 given via 30-gauge needle posteriorly. A corneal traction suture is placed in partial thickness fashion inferiorly and passed beneath the lid speculum to rotate the eye downward and not distort the superior anatomy during deep dissection. A superior limbal peritomy of 6–8 mm is performed. Cautery should be minimized or avoided in CPST to preserve aqueous outflow veins on the scleral surface. Dissection of conjunctiva and Tenon's capsule is carried posteriorly 4–5 mm for CPST and 10–12 mm for NPDS. A superficial limbal-based scleral flap is fashioned in partial thickness. For CPST, a 4 × 4 mm parabolic flap is made at ~ 1/3 scleral depth (~200 µm) to achieve watertight closure. For NPDS, flap thickness is similar and shape is usually square at 4 × 4 mm. The flap may be outlined with a calibrated diamond blade or metal blade. Caution should be taken in highly myopic eyes where the sclera is thinner and SC is more posterior. The flap is then dissected toward the limbus using a diamond or metal blade and then 1–2 mm into clear cornea. If MMC is used, 0.2–0.4 mg/mL solution is placed on a saturated sponge beneath the superficial flap for 30–90 seconds. The sponge is then removed and the area is irrigated. The deep scleral flap is then outlined 1 mm inside the margins of the superficial flap and may be triangular, square, or parabolic. A parallel plane is started just superficial to the ciliary body. This dissection is carried anteriorly until SC is unroofed. If cataract surgery is planned simultaneously, temporal clear corneal phacoemulsification with IOL is completed, or phacoemulsification may be completed in its entirety prior to the NPGS. It is important to remove all viscoelastic to assess aqueous percolation later. In NPGS, the cataract incision should be sutured as the IOP may be quite low for the first day or two postoperative This is where the two procedures diverge.

## NPDS (Figs. 49-6A to E)

After opening SC, lower IOP via a paracentesis to avoid perforation of the TDW. Using gentle upward traction on the deep flap, sponges can be gently used to further bluntly dissect the TDW for 1–2 mm into clear cornea. A modified Drysdale spatula (Katena Products, Denville, NJ, USA) or Khan (Mastel Precision Surgical Instruments, Rapid City, SD, USA) dissector can facilitate this step as well. The sides of the flap are then cut with sharp dissection taking care not to perforate the anterior chamber. Scissors or a diamond Zip blade (Mastel Precision Surgical Instruments, Rapid City, SD, USA) can make this easier. The deep flap is then excised with scissors or a blade, again with caution not to torque the flap and perforate the TDW. During canaloplasty, the deep flap may be removed after suture tightening or before. Fine-tipped forceps (Mermoud; Huco, Switzerland or Ahmed, MST, Redmond, WA, USA) are then used to strip the inner wall of the canal and aqueous percolation is noted. This may be more difficult after ALT, and it is vital for the success of the procedure to get flow at this step. If no flow is observed, restripping may be attempted, or polishing the canal area gently with a diamond burr is performed. If there is still no flow, plan for future laser goniopuncture, or consider using a 30-gauge needle to make two to three tiny perforations anteriorly to prevent iris prolapse. If perforation of the TDW occurs, and there is significant iris prolapse, a small peripheral iridotomy is made. The procedure may still be completed. A spacer like the AquaFlow is then sutured to the deep scleral bed of the dissection, butting the anterior edge of the implant anteriorly against the excised deep dissection. If there is no perforation of TDW, the superficial flap is then closed with two 10-0 nylon sutures with an attempt to reapproximate the tissue to avoid induced astigmatism. If a perforation of TDW occurs, additional sutures are required with tighter closure of the flap. Aqueous outflow should be titrated to desired IOP. Conjunctiva is then closed in watertight fashion with absorbable 8-0 or 9-0 polygalactan suture. The corneal traction suture is removed and antibiotic/steroid drops are given, followed by placement of an eyeshield.

## CPST (Canaloplasty) (Figs. 49-7A to N)

After unroofing the canal, it is important to lower IOP via paracentesis to avoid perforation of the TDW. The iTrack microcatheter is then primed with HVSH, connected to the light box, and brought into the surgical field. The iTrack catheter is then placed into the open ostium of the canal and advanced 360° until the catheter appears from the other ostium. The 10-0 or 9-0 polypropylene suture is tied to the distal tip of the iTrack and in a single smooth motion, the catheter is withdrawn thus placing the suture in the canal. While withdrawing the iTrack, small aliquots of HVSH are injected into the canal by the assistant who "clicks" the calibrated delivery syringe every 2 clock hours, to further dilate the canal and collector system. The suture is then cut off the tip of the iTrack, and the ends pushed to the sides of the scleral bed. The TDW is then completed as described above for NPDS and the deep flap excised. The suture(s) is then tied in adjustable fashion using a slip-knot, then tensioned, and gently "flossed" in the canal to position the suture as anteriorly as possible. The knot is then locked and ends trimmed. The superficial flap is then closed in watertight fashion with 10-0 nylon, polypropylene, or mersilene. Just prior to closing the flap, HVSH is placed into the intrascleral space or "lake" to maintain the space and possibly reduce inflammation and scarring. The conjunctiva is then closed in a watertight fashion and the case is completed as in NPDS.

## Mechanism of Action NPDS

Filtration is achieved via the TDW beneath the scleral flap into the subconjunctival space. This is facilitated long term by the spacer device, which in the case of collagen may take 6–9 months to resorb. MMC prevents scarring. There may also be a component of supraciliary filtration as occasionally a small, localized effusion is noted by ultrasound biomicroscopy (UBM) or ocular coherence tomography (OCT) beneath the spacer. In addition, there may be enhanced flow into the collector system through the cut ends of SC. Usually with NPDS, there is a low-lying vascularized bleb.

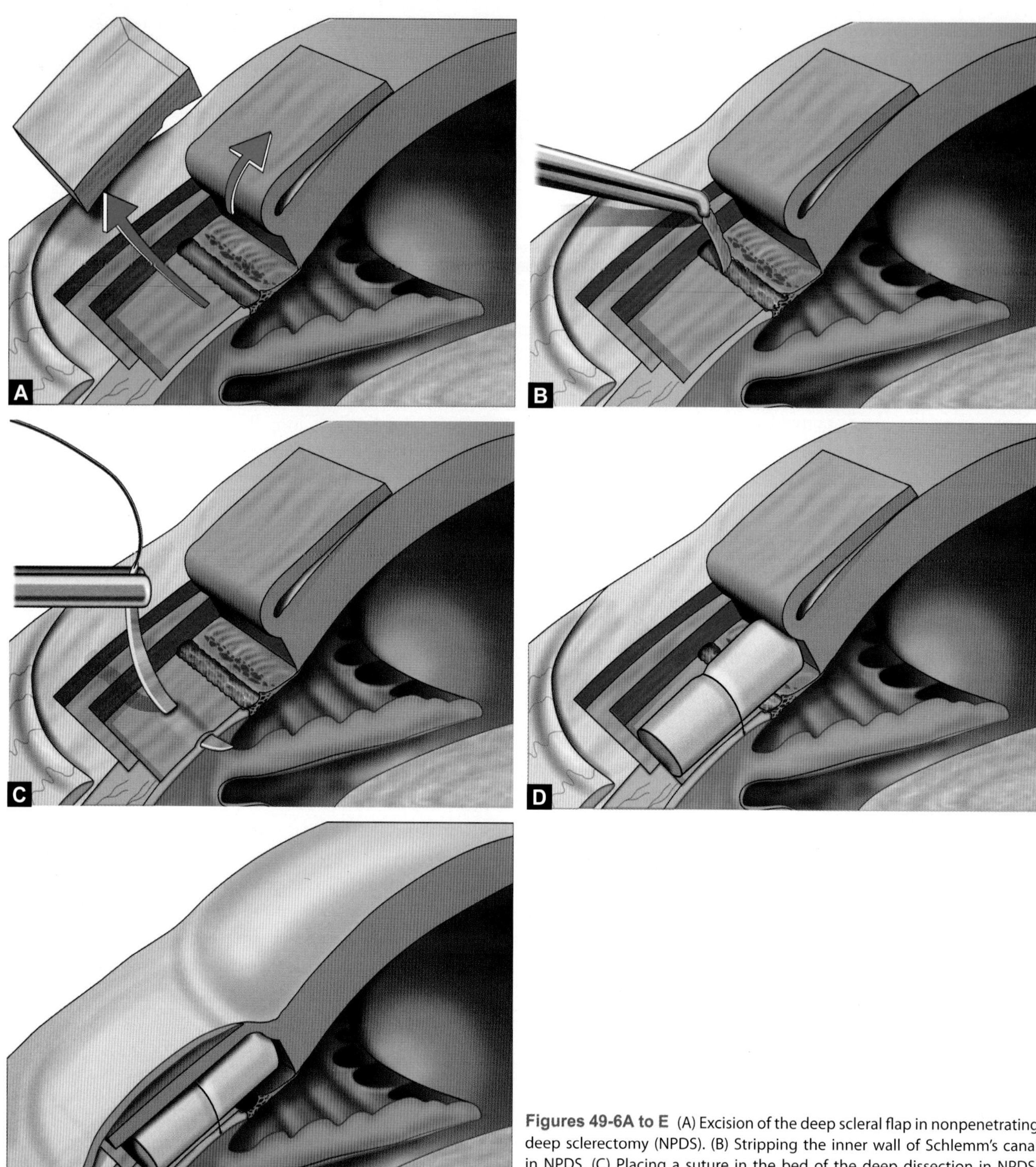


**Figures 49-6A to E** (A) Excision of the deep scleral flap in nonpenetrating deep sclerectomy (NPDS). (B) Stripping the inner wall of Schlemm's canal in NPDS. (C) Placing a suture in the bed of the deep dissection in NPDS. (D) Collagen implant sutured in place in NPDS. (E) Completed NPDS with closure of superficial scleral flap and conjunctiva.

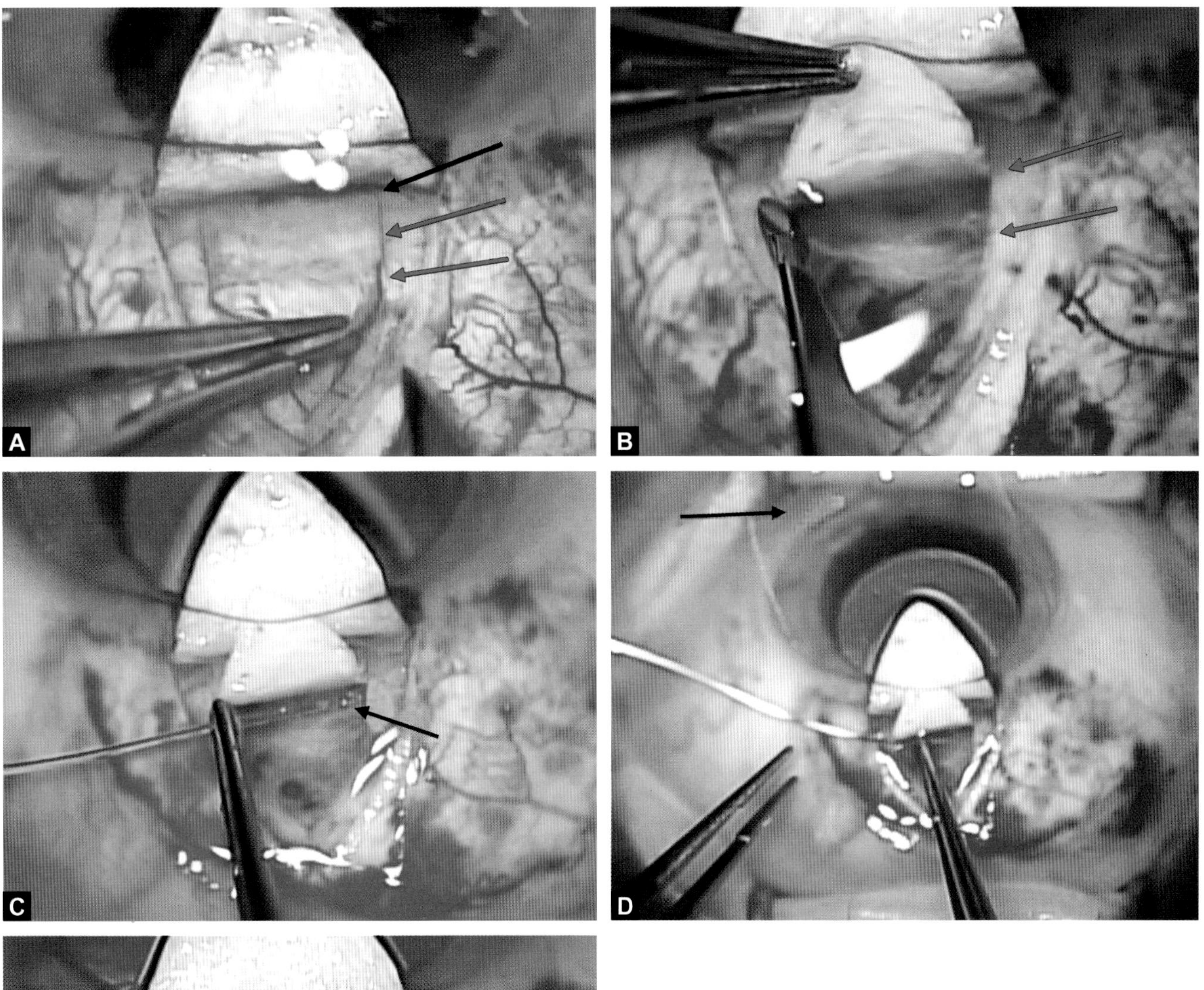


**Figures 49-7A to E** (A and B) Outline deep flap and unroof Schlemm's canal after outlining the deep flap, note the limbal landmarks, the black arrow denotes the anterior limbal border, the green arrow the posterior limbal border, and the blue arrow is the midlimbus. The key is to remember that underneath the blue arrow is Schwalbe's line and below the green arrow is the approximate location of Schlemm's canal. With the proper deep flap plane, the anterior dissection will unroof Schlemm's canal. Delicate dissection of the edges of the flap over the canal with a radial-upward movement (B) is necessary to completely unveil the canal. The blue and green arrows remain in the same position. The deep flap is then pinned under the traction suture to improve visibility of limbal structures. (C to E) iTrack cannulation, viscodilation, and delivery of suture. The illuminated microcatheter is directed into Schlemm's canal (C) and advanced for 360° (D and E). The black arrow in (D) points to the illuminated tip in the canal as it progresses around the canal. The iTrack tip is externalized as seen in (E), ready for the suture to be tied.

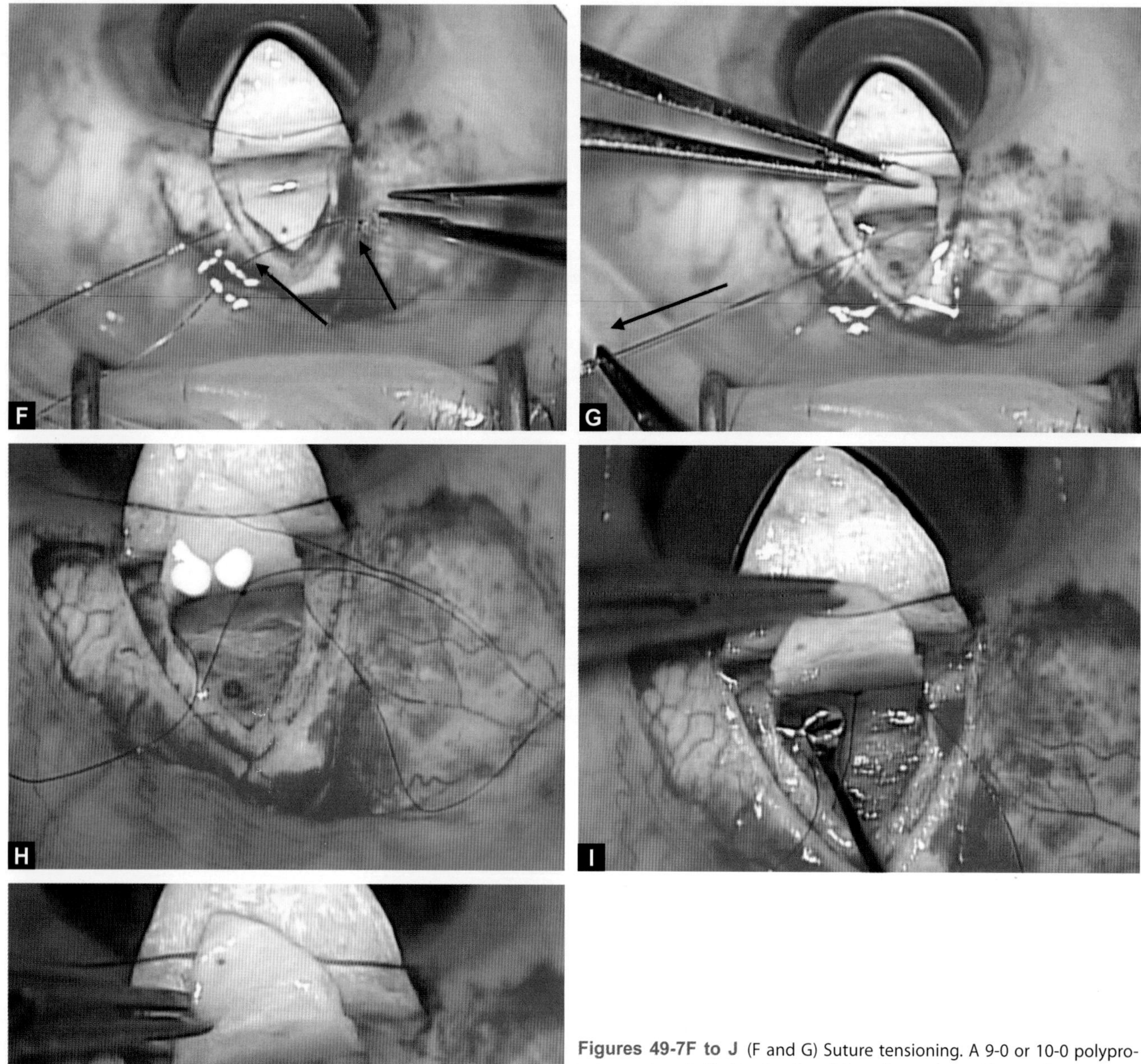


**Figures 49-7F to J** (F and G) Suture tensioning. A 9-0 or 10-0 polypropylene suture is tied to the tip of the microcatheter. Two prolene sutures are tied to the tip, a second is available if the knot breaks or is defective. The black arrow in (G) denotes the direction the iTrack is pulled to retract it and retrieve the polypropylene suture. As the iTrack is retrieved, viscoelastic is injected into the canal at 2-clock hour intervals to dilate the canal. (H) Suture tie. After retrieving the iTrack, the suture is cut from the catheter, the catheter is discarded and the suture ends tied with definite tension to create a tightening of the canal. (I and J) Advancement of deep flap. A spatula is used to further separate the flap from Descement's membrane and the ends of the flap are dissected anteriorly over clear cornea to create a large trabeculodescemetic membrane.

## Mechanism of Action CPST

Many studies have been done to try to elucidate the mechanism of action, and all mechanisms are not entirely understood. Several things are occurring simultaneously. Viscodilation and catheterization of the canal has been shown to create microtears in it along with the juxtacanalicular meshwork, increasing its permeability and thereby decreasing the

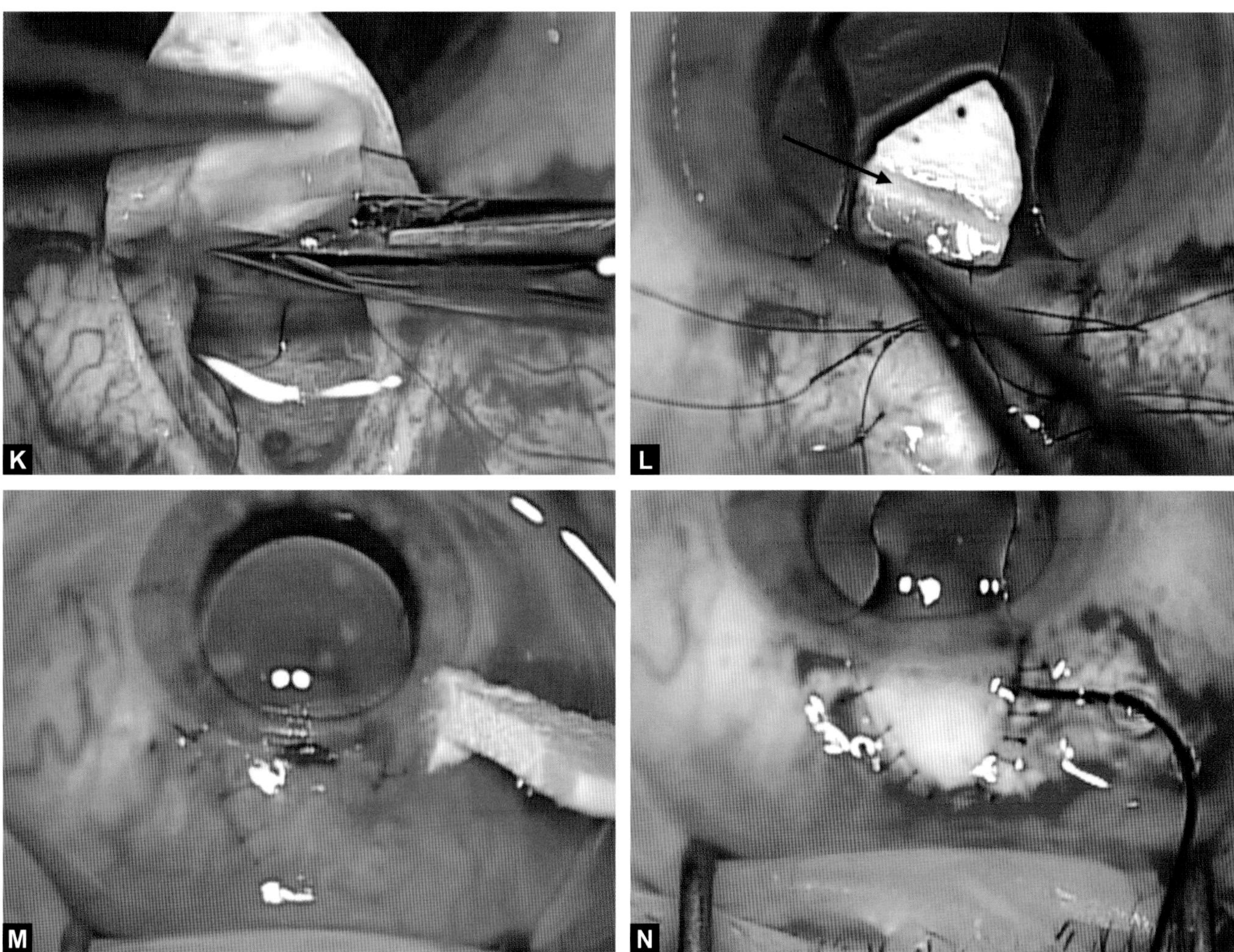


**Figures 49-7K to N** (K) Deep sclerectomy. Vannas scissors are used to carefully remove the deep flap. (L) Inspection of deep flap. The black arrow denotes a groove in the tissue, which is the anterior roof of Schlemm's canal. (M) Closure of superficial flap with injection of viscoelastic. This flap must be closed in a watertight fashion to encourage aqueous to flow into the canal, not under the conjunctiva. Viscoelastic is injected into the potential lake to discourage bleeding and help maintain the space. (N) Conjunctival closure. Even the conjunctiva is closed in a watertight fashion for it is not uncommon to have a bleb for the first week.

resistance to outflow as in a minitrabeculotomy.[a] The suture or stent, which is tensioned, has also been shown to facilitate this outflow and flow is tension dependent. Overtensioning can however lead to less flow. This has been demonstrated in Grant perfusion models. Viscodilation may improve the collector channel system, opening previously poor functioning channels and allowing for increased outflow via this system. There is egress of aqueous from the TDW into the intrascleral lake. It may then go into the canal or may drain to some extent by the suprachoroidal route as described above. MMC may aid the prevention of scarring in this area.

## POSTOPERATIVE CARE

Similar for both procedures. Topical antibiotics are used qid (four times a day) for 1 week. Topical nonsteroidal anti-inflammatory drugs are used bid (twice a day)–qid for 4 weeks. Topical steroids are used four to six times daily for 4–6 weeks and then tapered. If the IOP begins to exceed target, and at least 3 weeks has elapsed, Nd:YAG goniopuncture is a useful adjunct to both procedures and is performed similarly. If additional IOP lowering is needed, laser suture lysis may be used in CPST to convert the procedure into a guarded filtration procedure. Needling with MMC can provide even further IOP reduction

[a]Johnson DJ, Johnson M. How does Nonpenetrating glaucoma surgery work? Aqueous outflow resistance and glaucoma surgery. J Glaucoma. 2001;10:55-67.

with NPDS. Steroid response may occur with either procedure and should be treated by reducing steroids and treating the IOP.

## SPECIFIC INSTRUMENTATION

- *Both procedures*: Blades for dissecting superficial and deep flaps. Dissector for enlarging TDW. Blade for dissecting sides of TDW. Forceps for stripping TDW
- *NPDS*: Spacer device of choice
- *CPST*: Ellex/iScience, iLumen, and iTrack catheter kit. Healon GV (AMO, CA, USA).

## COMPLICATIONS

- Both procedures:
  - Rupture of TDW
  - Avulsion of superficial flap
  - Transient hyphema
  - Iris incarceration into TDW.
- NPDS:
  - Hypotony
  - Bleb leak.
- CPST:
  - Descemet's detachment (serous or hemorrhagic)
  - Goniotomy, partial or complete.

## SURGICAL OUTCOMES: SCIENTIFIC EVIDENCE/META-ANALYSES

Numerous publications in peer-reviewed journals on these procedures exist. In one long-term study, at a mean of 64-month study, Shaarawy et al. found a complete success rate of 57% and a qualified success rate of 91% with an IOP ≤21 mm Hg with deep sclerectomy collagen implant. Goniopuncture was necessary in 51% of eyes. Most studies show comparable success rates to trabeculectomy, with a reduction in complications and usually the filter lowers IOP slightly better[18-20] with similar findings for phacocanaloplasty[21] Canaloplasty takes longer to perform than a filter; however, the postoperative care after trabeculectomy is much more labor intensive with typically a mean of four visits for a canaloplasty and nine for a filter.[22] Goniopuncture may be necessary after any nonpenetrating procedure, and careful gonioscopy is critical in making the decision to open the TDM.[23]

## PLACE OF THE TECHNIQUE IN SURGICAL ARMAMENTARIUM

Nonpenetrating surgeries typically do not penetrate into the anterior chamber and are safer than standard trabeculectomy. However, the IOP is typically not as low as a standard trabeculectomy, the nonpenetrating procedure may require longer surgical time, and both the procedures are performed in tandem with cataract extraction. Canaloplasty is especially helpful when a bleb is to be avoided such as patients at high risk for hypotony such as myopes, or patients with ocular surface disease when a bleb is to be avoided, or patients whose occupation requires them to be outside exposed to environmental pollutants or dust. CPST and NPDS may be used when target IOP is in the mid-teens. The author prefers MMC-trabeculectomy when single digit to low teens IOP is required.

## PEARLS AND PITFALLS

- *Both procedures:*
  - Use of high magnification is helpful for correctly identifying anatomic structures.
  - To find the correct plane for dissection, a posterior tip of the deep flap is incised to expose the ciliary body (CB), then a parallel plane is started just superficial to the CB.
  - After opening SC, lower IOP via paracentesis to avoid perforation of the TDW.
- *NPDS:*
  - If perforation of the TDW occurs, suture the spacer to tamponade the rupture.
  - When suturing the superficial flap, reapproximate the tissue to minimize astigmatism.
- *CPST:*
  - If a pause occurs during this withdrawal of the catheter, a focal Descemet's detachment can occur and may become hemorrhagic. The inferonasal quadrant is particularly vulnerable. Smooth motion helps.
  - Wetting the catheter and suture on the drape can prevent excess tension on the canal, to prevent goniotears.
  - Watch for postop IOP elevation due to steroid responders.

## REFERENCES

1. Epstein E. Fibrosing response to aqueous: its relation to glaucoma. Br J Ophthalmol. 1959;43:641-7.
2. Walker WM, Kanagasundaram CR. Surgery of the canal of Schlemm. Trans Ophthalmol Soc UK. 1964;84:427-42.
3. Krasnov MM. Externalization of Schlemm's canal (sinusostomy) in glaucoma. Br J Ophthalmol. 1968;52:157-61.
4. Zimmerman TJ, Kooner KS, Ford VJ, et al. Effectiveness of nonpenetrating trabeculectomy in aphakic patients with glaucoma. Ophthalmic Surg. 1984;15(1):44-50.
5. Zimmerman TJ, Kooner KS, Ford VJ, et al. Trabeculectomy vs. non-penetrating trabeculectomy: a retrospective study of two procedures in phakic patients with glaucoma. Ophthalmic Surg. 1984;15(9):734-40.

6. Fyodorov SN, Ioffe DI, Ronkina TI. Deep sclerectomy: technique and mechanism of a new glaucomatous procedure. Glaucoma. 1984;6:281-3.
7. Koslov VI, Bagrov SN, Anisimova SY, et al. Nonpenetrating deep sclerectomy with collagen. Ophthalmic Surg. 1990;3:44-6.
8. Stegmann R, Pienaar A, Miller D. Viscocanalostomy for open-angle glaucoma in black African patients. J Cataract Refract Surg. 1999;25(3):316-22.
9. Shaaraway T, Karlen M, Schnyder C, et al. Five-years results of deep sclerectomy with collagen implant. J Cataract Refract Surg. 2001; 27:1770-8.
10. Sourdille P, Santiago P-Y, Villain F, et al. Reticulated hyaluronic acid implant in nonperforating trabecular surgery. J Cataract Refract Surg. 1999;25:332-9.
11. Mousa, ASG. Preliminary evaluation of nonpenetrating deep sclerectomy with autologous scleral implant in open-angle glaucoma. Eye. 2007;21:1234-38.
12. Dahan E, Ravinet E, Ben-Simon GJ, Mermoud A. Comparison of the efficacy and longevity of nonpenetrating glaucoma surgery with and without a new, non-absorbable hydrophilic implant. Ophthalmic Surg Lasers Imag. 2003;34(6):457-63.
13. A Basso, S Roy, A Mermoud. Biocompatibility of an x-shaped zirconium implant in deep sclerectomyin rabbits. Graefe's Arch Clin Exp Ophthalmol. 2008;246(6):849-55.
14. Kozobolis VP, Christodoulakis EV, Tzanakis N, Zacharopoulos I, Pallikaris IG. Primary deep sclerectomy versus primary deep sclerectomy with the use of mitomycin C in primary open-angle glaucoma. J Glaucoma. 2002;11:287-93.
15. Cameron B, Field M, Ball S, Kearney J. Circumferential viscodilation of Schlemm's canal with a flexible microcannula during non-penetrating glaucoma surgery. Digit J Ophthalmol. 12(1). http://www.djo.harvard.edu/site.php?urlZ/physicians/oa/929. 2006:1-10, last accessed 2/20/13.
16. Lewis RA, von Wolff K, Tetz M, et al. Canaloplasty: three-year results of circumferential viscodilation and tensioning of Schlemm's canal using a microcatheter to treat open-angle glaucoma. J Cataract Refract Surg. 2011;37:682-90.
17. Barnebey, H. Canaloplasty with intraoperative low dosage mitomycin C: a retrospective case series. J Glaucoma. 2013;22:201-4.
18. Shaarawy T, Mansouri K, Schnyder C. et al. Long-term results of deep sclerectomy with collage implant. J Cat Refract Surg. 2004;30:1225-31.
19. Cillino S, Di Pace F, Cillino G, et al. Deep sclerectomy versus trabeculectomy with low dose mitomycin C: a 4-year follow-up. Ophthalmologica. 2008;222:81-7.
20. Ambresin A, Shaarawy T, Mermoud A. Deep sclerectomy with collagen implant in one eye compared with trabeculectomy in the other eye of the same patient. J Glaucoma. 2002;11:214-20.
21. Schoenberg ED, Chaudhry AL, Chod R. Comparison of surgical outcomes between phacocanaloplasty and phacotrabeculectomy at 12 months' follow-up: a longitudinal cohort study [published online ahead of print November 14, 2013]. J Glaucoma.
22. Brüggemann A, Despouy JT, Wegent A, et al. Intraindividual comparison of canaloplasty versus trabeculectomy with mitomycin C in a single-surgeon series. J Glaucoma. 2013;22(7): 577-83.
23. Tam DY, Barnebey HS, Ahmed IIK. Nd: YAG laser goniopuncture: indications and procedure. J Glaucoma. 2013;22(8):620-5.

# Section 6

# Oculoplastic, Orbital and Lacrimal Surgery

*Section Editor* Santosh G Honavar

CHAPTER

50

# Anatomical and Radiological Considerations

Jonathan J Dutton

## INTRODUCTION

Evaluation of orbital disease requires a firm understanding of normal orbital anatomy and function. The human orbit contains a complex array of closely packed structures mostly subserving visual function. Orbital fat, surrounded by an extensive network of connective tissue fascia, fills the spaces between structures and provides structural support and helps maintain alignment of muscles during ocular movement.[1]

The major anatomic systems in the orbit consist of bones, muscles, nerves, vascular elements, and connective tissue,[2] all of which can be involved in pathological processes, either primarily or secondarily. Clinical evaluation of the patient is enhanced by combining knowledge of these anatomical relations along with simultaneous radiologic imaging. Taken together, these allow the creation of a differential diagnosis that often permits more refined evaluation and the determination of a more specific diagnosis.

Radiographic examination of the orbit is an important adjunct to the clinical evaluation of any patient with suspected orbital disease. It can confirm normal anatomy or demonstrate a variety of pathologic processes.[3,4] A carefully selected imaging sequence not only contributes to narrowing the differential diagnosis, but it can provide guidance in planning appropriate medical or surgical therapy. Radiologic imaging should never take the place of a thorough clinical examination, but it should be undertaken to confirm or narrow the possible diagnostic possibilities. Computerized tomography (CT) and magnetic resonance imaging (MRI) are the mainstay of modern imaging techniques, but newer technologies, such as positron emission tomography, especially when combined with CT, can add useful information.[5] Each provides some distinctive types of information not available on the others, so that a differential diagnosis established from the clinical examination is essential so that the most appropriate imaging technique can be selected.[6] For example, if a bony process is suspected such as a fracture, sinus mucocele, erosion from a malignant tumor, fibrous dysplasia, etc, a CT scan with bone window settings is ordered to evaluate bone detail that would not be visible on MRI. On the other hand, an optic nerve lesion such as a glioma, or inflammatory perioptic neuritis will be better imaged on MRI than on CT with tissue settings, even after contrast enhancement. MRI is also superior for imaging the orbital apex and cavernous sinus where the proximity of bony structures obscures soft tissue details on CT.

## ORBITAL BONES

The orbit is composed of seven bones that surround the eye and soft tissue structures, which serve visual function.[2] Except for a series of canals, fissures, and foramina that communicate with extraorbital compartments, the orbit is a closed space with a broad opening anteriorly (Fig. 50-1). This explains the

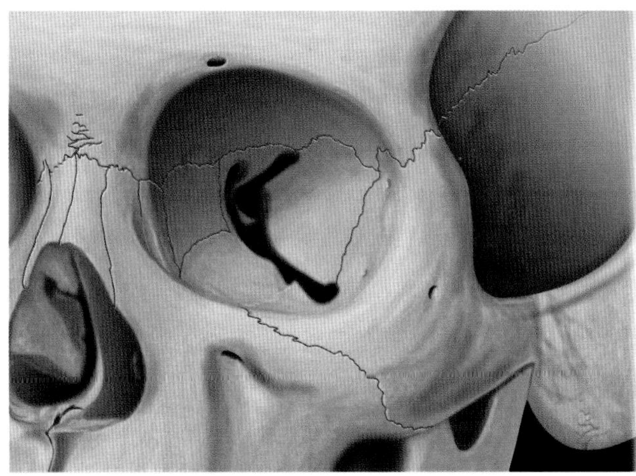

**Figure 50-1** Orbital bones from frontal view.

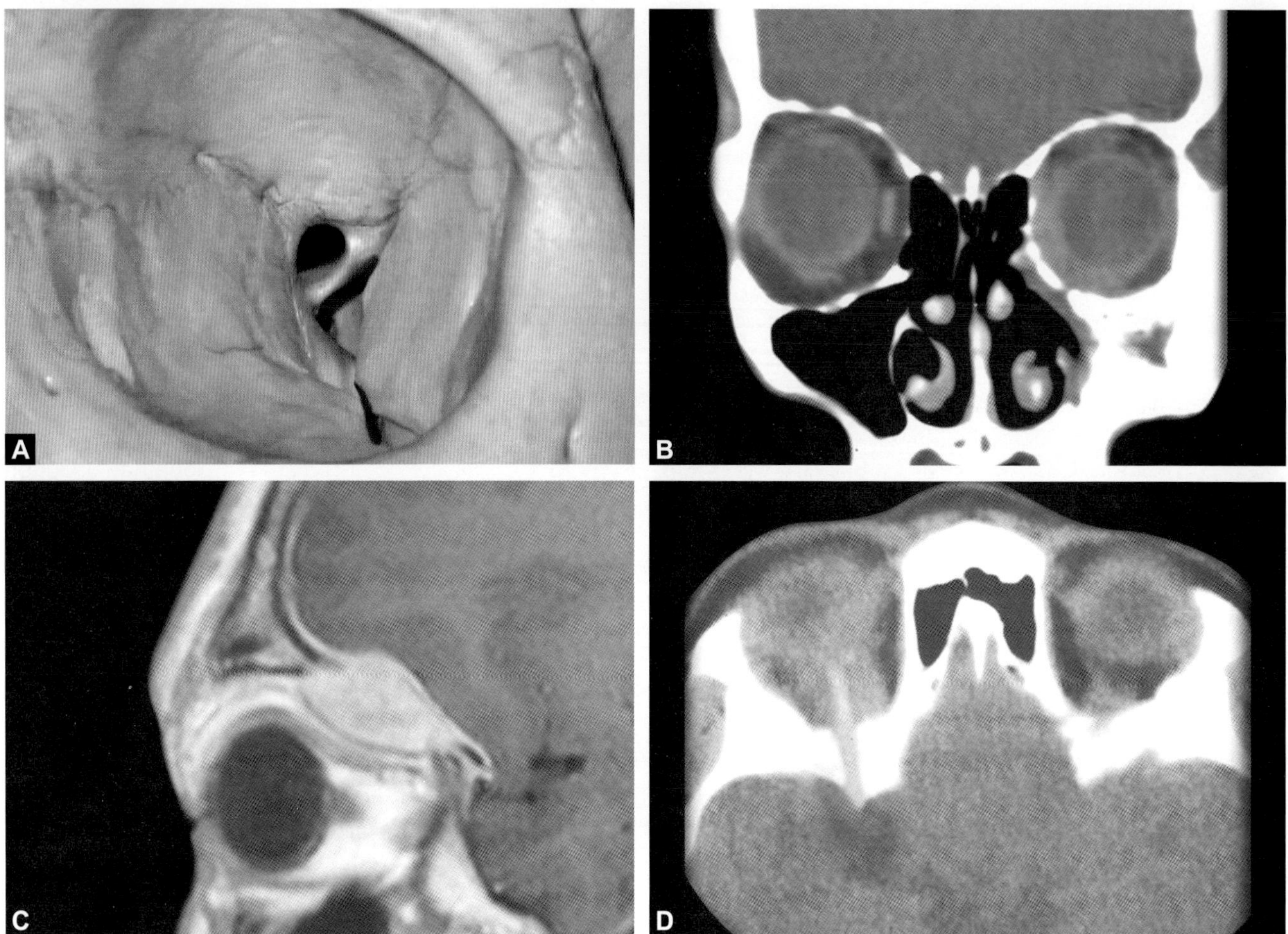


**Figures 50-2A to D** The orbital roof. (A) Frontal view of the orbit showing the roof sloping back and down from the superior rim to the optic canal. (B) Coronal section on CT scan the orbital roof appears as a thin undulating plate of the frontal bone. (C) Magnetic resonance imaging showing an orbital tumor eroding through the roof. (D) Axial cut on CT Scan with a wooden foreign body penetrating the orbit roof.

frequent development of proptosis as a clinical sign, even in early stages of orbital disease. Bones can be the site of many orbital disorders, and these can also involve the adjacent cranial vault, or paranasal sinuses. Since CT is based on the passage of X-rays through tissues of varying densities, it cannot easily distinguish between two tissues of equal density. However, bone is very dense and typically images appear white without any detail. Bone window settings adjust the image contrast level closer than that of bone and so offer excellent detail such as erosion or subtle areas of destruction. MRI, on the other hand, relies on the movement of protons within a magnetic field to image tissues based on their biochemical properties. Since there are very few protons in bone, it does not image on MRI.

## Orbital Roof

The orbital roof is composed of the orbital plate of the frontal bone with a small contribution from the lesser wing of the sphenoid at the apex. The roof slopes backward and downward towards the orbital apex, where it ends at the optic canal and superior orbital fissure (Fig. 50-2A). On CT, the roof appears as a thin, bone density line arching over the orbit, separating it from the anterior cranial fossa (Fig. 50-2B). On the cranial side, the surface is gently undulating reflecting the sulci and gyri of the overlying brain. Anteriorly, the paired frontal sinus can be seen within the roof. Mass lesions in the superior orbit can deform the roof shape if long standing, or erode the roof forming a dehiscence into the anterior cranial fossa (Fig. 50-2C). Bone destruction is a sign of malignancy or significant inflammatory reaction. The roof is a common site for penetration of orbital foreign bodies (Fig. 50-2D), and it is best evaluated with CT.[7]

## Lateral Orbital Wall

The lateral wall is formed by the greater wing of the sphenoid bone posteriorly and by the zygomatic process of the frontal

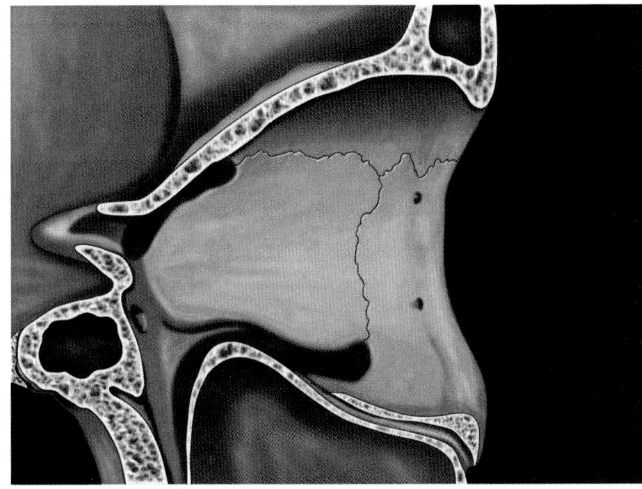

Figure 50-3 Sagittal section through the orbit showing the bones of the lateral wall.

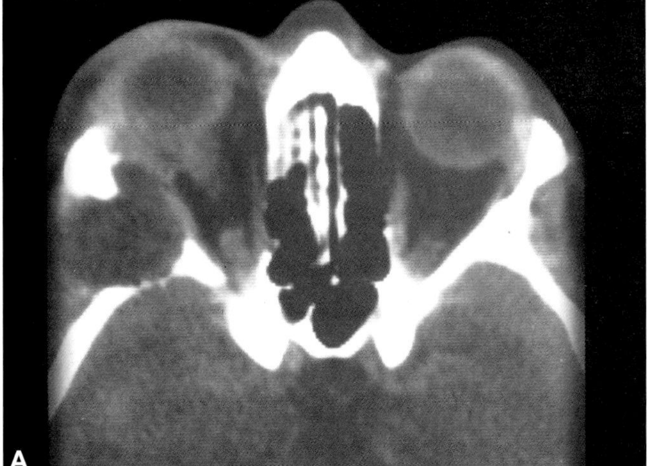

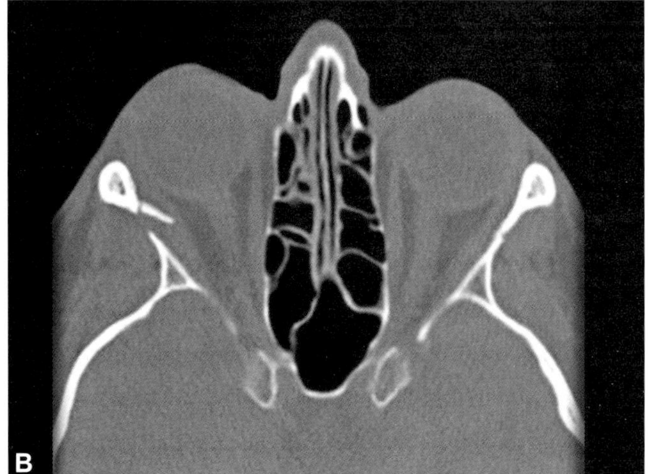

Figures 50-4A and B The lateral orbital wall. (A) Congenital dermoid cyst with a defect in the right zygomatic bone on computerized tomographic (CT) scan. (B) Traumatic fracture of the lateral wall through the greater sphenoid wing on bone window CT.

bone and the orbital process of the zygomatic bone anteriorly along the lateral rim (Fig. 50-3). The lateral wall is bounded below by the inferior orbital fissure and medially by the superior orbital fissure. Behind the lateral orbital rim, the wall becomes quite thin where the zygomatic bone joins the greater sphenoid wing. During lateral orbitotomy surgery, cutting the rim through to this thin plate allows easy outward fracture of the bone. The convoluted frontozygomatic suture line runs approximately horizontally and crosses the superotemporal rim near the lacrimal gland fossa. About 5–15 mm above this line, the frontal bone widens as it passes around the front end of the middle cranial fossa and the temporal lobe of the brain. Pathology involving the lateral wall is uncommon. It can be eroded by tumors of the lacrimal gland or shows defects from congenital lesions such as a dermoid cyst (Fig. 50-4A),[8] or it can be distorted by fractures across the lateral rim that may impinge on the lateral rectus muscle (Fig. 50-4B).

## Orbital Floor

The floor is the shortest of the orbital walls. It is composed primarily of the maxillary bone, with the zygomatic bone forming the anterolateral portion, and the palatine bone lying at its posterior extent. The floor ends at the posterior limit of the maxillary sinus and, therefore, does not extend to the orbital apex (Fig. 50-5). On CT scans, the floor appears as a thin plate of bone separating the orbit from the maxillary sinus. The latter usually images black when it contains air. The infraorbital neurovascular canal runs anteroposteriorly within the central portion of the floor and images as an oval-shaped density in the floor on coronal images. The orbital floor is thinnest just medial to the canal so that it is the most common site for blowout fractures.[9] These frequently show displacement of bony fragments and orbital tissue into the maxillary sinus (Fig. 50-6A), and the sinus may be opacified

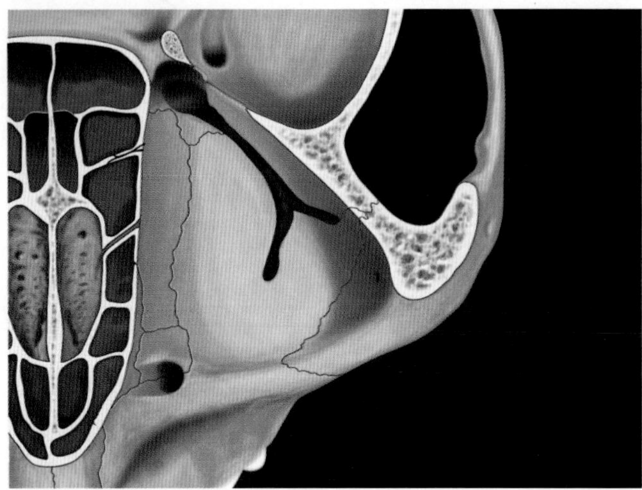

**Figure 50-5** Axial section through the orbit showing the anatomy of the maxillary bone forming the floor.

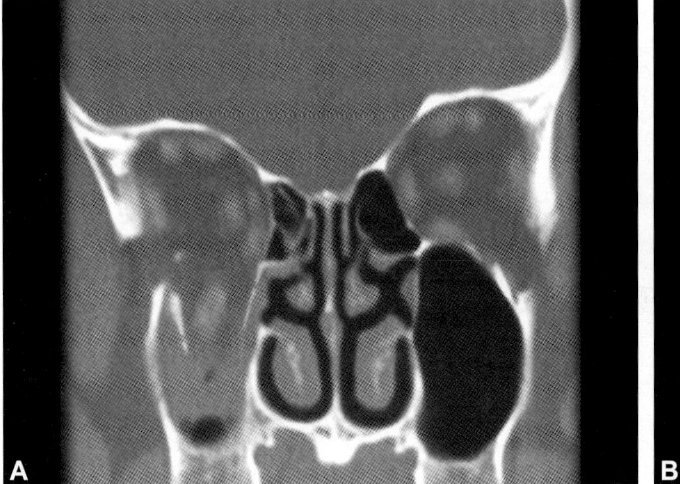


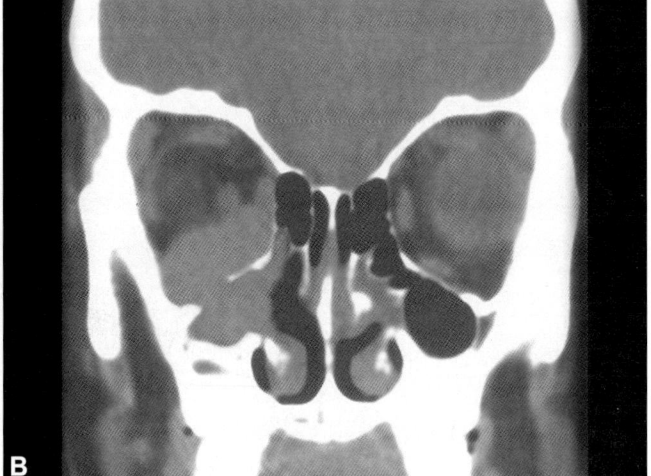


**Figures 50-6A and B** (A) Computerized tomographic (CT) bone window scan with a blowout fracture of the orbital floor; bone fragments and the inferior rectus muscle are displaced into the maxillary sinus. (B) Tissue window CT with a maxillary sinus tumor eroding through the floor into the inferior orbit.

from blood. Evaluation is best with coronal CT using bone window settings.[10] Vertical elongation of the inferior rectus muscle toward the bony fragments suggests entrapment within the fracture site. This usually correlates clinically with persistent diplopia. Maxillary sinusitis or tumors may erode upward through the floor into the inferior orbit (Fig. 50-6B).

## Medial Orbital Wall

The medial walls of the orbits are approximately parallel to each other and to the midsagittal plane. They are composed largely of the very thin lamina papyracea of the ethmoid bone that separates the orbit from the ethmoid sinus air cells (Fig. 50-7). It is a frequent site of fracture in orbital trauma where the lamina and orbital tissues are displaced into the ethmoid sinus (Fig. 50-8A).[11] The medial rectus muscle can be entrapped within these bony fragments. The lamina papyracea offers little resistance to expanding ethmoid sinus mucoceles, which slowly expand into the medial orbit displacing the medial rectus muscle and sometimes even the optic nerve (Fig. 50-8B). Inflammatory sinusitis can be transmitted through the lamina papyracea or the ethmoidal foramina, forming a subperiosteal abscess in the orbit (Fig. 50-8C). In orbital decompression surgery for thyroid eye disease, the lamina papyracea is removed to allow the medial rectus muscle and orbital fat to prolapse into the ethmoid sinus, thus reducing proptosis (Fig. 50-8D).[12]

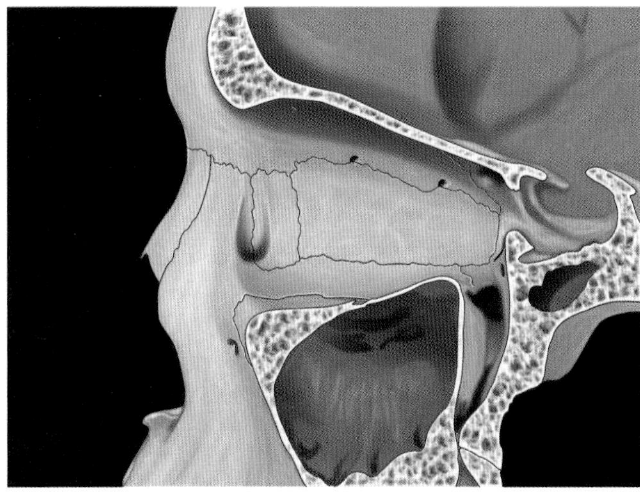

**Figure 50-7** Sagittal section through the orbit showing the medial wall with lamina papyracea of the ethmoid bone and the lacrimal bone anteriorly.

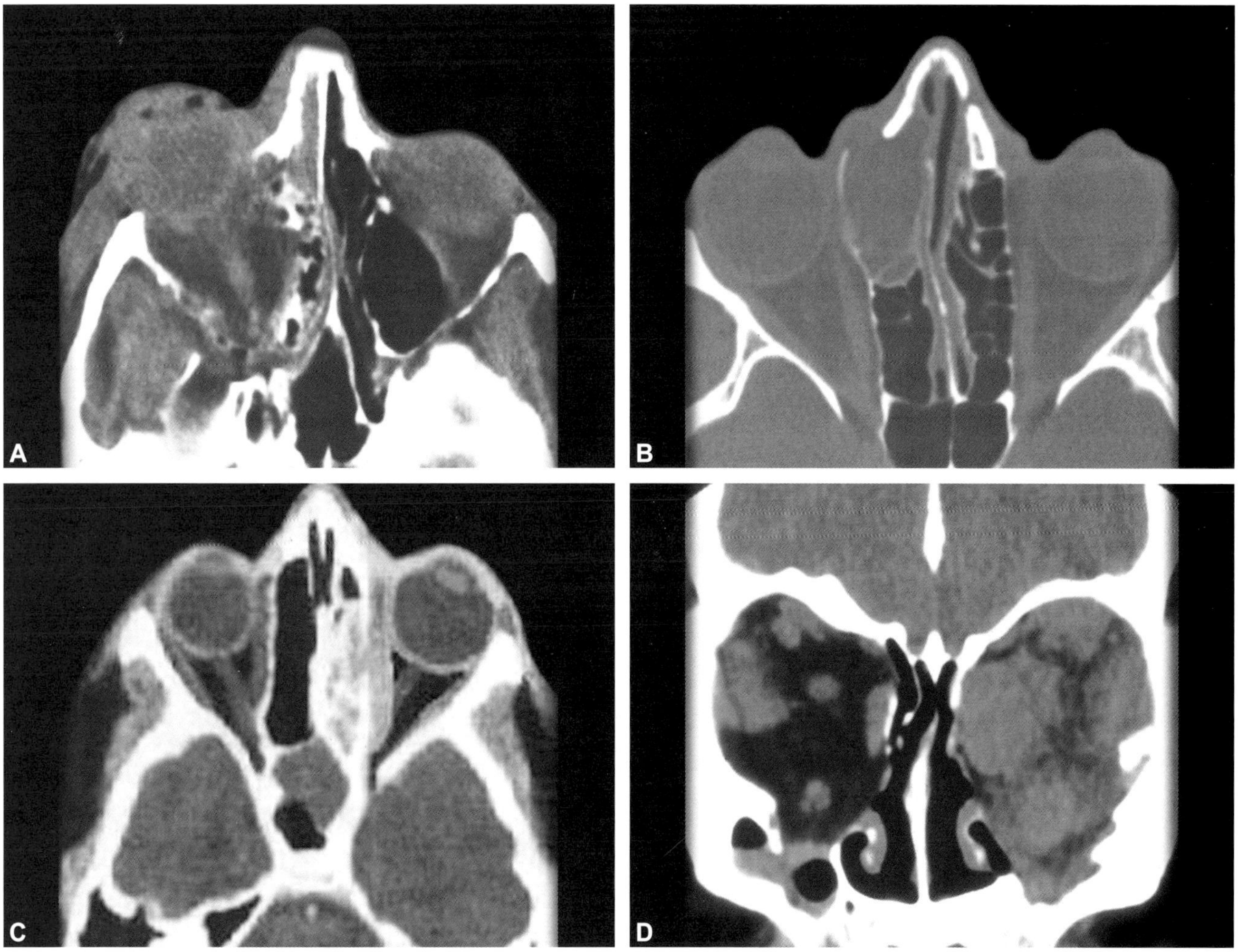

**Figures 50-8A to D** (A) Computerized tomographic (CT) scan showing a right ruptured globe with blow-out fracture of the medial wall. (B) Ethmoid sinus mucocele with expansion of the lamina papyracea into the medial orbit on bone window CT. (C) CT with ethmoid sinus sinusitis associated with a medial orbital subperiosteal abscess. (D) Prolapse of the medial rectus muscle into the ethmoid sinus on CT after orbital decompression for thyroid eye disease.

## MUSCLES OF OCULAR MOTILITY

The eye is an approximate sphere normally measuring about 24 mm in diameter and is situated in the anterior one-half of the orbit. Attached to it are the six striated extraocular muscles of ocular motility (Fig. 50-9). Four rectus muscles arise at the orbital apex from the annulus of Zinn, a fibrous band continuous with periorbita and dura at the optic foramen and superior orbital fissure. The muscles run forward with a layer of extraconal fat separating them from periorbita along the orbital walls. Anteriorly, they pass through Tenon's capsule to insert onto the sclera about 6–8 mm behind the corneal limbus.[2] On both CT and MRI scans, the rectus muscles appear as slightly fusiform straps of moderate tissue density, thickest at the bellies and thinnest at the tendons of insertion (Figs. 50-10A and B). Structures within the imaginary cone formed by the rectus muscles are said to be intraconal, and those between the muscles and the orbital walls are extraconal.

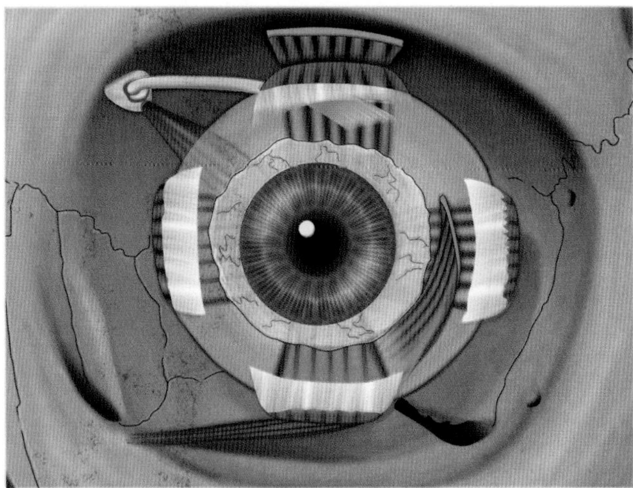

Figure 50-9 Anatomy of the extraocular muscle in frontal view.

The superior oblique muscle arises above the annulus, just superior and medial to the optic foramen. It runs forward along the superomedial orbital wall to the cartilaginous trochlea at the superior medial corner of the orbit. The tendon of this muscle slides through the trochlea before turning sharply posterolaterally to insert on the superoposterior aspect of the globe.

The inferior oblique muscle takes its origin in the anterior orbit from a small depression on the maxillary bone, below, and lateral to the lacrimal sac fossa. It passes laterally and slightly backward beneath the inferior rectus muscle to insert on the inferoposterior surface of the globe near the macula. Anteriorly, the sheath of the inferior oblique muscle joins that of the inferior rectus muscle and Tenon's capsule just behind the orbital rim to form Lockwood's inferior suspensory ligament. During surgery in the inferior orbit, care must be taken not to injure this muscle since it lies immediately behind the orbital rim.

Numerous diseases can affect the extraocular muscles. In thyroid eye disease multiple muscle bellies are usually enlarged by infiltration of glycosaminoglacans, but the tendons of insertion are typically normal (Fig. 50-11A). Most commonly, the inferior and medial rectus muscles are involved, although any muscle can be enlarged.[13] Orbital myositis is an idiopathic disorder characterized by inflammatory infiltration into one or more muscles, involving both the belly and the tendon (Fig. 50-11B). Metastatic tumors frequently localize in

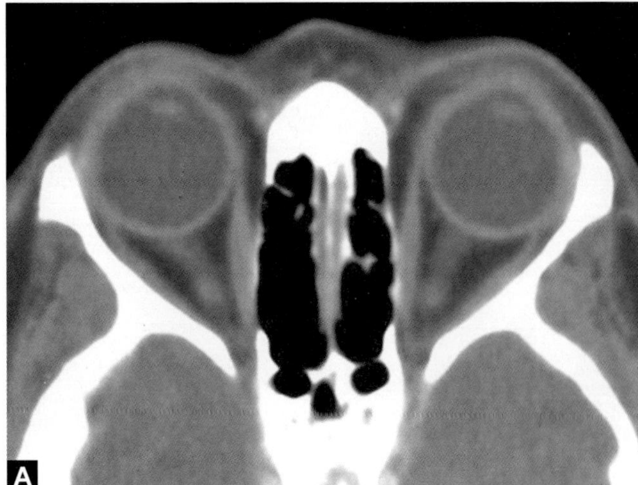

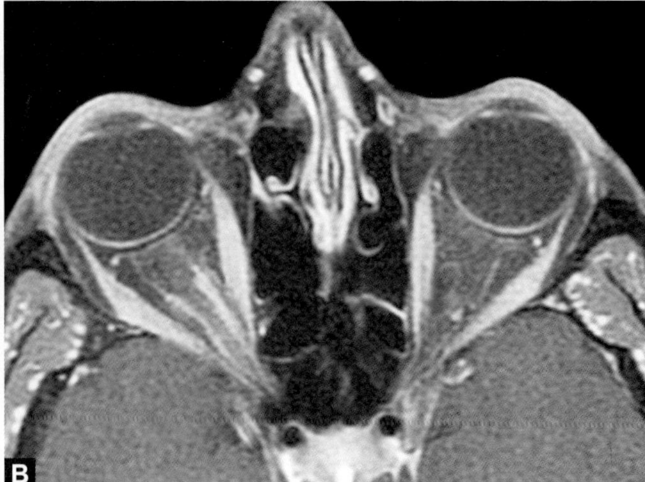

Figures 50-10A and B (A) Normal extraocular muscles on computerized tomographic scan. (B) Normal extraocular muscles on magnetic resonance imaging.

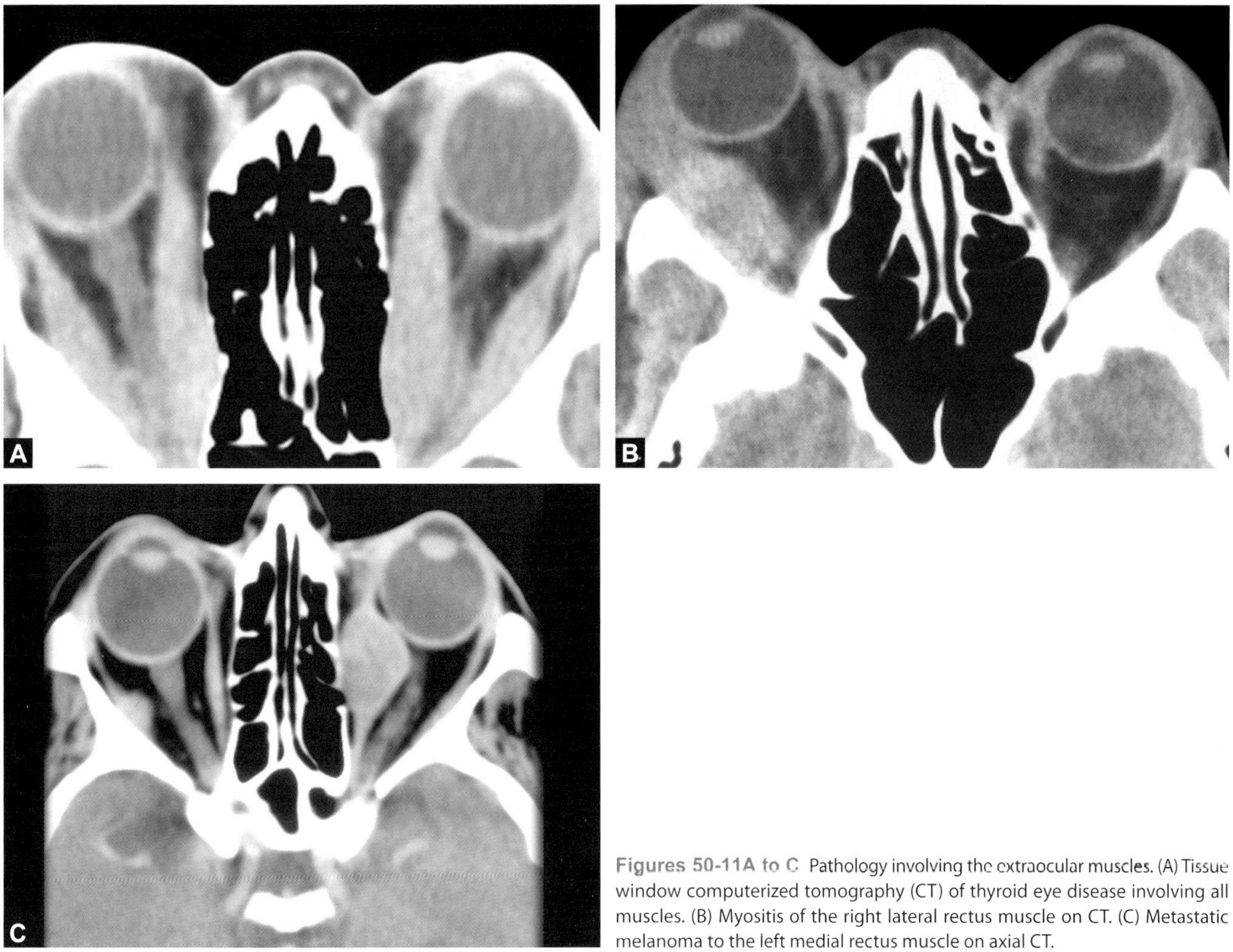

**Figures 50-11A to C** Pathology involving the extraocular muscles. (A) Tissue window computerized tomography (CT) of thyroid eye disease involving all muscles. (B) Myositis of the right lateral rectus muscle on CT. (C) Metastatic melanoma to the left medial rectus muscle on axial CT.

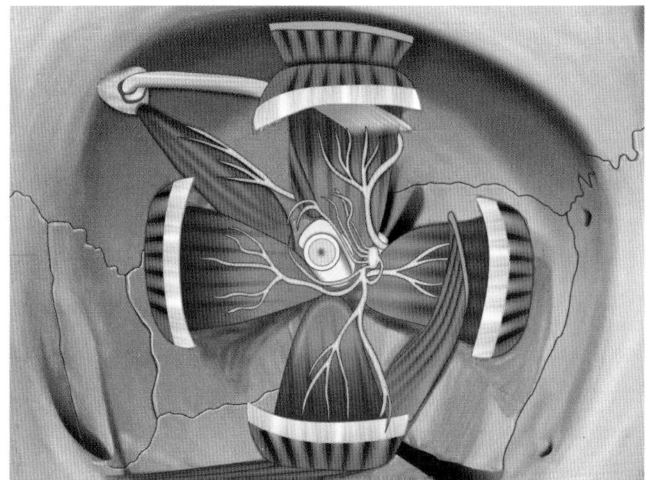

**Figure 50-12** Anatomy of the motor nerves to the muscles of ocular motility in frontal view.

the extraocular muscles due to their extensive vascular supply and may appear as a focal nodular enlargement in one or sometimes several muscles (Fig. 50-11C).[14] With orbital wall fractures, the muscle often shows a more rounded contour from edema or hemorrhage. It can also be entrapped, pulled into the bony fragments, and it appears elongated toward the fracture site (*see* Fig. 50-6A).

## MOTOR NERVES OF THE ORBIT

The extraocular muscles are innervated by the third, fourth, and sixth cranial nerves (Fig. 50-12). The oculomotor nerve (N.III) enters the orbit from the cavernous sinus as two branches. The superior branch innervates the superior rectus and levator muscles. The inferior branch sends fibers to the inferior rectus, the medial rectus, and the inferior oblique muscles on the conal surfaces. The trochlear nerve (N.IV)

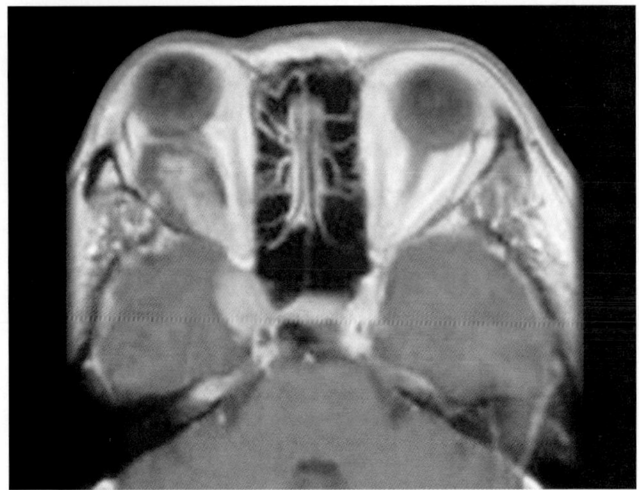

**Figure 50-13** Tumor of the right orbital apex and cavernous sinus causing ophthalmoplegia on axial magnetic resonance imaging.

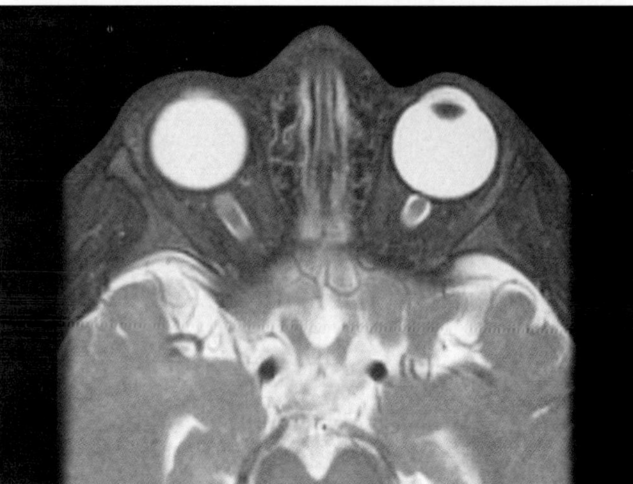

**Figure 50-14** Axial magnetic resonance imaging showing the optic nerves and the optic chiasm.

enters the orbit through the superior orbital fissure above the annulus of Zinn. It crosses over the superior rectus and levator muscle complex, in the extraconal space adjacent to the orbital roof, and runs along the external surface of the superior oblique muscle before penetrating its substance in the posterior third of the orbit. In this position against the orbital roof, the trochlear nerve is easily damaged during blunt trauma and can be injured with displacement of periorbita during deep superior orbital surgery. The abducens nerve (N.VI) enters the orbit through the superior orbital fissure and annulus of Zinn. It runs in the lateral intraconal space to supply the lateral rectus muscle.

Pathology in the posterior orbit can affect any of these nerves to the extraocular muscles.[15] This can result in motility disturbance with characteristic ocular deviation depending on the nerves involved. Injury to the superior branch of the oculomotor nerve often causes ptosis of the upper eyelid. All three nerves are usually affected simultaneously from lesions located in the orbital apex or the cavernous sinus (Fig. 50-13).[16]

## SENSORY NERVES OF THE ORBIT

The optic nerve (N.I) is technically not a sensory nerve, but a central nervous system tract arising from the retinal ganglion cells. Nasal fibers from each eye decussate in the optic chiasm and continue in the optic tracts to synapse in the lateral geniculate nuclei. From here, they radiate to the occipital cortex. The orbital portion of the optic nerve measures about 3 cm in length and is somewhat undulating and redundant to allow for ocular movement. It passes back through the optic canal in close approximation to the ophthalmic artery. On CT and MRI images the optic nerve runs through the canal to the optic chiasm just posterior to the pituitary stalk (Fig. 50-14). Since the nerve measures only about 3 mm in diameter, high-resolution thin section scans are necessary to image adequately the optic nerve. Lesions involving the nerve can cause enlargement, typically fusiform with optic nerve gliomas (Fig. 50-15A), or tubular with optic nerve sheath meningiomas.[17] In the latter case, the central nerve remains low density while the sheath enhances to produce the classic tram-tracking sign (Fig. 50-15B). Inflammatory perioptic neuritis appears as thickening with a shaggier surface (Fig. 50-15C).

Sensory innervation to the orbit is primarily from the ophthalmic division of the trigeminal nerve (N.V). The ophthalmic division divides within the cavernous sinus just as it passes into the superior orbital fissure. These branches are the lacrimal, frontal, and nasociliary nerves (Fig. 50-16A). The lacrimal nerve enters above the annulus of Zinn into the extraconal space and proceeds forward to the lacrimal gland and upper eyelid. The frontal nerve runs forward between the levator muscle and the superior periorbita and exits the orbit at the supraorbital notch or foramen at the superior orbital rim. The nasociliary nerve is the only branch that enters the orbit through the annulus of Zinn into the intraconal space. It crosses from lateral to medial over the optic nerve after sending small sensory branches that pass through the ciliary ganglion to the globe as the short ciliary nerves. As the nasociliary nerve passes to the medial side of the orbit it gives off the long posterior ciliary nerves, which extend to the posterior globe. The nasociliary nerve continues forward in the medial

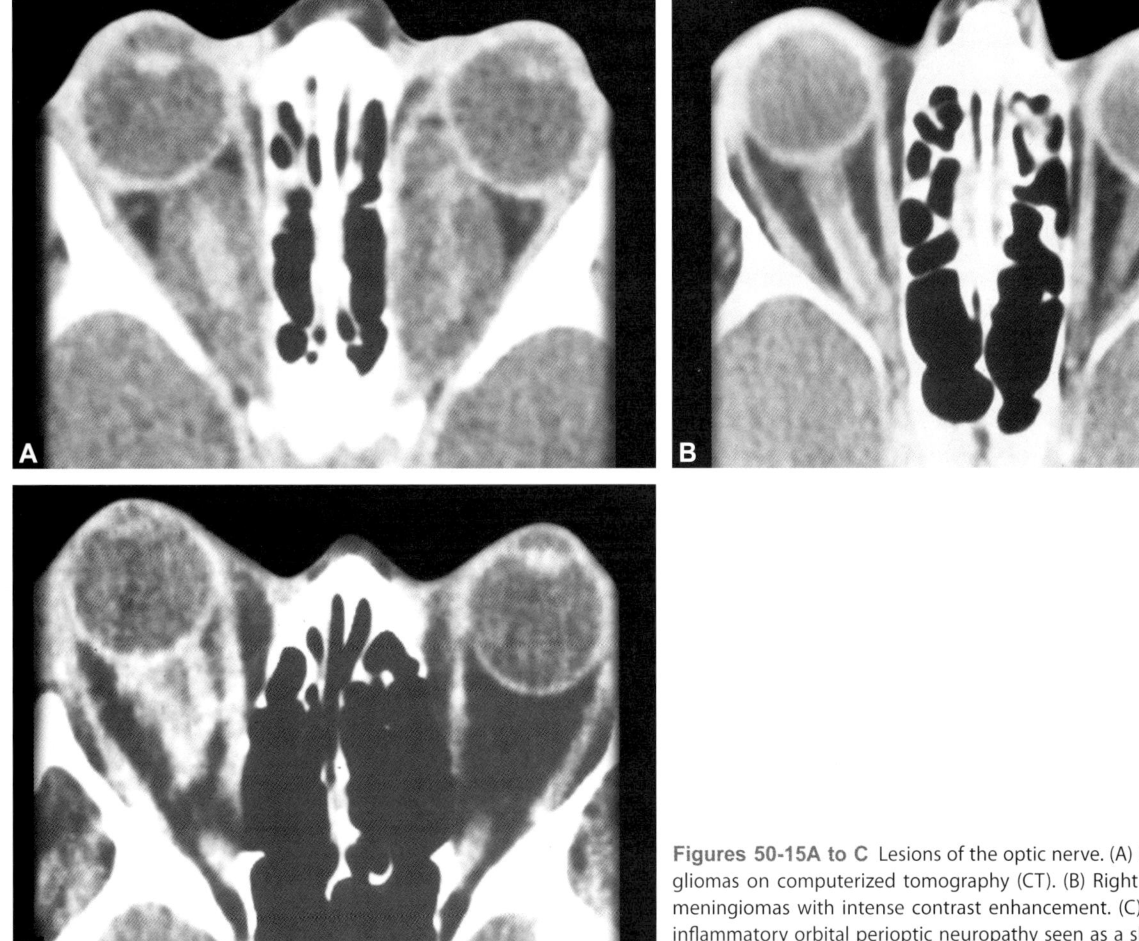


**Figures 50-15A to C** Lesions of the optic nerve. (A) Bilateral optic nerve gliomas on computerized tomography (CT). (B) Right optic nerve sheath meningiomas with intense contrast enhancement. (C) CT with idiopathic inflammatory orbital perioptic neuropathy seen as a shaggy infiltration of the nerve sheath.

where it gives off the anterior and posterior ethmoidal nerves and exits the orbit anteriorly as the infratrochlear nerve. Sensory nerves can be affected by inflammations or tumors. Paresthesias of the upper eyelid and forehead should alert the clinician to the possibility of an apex or cavernous sinus lesion. Within the orbit, neural tumors, such as neurofibromas and schwannomas, may be seen in the superior orbit where they more commonly affect sensory nerves (Fig. 50-16B).

## ARTERIAL SUPPLY TO THE ORBIT

The arterial supply to the orbit is from the internal carotid system through the ophthalmic artery (Fig. 50-17). The ophthalmic artery enters the orbit through the optic canal inferotemporal to the optic nerve and gives off branches to orbital structures.[18,19] The central retinal artery is usually the first branch. It runs along the inferior aspect of the optic nerve to penetrate the dura about 1 cm behind the globe. The lacrimal artery generally arises next and courses upward and forward extraconally to the lacrimal gland. The lateral and medial long posterior ciliary arteries arise on either side of the lacrimal artery and run forward to the globe parallel to the optic nerve.[20]

As the ophthalmic artery passes toward the medial orbit, it gives rise to the various muscular arteries that enter the conal surfaces of the rectus and oblique muscles. The supraorbital branch runs along in the superior extraconal space orbit to exit via the supraorbital foramen or notch. The ophthalmic artery then continues forward as the nasofrontal artery to exit just above the medial canthus. Here, it terminates as the supratrochlear and dorsal nasal arteries, which anastomose with facial arteries from the external carotid system.

On a normal CT or MRI, the ophthalmic artery is seen as a vessel entering the orbit just lateral and inferior to the optic nerve. It crosses over the optic nerve from lateral to medial near the orbital apex (Fig. 50-18). It can sometimes be seen running anteriorly just medial to the medial rectus muscle.

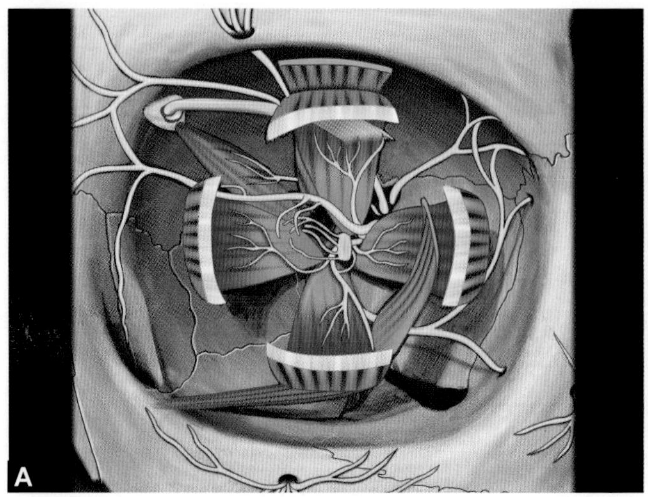


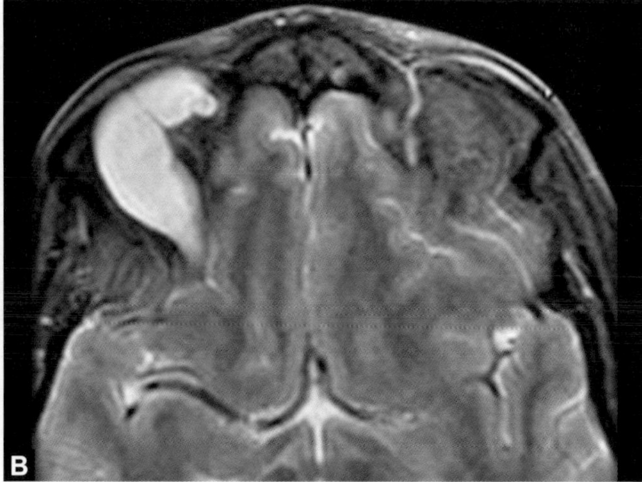


**Figures 50-16A and B** (A) Anatomy of the sensory branches of the ophthalmic division of the trigeminal nerve, in frontal orbital view. (B) Schwannoma of the ophthalmic division of the trigeminal nerve in the superior orbit.

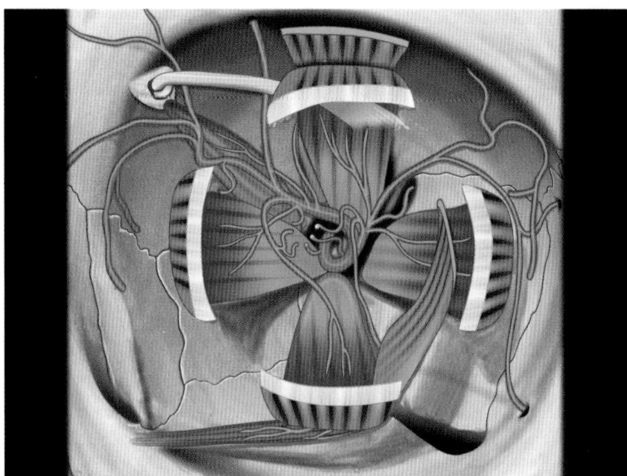

**Figure 50-17** Anatomy of the orbital branches of the ophthalmic artery, in frontal orbital view.

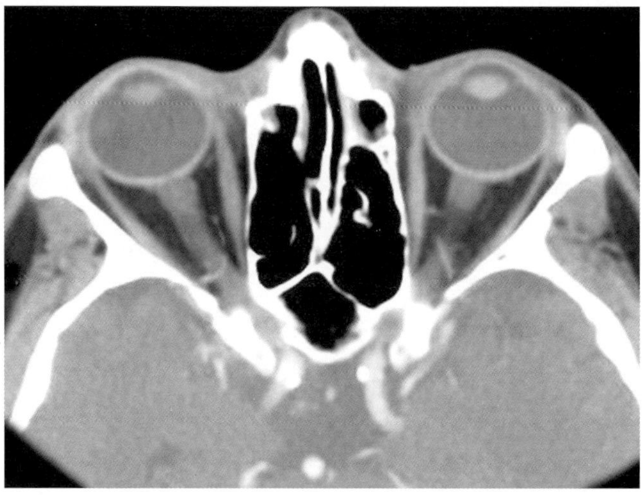

**Figure 50-18** Axial magnetic resonance imaging with the ophthalmic arteries seen cross the optic nerves in the orbital apex.

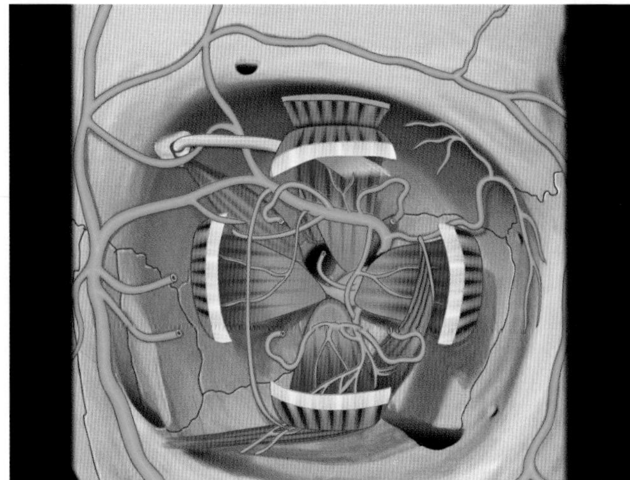

**Figure 50-19** Anatomy of the orbital veins seen in frontal orbital view.

The ophthalmic artery only rarely is involved directly with orbital pathology. Aneurysms are occasionally seen, as are arteriovenous malformations that appear as a tangle of dilated vessels best seen on angiography.

## VENOUS DRAINAGE FROM THE ORBIT

Venous drainage from the orbit is through the superior and inferior ophthalmic veins and their tributaries that drain backward into the cavernous sinus (Fig. 50-19).[21] The superior ophthalmic vein originates at the superomedial orbital rim from branches of the angular, supratrochlear, and supraorbital veins of the facial system. As it passes backward crossing from medial to lateral over the optic nerve in the superior mid orbit it is joined by the superior vortex veins, the anterior ethmoidal vein, collateral branches from the inferior ophthalmic vein,

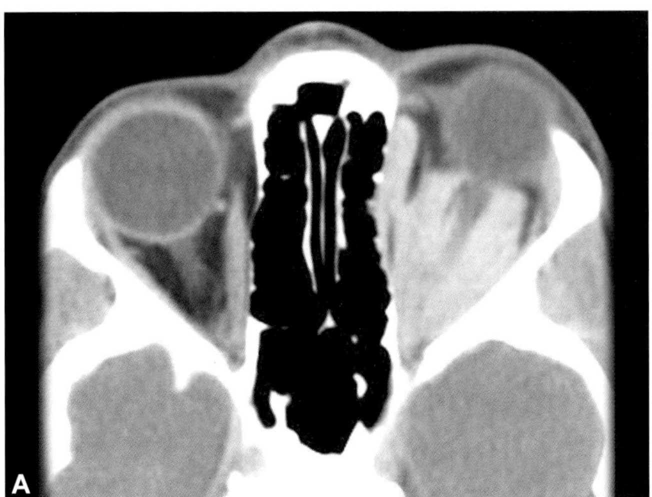


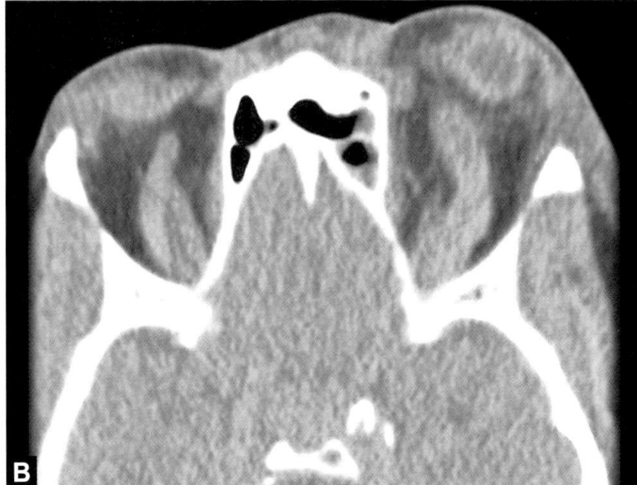


**Figures 50-20A and B** Pathology of the orbital venous system. (A) Orbital computerized tomography with a varix filing much of the left orbit. (B) Carotid–cavernous fistula with bilaterally dilated superior ophthalmic veins on axial magnetic resonance imaging scan.

branches from the extraocular muscles, and the lacrimal vein. It continues posteriorly to enter the cavernous sinus through the superior orbital fissure.

Ophthalmic veins not uncommonly show pathologic processes such as orbital varices that appear on imaging as irregular masses, sometimes with dilated vascular channels (Fig. 50-20A). A dilated superior ophthalmic vein (Fig. 50-20B) is suggestive of a carotid–cavernous or dural–cavernous fistula with increased venous pressure and often correlates with congested extraocular muscles.[22]

## KEY POINTS

- The orbit is composed of a complex tightly compacted array of various anatomic elements.
- Soft tissue elements are juxtaposed into a bony compartment close on all sides except anteriorly.
- Evaluation of orbital disease demands a thorough knowledge of anatomy, distorted by pathologic structures, and confirmed with radiographic imaging.
- Radiologic imaging is an important adjunct to the evaluation of any orbital disease.
- Orbital imaging should not replace a careful physical examination to establish a differential diagnosis.
- CT utilizes X-rays to create a two-dimensional image in any plane; this is a uniparametric modality based only on tissue transparency to the passage of X-rays.
- MRI is a multiparametric modality that utilizes atomic characteristics of tissue protons and their behavior in an external magnetic field; the image therefore reflects biochemical differences between tissues based on the molecular environment in which the proton is situated.

## REFERENCES


1. Koornneef L. Orbital septa: anatomy and function. Ophthalmology. 1979;86:876-80.
2. Dutton JJ. Atlas of clinical and surgical orbital anatomy, 2nd edn. London: Elsevier Saunders; 2011:262.
3. Aviv RI, Casselman J. Orbital imaging: part 1. Normal anatomy. Clin Radiol. 2005;60:279-87.
4. Aviv RI, Miszkiel K. Orbital imaging: Part 2. Intraorbital pathology. Clin Radiol. 2005;60(3):288-307.
5. Gayed I, Eskandari MF, McLaughlin P, et al. Value of positron emission tomography in staging ocular adnexal lymphomas and evaluating their response to therapy. Ophthal Surg Lasers Imaging. 2007;38:319-25.
6. Dutton JJ. Introduction to orbital imaging. In: Dutton JJ, Byrne SF, Proia AD (eds), Diagnostic Atlas of orbital diseases. Philadelphia, PA: WB Saunders; 2000:31-41.
7. Pinto A, Brunese L, Daniele S, et al. Role of computed tomography in the assessment of intraorbital foreign bodies. Semin Ultrasound CT MR. 2012;33:392-5.
8. Qin W, Chong R, Huang X, et al. Adenoid cystic carcinoma of the lacrimal gland: CT and MRI findings. Eur J Ophthalmol. 2012;22:316-9.
9. Jo A, Rizen V, Nikolic V, et al. The role of orbital wall morphological properties and their supporting structures in the etiology of "blow-out" fractures. Surg Radiol Anat. 1989;11:241-8.
10. Caranci F, Cicala D, Cappabianca S, et al. Orbital fractures: role of imaging. Semin Ultrasound CT MR. 2012;33:385-91.
11. Song WK, Lew H, Yoon JS, et al. Role of medial orbital wall morphologic properties in orbital blow-out fractures. Invest Ophthalmol. 2009;50:495-9.
12. Borumandi F, Hammer B, Noser H, Kamer L. Classification of orbital morphology for decompression surgery in Graves' orbitopathy: two-dimensional versus three-dimensional orbital parameters. Br J Ophthalmol. 2013;97:659-62.

13. Müller-Forell W, Kahaly GJ. Neuroimaging of Graves' orbitopathy. Best Pract Res Clin Endocrinol Metab. 2012;26:259-71.
14. Gupta P, Singh U, Singh SK, et al. Bilateral symmetrical metastasis to all extraocular muscles from distant rhabdomyosarcoma. Orbit. 2010;29:146-8.
15. Adams ME, Linn J, Yousry I. Pathology of the ocular motor nerves III, IV, and VI. Neuroimag Clin N Am. 2008;18:261-82.
16. Korchi AM, Cuvinciuc V, Caetano J, et al. Imaging of the cavernous sinus lesions. Diagn Interv Imaging. 2013;S2211-5684.
17. Lee AG, Johnson MC, Policeni BA, et al. Imaging for neuro-ophthalmic and orbital disease – a review. Clin Experiment Ophthalmol. 2008;37:30-53.
18. Hayreh SS, Dass R. The ophthalmic artery, II. Intra-orbital course. Br J Ophthalmol. 1962;46:165-85.
19. Hayreh SS. The ophthalmic artery, III. Branches. Br J Ophthalmol. 1962;46:212-47.
20. Erdogmus S, Govsa F. Anatomic characteristics of the ophthalmic and posterior ciliary arteries. J Neuroophthalmol. 2008;28:320-4.
21. Brismar J. Orbital phlebography, III. Anatomy of the superior ophthalmic vein and its tributaries. Acta Radiol (Diagn) (Stockh). 1974;15:481-96.
22. Miller NR. Dural carotid-cavernous fistulas: epidemiology, clinical presentation, and management. Neurosurg Clin N Am. 2012;23:179-92.

CHAPTER

# 51

# Basic Instrumentation and Techniques

Charles Kim, Gary J Lelli, Jr

## INTRODUCTION

Achieving successful results in ophthalmic plastic and reconstructive surgery is predicated on a wide range of factors, including a detailed understanding of fundamental surgical principles as well as an appreciation of the anatomy and pathophysiology pertinent to the case. Of particular importance is a familiarity with the wide array of surgical instruments that are available for oculoplastic procedures. The ability to implement these instruments in a controlled and consistent manner provides the surgeon with predictability and prepares him/her to address any potential intraoperative complications, thereby optimizing surgical outcomes.

This chapter will provide an overview of the instruments commonly utilized by oculoplastic surgeons, highlighting their specific uses and proper techniques.

## OCULOPLASTIC SURGICAL TRAY

Table 51-1 is a compilation of instruments found in a standard oculoplastics tray, many of which are depicted in Figure 51-1. The specific contents will vary according to the nature of the proposed procedure as well as surgeon's preference.

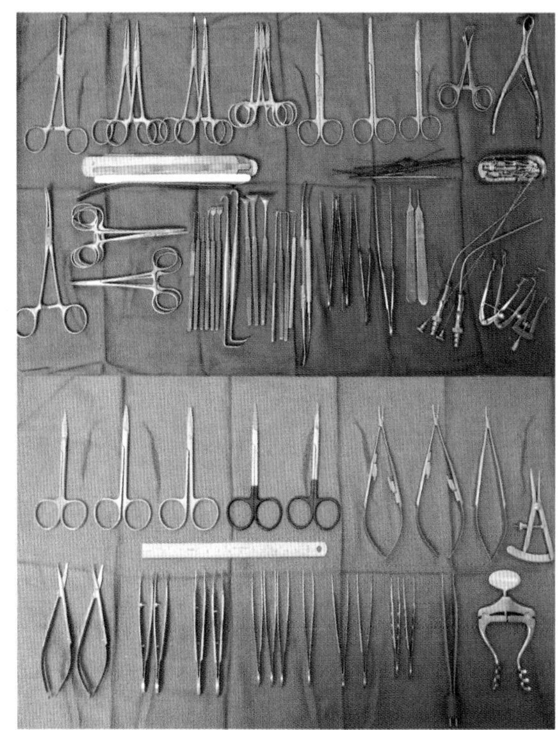

**Figure 51-1** A representative compilation of surgical instruments found in a standard oculoplastics tray.

**TABLE 51-1** Contents of standard oculoplastics tray

| | | | | |
|---|---|---|---|---|
| Mosquito clamps (4) | 0.3-mm forceps (2) | Senn retractor, blunt | Suction tube [7FR, 8FR, 9FR] | Adson dressing forceps |
| Iris scissors, straight | 0.5-mm forceps (2) | Senn retractor, sharp | Desmarres retractors [0,1,2,3] | Adson tissue forceps (2) |
| Iris scissors, curved | Westcott scissors, sharp (2) | Webster needle holder | Allis clamps | Brown–Adson forceps (2) |
| Jameson muscle hook | Westcott scissors, blunt (2) | Castroviejo needle holder | Ruler | Stevens scissors, straight |
| Blair retractor, sharp (2) | Bayonet forceps | Skin hook (2) | Periosteal freer elevator | Stevens scissors, curved |
| Knapp retractor, blunt (2) | Orbital retractor, small (2) | Mayo scissors | Jewelers forceps | Bipolar forceps |
| Wire speculum | Orbital retractor, large (2) | Nasal speculum | Bard-Parker handle (2) | |

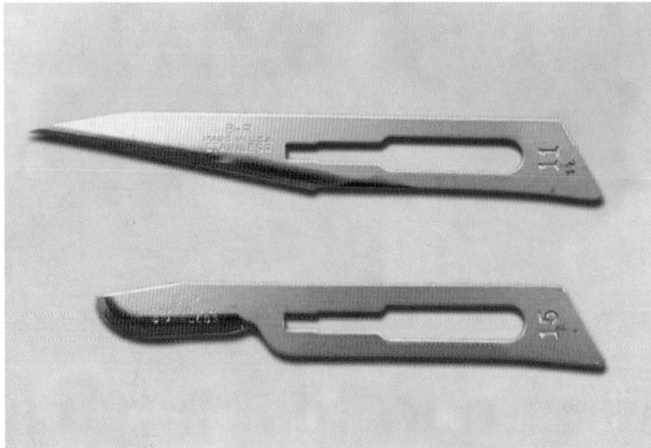

Figure 51-2 Both the #11 blade (top) and #15 Bard-Parker blade (bottom) are commonly employed by ophthalmic plastic surgeons.

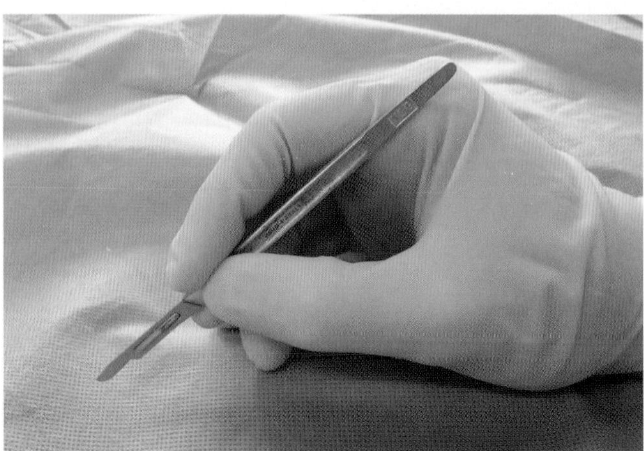

Figure 51-3 Conventional three-point fixation technique used to grip a scalpel, with the instrument held between the thumb and index and middle fingers.

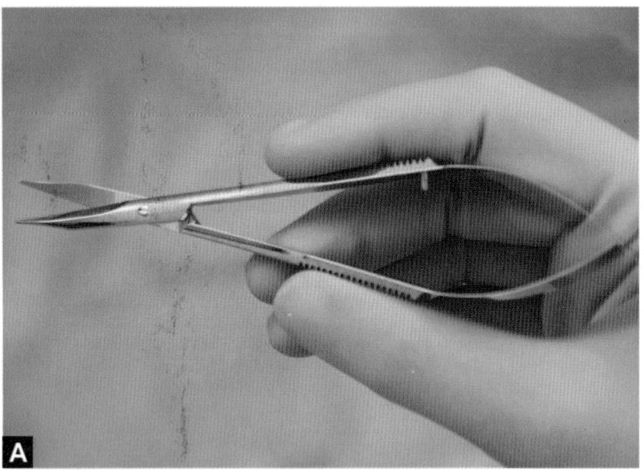

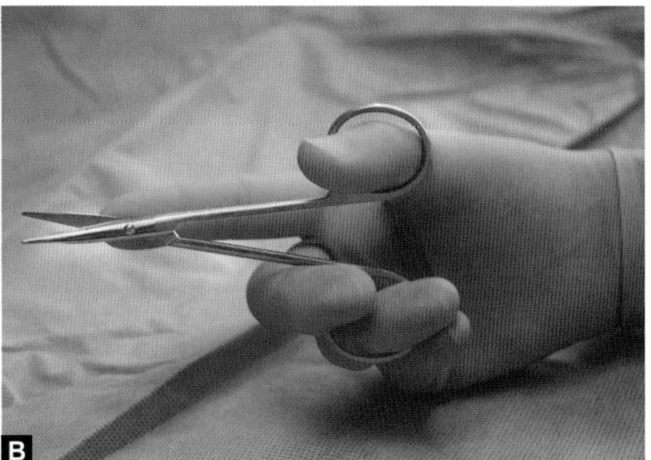

Figures 51-4A and B (A) Westcott and (B) Stevens scissors can be used for the cutting and dissection of tissue.

## INCISIONS

While a variety of scalpel blades can be used to create skin incisions, the most commonly used is the #15 Bard-Parker blade, which is ideal for straight and curvilinear patterns. By comparison, the #10 blade has a larger belly, making it particularly useful for large facial incisions, flap formations, and the harvesting of dermis fat grafts. The #11 scalpel blade, which is tapered to a fine point, is preferred for the removal of small lesions or the creation of stab incisions, as required in chalazion excision (Fig. 51-2). Similarly, Beaver #57 blades are also used to excise smaller lesions.

Stylistic variation aside, the standard technique for gripping a scalpel involves three-point fixation between the thumb, index finger, and middle finger (Fig. 51-3). It is important to note that the belly of the blade–as opposed to its point–should be used to create the incision. Hand tremors can be minimized by avoiding excessive grip pressure and by stabilizing the forearms on a solid interface.

In addition to scalpel blades, skin incisions can also be made using sharp scissors, which are useful when working with the thin skin of the eyelid (Figs. 51-4A and B). Additional modalities for creating incisions include electrocautery and carbon dioxide ($CO_2$) laser, although these techniques can be limited by thermal damage to adjacent tissue and subsequent adverse effects on wound healing.[1]

## TISSUE DISSECTION

Once the incision has been made and the appropriate plane has been identified, tissue can be dissected using either blunt-tipped Stevens or Westcott scissors. Metzenbaum scissors

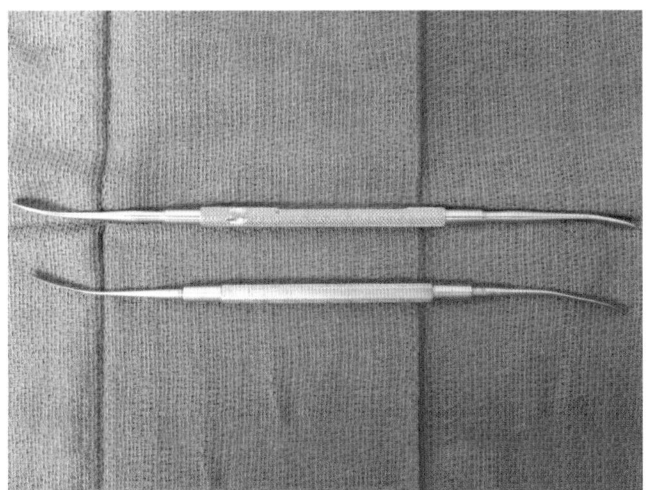

Figure 51-5 Periosteal elevators can serve multiple functions during orbital surgery.

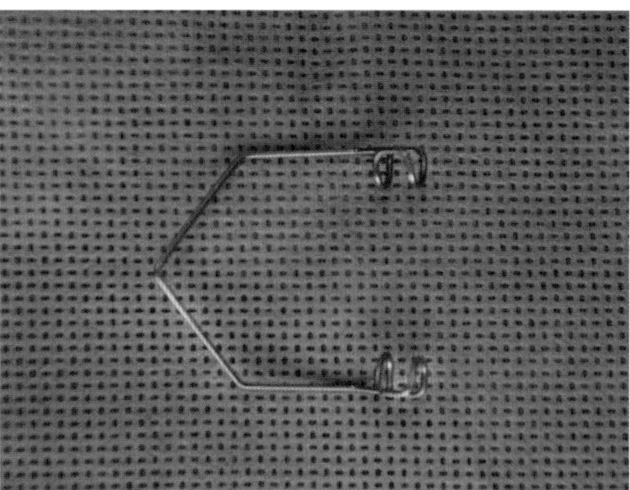

Figure 51-6 Eyelid speculums are used to keep the operative eye open and provide adequate exposure for surgery.

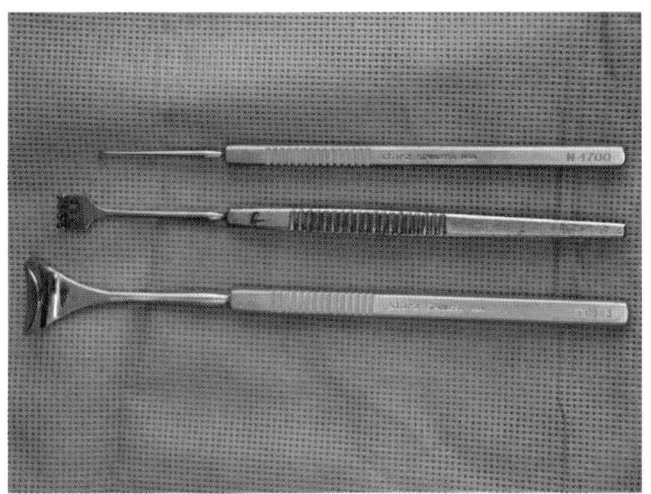

Figure 51-7 Desmarres retractor (left), skin rake (middle), and skin hook (right).

may be helpful in areas of denser tissue. These scissors can also be used to directly lyse connective tissue bands that are encountered during dissection.

Within the orbit, blunt dissection can be performed with a periosteal freer elevator, which can also be used to release the periosteal layer from bone, as well as the retraction and repositioning of soft tissues (Fig. 51-5). Alternatively, neurosurgical cottonoids and cotton-tipped applicators can also be used for orbital dissection.

## EXPOSURE OF THE SURGICAL FIELD

Choosing the appropriate modality for exposure is dependent on a number of different factors, including surgical site, surgeon's preference, and assistant availability. Mechanical devices such as the lacrimal speculum, eyelid speculum, and the Kennerdell–Maroon and Greenberg orbital systems are popular options (Fig. 51-6). For most aesthetic and reconstructive eyelid surgeries, any combination of skin hooks and rakes, Desmarres retractors, and lid margin sutures can be used (Fig. 51-7). Orbital cases can be greatly aided by the use of malleable retractors, which can provide access to deeper fields. However, great care must be utilized when positioning these retractors to prevent tissue damage. Desmarres, Converse, and Senn retractors are also commonly used for orbital procedures.

## HEMOSTASIS

Discontinuing anticoagulation prior to surgery should be considered in the appropriate clinical context and must be coordinated with the patient's primary care physician. If the decision is made to hold anticoagulants, aspirin should be stopped for 10–14 days, warfarin for 5 days, and nonsteroidal anti-inflammatory agents for 3–5 days before surgery.

In the operating room, the injection of local anesthetic containing epinephrine (1:100,000) into the surgical site is an imperative initial step. Intraoperatively, bleeding from large vessels typically requires ligation, whereas hemorrhages from smaller vessels can be controlled using direct pressure (tamponade). Alternatively, thrombin and microfibrillar collagen products may be applied directly onto sites of active bleeding.

Electrocautery is frequently implemented for hemostasis during surgery (Fig. 51-8). The most common mode is the Bovie, which can also be used for the cutting and fulguration

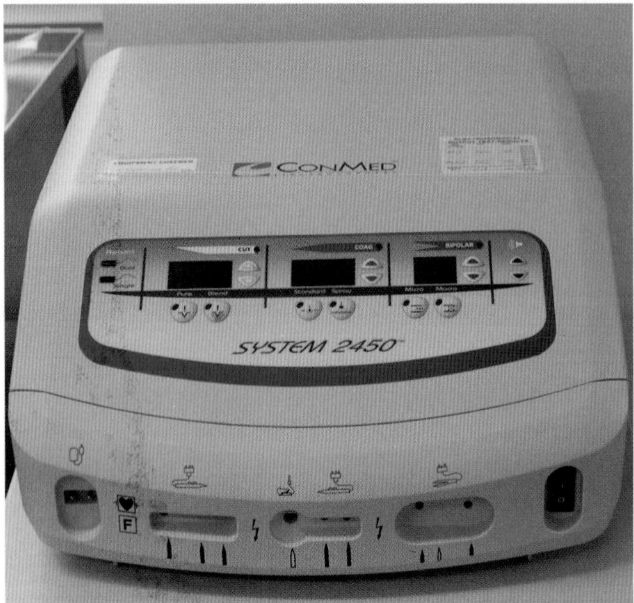


**Figure 51-8** Standard electrocautery unit, featuring cut, coagulation, and bipolar settings.

of tissue. Bovie cautery is monopolar and therefore requires a reference electrode that is placed on the back or thigh of the patient. Special consideration must be given to patients with pacemakers, as the monopolar current can disable the defibrillator or cause it to discharge inappropriately. As such, a limit of 30 seconds per discharge should be enforced, in conjunction with careful cardiac monitoring by an anesthesiologist.[2]

In contrast, bipolar cautery incorporates both the active and reference electrodes, typically in the parallel tines of a pair of forceps. As a result, current is only passed through tissue held between the electrodes, eliminating the aforementioned risk in patients with pacemakers and providing a controlled area of coagulation with minimal damage to adjacent tissue. However, bipolar cautery can take longer for hemostasis due to its reduced power settings and may also tear blood vessels due to its tendency to adhere tightly to tissue.

If the measures described above are inadequate, placement of the Hemovac drainage system, Jackson Pratt, or Silastic tubing into the surgical wound may be required. These devices drain into vacuum test tubes and are typically removed during the postoperative period.

## SUTURING

A variety of sutures–which vary according to composition and absorbability–are available to the oculoplastic surgeon. Sutures can be composed of either natural or synthetic materials, consisting of a single-strand (monofilament) or multiple-braided strands (multifilament). Monofilaments inherently cause less tissue reaction, whereas multifilaments are capable of maintaining greater tension on wounds. Absorbable sutures include gut (fast absorbing, plain, and chromic), Vicryl, Dexon, Monocryl, and polydioxanone (PDS), which vary in degradation time. Permanent sutures include nylon, polyester, Prolene, and stainless steel.

The needles attached to sutures are distinguished by their shape, size, and point. The most common varieties are the 3/8 circle needle, which can be used under a wide range of conditions, and the reverse cutting needle, which can be pushed through tissue without enlarging the needle tract due to the presence of sharp edges on its outer curvature.

The Castroviejo and ring handle needle holders are preferred by most surgeons for suturing. While the former are held using a conventional pencil grip, the latter are held with the thumb in one ring and the ring finger in the other (Figs. 51-9A and B).

## SOFT TISSUE GRAFTS

Dermatomes can be used to produce the large split-thickness skin grafts typically required for socket reconstruction–these grafts can be further expanded using meshing instruments. Similarly, mucous membrane grafts are harvested with mucotomes and microdermatomes, which permit mucosal regeneration and allow the grafts to be reharvested as needed. In contrast, hand cutting of full-thickness skin grafts remains the favored approach in eyelid surgery.

Given its wide availability, ease of use, and inherent anti-inflammatory and antivascular properties, amniotic membrane is a popular substrate for forniceal reconstruction.[3] Hard palate grafts provide rigidity and flexibility to the eyelid, serving as viable substitutes for the posterior lamella in cases of eyelid malpositioning. These grafts also avoid morbidity to the contralateral eye, as encountered during the harvesting of autogenous free tarsal grafts. However, the keratinized mucosa of the hard palate can be irritating to the cornea, and significant complications can develop at the donor site over time.[4]

Synthetic agents such as AlloDerm (Lifecell Corp, Woodlands, TX, USA), an acellular human dermis derived from cadavers, can serve as an alternative to autologous grafts in eyelid reconstruction. AlloDerm is immunologically inert, rigid and provides the necessary substrate for conjunctival epithelial migration and repopulation of the graft surface.[5]

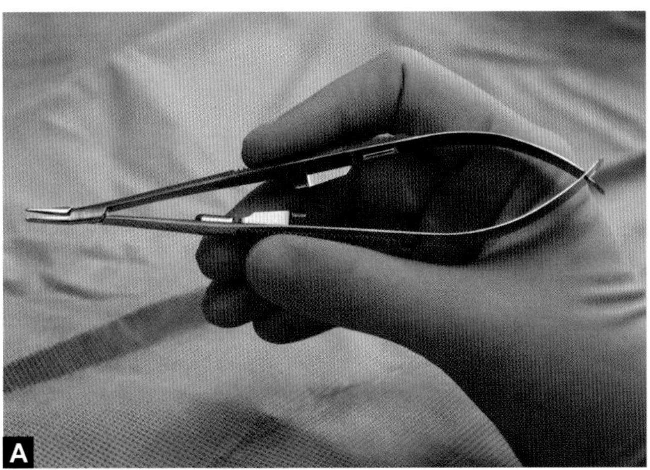
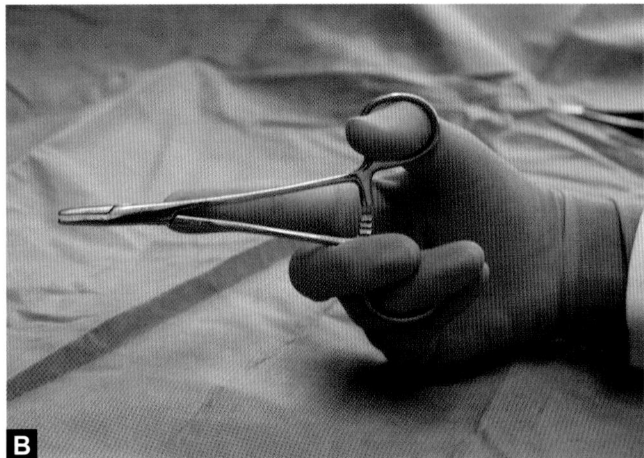

**Figures 51-9A and B** Proper grip technique for using the (A) Castroviejo and (B) ring handle needle holders.

**TABLE 51-2** Summary of autologous and alloplastic substrates available for orbital reconstructive surgery

| Autologous | Alloplastic | |
|---|---|---|
| Bone | Nonporous | Porous |
| Cartilage | Silicone polymer | Hydroxyapatite |
| | Polyurethane | Methyl methacrylate |
| | Aluminum oxide ceramic | Gore-Tex (expanded polytetrafluoroethylene) |
| | Teflon (polytetrafluoroethylene polymer) | Gelatin film |
| | Supramid (polyamide) | Polyvinyl sponge |
| | Nylon foil (SupraFOIL) | Vicryl mesh (polyglactin) |
| | Titanium mesh | Polylactide plates |
| | Vitallium mesh | Porous polyethylene (Medpor) |
| | Polydioxanone plates | |

Nevertheless, many surgeons continue to prefer hard palate grafts for eyelid reconstruction due to their proven longevity.[6,7]

## BONE AND CARTILAGE

Manipulation of bone is a requisite component of orbital fracture repair, orbital surgery, and dacryocystorhinostomy (DCR). Small-tipped osteotomes and mallets can be used to create controlled bone fractures, whereas biting instruments such as rongeurs can remove bone and widen osteotomies. Long-handed Kerrison rongeurs are able to reach deep bone, which can be particularly useful during orbital decompression and DCR. Rongeurs must be used in a gentle side-to-side motion to prevent inadvertent posterior extension of the fracture.

Air powered drills and saws can also create controlled osteotomies. In addition, these drills are used to create the holes required for the placement of screws, sutures, and wires. Cutting bits can be attached for the contouring and sculpting of bone, as required for lateral orbital decompressions. Oscillating saws can be employed during lateral orbitotomies to form bony windows for improved visualization. The blade of the saw should be in motion prior to the initial cut, held firmly against the bone during cutting, and withdrawn from the osteotomy while still in motion. During creation of an osteotomy, the orbital contents are protected using malleable retractors, and the bone is irrigated with saline to prevent bone necrosis.

Cartilage knives, nasal speculums, and nasal scissors can be used to harvest cartilage grafts from the nasal septum, external ear, or the rib.

## ORBITAL IMPLANTS

### Repairing Orbital Fractures

Many different autogenous tissues and alloplastic materials are available for orbital reconstruction (Table 51-2). Over the years, alloplastic materials have become increasingly favored over autogenous bone grafts, which can have variable rates of resorption. Alloplastic implants can be grouped into nonporous and porous varieties. Nonporous implants provide excellent structural support but typically do not allow vascular ingrowth, leading to capsule formation at the graft–host interface. Examples include Teflon, nylon foil (SupraFOIL), silicone (Silastic), and titanium mesh. Titanium provides excellent structural support despite its easy manipulability, is chemically inert, and can undergo osseointegration.

In contrast, porous implants such as Medpor (porous high-density polyethylene) allow for vascular and osseous ingrowth, leading to even greater biocompatibility. The large pore size (100–200 μm) prevents capsule formation, maintains the host immune response, and minimizes infection.[8] However, Medpor is not as malleable as titanium and is not well visualized on imaging studies. As a result, porous polyethylene implants with embedded titanium mesh have been developed. These implants provide excellent structural support and malleability while allowing rapid host integration and resistance to infection.[9,10]

### Orbit Volume Enhancement

Spherical implants are used within the orbit to replace intraorbital volume loss and impart motility to an ocular prosthetic after globe removal. These alloplastic implants are composed of either integrated or nonintegrated materials.

Nonintegrated implants are single spheres composed of inert substances such as silicone, acrylic, or polymethylmetacrylate. Because these implants do not allow the integration of extraocular muscles, imbrication of the muscles is needed to provide motility to the implant and overlying prosthesis.

In contrast, integrated implants such as hydroxyapatite and Medpor permit fibrovascular ingrowth and subsequent incorporation of the implant into the orbit, providing a multitude of benefits over the nonporous variety. Hydroxyapatite is a calcium phosphate salt that is naturally present in human bone. As a result of its inherently rough surface, hydroxyapatite has a propensity to erode through overlying soft tissue. Consequently, wrapping material, such as donor sclera, fascia lata, and synthetic materials, is typically used to encapsulate the implant prior to placement and ultimately serves as the substrate onto which the extraocular muscles are sutured.

As detailed above, Medpor is another commonly utilized integrated implant that allows fibrovascular ingrowth, albeit at a slower rate than hydroxyapatite. Extraocular muscles can be directly attached to Medpor implants, although they can be wrapped as well.

Integrated implants can be attached to pegs to create a fixed interface between the implant and prosthesis. While pegs have been associated with high complication rates,[11] they allow for smaller and lighter prostheses, thereby reducing the risk of lower eyelid displacement over time.

### Orbital Tissue Expanders

Anophthalmia is a congenital condition in which some or all of the ocular tissues fail to develop properly, resulting in microorbitism and microblepharon. As a result of stunted bony orbital growth, the entire hemiface also remains underdeveloped. By convention, the implantation of progressively larger conformers and spherical orbital implants has been used for orbital and periocular soft tissue expansion. More recently, however, hydrogel tissue expanders composed of highly hydrophilic polymers capable of self-expansion have been produced. These expanders exert constant hydrostatic pressure designed to stimulate orbital growth. In addition, the use of integrated orbital tissue expander models has also been described in the literature.[12–14]

## PTOSIS SURGERY

Suspension during frontalis sling ptosis surgery can be achieved via simple sutures (e.g. 4-0 Supramid on a ski needle), silicone bands (e.g. #240 used for scleral buckling), 1-mm silicone rods (Dow Corning Corp, Midland, MI, USA), fascia lata strips, or banked fascia lata and tendon transfers.[15–17]

Ptosis repair via Muller's muscle-conjunctival resection can be greatly facilitated with the use of the Putterman clamp, which allows for efficient and accurate tissue removal. Of note, fibrant sealant (Tisseel) can be used effectively during this procedure for wound closure.[18]

## CANALICULAR LACERATION REPAIR

Any canalicular or nasolacrimal probing that may involve silicone intubation requires perioperative nasal packing with neurosurgical cottonoids soaked in a vasoconstrictor (e.g. Afrin, phenylephrine, cocaine) using a nasal speculum and Bayonet instrument.

If the proximal end of the lacerated canaliculus cannot be located directly, a pigtail probe can be used to intubate the intact side of the lacrimal system. The probe will ultimately enter the distal end of the torn canaliculus and exit within the wound.

## CANALICULAR STENTS

Although a variety of methods to stent the canaliculi have been reported, bicanalicular and monocanalicular silicone

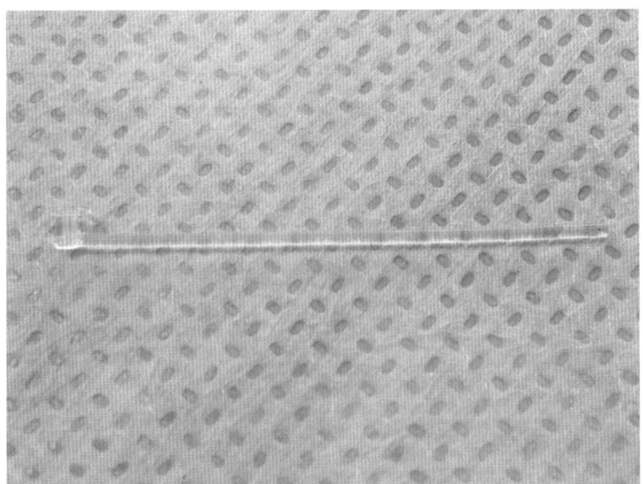

Figure 51-10 Mini Monoka tubes are used to stent the canalicular portion of the lacrimal drainage system.

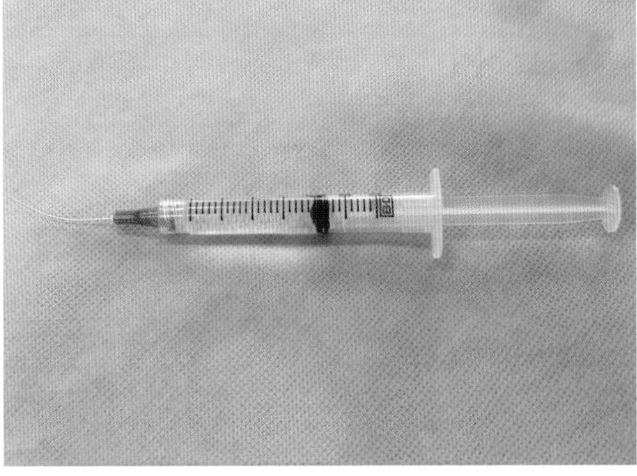

Figure 51-11 Syringes outfitted with irrigation cannulas are used to probe and irrigate the lacrimal drainage system in cases of suspected nasolacrimal duct obstruction.

stents are used most commonly. The "Mini Monoka" tube is used in the setting of single canalicular lacerations and is designed to fit the ampulla with its plug and collarette lying flush against the eyelid margin (Fig. 51-10). Variants of this system include tubes with perforated plugs that keep the punctum open and allow it to drain tears.[19]

## LACRIMAL SYSTEM OBSTRUCTION

Investigation of patients with suspected obstruction of the lacrimal drainage system typically involves probing and irrigation (Fig. 51-11). The location and degree of saline reflux be used to identify the site of obstruction. Probing can confirm obstruction of the punctum, canaliculus, or lacrimal sac.

First introduced by Becker and Berry in 1989, balloon dacryoplasty has been used to dilate the nasolacrimal duct in the setting of congenital obstructions.[20] It is typically implemented as a primary procedure in children over the age of 12 months and as a secondary measure following failed probing or silicone intubation. More recently, balloon canaliculoplasty has been used to treat cases of canalicular stenosis and obstruction.[21,22]

## ENDOSCOPIC SURGERY

The use of endoscopes is becoming increasingly popular among oculoplastic surgeons for both forehead rejuvenation surgery (brow lifting) and DCR. Endoscopes provide adequate visualization while minimizing the use of incisions. Rigid endoscopes are typically 4.5 mm in diameter, range 18–23 cm in length, and incorporate a 0–30° lens. Illumination is provided by a halogen or xenon light source. The endoscopy system is equipped with a coupling device that projects the images onto a video monitor.

### Endoscopic Brow Lifting

Endoscopy can provide safe and effective visualization during brow resuspension. The paramedian forehead and temporal hairline incisions are minimal, leading to quicker healing times and greater postoperative comfort compared with the conventional method.

Specialized instruments for brow lifting include angled endoscopic sheaths, which extend beyond the scope tip and allow for improved visualization during bimanual dissection. In addition, the surgeon should have straight and curved periosteal elevators available, as well as sharp and blunt-tipped elevators to break periosteal adhesions.

The brow can be resuspended using a variety of methods, including bone tunnel sutures, screw fixation, the Mitek 2.0-mm Quick anchor screw (Ethicon, Norwood, MA, USA), and the Endotine Forehead devices (Coapt Systems, Inc, Palo Alto, CA, USA).[23,24]

### Endoscopic DCR

Endoscopes can be used in DCR to visualize the paranasal sinuses, thereby obviating the need for an external incision. Reports have estimated success rates of endoscopic DCR around 90%, which is at least comparable with the rates associated with the external approach.[25]

Takahashi and Blakesley forceps, typically found in an ENT sinus tray, are used to grasp mucosa and bone fragments. A fiberoptic light pipe (20-gauge diameter) can be cannulated through the upper canaliculus to provide transillumination of the osteotomy site.[26,27]

## REFERENCES


1. Liboon J, Funkhouser W, Terris DJ. A comparison of mucosal incisions made by scalpel, $CO_2$ laser, electrocautery, and constant-voltage electrocautery. Otolaryngol Head Neck Surg: official journal of American Academy of Otolaryngology-Head and Neck Surgery. 1997;116(3):379-85. Epub 1997/03/01.
2. Sherman DD, Dortzbach RK. Monopolar electrocautery dissection in ophthalmic plastic surgery. Ophthal Plast Reconstr Surg. 1993;9(2):143-7. Epub 1993/06/01.
3. Solomon A, Espana EM, Tseng SC. Amniotic membrane transplantation for reconstruction of the conjunctival fornices. Ophthalmology. 2003;110(1):93-100. Epub 2003/01/04.
4. Cohen MS, Shorr N. Eyelid reconstruction with hard palate mucosa grafts. Ophthal Plast Reconstr Surg. 1992;8(3):183-95. Epub 1992/01/01.
5. Pushpoth S, Tambe K, Sandramouli S. The use of AlloDerm in the reconstruction of full-thickness eyelid defects. Orbit. 2008;27(5):337-40. Epub 2008/10/07.
6. Rubin PA, Fay AM, Remulla HD, et al. Ophthalmic plastic applications of acellular dermal allografts. Ophthalmology. 1999; 106(11):2091-7. Epub 1999/11/26.
7. Lee S, Maronian N, Most SP, et al. Porous high-density polyethylene for orbital reconstruction. Arch Otolaryngol Head Neck Surg. 2005;131(5):446-50. Epub 2005/05/18.
8. Romano JJ, Iliff NT, Manson PN. Use of Medpor porous polyethylene implants in 140 patients with facial fractures. J Craniofac Surg. 1993;4(3):142-7. Epub 1993/07/01.
9. Ellis E, 3rd, Messo E. Use of nonresorbable alloplastic implants for internal orbital reconstruction. J Oral Maxillofac Surg: official journal of the American Association of Oral and Maxillofacial Surgeons. 2004;62(7):873-81. Epub 2004/06/26.
10. Garibaldi DC, Iliff NT, Grant MP, et al. Use of porous polyethylene with embedded titanium in orbital reconstruction: a review of 106 patients. Ophthal Plast Reconst Surg. 2007;23(6):439-44. Epub 2007/11/22.
11. Moshfeghi DM, Moshfeghi AA, Finger PT. Enucleation. Surv Ophthalmol. 2000;44(4):277-301. Epub 2000/02/10.
12. Mazzoli RA, Raymond WR, 4th, Ainbinder DJ, et al. Use of self-expanding, hydrophilic osmotic expanders (hydrogel) in the reconstruction of congenital clinical anophthalmos. Current opinion in ophthalmology. 2004;15(5):426-31. Epub 2005/01/01.
13. Tse DT, Pinchuk L, Davis S, et al. Evaluation of an integrated orbital tissue expander in an anophthalmic feline model. Am J Ophthalmol. 2007;143(2):317-27. Epub 2006/12/16.
14. Gundlach KK, Guthoff RF, Hingst VH, et al. Expansion of the socket and orbit for congenital clinical anophthalmia. Plast Reconstr Surg. 2005;116(5):1214-22. Epub 2005/10/12.
15. Park S, Shin Y. Results of long-term follow-up observations of blepharoptosis correction using the palmaris longus tendon. Aesthetic Plast Surg. 2008;32(4):614-9. Epub 2008/05/01.
16. Leibovitch I, Leibovitch L, Dray JP. Long-term results of frontalis suspension using autogenous fascia lata for congenital ptosis in children under 3 years of age. Am J Ophthalmol. 2003;136(5):866-71. Epub 2003/11/05.
17. Esmaeli B, Chung H, Pashby RC. Long-term results of frontalis suspension using irradiated, banked fascia lata. Ophthal Plast Reconstr Surg. 1998;14(3):159-63. Epub 1998/06/05.
18. Foster JA, Holck DE, Perry JD, et al. Fibrin sealant for Muller muscle-conjunctiva resection ptosis repair. Ophthal Plast Reconstr Surg. 2006;22(3):184-7. Epub 2006/05/23.
19. Reifler DM. Management of canalicular laceration. Surv Ophthalmol. 1991;36(2):113-32. Epub 1991/09/01.
20. Becker BB, Berry FD. Balloon catheter dilatation in lacrimal surgery. Ophthal Surg. 1989;20(3):193-8. Epub 1989/03/01.
21. Zoumalan CI, Maher EA, Lelli GJ, Jr, et al. Balloon canaliculoplasty for acquired canalicular stenosis. Ophthal Plast Reconstr Surg. 2010;26(6):459-61. Epub 2010/09/28.
22. Yang SW, Park HY, Kikkawa DO. Ballooning canaliculoplasty after lacrimal trephination in monocanalicular and common canalicular obstruction. Jpn J Ophthalmol. 2008;52(6):444-9. Epub 2008/12/18.
23. Romo T, 3rd, Zoumalan RA, Rafii BY. Current concepts in the management of the aging forehead in facial plastic surgery. Curr Opin Otolaryngol Head Neck Surg. 2010;18(4):272-7. Epub 2010/06/15.
24. Chowdhury S, Malhotra R, Smith R, et al. Patient and surgeon experience with the endotine forehead device for brow and forehead lift. Ophthal Plast Reconstr Surg. 2007;23(5):358-62. Epub 2007/09/21.
25. Yung MW, Hardman-Lea S. Analysis of the results of surgical endoscopic dacryocystorhinostomy: effect of the level of obstruction. Br J Ophthalmol. 2002;86(7):792-4. Epub 2002/06/27.
26. Codere F, Denton P, Corona J. Endonasal dacryocystorhinostomy: a modified technique with preservation of the nasal and lacrimal mucosa. Ophthal Plast Reconstr Surg. 2010;26(3):161-4. Epub 2010/05/22.
27. Tsirbas A, Davis G, Wormald PJ. Mechanical endonasal dacryocystorhinostomy versus external dacryocystorhinostomy. Ophthal Plast Reconstr Surg. 2004;20(1):50-6. Epub 2004/01/31.

CHAPTER

# 52

# Upper and Lower Eyelid Entropion

Christoph Hintschich

## INTRODUCTION

The eyelids protect the eye and keep the ocular surface moist. Eyelid malpositions can cause ocular surface disease (OSD) and threaten sight. This is in particular true for any eyelid entropion, which probably is the most common eyelid malposition. This chapter deals with the different forms of upper and lower eyelid entropion and their adequate therapies.

## DEFINITION

Entropion is defined as an eyelid malposition, where the lid margin is inverted and directed toward the globe. The lid margin with or without lashes rubbing against the conjunctiva, and the cornea causes foreign body sensation, pain, and leads eventually to epithelial defects, ulceration, and finally to corneal scarring (Figs. 52-1A and B). Entropion should be distinguished from trichiasis and distichiasis, which present with similar symptoms, but usually need different therapy. If there is entropion of the lid margin, this must be treated first before the treatment of eyelash abnormality.

## CLASSIFICATION OF ENTROPION

Different types of entropion can be distinguished according to the underlying etiology:

- Congenital entropion
  - Entropion (lower eyelid)
  - Epiblepharon (lower eyelid)
  - Tarsal kink syndrome (upper eyelid)
- Acquired entropion
  - Involutional entropion (lower eyelid)
  - Cicatricial entropion (upper and lower eyelid)
  - Acute spastic entropion (lower eyelid).

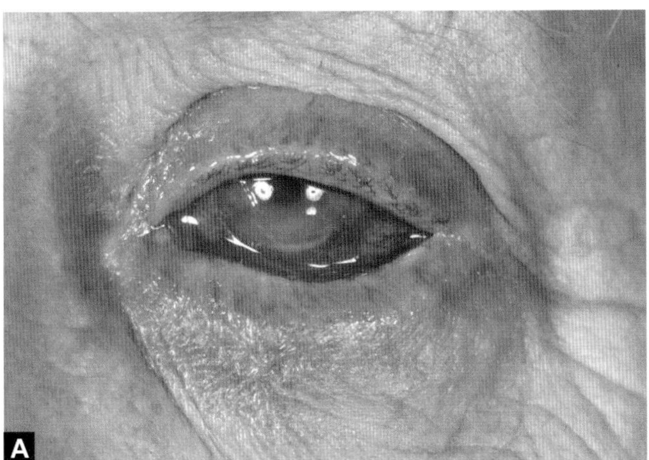


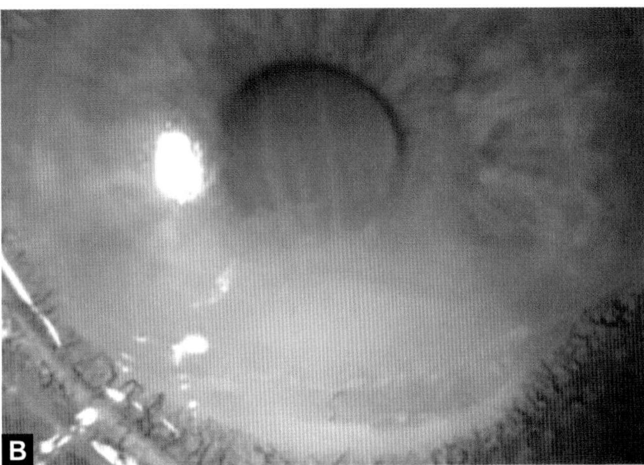


**Figures 52-1A and B** (A) Involutional lower eyelid entropion. (B) Ocular surface disease with corneal ulceration caused by involutional lower eyelid entropion (same patient).

## ANATOMICAL CONSIDERATIONS

Anatomically, in both upper and lower eyelids, an anterior lamella can be distinguished from a posterior lamella. The anterior lamella consists of skin and orbicularis muscle, the posterior lamella of the tarsal plate, and the conjunctiva covering its posterior surface. Both lamellae can be shifted against each other, as done in the "anterior lamellar repositioning"-procedure to evert the upper eyelid margin for the correction of minimal to moderate upper eyelid entropion.

Medially and laterally, the canthal tendons fixate the lids to the medial and lateral orbital walls. For any surgical procedure at the canthi, it is mandatory to follow the principle that the vector of the deep canthal fixation is orientated posteriorly into the orbit. Only this ensures a proper apposition of the eyelid margin toward the globe.

## INDICATIONS FOR SURGERY

Surgical correction of an eyelid entropion is indicated when the patient has discomfort and/or OSD developed. In addressing the patient with lid margin malposition, it is important to first decide whether the condition is disturbing the normal lid function and surgery is indicated without unnecessary delay to prevent further damage to the ocular surface or if it is mainly an esthetic problem for which surgery is elective.

## CLINICAL EXAMINATION

The choice of procedure depends on the clinical findings and anatomical changes in the eyelids; therefore, it is advisable to assess these conditions systematically:

First, exclude cicatricial changes in the posterior lamella by everting the eyelids.

What is the position of the lid margin in the primary position and on up- and downgaze? This defines the condition and the tightness of the lid retractors.

Then check for horizontal lid laxity by pulling the lower lid down with a thumb–allow it to return to the eye and watch the speed of return: if it "snaps back" there is minimal laxity; if it returns slowly there is mild laxity; if it returns completely but only after the patient blinks, there is moderate laxity; if it does not return completely even after a blink there is marked laxity (Figs. 52-2A to C).

Are the canthal tendons elongated? Check the medial and lateral canthal tendons by pulling the lids gently medially, then laterally. Laxity in the medial canthal tendon is present if the punctum moves more than about 3 mm laterally. Laxity of the canthal tendons needs correction at the canthi (Figs. 52-3A and B).

Is there overaction or malposition of the orbicularis muscle? Upward displacement of the orbicularis muscle is a typical sign of involutional "spastic" entropion.

Is the skin tight or loose? Shortage of skin needs a skin replacement, with significant redundancy careful resection can be performed.

Are there signs of OSD like conjunctival redness, corneal epithelial damage, or even ulceration?

## ANESTHESIA

The majority of surgical procedures can be performed under local anesthesia, using 2% Xylocaine (lidocaine, lignocaine) or 0.5% bupivacaine with 1:200.000 Adrenaline. Some surgeons add hyaluronidase to the solution to get a faster effect. Claustrophobic or psychologically instable patients usually prefer intravenous sedation or general anesthesia, the latter being mandatory for infants and children.

## LOWER EYELID ENTROPION

### Congenital Entropion

Congenital entropion is rare and should not be confused with epiblepharon. In congenital entropion, the eyelid in its whole horizontal extension is involved and the eyelashes are directed toward the eye (Fig. 52-4), but in epiblepharon they are orientated more vertically (Figs. 52-5A and B). Congenital entropion tends to persist and cause keratopathy, whereas epiblepharon often resolves spontaneously.

### Epiblepharon

Epiblepharon is characterized by an apparent over-riding of the pretarsal orbicularis muscle and skin over the eyelid margin, causing the eyelashes to assume a vertical position. It most commonly occurs in Asians and affects the medial part of the lower eyelids. Not every child presenting with an epiblepharon, even when the lashes come into contact with the cornea, needs immediate surgery. Often, this resolves spontaneously during the first years of life. If this fails to resolve or if corneal irritation occurs, surgery is indicated. Recurrent attacks of conjunctivitis and persistent photophobia in children are indicators for symptomatic OSD.

### Principles of Surgical Therapy

Surgical repair can be performed with the Hotz procedure[1] and consists of circumscribed anterior eyelid lamellar shortening and tarsal fixation. An elliptical strip of skin and underlying orbicularis muscle is excised below and lateral the inferior

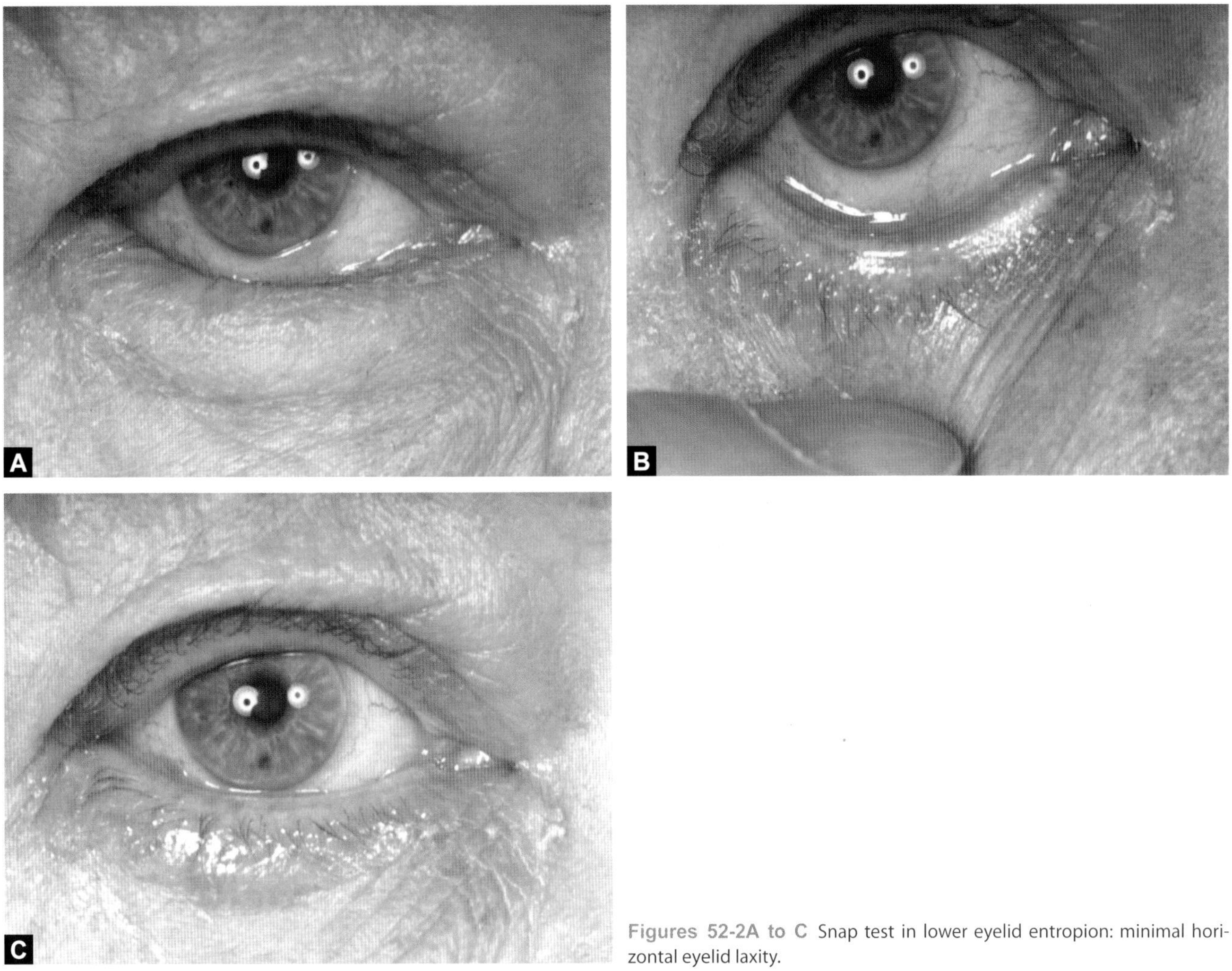

Figures 52-2A to C Snap test in lower eyelid entropion: minimal horizontal eyelid laxity.

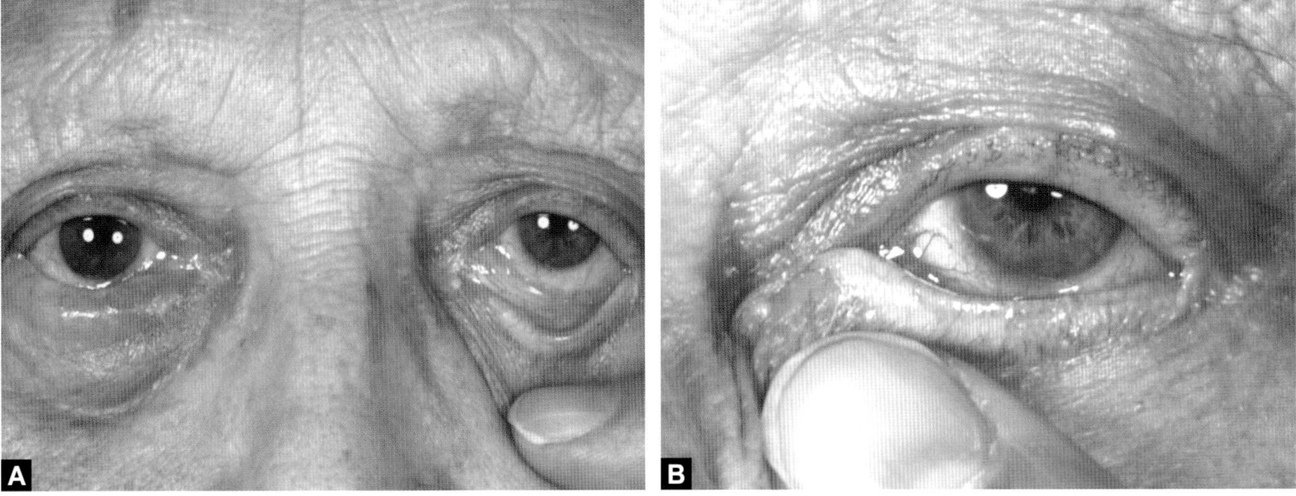

Figures 52-3A and B (A) Involutional lower eyelid entropion with marked horizontal eyelid laxity. (B) Involutional lower eyelid entropion with stable lateral canthal tendon.

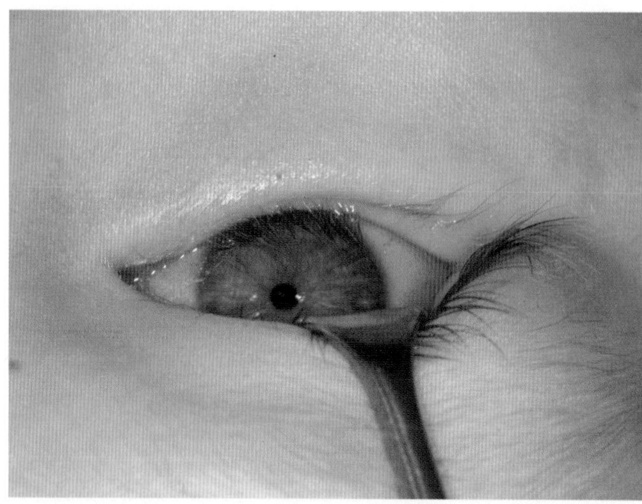

**Figure 52-4** Congenital entropion showing the whole lower eyelid margin directed toward the eye.

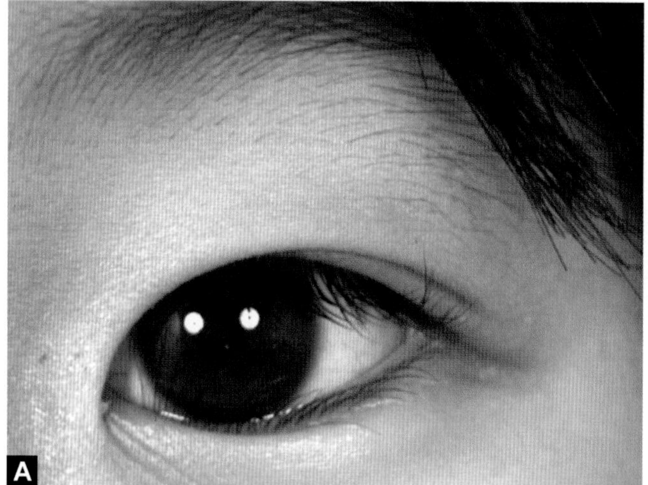

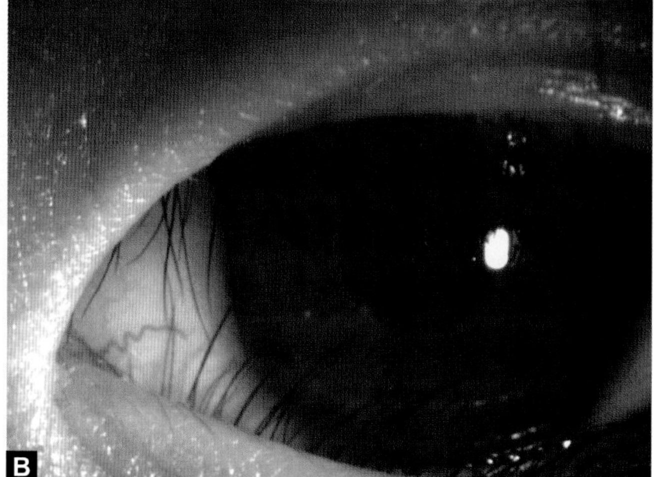

**Figures 52-5A and B** (A) Epiblepharon in an Asian girl. (B) Epiblepharon (same patient) causing already ocular surface disease. Adapted with permission from Collin.[13]

punctum. The skin edges are sutured to the lower border of the tarsal plate or the eyelid retractors with absorbable sutures to prevent the orbicularis from over-riding the lid margin (Figs. 52-6A to C). The cosmetic results are better, when the procedure is performed symmetrically on both sides. The vertical amount of skin excision should be moderate enough to prevent iatrogenic medial lower eyelid retraction causing ectropion and an eversion of the lacrimal punctum.

### *Hotz Procedure—Technique*

The skin below the everted lid margin and punctum in the nasal third of the eyelid is excised with underlying orbicularis muscle in an ellipsoid fashion (Figs. 52-7A to H). The amount of skin excised depends on the amount that can be picked up to just turn the lid margin into the correct position, usually not exceeding a few millimeters; if too much skin is taken, a secondary ectropium will result. Three to four single 6-0 absorbable sutures are passed through the skin, picking up the lower lid retractors just at the lower border of the tarsal plate and passed back through the skin. They can stay in place until they are spontaneously resorbed, but they may be removed after 10–14 days if necessary.

Real congenital entropion (*see* above) can be corrected with a lower eyelid retractor shortening (i.e. Jones procedure).

## Acquired Entropion

Acquired entropion can be either involutional or cicatricial. In addition, a form of acute spastic entropion can be defined in susceptible individuals with blepharospasm that has been induced by ocular irritation.

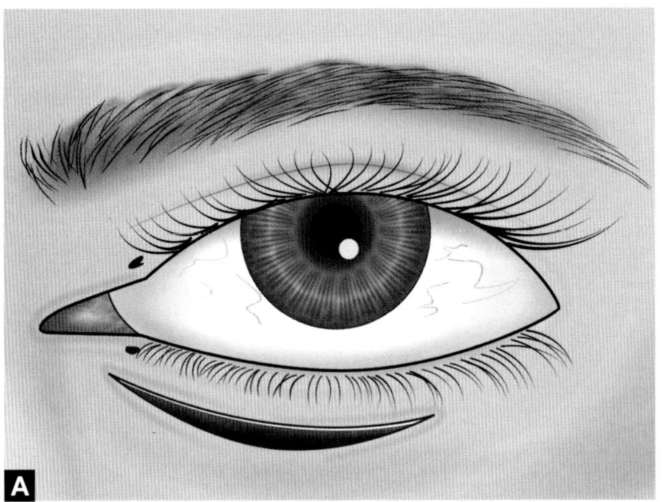

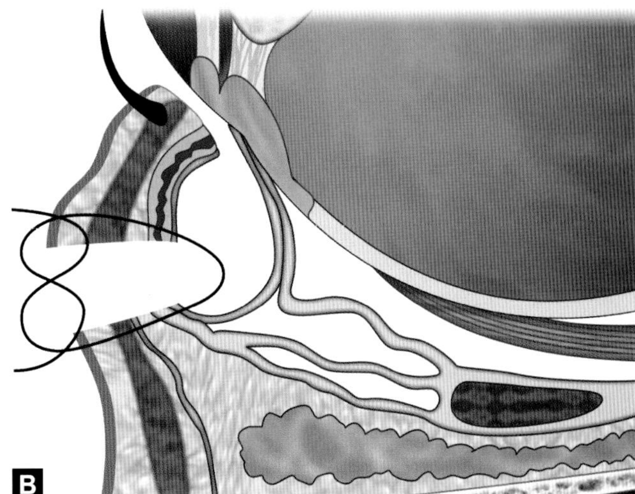

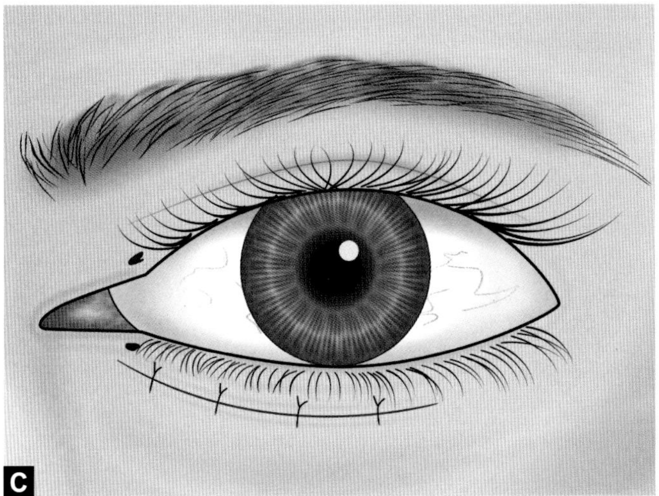

Figures 52-6A to C Surgical correction of epiblepharon (Hotz procedure), schematic.

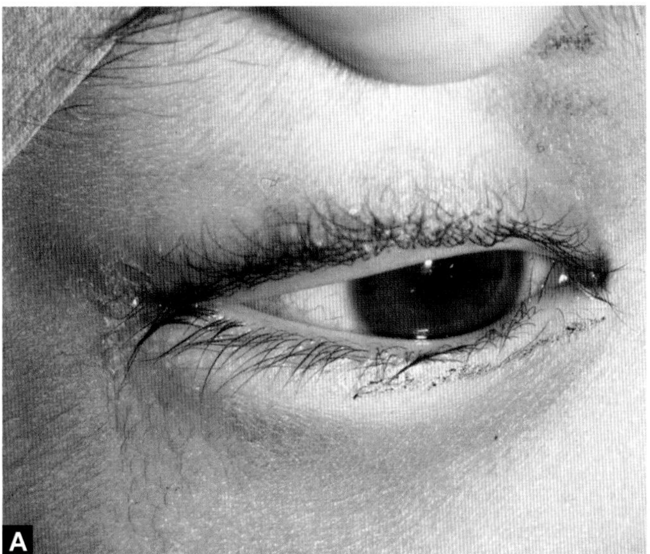

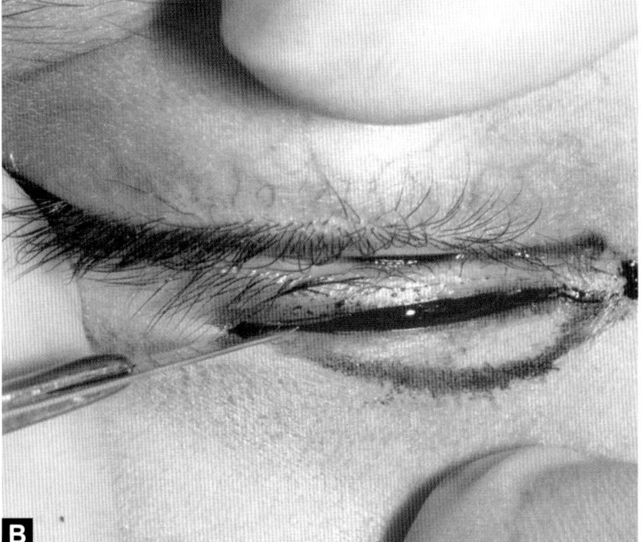

Figures 52-7A and B Hotz procedure, intraoperative steps. (A) Incision line, (B) skin incision.

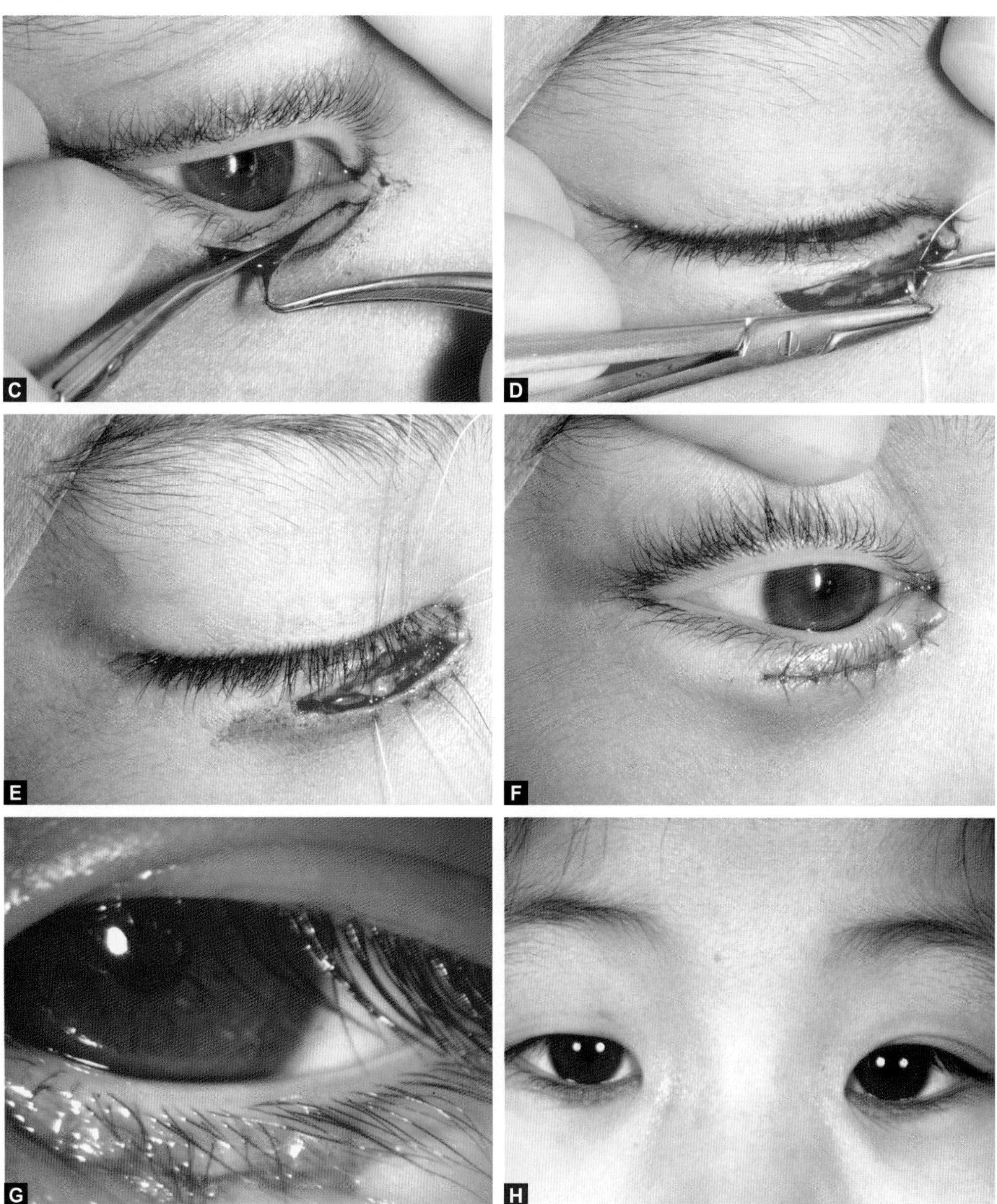


**Figures 52-7C to H** Hotz procedure, intraoperative steps. C) skin and orbicularis muscle excision, (D) first 6-0 Vicryl-suture skin-lower eyelid retractor skin, (E) four everting 6-0 Vicryl-sutures, (F) after wound closure, (G) 1 day postoperatively, (H) 6 weeks postoperatively.

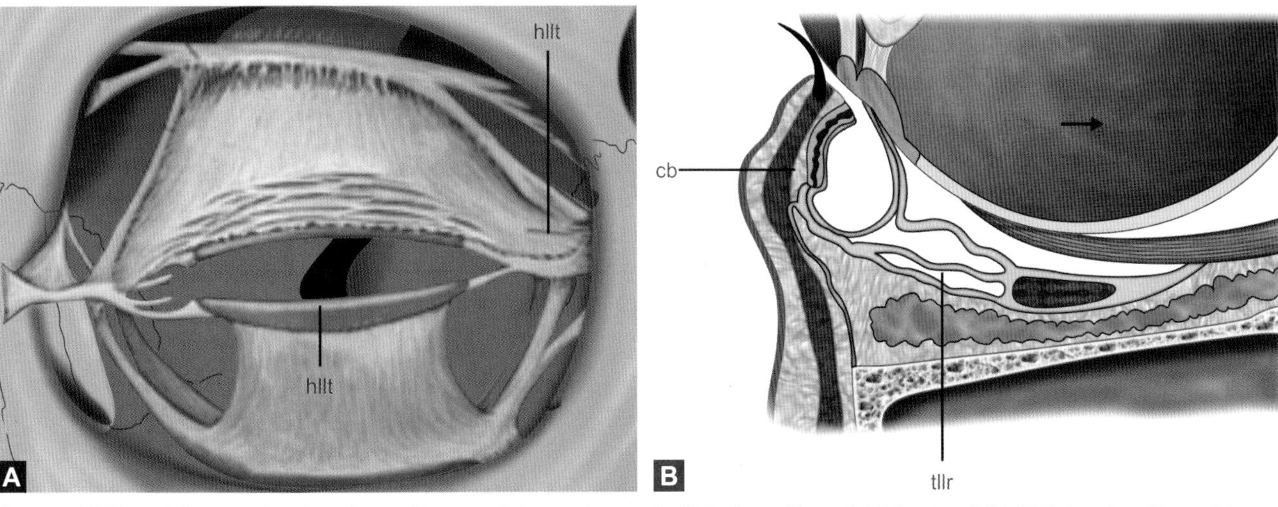


**Figures 52-8A and B** Principles of involutional lower eyelid entropion repair. (A) Horizontal lower lid tightening (hllt). (B) Tightening of lower lid retractors (tllr) and cicatricial barrier (between pretars. u. presept. orbicularis m.) (cb).

## Involutional Entropion

Involutional entropion is the most common form of all entropia, and it is probably the most common eyelid malformation. Since involutional changes of the eyelid anatomy are responsible for this kind of entropion, the incidence is increasing in elderly patients. A combination of factors has been advocated to account for this kind of eyelid malposition.[2,3] This includes the following features:

- Horizontal eyelid laxity (desinsertion of lateral and medial canthus and/or tarsal plate laxity)
- Laxity and/or desinsertion of lower lid retractor complex
- Over-riding of the preseptal orbicularis muscle over the pretarsal orbicularis.

Enophthalmos due to orbital fat atrophy might aggravate the pathogenesis of involutional lower eyelid entropion, but it is no longer considered a significant factor in its etiology.

Any surgical treatment should address these factors.

## Therapy

The use of tape or therapeutic contact lenses temporarily can help reduce bulbar irritation. Eventually, surgical intervention is the only effective way to correct this eyelid malposition.

To achieve a long-lasting effect, all pathogenic features should be addressed. This includes horizontal lid laxity, vertical lid laxity, and eyelid lamella dissociation (Figs. 52-8A and B). In the following a small number of procedures are described, which will allow one to correct the majority of involutional entropia.

## Procedures Addressing Lower Eyelid Horizontal Laxity

### *Horizontal Lid Shortening and Skin Excision (Kuhnt–Szymanowski)*

If horizontal lower lid laxity and an abundance of skin is present while the medial and lateral canthal tendons are firm, the lid can be tightened by a pentagonal posterior lamellar excision and the skin excess reduced via a subciliary incision.

*Technique:* A skin incision is made just below the lash line. The incision is extended over the lateral canthal region in the lateral skin crease. A skin–muscle flap is raised laterally and superiorly. A full thickness pentagonal excision of the lid is performed in the lateral third of the lid margin with straight scissors or a #11 blade. The wound is closed with two or three intertarsal 6-0 Vicryl sutures and two eyelid margin sutures (6-0 silk), placed to adjust and slightly evert the gray line. The sutures are left long and buried later under the 6-0 silk skin sutures. While the patient opening his mouth and looking upward, the amount of skin–muscle tissue that can be resected without risking an overcorrection is marked and resected. The skin is then closed with cutaneous running 6-0 silk sutures

### *Lateral Tarsal Strip Procedure (Lateral Canthal Sling)*

This procedure is an excellent and very versatile way to correct any horizontal lower lid laxity. It is the author's first choice and can be used for entropion and also ectropion repair.[4] It might be combined with everting procedures, depending on

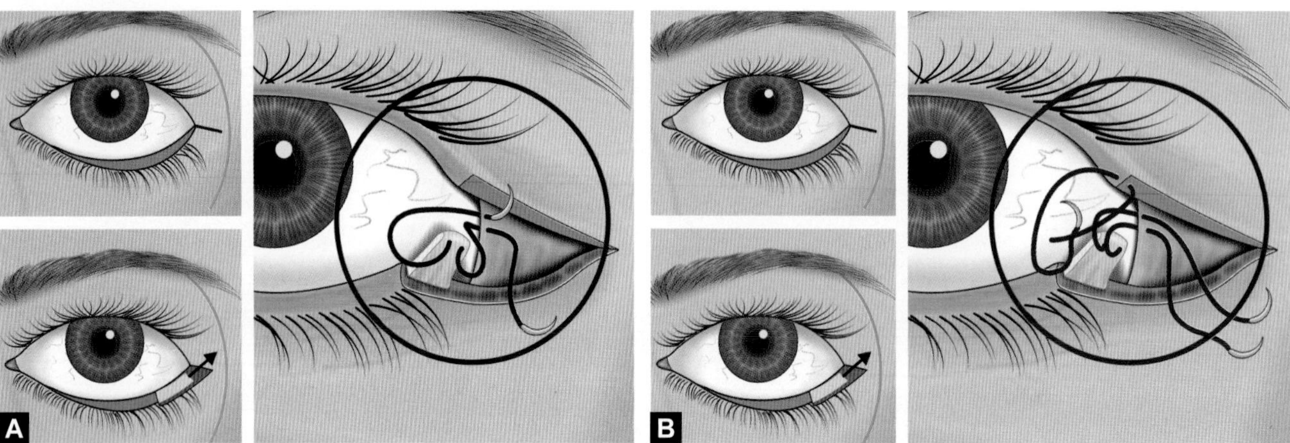


**Figures 52-9A and B** (A) Lateral canthal sling procedure (attachment of the lateral part of the tarsal plate to the periorbit at the anterior bony orbital wall (behind the orbital rim). (B) Restoration of the lateral canthus with hidden 6-0 Vicryl suture.

the underlying pathology. If there is significant medial canthal laxity and the procedure would cause an unacceptable lateral displacement of the punctum, a lateral tarsal strip procedure should not be used (or only in combination with a medial tendon reinforcement).

*Principles of surgical therapy:* The principle of this procedure is based on a (re)attachment of the lateral part of the tarsal plate to the periorbit at the anterior bony orbital wall (behind the orbital rim). To attain a good result it is mandatory to free the lateral end of the tarsal plate from any epithelial tissues and to suture it as posterior as feasible inside the orbital rim. This is necessary to firstly avoid the complication of inclusion cysts and secondly to reach the best alignment of the lid margin to the globe (Figs. 52-9A and B).

*Technique:* The lateral canthal area and the zygomatic bone are approached by a 10-mm horizontal skin incision starting at the lateral canthus. The lower limb of the lateral canthal tendon is cut. The lateral part of the lower lid tarsal plate is completely denuded by removing the lid margin with all lash roots, the orbicularis muscle, and the conjunctiva. In cases of a stretched tarsal plate causing marked laxity, a few millimeters of tarsus can be resected. If the tarsal plate is too short to be attached to the periorbit, a periosteal flap can be formed. Such a flap can easily be dissected by incising the periosteum in a door-shaped manner at the outer surface of the zygomatic bone, leaving the junction to the inner part of the arch intact. The lateral tarsal strip is sutured with a double-armed 5-0 suture to either the periorbital tissue behind the orbital rim or the periosteal flap. The lateral canthus is restored with a hidden simple suture and the skin is closed. Usually, monofile nonabsorbable sutures, like 6-0 Prolene, are used; the author prefers long-acting absorbable sutures, as 5-0 Vicryl.

## Procedures Addressing Lower Eyelid Retractors (Tightening and/or Shortening)

### *Transverse/Everting Sutures*

This simple, quick, and everywhere (e.g. at the bedside) applicable procedure can correct involutional entropion in the absence of significant lower lid laxity. Temporary cure for up to 6 months can be expected, making it particularly helpful in geriatric patients.[5]

Transverse sutures prevent the preseptal orbicularis muscle from over-riding the pretarsal part and are placed horizontally through the lid just below the tarsal plate.[6] Everting sutures are placed more obliquely through the lid to tighten the lower lid retractors and transfer their pull to the lid margin.[7]

*Technique:* For transverse sutures 3 double-armed 5-0 Vicryl sutures are passed through the lid from the conjunctiva to the skin in the lateral two thirds of the lid, starting from just below the tarsal plate with transverse sutures and emerging through the skin just above that level in a distance of about 2 mm from each other (Figs. 52-10A to D). Everting sutures run more obliquely and start lower in the fornix and emerge nearer to the lashes. The sutures are tied tightly and can be removed, if an overcorrection is present. Usually, they are left for spontaneous resorption.

### *Wies Procedure*

The Wies procedure consists of a transverse lid split combined with everting sutures.[8] By performing a horizontal full-thickness lid split a fibrous tissue scar is induced, which permanently prevents an over-riding of the preseptal orbicularis muscle. This is combined with everting sutures to tighten the

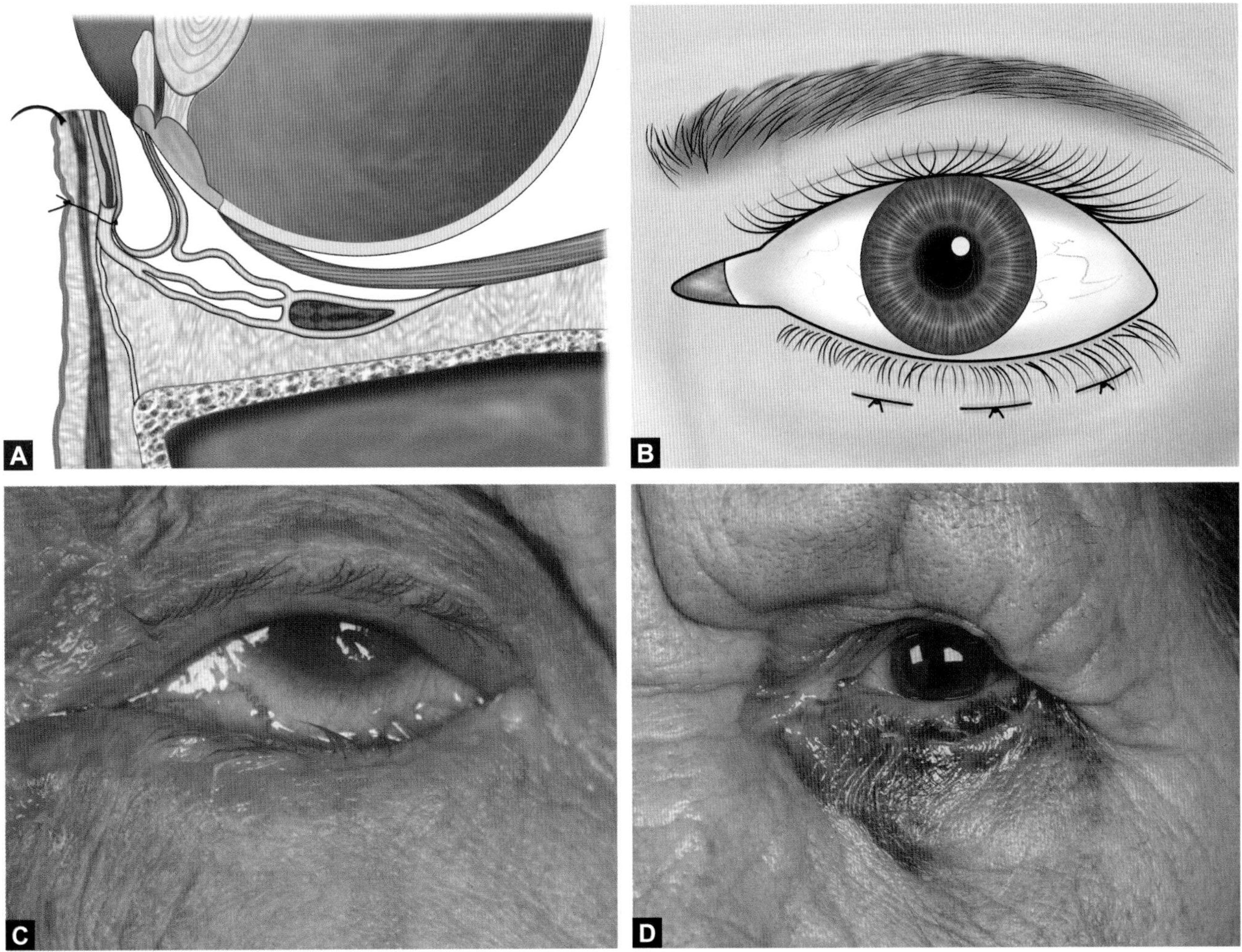


**Figures 52-10A to D** Lower lid retractor tightening with transversal/everting sutures (A and B) principle. Adapted from Collin.[13] (C and D) pre-/post-operatively.

lower eyelid retractors and increase their pull to the lid margin. This procedure gives good long-term results, if no horizontal lid laxity is present.

*Technique:* The technique consists of a horizontal full-thickness transsection of the whole of the lower eyelid about 4–5 mm below the lash line. The cut should be as horizontal as possible, medially not as far as the punctum. Three double-armed 5-0 Vicryl sutures pick up the conjunctiva (and with it the underlying lower lid retractors) below the transsection and passed through the pretarsal orbicularis muscle to the skin. The needles should start 1–2 mm from the conjunctival cut and emerge through the skin 1–2 mm below the lash line and about 2 mm apart. Before tying the everting sutures, the horizontal skin incision can be closed with a running 6-0 silk suture. Skin sutures are removed after 1 week. The everting sutures usually are left for spontaneous resorption, unless there is marked overcorrection, which in most cases is due to pre-existing horizontal laxity.

### Jones Procedure

In lower eyelid entropion recurrences with absent horizontal laxity, and in cases, where surgical trauma to the conjunctiva should be avoided, the lower lid retractors plication through an anterior skin approach is indicated. This is in particularly helpful in lower eyelid cicatricial entropion due to ocular pemphigoid, when any surgical trauma to the conjunctiva should be avoided to prevent an exacerbation of the disease.

With the Jones procedure the lower eyelid retractors are exposed via a skin approach, shortened, and the sutures used to create a barrier to prevent the preseptal orbicularis from

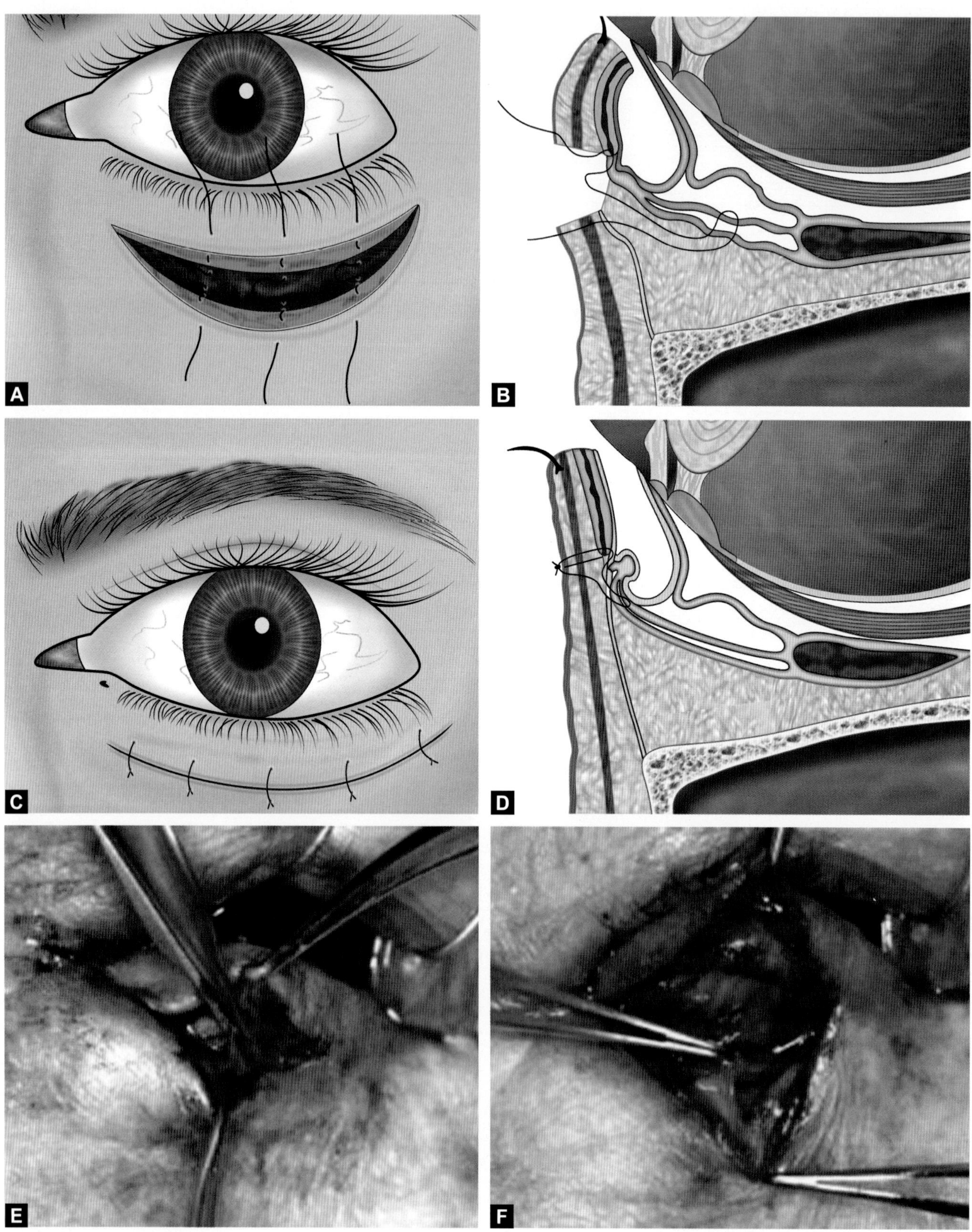


Figures 52-11A to F (A to D) Lower eyelid retractor tightening (principle). (E) opening of the septum. (F) exposing lower eyelid retractors.

over-riding the pretarsal part[9] (Figs. 52-11A to C). In the presence of additional lower eyelid laxity, particularly in the lateral canthal tendon, this procedure can be combined with a lateral tarsal strip procedure to tighten and shorten the lower eyelid.

The Jones procedure needs more dissection in the lower lid and somehow better knowledge of the anatomy.

## Procedures Addressing Over-Riding of the Preseptal Orbicularis Muscle

This principle applies for all procedures inducing a scar formation between the pretarsal and the preseptal orbicularis muscle, as in the Wies procedure or the Jones procedure. This is even one aspect of the transverse sutures.

## Procedures Combining Different Principles

### *Quickert Procedure*

In most cases of involutional entropion, horizontal lid laxity is present. In these cases, an additional horizontal eyelid shortening is indicated (nowadays horizontal tightening usually is achieved with a lateral canthal sling). Alternatively, a Quickert procedure,[10] which is a Wies procedure combined with a horizontal full-thickness eyelid resection, can be performed. The horizontal full-thickness lid split induces a fibrous tissue barrier to prevent the preseptal orbicularis muscle from overriding, the everting sutures tighten the lower eyelid retractors and increase their pull to the lid margin, and the horizontal lid shortening corrects lower lid laxity and stabilizes the lid.

*Technique:* A horizontal skin incision is made 4–5 mm from the lash line in the whole of the lower lid. Then a vertical full-thickness eyelid incision is performed 5 mm apart from the lateral canthus, down to the horizontal skin incision. Directed medially and laterally of the vertical incision, a horizontal full-thickness transsection along the skin incision–as in a Wies procedure–is done. Finally a full-thickness resection of excess lid margin/tarsal plate is performed. The amount of excess tissue is estimated by overlapping the medial and the lateral end of the lid margin under slight tension. Three double-armed 5-0 Vicryl sutures are positioned in the lower conjunctival wound edge (as in the Wies procedure) before readapting the two ends of the lid margin with tarsal (6-0 Vicryl) and lid margin (6-0 silk) sutures. Surgery is continued and finished as in the Wies procedure. All silk sutures are removed after 1 week, the everting sutures left for spontaneous resorption.

The results after a Quickert procedure usually are good, the recurrence rate is as low as 3.7%.[3]

### *Lateral Tarsal Strip Procedure and Transverse/Everting Sutures*

The lateral tarsal strip procedure [*see* section Lateral Tarsal Strip Procedure (Lateral Canthal Sling)] can easily be combined with transvers/everting sutures (*see* section Transverse/Everting Sutures). This is a simple and very efficient way to correct even marked and long-existing involutional entropion.

### *Lateral Tarsal Strip Procedure and Jones Procedure*

This combination is an excellent and highly efficient procedure to correct difficult conditions, like recurrences with residual lower eyelid laxity.

## Cicatricial Entropion

Cicatricial entropion is due to a shortage of the posterior lid lamella following tissue contraction. Severe posterior lamellar cicatrization often leads to additional eyelid retraction. Causes for cicatricial entropion include mechanical and chemical trauma, burns, trachoma infection (particularly in the upper eyelid), and cicatrizing conjunctivitis like topical glaucoma medication, herpes infection, Stevens–Johnson syndrome and ocular cicatricial pemphigoid. It occurs both in upper and lower eyelids. Before surgical therapy, any possibly ongoing cicatrizing disease, like ocular pemphigoid, should be ruled out, or if present, treated accordingly.

## Surgical Therapy

The choice of surgical procedures to correct lower eyelid cicatricial entropion is dictated by the severity of the entropion, the degree of retraction, and the underlying cause. In ocular cicatricial pemphigoid, surgery should be confined to the anterior lamella whenever possible to avoid exacerbating the conjunctival disease. A retractor tightening procedure like the Jones procedure (*see* above) would be the method of choice (Table 52-1).

## Z-Plasty/Mucous Membrane Grafts

Circumscribed conjunctival scars can be excised and corrected with a Z-plasty. Moderate degrees of cicatricial entropion with a minor degree of lid retraction can be managed with a "tarsal fracture" procedure. A horizontal incision is made through the whole length of the tarsus just below its center down

**TABLE 52-1** Compendium of surgical procedures to correct involutional lower eyelid entropion.

| Procedure | Indication |
|---|---|
| Transverse/ everting sutures | Involutional entropion without horizontal laxity |
| Wies | Involutional entropion without horizontal laxity |
| Quickert | Involutional entropion with horizontal laxity |
| Lateral tarsal strip + everting sutures | Involutional entropion with horizontal laxity |
| Jones | • Involutional entropion without horizontal laxity<br>• Recurrence without horizontal laxity<br>• Mild to moderate cicatricial entropion with pemphigoid |
| Jones + lateral tarsal strip | Recurrence with horizontal laxity |

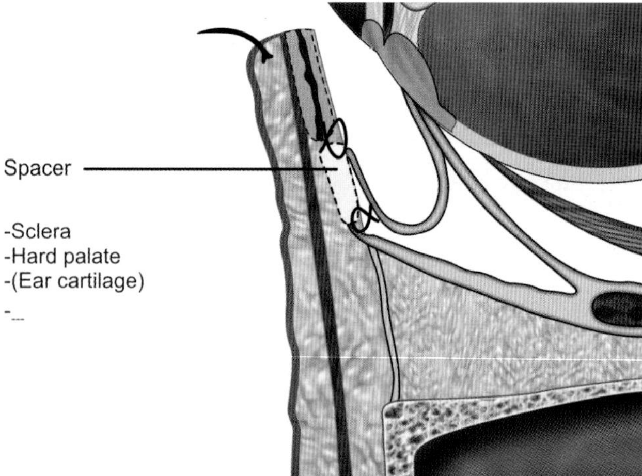


**Figure 52-12** Correction of lower eyelid cicatricial entropion with spacer.

to the orbicularis muscle. Three double-armed 5-0 Vicryl sutures are passed from the lower fragment just below the incision and out through the skin immediately below the lash line. The sutures are tied to produce a mild overcorrection and removed after 2 weeks.

In severe cicatricial lower lid entropion with more severe degree of lid retraction, a posterior lamellar graft is indicated. The tarsoconjunctiva is lengthened with a graft, which is inserted near the lid margin to allow eversion. A piece of full-thickness buccal mucosa, tarsal plate, hard palate, or donor sclera is sutured with running 6-0 Vicryl sutures between the superior and inferior fragment of the horizontally divided lower tarsal plate (Fig. 52-12). The lid margin is hold everted and the graft against its bed with everting sutures passed through the graft and tied on the skin just below the lashes.

**TABLE 52-2** Causes of upper eyelid cicatricial entropion.

| |
|---|
| Trachoma |
| Chronic blepharoconjunctivitis |
| Erythema multiforme |
| Chemical/thermic burn |
| Postoperative (s/p reconstructive surgery) |
| Pemphigoid |
| Stevens–Johnson/Lyell syndrome |
| Postenucleation socket syndrome |
| Herpes infection |
| Idiopathic/unknown |

### Acute Spastic Entropion

Topical therapy of the underlying cause of ocular irritation may reverse the eyelid malposition. If this is not the case, a permanent entropion with usually involutional components may ensue, which will require surgical intervention according to the rules given before.

## UPPER EYELID ENTROPION

Upper eyelid entropion is an eyelid malposition in which the upper eyelid margin is turned inward against the globe. It can be responsible for severe OSD and ocular morbidity. It is relatively uncommon in the Northern Hemisphere in contrast to a number of countries in more arid areas of the world, where trachoma is endemic.

The condition can be congenital, which is rather rare, but is mainly caused by cicatricial changes of the posterior upper eyelid lamella. Any trauma, either mechanical or chemical, and infection to the conjunctiva can cause an upper eyelid entropion. Worldwide, trachoma (Figs. 52-13A and B) is the most common cause of this upper eyelid malposition. More causes are listed in Table 52-2. In addition to careful history, a complete ocular examination with eversion of the posterior lamella and the superior fornix is essential to determine the etiology. It is important to establish the diagnosis of upper eyelid entropion and differentiate this from simple trichiasis—this helps avoid unnecessary and often useless epilation procedures of the upper eyelid lashes.

Upper eyelid trachoma may be further classified according to its severity as mild, moderate, or severe. This is essential in regard of choosing the most appropriate surgical procedure.

### Principles of Surgical Therapy

The concept of surgical therapy is to evert the lid margin to prevent it from rubbing against the ocular surface. In cases,

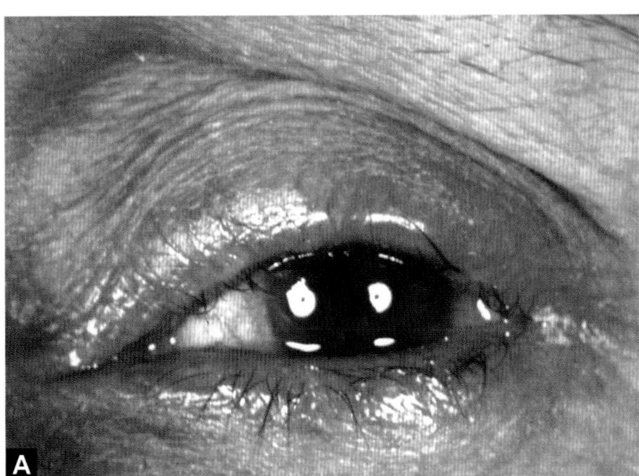


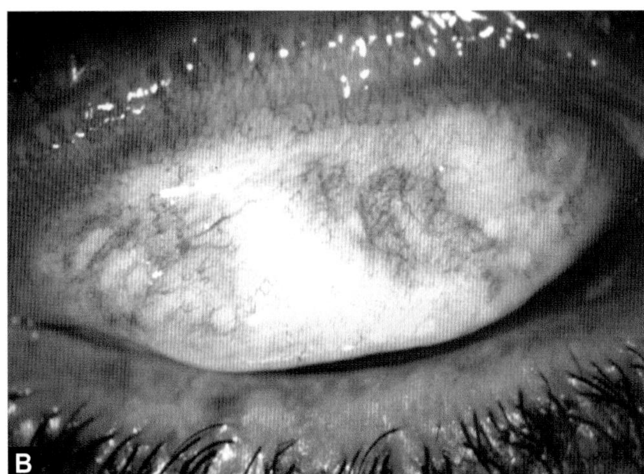


**Figures 52-13A and B** (A) Upper eyelid cicatricial entropion due to trachoma, (B) everted upper eyelid with scarred tarsal plate.

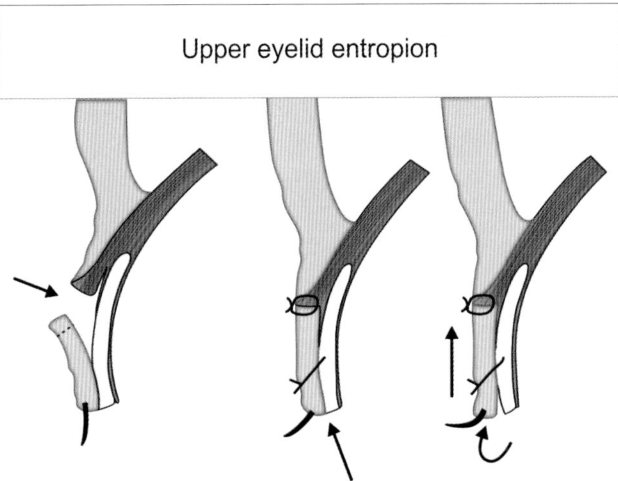


**Figure 52-14** Anterior lamellar repositioning with lid split (principle).

where significant keratinization and scar formation at the eyelid margin or tarsal plate is present, this must be resected and replaced by mucous membrane grafts.

## Anterior Lamellar Repositioning

This procedure is indicated in mild to moderate forms of upper eyelid entropion. It is easy to perform, safe, and corrects the majority of upper lid entropia in the Northern Hemisphere.[11] The surgery is based on dividing the anterior from the posterior lamella of the upper eyelid, reposition the anterior lamella superiorly and suture it to the tarsal plate at a higher level. This is often combined with a lid split at the gray line of the lid margin, which enhances the everting effect to the lid margin. This procedure requires a stable upper tarsal plate.

### *Technique*

The superior tarsal plate is completely freed from the overlying orbicularis muscle down to the roots of the lashes through a skin crease incision. The lid margin is split in its entire length at the gray line, just anteriorly to the orifices of the meibomian glands, to a depth of 1–2 mm. Five to six 6-0 double-armed Vicryl sutures are anchored in the upper third of the tarsal plate and then passed out through orbicularis and skin, just above the lash line (Fig. 52-14). By closing these sutures, the anterior lamella is lifted and the lash-bearing part of the lid margin is everted. The split is allowed to granulate, the sutures left for spontaneous resorption.

### *Other Procedures*

In more severe forms of upper eyelid entropion, a tarsal wedge resection or a rotation of the terminal tarsus can be performed.[12,13] In cases of post-traumatic upper eyelid entropion, particularly after severe burns, the tarsal plate tends to be thin and unstable. This situation often is combined with upper lid retraction, conjunctival scarring, and an upper fornix shortening. Under such condition none of the aforementioned techniques are applicable. A posterior lamellar graft is then indicated to stabilize and lengthen the upper eyelid. An autologous graft is put between the upper eyelid margin or the remnant of the tarsal plate and the recessed upper lid retractors (Fig. 52-15). A graft from the hard palate is favorable, because it combines some stiffness with mucous membrane lining and is ideal for this kind of upper eyelid correction. Sutures and knots always should be covered by tissue to avoid corneal damage. Any aberrant or misdirected lashes and lid margin malpositions can be corrected at the same time, if necessary, by a full-thickness wedge excision.

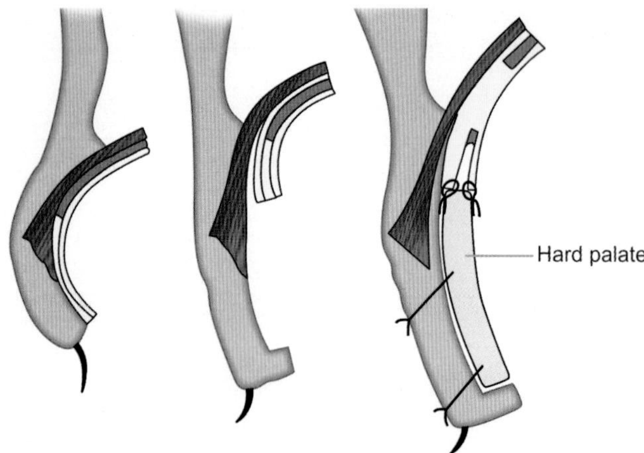


**Figure 52-15** Upper eyelid entropion correction with hard palate grafting and anterior lamellar repositioning.

## Tarsal Wedge Resection

If the tarsal plate is thick, the effect of everting an upper lid entropium by everting sutures and a marginal lid split will be better stabilized by excising a wedge from the anterior portion of the tarsal plate.

### *Technique*

A horizontal incision is made in the upper lid crease and the tarsal plate exposed by blunt dissection. The lash roots should not be exposed. Two incisions at a 90° angle to each other are made along the tarsal surface, in the area of maximal thickening, and the resulting wedge of tarsus is removed. It will be necessary in most cases to incise the insertion of Muller's muscle fibers at the upper border of the tarsal plate to advance the posterior lamella of the lid sufficiently. Three to four double armed 6-0 silk sutures are passed through the inferior part of the tarsus, onto the superior part, and then out through the skin above the lash roots. A marginal split is done like in an anterior lamella repositioning procedure. The knots are tied and the lid will evert when the wound edges of the tarsal wedge resection are brought together (the marginal split will open and the anterior lamella will be repositioned). Any excess lid skin can now be removed and the wound closed with interrupted sutures or a running suture. Skin sutures are removed after 1 week. Everting sutures should be left longer, i.e. 3–4 weeks. Long-acting absorbable sutures can be left until they disintegrate spontaneously.

## Posterior Lamella Advancement

Severe upper lid entropium with a thin tarsus is not suitable for a tarsal wedge resection. If the tarsoconjunctiva is intact and there is no or only minimal keratinization of the lid margin, the posterior lamella can be advanced by a lid split and the resulting anterior tarsal wound can be covered by a mucous membrane graft.

### *Technique*

The lid is split with a knife into an anterior lamella and posterior lamella. The cut is made anterior to the glands of Meibom and the posterior lamella is freed upward the fornix; Mueller's muscle will have to be horizontally dissected to allow vertical stretching of the posterior lamella. It can then be advanced until the lids close easily. To hold the posterior lamella advanced in relation to the anterior lamella, several double-armed 5-0 long-acting absorbable sutures are placed at the upper border of the tarsal plate and passed through the skin crease. The sutures should be passed through the skin somewhat lower than the upper tarsal border to hold the lashes everted. The lower border of the anterior lamella is fixed to the tarsus with interrupted 6-0 absorbable sutures. A strip of full-thickness mucous membrane graft is fixated with a 6-0 or 7-0 absorbable running suture. The sutures can be removed after 10–14 days.

It is important to correct cicatricial upper eyelid entropion before starting with any visual rehabilitative procedures, such as keratoplasty. Otherwise, the continuing mechanical stress to the ocular surface caused by the lid malposition will jeopardize the result of any of these procedures. In consequence, one might be forced to perform lid surgery earlier than 6 months after a trauma to prevent ongoing damage to the ocular surface, although this can be associated with a higher failure rate of the surgery. Usually, one waits for at least 6–9 months until healing and scarring is completed before corrective and reconstructive procedures are performed.

## Tarsal Kink Syndrome

Tarsal kink is a rare condition in which the upper eyelid tarsus is completely folded horizontally and the lid margin is inverted.[14] As a result, the lashes are not visible and severe corneal ulceration occurs. Newborns present with severe blepharospasm, lacrimation, photophobia, and seemingly absent lashes. Immediate correction is mandatory to prevent loss of visual development.[15] To obtain a normal tarsal plate, the kink in the tarsal plate has to be completely corrected. This can be done by a simple repositioning of the anterior lamella if the kink is not complete or the patient presents too late. In the latter case, marked entropion will be manifest, with an inward fold just above the lid margin and the remaining tarsal plate will be thickened and inflamed. If the patient is seen early, the tarsal plate can be reconstructed by a transconjunctival or transcutaneous approach.

### Horizontal Tarsal Reconstruction

The tarsal plate is exposed via an incision in the lid crease. The kink in the tarsal plate is identified and the tarsus cut exactly along this "fold". The resulting two parts of the tarsal plate can now be repositioned and sutured with a 6-0 absorbable suture. If the lid margin is still inverted, everting sutures can be placed. If the lid margin is correctly repositioned after adjustment of the tarsal plate, it can be secured by placing three 6-0 silk sutures transcutaneously through the lower and upper part, pass them through the skin at a superior level and tie them over a bolster.

The skin can be closed by an absorbable suture that is left to dissolve or can be removed after a week.

## PEARLS AND PITFALLS

- *In epiblepharon*: Only perform surgery, when complaints due to OSD are present.
- *In acquired entropion*: First rule out cicatricial causes.
- *If horizontal eyelid laxity is present*: Always tighten lid horizontally, because if horizontal eyelid laxity is present, lower eyelid retractor tightening causes iatrogenic ectropion formation.
- *For lateral tarsal strip-procedure*: The vector of the deep canthal fixation is orientated posteriorly into the orbit.
- *Irritated eye in a newborn and upper eyelid with apparently no lashes*: Think of a "tarsal kink syndrome".

## REFERENCES


1. Hotz F. Eine neue Operation für Entropium und Trichiasis. Arch f Augenheilkunde. 1879;9:68.
2. Jones L. The anatomy of the lower eyelid and its relation to the cause and cure of entropion. Am J Ophthalmol. 1960;49:29-36.
3. Collin JRO, Rathburn JE. Involutional entropion. A review with evaluation of a procedure. Arch Ophthalmol. 1978;96:1058-64.
4. Anderson R, Gordy D. The tarsal strip procedure. Arch Ophthalmol. 1979;97:2192-6.
5. Wright M, Bell D, Scott C, et al. Everting suture correction of lower lid involutional entropion. Br J Opthtalmol. 1999;83:1060-63.
6. Schöpfer O. Über einen einfachen Eingriff zur Behandlung des Entropiums. Klin Monatsbl Augenheilk. 1949;115:40-2.
7. Feldstein M. A method of surgical correction of entropion in aged persons. Eye Ear Nose Throat Mon. 1960;39:730.
8. Wies F. Surgical treatment of entropion. J Int Surg. 1954;21:758-60.
9. Jones L, Reeh M, Wobig J. Senile entropion: a new concept for correction. Am J Ophthalmol. 1972;74:327-9.
10. Quickert M, Rathburn E. Suture repair of entropion. Arch Ophthalmol. 1971;85:304-5.
11. Hintschich CR. "Reposition der vorderen Lidlamelle" zur Korrektur des Oberlidentropiums. Ophthalmologe. 1997;94:436-40.
12. Trabut G. Entropion-Trichiasis en Afrique du Nord. Arch d´ Ophthalmol. 1949;9:701.
13. Collin JRO. A manual of systematic eyelid surgery. Edinburgh: Churchill Livingstone; 1989:7-108.
14. Briglan A. Buerger GJ. Congenital horizontal tarsal kink. Am J Ophthalmol. 1980;89:522-4.
15. Sires B. Congenital horizontal tarsal kink: clinical characteristics from a large series. Ophth Plast Reconstr Surg. 1999;15:355-9.

CHAPTER 53

# Surgical Techniques for Upper and Lower Eyelid Ectropion

Steven M Couch, Philip L Custer

## INTRODUCTION

Eyelid ectropion is present when the eyelid margin is rotated outward, no longer being apposed to the globe. Ectropion most commonly affects the lower eyelid but rarely occur in the upper eyelid. It is important to differentiate ectropion from other malpositions, including eyelid retraction and entropion. Eyelid retraction refers to inferior displacement of the margin, but unlike ectropion, the margin remains apposed to the ocular surface. Typically, the square-shaped eyelid margin rests against the ocular surface within 1 mm of inferior corneal limbus. Eyelid entropion refers to internal rotation of margin such that the eyelashes are directed toward the globe.

Clinically, it is important to distinguish between the common etiologies of ectropion, including involutional, cicatricial, paralytic, mechanical, and rarely congenital. Multiple causes may be present in selected patients. Anatomic conditions contributing to the development of ectropion include horizontal eyelid laxity, lower eyelid retractor dehiscence, anterior lamellar shortening, orbicularis weakness, and mechanical distraction. Surgical decision making is based on the identification and repair of the underlying etiology.

## INDICATIONS

- Corneal exposure (dry eye, superficial keratitis)
- Conjunctival keratinization (redness, discharge, occasionally bleeding)
- Tearing
- Aesthetic concerns.

## CONTRAINDICATIONS

- Rarely systemic comorbidities may preclude surgery.

## SURGICAL TECHNIQUE DEFINED BY ETIOLOGY

### Involutional Ectropion

Involutional ectropion typically first affects the medial eyelid. As the disorder progresses, the lid eversion extends laterally in varying degrees depending on degree of retractor dehiscence and horizontal laxity. Mild medial ectropion without significant horizontal laxity can be corrected with the medial spindle procedure. Patients with horizontal eyelid laxity usually require some form of eyelid tightening. The lateral tarsal strip is often most ideal, since this procedure also repositions a displaced canthus and minimizes the complications of noticeable scarring and trichiasis. Alternatively, a full-thickness block resection may be indicated in those patients with an area of pre-existing marginal scarring. Commonly, a medial spindle and lateral tarsal strip are performed simultaneously when the entire lid is ectropic.

#### *Lateral Tarsal Strip*

The goal of the lateral tarsal strip procedure is to re-establish lateral fixation of the lower eyelid and lateral canthus.[1] The eyelid is fixated inside the orbital rim periosteum. The lateral tarsal strip is created after separation of the anterior and posterior lamellae; removal of the eyelash follicles, mucocutaneous junction, and conjunctival epithelium; and release of eyelid retractors. The length of the strip is determined by the degree of eyelid laxity. Excessive tightening should be avoided, particularly in patients with prominent globes.

Steps:

- Lateral canthotomy, identification of the inferior crus of the canthal tendon, and inferior cantholysis (Fig. 53-1A)

- Exposure of the lateral orbital rim periosteum
- Determine length of lateral tarsal strip and degree of lid tightening by manually directing the lower eyelid laterally to the desired tension (Fig. 53-1B)
- Subciliary incision along the desired length of the strip. Elevate small skin flap (Fig. 53-1C)
- Incision along the gray line followed by excision of remaining anterior lid margin and eyelash follicles (Fig. 53-1D)
- Excision of mucocutaneous epithelium of posterior lid margin
- Release of conjunctiva and eyelid retractors at the tarsal base
- Superficial cauterization or scrapping of tarsal conjunctival epithelium (Fig. 53-1E)
- Dissection of preperiosteal pocket medial to upper crus of lateral canthal tendon, designed to receive the tarsal strip
- Secure tarsal strip to periosteum along inside of orbital rim using a mattress 5-0 Prolene (polypropylene filament) suture [other surgeons have used 5-0 Vicryl (polyglactin 910), Mersilene (polyester), or PDS (polydioxanone)]. It is important to direct the strip into the previously designed preperiosteal pocket. Evaluate lid contour and tension (Fig. 53-1F)
- Lateral canthal angle reformation and orbicularis closure using 6-0 Vicryl suture
- Skin rearrangement and closure with 6-0 gut suture.

### *Medial Spindle Procedure with Rotational Suture*

When retractor dehiscence causes medial ectropion that is not fully correctable with horizontal tightening of the eyelid, a medial spindle procedure can also be performed.[2] Isolated medial spindle can be an effective method of ectropion repair in those patients with retractor dehiscence without eyelid laxity. After excision of redundant conjunctiva and subconjunctival tissue, full-thickness mattress sutures are placed to advance the eyelid retractors and rotate the lid margin inward.

Steps:

1. Confirm the medial palpebral conjunctiva is redundant. An elliptical resection of redundant conjunctiva and subconjunctival tissue is performed just inferior to tarsus and punctum (Figs. 53-2A to C)
2. Advancement of the eyelid retractors is performed with a full-thickness mattress double-armed 5-0 chromic gut suture. Each arm is initially passed through the inferior edge of the tarsus, then through the lower eyelid retractors, that are located just inside the inferior conjunctival incision. The suture arms are then directed through the anterior eyelid lamella, so that they are externalized on the skin surface at a point lower than their initial tarsal bite (Fig. 53-2D). The conjunctival wound should close and the lid margin rotate inward as the sutures are tied (Fig. 53-2E)

### *Retractor Reconstruction*

In advanced involutional ectropion, marginal external rotation increasingly extends laterally secondary to progressive retractor dehiscence.[3] As the ectropion extends laterally, graded repair of the eyelid ectropion may be required.

Steps:

- Transconjunctival incision along the length of eyelid where retractor advancement is required
- Excision of redundant conjunctiva and subconjunctival tissue
- Advancement of the retractors is performed using multiple full-thickness horizontal mattress double-armed 5-0 chromic gut suture placed similarly in orientation to medial spindle sutures.

## Cicatricial Ectropion

Shortening of the lower eyelid anterior lamella can occur after actinic skin damage, trauma, and surgical procedures including blepharoplasty. Occasionally, infiltrating cutaneous malignancy can cause cicatrization and biopsies should be performed prior to repair in suspected cases. Long-standing eyelid malposition either from involutional or paralytic etiologies can also lead to cicatricial changes. Scarring of the eyelid can occur in segmental fashion or be present along the entire length of the eyelid.

### *Local Skin Flaps*

When segmental eyelid scarring causes eyelid ectropion, Z-plasty or other local flaps may be effective in relieving the skin tension upon the lid margin. In patients with mild skin shortage and cheek descent, mid-face lifting procedures can be performed to augment vertical anterior lamellar height.

### *Full-Thickness Skin Grafts*

When significant anterior lamellar scarring or vertical shortage occurs, skin grafting may be necessary. It is important to consider the th patients with cicatricial changes also have significant horizontal laxity requiring simultaneous treatment with tarsal strip procedures.

Steps:

- *Incision planning*: When a cicatrix is present, the incision is frequently placed at the superior edge of the scar.

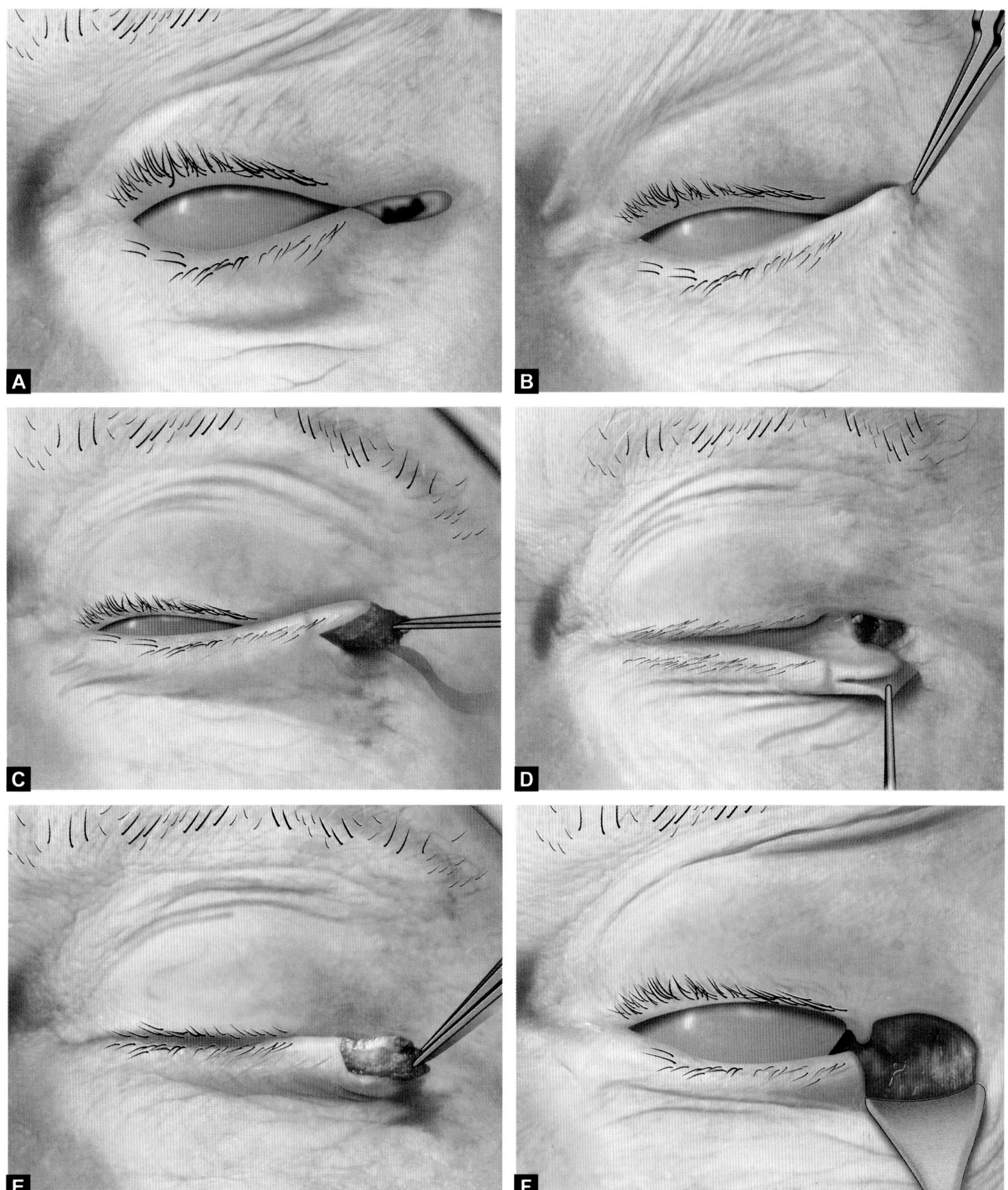


**Figures 53-1A to F** (A) Lateral canthotomy and inferior cantholysis is performed. (B) The proposed new canthal angle is marked after appropriate horizontal tension is determined. (C) Subciliary incision is made and small skin–muscle flap is elevated. (D) Incision is made down the gray line prior to excision of the pilosebaceous units. (E) Cautery is applied to the posterior lamella to remove conjunctival cells. (F) The tarsal strip is fixated into the inside of the orbital rim.

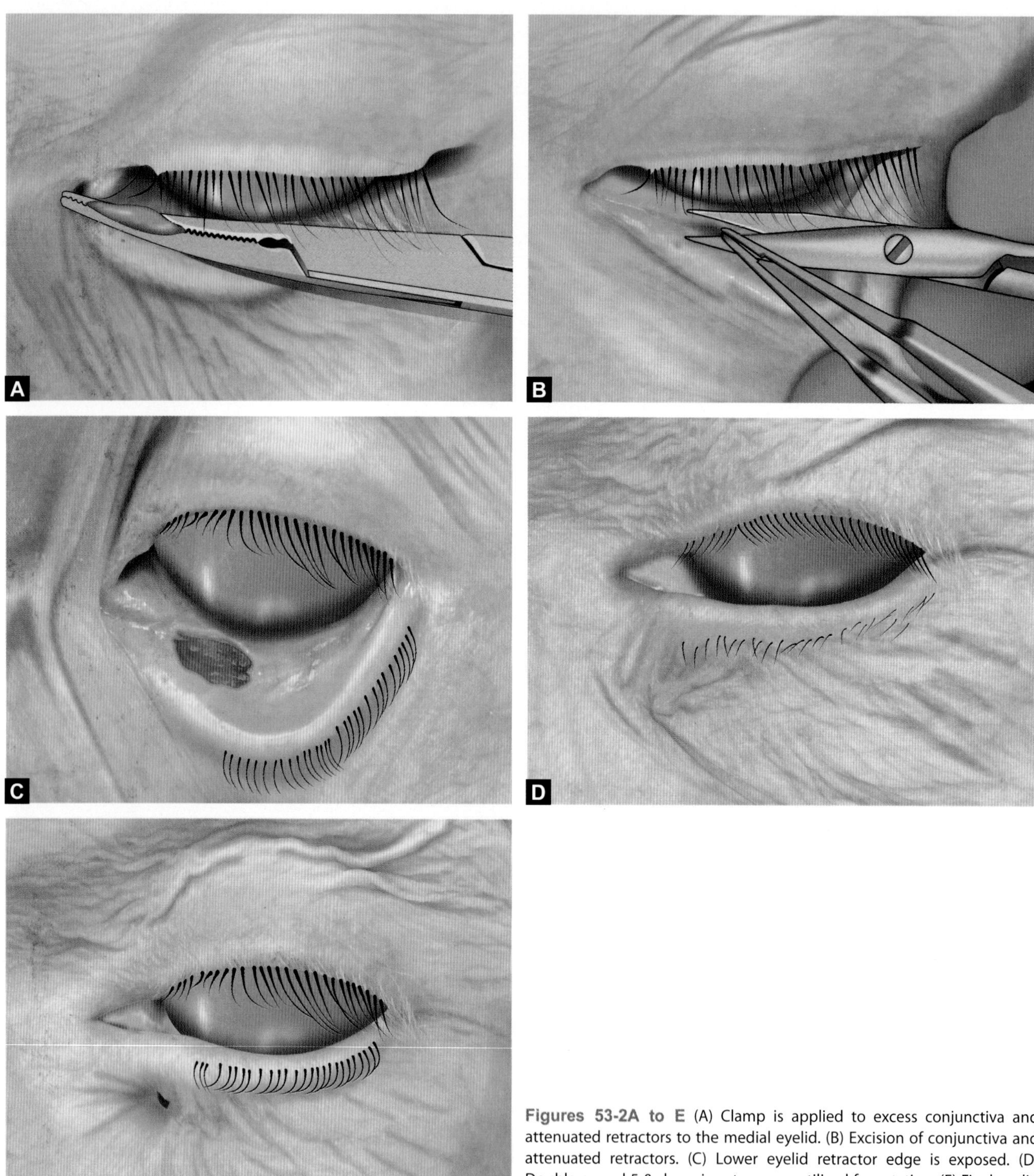


**Figures 53-2A to E** (A) Clamp is applied to excess conjunctiva and attenuated retractors to the medial eyelid. (B) Excision of conjunctiva and attenuated retractors. (C) Lower eyelid retractor edge is exposed. (D) Double-armed 5-0 chromic sutures are utilized for rotation. (E) Final eyelid position.

A subciliary incision is typically used in those patients with generalized skin shortage without pre-existing scars. Subcutaneous dissection is performed in a fashion to release deeper cicatrix while developing a smooth recipient bed for the graft

- Measurement of skin defect with eyelid in normal position

- Incision, dissection, and closure of skin graft donor site
- Skin graft thinned of excess subcutaneous tissue and fat
- Skin graft is placed in position, precisely trimmed and sutured in place with 6-0 gut sutures
- When possible, bolster placement using a nonadherent dressing and tie-down sutures will prevent graft dislodgement and fluid collection under graft.

## Paralytic Ectropion

Contracture of an intact orbicularis muscle is required to maintain lid position and function. When the orbicularis muscle is weak, horizontal eyelid laxity can be exaggerated. Surgical repair of horizontal laxity is usually performed with the lateral tarsal strip procedure, which also helps suspend the paralytic eyelid. Other common treatments include medial canthoplasty and limited lateral tarsorrhaphy (discussed in Chapter 55).

### *Medial Canthoplasty*

Commonly, when orbicularis muscle weakness is the main cause of eyelid ectropion, there is also retraction of the medial eyelid and gaping of the canthus. Medial canthoplasty procedure involves closure of the medial canthal angle to improve exposure and medial eyelid apposition.
Steps:

- Bowman probe placement in the superior and inferior canliculus
- Skin incisions along the mucocutaneous junction of each eyelid, extending from the canthal angle to within 1–2 mm of the puncta
- Elevation of skin flaps superiorly and inferiorly for several millimeters from each incision
- Excision of palpebral conjunctiva adjacent to each incision, staying superficial to the underlying canthal tendons and canaliculi
- Closure of the medial canthal angle is then achieved with precise placement of 7-0 Vicryl interrupted sutures, engaging the superficial orbicularis muscles and canthal tendons while avoiding the canalicular system
- Confirmation of no canalicular disruption is performed with Bowman probes
- Skin closure is performed using 6–0 gut suture.

## POSTOPERATIVE CARE

After the procedure, appropriate wound and suture care with mild topical antibiotic ointment is necessary. Suture removal may be performed 1 week after surgery should gut sutures not be fully degraded. Rotational chromic sutures are usually left intact for several weeks. If skin grafting is performed, bolster removal can occur within the first 5–8 days. Lubrication of graft before and after bolster removal is imperative for graft health and survival.

## SPECIFIC INSTRUMENTATION

Standard eyelid instruments are required. Exposure of the lateral orbital rim can be aided with the use of Ragnell retractor.

## COMPLICATIONS

- Lateral tarsal strip:
  - Incorrect eyelid tension (over or under tightening)
  - Canthal malposition, poor alignment of lids at canthus
  - Chemosis.
- Medial spindle with rotational suture/retractor reconstruction:
  - Incorrect eyelid margin position (persistent ectropion or entropion)
  - Lacrimal system damage
  - Excessive conjunctival resection.
- Local skin flaps:
  - Persistent cicatricial change with eyelid malposition
  - Scarring
  - Flap necrosis.
- Full-thickness skin graft:
  - Graft contracture
  - Poor skin color match
  - Graft necrosis/infection
  - Donor site complications.
- Medial canthoplasty:
  - Lacrimal system damage.

## PLACE OF THE TECHNIQUE IN SURGICAL ARMAMENTARIUM

The most important consideration when choosing surgical therapy for ectropion is identification and targeted treatment of the primary etiology for the ectropion. Each technique described addresses specific anatomical issues known to cause ectropion and should be chosen based on physical examination findings and historical information.

## PEARLS AND PITFALLS

- If the punctum is visible on casual observation of the resting eyelid, ectropion is present.

- Appropriate eyelid tension with the eyelid comfortably resting against the globe is ideal. The tendency for surgical over tightening is common and should be avoided.
- Persistent or recurrent ectropion after initial repair is seldom caused by eyelid laxity. More commonly, there is residual retractor dehiscence, skin shortage, or orbicularis weakness.
- Chronic ectropion may cause marginal eyelid inflammation and contracture with upward rotation of the eyelashes. Symptomatic trichiasis may develop when the lid is surgically repositioned. Cilia epilation or ablation may be required after ectropion repair.
- Chronic involutional ectropion can lead to shortening of the anterior lamella.
- Vertical rhytids in the medial eyelids may indicate there is mild skin shortage and the need for a small skin graft.
- Inadequate eyelid skin can also be identified by induced eyelid ectropion with upgaze or wide mouth opening.
- Tearing in the setting of paralytic ectropion is multifactorial including punctal malposition, reflex tearing from dryness, and lacrimal pump dysfunction.
- Allergic blepharitis is a common cause of cicatricial ectropion. Treatment of the underlying etiology frequently results in full or partial resolution of the lid malposition without surgery.

## CONCLUSION

Ectropion is a common eyelid malposition that most frequently affects the lower eyelid. Careful historical and clinical information must be collected for surgical planning. A variety of surgical techniques can be utilized to treat the underlying mechanisms for eyelid ectropion.

## REFERENCES

1. Anderson RL, Gordy DD. The tarsal strip procedure. Arch Ophthalmol. 1979; 97;2192.
2. Nowinski TS, Anderson RL. The medial spindle procedure for involutional medial ectropion. Arch Ophthalmol. 1985;103(11): 1750-3.
3. Tse DT, Kronish JW, Buus D. Surgical correction of lower-eyelid tarsal ectropion by reinsertion of retractors. Arch Ophthalmol. 1991;109(3):427-31.

CHAPTER

# 54

# Abnormalities of the Eyelashes

Alexander Foster, Bradford W Lee, Don O Kikkawa, Bobby S Korn

## INTRODUCTION

Eyelashes are thick, curved hair at the margins of the eyelids that serve to protect the ocular surface. They are formed by keratinocytes of the hair bulb, are composed of hard keratin, and number approximately 100–150 cilia per lid.[1] Their protective function is facilitated by the low excitatory threshold of their associated nerve plexus, which produces a brisk blink reflex with stimulation. Sebaceous glands contained within the hair follicle secrete sebum that tracks up the lash to lubricate the eye. Thus, any disease that affects the eyelashes may ultimately result in damage to the ocular surface.

Trichiasis is misdirection of the eyelashes normally growing from the anterior lamella of the eyelid in the setting of normal eyelid position[2] (Fig. 54-1). This is typically an acquired entity, and etiologies include mechanical disruption (such as trauma or adverse healing of a prior incision) and cicatrizing processes such as chemical burns, Stevens–Johnson syndrome, chronic blepharitis, or trachoma. Eyelashes may be involved in isolated, segmental, or diffuse patterns.

Distichiasis refers to abnormal lashes growing posterior to the normal lashes (Fig. 54-2). These abnormal lashes emanate from the tarsal portion of the lid in which the meibomian glands normally reside. The condition is either congenital or acquired. Congenital distichiasis results from abnormal differentiation of embryonic pilosebaceous units into hair follicles rather than meibomian glands.[2] Acquired distichiasis occurs in processes that induce metaplasia of the meibomian glands, such as chemical injury, Stevens–Johnson syndrome, blepharitis, ocular pemphigoid, and other chronic inflammatory entities.[1]

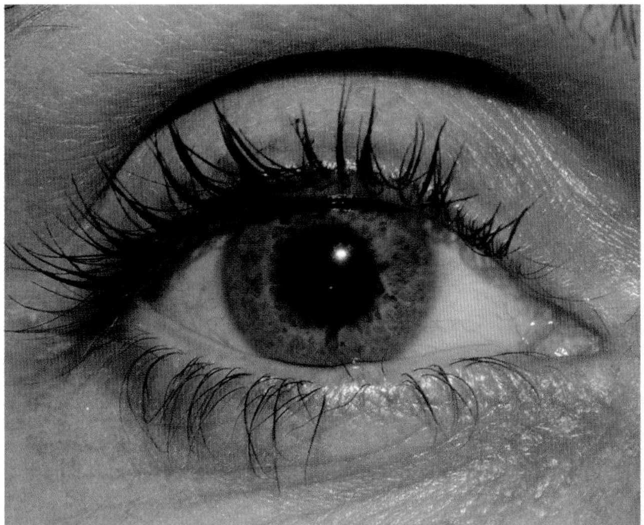

**Figure 54-1** Right lower eyelid trichiasis.

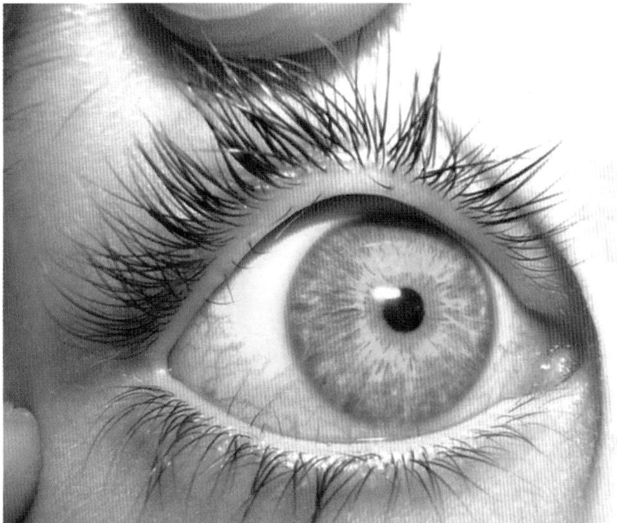

**Figure 54-2** Right upper and lower eyelid distichiasis.

## INDICATIONS

- Symptomatic ocular surface irritation
- Conjunctival and/or corneal abrasion, vascularization, scarring, ulceration
- Secondary epiphora.

## CONTRAINDICATIONS

- Medical contraindications to specific treatment modalities
- Caution when using electrocautery in patients with implanted cardiac devices.

## SURGICAL TECHNIQUES

### Mechanical Epilation

In cases that involve relatively few trichiatic eyelashes, mechanical epilation may be performed with forceps. Regrowth is common and recurrence occurs within 3–8 weeks. When performing mechanical epilation, it is essential to remove the entire follicle to its root as broken cilia and short, regrowing cilia can be more irritating to the cornea than mature lashes.

### Electrolysis and Radiofrequency Ablation

For a more definitive treatment of misdirected lashes, low-powered electrolysis/hyfrecation or radiofrequency ablation of the follicle base can be employed to treat a limited number of misdirected lashes.[3,4] The procedure is best performed with local anesthetic and aims to selectively destroy the follicular stem cells responsible for regrowth of eyelashes. Electrolysis can be performed using various types of instrument tips. The needle-style tip works particularly well for electrolysis of eyelashes. The tip is directed parallel to the base of the follicle, and in some cases, the tip must be obliquely oriented because of a lash's aberrant direction of growth. Once the tip is properly oriented, energy is applied and bubbles can be seen emerging from the base of the lash. If done properly, the lash can be easily removed without resistance using jeweler's forceps. If there is resistance to epilation, the placement of the probe may be suboptimal or the treatment power may be inadequate. In such cases, re-treatment may be performed to improve the success of treatment. Care should be taken to avoid multiple treatments, as this may lead to scarring of eyelid margin tissue that can exacerbate pre-existing trichiasis.

### Cryotherapy

More widespread and recalcitrant trichiasis may be treated with cryotherapy under local anesthesia. A double freeze-thaw technique is employed by freezing the involved area once for 25 seconds, allowing thawing, and then refreezing for an additional 20 seconds.[5] Lashes are subsequently mechanically removed. Adverse reactions include unwanted loss of lashes adjacent to the treatment area, depigmentation of eyelid skin, exacerbation of pre-existing eyelid cicatrization, eyelid necrosis, and depressed scarring of the eyelid margin (Fig. 54-3). Due to the risk of disfiguring skin depigmentation, cryotherapy is not advised in patients with darker skin pigmentation.

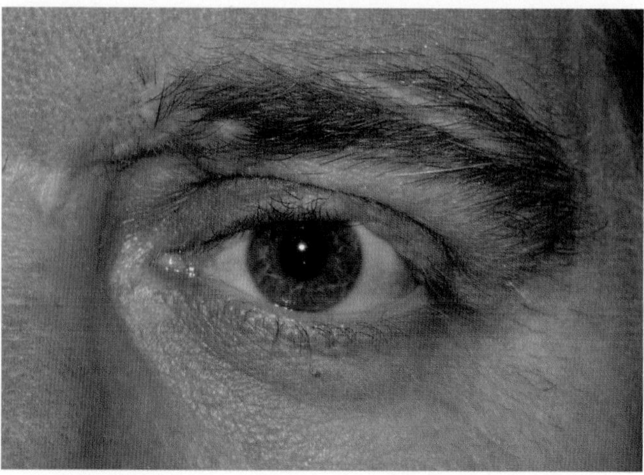

**Figure 54-3** Right upper eyelid madarosis and eyelid notching after cryotherapy for trichiasis.

### Argon Laser Ablation

Argon laser photocoagulation can be used effectively in treating trichiasis particularly after multiple treatments. With the patient sitting at the slit lamp, the lid is everted such that the eyelash root is coaxial with the laser beam. A 50- to 200-μm spot size with power ranging from 0.2 W to 1.5 W is used. More recently, yttrium aluminium garnet and diode lasers have been shown to provide better penetration than argon.[6] This therapy is preferable in cases of limited trichiasis; more widespread disease is more amenable to definitive surgical treatment. Placement of a corneal shield prior to treatment is strongly recommended.

### Eyelash Trephination

For isolated trichiasis, a lacrimal trephine can be used to remove the errant eyelash. In this procedure, the trephine is directed parallel to the misdirected eyelash. A cylindrical core of the tarsal plate encompassing entire lash is removed as a single unit. The procedure can be rapidly performed in the office setting with local anesthetic with low morbidity.[7]

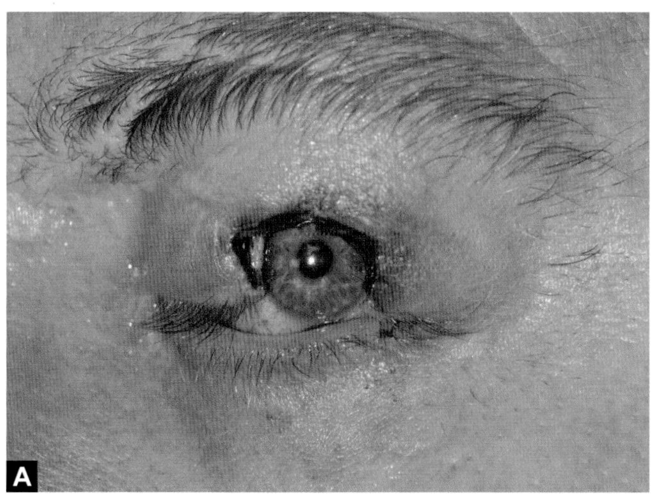


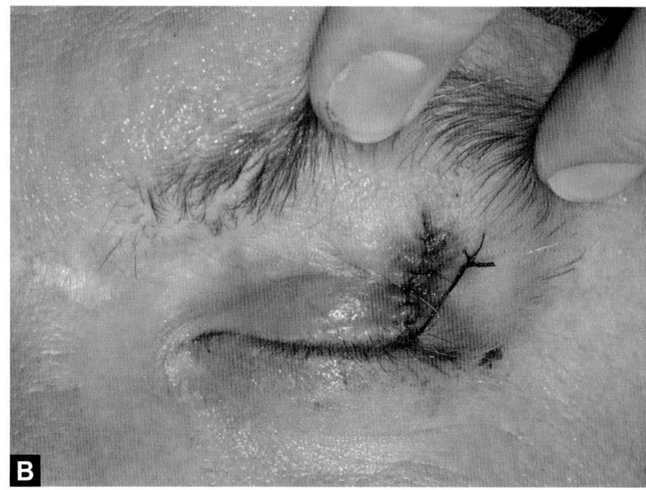


Figures 54-4A and B (A) Full-thickness wedge excision of left upper eyelid for recalcitrant trichiasis. (B) Primary closure of left upper eyelid after full-thickness wedge excision.

### Full-Thickness Eyelid Wedge Resection

Definitive treatment of misdirected eyelashes can be achieved with segmental wedge resection. A full-thickness pentagonal wedge of eyelid is excised that includes the area of involvement (Fig. 54-4A). Primary eyelid reconstruction is attempted first with three 6-0 silk sutures that are used to reapproximate the lash line, gray line, and mucocutaneous junction. The tarsus is united with 7-0 polygalactin sutures in a lamellar fashion and the skin is closed with 6-0 fast absorbable gut or 6-0 polypropylene sutures (Fig. 54-4B). If insufficient eyelid laxity is present, a lateral canthotomy or a semicircular rotational flap can be performed concurrently.

## POSTOPERATIVE CARE

Postoperative care varies based on the invasiveness of each procedure. For mechanical epilation, electrolysis, radiofrequency, laser photocoagulation, or cryotherapy without lid splitting, conservative management with topical lubrication, and oral analgesia (e.g. acetaminophen) is sufficient. When an incisional approach is employed such as cryotherapy with lid margin splitting or full-thickness wedge resection, an ophthalmic antibiotic–steroid ointment is applied topically two times per day for 14 days. Oral antibiotics are rarely used. Silk sutures placed for lid margin repair are removed at 14 days after surgery.

## COMPLICATIONS

The most common complication in the treatment of misdirected eyelashes is recurrence, and patients should be appropriately counseled about the likely need for retreatment. Recurrence occurs most commonly with mechanical epilation and less commonly when thermal energy is applied to the lash root. To reduce the risk of corneal injury associated with many of these procedures, a corneal shield can be used to protect the ocular surface. Multiple or overly aggressive treatments can lead to scarring, notching, and frank ulceration of the eyelid margin. Excessive madarosis can also result, particularly with cryotherapy. Lid margin necrosis can rarely occur if the marginal vascular arcade is significantly disrupted.

## SURGICAL RESULTS: SCIENTIFIC EVIDENCE/META-ANALYSIS

No level I scientific studies have been reported for the treatment of trichiasis, and most studies are level II or higher. Of note, for radiofrequency ablation, Kormann and Moreiera treated 54 eyelids of 34 patients with trichiasis with radiofrequency ablation. Cure was achieved following a single treatment in 22 patients, and the remaining 12 required one or two additional sessions. No complications were reported in this series.[4] With respect to cryotherapy, Khafagy et al. demonstrated that an approach combining lid margin splitting with subsequent cryotherapy was effective, with a 90% treatment success rate and 10% rate of recurrence across 20 total eyelids treated.[5]

## REFERENCES

1. American Academy of Ophthalmology. Basic and clinical science course section 7: orbit, eyelids, and lacrimal system. San Francisco: American Academy of Ophthalmology; 2013.

2. Choo PH. Distichiasis, trichiasis, and entropion: advances in management. Int Ophthal Clin. 2002:42(2):75-87.
3. Vaugn GL, Dortzbach RK, Sires BS, et al. Eyelid splitting with excision or microhyfrecation for distichiasis. Arch Ophthalmol. 1997;115:282-4.
4. Kormann RB, Moreiera H. Treatment of trichiasis with high-frequency radio wave electrosurgery. Arg Bras Oftamol. 2007; 70(2):276-80.
5. Khafagy A, Mostafa M, Fooshan F. Management of trichiasis with lid margin split and cryotherapy. Clin Ophthalmol. 2012; 6:1815-7.
6. Basar E, Ozdemir H, Ozkan S, et al. Treatment of trichiasis with argon laser. Eur J Ophthalmol. 2000;10:273-5.
7. McCracken MS, Kikkawa DO, Vasani SN. Treatment of trichiasis and distichiasis by eyelash trephination. Ophthal Plast Reconstr Surg. 2006;22(5):349-51.

CHAPTER

55

# Management of Facial Palsy

Sally L Baxter, Richard L Scawn, Bobby S Korn, Don O Kikkawa

## INTRODUCTION

Facial palsy is characterized by both functional and aesthetic deficits (Fig. 55-1) occurring secondary to multiple causes (Table 55-1). The facial nerve innervates the orbicularis oculi, the primary protractor muscle in eyelid closure. In addition to gravitational factors, a paretic orbicularis allows the eyelid retractors to act unopposed, causing upper and lower eyelid retraction and compounding the potential for lagophthalmos and exposure keratopathy. Other clinical features include brow ptosis, both lower lid ectropion and epiphora can occur secondary to lacrimal pump failure, lower lid retraction, loss of the nasolabial fold, and facial descent.[1-3]

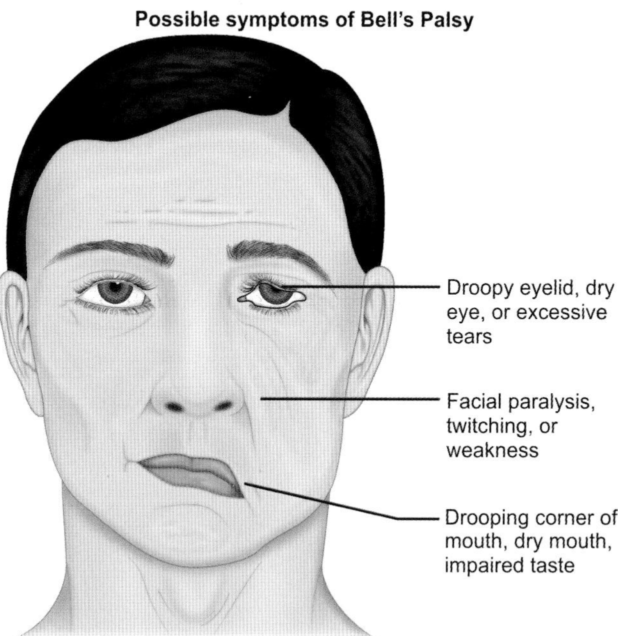


**Figure 55-1** Changes caused by facial nerve palsy. Several changes may result from facial palsy, including smoothing of the forehead, brow ptosis, upper and lower eyelid retraction, lagophthalmos, lower lid ectropion, midface descent, flattened nasolabial fold, and drooping of the corner of the mouth.

**TABLE 55-1** Causes of facial palsy.

| Category | Example(s) |
|---|---|
| Idiopathic | Bell's palsy |
| Traumatic | Zygomatic and temporal bone fractures (e.g. from blunt trauma or from gunshot wounds), iatrogenic injury during surgery |
| Infectious | Herpes simplex virus, Ramsay–Hunt syndrome (herpes zoster), Lyme disease, tuberculous chronic HIV, polio, mumps, leprosy, otitis media |
| Neoplastic | Acoustic neuroma, facial schwannoma, parotid neoplasms |
| Congenital | Mobius syndrome, Goldenhar syndrome, DiGeorge syndrome, CHARGE syndrome, birth trauma |
| Systemic | Diabetes mellitus, hypertension, amyloidosis, sarcoidosis |
| Neurologic | Multiple sclerosis, Guillain–Barre syndrome, myasthenia gravis, cerebrovascular accident |

Facial palsy has the potential to cause sight-threatening keratopathy, so the primary goal of treatment is corneal protection. Secondary goals include addressing cosmesis, epiphora, and complications from paretic musculature and aberrant regeneration when reinnervation occurs. The prognosis for recovery from facial palsy is variable with no reliable early prognostic indicators. Likelihood of recovery is lower in cases of tumor infiltration compared with those deriving from a presumed viral etiology such as Bell's palsy. Initial treatments consist of supportive measures, including lubricating eye ointments and drops, eyelid taping, moisture chambers,

**TABLE 55-2** Surgical techniques for management of facial palsy

- Upper and lower eyelid complex:
  - Tarsorrhaphy
- Upper eyelid procedures:
  - Gold or platinum weight implantation
  - Palpebral spring placement
- Lower eyelid procedures:
  - Lower lid shortening and tightening
    - Lateral tarsal strip
    - Medial lid tightening: transcaruncular medial, canthopexy, medial spindle
  - Spacer grafting
  - Subperiosteal midface elevation/suborbicularis oculi fat lift
  - Lower lid fascial suspension
- Adjunctive techniques:
  - Brow ptosis correction
  - Upper eyelid blepharoplasty
  - Upper eyelid retraction surgery (levator recession and mullerectomy)
  - Neurotoxin injections
  - Facial reanimation procedures

environmental humidification, and soft contact or scleral lenses.[2,4,5] However, if a patient shows no signs of spontaneous recovery within 6–12 months, or sight-threatening exposure keratopathy ensues, surgical intervention may be indicated.[3,6] This chapter describes the surgical treatment of facial palsy with a focus on the upper and midface (Table 55-2).

## INDICATIONS

- Exposure keratopathy despite maximally tolerated medical therapy
- Facial palsy without signs of recovery within 6–12 months
- Neurotrophic keratitis and reduced or absent Bell's phenomenon make early surgical intervention more likely
- Vision compromize secondary to brow ptosis and dermatochalasis
- Aesthetic concerns
- Epiphora

## CONTRAINDICATIONS

Medically unfit for surgery, although some procedures can be performed at the bedside under local anesthesia.

## SURGICAL TECHNIQUES AND MECHANISMS OF ACTION

### Upper and Lower Eyelid Complex

#### *Tarsorrhaphy*

Tarsorrhaphy (Figs. 55-2A and B) involves reducing the horizontal and vertical palpebral aperture. It may be performed laterally, medially, or both. Tarsorrhaphy may be temporary or permanent. In a permanent tarsorrhaphy, an incision is made at the gray line in corresponding segments of the upper and lower eyelids along the intended tarsorrhaphy length. The anterior and posterior lamellar layers are separated. The mucocutaneous junctions of the upper and lower posterior lamellar flaps are excised, exposing the tarsal plates and creating fresh de-epithelialized surfaces. The lateral canthal angle should be preserved to allow reversal without permanent horizontal fissure shortening.[7] The tarsal flaps are approximated using multiple 7-0 Vicryl sutures with partial thickness bites. The anterior lamella flaps are then closed with 6-0 fast-absorbing gut sutures in a horizontal mattress fashion to evert the lashes. Another option for permanent tarsorraphy is a conjunctival pillar tarsorrhaphy. A 3–4 mm tarsoconjunctival flap is raised, based in the upper fornix. This pillar is then secured to the conjunctiva of the lower lid. The advantage of this approach is that it spares the lid margin and does not narrow the horizontal palpebral fissure.

In a temporary tarsorrhaphy, the epithelium is not denuded and the gray line is maintained. Nonabsorbing 6-0 Prolene sutures are placed in a horizontal mattress fashion through the skin, emerging at the gray line and back through the gray line of the opposite eyelid to exit the skin. Bolsters are used to prevent suture "cheese wiring".

Permanent lateral tarsorrhaphy was traditionally a first-line surgical treatment. Due to its static nature, poor cosmesis, peripheral field constriction, and often inadequate central cornea protection, an upper lid weight is preferred by some surgeons.[2,3,8] However, tarsorrhaphy may be useful for those who have not responded well to other procedures, are unable to comply with supportive therapy, and lack adequate follow-up care.[2,6]

### Upper Eyelid

The downward excursion of the upper eyelid is largely responsible for eyelid closure and is a key area of focus for the management of facial palsy.

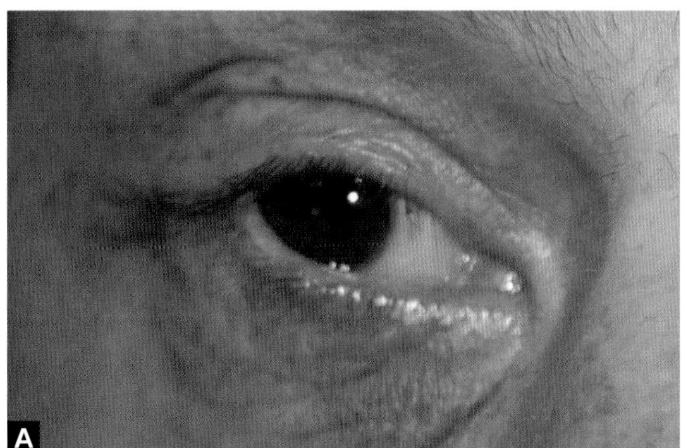
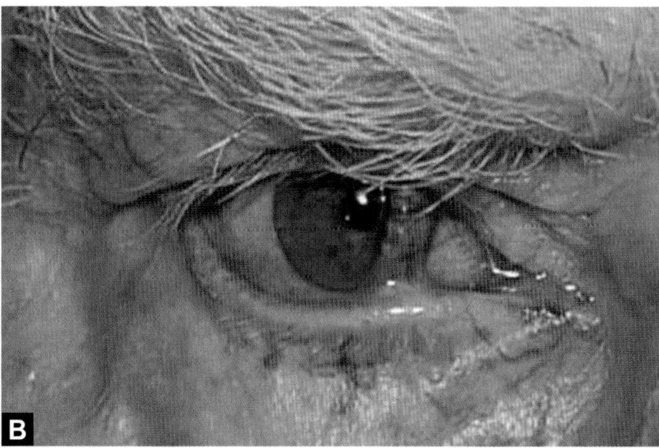

**Figures 55-2A and B** Tarsorrhaphy. (A) Depicts a patient who has undergone lateral tarsorrhaphy, which brings the lateral aspect of the tarsus and anterior lamella into apposition. This shortens the horizontal and vertical palpebral aperture, which improves corneal protection, but may also limit peripheral vision. (B) Shows a patient with a pillar tarsorrhaphy, which shortens the vertical but not the horizontal aperture while preserving the lid margin.

### *Lid Loading*

Implantation of a weight in the upper eyelid (Figs. 55-3A to D) is a commonly used procedure in paralytic lagophthalmos and upper eyelid retraction.[1,9] Although gold weights have traditionally been used, our preferred material is platinum. Platinum can be used in patients with gold allergy, offers a thinner profile due to its higher specific gravity, is magnetic resonance imaging compatible and may be associated with lower rates of capsule formation and extrusion.[10]

During preoperative planning, trial weights are placed on the patient's upper eyelid skin to determine the ideal weight allowing for corneal protection but minimizing mechanical ptosis. Typically, a 1.0–1.6 g weight is sufficient to achieve complete eyelid closure.[2] A lid crease incision is made, and dissection exposes the superior tarsal border. A pretarsal orbicularis pocket is created, but the lid margin orbicularis is left intact to avoid extrusion. The weight is placed between the orbicularis and the tarsus and is secured to the tarsus with partial thickness 7-0 Vicryl.[2,4] The lid should be everted after suture placement to check that the conjunctiva has not been incorporated.[3] The orbicularis is closed with 7-0 Vicryl and the skin closed with 6-0 fast-absorbing gut or Prolene sutures. Options to minimize extrusion in patients with thin anterior lamella include placing fascia superficial to the implant and retrolevator and supratarsal placement of the weight.[2,4]

Success of weight implantation depends on gravitational force, so globe size and position may influence effectiveness, with smaller and more recessed globes conferring maximal gravitational benefit.[3] In the supine position, despite weight placement, incomplete closure may still exist, necessitating lubrication or eyelid taping.[5]

### *Palpebral Spring Procedure*

An alternative to weight placement is dynamic eyelid reanimation using a palpebral spring (Fig. 55-4).[1,5,11] The spring is pre-bent to a certain tension allowing the eyelid to completely close. With elevation of the upper eyelid, the tension increases, leading to lid closure with relaxation.[11] Because it does not depend on gravitational forces, the patient is able to have a more natural appearing blink, and adequate eyelid closure can also be achieved in the supine position.[3,12] Although they are highly effective in some cases, palpebral springs are less commonly used due to their higher frequency of complications and revisions.

## Lower Eyelid

Paralysis of the lower eyelid can lead to lower eyelid retraction, compounding lagophthalmos. Lacrimal pump failure and frank ectropion often ensue.[13] Multiple techniques exist to assist elevation and reapproximation of the lower eyelid to improve both function and cosmesis. It is important to counsel patients that initial overcorrection is desired, as gravity and lack of muscle tone typically leads to descent and relaxation over time.

### *Lower Lid Shortening and Tightening*

The lateral tarsal strip procedure (Figs. 55-5A and B) is the most common lower lid-shortening procedure for treatment of facial palsy in mild to moderate cases of eyelid laxity.[14] After a lateral canthotomy and inferior cantholysis, the degree of lid shortening to provide adequate tightening is determined. The skin and orbicularis muscle are dissected from the tarsus,

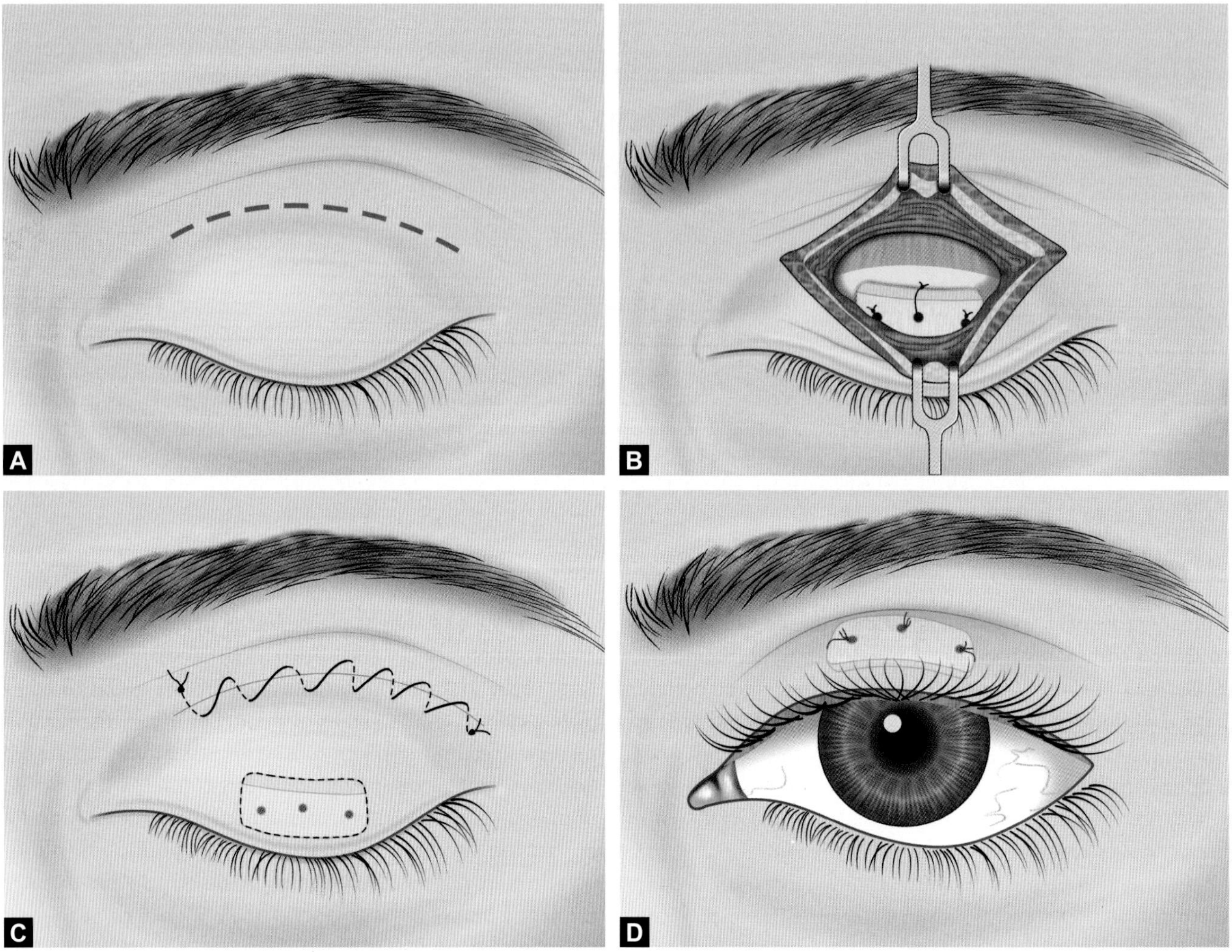

**Figures 55-3A to D** Gold weight implantation in the upper eyelid. This illustration depicts the surgical technique for lid loading in the upper eyelid with a weight for treatment of paralytic lagophthalmos. An incision is made in the upper eyelid crease (A), through which dissection is carried to expose the superior tarsal border. The gold weight is placed between the orbicularis and the tarsal plate (B). After orbicularis and skin closure (C), the weight should allow the patient to achieve full eyelid closure with minimal or no mechanical ptosis (D).

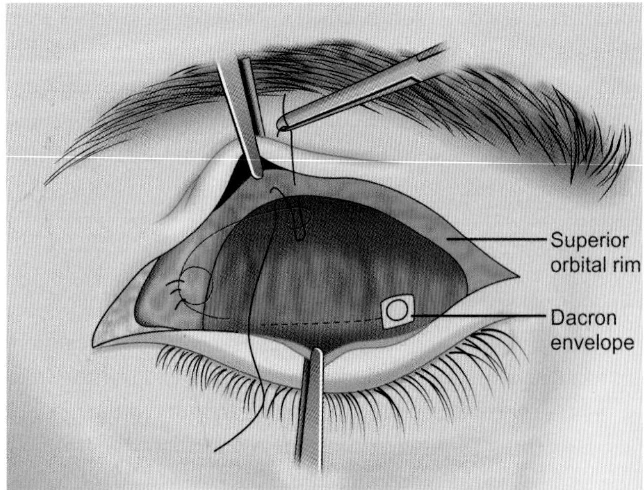


**Figure 55-4** Palpebral spring procedure for the upper eyelid. This diagram shows the position of the palpebral spring. Note that the fulcrum is anchored to lateral orbital rim. The tension is adjusted at the fulcrum using metal memory, with the goal of making the palpebral aperture symmetric with the opposite side.

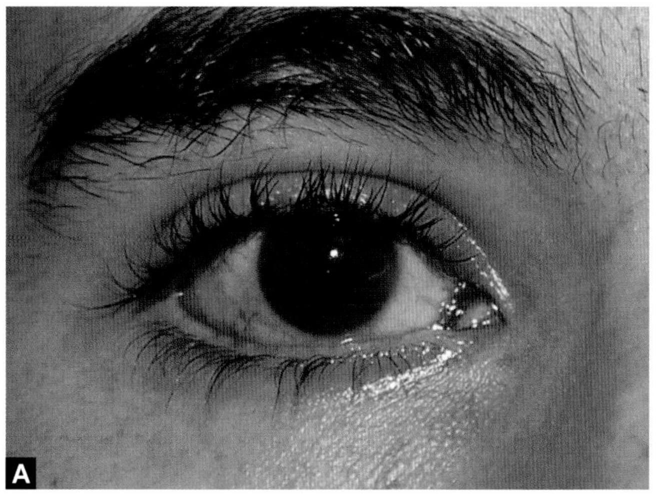

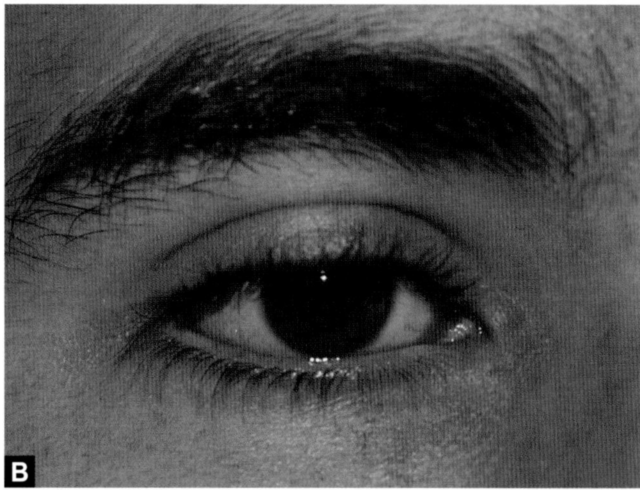

Figures 55-5A and B Lateral tarsal strip procedure for the lower eyelid. This patient has horizontal lower lid laxity and sagging due to facial palsy (A). (B) Demonstrates the lower lid shortening and elevation achieved after undergoing the lateral tarsal strip procedure.

the conjunctiva is denuded, and the tarsal strip is sutured to the lateral orbital rim periosteum, resulting in horizontal tightening and elevation of the lateral portion of the lower eyelid.[1-3] To address medial lower lid laxity, medial lid tightening techniques include retrocaruncular medial canthal tendon plication to the posterior lacrimal crest and the medial spindle procedure.[2]

### *Posterior Lamellar Grafts*

Posterior lamellar grafts can be placed to vertically lengthen the lower lid and increase stability.[2,3] Posterior lamella grafting is typically combined with anterior lamellar elevation with periosteal or rigid fixation. Hard palate grafts (HPGs) (Figs. 55-6A to C) are commonly used,[3,15] but alternative materials, such as a porcine-derived acellular dermis (EnduraGen; Stryker Corp, Kalamazoo, MI, USA), can be used as an alternative to avoid HPG donor-site complications.[1-3] After canthotomy and cantholysis, an infratarsal incision is made through the conjunctiva and lower lid retractors, extending from below the punctum to the lateral canthus. The graft is secured between the inferior border of the tarsus and the recessed inferior retractors using 6-0 absorbable sutures.[15] EnduraGen acts as a scaffold and is populated with conjunctival epithelium, so no mucous membrane graft is required. This procedure is usually combined with suborbicularis oculi fat (SOOF) or midface elevation.

### *Subperiosteal Midface Elevation/SOOF Lift*

Lid-shortening procedures address horizontal laxity and provide some lower lid elevation, but they do not address midface descent. Elevating the SOOF pad supports the inferior periorbital skin and soft tissues, thereby counteracting inferior vectors on the lower lid and improving cosmesis and function[16,17] (Figs. 55-7A to C). After lateral canthotomy and inferior cantholysis, a transconjunctival incision is made 6–8 mm below the inferior tarsal border. Dissection is carried anteriorly along the lateral aspect of the inferior orbital rim, liberating the attachments of the orbitomalar ligament. A subperiosteal release can be performed, followed by fixation of the midface with 4-0 polygalactin suture to the periosteum.[7]

### *Lower Lid Suspension Sutures*

A temporary suspension suture (Frost) is a useful adjunct to lower lid surgery to reduce traction, especially in the early postoperative period when tissue swelling is most pronounced. 6-0 Prolene tied over bolsters through upper and lower eyelid margins are secured above the brow and can be removed in the clinic within the first postoperative week.

## Adjunctive Techniques

### *Brow Ptosis Correction*

A brow lift may be a useful ancillary procedure to provide a more symmetrical appearance and increase the visual field, especially when combined with an upper lid blepharoplasty.[12,18] Options include a direct (coronal, midforehead, or brow incision), an endoscopic, or a minimally invasive temporal brow lift using a biodegradable stabilization device (ENDOTINE, Coapt Systems Inc, Palo Alto, CA, USA).[19] Brow ptosis is often marked in facial palsy, so a direct brow lift with

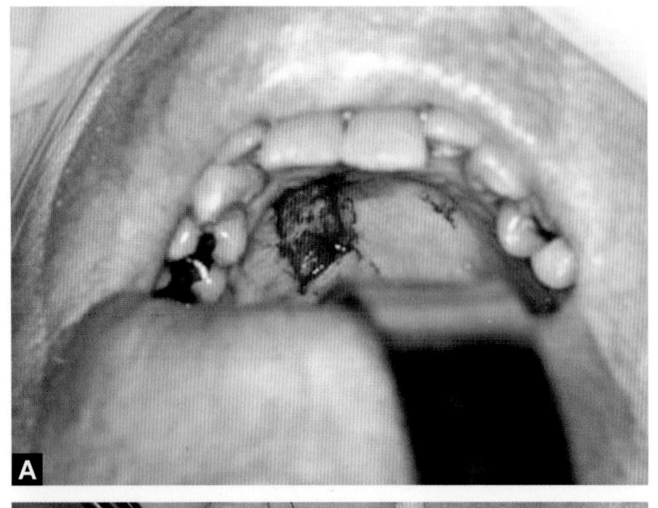


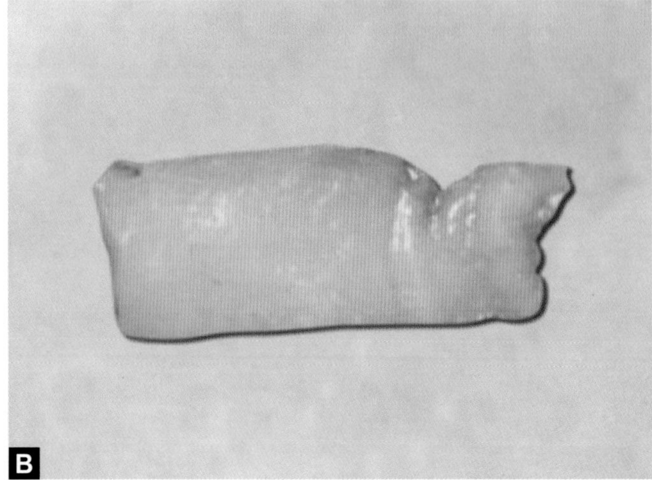


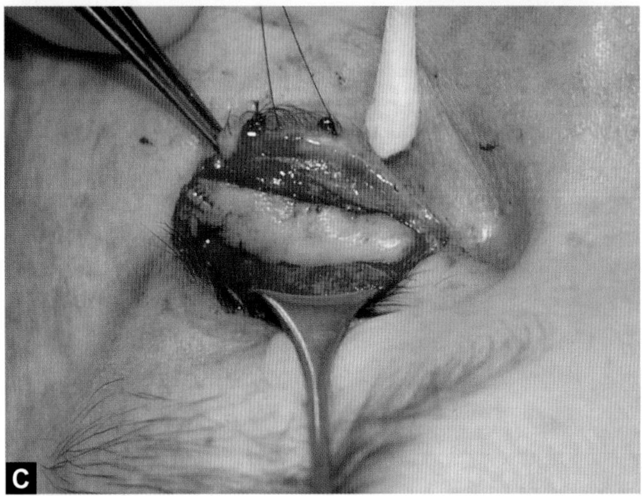


**Figures 55-6A to C** Hard palate graft (HPG) for lower eyelid support. HPG can be used as spacer material for lower lid elevation and additional vertical support. (A) Shows the HPG harvest site. Once the graft (B) is harvested, it is thinned and placed in the lower lid between the lower lid retractors and the tarsal plate (C).

fixation to the periosteum is commonly favored, especially in male patients. Slight overcorrection is typically desirable to account for postoperative descent.

## *Upper Eyelid Blepharoplasty*

Dermatochalasis is common in facial palsy and often coexists with brow ptosis. Removal of the excess skin in the upper eyelids can improve the superior visual field for these patients,[1] but careful preoperative surgical planning is necessary to determine the relative contribution from the dermatochalasis versus brow ptosis before excising excessive eyelid skin.

## *Upper Eyelid Retraction Surgery*

Upper eyelid retraction may be present in facial nerve palsy due to unopposed levator action. Levator or Mueller's recession could be considered if eyelid retraction is contributing to lagophthalmos.[12]

## *Injection of Botulinum Toxin*

Botulinum toxin type A can be used to induce levator paralysis, causing complete upper eyelid ptosis and affording temporary corneal protection, with effects typically lasting 3 months. This may be used as an adjunct in nonhealing epithelial defects or corneal ulcers.[2,12] A transcutaneous or transconjunctival approach can be used. Transcutaneous injections are typically given in the pupillary line at the midpoint of the superior orbital rim and the lid crease.[20] An unintended side effect is local diffusion inducing superior rectus paresis, thereby diminishing Bell's phenomenon and potentially worsening exposure.

Botulinum toxin is also used in aberrant facial nerve regeneration, which can cause eyelid or facial dystonias and lacrimation evoked by gustatory stimulation ("crocodile tearing").[21,22] Selective injections of botulinum toxin can alleviate synkinetic movements[21] (Figs. 55-8A and B) and mitigate excess

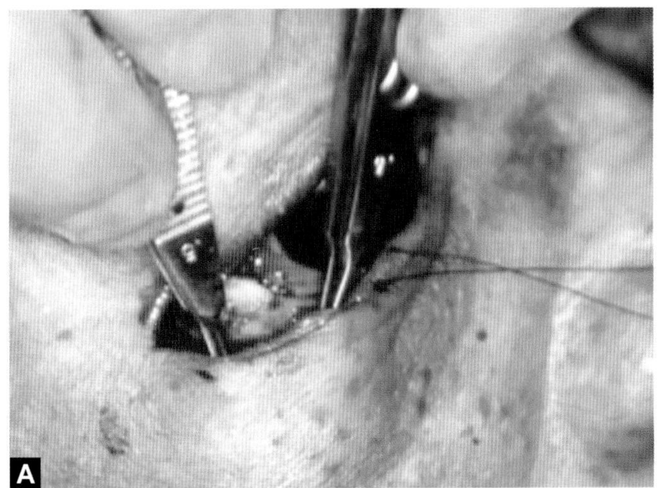

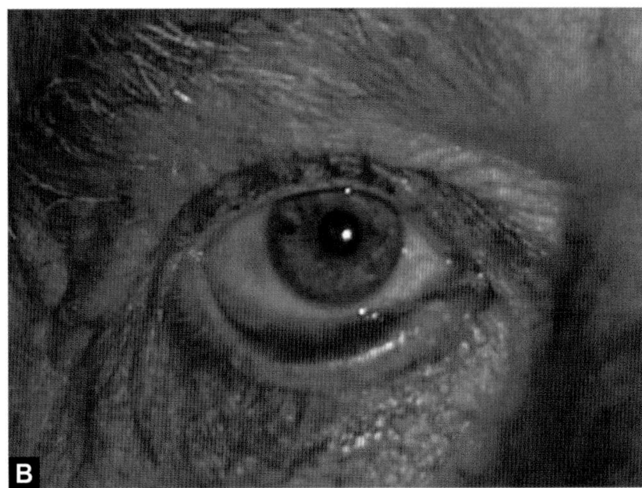

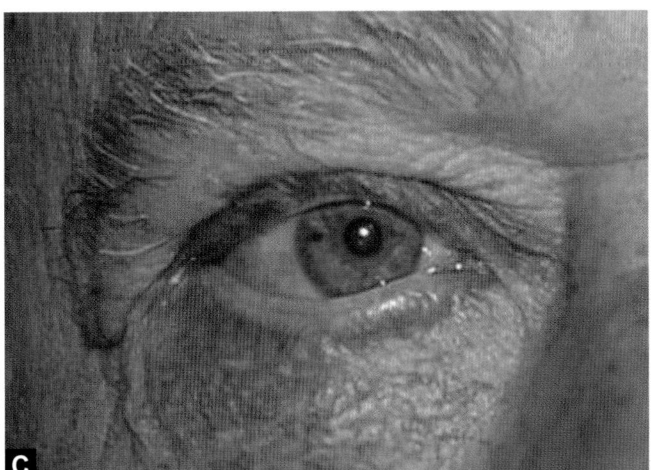

**Figures 55-7A to C** Suborbicularis oculi fat pad (SOOF) lift. A SOOF lift is often performed in conjunction with the lateral tarsal strip procedure and lower lid retraction repair surgery to address midface descent and provide adequate tissue elevation to support the lower eyelid. (A) Demonstrates intraoperative manual elevation of SOOF plane with forceps. This plane is then rigidly fixated to the lateral orbital rim. The preoperative photograph of this patient with facial palsy demonstrates lower eyelid retraction (B), with substantial improvement following a SOOF lift (C).

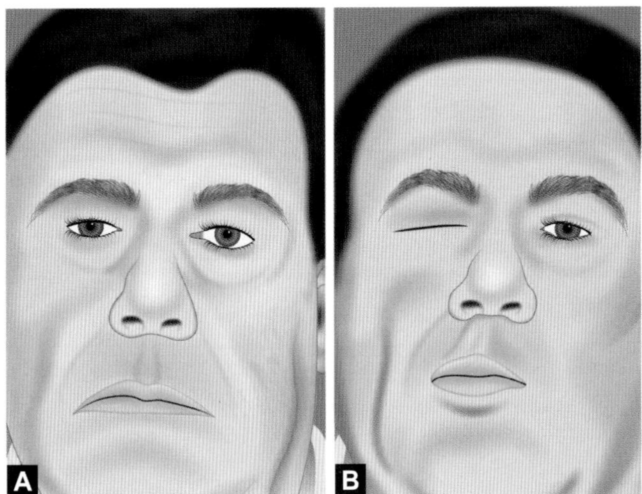

**Figures 55-8A and B** Synkinetic movements resulting from aberrant facial nerve regeneration. In aberrant facial nerve regeneration, fibers innervating other facial musculature, such as the orbicularis oris may be misdirected into the orbicularis oculi, causing synkinetic movement. Targeted neurotoxin injections can help relieve these synkinetic movements.

tearing. Treatment of crocodile tears entails a transconjunctival injection of 2.5 units into the palpebral lobe of the lacrimal gland.[23]

## *Facial Reanimation*

If the facial nerve is transected during surgery, a primary end-to-end anastomosis or nerve grafting can be performed intraoperatively to allow optimal functional recovery.[1,5] A hypoglossal–facial nerve (XII–VII) anastomosis can be considered in the early stages if the proximal facial nerve segment is not available or unsuitable for anastomosis.[24] Other possible nerve transfers include transferring the motor branches of the fifth cranial nerve[25] and cross-facial nerve grafting, which can be performed in isolation or combined with free muscle transfer.[26] Free muscle transfer, such as the temporalis or gracilis, may be considered if muscle fibrosis or atrophy is present.[1,5,26,27] Additional procedures for lower facial reconstruction include facial slings with fascia, rhytidectomy, and temporalis tendon transfer to the oral commissure.

**Flowchart 55-1** Clinical algorithm for treatment of facial palsy. This outlines the general approach to management of facial palsy at our center.

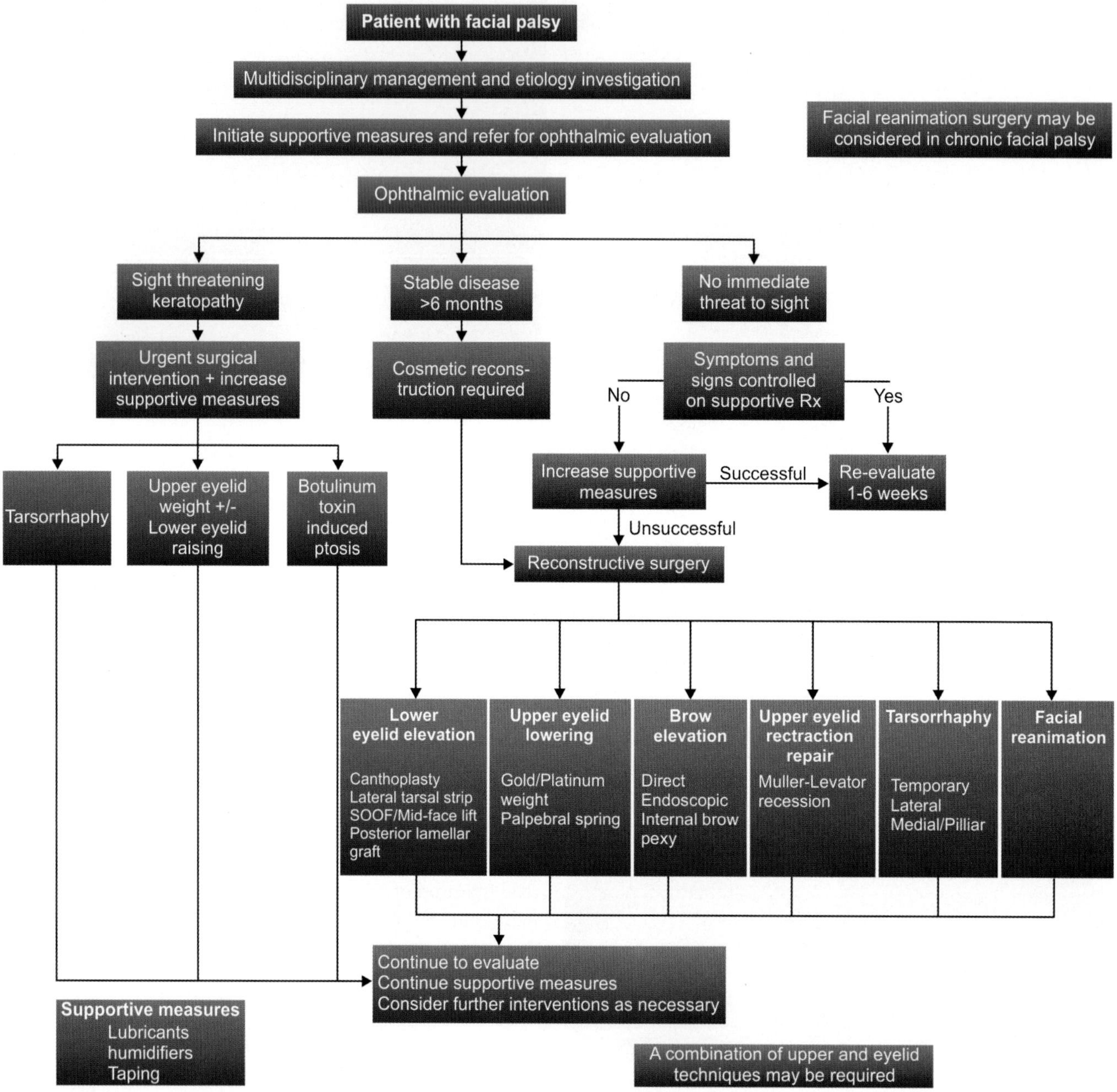

Patient with facial palsy
Multidisciplinary management and etiology investigation
Initiate supportive measures and refer for ophthalmic evaluation
Facial reanimation surgery may be considered in chronic facial palsy
Ophthalmic evaluation
Sight threatening keratopathy
Stable disease >6 months
No immediate threat to sight
Urgent surgical intervention + increase supportive measures
Cosmetic reconstruction required
Symptoms and signs controlled on supportive Rx
No
Yes
Tarsorrhaphy
Upper eyelid weight +/- Lower eyelid raising
Botulinum toxin induced ptosis
Increase supportive measures
Successful
Re-evaluate 1-6 weeks
Unsuccessful
Reconstructive surgery
**Lower eyelid elevation** Canthoplasty, Lateral tarsal strip, SOOF/Mid-face lift, Posterior lamellar graft
**Upper eyelid lowering** Gold/Platinum weight, Palpebral spring
**Brow elevation** Direct, Endoscopic, Internal brow pexy
**Upper eyelid rectraction repair** Muller-Levator recession
**Tarsorrhaphy** Temporary, Lateral, Medial/Pilliar
**Facial reanimation**
Continue to evaluate
Continue supportive measures
Consider further interventions as necessary
**Supportive measures** Lubricants, humidifiers, Taping
A combination of upper and eyelid techniques may be required

## POSTOPERATIVE CARE

Postoperative care for these procedures may vary slightly depending on technique and surgeon's preference, but generally include continuation of eye lubrication, topical antibiotics, and topical steroid ointment. Bandage contact lenses may be helpful particularly after posterior lamella grafts. We do not routinely use oral antibiotics. Analgesic requirement for most upper and superficial lower eyelid procedures is usually minimal, and acetaminophen or ibuprofen will suffice. Bone or deep tissue surgery may require a mild oral opiate for 3–5 days.

## COMPLICATIONS

In general, surgical treatments of facial palsy are well tolerated. For any procedure that involves implantation of a foreign material into the eyelid (e.g. gold or platinum weight,

TABLE 55-3 Key points in the management of facial palsy.

| Key points |
|---|
| • Patients with absent corneal sensation and/or absent Bell's phenomenon are at greatest risk of keratopathy |
| • Management should begin with conservative measures to lubricate the eye and protect the cornea |
| • Injections of botulinum toxin can also be an effective temporizing measure by inducing a protective ptosis |
| • For patients who show evidence of having long-term paralysis (i.e. no spontaneous nerve recovery after 6 months) surgical intervention may be indicated |

palpebral spring, or spacer/graft material), there is a risk of infection, migration, and/or extrusion. Palpebral springs in particular often require multiple revisions. Refractive change after weights and palpebral springs has been described. Management of patient expectations is important. Patients should be aware that perfect symmetry is unrealistic, and diminished symptoms and enhanced aesthetics is the goal. Despite good surgical results, ocular lubricants are usually still required. Patients should also be counseled that elevating procedures will tend to regress with time, and repeated interventions may be required in the long term.

## SURGICAL RESULTS AND DECISION MAKING

The techniques described in this chapter have been shown to be effective in mitigating the features of facial palsy. The efficacy of individual techniques over others is difficult to determine because most published studies involve retrospective case series, variable etiologies, and surgeon procedure preferences. Both the art and science of medicine are required to achieve satisfactory final outcomes.

Key points regarding surgical management are outlined in Table 55-3. A number of clinical algorithms have been proposed to guide the surgical management of facial palsy. Although there is no consensus regarding the ideal systematic approach, we have found the procedures listed to be the most useful in our practice. The algorithm used at our center is outlined in Flowchart 55-1.

## REFERENCES


1. Mehta RP. Surgical treatment of facial paralysis. Clin Exp Otorhinolaryngol. 2009;2(1):1-5.
2. Bhama P, Bhrany AD. Ocular protection in facial paralysis. Curr Opin Otolaryngol Head Neck Surg. 2013;21(4):353-7.
3. Momeni A, Khosla RK. Current concepts for eyelid reanimation in facial palsy. Ann Plast Surg. 2012.
4. Amer TA, El-Minawi HM, El-Shazly MI. Low-level versus high-level placement of gold plates in the upper eyelid in patients with facial palsy. Clin Ophthalmol (Auckland, NZ). 2011;5:891-5.
5. Liu JK, Saedi T, Delashaw JB, Jr, McMenomey SO. Management of complications in neurotology. Otolaryngol Clin N Am. 2007;40(3):651-67, x-xi.
6. Bergeron CM, Moe KS. The evaluation and treatment of upper eyelid paralysis. Facial Plast Surg: FPS. 2008;24(2):220-30.
7. Korn BS, Kikkawa DO. Video atlas of oculofacial plastic and reconstructive surgery. Edinburgh: Elsevier Saunders; 2011.
8. Boerner M, Seiff S. Etiology and management of facial palsy. Curr Opin Ophthalmol. 1994;5(5):61-6.
9. O'Connell JE, Robin PE. Eyelid gold weights in the management of facial palsy. J Laryngol Otol. 1991;105(6):471-4.
10. Silver AL, Lindsay RW, Cheney ML, et al. Thin-profile platinum eyelid weighting: a superior option in the paralyzed eye. Plast Reconstr Surg. 2009;123(6):1697-703.
11. Demirci H, Frueh BR. Palpebral spring in the management of lagophthalmos and exposure keratopathy secondary to facial nerve palsy. Ophthalm Plast Reconstr Surg. 2009;25(4):270-5.
12. Sadiq SA, Downes RN. A clinical algorithm for the management of facial nerve palsy from an oculoplastic perspective. Eye (London, England). 1998;12 ( Pt 2):219-23.
13. Terzis JK, Kyere SA. Minitendon graft transfer for suspension of the paralyzed lower eyelid: our experience. Plast Reconstr Surg. 2008;121(4):1206-16.
14. Tucker SM, Santos PM. Survey: management of paralytic lagophthalmos and paralytic ectropion. Otolaryngol Head Neck Surg: official journal of American Academy of Otolaryngology-Head and Neck Surgery. 1999;120(6):944-5.
15. Wearne MJ, Sandy C, Rose GE, et al. Autogenous hard palate mucosa: the ideal lower eyelid spacer? Br J Ophthalmol. 2001; 85(10):1183-7.
16. Hoenig JA, Shorr N, Shorr J. The suborbicularis oculi fat in aesthetic and reconstructive surgery. Int Ophthalmol Clin. 1997; 37(3):179-91.
17. Olver JM. Raising the suborbicularis oculi fat (SOOF): its role in chronic facial palsy. Br J Ophthalmol. 2000;84(12):1401-6.
18. Shindo M. Management of facial nerve paralysis. Otolaryngol Clin N Am. 1999;32(5):945-64.
19. Meltzer NE, Byrne PJ. Management of the brow in facial paralysis. Facial Plast Surg: FPS. 2008;24(2):216-9.
20. Yucel OE, Arturk AN. Botulinum toxin-A-induced protective ptosis in the treatment of lagophthalmos associated with facial paralysis. Ophthal plast Reconstr Surg. 2012;28(4):256-60.
21. Alsuhaibani AH. Facial nerve palsy: providing eye comfort and cosmesis. Middle East Afr J Ophthalmol. 2010;17(2):142-7.

22. Nava-Castaneda A, Tovilla-Canales JL, Boullosa V, et al. Duration of botulinum toxin effect in the treatment of crocodile tears. Ophthal Plast Reconstr Surg. 2006;22(6):453-6.
23. Wojno TH. Results of lacrimal gland botulinum toxin injection for epiphora in lacrimal obstruction and gustatory tearing. Ophthal Plast Reconstr Surg. 2011;27(2):119-21.
24. Julian GG, Hoffmann JF, Shelton C. Surgical rehabilitation of facial nerve paralysis. Otolaryngol Clin N Am. 1997;30(5): 701-26.
25. Wang W, Yang C, Li W, et al. Masseter-to-facial nerve transfer: is it possible to rehabilitate the function of both the paralyzed eyelid and the oral commissure? Aesth Plast Surg. 2012; 36(6): 1353-60.
26. Manktelow RT, Zuker RM. Muscle transplantation by fascicular territory. Plast Reconstr Surg. 1984;73(5):751-7.
27. Ueda K, Harii K, Yamada A, et al. A comparison of temporal muscle transfer and lid loading in the treatment of paralytic lagophthalmos. Scand J Plast Reconstr Surg Hand Surg/Nordisk plastikkirurgisk forening [and] Nordisk klubb for handkirurgi. 1995;29(1):45-9.

CHAPTER

56

# Eyelid Tumor Surgery

Roshmi Gupta, Santosh G Honavar

## INTRODUCTION

Surgery is the most widely practiced treatment modality for eyelid tumors, both benign and malignant. The treatment principles include complete excision of tumor with margin clearance, minimizing the chance of recurrence and reconstruction, preserving the function and cosmesis for the eyelid.

## SURGICAL TECHNIQUES

### Shave Excision

A benign tumor involving the eyelid margin may be excised for cosmesis. In shave excision, the eyelid is placed stretched against a lid guard, and with a #15 Bard-Parker blade, the tumor is excised flush to the lid margin contour. The eyelash line is spared. If a part of the lesion involves the base of the eyelashes, it is left behind. No suturing is required. This technique is unsuitable where there is any suspicion of malignancy (Figs. 56-1A and B).

### Excision of Cystic Lesions of the Eyelid

Several varieties of retention cysts may arise from the various glands on the eyelids. The cystic natures of most are evident on clinical examination. Cysts containing clear fluid transilluminate on examination. In most, the overlying skin is freely mobile over the cyst. An incision is placed at the margin of the lesion, taking care to incise the skin alone. The location of the incision is preferably in a skin crease, or along relaxed skin tension lines. Fine scissors are spread to dissect in between the skin and the lesion, severing the tissue attachments by stretching the surrounding tissue away from the lesion. The dissection reaches the circumference of the lesion

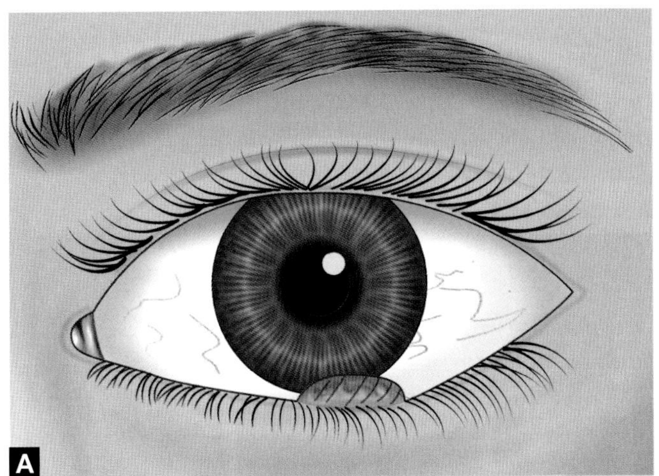


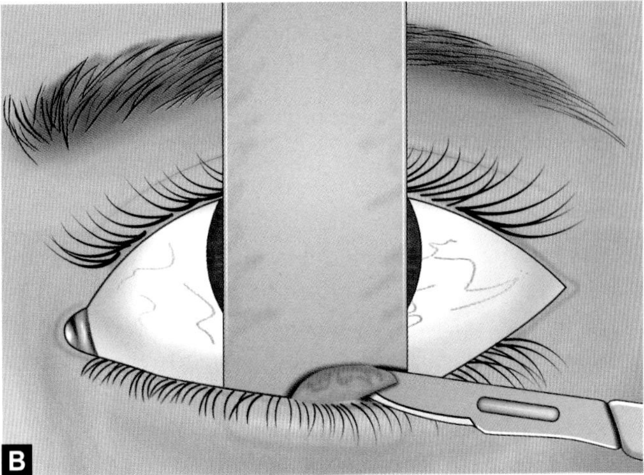


**Figures 56-1A and B** (A) A lesion on the lid margin (B) Lesion removed flush to the margin, sparing the lash line.

and continues deep to it, separating it from the underlying tissue. We avoid grasping the thin wall of the cyst with forceps and aim to remove the wall in toto. The overlying skin is often found stretched. Redundant skin may be excised from the edge of the incision, such that a smooth closure of the incision is possible.

## Complete Excision of Tumors with Margin Clearance

Any eyelid tumor suspected of malignancy requires particular attention. A complete excision with histopathologic examination is mandatory, along with verification of tumor-free edge and base of the excised area. This can be achieved by direct excision and verification of edge clearance by frozen section, or by Mohs' micrographic surgery.[1] In the eyelids, it is not feasible to obtain the wide margins available elsewhere in the body; tumor-free margin of 4–5 mm is considered adequate. Tumors that do not have a clear circumference pose a particular challenge, as in cases of pagetoid spread or skip lesions of sebaceous carcinoma, or morpheaform basal cell carcinoma.

## Direct Excision and Examination of Fresh Frozen Tissue

### *Tumors Involving the Anterior Lamella*

The incision line is marked with a 4–5 mm clinically free margin around the tumor, before any infiltration anesthesia is used. With a sharp Bard-Parker blade, incision is made to the full thickness of the skin, and scissors are used to dissect the tumor off the posterior lamella. This method is particularly suitable for the tumors which are less likely to involve full-thickness eyelid, for instance, basal cell carcinoma.

### *Full-Thickness Excision of Tumor*

The incision line is marked clearly leaving a 4–5 mm clinically tumor-free margin. A corneal protector shield or a lid guard is placed behind the eyelid, protecting the globe. The lid margin is placed on traction, and with sharp Bard-Parker knife, the incision line and the marginal incisions are made. The lid margin and the blade are carefully oriented to ensure that incisions are made at right angles to the lid margin. The excision is completed with sharp straight scissors. Curved scissors may cause a sloping of the tissue between the different layers, causing unequal margins on the skin and the conjunctival aspects. We avoid heavy use of electrosurgical units to reduce burn artifacts on the margins and ensure the instruments are sharp to avoid crush artifacts.

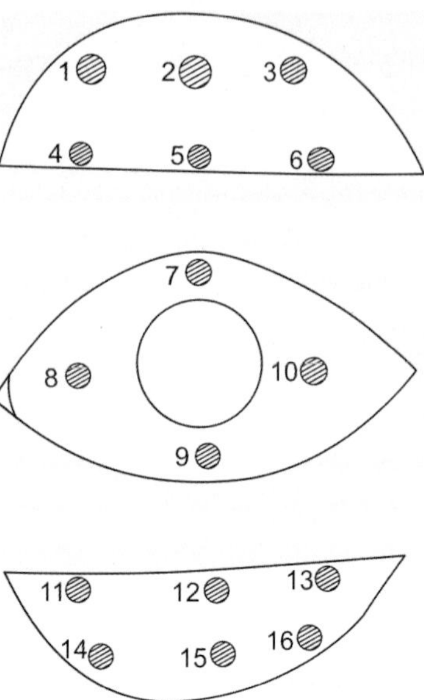


**Figure 56-2** Map biopsy specimens are placed on a filter paper with a drawing of the eye indicating location of each specimen.

### *Map Biopsy of the Conjunctiva*

Sebaceous carcinoma is known for pagetoid spread on the conjunctiva; the reported rates are as high as 44–80%.[2,3] At the time of removing the sebaceous carcinoma, a map biopsy is also performed for the conjunctiva. Small samples of tissue are excised from the conjunctiva in various quadrants and mounted on a filter paper with a diagram indicating the location (Fig. 56-2). Each sample is labeled. The pathologist is able to report back the exact location of the tumor positive sample.

### *Marking the Tissue for Orientation*

The excised eyelid tumor is attached to a filter paper, along with a free-hand diagram indicating the location of the tumor. The thin margins are excised, and mounted separately, clearly labeled nasal, temporal, inferior, or superior (Figs. 56-3A to D). The fresh tissue is transported to the laboratory; it is important to communicate clearly with the pathologist regarding the provisional clinical diagnosis.

### *Frozen Section*

The fresh excised tissue is transferred to the pathology lab. It is frozen in a cryostat machine, and the pathologist comments on the presence or absence of tumor cells in the excised margins and base. The markings for orientation help localize the area of interest. If indicated, further strips of tissue are excised, and the process repeated till a free margin is achieved; the surgeon then proceeds with reconstruction. The pathologist

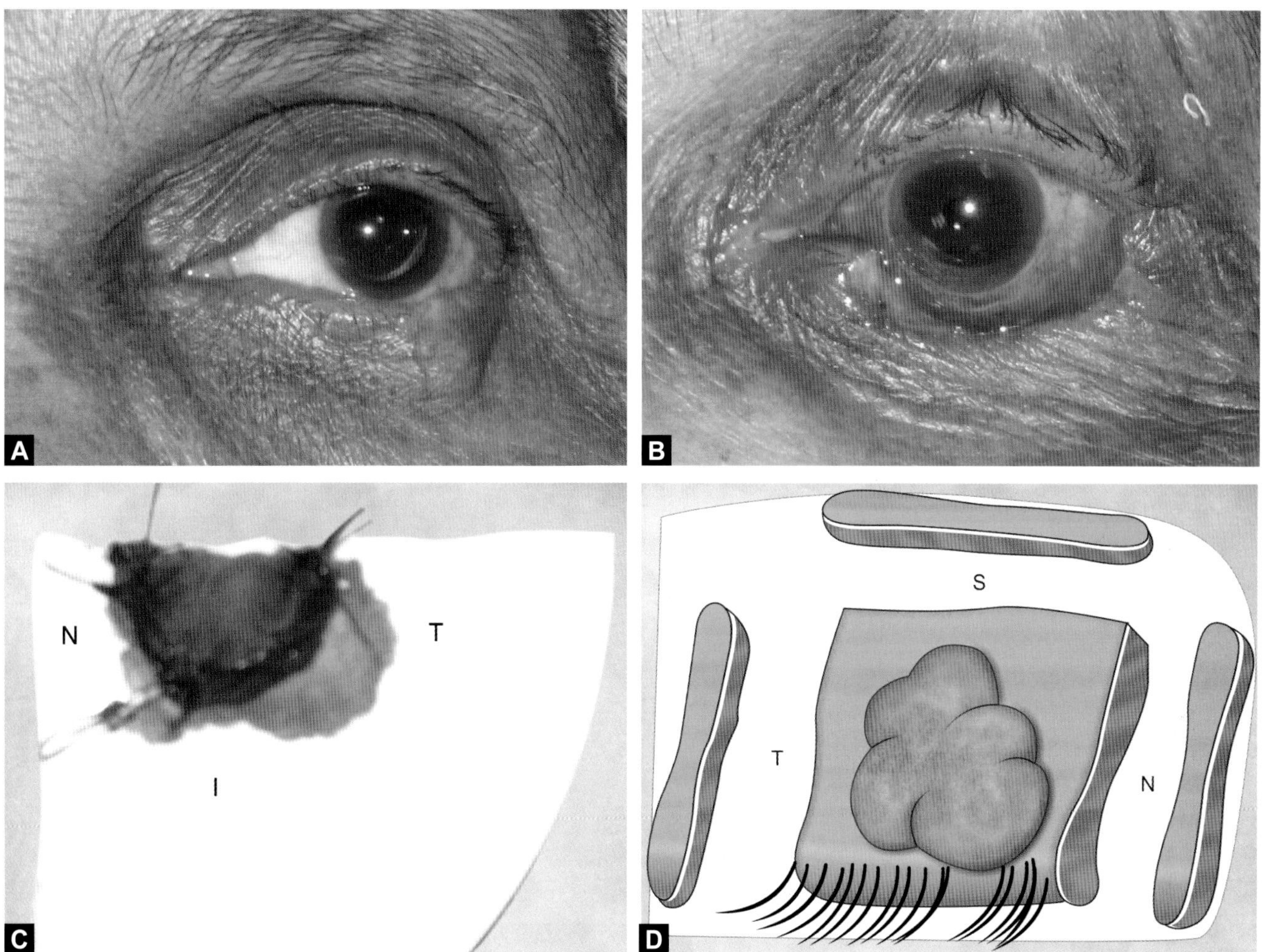


Figures 56-3A to D (A) Lower lid sebaceous carcinoma. (B) Excision with clear margins. (C) Mounting the specimen on filter paper with markings. (D) Eyelid specimen with margin specimen taken separately, marked for orientation.

will also perform a detailed histopathologic examination on the permanent sections.

In a location where frozen section pathology is unavailable within easy distance, tumor-free incision margin should still be verified. After excision, the eye is patched while the tissue is transported to the pathologist in 10% formalin, with the markings for orientation. The results of the histopathologic examination on permanent sections are known in 2–3 days, and the lid reconstruction can proceed. The delayed reconstruction does not cause any significant adverse outcome.[4,5]

## *Mohs' Micrographic Surgery*

Mohs' micrographic surgery is performed by a Mohs' surgeon who also examines the histopathology. The original surgery described by Frederick Mohs comprised in vivo fixation of the tumor tissue, and excision in layers, with several days intervals between layers. Currently, the fresh tissue technique is used for Mohs' surgery.[6,7]

The surgery is performed under local anesthesia. The tumor is debulked either with a scalpel, or a curette in case of a softer consistency. A one millimeter margin is taken around the circumference of the tumor, and a scalpel is held at 45° to make the incisions (Fig. 56-4A). Finally, the base is excised by holding the blade of the scalpel flat. If the layer removed is small enough to fit on a slide, it is examined as a whole. Otherwise, segments are placed on a slide separately, each clearly numbered. Each layer is divided into sections, and the sections are color coded using permanent tissue inks. The rule followed is that for each section, the sections on either side of it have different colors; this allows accurate identification of each location. An exact diagram of the lesion is made to help in orientation.

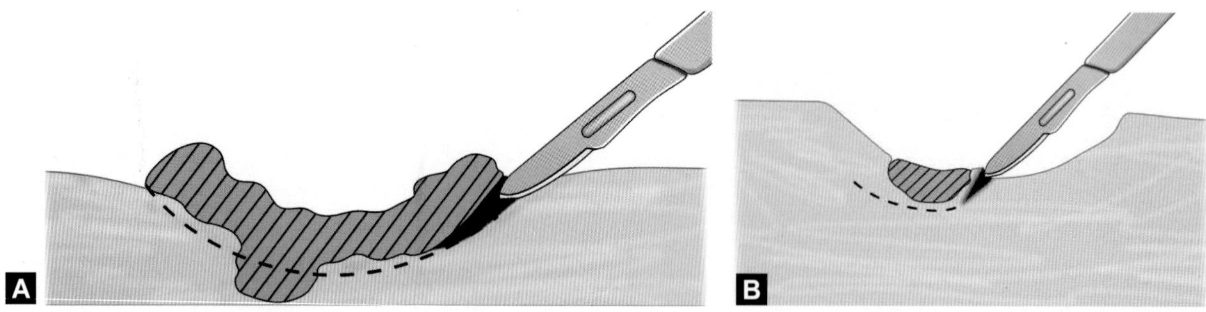


**Figures 56-4A and B** (A) First-layer excision in Mohs' surgery. (B) Second-layer excision: only the tumor-positive area is removed.

Each segment is placed on a slide and flattened so that the base and the edges lie on the same plane. Ornithine carbamoyltransferase is applied to the tissue, and the entire piece is frozen solid in the cryostat. Sections are cut with a microtome and stained with hematoxylin and eosin. Each section is examined, and if tumor tissue is seen, it is marked on the glass slide itself. Finally, the tumor-positive areas are marked on the initial diagram; the color coding helps in identifying the exact location. The next layer is excised for only the areas testing positive for tumor cells (Fig. 56-4B). The process is repeated till the base and edged are free of pathology.

The reconstructive surgeon repairs the surgical area the same day, or the next day. The plan of repair is made after the extent of the final defect is known.

### *Lymph Node Biopsy*

Lymph node biopsy for eyelid tumors includes needle biopsy of clinically suspected draining lymph nodes and sentinel node biopsy.

Fine-needle aspiration biopsy of clinically involved lymph node in preauricular and cervical locations may reveal presence of metatstases in lymph nodes.[8]

Sentinel node biopsy is a recent technique based on the premise that the first lymph node providing lymphatic drainage to the affected eyelid can indicate whether the rest of the lymphatic chain needs radical dissection and excision.[9] The area of the eyelid surrounding the tumor is injected with 0.2-mL isosulfan blue and 0.2-mL radioactive Tc 99m sulfur colloid. After an interval the area of the draining lymph nodes is explored. The bluish color or trace radioactivity on the handheld gamma probe can identify the first lymph node. This node is then dissected out and examined for lymph-borne metastasis. If it tests positive, the rest of the lymphatic chain is dissected. Sentinel node biopsy holds significance in eyelid tumors that have metastatic potential, such as sebaceous carcinoma or malignant melanoma.

## POSTOPERATIVE CARE

A light dressing is placed over the surgical area. A systemic antibiotic and an analgesic are prescribed. The dressing is removed the day after surgery, and an antibiotic ointment is applied. The patient returns for review at 1 week; at this visit the histopathologic report from the permanent sections is available, and any further management is planned.

## COMPLICATIONS

Surgical complications after eyelid tumor surgery are very rare. Wound infection happens very rarely. Wound dehiscence after repair would indicate inappropriate technique and closure of wound under excessive tension. A lesion extending close to the lid margin may later cause misdirected eyelashes. Scarring may have implications for both function and cosmesis of the eyelids.

## SURGICAL OUTCOMES

Achieving a tumor-free surgical margin reduces the metastasis and mortality for eyelid malignancies. Prior to the standard use of margin verification techniques, the metastasis and mortality form eyelid malignancies ranged from 2% to 36%.[10] After the techniques have been modified, the mortality and metastases have been reduced to 1–2% for squamous cell carcinoma and basal cell carcinoma, and 11% for sebaceous carcinoma.[11-14]

The largest series of eyelid tumors treated by Mohs' micrographic surgery or frozen-section control included basal cell carcinoma and squamous cell carcinoma. Sebaceous carcinoma and malignant melanoma of eyelid are rarer entities. Mohs' micrographic surgery gave the lowest recurrence rate for eyelid tumors, 1% for basal cell carcinoma and 1.9% for squamous cell carcinoma.[11,15] Frozen-section control is also recommended with Level 1 evidence, with recurrence rates of 1.6–2% for basal cell carcinoma.[1,4,16]

The outcomes for sebaceous carcinoma and malignant melanoma of eyelid come from retrospective studies, giving Level II evidence. However, for sebaceous carcinoma and malignant melanoma as well, either frozen-section control or Mohs' micrographic surgery is the surgical method preferred.[1] Map biopsy has been recommended to check for pagetoid spread of sebaceous carcinoma; this recommendation has Level 1 rating for evidence-based eyelid tumor management.[1,3,17] Pagetoid spread is found more commonly in superior tarsal and forniceal conjunctiva. Identification of such disease helps plan further management, such as cryotherapy, excision, or topical chemotherapy.

Sentinel lymph node can test positive for 20–33% of patients with ocular adnexal sebaceous carcinoma and malignant melanoma. Initial studies showed 20–25% false-negative results, which have improved subsequently.[18] Sentinel lymph node biopsy is currently recommended for eyelid malignant melanoma >1 mm in thickness, >1 mitotic figure/HPF, sebaceous carcinoma >10 mm in diameter, and all Merkel cell carcinoma.[19,20]

## LIMITATIONS OF TECHNIQUES

Excision with frozen-section edge control is easily available and widely practiced. However, with standard histopathologic techniques, presence of tumors cells in one particular region of the margin may be missed.

Mohs' micrographic surgery combines conservation of tissue with excision of all tumor cells from the margins. Since the Mohs' surgery and reconstruction are performed by different surgeons at different sittings, there is less conflict of interest, and operating room time is better utilized.

However, Mohs' micrographic surgery has certain limitations.[6] Tumors with noncontiguous growth patterns may not be adequately cleared by Mohs' micrographic surgery, for instance sebaceous carcinoma. A tumor difficult to interpret from frozen sections, or a tumor-associated inflammatory cells may not be distinguished well.

## CONCLUSION

Eyelid tumors are in a location where there can be diagnosed early. The paucity of tissues in the eyelid precludes excision of such wide margins as elsewhere in the body. Appropriate technique for management can reduce both recurrence and mortality.

## REFERENCES


1. Cook BE, Jr, Bartley GB. Treatment options and future prospects for the management of eyelid malignancies: an evidence-based update. Ophthalmology. 2001;108(11):2088-100.
2. Rao NA, Hidayat AA, McLean IW, et al. Sebaceous carcinomas of the ocular adnexa: a clinicopathologic study of 104 cases with five-year follow-up data. Hum Pathol. 1982;13(2):113-22.
3. Shields JA, Demirci H, Marr BP, et al. Conjunctival epithelial involvement by eyelid sebaceous carcinoma. The 2003 J. Howard Stokes lecture. Ophthal Plast Reconstr Surg. 2005;21(2): 92-6.
4. Hamada S, Kersey T, Thaller VT. Eyelid basal cell carcinoma: non-Mohs excision, repair, and outcome.Br J Ophthalmol. 2005; 89(8):992-4.
5. Hsuan JD, Harrad RA, Potts MJ, Collins C. Small margin excision of periocular basal cell carcinoma: 5 year results. Br J Ophthalmol. 2004; 88(3):358-60.
6. Odland P, Whitaker DC. Mohs micrographic surgery. In: Tse D (ed), Colour Atlas of oculoplastic surgery, 2nd edn. Philadelphia, PA: Lippincott Williams & Wilkins; 2011:196-201.
7. Rivlin D, Moy RL. Mohs' surgery for periorbital malignancies. In: Bosniak S (ed), Ophthalmic plastic and reconstructive surgery. Philadelphia, PA: WB Saunders; 1996:352-5.
8. Goyal S, Honavar SG, Naik M, Vemuganti GK. Fine needle aspiration cytology in diagnosis of metastatic sebaceous gland-carcinoma of the eyelid to the lymph nodes with clinicopathological correlation. Acta Cytol. 2011;55(5):408-12.
9. Golio D, Esmaeli B. Sentinel lymph node biopsy for conjunctival and eyelid malignancies. In: Guthoff R, Katowitz J (eds), Essentials in ophthalmology: oculoplastics and orbit. Heidelberg, Berlin: Springer-Verlag; 2006:38-46.
10. Payne JW, Duke JR, Butner R, Eifrig DE. Basal cell carcinoma of the eyelids. A long-term follow-up study. Arch Ophthalmol. 1969;81(4):553-8.
11. Mohs FE. Micrographic surgery for the microscopically controlled excision of eyelid cancers. Arch Ophthalmol. 1986;104(6): 901-9.
12. Kass LG, Hornblass A. Sebaceous carcinoma of the ocular adnexa. Surv Ophthalmol. 1989;33(6):477-90.
13. Shields JA, Demirci H, Marr BP, et al. Sebaceous carcinoma of the ocular region: a review. Surv Ophthalmol. 2005;50(2): 103-22.
14. Shields JA, Demirci H, Marr BP, et al. Sebaceous carcinoma of the eyelids: personal experience with 60 cases. Ophthalmology. 2004;111(12):2151-7.
15. Downes RN, Walker PJ, Collin JRO. Micrographic (MOHS') surgery in the management of periocular basal cell epitheliomas. Eye. 1990;4(Pt 1):160-8.
16. Frank HJ. Frozen section control of excision of eyelid basal cell carcinomas: 8 1/2 years' experience. Br J Ophthalmol. 1989; 73(5):328-32.
17. Putterman AM. Conjunctival map biopsy to determine pagetoid spread. Am J Ophthalmol. 1986;102(1):87-90.
18. Ho VH, Ross MI, Prieto VG, et al. Sentinel lymph node biopsy for sebaceous cell carcinoma and melanoma of the ocular adnexa. Arch Otolaryngol Head Neck Surg. 2007;133(8):820-6.
19. Pfeiffer ML, Savar A, Esmaeli B. Sentinel lymph node biopsy for eyelid and conjunctival tumors: what have we learned in the past decade? Ophthal Plast Reconstr Surg. 2013;29(1):57-62.
20. Esmaeli B, Nasser QJ, Cruz H, et al. American Joint Committee on Cancer T category for eyelid sebaceous carcinoma correlates with nodal metastasis and survival. Ophthalmology. 2012; 119(5):1078-82.

CHAPTER

57

# Techniques in Eyelid Reconstruction

Samuel Baharestani, Jonathan Pargament, Jeffrey Nerad

## INTRODUCTION

Eyelid reconstruction may be required following soft tissue trauma or tumor excision. Restoration of normal anatomy and function is always the goal regardless of the indication. There are many different eyelid repair techniques, the choice of which depends on the size, location, and depth of the eyelid defect. The most accurate determination of these variables requires a thorough understanding of eyelid and periocular anatomy. We will begin this chapter with a review of the relevant anatomical principles and use these fundamentals to discuss how to describe the eyelid defect. Then we will explore the advantages, disadvantages, and step-by-step process of each eyelid reconstruction technique.

### Eyelid Anatomy

The eyelid serves multiple functions, most importantly, protection of the eye. However, maintenance of normal lid anatomy is essential for the distribution of tears over the surface of the eye and facilitation of tear drainage. Fundamentally, the structure of the eyelid can be divided into the margin, anterior, and posterior lamellae and lateral and medial canthi.[1]

#### *Eyelid Margin*

The architecture of the eyelid margin can be described as a flat platform with angled anterior and posterior edges. The posterior edge of the margin is referred to as the mucocutaneous junction. Moving anteriorly, the structures encountered are the meibomian gland orifices, the gray line, and eyelash follicles (Fig. 57-1). Precise alignment of these structures is essential to restoring anatomy and function.

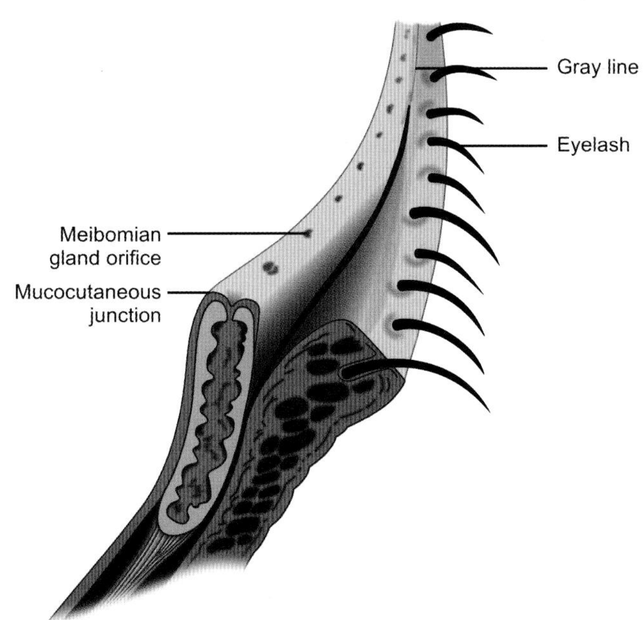


**Figure 57-1** Anatomy of the lower eyelid.

#### *Anterior and Posterior Lamellae*

Division of the eyelid into the anterior and posterior lamellae is a helpful concept.[2] The anterior lamella consists of the skin and orbicularis muscle. The posterior lamella is composed of the tarsus and tarsal conjunctiva. The gray line of the eyelid margin divides the anterior and posterior lamellae. As we will describe, defects of the anterior lamella are repaired differently from defects of the posterior lamella.

#### *Lateral Canthus*

The lateral canthal tendon is formed from the confluence of the upper and lower crura extending from each tarsal plate.

The tendon inserts at Whitnall's tubercle on the inner aspect of the lateral orbital rim approximately 10 mm below the frontozygomatic suture. Additional lateral support of the eyelid is provided by contributions from the orbicularis muscle, orbital septum, levator aponeurosis, and lower lid retractors. Reconstruction of the lateral canthus is relatively straightforward and requires reattachment of the remaining lateral tissues to the inside of the lateral orbital rim to achieve apposition of the lid against the globe.

### *Medial Canthus*

The medial canthal tendon is divided into the anterior and posterior limbs, which surround the lacrimal sac. The anterior limb attaches to the frontal process of the maxilla, while the posterior limb inserts on the posterior lacrimal crest. Surrounding the lacrimal sac is a tough layer of tissue called the lacrimal fascia, which fuses with the periosteum of the orbital rim and periorbita of the orbital walls. As a result, defects of the posterior limb may result in impaired apposition of the medial lower lid against the globe.

## Description of Eyelid Defect

The first step in describing the eyelid defect is a thorough examination to determine what structures are involved. It is especially important to evaluate for involvement of canalicular structures, canthal tendons, and the orbital septum. Next, depth of the defect is assessed. Depth can be described as partial thickness, including anterior or posterior lamellar, and full-thickness, involving all layers of the lid. The final step is to estimate the size in terms of percentage eyelid missing. An effective description of the eyelid defect provides the surgeon with the information needed to determine the most appropriate eyelid reconstruction technique.

# ANTERIOR LAMELLAR DEFECTS

Eyelid defects involving the skin and muscle anterior to the tarsal plates are referred to as anterior lamellar defects. However, we will use the same term to describe skin and muscle defects superior and inferior to the tarsal plates where no posterior lamella exists. Multiple options exist for repair of anterior lamellar defects including healing by granulation, primary closure with or without undermining, free skin graft, and myocutaneous advancement flap. Each of these techniques has advantages and disadvantages and may be combined with each other for the best result.

## Healing by Granulation

Healing by granulation is an option for small defects away from the eyelid margin. Completion of the healing process is prolonged and may result in scar formation. Granulation causes tissue contraction, which can alter normal anatomy and function. Canthal defects that occupy equal defects superior and inferior to the tendon may represent opportunities for healing by granulation.

## Primary Closure with or Without Undermining

Primary closure with or without undermining is an excellent technique for repair of small or moderate size anterior lamellar defects. If the patient has an abundance of redundant skin, primary closure can be performed without undermining. The lower eyelid and medial canthus normally have the least amount of redundant skin while the glabella, upper eyelid, and temple typically have more redundant tissue.

Undermining may be utilized to minimize tension on the skin closure of an anterior lamellar defect away from the eyelid margin. However, it is essential to have a thorough understanding of the tissue plane being mobilized to avoid damage to underlying nerves and blood vessels. For example, as the facial nerve courses from the tragus of the ear to the lateral eyebrow, its most superficial course is over the zygomatic arch. Undermining should be performed superficial to the nerve in the subcutaneous fat. Undermining in the eyelid should occur under the orbicularis muscle. In contrast, undermining outside of the orbital rim should be performed within the subcutaneous tissue. It is helpful to remember that tissue is most easily mobilized when the undermining is performed 90° from the natural skin crease. Orientation of the reconstruction with the skin crease minimizes tissue distortion and helps camouflage the scar. However, when repairing a lower lid defect, the surgeon must leave a vertical scar to minimize vertical traction and reduce the risk of ectropion or eyelid retraction.

After adequate undermining has been performed, anchoring sutures may be used to support the deep tissues and to take additional tension off of the final closure. Anchoring sutures secure the deep tissues to the periosteum along the inferior and lateral orbital rims or to the deep temporalis fascia. Anchoring sutures in lower eyelid reconstruction help prevent lower eyelid retraction or ectropion. Interrupted deep layer closure is utilized after tension is taken off of the edges of the defect. Routine skin closure can then be performed with interrupted sutures to provide slight eversion of wound edges without tension on the final wound closure.

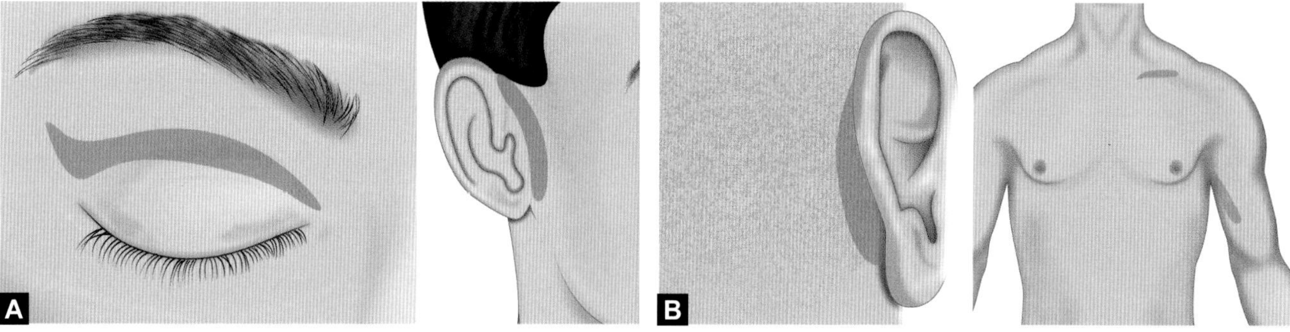


**Figures 57-2A and B** Donor sites to replace anterior lamella during eyelid reconstruction.

## Free Skin Grafts

Free skin grafts are used to repair an anterior lamellar defect. However, they usually result in an inferior cosmetic result compared with myocutaneous advancement flaps. Free skin grafts may be full or split thickness. Full-thickness graft donor sites require closure, whereas split-thickness grafts heal without closure and new skin grows over the defect. Both types of grafts are harvested from a donor site and used to fill the anterior lamellar defect. Graft survival is dependent on an adequate vascular supply provided by the recipient site. Full-thickness grafts are used commonly in eyelid reconstruction. Due to graft shrinkage and poor match in color, texture, and thickness, split-thickness grafts are utilized only when the defect is too large for a full-thickness graft and a myocutaneous flap is not possible. This discussion will focus on the full-thickness skin graft.

The first step of a full-thickness skin graft is choosing a donor site with the most similar color, texture, and thickness as the area surrounding the defect. Donor sites include skin of the upper eyelid, retro- or preauricular areas, supraclavicular area, or the upper inner arm (Figs. 57-2A and B). The upper eyelid skin is considered the best donor site, but the risk of asymmetry and lagophthalmos should be considered. Preauricular skin is an excellent option because of its character and accessibility. Retroauricular grafts provide excellent coverage, but harvesting and closure can be more difficult than any other donor sites.

## Myocutaneous Advancement Flaps

Myocutaneous advancement flaps are the best option for large anterior lamellar defects. They are created by dissecting the anterior lamellae overlying the orbital septum surrounding the defect and then stretching it into position over the defect. Use of the surrounding tissue means an excellent match for color and texture. Other advantages include preserved motor and sensory innervation, a rich blood supply, and near normal rates of postoperative functioning. Myocutaneous flaps may also be used to cover bare bone, because they bring their own blood supply.

Creation of the myocutaneous flap begins with an incision in a natural skin crease. When developing the flap, remember the principles emphasized in the discussion of primary closure with undermining. It is important to know the planes that are being mobilized and to avoid the facial nerve coursing lateral to the brow and superficially over the zygomatic arch. The surgeon should strive for horizontal tension as vertical tension may cause eyelid retraction or ectropion. As the flap is developed, periodically pause and check to see if enough tissue has been mobilized to cover the defect without tension. A small amount of contraction always occurs during healing so when in doubt dissect further. Once the flap is sufficient to cover the defect, anchoring sutures are placed from the undersurface of the flap to the periosteum at the orbital rim to support the flap and reduce tension on the skin closure. A small overcorrection of the vertical height of the flap at the lateral canthus will prevent lid retraction and lateral canthal dystopia. There should be a low threshold for a concomitant lateral tarsal strip when closing anterior lamellar defects under tension to avoid posterior lamellar laxity.

# REPAIR OF FULL-THICKNESS EYELID DEFECTS UP TO 25%

## Primary Eyelid Margin Repair

There are multiple techniques to repair a full-thickness eyelid defect. Classically, it has been taught that the technique utilized to repair the eyelid is chosen based on the percentage defect. However, interpatient differences in tissue laxity and character means that the most effective repair may not correlate with a given percentage defect. The best approach is to try to pull the defect together and then choose the simplest technique to close the defect without tension. The primary eyelid margin repair technique is utilized if the defect can be closed without undue tension.

The first step in the primary eyelid margin repair is identification of the pertinent anatomic structures. Local anesthetic with epinephrine is injected into the wound margins, and topical anesthetic is instilled into the eye. Using vertical mattress (7-0 Vicryl) sutures passed through the meibomian gland orifices, the margin is aligned and everted. It is helpful to keep this suture long for eyelid traction. With the margin aligned, the tarsal plate is sutured using two or three interrupted 5-0 Vicryl sutures in a lamellar fashion. These sutures are important because they provide the strength of the closure. Next, an additional vertical mattress suture is passed anterior to the gray line, which should align the eyelashes and provide further eyelid eversion. Finally, the skin is reapproximated with interrupted simple or vertical sutures using permanent or absorbable stitches.

### Lateral Canthal Defects of < 25%

Small defects involving the lateral canthus can be repaired using the lateral tarsal strip procedure.[3] First, a strip is formed from the remaining tarsus and sutured to the periorbita on the inner aspect of the lateral orbital wall. Use of the P-2 small circle needle will ease anchoring of the tarsal strip. If the periosteum of the lateral orbital rim must be sacrificed, as in a tumor excision, two holes should be drilled in the lateral orbital rim to serve as anchoring points for the reattachment of the tarsus.

In cases where the full-thickness defect is large and the remaining tarsus cannot stretch to the orbital rim, a 5-mm periosteal strip from the superolateral rim may be created and sutured to the cut end of the tarsus. The anterior lamellae will need to be repair using the myocutaneous flap discussed above. If the defect is too large and the periosteal strip is insufficient, use of a free tarsal graft or a Hughes flap may be required. These techniques will be discussed below. In some cases, combinations are required.

### Medial Canthal Defects of <25%

Eyelid defects involving the medial canthus are complicated by involvement of the lacrimal drainage system and the difficult reattachment of the eyelid to the posterior lacrimal crest.[4] If the lacrimal drainage system is involved, canalicular reconstruction can be attempted with a pigtail probe or Crawford/Monoka stents. A more anatomic reattachment of the medial canthus may be achieved if the canaliculus is not reconstructed. First, Wescott scissors are used to incise the conjunctiva between the plica and caruncle. Blunt dissection using Stevens scissors is then performed to access the medial orbital wall. Next, a permanent suture is used to reattach the cut end of the tarsus to the posterior lacrimal crest. A canthotomy and cantholysis may be required to allow the eyelid to move laterally if the defect will not stretch to the medial orbital wall. If removal of a tumor requires sacrifice of the entire lacrimal system, periosteum and canthal tendons, a Y-shaped microplate is the best option to reattach the remaining eyelid. The plate is attached to the maxillary process of the frontal bone. A slight overcorrection of the height and posterior position of the microplate will help achieve an optimal result. A Prolene suture on a free needle is used to suture the remaining lid tissue to the plate.

## REPAIR OF FULL-THICKNESS EYELID DEFECTS OF 25 TO 50%

### Canthotomy, Cantholysis, and Eyelid Margin Closure

Full-thickness eyelid defects that are too large to be repaired with primary closure require a canthotomy and cantholysis.[5-7] This technique involves advancement of a small amount of skin medially over the lateral orbital rim to become part of the lateral lid margin. First, local anesthetic with epinephrine is injected under the skin of the lateral canthus and conjunctiva. The canthotomy is created using Wescott scissors, Stevens scissors, or a Colorado needle to open the lateral canthus for 1 cm (Figs. 57-3A to D). The cantholysis is performed using scissors turned 90° to the eyelid margin to 'strum' the deep tissues to find the crus. Once the crus is found, the tissue is cut until the lid is released from the rim. If a canthotomy and cantholysis does not mobilize the tissue enough to allow for closure without tension, the canthotomy should be extended to perform a Tenzel flap procedure. This technique will be described below.

## REPAIR OF LID DEFECTS OF 50 TO 75%

### The Tenzel Flap

A Tenzel flap allows for closure of a marginal eyelid defect that involves 50% of the lid in a single-stage procedure.[8-11] This procedure involves performing a lateral canthotomy and inferior cantholysis to form a long-arched incision toward and often past the lateral orbital rim. The mobilization of this rotational flap provides good donor tissue for closing larger

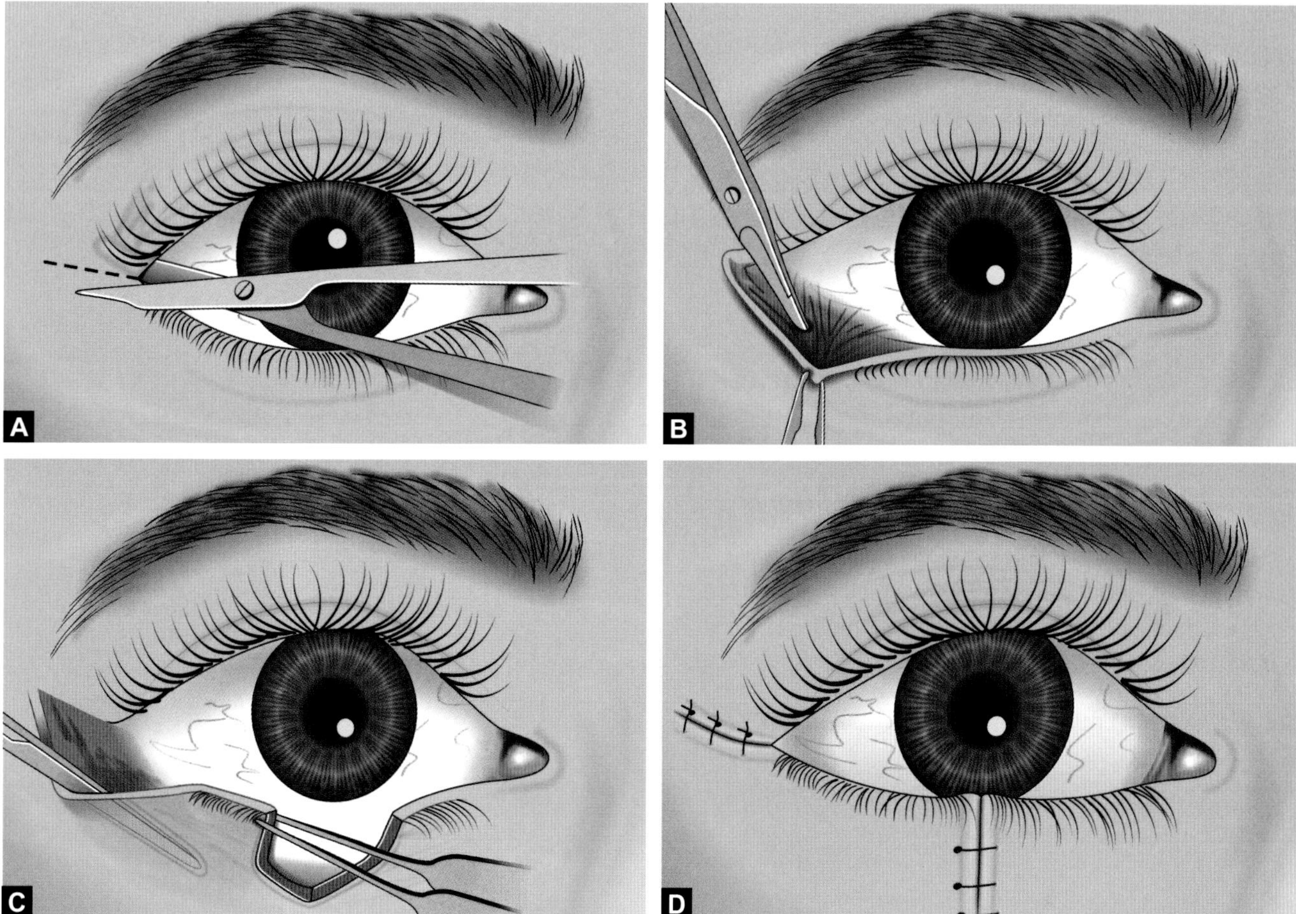


Figures 57-3A to D Lateral canthotomy and inferior cantholysis to recruit and mobilize the lateral eyelid to achieve reapposition of the eyelid margin.

eyelid defects and can be thought of as the beginning of a larger rotational flap called the Mustarde cheek rotation.

It is important to note that the frontal branch of the facial nerve passes in this region, thus it is important to keep the incision superficial to avoid inadvertent injury. After the flap has been created, it may be necessary to intermittently check the tension on the wound edges so that the perfect match between lateral canthal incision and wound apposition can be made. Once noted to be in good position, the eyelid margin may be repaired in the standard fashion as described earlier.

## REPAIR OF LOWER LID DEFECTS OF 75% OR GREATER

### The Hughes Procedure

The Hughes procedure is used to reconstruct the posterior lamella of a full-thickness lower eyelid defect that is too large for the use of a Tenzel flap.[12] This procedure replaces the missing tarsus and conjunctiva of the lower eyelid by borrowing it from the upper lid. By remaining attached to its vascular pedicle after primary repair, the tarsoconjunctival flap renders the patient monocular until division.

After measuring the lower eyelid defect, the Hughes flap is harvested from the upper eyelid. Classically, up to 20 mm of tarsus can be moved down to the lower eyelid and 3 mm of tarsus must be left in the upper lid to prevent entropion. The graft is secured to the remaining lower eyelid tarsus and overlying anterior lamellar repair can be done using the techniques above. Division of the eyelids is generally done after 3–4 weeks, re-establishing binocularity. As one would imagine, this procedure would be a suboptimal choice in the monocular patient.

### Free Tarsal Graft

A free tarsal graft can be harvested from the contralateral upper eyelid to replace missing posterior lamellae of a lower eyelid defect.[13] The advantage of a free tarsal graft is that it requires only a single procedure. However, the free tarsus does not have its own blood supply, thus must be covered by a myocutaneous advancement flap. Similar to a Hughes procedure except for the severing of the graft, a free tarsal graft provides an excellent option for large posterior lamellar reconstruction when adequate anterior lamella exists for an overlying advancement flap.

## SUMMARY

Eyelid reconstruction after an acquired defect is a common challenge to the ophthalmic plastic surgeon that can be approached in a step-wise fashion to achieve both a functionally and cosmetically acceptable result. The choice of procedure depends on the degree of eyelid laxity, quality of eyelid skin, location and size of the defect, and the surgeon's experience. Restoration of eyelid anatomy and dynamic function can be achieved through the recruitment of local tissues or harvesting of remote grafts to reconstruct eyelid defects of any size.

## REFERENCES


1. Orbit, eyelids, and lacrimal system. BCSC Section 7. American Academy of Ophthalmology; 2008.
2. Jeffrey A. Nerad. Techniques in ophthalmic plastic surgery with DVD: a personal tutorial. Philadelphia, PA: Saunders; 2010.
3. Anderson, RL, Gordy, DD: The tarsal strip procedure. Arch Ophthalmol. 1979;97:2192-6.
4. Daily RA, Habrich D. Medial canthal reconstruction. In: Bosniak S (ed), Principles and practice of ophthalmic plastic and reconstructive surgery, Vol 2. Philadelphia, PA: WB Saunders; 1996:387-99.
5. Jackson IT (ed). Local flaps in head and neck reconstruction. St. Louis: CV Mosby; 1985.
6. McCord CD. System of repair of full-thickness eyelid defects. In: McCord CD, Tannenbaum M, Nunery WR (eds), Oculoplastic surgery, 3rd edn. New York: Raven Press; 1995:85-97.
7. McCord CD, Nunery WR, Tanenbaum M. Reconstruction of the lower eyelid and outer canthus. In: McCord CD, Tannenbaum M, Nunery WR (eds), Oculoplastic surgery, 3rd edn. New York: Raven Press; 1995:119-44.
8. Patrinely JR, Marines HM, Anderson, RL. Skin flaps in periorbital reconstruction. Surv Ophthalmol. 1987;31(4):249-61.
9. Wesley RE, McCord CD. Reconstruction of the upper eyelid and medial canthus. In: McCord CD, Tannenbaum M, Nunery WR (eds), Oculoplastic surgery, 3rd edn. New York: Raven Press; 1995:99-117.
10. Shinder R, Esmaeli B. Eyelid and ocular adnexal reconstruction. In: Black EH, Nesi FA, Calvano CJ, Gladstone, GJ, Levine MR (eds), Smith and Nesi's ophthalmic plastic and reconstructive surgery, 3rd edn. New York: Springer; 2012:551-70.
11. Tenzel RR, Stewart WB. Eyelid reconstruction by the semicircle flap technique. Ophthalmology. 1978;85(11):1164-9.
12. Hughes WL. Total lower lid reconstruction: technical details. Trans Am Ophthalmol Soc. 1976;74:321-9.
13. Stephenson CM, Brown BZ. The use of tarsus as a free autogenous graft in eyelid surgery. Ophthal Plastic Reconstr Surg. 1985;1(1):43-50.

CHAPTER

58

# Botulinum Toxins Injections—Functional and Aesthetic

Shubhra Goel, Cat Nguyen Burkat

## INTRODUCTION

Injection of botulinum toxin A is one of the most popular noninvasive facial rejuvenation techniques in the modern world. Although originating as a potentially lethal substance, its history within the fields of ophthalmology, oculoplastics, and facial cosmetics has been very fascinating.

The history of botulinum toxin can be traced back to 800 AD when it was referred to as "sausage poison", as the bacterium was believed to grow from improperly handled meat products. In 1822, Kerner published his ideas for therapeutic uses of botulinum toxin to treat neurological disorders.[1] Later in 1949, Burgen made the landmark discovery that botulinum toxin blocks the neurotransmitter at the neuromuscular junction.[2] Subsequently, Alan Scott, in 1970, became one of the first to utilize botulinum toxin in patients with strabismus. Food and Drug Administration (FDA) approval for human use was granted in 1978, and since then botulinum toxin was used therapeutically to treat esophageal achalasia, eyelid blepharospasm, and other facial dystonias.[3] In 1992, Carruthers and Carruthers published the use of botulinum toxin to alleviate facial wrinkles. Allergen purchased the rights in 1988 to use the toxin for clinical trials, and in 1989[3-6] the FDA-approved botulinum toxin for the treatment of strabismus, blepharospasm, and hemifacial spasm associated with dystonia in patients ≥12 years of age. In 1991, botulinum toxin achieved its trade name, BOTOX.[3] Molecular analysis and categorization into A–C types emerged thereafter. In 1997, the FDA approved a new bulk toxin source for use in the manufacture of botulinum toxin A, or BTX-A. The new product, known as BOTOX, was comparable in clinical efficacy to the "original" BOTOX, but it had a significant decrease in neurotoxin protein thus resulting in less antibody production.

In 2000, the FDA approved BOTOX (Allergen, botulinum toxin type A) and Myobloc (Elan Pharmaceuticals, botulinum toxin type B) for the treatment of cervical dystonia. In the ensuing years, BOTOX expanded in both functional applications, such as for hyperhidrosis and migraine headaches, and cosmetic applications when it was FDA approved in 2002 for the treatment of glabellar wrinkles.

The clinical uses of botulinum toxin are still emerging throughout all fields of medicine. It has undoubtedly become one of the most desirable nonsurgical treatment modalities in the aesthetic oculofacial field. Therefore, the physician must be thoroughly knowledgeable in the facial anatomy, indications, techniques, and individual variations to avoid undue complications.

## INDICATIONS IN OPHTHALMOLOGY AND OCULOPLASTIC SURGERY

### Functional

- Blepharospasm is a focal dystonia of the orbicularis oculi muscles, manifested by the involuntary closure and exaggerated blinking of the eyelids. On average, 12.5–25 units (U) per side can be injected just beneath the skin over or into the orbicularis muscle.[3-7] A common injection pattern is injecting the medial and lateral orbital orbicularis oculi muscles (above and below the medial and lateral eyebrows), and along the lateral canthus and inferior orbital rim. In general, placement of botulinum toxin closer to the lid margin into the preseptal and pretarsal orbicularis would increase the risk of lower lid ectropion. Rarely, if necessary, the medial and lateral portions of the pretarsal orbicularis may be injected, avoiding the central lid region to minimize the risk of ptosis[4] (Fig. 58-1).

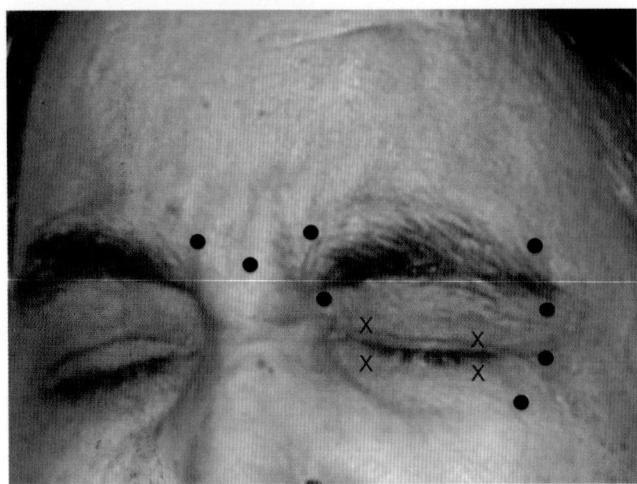


**Figure 58-1** Patient with bilateral blepharospasm. The glabellar muscle complex will often spasm in addition to the orbicularis oculi muscle; therefore, injection sites should include the corrugator, procerus, and the medial and lateral orbital orbicularis muscles (above and below the brow hairs). Pretarsal orbicularis oculi injections should be preserved for those with inadequate results, or apraxia of lid opening.

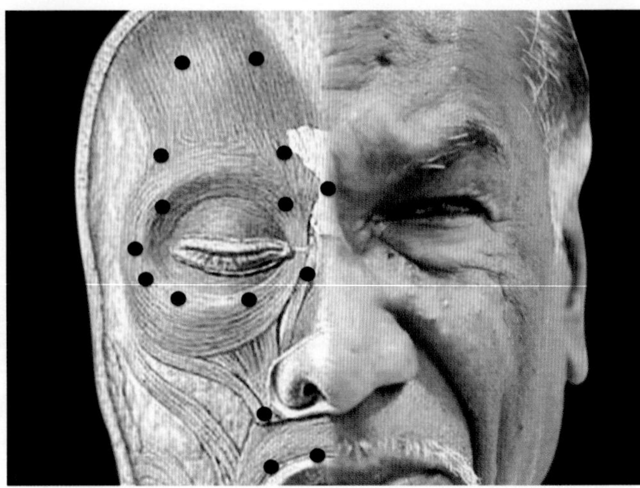

**Figure 58-2** Patient with left-sided hemifacial spasm. The injection sites target the affected forehead, periocular, and lower facial muscles [levator labii (top of the nasolabial fold), depressor anguli oris (below angle of the mouth), mentalis (middle of lower chin), orbicularis oris]. Chemodenervation of the platysma muscle may also be indicated.

- Apraxia is an inability to perform learned complex movements in the absence of paralysis, sensory loss, or disturbance of coordination. Eyelid apraxia, or apraxia of lid opening, refers to the nonparalytic inability to raise the upper eyelid in the absence of levator muscle injury. Apraxic-like eyelids have been associated with disorders such as dystonic Parkinson syndrome, progressive supranuclear palsy, and isolated loss of levator muscle control. Apraxia of lid opening seen in benign essential blepharospasm is important to note on examination, as the injection pattern may include placement of 1.25–2.5 U botulinum toxin into the pretarsal orbicularis oculi portion to help eyelid opening.[6] In some cases, patients with lid apraxia have been found to have less optimal results with chemodenervation and may progress to orbicularis myectomy surgery sooner.
- Hemifacial spasm refers to involuntary large muscle spasms of one half of the face, from the forehead frontalis muscle down to the platysma of the neck. Complete neurological evaluation must include imaging of the cerebellopontine angle of the brainstem to rule out a tumor mass compressing the facial nerve. If the patient is not a candidate for decompression surgery of the facial nerve, the spasms may be alleviated dramatically by botulinum injection to the periorbital region, as described above for blepharospasm, along with injection to the middle and lower face if indicated. Some potential sites of injection if spasms are prominent include the top of the nasolabial fold, the angle of the mouth, the depressor anguli oris along the mandible, the mentalis muscle, and the platysmal bands[4] (Fig. 58-2).
- Facial synkinesis following facial nerve paralysis—facial nerve palsy can result in permanent motor dysfunction and may manifest as increased blinking and eyelid spasms on either the paretic or the nonparalytic side. This may result from increased excitability of facial motor neurons mediating trigeminal reflexes. Significant synkinesis can result in facial deformity, inappropriate eyelid closure, drooling, and facial twitching mimicking hemifacial spasm. Use of botulinum toxin in an injection pattern similar to hemifacial spasm can effectively reduce discomfort, social embarrassment, and facial asymmetry.
- Therapeutic chemical tarsorrhaphy—blepharoptosis can be a potential side effect of botulinum injection in the periorbital area due to the inadvertent spread of toxin into the levator aponeurosis. This complication is typically cosmetically unacceptable to the patient. However, this induced ptosis can be beneficial in patients with poor blink reflex, lagophthalmos, or nonhealing corneal ulcers. One to three injections of 2.5 to 5 U of botulinum toxin injected directly into the levator or Müller's muscle can result in a chemical tarsorrhaphy in select patients. This allows improved corneal protection for healing while simultaneously permitting frequent examinations with ease. The injections can be placed transcutaneously above the superior tarsal level, or transconjunctivally superior to the tarsus with the lid

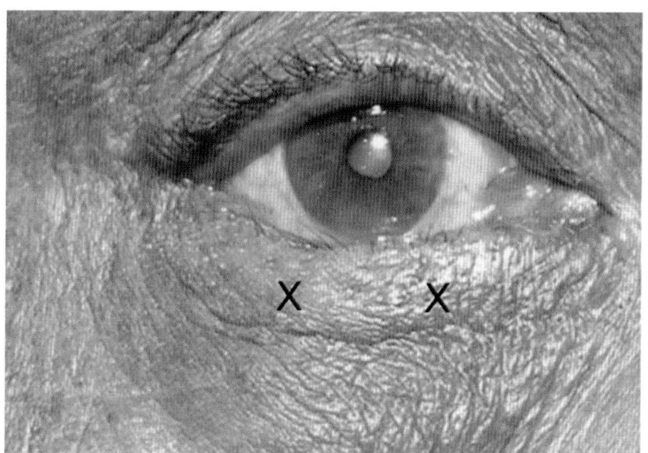


**Figure 58-3** Typical injection sites for correction of lower lid spastic entropion. The injections are placed subcutaneously in the preseptal orbicularis oculi muscle.

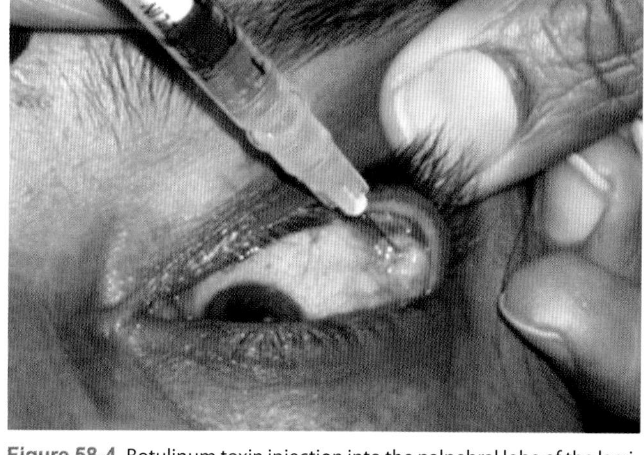

**Figure 58-4** Botulinum toxin injection into the palpebral lobe of the lacrimal gland. It is important to direct the needle away from the globe to avoid inadvertent perforation.

everted. Take care to avoid injecting too superficially in the orbicularis oculi muscle as this could result in weakened eyelid closure, thus exacerbating the corneal exposure.[6]

- Lid retraction—upper eyelid retraction in patients with thyroid eye disease can often be cosmetically objectionable, and it may also lead to corneal exposure and secondary tearing or dry eyes. Botulinum toxin can be a simple, albeit temporary, office alternative for patients who are not undergoing surgical intervention, have residual retraction after surgical retraction repair, or are still in the active stage of thyroid eye disease. Small doses of toxin are usually injected at 1–3 sites across the lid into the levator or Müller's muscle, performed transcutaneously or transconjunctivally, as described above.
- Lower lid entropion—spastic lower lid entropion occurs when there is any ocular surface irritation that results in preseptal orbicularis override of the pretarsal orbicularis oculi muscle. The eyelid margin rotation causes the eyelashes to rub the corneal surface, which further precipitates more lid squeezing and entropion. This spastic cycle can be temporarily relieved by weakening the lower lid muscle tone with 2.5-U botulinum toxin injected subcutaneously at 2–3 sites along the preseptal orbicularis oculi muscle. Placement too high into the pretarsal orbicularis muscle, or large doses of botulinum toxin (particularly if there is pre-existing horizontal lid laxity), could potentially result in iatrogenic lid margin ectropion. Proper technique could thus achieve symptomatic relief in patients suffering from keratitis due to eyelash trichiasis, without the need for surgical intervention (Fig. 58-3).
- Hyperlacrimation—primary lacrimal gland hypersecretion and gustatory epiphora are both extremely rare, but like severe reflex lacrimation, can lead to constant irritation, tearing, and periocular dermatitis. A total of 2.5–5 U of botulinum toxin can be injected into the palpebral lobe of the lacrimal gland to effectively reduce tear production[3] (Fig. 58-4).
- Dry eye—standard treatments for chronic dry eye syndrome, such as punctal cautery, punctal plugs, autologous serum, and lubricating eye drops, can often be insufficient for relief of symptoms. A small injection of botulinum toxin into the medial portion of the pretarsal orbicularis muscle of the lower lid, or to both the upper and lower lids, reduces the effectiveness of the orbicularis muscle pump mechanism surrounding the canaliculi. In conjunction with conservative medical therapy, this can provide significant symptomatic improvement.
- Wound healing, trauma, and eyelid reconstruction—use of botulinum toxin in wound healing is a relatively new modality of treatment. In general, wounds that are repaired along relaxed skin tension lines, under minimum tension, are more stable and heal with minimal scarring. Incisions under tension develop wider, thicker, and more hypertrophic scars. Botulinum toxin can be an adjunct to minimize wound tension by temporarily weakening the surrounding muscles that are inducing tension.

## Cosmetic

- Wrinkle reduction—botulinum toxin is the most popular nonsurgical facial rejuvenation procedure and treats dynamic facial rhytids as apposed to static creases. While FDA approval in 2002 was only for the correction of glabellar lines, the off-label use of BOTOX. Cosmetic in cosmetic facial rejuvenation has been in practice for many years. Some practical pearls for the use of BOTOX. Cosmetic throughout the face will be highlighted in the techniques section below.

- Brow elevation—nonsurgical correction of lateral brow ptosis can be achieved by injection of botulinum toxin into the orbital portion of the orbicularis oculi muscle over the superolateral rim, just inferior to the brow tail.[5,8-10]
- Neck rejuvenation—vertical neck bands, or platysmal ridges, can be softened with the use of botulinum injections at several sites along the length of the band. Even small amounts of toxin, placed 1–3 cm apart along the ridges, can effectively weaken the platysma muscle contraction, and thus create a smoother neck contour. Aggressive injection can affect the ability to swallow.[5,8-10]
- Acne—Although there are no long-term studies to support the efficacy of botulinum toxin for this indication, it has shown promising results in patients with active acne. Botulinum toxin is believed to decrease sebum secretion by blocking the chemical acetylcholine, which stimulates oil production, and secondly by paralyzing the small muscles that surround pores to prevent them from expanding.
- Axillary hyperhydrosis—treatment of severe axillary hyperhydrosis with botulinum toxin was FDA approved in 2004. Botulinum toxin decreases secretion by targeting the postganglionic sympathetic cholinergic nerves to eccrine sweat glands. Typically, a grid pattern of many small injections is spread diffusely over the axilla, with each site typically starting at 2.5 U. Significant improvement in sweating can occur within a few weeks.

## CONTRAINDICATIONS

- Prior allergic reaction to Botox, Myobloc, Dysport, or Xeomin, or albumin (eggs).
- Pregnancy.
- Lactating/breastfeeding.
- Diseases of the neuromuscular junction (e.g. myasthenia gravis, amyotropic lateral sclerosis), as underlying systemic weakness can be exacerbated.
- Use of medications, such as aminoglycosides, penicillamine, quinine, and calcium channel blockers, that further decrease neuromuscular transmission.
- Infection at injection site; a careful history of herpetic infections should also be taken.

## RELATIVE CONTRAINDICATIONS

- Use of chronic anticoagulants
- Aspirin, nonsteroidal anti-inflammatory drugs such as ibuprofen, vitamin E, ginger, gingko biloba, ginseng, and garlic should ideally be discontinued 7–14 days prior to the procedure to minimize bleeding and bruising
- Unrealistic expectations.

## STRUCTURE AND RECONSTITUTION

Botulinum toxin exists as seven distinct serotypes, A–G, each with different terminal binding configurations. The neurotoxin molecule is synthesized by the clostridium bacterium and acts on cholinergic nerve terminals. The fundamental mechanism of action of botulinum toxin is to inhibit the extracellular release of acetylcholine at the neuromuscular junction, thus lowering the probability that an action potential will propagate and result in muscle fiber contraction. This results in local chemodenervation of the muscle and paralysis of the target muscle. Inhibition of acetylcholine exocytosis by botulinum toxin is temporary, and neurotransmission is eventually restored in weeks to months. This functional recovery is thought to be secondary to noncollateral sprouting of nerve fibers from the terminal axon.[3-6]

The potency of botulinum toxin is expressed in terms of units (U). One U is defined as the amount of toxin that is lethal in 50% of female Swiss-Webster mice following intraperitoneal injection, also called the mouse LD50. BOTOX Cosmetic is available in the lyophilized freeze-dried form, in 50/100/200 Unit vials. The vials are vacuum sealed and contain 0.5 mg of human albumin and 0.9 mg of preservative-free sodium chloride. Prior to use, reconstitution with 0.9% preservative or nonpreservative normal saline is required to formulate concentrations of 2–10 U/0.1 mL. For instance, reconstitution with 4 mL of normal saline yields a concentration of 2.5 U/0.1 mL botulinum toxin, whereas 2 mL of diluent would yield a concentration of 5 U/0.1 mL (Tables 58-1 and 58-2). The cap on the vial should be cleansed with 70% alcohol before adding the diluent. According to the manufacturer's directions for use, a vial should be discarded if the vacuum does not pull the diluent into the vial. However, the plunger of the syringe should be held prior to the addition of saline and slowly released with the diluent running along the

**TABLE 58-1** Storage recommendations on the use of botulinum toxin type A in facial aesthetics

| Parameter | Recommendation |
|---|---|
| Storage<br>Before reconstitution | 2°C to 8°C for up to 24 months |
| After reconstitution | 4 hours at 2°C to 8°C<br>Up to 6 weeks at 4°C |
| Handling | Special precautions not required |

**TABLE 58-2** Reconstitution recommendations on the use of botulinum toxin type A in facial aesthetics

| Parameter | Recommendation | |
|---|---|---|
| Diluent | Preserved 0.9% saline (preferred)<br>Nonpreserved 0.9% saline | |
| Concentration | 2.5 U/0.1 mL starting dose, up to 4, 5, or 10 U/0.1 mL as deemed necessary to optimize higher concentration of botulinum toxin into smaller volumes, as this minimizes large volume injections that increase diffusion into surrounding tissues and muscles | |
| Dilution | **Dilution for 100 U vial addition of mL of normal saline** | **Dose in units per 0.1 mL** |
| | 1.0 | 10 |
| | 2.0 | 5 |
| | 4.0 | 2.5 |
| | 8.0 | 1.25 |
| | 10.0 | 1.0 |

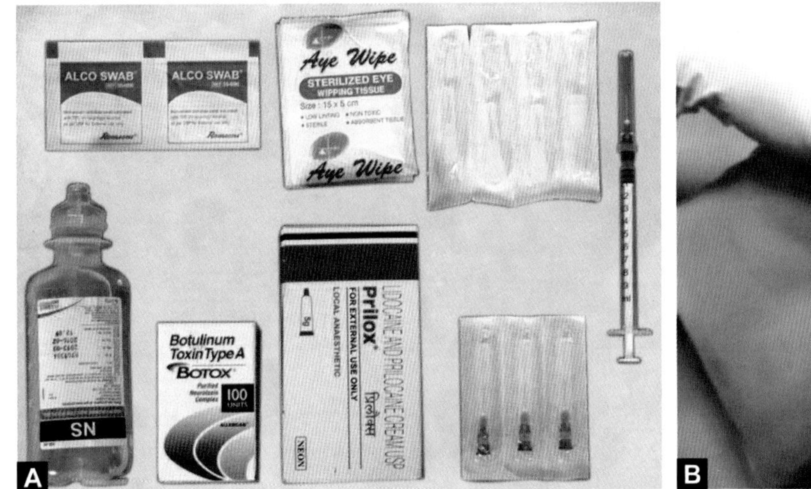


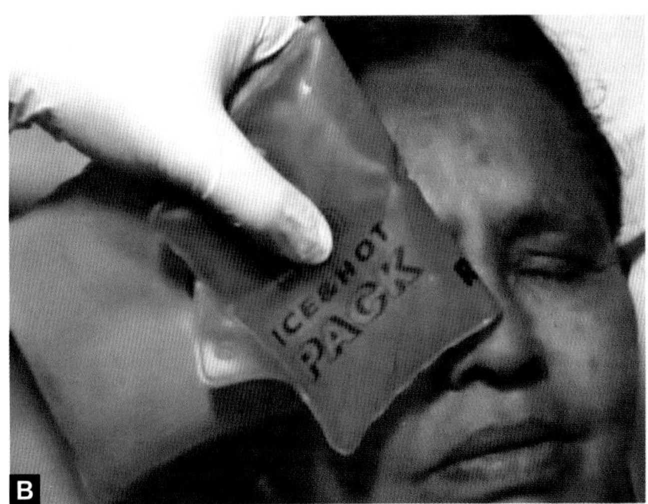


**Figures 58-5A and B** Basic tools for Botox injections include: vacuum-sealed 100-U Botox vial, 0.9% normal saline for sterile diluent, 30- or 32-gauge needles for injection, 1-cc syringe, sterile gauze, alcohol pads, 1% topical lidocaine cream, and ice packs.

inside wall of the vial, to avoid agitation of the toxin. Turbulent injection of diluent into the vial, or vigorous shaking of the vial when mixing, is discouraged as these could result in protein denaturation and thus render the toxin less effective. The vial may then be gently rolled several times to ensure proper homogenization of the mixture. The solution should be clear, homogeneous, colorless, without air bubbles, and free of particles. A 1-mL insulin or tuberculin syringe, with a 30- or 32-gauge needle, is most optimal for injection, as the injected 0.05 or 0.1 mL amounts can be more accurately achieved (Fig. 58-5). On average, the time of onset of clinical effectiveness is generally 3–5 days, with a peak at 2–4 weeks, and duration of 3–4 months.

Reconstitution releases the toxin from the protein complex. Although company guidelines suggest using the drug within 4 hours of preparation, many clinical practices use reconstituted vials safely for up to 4–6 weeks with only minimal loss of potency, if stored properly at 4°C.

There are also different clinical forms of botulinum toxin (type A, B) available for clinical use, which vary in the manufacturing process and the amount of associated protein. Some popular variations of type A botulinum toxin are PurTox, Xeomin, BTX-A, and Dysport. Type B botulinum toxin is structurally and functionally similar to type A but differs in molecular size and cellular constitution. It is available as a liquid formulation without the need for reconstitution. With a pH of 5.6, it has a long shelf-life that can be used for up to 9 months.[3-6]

When using botulinum toxin in facial aesthetics, any range of dilution and volume is acceptable and depends primarily on the site to be injected, the strength of the dynamic rhytids, and practitioner's preference. Recommendations for reconstitution and handling are summarized in Tables 58-1 and 58-2. The approved package inserts are also a useful guideline when beginning the use of botulinum toxin. The recommended diluent for reconstitution is 0.9% sterile saline, either with or without preservatives.

## INJECTION TECHNIQUE

As with any procedure, patients expect maximum benefits with minimum side effects. It is advisable to perform a thorough facial examination, develop realistic expectations with the patient, and counsel the patient about the mechanism of action of botulinum toxin, its longevity, and expected side effects. It is advisable to instruct patients to discontinue anticoagulants at least 1 week prior to treatment if possible. Because Botox uses albumin as the excipient vehicle, it should not be administered to individuals with a history of allergy or intolerance to the ingredient. Botox should also be avoided in patients with a history of systemic muscle weakness, as mentioned earlier. An informed consent should be signed, and the lot number and expiration date of the vial recorded. A facial map is often useful to record the site, dose (in number of units), and pattern of injections given during each visit. Pre- and post-treatment pictures can also be taken.

Although normally not necessary, topical anesthesia creams with 1% lidocaine (EMLA, Prilox) can significantly reduce discomfort, especially in patients who may be anxious or having injections for the first time. These can be applied at least 10 minutes or more before injection. The smaller 30- or 32-gauge needles have been reported to cause less discomfort and bruising. Alcohol to clean the skin may be used, but it should be dried completely because of toxin lability. Some physicians prefer ice as a topical anesthetic agent, as well as for vasoconstriction in the periorbital region.

The precise treatment plan both in functional and cosmetic patients depends on a thorough understanding of the variables constituting the facial framework. The number of units per site to be injected is dependent upon the area injected, muscle thickness, skin thickness, gender variations, and patient's expectations. Injection is perpendicular to skin for placement of the botulinum toxin just above, or into, the targeted muscle belly. Injecting directly into the muscle may increase the chance of ecchymosis, however. The skin around the eyes and lips is thin, and injections should remain superficial in the subcutaneous plane. The general pattern and dosage of Botox in popular areas of cosmetic concerns are summarized in Figs. 58-6 to 58-11.

Important considerations prior to cosmetic injection of botulinum toxin include:

- Assess facial expression at rest and during animation and evaluate the range of motion of the involved musculature.
- Static rhytids may need correction with soft-tissue augmentation and/or skin resurfacing.
- Palpate the muscles and note asymmetries and variations before injecting. For instance, the tail of the corrugator supercilii muscle may extend anywhere from midbrow to lateral brow, and the injection site should vary accordingly.
- The muscle bellies are largest on either side of a crease, as opposed to under the crease, and therefore, injections should be placed in these sites. If beginning, facial topography and the areas to be treated should be studied through clinical pictures.
- Exercise caution in patients who have undergone surgery that may have altered the underlying anatomy.
- Begin with conservative low doses and add additional units or sites if there is still insufficient effect after at least two weeks.
- Higher concentrations of Botox in a smaller volume is preferable over a larger volume of lower concentration. toxin, as this allows for more accurate placement of injection without unwanted diffusion that could result in complications.
- Injection of the frontalis muscle should start at a level at least halfway up between the eyebrows and hairline, to avoid brow ptosis.
- Injecting the lower lid preseptal creases and perioral lip lines are advanced techniques and should be performed after sufficient expertise.
- Avoid the unnatural appearance of completely paralyzed facial muscles.
- Asking the patient to animate can help localize the target creases and muscles before each injection for optimal individualization.
- Appropriate lighting and magnification may help avoid intravascular injection.
- Applying ice before and/or after injection can minimize ecchymosis.
- Facial rhytids should typically be treated symmetrically.

## COMPLICATIONS

There are many potential side effects of botulinum toxin injections. However, most are of mild degree and transient, due to either excessive chemodenervation of target muscles, or due to diffusion of toxin to surrounding muscles. The majority of these side effects can easily be avoided with excellent technique.[3-7]

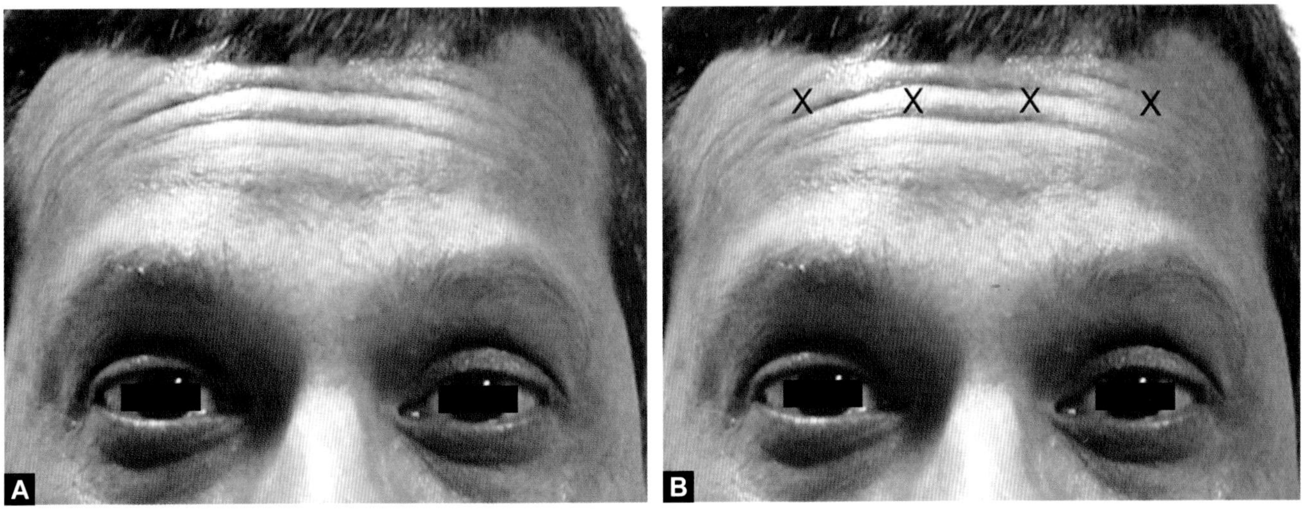

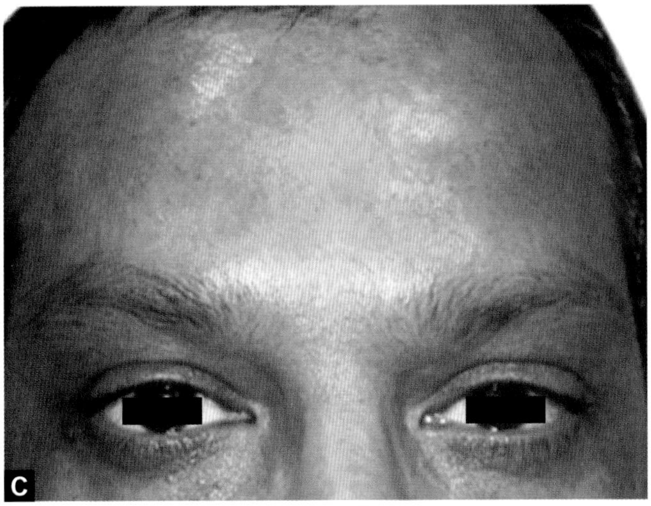

**Figures 58-6A to C** Horizontal forehead rhytids. (A) Prominent horizontal dynamic creases due to frontalis muscle overaction, (B) Typical sites for injection at least 2 cm away from the brow area, or above the midforehead level; (C) Postinjection smoothing of the rhytids.

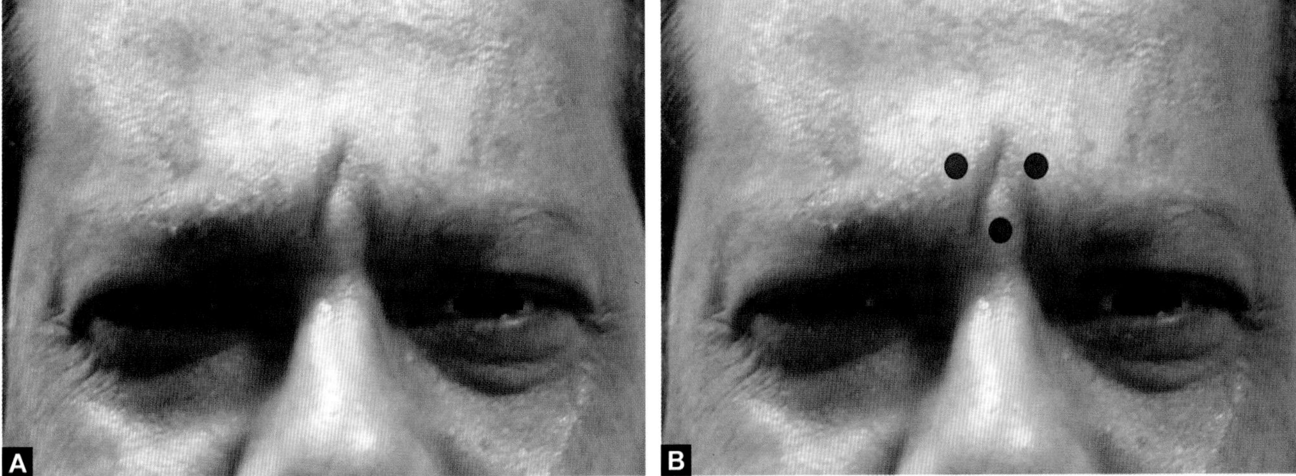

**Figures 58-7A and B** Vertical glabellar rhytids. (A) Vertical, or oblique, glabellar creases created by overacting corrugator supercilii and procerus muscles give the patient an angry appearance. (B) Typical sites for injection targeting the muscles in the medial brow and central glabella. If the lateral extent of the corrugator muscle is very strong, creating a pulling or dimpling appearance to the skin above the mid to lateral brow then a small dose can be placed here.

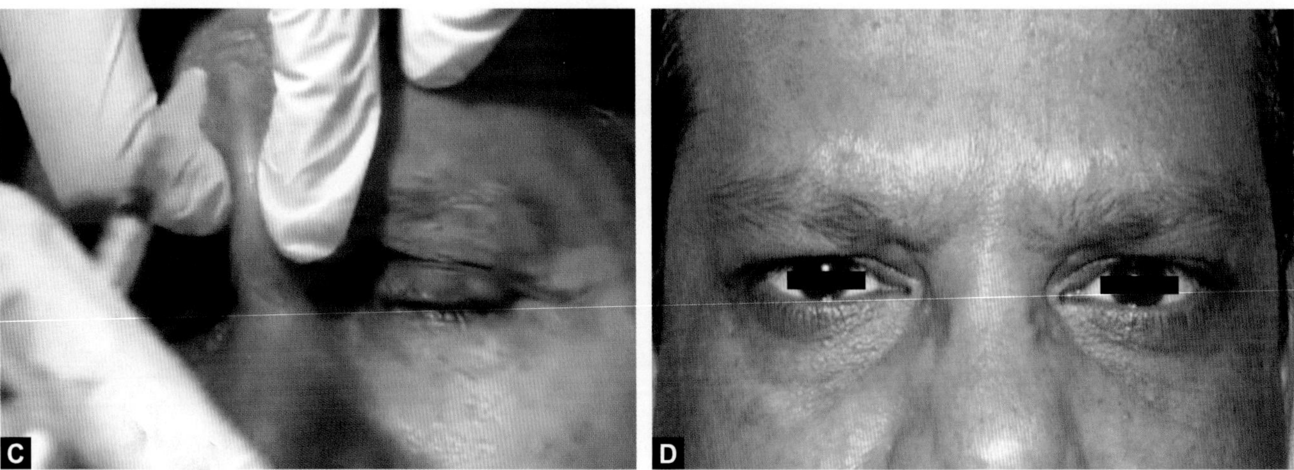


**Figures 58-7C and D** Vertical glabellar rhytids. (C) The muscle can be pinched during injection to minimize pain, as well as to limit dispersion. (D) Improvement of vertical rhytids after 1 week.

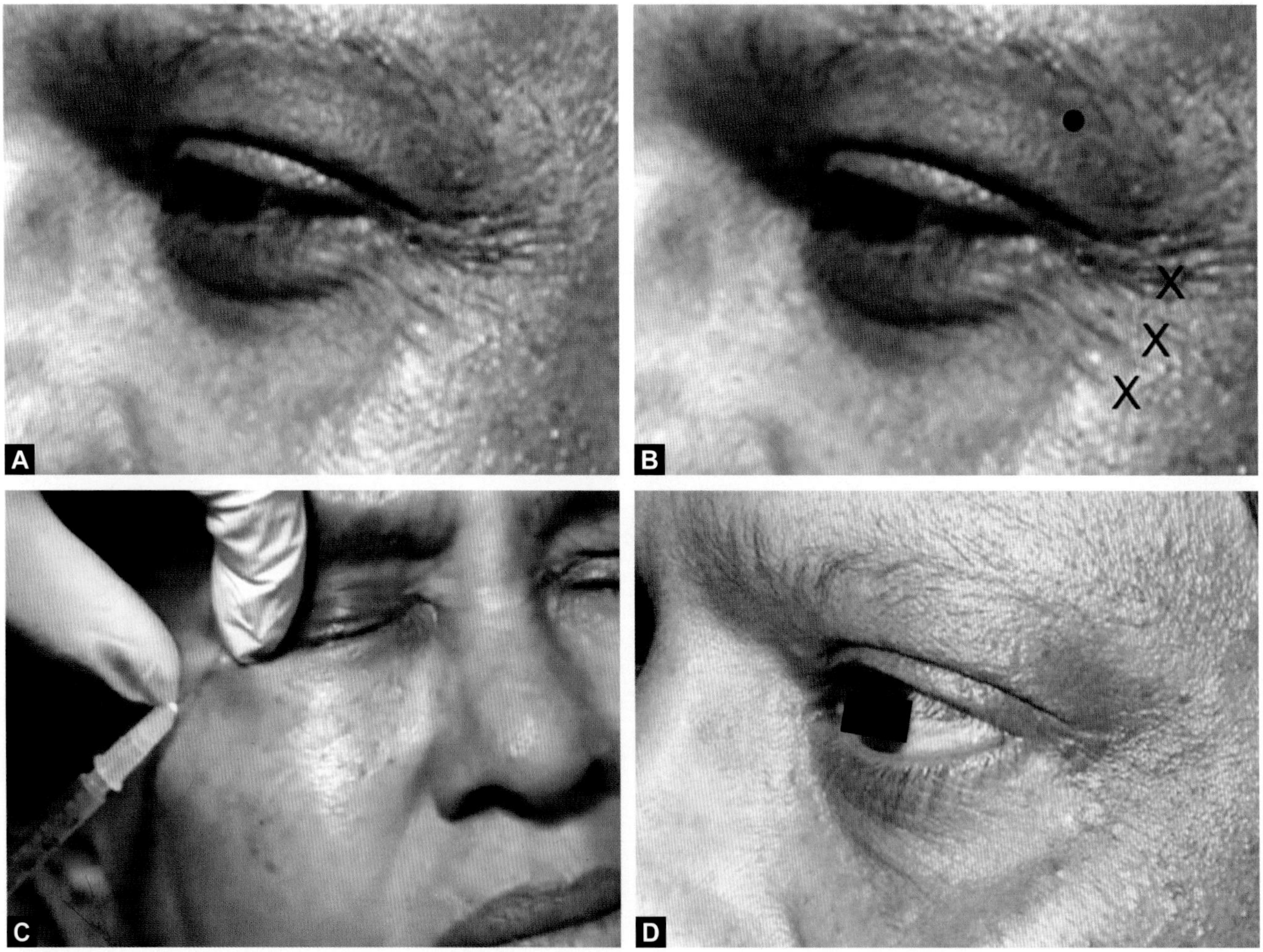

**Figures 58-8A to D** Periocular crow's feet or smile lines. (A) Lateral orbital crow's feet wrinkles result from contraction of the vertical fibers of the orbital orbicularis muscle. (B) Subcutaneous injection sites can range from 1 outside the lateral canthus for minimal creases, to several more sites depending on the degree and spread of dynamic lines. (C) The index finger can be placed inside the lateral orbital rim while injecting to avoid globe injury and diffusion into the upper lid. (D) Postinjection resolution of lateral rhytids.

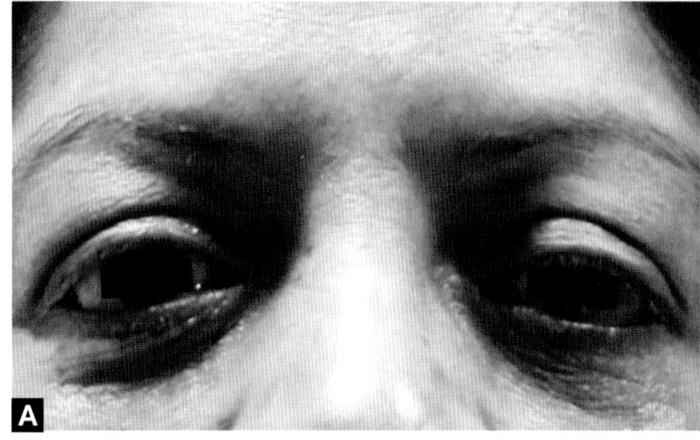


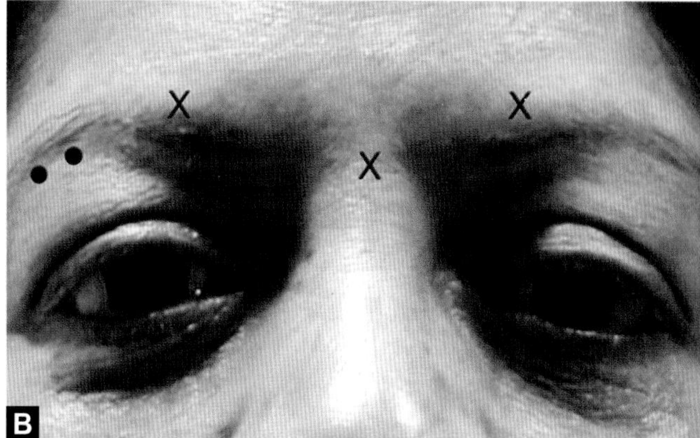


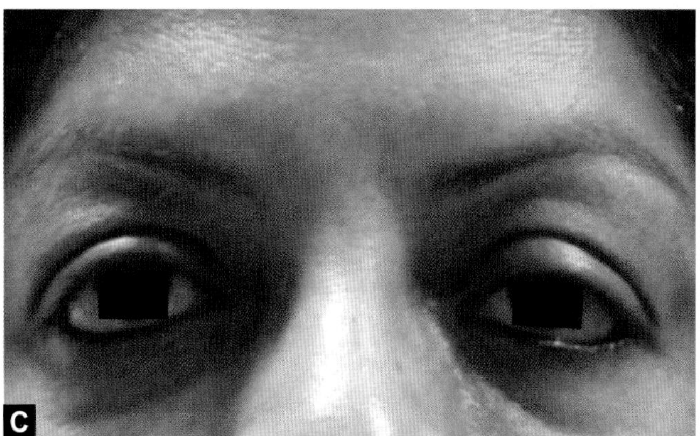


**Figures 58-9A to C** Botulinum toxin brow lift. (A) Patient with mild lateral brow ptosis and dermatochalasis. (B) Injection sites target the corrugator supercilii (medial brow depressor, X) and the orbital portion of the supero-lateral orbicularis oculi muscle (lateral brow depressor, •). (C) Postinjection appearance demonstrates a natural elevation of the lateral brow, and a subtle decrease in pseudodermatochalasis.

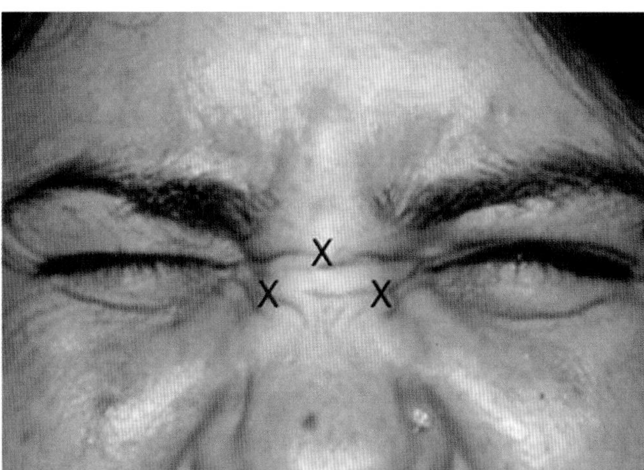


**Figure 58-10** Correction of nasal "bunny lines"—horizontal creases on both sides of the nose.

Potential side effects include:

- Local pain
- Ecchymosis
- Inadequate result
- Asymmetry
- Ptosis
- Epiphora
- Dry eyes
- Diplopia
- Ectropion
- Entropion
- Facial weakness
- Lagophthalmos
- Mouth droop, drooling, weak lip pursing
- Facial numbness
- Allergic reaction
- Death

Almost all patients experience mild local discomfort and burning with the injection and infiltration of toxin. Bruising is also not uncommon, particularly in the periocular region due to the thin skin and high concentration of vessels. Ptosis has been reported to occur in up to 13.4% patients. Ptosis may be minimized by avoiding injection into the central upper lid near the levator muscle and staying 1 cm outside the lateral and superior orbital rim when treating the crow's feet wrinkles and lifting the lateral brow, respectively. Aggressive injections above the eyebrows also create heaviness to the lids and should be limited to sites just above the medial brow and the tail of the corrugator muscle if very prominent. Injecting

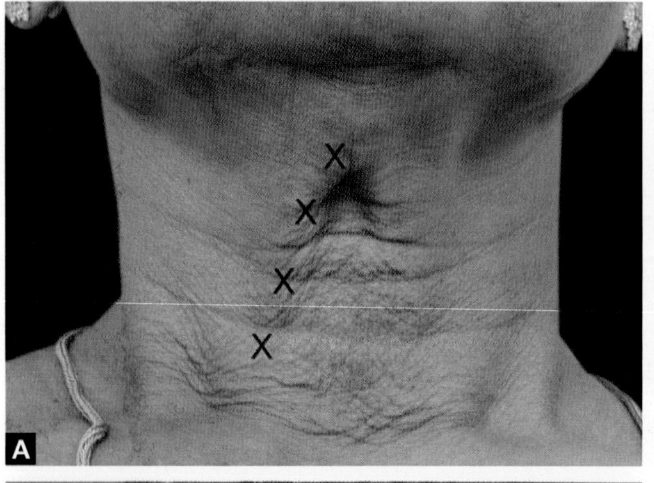


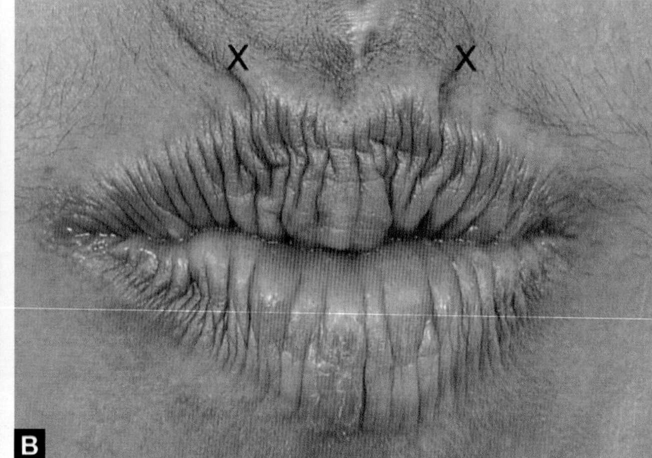


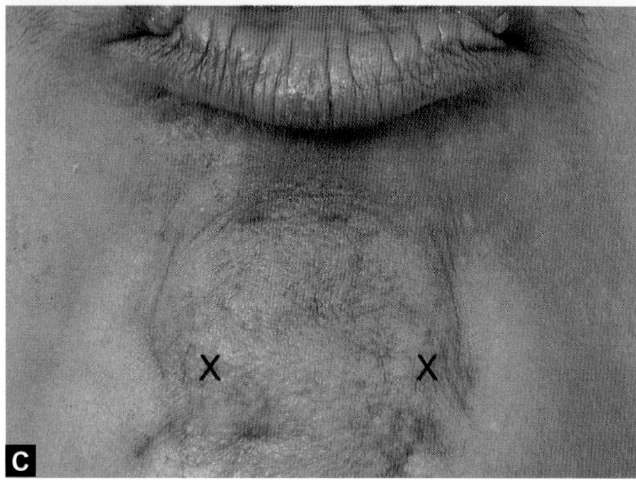


**Figures 58-11A to C** Botulinum toxin for lower face and neck dynamic rhytids. (A) Vertical neck bands result from loss of elasticity of the platysma muscle. Injections should be placed subcutaneously along each band, with each site 1–3 cm apart, using low concentrations of 1–4 U per site initially. (B) Treatment of vertical upper or lower lip lines should be conservative at first, as this carries a higher risk of complications and weakness of the mouth. A 1–2 U per site into the orbicularis oris is reasonable. It is better to treat with very low doses initially, and re-evaluate the patient in several weeks for additional treatment if needed. (C) Chin dimpling, like a 'peau d'orange,' can be smoothed nicely with 1 central site, or 2 sites of botulinum toxin into the mentalis muscle. Avoid placing the injections laterally as the depressor labii inferioris could be inadvertently affected.

the frontalis muscle below the midforehead level (or within a 2-cm region above the eyebrows), or using doses such as 5 U per site, could also result in significant forehead and lid ptosis. In patients with mild to moderate horizontal forehead rhytids, or in whom treatment is being initiated, low doses of even 1.25–2.5 U per site along 4–5 sites across the forehead can be extremely effective. In patients with a high forehead, the superior half of the forehead and the hairline may still have residual movement, and in these patients, a second row of small injections can be placed higher up in the pretrichial region, without resulting in eyelid or brow ptosis. Keep in mind that if the frontalis muscle is treated, there is unopposed brow depressor action, and the lateral orbital orbicularis oculi muscle may need to be treated just under the tail of the brow to help lift the lateral brow.

Approximately 60–5% of patients have been reported to have an impaired blink with lagophthalmos from orbicularis oculi muscle weakening, mainly after functional treatment for blepharospasm. Therefore, if the upper lid requires treatment to improve apraxia of lid opening, very small 1–2 U per site injections should be placed superficially (subcutaneous) to minimize this risk. Directing the needle tip away from the orbit is always important as well to avoid globe injury.

The incidence of mouth droop and drooling has been reported as high as 12% when injecting in the midface and lower face for hemifacial spasm and oromandibular dystonia, as well as for cosmetic rejuvenation. It is important to keep dosages to 1–2 U per site and to inject very superficially around the mouth. Upper and lower lip vertical lines should be treated with a maximum of four sites in the upper lip, and four in the lower lip at first. The patient can then return in 2 weeks to assess the need for additional small injections slightly higher up along the vertical lines if needed. Knowledge of the anatomy is important to avoid mouth droop, which results from injecting the wrong perioral muscle. In cases of hemifacial spasm, the patient should be counseled about the possibility of facial asymmetry secondary to the treatment of one half of the facial musculature. They may thus opt for cosmetic treatment of the contralateral rhytids to maintain symmetry.

## POST PROCEDURE CARE

- Avoid strenuous physical activities for 24 hours following the procedure
- Avoid applying pressure or massaging the treated areas for 24 hours after injection, as this may disperse the botulinum toxin into undesired areas
- Avoid lying down on the face for 24 hours
- Minimize alcohol consumption for the remainder of the day
- Facial massages should be avoided for 24–48 hours
- Cold compresses may be used for discomfort and bruising
- Anticoagulant medications may be resumed the following day.

## CONCLUSION

Botulinum toxin has evolved into one of most common, and effective, noninvasive treatments in the realm of functional and cosmetic oculoplasty. Understanding the facial muscle anatomy is mandatory to be able to individualize treatment for each patient, as well as to avoid undesirable complications. When properly administered, botulinum toxin can provide safe and highly gratifying results for both the patient and physician.

## REFERENCES


1. Kerner-Erbguth FJ, Naumann M. On the first systematic descriptions of botulism and botulinum toxin by Justinus Kerner (1786-1862). J Hist Neurosci. 2000 Aug;9(2):218-20.
2. Burgen AS, Dickens F., Zatman LJ.The action of botulinum toxin on the neuro-muscular junction. J Physiol. 1949 Aug;109 (1-2):10-24.
3. Dutton JJ, Fowler AM. Botulinum toxin in ophthalmology. Major review. Surv Ophthalmol. 2007;52(1):13-21.
4. Carruthers JD1, Carruthers JA. Treatment of glabellar frown lines with C. botulinum-A exotoxin. J Dermatol Surg Oncol. 1992 Jan;18(1):17-21.
5. Said SZ, Meshkinpour A, Carruthers A, et al. Botulinum toxin A. Its expanding role in dermatology and esthetics. Am J Clin Dermatol. 2003;4(9):609-16.
6. Carruthers J, Fagien S, Matarasso SL, the Botox Consensus Group. Consensus recommendations on the use of botulinum toxin type A in facial aesthetics. Plast Reconstr Surg. 2004; 1S-20S.
7. Lee C, Kikkawa DO, Pasco NY, et al. Advanced functional oculofacial indications of botulinum toxin. Int Clin Ophthalmol. 2005;45(3):77-91.
8. Kalra HK, Magoon EH. Side effects of use of botulinum toxin for treatment of benign essential blepharospasm and hemi facial spasm. Ophthal Surg.1990;21(5):335-8.
9. Faigen S, Brandt FS. Primary adjunctive use of botulinum toxin type A in facial aesthetic surgery. Beyond Glabella. Non operative techniques for facial rejuvenation, Part II. Clin Plast Surg. 2011;28(1):127-4.
10. Ascher B. Injection treatment in cosmetic surgery. New York: Taylor & Francis; Informa UK Ltd; 2009.

CHAPTER

59

# Periocular Fillers

Andre S Litwin, Raman Malhotra

## INTRODUCTION

The last 10 years have witnessed a revolution in the field of cosmetic surgery. The current top nonsurgical cosmetic procedures are botulinum toxin injections and hyaluronic acid (HA) fillers.[1] This is a dramatic change from 15 years ago when the majority of aesthetic procedures were surgical.[2] The shift has been based on our recognition that the aging face does not revolve around the effects of gravity, but instead, volume loss. This, combined with a quest for less invasive more predictable procedures while achieving a natural result, helps to explain the current popularity of fillers in facial aesthetic treatment.

Volume loss has increasingly been recognized as an important aspect of facial aging and this is especially true of the periocular region.[3-5] As volume is lost through either atrophy or excision, the bony orbit becomes more visible and the eyes appear more rounded and hollow. The increased definition of the periorbital area resulting from conventional, excision- or tightening-based surgical philosophy can often result in quite the opposite of a younger looking eyelid appearance.[6] Restoration of this lost volume can be achieved through placement of fillers, an example of the technologically driven shift in aesthetic rejuvenation.[7] The periorbital complex consists of the temples, brow, superior orbital rim, upper eyelid, lateral canthus, lower eyelid, inferior orbital rim, and cheek. Repositioning more so than removing tissue, combined with adding volume, is nowadays considered the more tailored approach toward improving the appearance around the eye.

Approaching the aging face from the standpoint of volume loss changes the paradigm of rejuvenation to now include "filling", or rather "reinflating" the face in addition to simply excising and lifting tissues. It has been said that "looking tighter does not necessarily mean looking younger or healthier". The periorbital area represents a focal point of attraction in a youthful face, which consists of intricate contours of varying convexities. These smooth convexities are the foundation for a soft, natural, youthful, and healthy-looking appearance.

## TEMPORARY FILLERS

### Collagen

Collagen can be obtained from various sources, each with its own characteristics. These products have, however, fallen out of favor with concerns regarding transmission of prion disease as well as inaccurate or uneven filler placement.

### Hyaluronic Acid

HA is unique in that it is found natively in the intracellular matrix of the dermis of all mammalian species in an identical form. HA is a disaccharide unit containing glucuronic acid and *N*-acetylglucosamine. These are joined together forming a uniform, linear polysaccharide molecule. Exogenous HA is rapidly eliminated with a tissue half-life of only 1–2 days; modification by cross-linking allows longer lasting results.[8] These new products can last many months and sometimes even years.[9]

HA (e.g. Restylane, Perlane, Juvederm, Captique, Hydra-Fill, Purogen, and Hylaform) is used for patients who do not have a severe degree of aging or those who wish to avoid the expense or recovery associated with more invasive procedures.[10] Restylane was the first HA to obtain Food and Drug Administration (FDA) approval; it has a good safety margin, as well as cost and beneficial effect.[11] Since its introduction, a wide range of other products have become available, each with slight differences, relating to the source derivation, the method, and amount of cross-linking and particle size. Understanding a product is essential to its efficacious use. Increasing particle size will increase its viscosity, reduce ease of injection, and increase longevity. Too small a particle will not yield a lasting result; too large a particle will not create the desired cosmetic result. Restylane, Perlane, and Skinboosters such as Vital and Vital light each have 20 mg/mL of nonanimal stabilized hyaluronic acid (NASHA). Perlane has a 1000 millimicron gel bead size and 10,000 units/mL, while Restylane has a 250 millimicron gel bead size and 100,000 units/mL.[12] Smaller particles are less persistent but are more applicable to superficial ritides, whereas larger particle formulations are longer lasting. Superficially placed products carry a higher risk of being visible or palpable.[11]

### Polylactic Acid

Polylactic acid (PLA) known as Sculptra is a synthetic biodegradable material. It is basically the same substance as that used in suture material. When injected into the deep dermis, it gradually stimulates collagen formation. After the three initial treatments (each approximately 6–8 weeks apart), the results are supposed to last for up to 2 years. PLA has FDA approval for use in patients with HIV-therapy-induced facial lipoatrophy.

## PERMANENT AND SEMIPERMANENT FILLERS

Nonbiodegradable fillers are also available. As well as being expensive, frequent injections can be quite tiresome for both the patient and the physician and so application of a nonbiodegradable or permanent filler may hold an appeal. It is important to remember that patients of all ages may be treated in aesthetic medicine and it can be very difficult to predict how permanent filler will appear with the passing of time.[13]

### Silicone

Injectable silicone is one of the oldest injectable filler materials used. As a result of severe adverse reactions, the FDA declared the use of injectable silicone illegal in 1991. It is not licensed for use within the EU either.[11]

### Calcium Hydroxylapatite

Calcium hydroxylapatite (e.g. Radiesse) is made from synthetically formed calcium phosphate pearls, a procedure that is classified as bioceramics and involves the ionic bonding of calcium and phosphate ions. When injected, they form a foundation within a matrix that allows the local cellular infiltration of fibroblasts. In contrast to the other fillers, it is visible on X-rays and patients should be informed of this.

### Polyacrylamide

Polyacrylamide (e.g. Aquamid) is composed of 97.5% water and 2.5% cross-linked polyacrylamide. It is recommended for folds, skin sculpturing and facial atrophy. It is not effective for fine wrinkles. Polyacrylamide should be injected deeply using a subcutaneous tunneling technique.

### Polyalkylamide

Polyalkylimide (e.g. Bio-alcamid) consists of alkylimide group networks (approximately 4%) and water (approximately 96%). The product is available at two different viscosities for lip and facial augmentation and is used for folds, skin sculpting (including the lips), and facial atrophy, but not for the treatment of fine lines. The material must be injected subdermally and according to the manufacturer's information is supposed to be easily removable when injected in larger volumes. Because of the hydrophilic and endoprosthetic nature of polyalkylimide 4%, migration of the product is unexpected. However, we have observed filler migration occurring after bimanual expression and manipulation of the product with disruption of the surrounding collagen capsule. Removal of polyalkylimide 4% is only achieved via aspiration and bimanual expression, which itself may precipitate long-term migration of the product.[14]

## INDICATIONS

Physicians who practice aesthetic medicine will know that many patients are unaware of what they really need. It is the physician who understands the anatomical basis of the aging process, who must then find a compromise between the expectations of the patient and what is possible. In order to understand how volume affects appearance, an understanding of the normal youthful appearance and the volume loss that occurs with aging is essential. Periorbital volume loss can present in a wide range of ways reflecting the many etiologies involved. Management of volume loss within the orbit and periorbital region first involves investigation and diagnosis of the underlying cause with treatment of any contributory factors. Only then volume replacement may be considered. Soft tissue atrophy due to aging is the most common cause of volume loss presenting to oculoplastic surgeons. Typical features are highlighted in Figure 59-1.

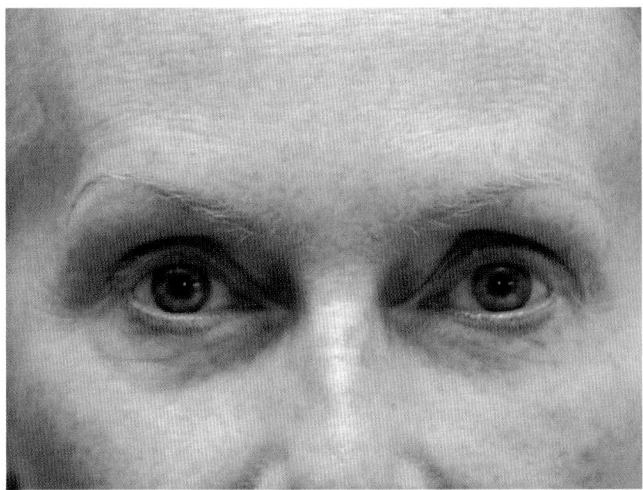

Figure 59-1 Volume loss in facial aging. Here we see in facial aging, volume loss manifests through unmasking of the lower eyelid fat pads and infraorbital rim both medially (tear trough) and laterally, superior sulcus hollowing and increased upper eyelid pretarsal show, brow descent and temple hollowing.

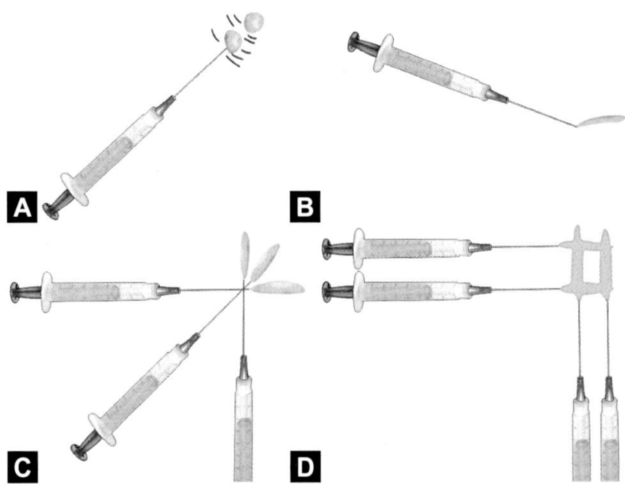


Figures 59-2A to D A variety of injection techniques can be employed, depending on the size of area to be filled. In serial puncture (A), the needle is inserted up to the appropriate depth and the product delivered in a small bolus to fill the defect. For superficial placement of fillers along a particular wrinkle, linear threading (B) is used. As the needle is withdrawn, the product is delivered in a slow, continuous stream. The fanning technique is similar, but the direction of the needle is continually changed in a radial fashion, without withdrawing the needle tip (C). Cross-hatching involves a series of threads injected in a perpendicular fashion to each other (D).

## CONTRAINDICATIONS

Patients with dysmorphism are preoccupied with real or imaginary defects. They may even take the mirror to point out a defect that has not been noted by the physician. The inability to deal with unavoidable scars is also a warning that dissatisfaction may arise after a cosmetic procedure. The presence of festoons or a history of fluid retention, seasonal allergies, previous lower lid, or midface surgery should warn the physician of the potential for persistent edema after filler injection.[15] One should be reluctant to inject patients with HA if they have strong tendencies toward periorbital edema.[16]

## SURGICAL TECHNIQUE

### Documentation

To ensure a safe and efficient procedure, a comprehensive documentation of all treatment is required. It is always advisable to document appearance by photography before and after treatment. In addition to being useful as legal documentation, these photographs will help to improve our communication with the patient. Patients should also be requested to provide old photographs of themselves, e.g. when teenagers, in their 20s and 30s in order to provide a reference point for assessing changes that have occurred and also a guide to where treatment should be directed. Patients need to sign and date a consent form for each procedure. This should be accompanied by a patient information brochure that includes all of the necessary information on the estimated efficacy and possible adverse events, including the remote risk of irreversible blindness.[17] Details of the product used should be attached to patient's records to allow some traceability in the event of adverse effects.[9]

### Injection Technique

Four commonly reported techniques are used for filler injection: serial puncture, threading, fanning, and cross-hatching (Figs. 59-2A to D). There is currently no algorithm for choosing an injection technique. While certain situations may lend themselves to a particular technique, this decision is typically surgeon dependent and related to experience, defect size and location, as well as the particular filler being used.[12,18] Although the needle utilized is generally the 30-gauge, half-inch needle, there are specific procedures for which alternative needle sizes are appropriate. Other needle adaptations may include using a longer needle (1 inch), using a finer gauge needle, or bending the needle to access particular contours of the face.[9]

The use of microcannulae rather than standard needles has now been described. Niamtu describes the use of a 0.9 mm (20-gauge) microinjection cannula (Tulip Medical, Inc.).[19] The perceived advantages are an atraumatic injection with reduced edema, bruising, and surface irregularity.[20] We reviewed our early experience using the Pix'L cannula through photographic assessment. We objectively found increased bruising immediately post-treatment in almost half of patients using the standard technique compared to <20% of patients with the Pix'L technique.[21]

## Bruising

Bruising occurs when the needle passes through the vascular orbicularis layer. Therefore, when multiple fanning passes are required to create a smooth contour, it is best to withdraw the needle just enough to change direction but not so much that it exits back through the orbicularis layer. In this way, the number of actual needle passes through the orbicularis can be minimized.[16] Minimizing the number of skin punctures also limits the associated trauma.[22] To reduce the risk of bruising, patients are advised to omit for 2 weeks prior to surgery: oily fish supplements, the 4 Gs (garlic, ginseng, ginko, ginger), and aspirin (where used for primary prevention and in consultation with their doctor). Patients are asked to have no alcohol on the day of treatment (to avoid being flushed) and to consider omitting SSRIs where safely possible for 1 week.[23]

## Pain

Several mechanisms can be used to diminish injection pain. Immediately before injection, cryoanalgesia with application of ice, or a tap distraction during injection can reduce discomfort.[24] The efficacy is predicated on the fact that vibratory sensation and sharp pain are transmitted through common neural pathways.[22] Nerve blocks were traditionally used for treating the cheek or even lips; however, recently, the introduction of fillers combining a local anesthetic (lidocaine) with HA in a single presentation has significantly improved patient experience during treatment. Juvederm was the first hyaluronic gel to be introduced to include lidocaine.[25] Our personal preference of filler material is NASHA including either Restylane with 0.3% lidocaine (Restylane-L) or Perlane with 0.3% lidocaine (Perlane-L Galderma UK), both of which are widely used.

# TEMPLE HOLLOWING

Temple hollowing is a common feature of the aging face, but rarely represents a specific concern of a patient seeking cosmetic consultation.[26] The area to be injected is cooled with ice packs for 2 minutes. The skin is prepared by cleaning with alcohol wipes. Patients are seated upright, with their head against a headrest. Injections are administered with the standard 27-gauge needle supplied or using a blunt-tip flexible cannula on a Luer-Lock vial. Avoid the superficial temporal artery and veins before needle entry. Injections are administered behind the zygomaticofrontal process so as to soften the bony contour of the lateral orbital rim. The skin over the temple is gently stretched perpendicular to the needle shaft, which is advanced bevel down to a subcutaneous plane within the superficial temporal fascia. When using a standard needle, the filler is administered via a serial puncture technique, with 3–5 injections, each delivering approximately 0.3 mL. Typical treatment volumes are 1 mL per side, although this can range up to 3 mL for profound hollowing. The aim is to soften the sharp demarcation from the prominent bony arch to the volume-deficient soft tissue of the temple. The filler was then molded to achieve the desired contour and reduce any prominent lumps (Fig. 59-3).[27]

# BROW DEFLATION

When evaluating and treating the upper eyelid and brow, it is useful to visualize a "periorbital frame" that is bordered by the eyebrows, glabella, temporal fossa, and superior midface. Over time the eyebrow tends to lose its lateral arch and appears somewhat flattened in older patients. Deflated brows have a reduced influence on dynamic changes of upper eyelid height and therefore often appear actively elevated ("brow compensation").[6]

When reinflating the brow, attention should be paid to maintaining a smooth continuum between the brow and temple. Therefore, it is usually necessary to extend filling to the temple and even lateral canthus, beyond the tail of the brow. Injection is deep to orbicularis and preperiosteal with small aliquots until brow fullness is restored. Do not inject below the inferior border of the superior orbital rim. The typical amount injected is 0.5–1 mL per brow. Most patients are satisfied with undercorrection.[6] Any unevenness or lumpiness in the brow is visible because of the relatively thinner skin in this area, particularly in older patients. Therefore, it is critical to "sculpt" the brow to achieve the desired look. The best perspective is that the brow is being filled-out rather than lifted-up.[9]

# UPPER EYELID

When treating patients who have upper eyelid hollowing, the concept of balanced proportions can be very helpful (Figs. 59-4A and B). Patients with either medial or generalized hollowing do very well with upper eyelid soft-tissue augmentation. Patients with combined dermatochalasis and sub-brow deflation usually do better with upper blepharoplasty, with or without brow lift and blepharoptosis surgery.

The thin upper eyelid skin calls for the use of a medium-low viscosity compound to prevent visible lumpiness. Filler

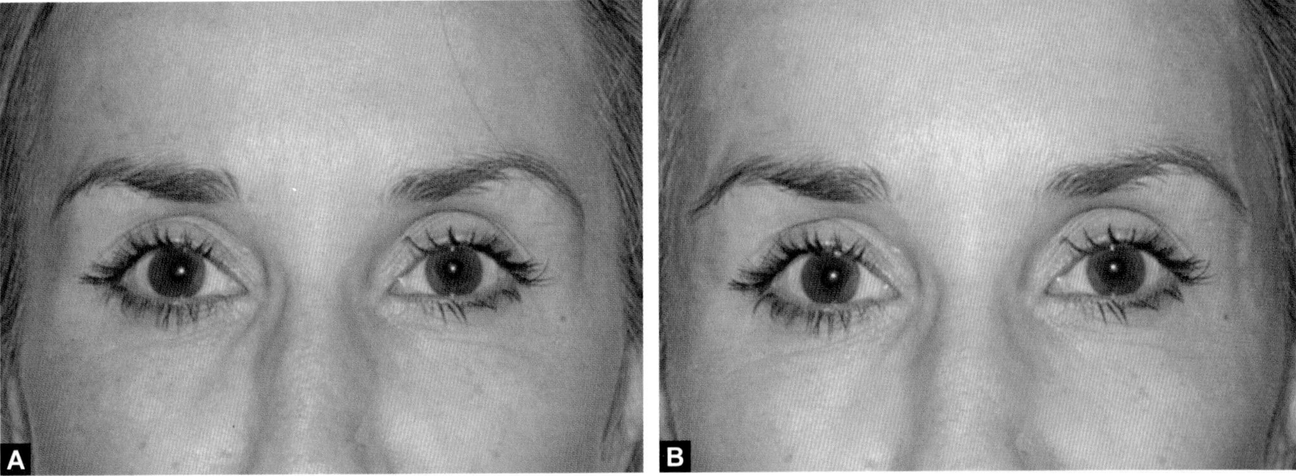

Figures 59.3A and B Avoid the superficial temporal artery and veins before needle entry. Injections are administered behind the zygomaticofrontal process so as to soften the bony contour of the lateral orbital rim. Note temple appearance before (A) and after (B) treatment.

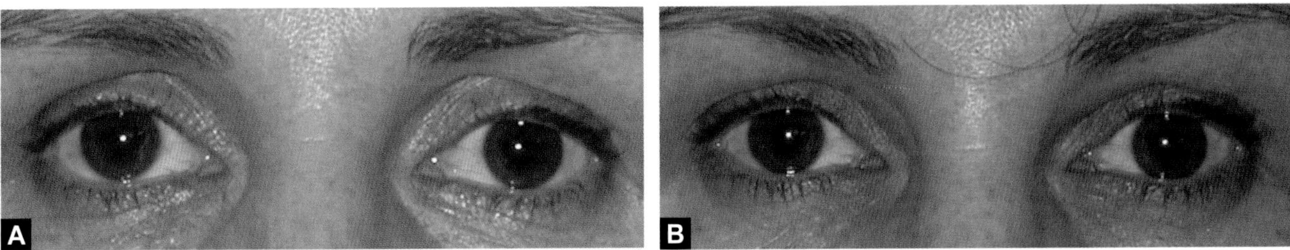

Figures 59-4A and B When treating patients who have upper eyelid hollowing, the concept of balanced proportions can be very helpful. The upper eyelid ratio compares the visible distance when looking straight ahead, of pretarsal show (distance between the lid margin and the upper eyelid skin fold), to preseptal show (distance between the skin fold and brow hair in a noncompensated brow). In general, the upper eyelid ratio increases from medial to lateral within the upper eyelid. Note appearance before (A) and after treatment (B).

placement should be as deep as possible within the preperiosteal plane to minimize this problem. The eyelid skin is numbed with ice and wiped with an alcohol swab. With the patient supine and the eyes in down gaze, the brow is manually raised and a needle puncture is created close to the junction of the lateral wall and roof. The needle or cannula tip is advanced in the suborbicularis plane until it reaches the inferior border of the superior orbital rim and 0.1 mL of filler is injected preperiosteally. The tip is then withdrawn and the raised bleb molded over the anterior aspect of the orbital rim in a medial direction to achieve a smooth contour. This process is repeated two to three times, using a serial puncture technique, with each injection progressing more medial, or using a cannula. In general, 0.4–0.5 mL of filler is suitable for treating each upper eyelid, although the range extends from 0.1 mL to 1 mL. The supraorbital notch is avoided to minimize trauma to the supraorbital neurovascular complex. With the brows relaxed, the upper eyelid contour must be reassessed to evaluate any residual irregularity.[28] Other authors have suggested administering filler by many small strokes in a fan-like fashion, using very small amounts in each pass, similar to the technique used for fat injections.[6]

## TEAR TROUGH AND EYELID-CHEEK JUNCTION

One of the most important areas of the facial ageing process is volume loss at the interface between the lower eyelid and upper cheek or midface,[10] the nasojugal groove.[29] The lateral half of the hollow that extends to the region of the lateral canthal tendon is referred to as the "lid-cheek junction", representing an arbitrary division between the lower eyelid and cheek, or malar fat pad (Figs. 59-5A to C).

A range of injection techniques have been described to treat tear trough filling.[29-31] A serial puncture or blunt-tip cannula technique are two main methods of treating this area. Injections are commenced medially, with the skin of the tear trough held taut while the 30-gauge needle is passed into

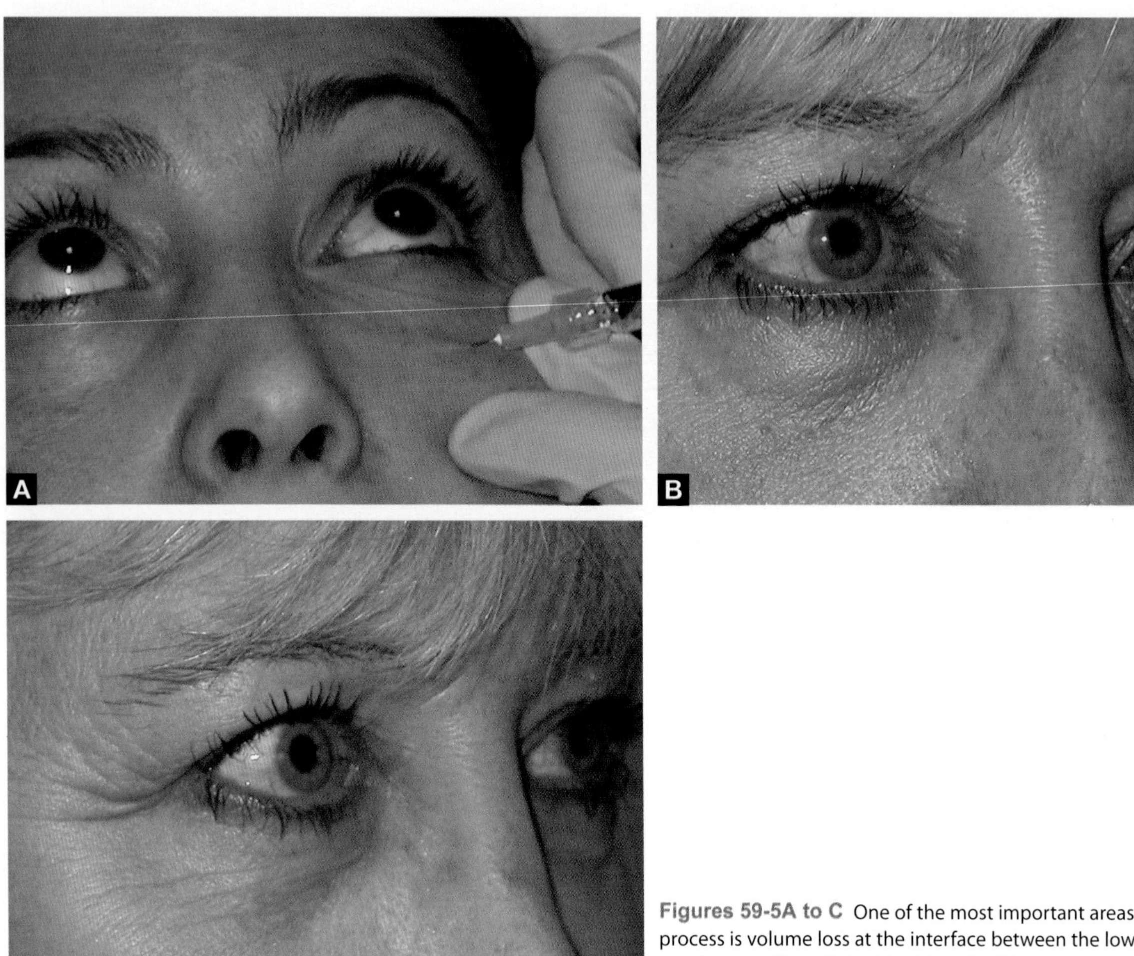

**Figures 59-5A to C** One of the most important areas of the facial ageing process is volume loss at the interface between the lower eyelid and upper cheek or midface. Note injection site (A), and appearance before (B) and after treatment (C).

the preperiosteal plane just anterior to the inferior orbital rim. A 0.1–0.2 mL aliquot of filler is injected, the needle is withdrawn and the filler molded against the bone to achieve the desired contour. The injections are repeated in successively more lateral locations along the tear trough. Usually 3–5 injections suffice. Care must be taken to avoid placement of more viscous gels in the preseptal lower eyelid location, as it is difficult to mold filler here and the very superficial position leads to prominent lumps or blue discoloration and subsequent patient dissatisfaction. Placement of filler extending out to the lateral zygomaticomalar region helps to achieve a smoother lower eyelid-cheek contour and often gives a better aesthetic result.

When using a blunt-tip cannula technique, a 21-gauge needle or importantly a needle larger than the 25-gauge Pix'L cannula is initially used to create a small stab entry laterally approximately 1 cm inferior and lateral to the inferolateral orbital rim, directly down to periosteum. The primed cannula is passed into this entry site to periosteum and a small aliquot of HA containing Lidocaine is injected in order to anesthetize this area before advancing the cannula tip in the suborbicularis plane. Prior to injection the microcannula is turned so that the aperture is aimed toward the periosteum as indicated by a mark at the base of the tip.

## OTHER PERIORBITAL USES OF INJECTABLE SOFT-TISSUE FILLERS

The advantages of injectable soft-tissue fillers have led to an expansion of their role in the periorbital area. Lower lid retraction has traditionally been managed through surgical intervention. Injectable tissue fillers can provide a temporary alternative, when used to create an adjustable tissue-expansion. Filler is placed in the suborbicularis plane in the preseptal region and adjacent to the orbitomalar ligament using a "haystack" approach. For 1 mL of HA placed in this manner,

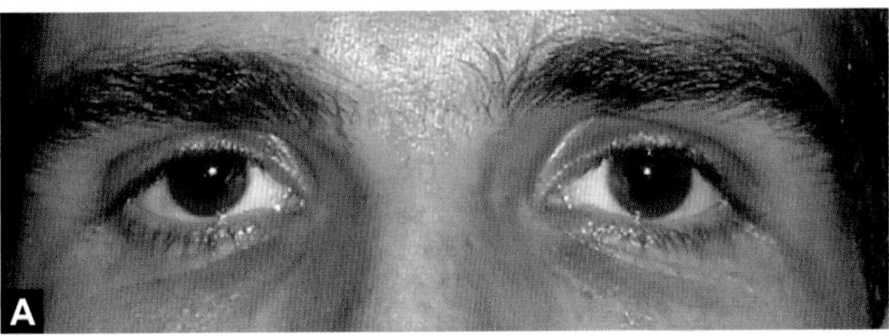


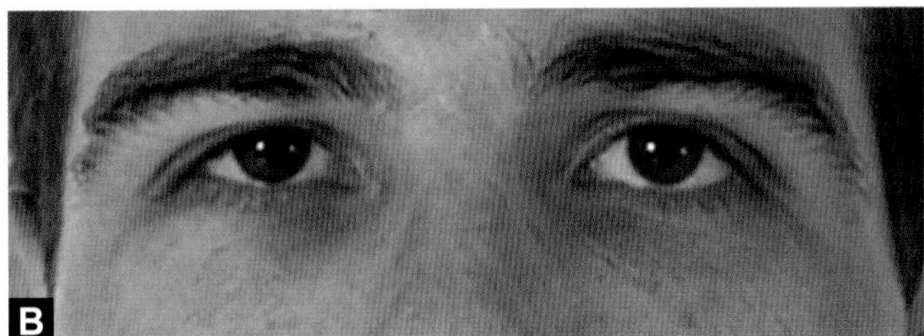


**Figures 59-6A and B** Two milliliter of a large gel particle size, viscous HA such as Restylane Sub Q administered into the posterior orbit via an inferotemporal peribulbar injection, placed posteriorly, can reduce enophthalmos by up to 2 mm and can reverse signs of periorbital volume deficiency. Note appearance before (A) and 12 months after treatment (B).

inferior scleral show typically improves by 1 mm. The effects of the filler are temporary, with one third of patients requiring a top-up by 4 months.[32]

HA has been used in both anophthalmic and sighted orbits to augment orbital volume loss. (Figs. 59-6A and B).[33] Reports have also emerged describing the use of HA for other periorbital pathologies, not always directly related to volume enhancement. Temporary upper eyelid loading with filler instead of implantation of either a gold or platinum weight has been described.[34] Lower eyelid cicatricial ectropion has also been treated with soft-tissue fillers by acting as a temporary tissue expander, stretching the deficient anterior lamella in that region.[35,36] In a similar manner, epiblepharon has also been treated.[37,38]

## POSTOPERATIVE CARE

To minimize potential for bruising, direct constant pressure with iced compress is applied to injection sites until there is no evidence of bleeding. Alcohol and exercise should be avoided for 24 hours. Ideally, sleep with head elevated for one night and over the counter pain medications or nonsteroidal anti-inflammatory drugs can be taken to alleviate minor discomfort and swelling. Skin care products can be resumed the same day. We do not recommend that patients self-mold any raised focal points until 1-week after treatment. A precise technique should be instructed.[9] Patients should allow 2 weeks before any important social or photographic events when planning injections.

## COMPLICATIONS

Overall, soft-tissue fillers have been shown to have an excellent safety record in the treatment of facial rhytids and wrinkles. Immediate complications are often related to injection technique. They include bruising, palpable or visible product resulting from superficial injection, uneven distribution, overcorrection, under correction and hypersensitivity.[39]

### Under Correction

Under correction is perhaps desirable and the easiest problem to correct. It should be the goal in every patient. All patients should be counseled on the likelihood that a second procedure may be needed to obtain the ideal result. Under correction with HA fillers can be touched up 2–4 weeks after initial treatment.

### Bruising

Although generally mild the main adverse effect reported by patients is bruising. Onset is usually within a day of treatment and lasts a median of 7 days.[30]

### Infection

Infection is rare but may occur between 2 days and a few weeks after treatment. Early inflammatory nodules are red and painful and should be treated as infected. If any fluctuation or impending skin erosion is present, incision and drainage with culture should be performed. Empiric antibiotic treatment should be continued for up to 4–6 weeks. If HA has been used then this should be dissolved using hyaluronidase. If no response is seen within 7–10 days, intralesional corticosteroid can be injected while continuing oral antibiotics. Active clinical reactions, presumed infected can flare up weeks, months or even years after initial surgery. When a filler becomes infected, antibiotic treatment can only mitigate the inflammatory process, and sooner or later, after discontinuation of medication, recurrence is inevitable. Therefore, it is necessary to remove or dissolve all infected material.[39]

Delayed hypersensitivity reactions to Restylane SubQ have been reported as a rare complication in patients receiving facial volume augmentation. Hypersensitivity reactions occur between 1 week and 4 months' post-treatment and can usually be successfully treated with hyaluronidase. Interestingly, all patients had previously (and some since) been treated with other NASHA products without adverse effect.[40]

### Overcorrection

Lumps occur as a result of too large a bolus of material or too superficial an injection. Dilute steroid injection and massage may treat these areas, but persistence may require direct surgical excision. Overcorrection is best avoided through a conservative product administration, especially when beginning. Hyaluronidase may be used in small quantities to enzymatically degrade the product, usually leading to a near complete return to the pretreatment appearance.[10] Two weeks is a reasonable follow-up time before doing anything about normally occurring areas of excess fullness and asymmetry, because they typically improve on their own.[9] Hyaluronidase at a concentration of 100–200 units/mL can be infiltrated directly below each area of persistent Restylane, using 0.025–0.05 mL (10–20 units) at each site.[29,41] In our experience hyaluronidase is effective in dissolving HA when used at concentrations of 150 IU/mL or above (1500 IU reconstituted in 10 mL saline for injection).

### Malar Edema

Malar edema lasting many weeks or even months can occur, particularly in patients with a tendency toward edema preoperatively (e.g. malar mounds before treatment).[16]

### Sight Loss Due to Central Retinal Artery Occlusion (CRAO) and Injection Site Necrosis

Injection into the glabellar region is the highest periorbital region at risk of arterial embolization or necrosis—injection into the supratrochlear artery or supraorbital artery. This is followed by the nasolabial fold, with injection into angular artery or lateral nasal artery. In the literature, most cases of iatrogenic CRAO were caused by autologous fat transfer, followed by injection of HA. Restylane has a gel particle size of 400 µm, whereas the lumen of the central retinal artery is only 160 µm, and the ophthalmic artery is 2 mm in diameter.[17] The proposed mechanism is a retrograde embolic mechanism and if an intravascular injection is recognized very early, flooding the area with hyaluronidase, topical nitroglycerin paste, and massage may be helpful.[39,42]

Inadvertent injection of the angular artery or supratrochlear artery can rarely induce an ischemic response with violaceous bluish gray discoloration, pain, erosion, and ulceration. Resolution without pain is routine except when a large bolus of material is injected, with ensuing full-thickness necrosis.[22]

### Late Change

Since the residence time and persistence for most fillers is greater the more superficially it is placed, when deeper product dissipates, the residual superficial component remains. This can become quite visible, despite an initially highly satisfactory result.[11]

## PLACE OF THE TECHNIQUE IN SURGICAL ARMAMENTARIUM

Soft tissue augmentation is a vital component of facial rejuvenation. The aesthetic market continues to be flooded with agents promising improvements. Newer is not always necessarily better and in aesthetic surgery, as in life, there is sometimes a place for subtlety. Counseling patients on their options will be one of the new challenges faced by physicians, reflecting the ongoing trend toward less invasive facial rejuvenation treatments.

## PEARLS AND PITFALLS

- Orbital or periorbital volume loss may be due to factors other than aging and should be investigated and treated first.
- There are rare but very serious complications of orbital and periorbital soft-tissue filler injections which patients need to be informed of (and agree to) before treatment.
- Never allow a patient to feel pain during an aesthetic procedure.
- Fillers can migrate over time despite manufacturer's claims.[43]
- Many surgeons routinely mix hyaluronidase with their local anesthetic during ophthalmic or facial surgery. It is now increasingly important to elicit an accurate history of prior HA injection in intended areas of surgery to prevent potential reversal of the filler's effect.
- Leftover filler should not be saved for use at a later date.

## REFERENCES

1. Wilson YL, Ellis DAF. Permanent soft tissue fillers. Facial Plast Surg. 2011;27:540-6.
2. Cohen JL, Dayan SH, Brandt FS, et al. Systematic review of clinical trials of small- and large-gel-particle hyaluronic acid injectable fillers for aesthetic soft tissue augmentation. Dermatol Surg. 2013;39(2):205-31.
3. Pessa JE. An algorithm of facial aging: verification of Lambros's theory by three-dimensional stereolithography, with reference to the pathogenesis of midfacial aging, scleral show, and the lateral suborbital trough deformity. Plast Reconstr Surg. 2000;106(2):479-88; discussion 489-90.

4. Pessa JE, Chen Y. Curve analysis of the aging orbital aperture. Plast Reconstr Surg. 2002;109(2):751-5.
5. Lambros V. Observations on periorbital and midface aging. Plast Reconstr Surg. 2007;120(5):1367-76.
6. Lambros V. Volumizing the brow with hyaluronic acid fillers. Aesthet Surg J. 2009;29(3):174-9.
7. Goldberg RA. The shift toward minimally invasive aesthetic facial rejuvenation. Arch Ophthalmol. 2010;128(9):1200-1201.
8. Rohrich RJ, Ghavami A, Crosby MA. The role of hyaluronic acid fillers (Restylane) in facial cosmetic surgery: review and technical considerations. Plast Reconstr Surg. 2007;120(6 Suppl): 41S-54S.
9. Matarasso SL, Carruthers JD, Jewell ML. Restylane Consensus Group. Consensus recommendations for soft-tissue augmentation with nonanimal stabilized hyaluronic acid (Restylane). Plast Reconstr Surg. 2006;117(3 Suppl):3S-34S.
10. Buckingham ED, Bader B, Smith SP. Autologous fat and fillers in periocular rejuvenation. Facial Plast Surg Clin North Am. 2010;18(3):385-98.
11. Fagien S, Klein AW. A brief overview and history of temporary fillers: Evolution, advantages, and limitations. Plast Reconstr Surg. 2007;120(6 Suppl):8S-16S.
12. Bosniak S, Cantisano-Zilkha M. Restylane and Perlane: a six year clinical experience. Operat Tech Oculoplas Orbital Reconstr Surg. 2001;4(2):89-93.
13. Broder KW, Cohen SR. An overview of permanent and semipermanent fillers. Plast Reconstr Surg. 2006;118(3 Suppl):7S-14S.
14. Ross AH, Malhotra R. Long-term orbitofacial complications of polyalkylimide 4% (bio-alcamid). Ophthal Plast Reconstr Surg. 2009;25(5):394-7.
15. Montes JR. Volumetric considerations for lower eyelid and midface rejuvenation. Curr Opin Ophthalmol. 2012;23(5): 443-9.
16. Goldberg RA, Fiaschetti D. Filling the periorbital hollows with hyaluronic acid gel: initial experience with 244 injections. Ophthal Plast Reconstr Surg. 2006;22(5):335-41; discussion 341-3.
17. Park SW, Woo SJ, Park KH, et al. Iatrogenic retinal artery occlusion caused by cosmetic facial filler injections. Am J Ophthalmol. 2012;154(4):653-62.e1.
18. Buck DW, Alam M, Kim JYS. Injectable fillers for facial rejuvenation: a review. J Plast Reconstr Aesthet Surg. 2009;62(1):11-8.
19. Niamtu J. Filler injection with micro-cannula instead of needles. Dermatol Surg. 2009;35(12):2005-8.
20. Berros P. Periorbital contour abnormalities: hollow eye ring management with hyalurostructure. Orbit 2010;29(2):119-25.
21. Malhotra R, Norris JH. Blunt tip PIXL® cannula for tear trough filler: patient experience. International Master Course on Aging Skin (IMCAS). 13th Annual meeting, Paris, France, 2011.
22. Alam M, Dover JS. Management of complications and sequelae with temporary injectable fillers. Plast Reconstr Surg. 2007;120(6 Suppl):98S-105S.
23. Hougardy DMC, Egberts TCG, van der Graaf F, Brenninkmeijer VJ, Derijks LJJ. Serotonin transporter polymorphism and bleeding time during SSRI therapy. Br J Clin Pharmacol. 2008;65(5):761-6.
24. Smith KC, Comite SL, Balasubramanian S, Carver A, Liu JF. Vibration anesthesia: a noninvasive method of reducing discomfort prior to dermatologic procedures. Dermatol Online J. 2004;10(2):1.
25. Weinkle SH, Bank DE, Boyd CM, et al. A multi-center, double-blind, randomized controlled study of the safety and effectiveness of Juvéderm injectable gel with and without lidocaine. J Cosmet Dermatol. 2009;8(3):205-10.
26. Rose AE, Day D. Esthetic rejuvenation of the temple. Clin Plast Surg. 2013;40(1):77-89.
27. Ross JJ, Malhotra R. Orbitofacial rejuvenation of temple hollowing with Perlane injectable filler. Aesthet Surg J. 2010;30(3): 428-33.
28. Morley AMS, Taban M, Malhotra R, et al. Use of hyaluronic acid gel for upper eyelid filling and contouring. Ophthal Plast Reconstr Surg. 2009;25(6):440-4.
29. Steinsapir KD, Steinsapir SMG. Deep-fill hyaluronic acid for the temporary treatment of the naso-jugal groove: A report of 303 consecutive treatments. Ophthal Plast Reconstr Surg. 2006;22(5):344-8.
30. Morley AMS, Malhotra R. Use of hyaluronic acid filler for tear-trough rejuvenation as an alternative to lower eyelid surgery. Ophthal Plast Reconstr Surg. 2011;27(2):69-73.
31. Griepentrog GJ, Lemke BN, Burkat CN, et al. Anatomical position of hyaluronic acid gel following injection to the infraorbital hollows. Ophthal Plast Reconstr Surg. 2013;29(1):35-9.
32. Goldberg RA, Lee S, Jayasundera T, et al. Treatment of lower eyelid retraction by expansion of the lower eyelid with hyaluronic acid gel. Ophthal Plast Reconstr Surg. 2007;23(5):343-8.
33. Malhotra R. Deep orbital sub-q restylane (nonanimal stabilized hyaluronic acid) for orbital volume enhancement in sighted and anophthalmic orbits. Arch Ophthalmol. 2007;125(12):1623-9.
34. Mancini R, Taban M, Lowinger A, et al. Use of hyaluronic acid gel in the management of paralytic lagophthalmos: The hyaluronic acid gel "gold weight". Ophthal Plast Reconstr Surg. 2009;25(1):23-6.
35. Taban M, Mancini R, Nakra T, et al. Nonsurgical management of congenital eyelid malpositions using hyaluronic acid gel. Ophthal Plast Reconstr Surg. 2009;25(4):259-63.
36. Kwong Q, Malhotra R, Morley AMS, et al. Use of dermal filler to improve exposure keratopathy in a patient with restrictive dermopathy. Orbit. 2013;32(1):70-2.
37. Almousa R, Nga M-E, Sundar G. Nonsurgical management of epiblepharon using hyaluronic acid gel. Ophthal Plast Reconstr Surg. 2010;26(3):205-6.
38. Naik MN, Ali MJ, Das S, Honavar SG. Nonsurgical management of epiblepharon using hyaluronic acid gel. Ophthal Plast Reconstr Surg. 2010;26(3):215-7.
39. Schütz P, Ibrahim HHH, Hussain SS, et al. Infected facial tissue fillers: case series and review of the literature. J Oral Maxillofac Surg. 2012;70(10):2403-12.
40. O'Reilly P, Malhotra R. Delayed hypersensitivity reaction to Restylane® subq. Orbit. 2011;30(1):54-7.
41. Soparkar CN, Patrinely JR, Tschen J. Erasing Restylane. Ophthal Plast Reconstr Surg. 2004;20(4):317-8.
42. Lazzeri D, Agostini T, Figus M, et al. Blindness following cosmetic injections of the face. Plast Reconstr Surg. 2012;129(4): 995-1012.
43. Malik S, Mehta P, Adesanya O, et al. Migrated periocular filler masquerading as arteriovenous malformation: a diagnostic and therapeutic dilemma. Ophthal Plast Reconstr Surg. 2013; 29(1):e18-20.

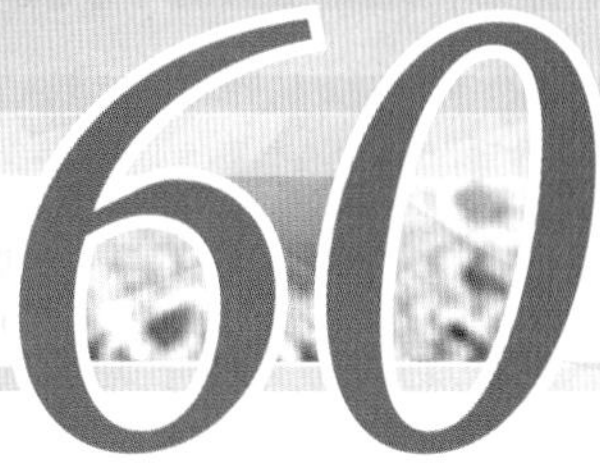

CHAPTER 60

# Lasers in Oculoplastic and Aesthetic Surgery

Cat Nguyen Burkat

## INTRODUCTION

Over the past years, aesthetic laser facial rejuvenation has achieved remarkable popularity due to a blossoming industry with newer products and devices, economic changes, decreased disposable income, and the desire to minimize time from work. While some lasers treat cutaneous vascular abnormalities and skin dyschromias, others are effective for cutaneous ablative resurfacing. The main target of laser procedures is to correct the spectrum of photoaging skin manifestations for a rejuvenated appearance. Despite the relative safety of these procedures in experienced hands, complications may include persistent erythema, postinflammatory hyperpigmentation and hypopigmentation, hypertrophic scarring, and bacterial or herpetic infections. Severe burns, lower lid cicatricial ectropion, corneal injuries, or ocular perforation are among the most severe complications. A thorough pretreatment skin evaluation, careful patient selection, informed consent, adequate training, and an individualized and conservative approach are necessary to obtain the greatest aesthetic outcomes while minimizing complications.

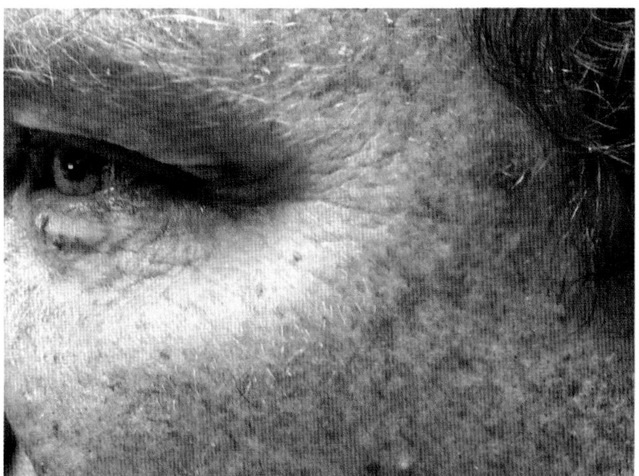

**Figure 60-1** Diffuse macular solar lentigines throughout the face.

## INDICATIONS

- Skin laxity
- Facial rhytids, fine lines
- Vascular lesions (hemangiomas, port-wine stains, telangiectasias)
- Rosacea flushing, "ruddy face", rhinophyma
- Senescent dyschromia, solar pigmentation (Fig. 60-1), melasma
- Pigmented lesions, nevi
- Periocular veins (Figs. 60-2A and B)
- Atropic acne scarring (Fig. 60-3)
- Benign eyelid lesions (milia, acrochordon, nevi, xanthelasma)
- Hypertrophic or erythematous scarring (after trauma, surgery, or resurfacing)
- Ecchymosis after cosmetic surgery, or after botulinum or filler
- Facial hair.

## CONTRAINDICATIONS

- History of poor wound healing
- Smoking
- Diabetes
- Recent oral retinoid (Accutane) use within the past year
- Active skin infection
- Personal history of abnormal scarring or keloids

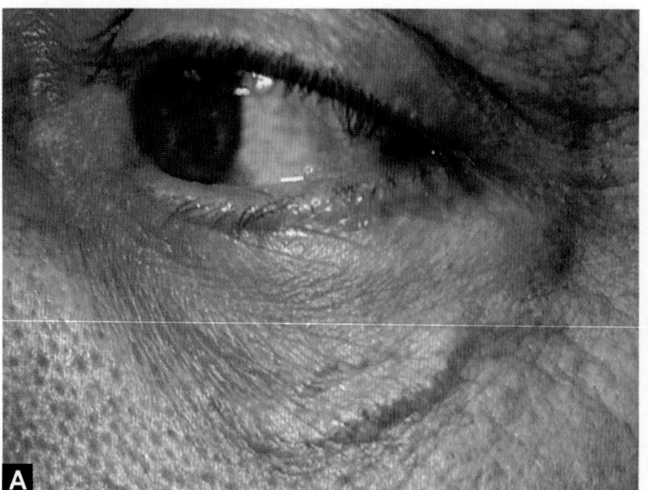


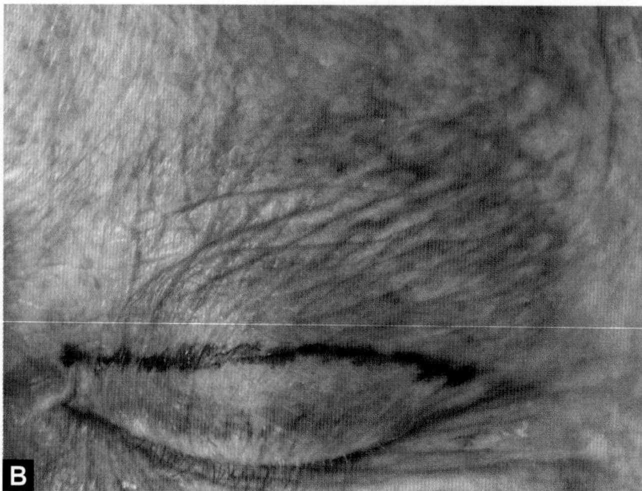


**Figures 60-2A and B** Prominent periocular veins common in the lower lid, lateral canthus, and upper lid.

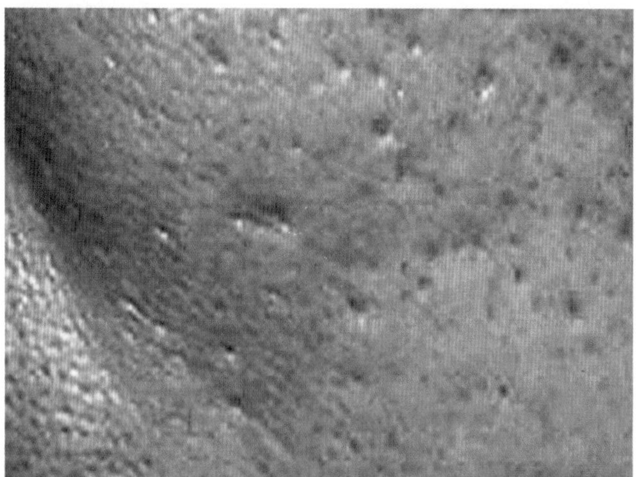

**Figure 60-3** Atrophic acne scarring of the cheek.

- Unrealistic expectations
- Pregnancy
- Other relative contraindications include vitiligo, history of deep peels or dermabrasion, history of skin radiation, eyelid malposition.

## RELEVANT ANATOMY

### Skin Anatomy

It is crucial for any physician performing laser rejuvenation to understand the layers of the skin, the thickness of each layer, and the depth of penetration necessary to induce certain changes within the skin. To review, the skin is composed of epidermis, dermis, and loose connective tissue with fat. The most superficial layer, the epidermis, is composed of four distinct layers: (1) keratinized and impermeable stratum corneum, (2) stratum granulosum, (3) vascular stratum spinosum, and (4) the cellular stratum basale (keratinocytes, melanocytes, fibroblasts). Although there is great variability in epidermal thickness based on anatomical site, it is approximately 100–200 μ deep (Table 60-1).

**TABLE 60-1** Average skin thickness based on facial region [in microns (μ)]

| Region | Epidermis (μ) | Dermis (μ) |
|---|---|---|
| Forehead | 202 | 969 |
| Glabella | 144 | 325 |
| Eyelid | 130 | 215 |
| Cheek | 145 | 909 |
| Nasal tip | 111 | 918 |
| Chin | 149 | 1375 |
| Neck | 115 | 158 |

The epidermis receives nutrition from the highly vascular papillary dermis, which is tightly adherent to the epidermis via the intervening basement membrane. $CO_2$ laser ablative resurfacing, for example, evaporates the epidermis and a portion of dermis using water as a chromophore.

The underlying dermis, measuring 500–1000 μ thick, provides structural support to the epidermis.[1] The dermis is subdivided into the superficial loose vascular connective tissue called the papillary dermis, and the deeper reticular layer rich in collagen and elastic fibers. The papillary dermis is approximately the same thickness as the epidermis, compared with the thicker reticular dermis. The major structural components of the dermis are collagen bundles and approximately 5% elastin fibers. As aging occurs, the skin degrades due to sun,

TABLE 60-2 Fitzpatrick Classification Scale

| Skin type | Skin color | Characteristics |
|---|---|---|
| I | Light, pale white; very fair; red or blond hair; blue eyes; freckles | Always burns, never tans |
| II | White; fair; red or blond hair; blue, hazel, or green eyes | Usually burns, tans with difficulty |
| III | Medium, white to olive; fair with any eye or hair color; very common | Sometimes mild burn, gradually tans |
| IV | Moderate brown; olive Mediterranean skin | Rarely burns, tans with ease |
| V | Dark brown; mid-eastern skin types | Very rarely burns, tans very easily |
| VI | Very dark brown to black | Never burns, tans very easily |

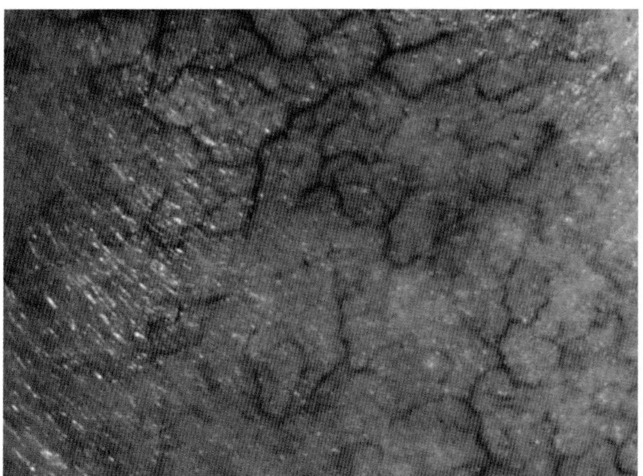

Figure 60-4 Facial telangiectasias, common on the cheeks and around the nasal ala, can be minimized with dermal treatments.

age, smoke, and other environmental pollutants. Although the body attempts to repair these aging changes within the skin, over time the normal architecture of collagen bundles breaks into fragmented bundles, and is manifested externally on the epidermal surface as the appearance of fine lines and deeper wrinkles, or rhytids. To optimally correct wrinkles and scars with skin rejuvenation procedures, the dermal layer needs to be targeted to the appropriate depth based on the structure to be treated. Vascular lesions like port-wine stains and telangiectasias are mainly dermal and can be minimized with dermal treatments (Fig. 60-4).

Regeneration of the epidermis with any form of treatment like dermabrasion, laser resurfacing, or chemical peels depends on the integrity and function of the dermal adnexal structures. The skin appendages, which include hair follicles, sebaceous glands, and sweat glands, arise within the deeper reticular dermis and subdermis and exit through the skin surface via epithelial-lined ducts. It is through the epithelium from these glands that re-epithelization occurs after the surface epithelium is completely removed via techniques such as ablative resurfacing. Areas that have a paucity of these appendage structures, such as the neck and anterior chest, are therefore less optimal candidates for laser resurfacing as poor healing and scarring may occur. The dermis is also highly vascular, which can serve as a useful endpoint during laser resurfacing to monitor the depth of treatment.

The subcutaneous layer located beneath the dermis comprised primarily of fat lobules. Its thickness and presence of robust fascial connections are vital to the youthful face and is therefore important in volumetric analysis of the aging face. The subcutaneous layer also functions as a buffer for skin trauma, as areas with abundant subcutaneous tissue often heal faster and with less scaring than areas with thin or no subcutaneous tissue. Therefore, deep dermal treatment in areas of the face with almost no subcutaneous tissue, such as the lips, jawline, and neck, should be carefully approached.

### Skin Type Classification

The provider must understand the importance of skin typing to perform aesthetic laser procedures, as this helps guide which type of laser treatment is most appropriate to use, and the parameters of the laser settings. The most commonly used scale is the Fitzpatrick Classification Scale, or Phototyping Scale, developed in 1975 by a Harvard Medical School dermatologist (Table 60-2).[2] This numerical scale classifies a person's skin color and their tolerance to sunlight. It helps determine how someone will respond or react to facial treatments, as well as how likely they are to develop skin cancer. Typically, patients with Fitzpatrick Type IV or darker should not undergo laser ablative techniques, or should be treated with extreme caution and expertise.

## MECHANISM OF ACTION

In laser resurfacing, the desired effects are epidermal ablation, heat-induced collagen shrinkage, and disruption of papillary dermis to induce collagen repair and re-epithelialization from hair follicles. Although detailed description of the physical properties of lasers and their mechanism of action is beyond the scope of this chapter, three basic laser–tissue interactions exist: photocoagulation, photodisruption, and photoablation.[3]

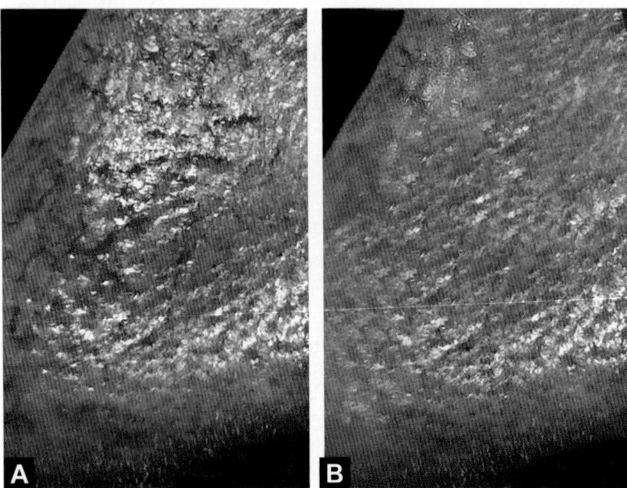


**Figures 60-5A and B** Nasal telangiectasias regress with a single treatment of intense pulsed light treatment (A) before treatment; (B) after one treatment).

Each laser modality may achieve one or several of these effects. In photocoagulation, laser light is absorbed by the tissue vessels or melanin, which generates heat that denatures or coagulates proteins. Photodisruption is largely a mechanical effect that produces a miniature lightning bolt that induces mechanical shock waves to disrupt tissue, such as seen with neodymium (Nd) and holmium:YAG lasers. These lasers may also induce photocoagulation, and as such can be used to treat periocular hemangiomas as well. Photoablation utilizes a sudden temperature rise beyond boiling point of intracellular water within the tissue, which results in vaporization. The $CO_2$ and erbium:YAG lasers cause photoablation and have therefore been highly popular for aesthetic skin resurfacing. $CO_2$ laser has a wavelength of 10,600 nm and is strongly absorbed by water, which is the main component of soft tissues. However, a variable amount of heat is also conducted to the surrounding tissues, which may cause lateral thermal damage and coagulative necrosis, which may ultimately result in scarring and healing complications. On the other hand, the surrounding tissue injury does induce the beneficial effects of thermal collagen contraction and remodeling. To minimize lateral thermal damage, the laser pulse duration should be shortened to less than the time needed for the tissue to irradiate and diminish its temperature to one half (thermal relaxation time).[4] Many modern lasers now have ultrapulsed or continuous mode systems that are able to deliver precise short-duration pulses at high irradiance, achieving tissue ablation with less depth of burn.[5] The erbium:YAG laser has a wavelength of 2940 nm and is more efficiently absorbed by water and collagen than the $CO_2$ laser, thus inducing less thermal damage. Nd:YAG lasers typically emit infrared light with a wavelength of 1064 nm and operate in both pulsed and continuous modes. The selective 1064-nm wavelength has strong absorption in oxyhemoglobin and melanin, resulting in selective heating of veins and hair follicles.

Pulsed dye laser, used extensively for capillary hemangiomas and port-wine stains in young children, uses a concentrated beam of yellow light that targets blood vessels in the skin while leaving the surrounding skin undamaged. Intense pulsed light (IPL), introduced in 1994, is a high-intensity polychromatic light source that emits pulsed light in a broadband of wavelengths between 400 and 1200 nm. Cutoff filters are available to narrow the bandwidth of emitted wavelengths to selectively target various structures at different depths within the skin. For example, filters may be changed to correspond to vessels of different depths and caliber, the hair follicle, or pigmented cells. It can target superficial vessels with shorter wavelengths while penetrating to deeper vessels with longer wavelengths and pulses. Between 75% and 100% of hemangiomas and telangiectasias (Figs. 60-5A and B) can clear after as few as one to three treatments. High cutoff filters can also be used to reduce melanin absorption and protect the epidermis in those with darker skin. Newer IPL devices have also demonstrated an excellent ability to treat rhytids as well, due to light-induced thermal denaturation of dermal collagen leading to reactive inflammation and collagen synthesis.

## TECHNIQUE

As there are a multitude of laser devices for cosmetic facial rejuvenation, all the various individual devices cannot be covered. The surgeon should review the instructions and parameters of the device being used and become familiar with its settings and achievable results through extensive practice, educational materials, and laser training conferences or seminars.

Regardless of the laser modality used, careful selection of ablation depth and energy is necessary to induce the desired changes while limiting complications. Several laser passes can be applied to the same areas to reach greater depths in the dermis and thus induce more collagen changes, and in general is useful for regions with deeper static rhytids. Each laser pass can be made, as needed, with the same or different settings. The number of passes over specific areas must be individualized for each patient, but conservative guidelines can be considered as: forehead = 2–3 passes; intraorbital eyelids = 1–2 passes; cheeks = 2–3 passes; perioral skin = 2–3 passes; jawline = 2 passes; upper neck skin = 1 pass; upper chest skin = 1 pass.

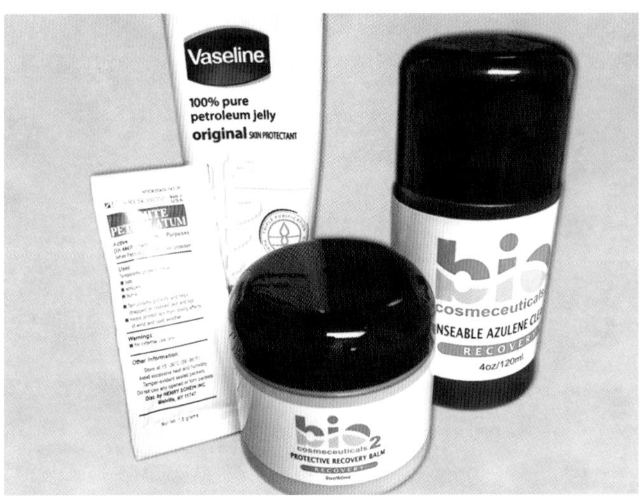


Figure 60-6 An occlusive barrier ointment should be applied immediately after ablative laser resurfacing.

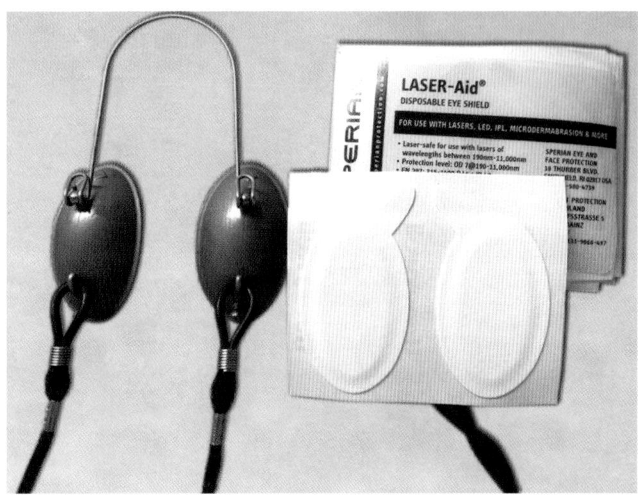


Figure 60-7 Eye shields to protect from ocular damage should be worn by the patient at all times.

## POST LASER CARE

Depending on the type of laser treatment, the patient is counseled that pain is typically minimal and easily controlled with over-the-counter analgesics. Cool soaks or compresses for the first 48 hours can help relieve discomfort, and the head of the bed should be elevated the first night to minimize facial edema. If ablative laser resurfacing has been performed, oral antibiotics or antivirals may be prescribed; these are not necessary after pulsed dye, IPL, microlaser peels (up to 50 μ), or skin-tightening lasers.

Topical soaks after ablative resurfacing with dilute vinegar solution (1 teaspoon white vinegar in 1 cup of water) can also help create a local environment that is weakly antibacterial and also undesirable to fungus. The soaks should be applied as "dripping wet" to the face several times a day, for 15–30 minutes at a time, and then the barrier ointment reapplied. In general, post laser skin infections can be avoided by keeping the treated surface clean and covered with a barrier environment. Petroleum ointment, Vaseline, or Aquaphor (Fig. 60-6) can be applied in a smooth layer over the face immediately after laser resurfacing and constantly reapplied as needed to keep the treated skin from drying out. Keeping the skin moist also promotes faster re-epithelialization. Topical antibiotics should be avoided during the early phase of wound healing after ablative laser procedures.

Depending of the depth of laser resurfacing, complete re-epithelialization should occur around 7–10 days, although it will take up to a month for the epithelium to regain full thickness and integrity. The patient should not pick or irritate any crusting present in the early healing phase as this could induce scarring.

Cosmetics and skin care regimens should be introduced gradually to avoid irritation, which could lead to contact dermatitis, acne, or poor healing. Oral minocycline or doxycycline may be prescribed if an acne flare is significant after treatment (10–15% incidence). The skin may remain slightly pink for several weeks to months, which may be camouflaged with makeup containing a yellow or green hue. Topical vitamin C in an aqueous formulation may also minimize the degree and duration of skin erythema. The use of broad-spectrum sunscreen (SPF 30 or higher) and minimizing sun exposure without protective head covering, both before and after laser treatments, will also limit ultraviolet stimulations of melanogenesis and hyperpigmentation issues. The effects of new collagen and elastin fiber production and tightening will continue to improve for up to 1 year after resurfacing.

## SPECIFIC INSTRUMENTATION

### Laser Safety

Appropriate and up-to-date education of all staff and providers is mandatory for the use of aesthetic lasers. The necessary checklist of safety precautions includes:

- Metal eye shields to protect patient from ocular damage (Fig. 60-7), applied with proparacaine and ophthalmic ointment
- Approved protective eyewear for staff (Fig. 60-8)
- Smoke/plume evacuator to remove viral and potentially mutagenic materials, gases, and blood-borne pathogens (Fig. 60-9)
- Avoid oxygen collection under facial drapes
- Use appropriate laser settings

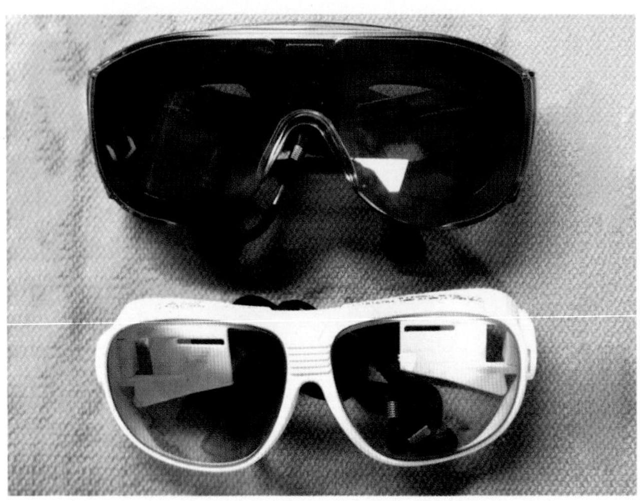

**Figure 60-8** Approved protective eyewear for staff is mandatory.

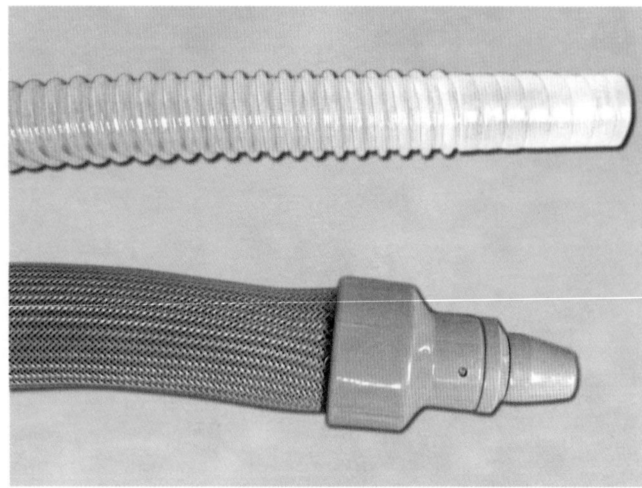

**Figure 60-9** A smoke or plume evacuator can remove viral and potentially mutagenic materials, gases, and pathogens.

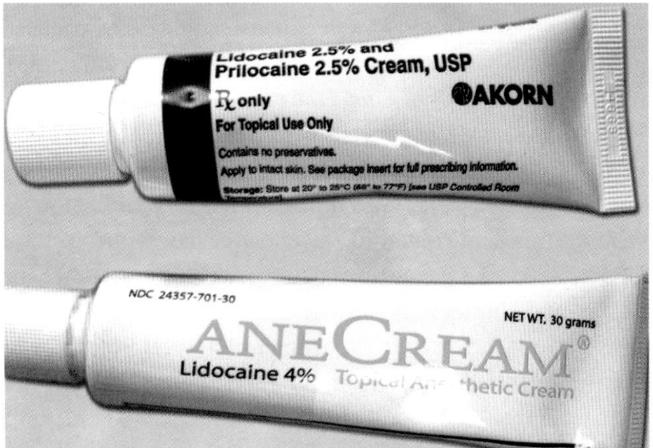


**Figure 60-10** Examples of topical anesthetic cream that can be applied 30–45 minutes prior to treatment.

- Topical anesthesia cream or nerve blocks (i.e. EMLA, LMX 4%) (Fig. 60-10)
- Facial masks, gloves
- Consider periprocedural antibiotics and antiherpetic medication.

## COMPLICATIONS

Despite the tremendous technical refinement of laser technology and its widespread popularity today, aesthetic facial and periocular laser procedures are not exempt from complications, some of which can be potentially severe.[6]

### Pigmentation Complications

Factors that affect healing include skin color and ethnicity, age, genetics, smoking, and other predisposing skin conditions. The treating physician should ask the patient about any issues with abnormal pigmentation changes or scarring from prior procedures or trauma. Excessive inflammation due to intense laser-induced thermal injury may cause significant lateral thermal tissue damage, which leads to persistent vasodilation, abundant melanin production, and transfer from the hair follicle melanocytes to the regenerated epithelial cells, causing increased pigmentation. Excess deposition of new collagen leads to hypertrophic scars or keloid formation.

Hyperpigmentation and hypopigmentation typically present in the first month and is most commonly seen in darker skin types (Fitzpatrick III to VI types) and in those patients with a prior history of postinflammatory dyschromia.[7,8] Often, the hyperpigmentation resolves without treatment but may take up to 6 months or more. Pretreatment with bleaching agents for 2–4 weeks, once or twice daily, may be recommended for patients at higher risk for postinflammatory hyperpigmentation. More common bleaching agents include topical hydroquinone 2–4% or kojic acid 2% (Fig. 60-11) and can be started anytime later if the dyschromia does not improve.[8] The concomitant use of tretinoin and a-hydroxy acids may facilitate penetration of these compounds and further stimulate collagen regeneration. In addition, sun avoidance and the use of broad-spectrum sunscreen, SPF 30 or higher, before and after laser treatment will limit ultraviolet stimulation of melanogenesis.[7,9]

Hypopigmentation after laser procedures is less common, but it may represent a loss of melanocytes due to deep thermal damage, or more rarely, an unmasking of vitiligo.[7] A histological study of skin after $CO_2$ laser resurfacing demonstrated dense subepithelial fibrosis and a decrease in the amount of epidermal melanin.[10] Previous cutaneous procedures such as

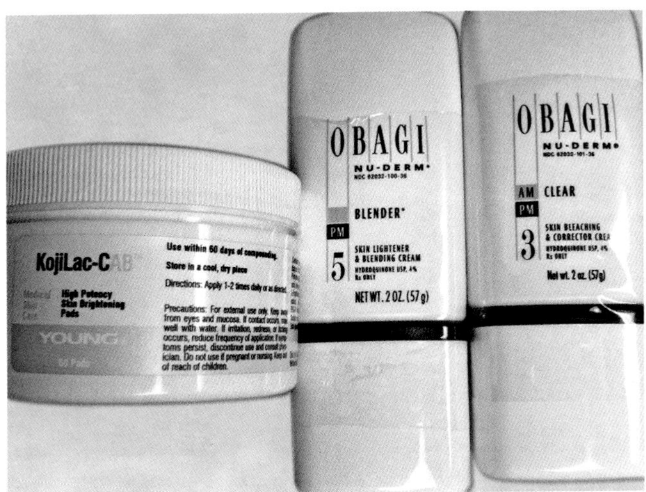


**Figure 60-11** Topical bleaching agents can minimize hyperpigmentation complications.

frequent dermabrasions, prior deep chemical peels, or topical 5-fluorouracil may increase the risk of post laser hypopigmentation.[10] Hypopigmentation is usually a late complication, and unfortunately, is best treated by camouflage with makeup. Studies have reported transient postinflammatory hyperpigmentation in up to 30% of patients after cosmetic laser resurfacing, whereas hypopigmentation was reported in only 1–3% of patients.[11]

## Hypertrophic Scarring

Several variables affect a patient's tendency to scar, with darker skin color and ethnicity in particular having a higher risk of hypertrophic scars and keloids. Hypertrophic scarring is a potentially devastating consequence of laser resurfacing, occurring in approximately 1% of patients.[11] Excessive thermal damage due to poor technique (inappropriate number of passes, excessive overlap between pulses, or overly aggressive depth of vaporization/ablation), infection, poor wound care, or patient-related risk factors, particularly keloid tendency, is among the most common causes. The periorbital region, particularly the medial lower lid, is at higher risk of developing hypertrophic scars after laser due to the extremely thin skin. Pretarsal and preseptal eyelid skin should therefore always be treated with caution. The patient should be instructed to avoid irritating, picking, or using nonprescribed topical agents on the treated area to prevent scarring. Hypertrophic scarring can also be minimized prior to laser treatments by pretreating the skin with a topical retinoid and bleaching agent, such as hydroquinone or kojic acid, 2-4 weeks prior. This is particular helpful when considering laser resurfacing in patients with Fitzpatrick skin types III or higher. Postlaser scarring should be treated as soon as it is detected with topical steroids and/or intralesional steroid injection, such as triamcinolone, alone or in combination with vitamin E gel, or silicone gel or sheets.[7] Dye laser treatment or fractionated $CO_2$ laser can also be helpful later to further debulk persistent scars.

## Prolonged Erythema

Prolonged erythema is one of the most common complications of laser rejuvenation and is due to vasodilation in the underlying dermis. Normal erythema may persist for minutes to several hours after IPL treatment for dyschromias or nonablative skin tightening lasers, and may persist several days following a microlaser peel. A general guideline is that for every 10 μ skin-depth treated, there may be a corresponding one day of mild erythema. With deeper laser ablation, the erythema is more intense and persists much longer, and on average lasts for 1–2 weeks with fractionated laser, or up to 3–4 months with complete laser ablation, depending on the depth of treatment. Prolonged or irregular erythema, despite preprocedure discussion of this possibility, may often lead to patient dissatisfaction despite good results. Although several factors including contact or irritant dermatitis, atopy, and superficial infections may lead to prolonged erythema, excess thermal damage and depth of tissue ablation are probably the most common causes and should be avoided by conservative settings until the patient has been shown to tolerate the laser treatment well.

In addition, prolonged erythema is a risk factor for hypertrophic scarring and atrophic textural changes. Topical steroid therapy may help improve erythema; however, due to the risk of atrophic changes or development of telangiectasias, they should be used for only a brief period of time. Aqueous topical vitamin C may also decrease the degree and duration of erythema after ablative laser resurfacing, and makeup foundation with a yellow or green tint can help mask the redness in the skin.[12]

## Infection

Infectious complications may present in the first 1–2 weeks particularly after deep ablative periocular and perioral laser resurfacing. Reports have shown a 6.5% incidence of bacterial infections, 1.7% incidence of herpes and other viral infections, and less commonly, fungal infections after periocular laser resurfacing.[11]

A primary herpes simplex virus outbreak or recurrence may occur in up to 9% after laser ablative resurfacing and may lead to undesirable scarring.[9] Herpetic lesions may appear as a cluster of small, raw, red lesions if they occur before complete

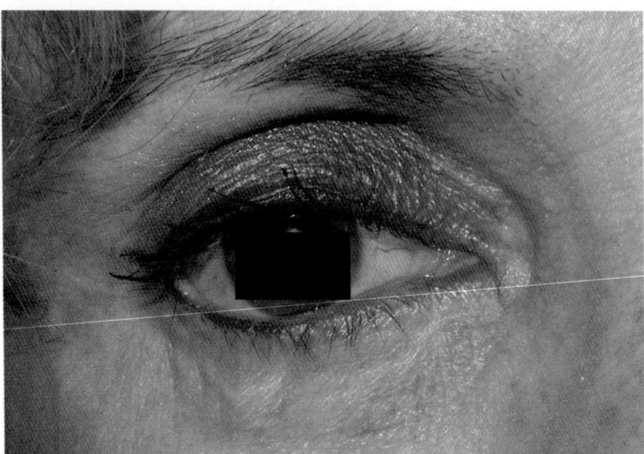

**Figure 60-12** Lower lid cicatricial ectropion and retraction after aggressive laser ablation.

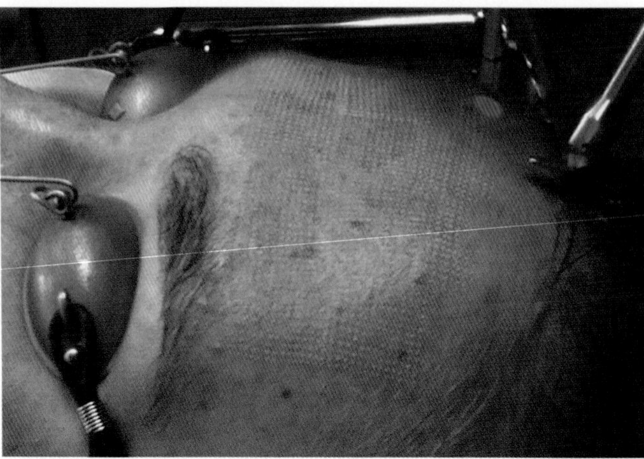

**Figure 60-13** At all times, adequate nonreflecting eye protective shields are mandatory to prevent corneal injury.

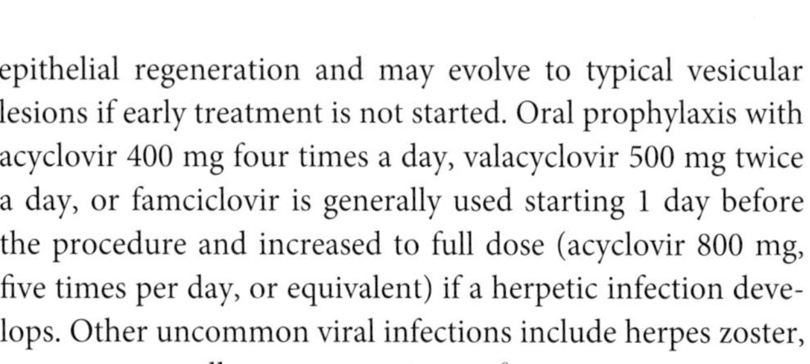

epithelial regeneration and may evolve to typical vesicular lesions if early treatment is not started. Oral prophylaxis with acyclovir 400 mg four times a day, valacyclovir 500 mg twice a day, or famciclovir is generally used starting 1 day before the procedure and increased to full dose (acyclovir 800 mg, five times per day, or equivalent) if a herpetic infection develops. Other uncommon viral infections include herpes zoster, verrucae, or molluscum contagiosum.[8]

The most common bacterial skin infection is impetiginization, which manifests as painless skin crusting, due to gram-positive cocci (*Staphylococcus pyogenes*, *S aureus*, or *S epidermidis*). Rarely, necrotizing fasciitis, pseudomonas, and other gram-negative infections may lead to more severe local and even systemic disease.[7,8,13] Oral prophylactic antibiotic therapy is recommended if resurfacing is moderate to extensive, typically for a duration of 5–7 days. The use of topical antibiotic ointment is discouraged due to the extremely high risk of contact dermatitis when applied to raw resurfaced areas. Occlusive dressings after resurfacing should also be avoided as they may predispose to bacterial or fungal infections.[9]

Superficial yeast infection may occur, especially in patients with a past history of vaginal candida infection, and manifests as erythematous areas, whitish plaques, pustules, or milia-like lesions. Oral fluconazole or ketoconazole may be useful prophylactically and postoperatively if needed.

### Skin Anterior Lamellar Shortening

Transient ectropion after laser lower lid blepharoplasty or resurfacing has been reported in 6% of patients and usually resolves when the edema improves. However, permanent cicatricial ectropion may occur in 0.4% and 0.1% after lower lid resurfacing and lower lid blepharoplasty, respectively, and can lead to cicatricial punctal ectropion due to severe anterior lamellar tightening (Fig. 60-12).[11] Risk factors for cicatricial ectropion after laser procedures include prior or simultaneous lower lid blepharoplasty or facelift, significant facial descent, and excessive lower lid or lateral canthal tendon laxity. Avoid ablative and aggressive laser resurfacing on the preseptal and pretarsal skin if possible, or consider performing a lateral canthopexy simultaneously if there is pre-existing lower lid laxity. Severe laser burns are fortunately rare, but may cause prolonged erythema, severe scarring, and permanent facial or eyelid contracture that may require skin grafting.

### Ocular Injury

At all times, the use of adequate nonreflecting eye protective shields is mandatory to prevent corneal thermal injury, globe perforation, or retinal injury during laser treatments (Fig. 60-13).

## PLACE OF THE TECHNIQUE IN AESTHETIC OCULOPLASTIC ARMAMENTARIUM

There are a multitude of laser applications in cosmetic periocular and facial rejuvenation, and they may be performed simultaneously during cosmetic surgery in most instances. This chapter focuses on the applications for cosmetic office procedures, with some of the most common uses in oculofacial practices directed to treat the following conditions:

### Skin Laxity

The goal of laser resurfacing is to induce significant improvement in the surface appearance of the skin. This is particularly useful in the periocular skin of the upper and lower eyelids, as surgical blepharoplasty alone may decrease the amount

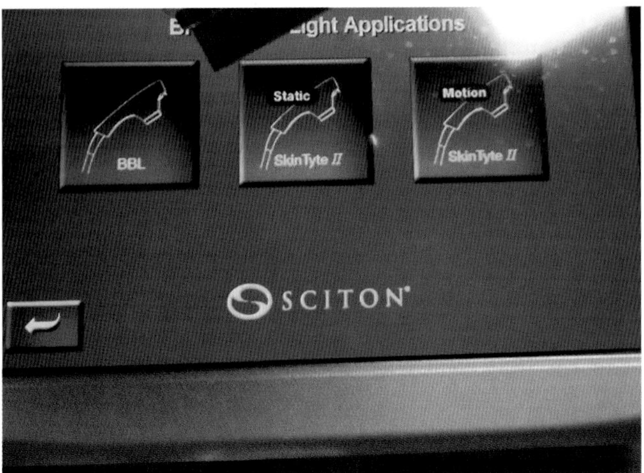


Figure 60-14 The Sciton Skintyte II may promote collagen contraction while protecting the epidermis.

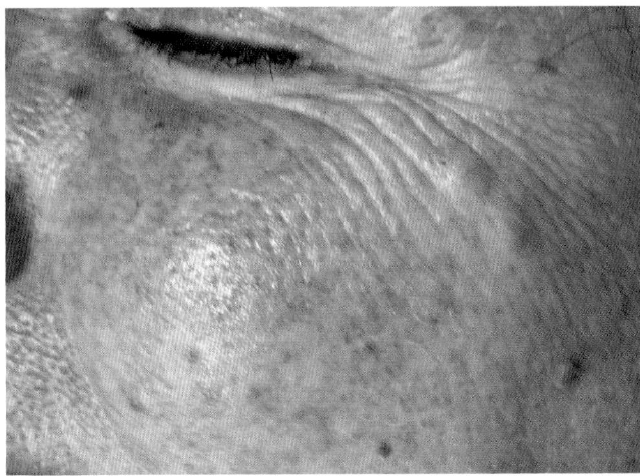

Figure 60-15 Prominent lateral eyelid and cheek wrinkles, "crow's feet," due to orbicularis oculi muscle contraction.

of redundant skin, but the remaining skin still maintains the pre-existing tone and laxity. In cases of younger patients or those with minimal skin excess, often laser resurfacing of the eyelid skin, with or without transconjunctival fat debulking, is the appropriate choice for tightening the skin. Some patients may also initially elect laser procedures to defer surgical options. Single or several passes of ablative resurfacing in the eyelid skin toward the eyelash line can result in significant rejuvenation and can be performed as minimal as 10 μ deep up to even 120 μ, depending on careful consideration of the patient skin and average skin thickness. This can also be combined with fractionated laser to a deeper depth of several hundred microns for even more dramatic improvement in the face, although this must be performed with caution to avoid complications of excessive tightening.

Other nonablative lasers, light sources, and radiofrequency devices also exist that may induce similar changes in the collagen of the papillary and reticular dermis without damaging the epidermis, which permits more rapid healing. With these devices, the laser or light energy is poorly absorbed by chromophores in the skin, and therefore most of the energy will pass through the epidermis to be scattered by the structures deeper in the skin. The thermal energy generated by this process is not sufficient to vaporize the tissue but still is able to devitalize the collagen and initiate a reparative process that will stimulate new collagen in the papillary and upper reticular dermis. Ideally, the epidermis is further protected by settings or instruments that cool the tissue. However, maximal results with nonablative devices may also take much longer, require multiple treatments and can be more subtle. One such device that is safe in all skin types is the Sciton Skintyte II that can firm or tighten any area of the body where improvement in skin texture laxity is desired, using infrared light technology to promote contraction and partial coagulation of the collagen (Fig. 60-14). The epidermis is continuously protected with an integrated sapphire contact cooling unit that precisely maintains temperatures between 0°C–30°C.

## Facial Rhytids and Fine Lines

In patients with "crow's feet" wrinkles (Fig. 60-15), laser ablation passes over the lateral periorbital lines (10–120 μ), with or without treatment with nonablative fractionated laser can diminish the lines. In those with more severe static lines, a deeper ablative treatment that removes the entire epidermis may be indicated, although the patient would need to be counseled that prolonged erythema and healing may take several months to resolve. In general, laser treatment with fewer passes results in more superficial resurfacing and less risk of complications, but it has the disadvantages of less dramatic improvement and more frequent sessions needed. In contrast, more aggressive treatment with more passes, deeper depth of ablation and penetration, multiple treatments, and longer downtime will often result in more dramatic eradication of severe rhytids and photodamage. Additional areas to target during facial rejuvenation with two to three more passes of deeper ablative or nonablative laser are the perioral vertical lip lines, nasolabial folds, chin lines and dimpling irregularities, and the glabellar and horizontal forehead rhytids.

## Vascular Lesions, Telangiectasias, and Rosacea

Pulsed dye laser, IPL, are excellent for treating vascular lesions such as hemangiomas, port-wine stains, facial and nasal telangiectasias (*see* Fig. 60-4), and rosacea. Treatment only takes a

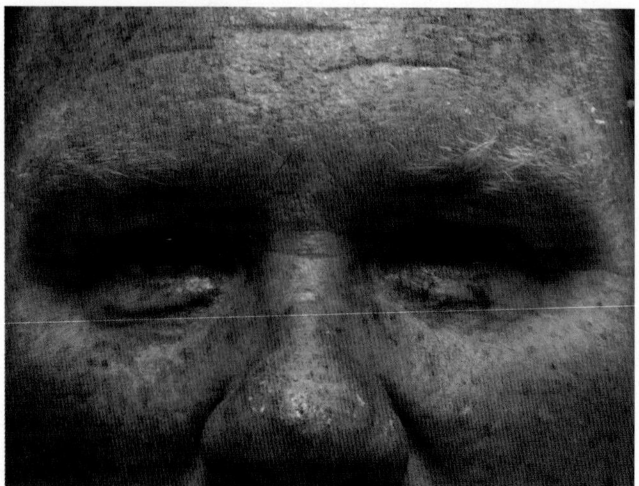

**Figure 60-16** The "ruddy" red facial appearance seen in rosacea, or in men, that can worsen and become uncomfortable with exercise.

few minutes, and most patients require between one and three treatments, depending on the extent of the lesion. When treating a vessel or telangiectasia, the laser should treat the entire vessel length without overlapping, as well as the trunk of the branching arterioles. As with any other treatment, incomplete response or recurrence may occur. Telangiectasias on the nose and around the nasal ala are often prominent and also respond very well to treatment (Fig. 60-5).

Patients with rosacea, or men or teenage boys, often complain of a constant "ruddy" appearance to the face that can worsen with exercise, stress, or alcohol (Fig. 60-16). The flushing in patients with rosacea can often be quite severe and painful as well, and may limit social activities. As with facial telangiectasias that can be directly treated with pulsed dye, broad-band light, or IPL treatments, the facial flushing or erythema can also improve with several sessions at 4–6-week intervals, although it may not improve as completely as do discrete telangiectasias.

## Senescent Dyschromia, Solar Pigmentation, Melasma

Macular brown spots are common on the aging or sunexposed face and can be treated with a variety of skin treatments. Ablative laser resurfacing to a more superficial depth or fractionated laser with or without epidermal ablation can yield significant improvement in solar lentigines, and also postpregnancy melasma. IPL has also been particularly excellent at removing these lesions scattered throughout the face, which typically involve not only the cheeks and nose, but also the forehead, pretrichial, and preauricular skin, jawline, and neck. The full extent of these dyschromias is sometimes not easily seen by the patient but contributes greatly to the overall dullness and uneven facial tone. A single full facial pass of pulsed light using a cut-off filter of 515 nm will target brown pigmentation in the skin and cause these to darken and eventually flake off within several days to a week (Figs. 60-17A and B). Larger lesions can be treated with another pass using higher energy and a focused spot adapter (Fig. 60-18). An additional side benefit is that the IPL also tends to improve overall skin texture, thus improving fine lines as well. Extremely dark lentigines may require more than one treatment. The patient should be aware that excessive sun exposure will lead to recurrence of pigmented lesions. Daily sunscreen and protective headwear, as well as possible hydroquinone or kojic acid products, can help slow the recurrence of solar lentigines. The patient should also avoid actively tanning for 1–2 weeks prior to treatment as the tanned skin may absorb more of the light energy and result in facial burns.

## Periocular Veins

Prominent periocular veins, primarily of the lower eyelid and lateral canthus more than the upper eyelid, are a relatively frequent cosmetic problem and may lead to the impression of dark circles around the eyes (Figs. 60-2 and 60-19). Laser treatment of periocular veins is an excellent treatment modality, with minimal side effects. The Nd:YAG 1064-nm laser is strongly absorbed by oxyhemoglobin and melanin, therefore selectively heating facial veins and hair follicles for reduction. On the Sciton machine, the ClearScan option is an excellent treatment modality for veins of varying caliber.

## Atrophic Acne Scarring

Atrophic acne scarring, or "pitting", is unfortunately common in younger and older patients and can be quite socially disruptive to the patient (Fig. 60-3). The skin defects may range from broad, atrophic shallowed scars, to fine-needle-tip deep pits or holes, scattered diffusely across the cheeks, jawline, or forehead. These manifestations can be extremely challenging to treat, and may require multiple treatments with a combination of surface ablation to even out the surface epithelium, and deep fractionated laser to stimulate new collagen formation that will remodel and elevate the atrophic scars from below. Deep scars can sometimes be discolored or erythematous, and therefore could also be treated with IPL to reduce redness or pigmentation.

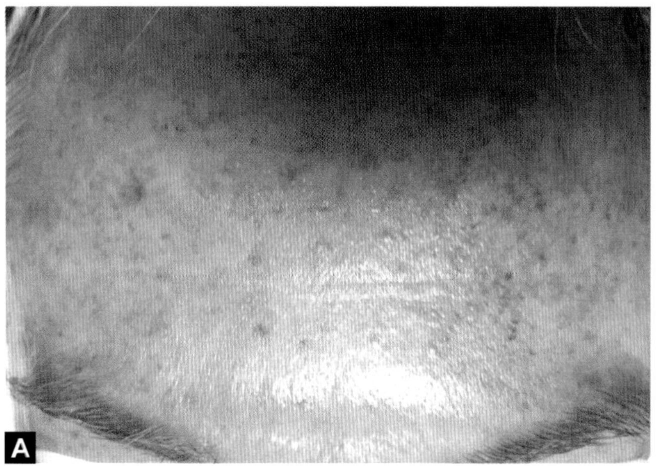


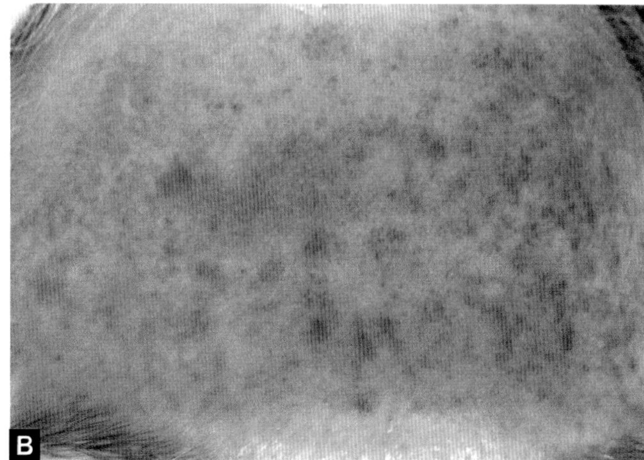


**Figures 60-17A and B** (A) Diffuse forehead pigmentation prior to pulsed light treatment. (B) The brown lesions are seen to darken immediately after treatment and will flake off in a week.

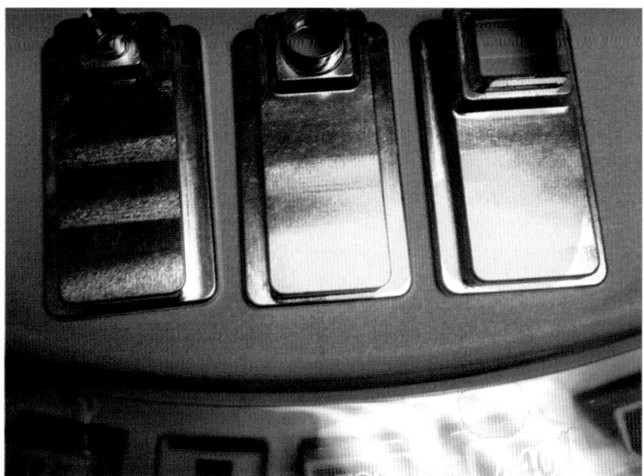

**Figure 60-18** Spot adapters can be used to focus the laser on specific lesions.

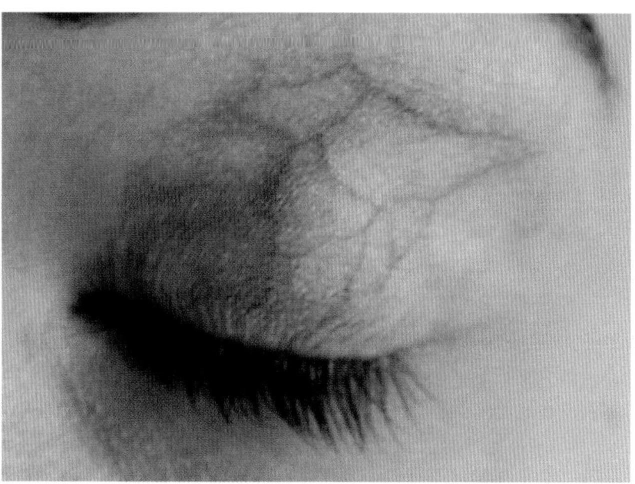

**Figure 60-19** Prominent periocular veins in the upper eyelid can be a frequent cosmetic concern.

## Eyelid Lesion Ablation (Milia, Acrochordon, Nevi, Xanthelasma)

Elevated skin lesions can often be removed with a single-spot laser, such as a 2- or 4-mm spot, to a desired depth of 10–50 μ or more, to ablate undesirable lesions without creating significant scar. Typically, patients with multiple facial pigmented or amelanotic nevi will prefer this treatment over shave excision.

## Laser Hair Removal

Unwanted facial hair may be a cosmetic issue or due to systemic conditions, such as hirsutism, and is an extremely popular niche for laser treatment. Careful patient selection and evaluation of skin type, hair color, and coarseness will determine which device is the most appropriate, as well as predict the response to treatment. The ideal candidate for laser hair removal is a patient with dark, coarse hair. White or very light hair or fine vellus hairs are much more difficult to treat, and the eyelid skin should be avoided to minimize complications. Suntanned patients should also avoid treatment until the tan has faded. Methods used for hair removal include ruby (694 nm), alexandrite (755 nm), pulsed diode laser (800 nm), long pulsed Nd:YAG lasers (1064 nm), IPL (590–1200 nm), all with potentially effective long-term results for hair removal via photothermal destruction of hair follicles. In general, ≥5 treatments performed at 1–3-month intervals are often necessary to achieve a reasonable reduction of excess hair.

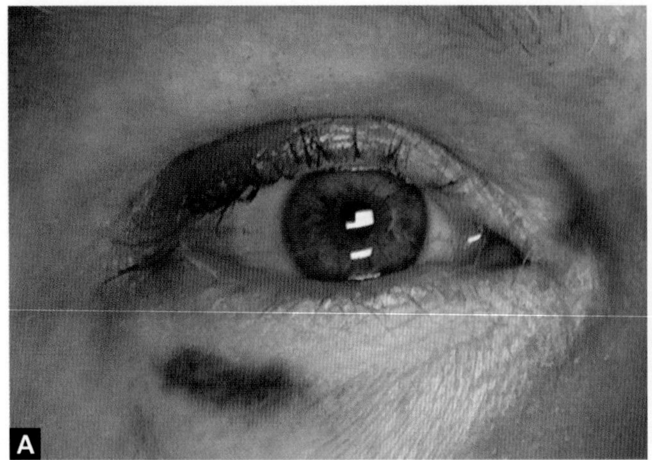


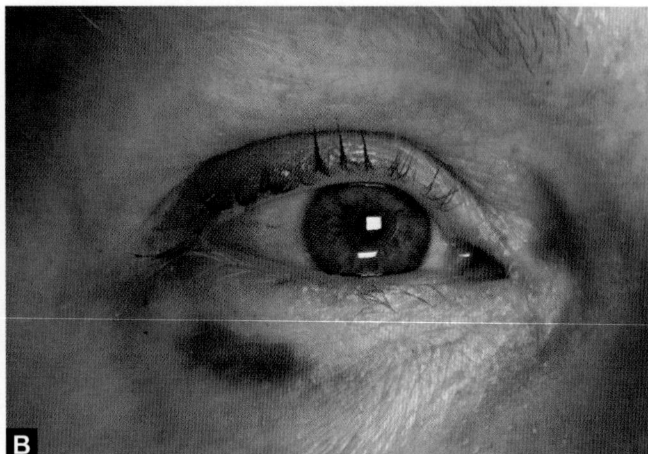


**Figures 60-20A and B** (A) Lower lid ecchymosis after cosmetic botulinum injection, not improved at 1 week. (B) Ecchymosis coagulated and much smaller, immediately after 560 filter pulsed light treatment.

## Hypertrophic or Erythematous Scarring (after Trauma, Surgery, or Resurfacing)

Pulsed dye laser or IPL can also be beneficial in improving the appearance of red scars or hypertrophic scars, which is helpful in the cosmetic patient who desires minimal downtime. A filter between 532 and 560 nm will direct the light to the vascular areas to cause immediate vasoconstriction of inflammatory telangiectasias and rapid improvement of erythema. This can be performed as early as several days to a week after surgery. Fractionated deep laser ablation can be used in several sessions for hypertrophic scars to break up the irregular collagen and stimulate new tissue remodeling that will flatten and blend the scar.

## Ecchymosis after Cosmetic Surgery or Cosmetic Injections

Unanticipated bruising at the sites of cosmetic injections, such as botulinum or soft tissue fillers, can sometimes occur and be bothersome to the patient. Pulsed light treatment using a filter in the 560 range can focus the light energy to the area of heme and cause almost complete resolution of ecchymosis within minutes to days after treatment. This is also an ideal cosmetic use after oculofacial surgery, such as cosmetic blepharoplasty, when the patient returns at the initial postoperative visit and has significant or persistent ecchymosis. Treating the areas with IPL can lessen the degree and duration of ecchymosis substantially, and thus provide greater patient satisfaction (Figs. 60-20A and B).

In conclusion, appropriate patient selection, adequate preoperative and prophylactic treatment, proper training and familiarity of the surgeon with the laser modalities and indications, and a cautious, conservative approach are strongly recommended to minimize complications after oculofacial laser rejuvenation.

## REFERENCES

1. Ruess W, Owsley JQ. The anatomy of the skin and fascial layers of the face in aesthetic surgery. Clin Plast Surg. 1987;14:677-82.
2. Glogau R. Physiologic and structural changes associated with aging skin. Dermatol Clin. 1997;15:555-9.
3. Thall EH. Ophthalmology. In: Yanoff M, Duker JS (eds), Principles of lasers. London, UK: Mosby; 1999:2.5.1–2.5.6.
4. Goldbaum AM, Woog JJ. The $CO_2$ laser in oculoplastic surgery. Surv Ophthalmol. 1997;42:255-67.
5. Grossman AR, Majidian AM, Grossman PH. Thermal injuries as a result of $CO_2$ laser resurfacing. Plast Reconstr Surg. 1998; 102:1247-52.
6. Blanco G, Soparkar CN, Jordan DR, et al. The ocular complications of periocular laser surgery. Curr Opin Ophthalmol. 1999; 10:264-9.
7. Linsmeier-Kilmer S. Laser resurfacing complications. How to treat them and how to avoid them. Int J Aesthet Restor Surg. 1997;5:41-5.
8. Khan JA. Millisecond $CO_2$ laser skin resurfacing. Int Ophthalmol Clin. 1997;37:29-67.
9. Nanni CA, Alster TS. Complications of cutaneous laser surgery. A review. Dermatol Surg. 1998;24:209-19.
10. Laws RA, Finley EM, McCollough ML, et al. Alabaster skin after carbon dioxide laser resurfacing with histologic correlation. Dermatol Surg. 1998;24:633-6.
11. Apfelberg DB. Summary of the 1997 ASAPS/ASPRS Laser Task Force Survey on Laser Resurfacing and Laser Blepharoplasty. Plast Reconstr Surg. 1998;101:511-8.
12. Alster TS, West TB. Effect of topical vitamin c on postoperative carbon dioxide laser resurfacing erythema. Dermatol Surg. 1998;24:331-4.
13. Jordan DR, Mawn L, Marshall DH. Necrotizing fasciitis caused by group A streptococcus infection after laser blepharoplasty. Am J Ophthalmol. 1998;125:265-6.

CHAPTER 61

# Ptosis Repair—Mullerectomy

Shubhra Goel, Cat Nguyen Burkat

## INTRODUCTION

With advancing knowledge and continuous refinement in oculofacial surgical techniques, there is an increasing demand for surgical approaches that avoid visible scars. As ptosis repair is one of the most common eyelid procedures, patients are becoming more aware of the less-invasive alternatives to conventional external levator repair.

First described in 1975 by Putterman and Urist, Müller's muscle conjunctival resection (MMCR), also known as conjunctivomüllerectomy or internal ptosis surgery, is an increasingly popular posterior-approach ptosis correction surgery. It is often performed in patients with mild to moderate ptosis.[1,2] When compared with external levator surgery, it is a faster procedure, with the advantages of less tissue dissection, better predictability, and reportedly less recurrences.

## PREREQUISITES

The MMCR is typically recommended in patients with mild ptosis (ptosis of ≤2–3 mm), good levator excursion (≥10 mm), positive phenylephrine test (Figs. 61-1A and B), and minimal skin excess.

## INDICATIONS

- Horner Syndrome
- Congenital ptosis with good levator excursion
- Acquired ptosis—aponeurotic dehiscence or attenuation due to involutional changes, residual ptosis after blepharoplasty surgery, chronic use of contact lens or prosthetic shell after traumatic eyelid injury
- Residual ptosis after conventional external ptosis surgery.

## CONTRAINDICATIONS

The MMCR is not recommended, or should be approached with expertise, in the following conditions:

- Myogenic ptosis
- Ptosis with decreased or poor levator excursion
- Ptosis with a negative phenylephrine test
- Severe ptosis.

## SURGICAL TECHNIQUE

A written informed consent should always be obtained from the patient. The patient is also requested to discontinue

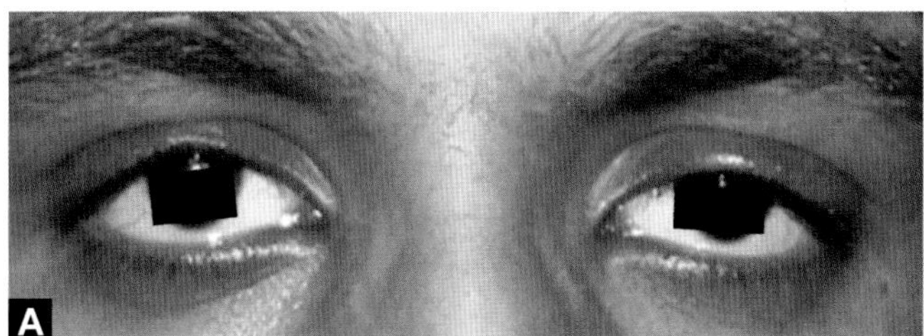


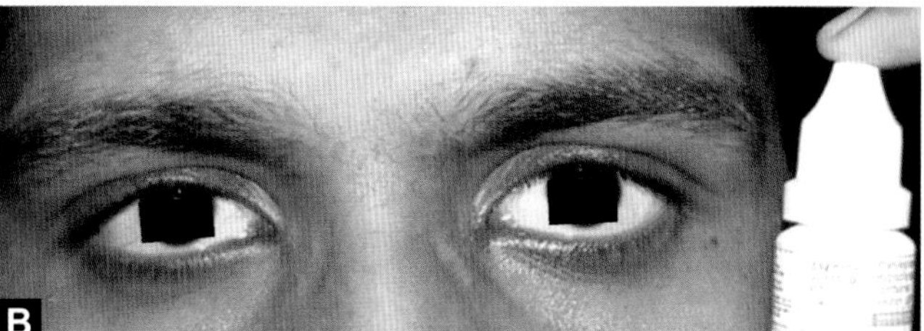


**Figures 61-1A and B** Phenylephrine test. (A) Left upper lid mild ptosis with margin-to-reflex distance (MRD1) of 3 mm on the right and 0 mm on the left. Levator excursion measures 12 mm. (B) Simulated correction of ptosis on the left following the phenylephrine test, with MRD1 of 3 mm on the right and 3 mm on the left.

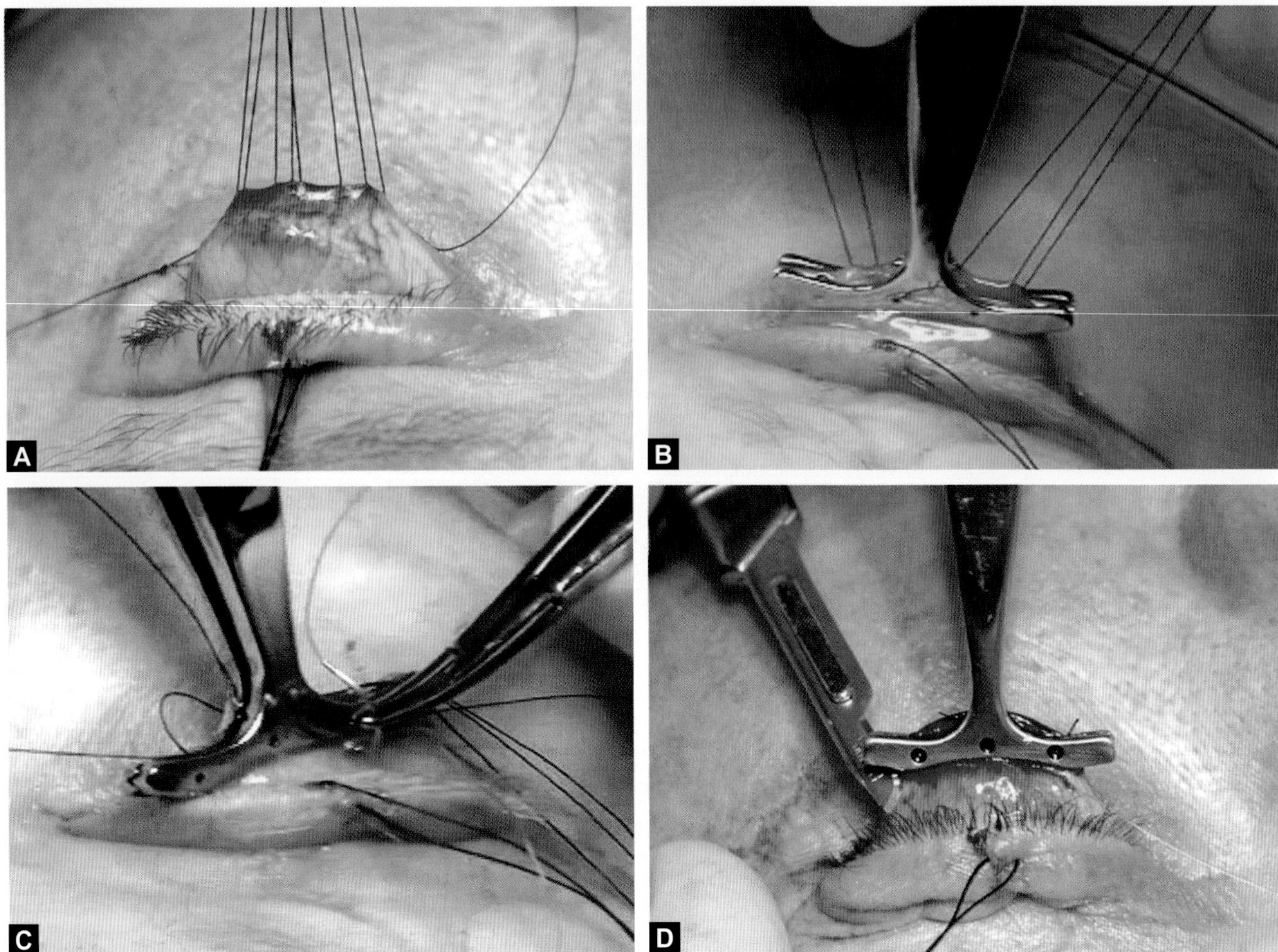

**Figures 61-2A to D** Surgical steps. (A) Calipers are used to measure half of the desired resection amount from the superior tarsus, with the lid everted over a Desmarres retractor. Silk sutures placed at three sites are elevated evenly in preparation for placement of the clamp. (B) The Putterman clamp encloses the elevated tissues up to the tarsal edge, which results in a total conjunctival and Muller's muscle resection that equals the preoperative calculated amount. (C) Running horizontal mattress sutures are passed just below the clamp, taking care to incorporate the superior tarsus. (D) The 15 blade scalpel is beveled toward the clamp while excising the enclosed tissues.

anticoagulants, aspirin, ibuprofen, vitamin E, fish oil, and garlic supplements approximately 1–2 weeks prior to surgery (Figs. 61-2A to D and 61-3A and B) .

- A surgical marking pen is used to mark the center of the pupil on the upper lid with the patient looking in primary gaze.
- A small amount (0.5–1 mL) of local infiltrative anesthesia (2% lidocaine with 1:100,000 epinephrine mixed in equal parts with 0.25–0.75% Marcaine) is administered to the upper lid near the margin.
- The face is prepped and draped in the usual fashion for ophthalmic plastic surgery.
- A 4-0 silk traction suture is placed near the central aspect of the upper lid margin, and the lid is everted over a small Desmarres retractor.
- One half of the intended excision measurement (precalculated as per the phenylephrine test results and the nomogram calculation) is made from the superior aspect of the tarsus toward the superior fornix. This is measured with compass point calipers and marked with a marking pen at three sites (central, medial, and lateral), taking care to follow the taper of the tarsus both medially and laterally. Another marking can be made further superiorly from the central marking, which would represent the total intended excision amount. A 6-0 silk suture is then passed in succession below all three markings, incorporating conjunctiva and Müller's muscle (MM). With equal elevation of the suture along the three sites, this results in the desired total excision amount (confirmed by the marking made above the central site). Measuring the half-markings

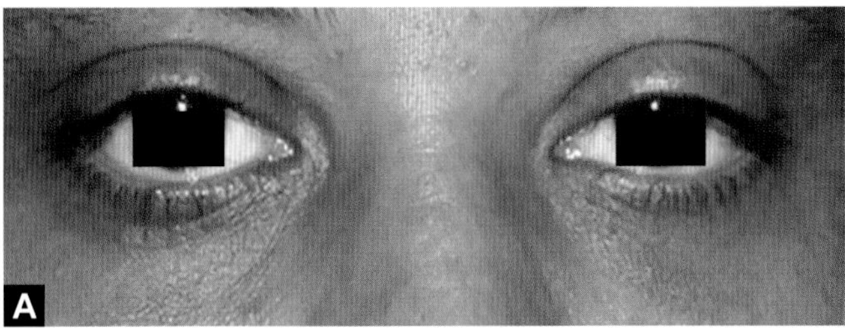


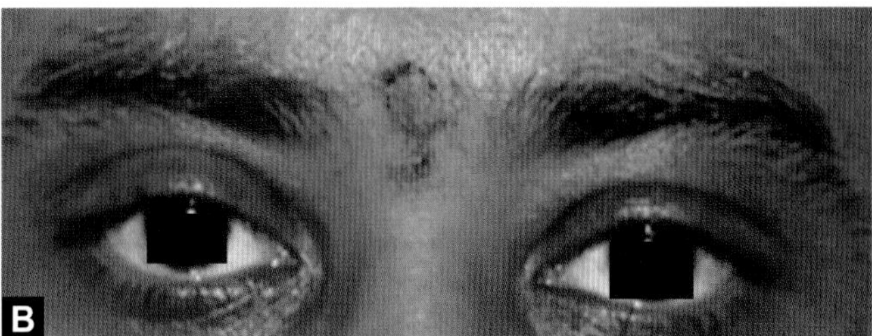


**Figures 61-3A and B** (A) Left upper lid ptosis correction 2 weeks after Müller's muscle conjunctival resection surgery. (B) Minimal edema and ecchymosis is seen.

is more accurate as the posterior conjunctival surface curves over the Desmarres retractor when everted, which may make a lengthy linear measurement less exact.

- With upward elevation on the silk traction suture (making sure to lift the medial and lateral ends equally), the Putterman clamp is closed over the conjunctival and MM layers, flush to the superior tarsal edge. Avoid incorporating tarsus, as this would result in a greater lift similar to a Fasanella–Servat technique.
- A 5-0 polypropylene suture is passed through the skin to the conjunctiva on one side, and then passed in serpentine fashion under the Putterman clamp, to exit out through the skin on the other side. Take care to pass the sutures at the same distance below the clamp at all times.
- The 15-blade is used to excise the clamped tissues, keeping the blade beveled toward the clamp to avoid cutting the suture.
- The suture is then tied over the skin, which closes the incision and results in imbrication of the overlying levator complex for correction of ptosis. Alternatively, an absorbable suture can be passed under the clamp as above, and then passed back after the tissues are excised in a running interrupted suture incorporating the superior conjunctiva and MM to the superior tarsal edge. The tied knot must be buried and rotated toward the skin surface to avoid corneal abrasions.
- The traction sutures are removed from the lid margin.
- Some surgeons may elect to place a bandage contact lens as a precautionary measure to avoid corneal irritation from the sutures.

## MECHANISM OF ACTION

The MM is the secondary elevator of the eyelid in addition to the levator palpebrae superioris muscle. It is innervated by the sympathetic nervous system and originates from the levator aponeurosis complex approximately 15 mm above the superior tarsus.[3] The MM is closely adherent to the underlying conjunctiva, but it is easily separable from the levator aponeurosis.[4] Some authors have postulated that the levator aponeurosis terminates 2–3 mm above the tarsal border and does not support the anterior lamella, and that the MM exerts the major pull on the superior tarsus.[5] Therefore, it is believed that MMCR surgery theoretically corrects ptosis via advancement of the anterior extensions of the levator aponeurosis to the tarsus to enhance its pull on the eyelid, as well as via vertical posterior lamellar shortening, wound cicatrization, and contraction.[1,6]

### What is the Phenylephrine Test?

Phenylephrine is a sympathomimetic drug and stimulates the MM, clinically demonstrated by an improvement in ptosis (secondary to the contraction of the smooth muscle fibers of MM). The phenylephrine test is commonly used preoperatively to predict the treatment response of MMCR surgery.

- Originally described by Putterman in 1975
- Determines if the patient is a candidate for conjunctivo-müllerectomy surgery
- May be used as a guide to determine the amount of conjunctival and MM resection
- Simulates the postoperative result for the patient and surgeon
- Unmasks latent contralateral ptosis due to Herring's effect.

### How is the Phenylephrine Test Performed?

- The margin-to-reflex distance ($MRD_1$) is measured with the frontalis muscle relaxed
- Topical proparacaine eye drops are applied to the ocular surface
- One to two drops of 2.5–10% phenylephrine are instilled into the superior conjunctival fornix of the ptotic eye with the patient looking in downgaze. Care should be used in patients with significant cardiac history
- The $MRD_1$ is remeasured at the end of 5 minutes. The process can be repeated if desired

**TABLE 61-1** Nomogram for Müller's muscle conjunctival resection surgery as proposed by Dresner

| Desired elevation (mm) | MMC resection (mm) |
|---|---|
| 1.0 | 4 |
| 1.5 | 6 |
| 2.0 | 8 |
| 3.0 | 10 |

- Document the presence of a Herring's effect, i.e. if improvement of ptosis in the eyelid results in contralateral ptosis that was initially absent
- An improvement in the $MRD_1$ of ≥ 1 mm is considered positive, and the patient may undergo MMCR surgery.

## CONSIDERATIONS IN SURGICAL PLANNING

There exist many different algorithms that may help guide the appropriate amount of MMCR in cases of mild to moderate ptosis. In general, for every 1 mm of desired elevation, 4 mm of resection has been advocated. It is important to stress that any algorithm should be adjusted for each individual surgeon.

- Weinstein and Buerger[7] in 1982 proposed 8-mm resection for 2-mm eyelid ptosis (+/- 1 mm for every 0.25-mm change)
- Putterman and Fett[2] in 1986 modified it to 8.25-mm resection (range 6.5- to 9.5-mm resection)
- Dresner[1] presented a nomogram in 1991 that is widely used and further modified by others. In this nomogram, 4 mm is resected to correct for 1 mm of ptosis, 6 mm for 1.5 mm ptosis, 10 mm for 2 mm ptosis, and 11 or 12 mm for >3 mm of ptosis (Table 61-1)
- Perry et al.[8] suggested an algorithm based on the hypothesis that the final lid height seen with maximal stimulation of MM with 10% phenylephrine eyedrops can be achieved by 9 mm of MM excision. Any residual undercorrection during phenylephrine testing can corrected with additional tarsal resection in a 1:1 ratio of eyelid elevation, up to a maximum of 2.5 mm (to avoid tarsal instability).

Working example (Table 61-2 and pictures (a) and (b) above the table): the nomogram by Dresner is used in planning the amount of MMCR in this patient.

## ADVANTAGES AND DISADVANTAGES

### Advantages[9-11]

- Lid contour and stability are not affected when compared to external levator repair and Fasanella–Servat techniques
- More predictable results
- Titration is based on severity of ptosis
- Minimal operative time
- No external incision, which results in no scar and more rapid recovery
- No intraoperative adjustments needed
- Can be safe in patients with filtering blebs
- Can be safe in patients with dry eyes
- Less reoperation rates when compared with external levator repair
- Can be performed in combination with blepharoplasty and other eyelid techniques.

### Disadvantages[12,13]

- Ocular surface irritation, or corneal abrasion
- Suture irritation and possible disturbance of filtering blebs
- Potential conjunctival forniceal shortening, although some studies have noted no change in fornix depth measurements following MMCR
- Caution in patients with anophthalmia and an ocular prosthesis
- Temporary effect on tear production due to excision of conjunctiva (with goblet cells) and damage to the accessory lacrimal glands (glands of Krause and Wolfring)
- Postoperative office adjustments for asymmetry are more difficult to perform in the early postoperative period
- Less ideal for patients with severe ptosis or decreased levator function.

## POSTOPERATIVE CARE

- Avoid strenuous activity, bending, or lifting heavy weights for 1 week
- Sleep with the head elevated at 30–45°, or on two pillows, for the next 72 hours
- Start cold, wet compresses immediately after surgery, and continue as much as possible for 48 hours to minimize bruising and swelling
- Clean the operated area gently with warm water and a clean cotton-tip applicator if necessary
- Use artificial tears as needed for lubrication as well as for mild surface irritation
- Consider a bandage soft contact lens if there is significant foreign body sensation
- Apply antibiotic ophthalmic ointment two to three times a day to the ocular surface if prescribed, which may also relieve discomfort

TABLE 61-2 Working example

| | Right (mm) | Left (mm) |
|---|---|---|
| Pretest margin-to-reflex distance (MRD1) | 1 | 3 |
| Post-test MRD1 | 3 | 3 |
| Amount of Müller's muscle-conjunctival resection surgery planned | 8 | |

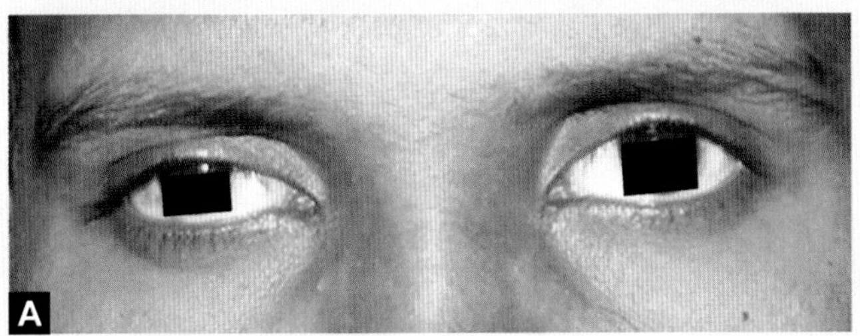


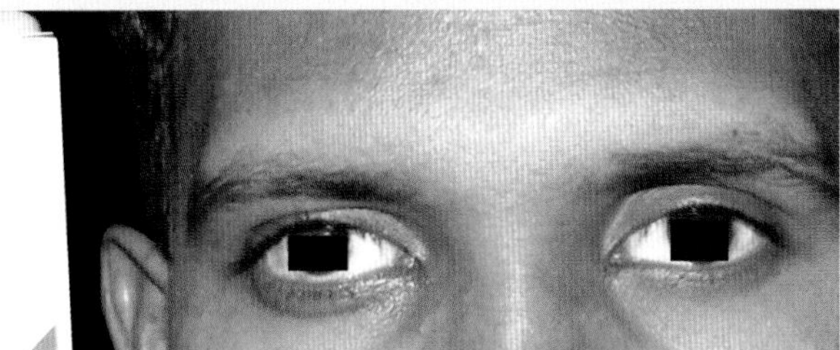


(A) Patient has a 2-mm mild right upper eyelid ptosis. (B) Phenylephrine testing was positive, and no Herring's effect was present. As per the nomogram by Dresner, 8 mm of resection is planned to correct for a 2-mm ptosis.

TABLE 61-3 Modified nomogram for Müller's muscle conjunctival resection surgery when performing concurrent blepharoplasty

| Ptosis amount (mm) | Resection amount (mm) |
|---|---|
| 1.0 | 5 |
| 1.5 | 7 |
| 2.0 | 9 |

- Resume normal activities after 1 week
- Sutures are removed at 1 week or will dissolve if absorbable sutures were used.

## ADDITIONAL PROCEDURES

Additional procedures, such as blepharoplasty, brow lifting, lacrimal gland resuspension, and ectropion repair, are often performed with MMCR. When performing concurrent blepharoplasty, a nomogram can be followed as a guideline[14] (Table 61-3).

## CONCLUSION

The MMCR surgery is an effective, reliable, and excellent alternative for ptosis correction in select patients with mild to moderate ptosis and good levator muscle function. It offers an easy, quick, and scarless surgical approach that can be highly desirable to many patients.

## REFERENCES


1. Dresner SC. Further modifications of the Muller's muscle-conjunctival resection procedure for the blepharoptosis. Ophthalmic Plast Reconstr Surg. 1991;7:114-22.
2. Putterman AM, Urist MJ. Müller muscle-conjunctiva resection. Technique for treatment of blepharoptosis. Arch Ophthalmol. 1975;93:619-23.
3. Beard C. Mullers superior tarsal muscle: anatomy, physiology, and clinical significance. Ann Plast Surg. 1985;14:324-33.
4. Chee-Chew Yip, Fong-Yee Foo, The role of Muller's muscle-conjunctiva resection (MCR) in the treatment of ptosis. Ann Acad Med. 2007;36(Suppl):10.
5. Collin JRO, Beard C, Wood I. Experimental and clinical data on the insertion of the levator palpebral superioris muscle. Am J Ophthalmol. 1978;85:792-801.
6. Buckman G, Jackobiec FA, Hyde K, et al. Success of Fasanella-Servat operation independent of Muller's muscle excision. Ophthalmology. 1989;96:413-8.
7. Weinstein GS, Buerger GF. The modifications of Muller's muscle conjunctival resection operation for blepharoptosis. Am J Ophthalmol. 1993;5:647-51.
8. Perry JD, Kadakia A, Foster JA. A new algorithm for ptosis repair using conjunctival Müllerectomy with or without tarsectomy. Ophthal Plast Reconstr Surg. 2002;18:426-9.
9. McCulley T, Kersten RC, Kulwin DR, et al. Outcome and influencing factors of external levator palpebral superioris aponeurosis advancement for blepharoptosis. Ophthal Plast Reconstr Surg. 2003;19:388-93.
10. Baroody M, Holds JB, Sakamoto DK, et al. Small incision transcutaneous levator aponeurotic repair for blepharoptosis. Ann Plast Surg. 2004;52:558-61.
11. Brown MS, Putterman AM. The effect of upper blepharoplasty on eyelid position when performed concomitantly with Müller muscle conjunctival resection. Ophthal Plast Reconstr Surg. 2000;16:94-100.
12. Jordan DR, Anderson RB, Mamalis N. Accessory lacrimal glands. Ophthalmic Surg. 1990;21:146-7.
13. Dailey RA, Saulny SM, Sullivan SA. Müller muscle-conjunctival resection: effect on tear production. Ophthal Plast Reconstr Surg. 2002;18:421-5.
14. Rose J, Lemke BN, Dresner SC, et al. Blepharoptosis treatment options during upper eyelid cosmetic blepharoplasty. Am J Cosmet Surg. 2003:20(1)73-8.

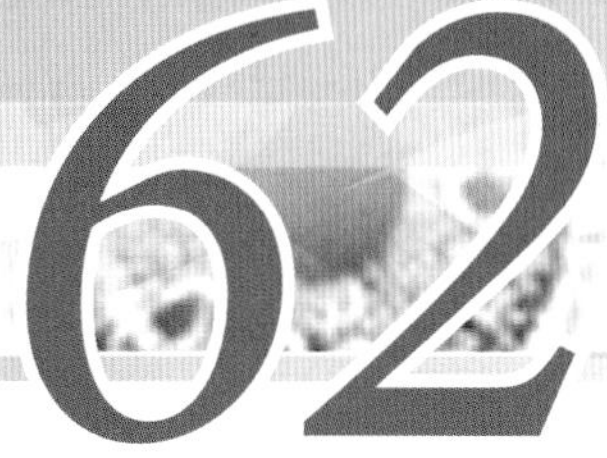


# Ptosis Repair—Fasanella Servat Procedure

Vikas Menon, Santosh G Honavar

## INTRODUCTION

Mild ptosis with good levator action poses a challenging situation for any oculoplastic surgeon. Treatment options include a small levator resection, conjunctivo–Müllerectomy, and Fasanella–Servat procedure. Although levator surgery is a bit difficult to titrate for mild ptosis and may require frequent postoperative adjustments, conjunctivo–Müllerectomy works by shortening the Müllers muscle and is best suited if the patient shows reasonably good response on being stimulated by phenylephrine. Fasanella and Servat described their technique for managing mild ptosis in 1961.[1] It is a relatively simple procedure to perform and does not require any specific instrumentation as sometimes required in other procedures.

Main criticism of Fasanella–Servat technique lies in the relatively low rate of success reported in literature (28–61%) and also frequent description of eyelid contour abnormalities. However, most authors have attributed these problems to poor patient selection and inappropriate technique.[2,3]

## INDICATIONS

- Mild congenital ptosis (<2.5 mm) with good levator action (>10 mm) (Fig. 62-1)
- Mild ptosis seen in Horner's syndrome
- Small degrees of involutional ptosis
- Small amount of asymmetry that may persist after primary ptosis repair.

## CONTRAINDICATIONS

A vertical tarsal height <8 mm is a relative contraindication, as a minimum of 4 mm of tarsus is required to prevent upper lid instability postsurgery.

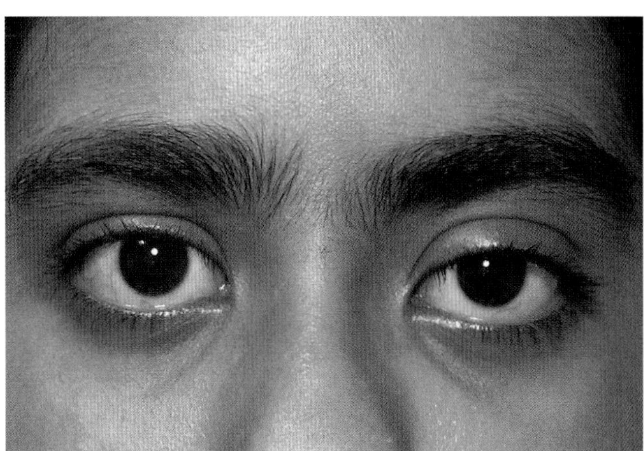

**Figure 62-1** A 12-year-old girl with mild (2 mm) congenital ptosis in the left eye. She has 12 mm levator action and 9 mm vertical tarsal height, an ideal setting for Fasanella–Servat surgery.

## SURGICAL TECHNIQUE

### Anesthesia

In older individuals, Fasanella–Servat surgery is preferably done under local anesthesia. Frontal nerve block supplemented with local infiltration of lignocaine is sufficient. However, general anesthesia is required in children.

### Surgical Procedure

Three 4-0 silk traction sutures are passed along the lid margin. The upper eyelid is everted over a Desmarre's retractor. Another set of 3, 4-0 silk sutures is passed about 1 mm away from the superior edge of tarsus for providing counter traction to the posterior lamella of lid during the procedure.

Two curved hemostats are applied to superior edge of tarsus and contiguous Müllers muscle and conjunctiva medially and laterally. A 6-0 running absorbable suture is passed just below the hemostats through tarsus and conjunctiva all along the length of the tarsus. Hemostats are then removed and tissues distal to the crush marks are excised. The preplaced running sutures are then tightened with knots exteriorized on the skin side.

Various modifications to the original technique have been described in literature. Since an inappropriate placement of hemostats can lead to a poor eyelid contour postoperatively, Samimi et al. have described a modified Müllerectomy clamp instead of the curved hemostats and reported better outcome with its use.[4] Betharia et al. have described a modified approach without the use of hemostats or Müllerectomy clamp.[5] The authors currently follow Dr Betharia's modified technique. In this method, the upper eyelid is everted and three traction sutures are passed through the everted superior edge of tarsus. Another set of three sutures are passed through the superior fornix to emerge just short of the eyelid margin. The purpose of these sutures is to advance the posterior cut edge of conjunctiva and prevent its retraction once the tarso-conjunctival excision is complete. Amount of tarsus to be excised is measured and marked in the centre of the eyelid. 2 mm of tarsus is excised to correct every 1 mm of ptosis. The marking follows the eyelid contour medially and laterally. Care must be taken to leave behind at least 4 mm of tarsal tissue intact to avoid lid instability post operatively. The tarso-conjunctivo-mullers complex beyond the markings made is excised. The pre-placed forniceal sutures are advanced and the cut edge of conjunctiva is sutured back to the edge of residual tarsus with continuous 6- 0 plain catgut sutures with knots exteriorized on skin surface (Figs. 62-2A to F). Bodian modified the technique by using 5-0 nylon sutures instead of absorbable sutures to reduce the incidence of suture-induced keratopathy.[6]

In recent times, conjunctivo-Müllerectomy has gained preference for management of mild ptosis over Fasanella–Servat procedure mainly due to the fact that it causes less disturbance to the upper lid skeleton giving a better final contour. As mentioned earlier, conjunctivo-Müllerectomy works best if phenylephrine test is positive, whereas Fasanella–Servat procedure has been seen to be independent of response to phenylephrine. A histopathologic study conducted on 40 surgical specimens of excised tissue obtained after Fasanella–Servat procedure concluded that success of Fasanella–Servat procedure does not depend on a Müllerectomy, but instead is probably due to a combination of (1) a vertical posterior lamellar shortening, (2) secondary contractile cicatrization of the wound, and (3) plication or advancement of the Müller's smooth muscle-levator aponeurosis complex on the tarsus.[7]

## POSTOPERATIVE CARE

Postoperative care includes oral antibiotics and anti-inflammatory-analgesics for a week. Topical antibiotic and steroid eye drops are initiated from the next day. Frequent instillations of topical lubricating eye drops and gel formulations are useful in early postoperative period. Cornea must be examined at frequent intervals to look for any suture-induced abrasion, and if found a soft bandage contact lens can be used for a short period.

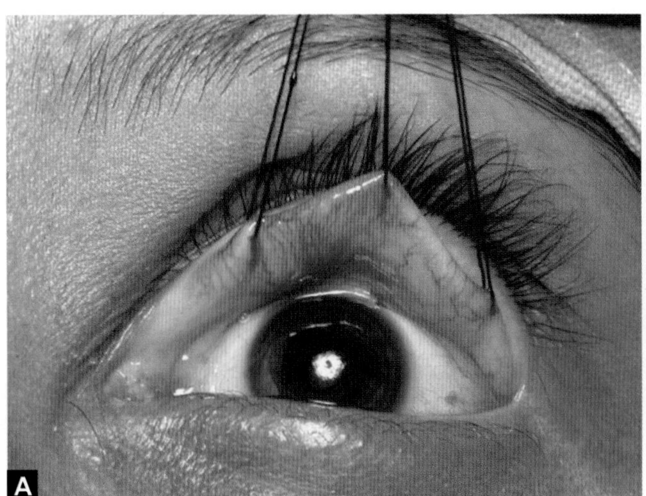


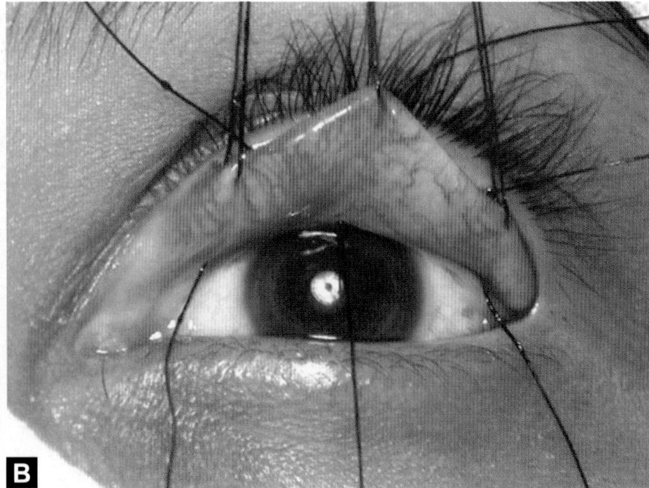


**Figures 62-2A and B** The surgical steps of Fasanella–Servat procedure: (A) A set of three traction sutures are passed through the everted tarsus. (B) Another set of three traction sutures are passed through the superior fornix, emerging just short of the eyelid margin.

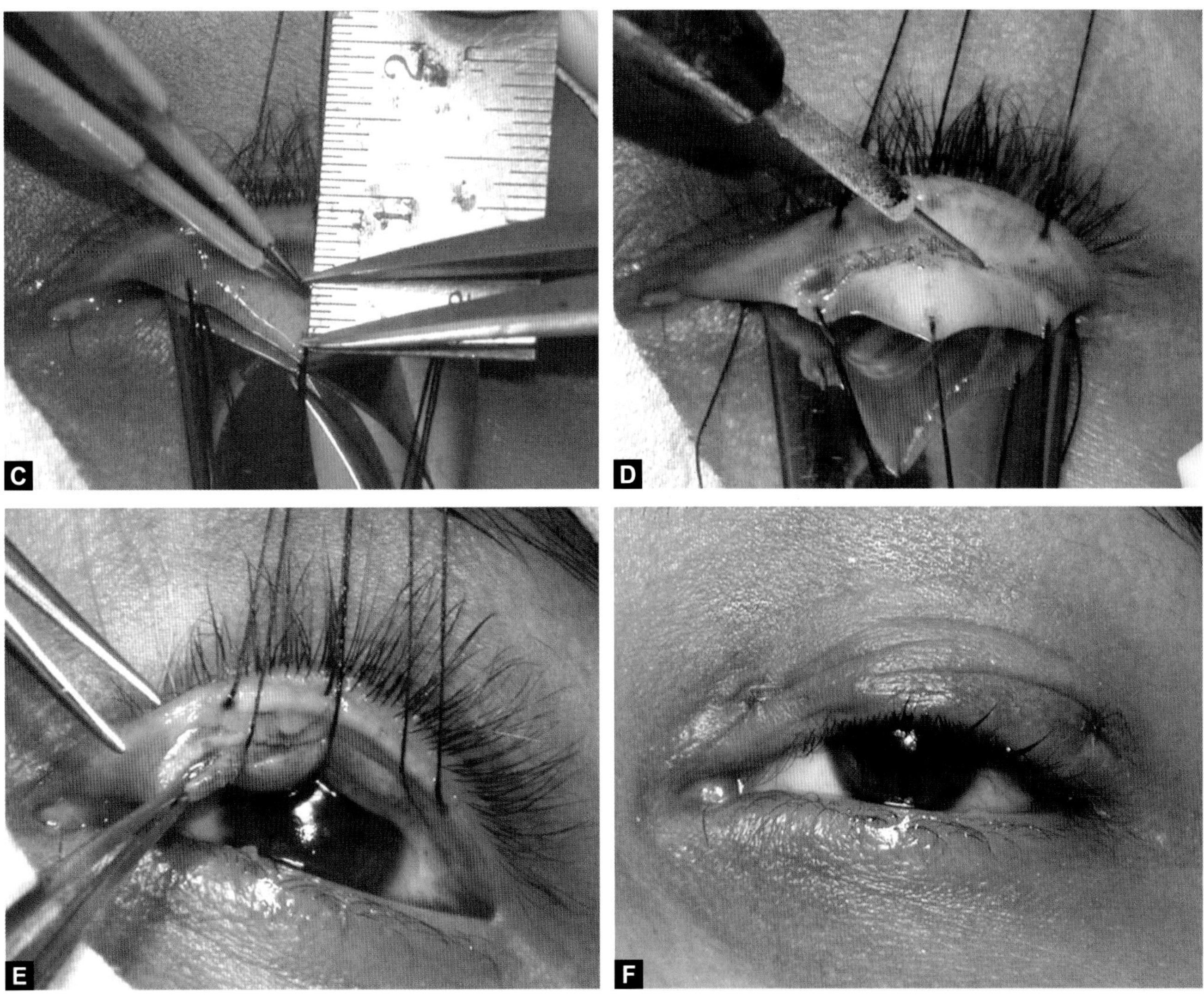


**Figures 62-2C to F** The surgical steps of Fasanella–Servat procedure: (C) Amount of tarsus to be excised is measured and marked in the center of the eyelid. The thumb rule is to excise 2 mm of tarsus for every 1 mm of ptosis—4 mm in this case for 2 mm ptosis. The mark follows the eyelid contour medially and laterally stopping short 5 mm from the medial and lateral canthus, respectively. (D) Controlled and blood-less excision of the tarsus along with the folded conjunctiva and Müllers is performed with a radio frequency-powered monopolar cutting tip. (E) The preplaced fornix suture bring into view the cut edge of the conjunctiva. (F) The cut edge of the conjunctiva is sutured back to the edge of the residual tarsus buried continuously with 6-0 plain catgut suture, with knots at both the edges exteriorized.

## COMPLICATIONS

*Eyelid height asymmetry*: Although Fasanella–Servat procedure is a very predictable procedure, undercorrection may occur at times if there was an error in the initial evaluation of the patient. Undercorrection can be managed by an anterior approach aponeurosis surgery. Overcorrection is even less common, and if seen is usually mild that can be managed by simple downward traction on the lid under local anesthesia in early postoperative stage or lid massage.

*Contour abnormality:* Contour disturbance can occur in the form of central peaking if excessive amount of tarsus is excised centrally. Tarsal instability can occur if < 4 mm of residual tarsus is left behind in the upper lid after excision of the tarsoconjunctivo Müller's segment.

*Lash ptosis:* It may be seen as a result of shortening of posterior lamella and may require excision of a small spindle of skin and orbicularis from anterior approach if significant.

Other minor complications like dry eyes, suture-induced keratopathy, entropion, dermatochalasis, hemorrhage, and infection are less common.

## PEARLS AND PITFALLS

- Fasanella–Servat procedure is an easy to learn, useful technique with fairly predictable outcome wherever indicated.
- Lid contour abnormalities can be prevented by avoiding any temptation to excise an excessive amount of tarsus.
- Postoperative care includes looking out for suture-induced corneal complications.

## REFERENCES

1. Fasanella RM, Servat J. Levator resection for minimal ptosis: another simplified operation. Arch Ophthalmol. 1961;65:493-6.
2. Carroll RP. Preventable problems following the Fasanella-Servat procedure. Ophthalmic Surg. 1980;11:44-51.
3. Sampath R, Saunders DC, Leatherbarrow B. The Fasanella-Servat procedure: a retrospective study. Eye (Lond). 1995;9 (Pt 1): 124-5.
4. Samimi DB, Erb MH, Lane CJ, et al. The modified Fasanella-Servat procedure: description and quantified analysis. Ophthal Plast Reconstr Surg. 2013;29(1):30-4.
5. Betharia SM, Grover AK, Kalra BR. The Fasanella-Servat operation: a modified simple technique with quantitative approach. Br J Ophthalmol. 1983;67(1):58-60.
6. Bodian M. A revised Fasanella-Servat ptosis operation. Ann Ophthalmol. 1975;7(4):603-5.
7. Buckman G, Jakobiec FA, Hyde K, et al. Success of the Fasanella-Servat operation independent of Müller's smooth muscle excision. Ophthalmology. 1989;96(4):413-8.

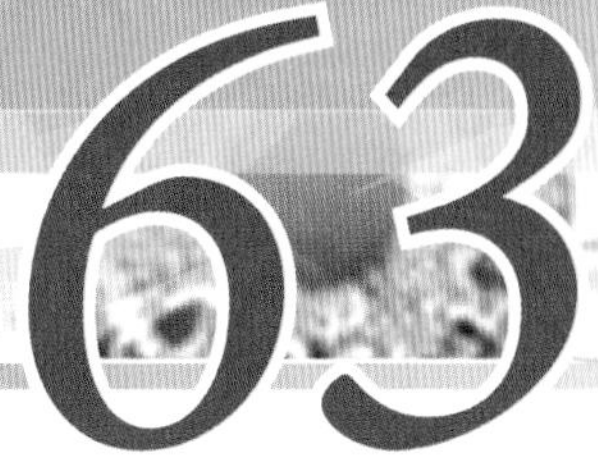


# Ptosis Repair—Levator Surgery (External Approach)

Vikas Menon

## INTRODUCTION

Levator surgery performed through anterior approach is one of the most commonly performed surgical procedures for ptosis correction. It is essential that the surgeon be familiar with anatomical relationship of levator to other vital tissues in the eyelid. Decision to proceed with levator surgery must be preceded by a detailed clinical evaluation of the patient. Everbusch is credited with the first description of anterior approach levator surgery by performing a tuck of the levator for ptosis correction.[1] His technique was modified by Wolff in 1896 by resecting the aponeurosis.[2] The technique has evolved over time and still remains one of the best methods for correction of ptosis. This chapter describes various surgeries performed on levator through the anterior or the cutaneous approach like standard levator resection, levator resection with adjustable sutures, levator excision, and aponeurotic repair surgery.

## INDICATIONS

- Congenital ptosis with moderate or good levator action (> 5474 mm)
- Congenital ptosis associated with synkinesis
- Involutional ptosis.

## CONTRAINDICATIONS

Although not an absolute contra-indication, levator surgery in a patient with poor levator action (< 4 mm) may result in under-correction, even after maximal resection. It may also lead to significant lagophthalmos and lid lag. Hence, such cases are better managed with other suitable techniques.

## SURGICAL TECHNIQUE

### Levator Resection

Anterior approach levator resection surgery is most commonly indicated in patients with congenital ptosis having fair or good levator function (> 4 mm).

#### *Anesthesia*

In older individuals, levator surgery is preferably done under frontal nerve block, as it keeps the motor part of levator functional and allows intraoperative adjustment of lid height. Frontal nerve block is given with a #26 needle, which is introduced just below the superior orbital rim in the midline and 0.5–1 mL of lidocaine is injected. This is supplemented with local infiltration of lidocaine along the eyelid crease. However, general anesthesia is required in children.

#### *Surgical Procedure*

The incision is given at the level of expected new eyelid crease. A fine-tip marking pen is advisable as a broad, wide marking can cause lid crease asymmetry by a few millimeters. In unilateral ptosis, the incision can be marked taking the contralateral eyelid crease position as a guide. In bilateral cases, the incision can be marked at about 10 mm above the eyelid margin in females and 1–2 mm lower down in males (Fig. 63-1).

A downward traction with a 4-0 silk suture is useful to keep the eyelid tissues taut. An upper eyelid crease incision is given through skin with a #11 or #15 surgical blade. A fine-cutting cautery can be used to deepen the incision through orbicularis maintaining a bloodless field. Orbicularis is then

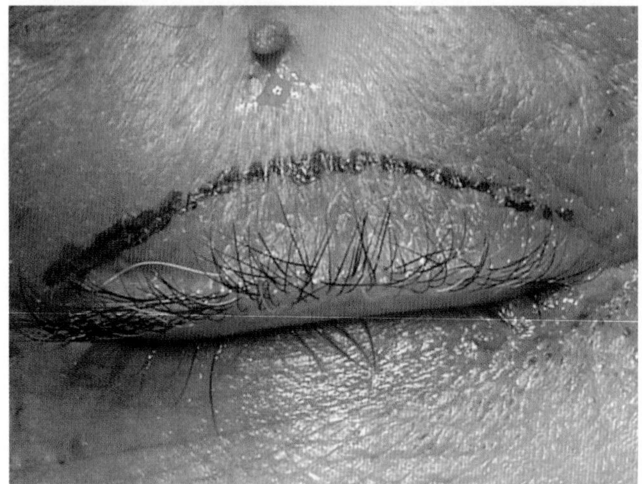

Figure 63-1 Marking the incision along eyelid crease.

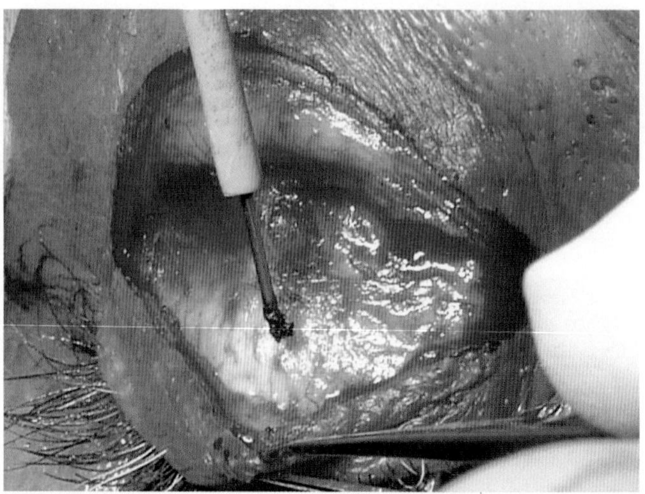

Figure 63-2 After making the incision through skin and orbicularis, the dissection is carried superiorly to expose the orbital septum and inferiorly to expose anterior surface of tarsus.

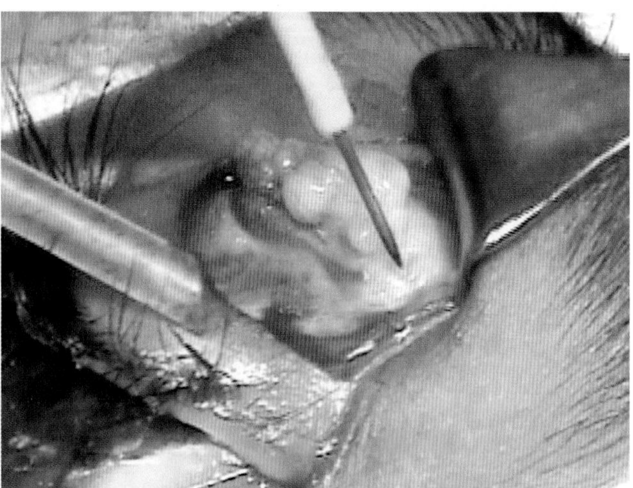

Figure 63-3 Incision on septum causes preaponeurotic fat to prolapse, an important anatomical landmark for identifying levator aponeurosis.

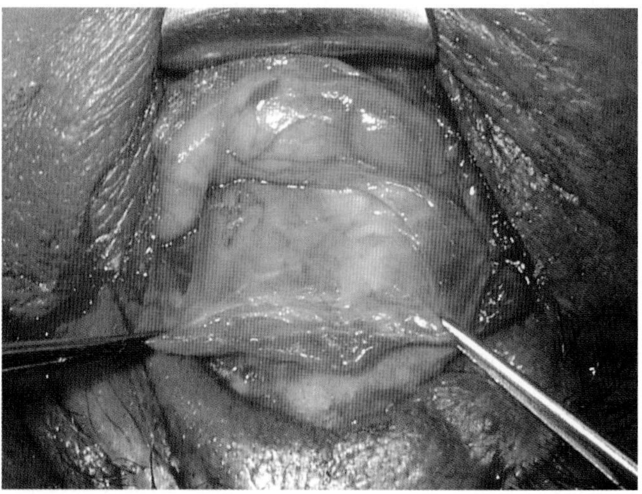

Figure 63-4 The levator aponeurosis appears as a broad whitish fibrous sheath under the preaponeurotic fat pads.

lifted up and dissected away from fibers of orbital septum. Dissection is then carried on inferiorly in the suborbicularis plane to expose the anterior surface of tarsal plate (Fig. 63-2). Care is taken not to go too close to the lid margin with cautery or lash roots may be affected. The proximal edge of skin-orbicularis flap is lifted up and retracted superiorly with a Desmarre's retractor while the multilayered orbital septum is incised. It can be incised with a cautery or manually cut with a Westcott scissors. Once the septum is incised, preaponeurotic fat starts prolapsing out (Fig. 63-3) and serves as an important landmark for identification of levator aponeurosis, which appears as a broad glistening white fibrous sheath just underneath the pad of fat (Fig. 63-4). Levator aponeurosis is then disinserted from its attachment on anterior surface of tarsus and separated from underlying conjunctivomullers complex by superiorly directed blunt dissection with a cotton-tipped applicator. Adequate countertraction on the lid in the downward direction is helpful to prevent button holing of the conjunctiva at this stage. Depending upon the amount of resection planned, medial and lateral horns of aponeurosis may be conservatively snipped to release more tissue. Care must be taken to free levator from all its septal attachments to reduce postoperative lagophthalmos without damaging Whitnall's ligament.

There are two commonly used nomograms based on which the amount of resection can be planned. Beard's method is

TABLE 63-1 Nomograms for Levator Resection

| *Berke's rule* | |
|---|---|
| Levator function | Intraoperative lid height |
| 2–3 mm | At upper limbus |
| 4–5 mm | 1–2 mm overlap |
| 6–7 mm | 2 mm overlap |
| 8–9 mm | 3–4 mm overlap |
| 10–11 mm | 5 mm overlap |
| ***Beard's rule*** | |
| **Preoperative margin-to-reflex distance** | **Amount of resection** |
| 3–4 mm | 10–13 mm |
| 2–3 mm | 14–17 mm |
| 1–2 mm | 18–22 mm |
| 0–1 mm | >23 mm |

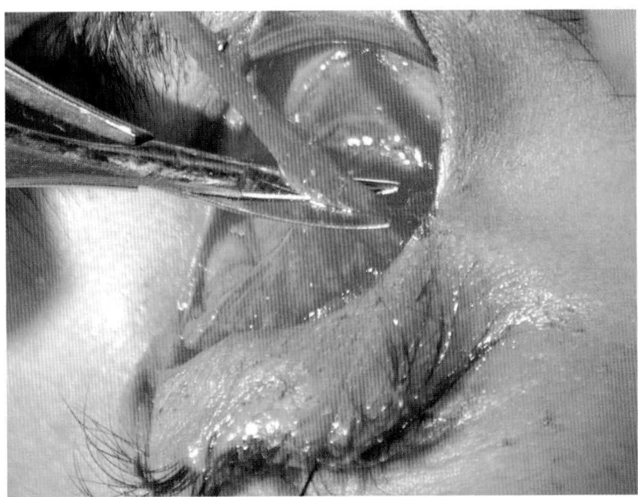

Figure 63-6 Redundant aponeurosis being excised after tightening the aponeurotic sutures once the desired lid height is achieved.

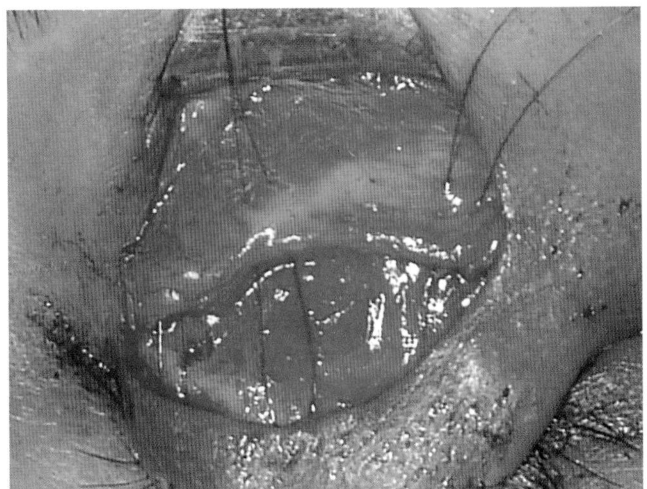

Figure 63-5 Medial, central, and lateral sutures are taken through anterior surface of tarsus and levator aponeurosis at the desired level.

based on the amount of levator that is excised[3] and Berke's method is based on intraoperative placement of the eyelid based on preoperative levator function[4] (Table 63-1). Berke's method has the advantage of not being affected by intraoperative stretch on aponeurosis. However, it should be understood that nomograms serve only as broad guidelines, and each surgeon ultimately adjusts his or her quantitative technique with experience.

Three double-armed partial thickness sutures (either absorbable or non-absorbable sutures can be used); central, medial, and lateral are passed through anterior surface of tarsus and then through aponeurosis at the desired level based on the method used for quantification of resection (Fig. 63-5). The central suture is tightened first with a single throw knot, if under-correction is noted, the suture is then passed through aponeurosis at a higher level. For over correction, the suture can be passed again at a lower level of aponeurosis or allowed to hang back by a few millimeters. Once satisfied with the amount of correction achieved, the central suture is tightened followed by tightening of the medial and lateral sutures taking care of the eyelid margin contour. Redundant levator aponeurosis beyond these sutures is then excised (Fig. 63-6).

Orbicularis is closed taking deeper bites through levator aponeurosis to form the lid crease with the help of absorbable polyglactin 6-0 sutures, followed by closure of skin with 6-0 polypropylene nonabsorbable suture. A frost suture is usually applied to the lower lid at the end of surgery. An antibiotic ointment is applied and a pad applied for 24 hours.

## Levator Resection with Adjustable Sutures

Results of standard levator surgery are often unpredictable, even in the hands of most expert surgeons. Many surgeons have described their experience with different techniques of using adjustable sutures in an attempt to overcome this problem and reduce the need of resurgeries.[5,6] The author prefers the technique described by Collins and O'Donnell.[6]

### *Surgical Procedure*

All the usual steps as for standard levator resection are carried on till separation of levator aponeurosis from tarsus and conjunctivomullers complex. Three double-armed sutures

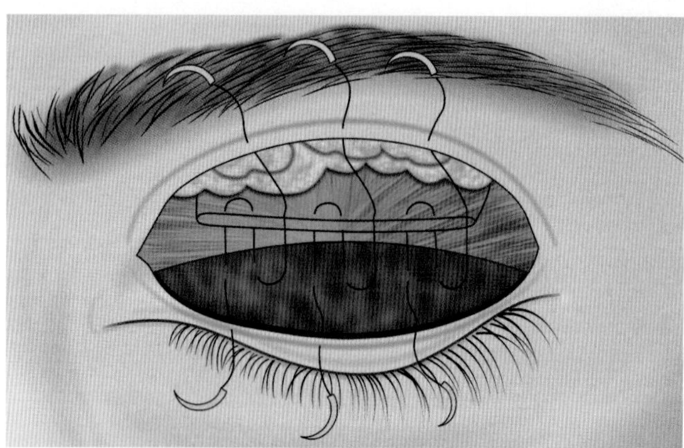

Figure 63-7 Adjustable sutures passed through tarsus, aponeurosis, and skin- orbicularis flaps.

are then passed from anterior surface of tarsus to levator aponeurosis at the desired level, but instead of tying the knots at this stage, each of the two suture ends are passed through free edge of skin-orbicularis flap of the lid crease incision and a single-throw bow knot is tied. which also closes the incision. Rest of the incision is closed in layers as usual (Fig. 63-7). The sutures can be tightened and lid height adjusted with the patient in sitting posture, and without taking the patient back to operation theater in the early postoperative period at about 3rd or 5th day once the edema is satisfactorily reduced.

## Aponeurotic Repair

Aponeurotic repair is indicated for patients with involutional ptosis where basic pathology is either an attenuation and elongation of levator aponeurosis or a complete disinsertion of the aponeurosis from its attachment to anterior surface of tarsus.[7]

These patients typically have a normal levator function, a higher eyelid crease, and a reduced lid lag on downgaze on the affected side.

Aponeurotic or involutional ptosis may present unilaterally or bilaterally, and though more common in elderly individuals, it can also occur in younger individuals as a consequence of trauma, surgery, or eyelid edema. Aponeurotic ptosis has rarely been reported congenitally.[8,9] Unlike congenital ptosis, where Beard's and Berke's nomograms are available, no such nomograms exist for aponeurotic ptosis surgery. Some surgeons use intraoperative lid height as a guide in performing aponeurotic surgery.[10]

### *Surgical Procedure*

A lid crease incision is given in accordance to the contralateral lid margin-crease distance in cases with unilateral ptosis or approximately 8–10 mm above the lid margin in bilateral cases. The incision is carried through orbicularis, and the orbital septum is opened up as described for standard levator resection. In cases where there is complete disinsertion of levator from tarsus, the superiorly migrated free edge of aponeurosis can be identified as a transverse whitish band visible after retracting the preaponeurotic fat pad. The free edge of aponeurosis can be advanced and sutured to anterior surface of tarsus with 6-0 polypropylene sutures about 3 mm below its superior edge.

In cases with just involutional attenuation or dehiscence of the aponeurosis, the technique is essentially similar to levator resection described previously. In involutional ptosis, it is relatively easier to separate the aponeurosis from Muller's muscle and conjunctiva. About 10 mm of resection is usually sufficient to raise the lid in most cases.

Lid height is adjusted on table in accordance with the contralateral lid in unilateral cases or kept 1–2 mm below the limbus in bilateral cases. Patient can be asked to sit up to have a better idea of the correction achieved. The suture can be loosened slightly for a hangback effect if over correction is noted or passed at a higher level through the aponeurosis if there is an under correction. Medial and lateral sutures are then passed through the tarsus and aponeurosis taking care of proper contour. Any redundant aponeurosis can be excised at this stage. Lid crease forming sutures are then passed, and skin closure is done as described previously.

## Levator Excision

Excision of levator is indicated in cases where there is an abnormal innervation of the levator leading to synkinesis, commonly seen in children with Marcus Gunn jaw winking phenomenon. This procedure is sometimes also indicated to relieve synkinesis secondary to aberrant regeneration following third nerve palsy.

Excision of levator leads to near complete ptosis, which subsequently needs to be corrected by frontalis suspension.

### *Surgical Procedure*

Levator is exposed through anterior approach as previously described. Whitnall's ligament, which appears as a shiny white transverse band at the junction of the muscular and aponeurotic portions of levator is identified. Whitnall's is retracted inferiorly and a muscle hook is passed underneath the levator above the level of Whitnall and pulled forward. Globe is moved gently to ensure that superior rectus is not caught in the muscle hook. Two hemostats are placed across

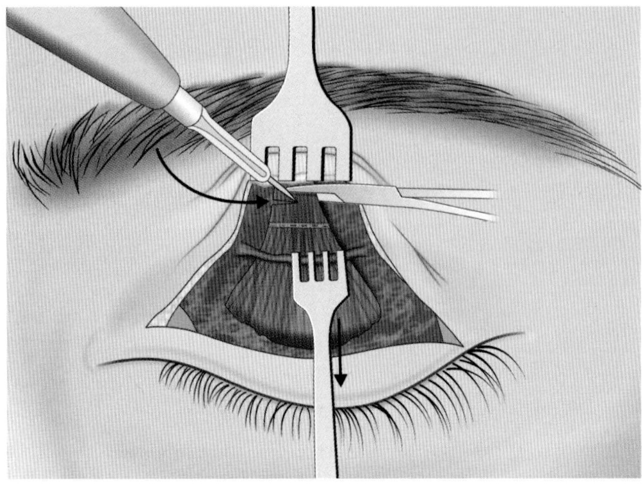

Figure 63-8 Excision of muscular part of levator in correction of synkinetic ptosis.

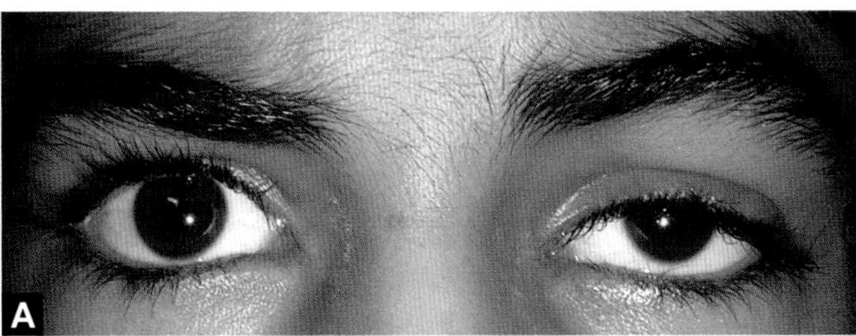

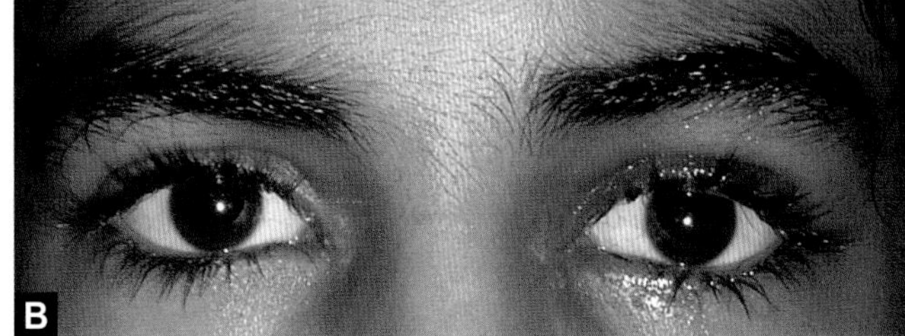

Figures 63-9A and B Pre- and postoperative result of anterior approach levator resection in moderate congenital ptosis.

the muscle approximately 5 mm apart in its proximal part, and the segment of muscle falling between the two hemostats is excised (Fig. 63-8). The proximal free edge can then be cauterized and either allowed to retract in the orbit or sutured to the periosteum. This method of limited levator excision helps to maintain some skeletal support in the upper lid by preserving aponeurosis.[11]

## POSTOPERATIVE CARE

Postoperative care includes oral antibiotics and anti-inflammatory analgesics for a week. Frequent instillations of topical lubricating eyedrops and gel formulations are useful in the early postoperative period. Proper application of frost suture at bedtime needs to be explained to the patient's family in cases of congenital ptosis, to avoid exposure keratopathy and related complications. Frost suture can be removed at 1 week in most cases if natural corneal protective mechanisms are good. Eyelid height usually stabilizes by 6 weeks (Figs. 63-9A and B).

### Complications

- Under-correction is usually a result of either suboptimal resection of levator aponeurosis or an attempt to correct ptosis by levator surgery in a patient with very poor levator action, where a procedure like frontalis suspension may be indicated (Figs. 63-10A to C).
- *Over-correction*: After levator surgery may be the result of inaccurate determination of levator function preoperatively, failure of applying proper technique, e.g. resecting the levator where only levator advancement was indicated (Fig. 63-11). If there is gross overcorrection then an early release of sutures with or without aponeurotic recession is indicated. A mild overcorrection in the early postoperative period can be managed by a downward traction under local anesthesia or even massaging the lid in a downward fashion. In patients who present late with an overcorrection require a levator recession procedure. A spacer graft may be required in very severe cases.
- *Lagophthalmos*: Some amount of lagophthalmos is invariably seen after most ptosis surgeries. Fortunately, the ocular surface can tolerate small amounts of lagophthalmos, but it can become troublesome in cases where the natural corneal protective mechanisms are deficient. Common causes of excessive lagophthalmos are incomplete separation of septal fibers from aponeurosis or excessive resection of aponeurosis

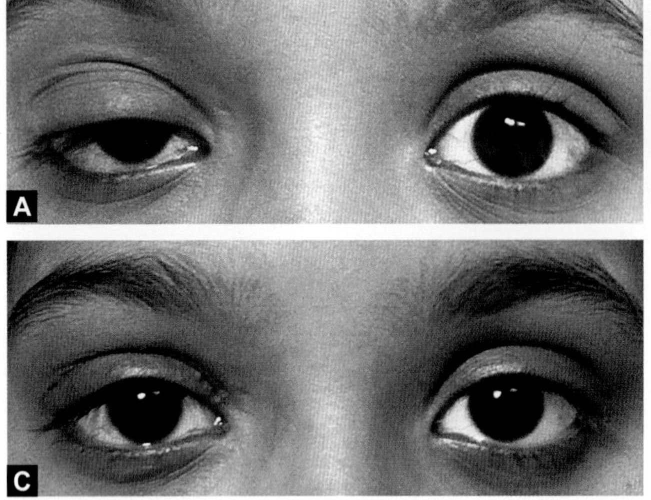


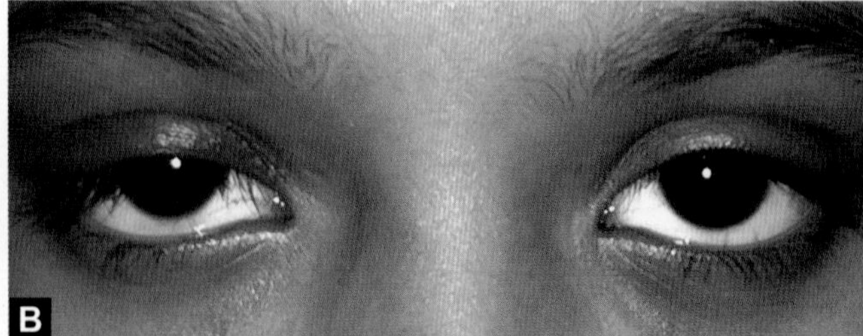


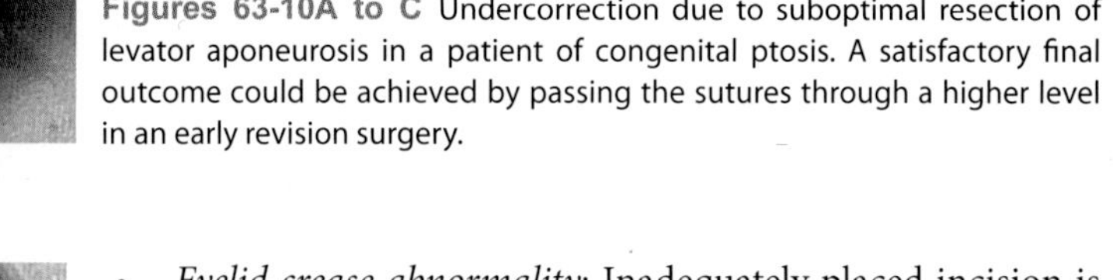

**Figures 63-10A to C** Undercorrection due to suboptimal resection of levator aponeurosis in a patient of congenital ptosis. A satisfactory final outcome could be achieved by passing the sutures through a higher level in an early revision surgery.

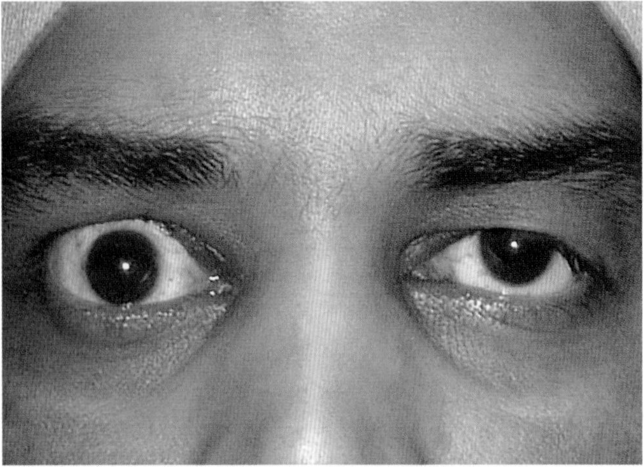

**Figure 63-11** Overcorrection after levator resection procedure.

- *Fornix prolapse:* Superior forniceal conjunctiva can prolapse if dissection of levator from conjunctiva is carried superiorly till the superior fornix, and all the forniceal attachments of conjunctiva are severed in the process. It is recommended to pass a blunt instrument to check and reposit any loose forniceal conjunctiva at the end of surgery. The prolapse can be managed by simple repositioning of the conjunctiva under topical anesthesia. In recalcitrant cases, fornix forming sutures usually resolve the problem
- *Contour abnormality*: Suboptimal contour after levator surgery usually results from inappropriate placement of sutures on the tarsal plate. It can also occur in patients with floppy eyelids and patients with prominent involutional lateral shift of tarsal plate
- *Eyelid crease abnormality*: Inadequately placed incision is the most common cause of lid crease asymmetry. It can also be seen if the lid crease forming sutures are passed too high through the levator. Occasionally, it is a result of postoperative contraction of the pretarsal skin. A fold of loose upper lid skin can also lead to an impression of asymmetrical lid crease; therefore, it is advisable to remove redundant upper lid skin at the time of surgery
- Other less common complications include extraocular muscle imbalance, lash ptosis, entropion, ectropion, hemorrhage, and infection.

## PEARLS AND PITFALLS

- Variety of procedures are available for ptosis correction, an accurate assessment of ptosis is vital toward choosing the most appropriate procedure in any patient and avoiding errors.
- The technique needs some experience to master. Under/overcorrections are not uncommon even in the hands of experts, but they can be managed rather easily with an early intervention.

## REFERENCES

1. Everbusch O. Zur operation der congenitalen blepharoptosis, Klin Monastbl Augenheilkd. 1883;21:100.
2. Wolff H. Die vorlagerung des Musc. levator palp. superioris mit Plurchttrengnung der Insertion. Zwei neue methoden gegen ptosis congenita. Arch Augenheilkd. 1896;33:125.
3. Beard C. The surgical treatment of blepharoptosis: a quantitative approach. Trans Am Ophthalmol Soc. 1966;64:401-87.

4. Berke RN. Results of resection of the levator muscle through a skin incision in congenital ptosis. AMA Arch Ophthalmol. 1959;61(2):177-201.
5. Hylkema HA, Koornneef L. Treatment of ptosis by levator resection with adjustable sutures via the anterior approach. Br J Ophthalmol. 1989;73(6):416-8.
6. Collin JRO, O'Donnell BA. Adjustable sutures in eyelid surgery for ptosis and lid retraction. Br J Ophthalmol.1994;78:167-74.
7. Fujiwara T, Matsuo K, Kondoh S, et al. Etiology and pathogenesis of aponeurotic blepharoptosis. Ann Plast Surg. 2001;46: 29-35.
8. Martin PA, Rogers PA. Congenital aponeurotic ptosis. Aust N Z J Ophthalmol. 1988;16(4):291-4.
9. Anderson RL, Gordy DD. Aponeurotic defects in congenital ptosis. Ophthalmology. 1979;86(8):1493-500.
10. Linberg JV, Vasquez RJ, Chao GM. Aponeurotic ptosis repair under local anesthesia. Prediction of results from operative lid height. Ophthalmology. 1988;95(8):1046-52.
11. McCord CD. Eyelid surgery. Principles and techniques. New York: Lippincott-Raven;1995:125-6.

CHAPTER

# 64

# Ptosis Repair—Levator Surgery (Internal Approach)

Andre S Litwin, Raman Malhotra

## INTRODUCTION

Involutional ptosis is the most commonly acquired ptosis requiring surgical correction and is defined by several well-known clinical features. These include constant ptosis, good levator function, a high or absent skin crease, increased lid excursion on down gaze, and a thinned eyelid.[1] Since the age of aponeurotic awareness[2-5] surgery for involutional ptosis has corrected the so-called anatomical defect while ignoring the contribution of involutional change such as volume deflation and fat atrophy.

The first descriptions of posterior-approach ptosis surgery were mainly excisional in nature, either tarsoconjunctival, Müller's muscle and conjunctiva, or Müller's muscle alone.[6-12] Removing structures that are not causing ptosis or are positively contributing to the tear film can be neither anatomically nor physiologically desirable.[13] Resection of posterior structures such as Müller's muscle leads to advancement and even plication of adjacent posterior and middle lamellar structures such as the levator aponeurosis.[14,15]

Early reports of posterior approach internal levator repair placed an incision through the superior tarsal plate, with subsequent creation of a conjunctivo-Müller flap.[10,16] The rolled white band of folded aponeurosis (white line) was then advanced.[10] Sutures were externalized and tied to form a skin crease. Although conjunctiva was largely preserved, the superior tarsus and the distal edge of Müller's muscle were excised. Other descriptions of posterior approach internal repair also placed the initial incision through the superior tarsus but went on to retract the preaponeurotic fat pad and expose the anterior surface of the levator complex before its advancement.[12,17] This effectively converted a posterior approach to the familiar anatomical view of an anterior approach ptosis repair without need for a skin incision.

Internal approach ptosis surgery has now been refined so that the levator aponeurosis can be advanced and plicated via a conjunctival approach with tissue preservation.[18] The so-called white-line advancement combines a predictable postoperative eyelid height with aponeurotic reattachment, and the normal eyelid contour seen with posterior-approach Müller's resection surgery[19] while avoiding any tissue excision. The plicated levator aponeurosis may contribute to volume enhancement[20] and tying of the sutures helps reform the natural skin fold, even in children. Whereas traditionally, internal approach levator surgery was reserved for those with minimal ptosis and a positive response to the phenylephrine test, these newer techniques have been shown to be effective in phenylephrine negative cases.[20,21]

## ANATOMY

Ptosis results from localized or generalized disinsertion or dehiscence of the aponeurosis from the tarsal plate. Retraction of the attenuated, dehisced, or detached aponeurosis, age-related soft tissue atrophy, combined retraction of orbital septum and preseptal orbicularis oculi muscle and stretching of the underlying Muller's muscle, all contribute to an increased translucency of the upper eyelid.[1] In a subset of patients there are also abnormalities of the levator muscle itself. The levator aponeurosis comprises two layers.[22] The anterior layer is thicker and reflects superiorly a few millimeters above the tarsus to become contiguous with the orbital septum. The posterior layer of aponeurosis is thinner with more smooth muscle fibers and becomes confluent with the lower third of the tarsal plate and subcutaneous tissues.[22] It remains controversial as to whether the deeper aponeurotic layer and Müller's muscle attach proximally at the superior tarsal border

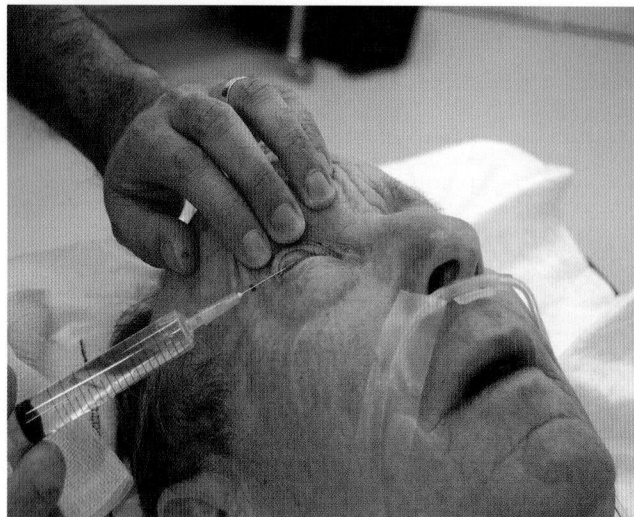

**Figure 64-1** Lid everted and subconjunctival injection of local anesthetic being administered.

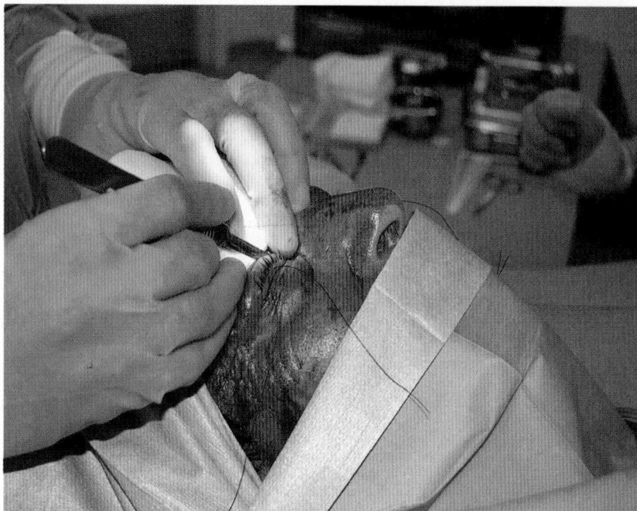

**Figure 64-2** A 4-0 silk traction suture placed through the gray line at the peak of the upper eyelid and skin incision for concurrent blepharoplasty being performed.

rather than at the lower third of the tarsus. A superior tarsal attachment also suggests that posterior surgical approaches that address Müller's muscle may involve resections in closer proximity to the aponeurosis than previously thought.[23]

## INDICATIONS

- Acquired involutional "aponeurotic" ptosis
- Mild-to-severe involutional ptosis
- Severe involutional ptosis with the "visible iris sign" present[1]
- Moderate to good levator function[18]
- Phenylephrine positive or negative[24]
- When an eyelid skin incision needs to be avoided
- Patients with dry eye who wish to have ptosis surgery. As no tarsal or conjunctiva is removed, goblet cells and accessory lacrimal glands are preserved and orbicularis oculi is not violated[25]
- Congenital ptosis with levator function greater than approximately 6 mm "levatorpexy".

## CONTRAINDICATIONS

- Levator function ≤ 4 mm
- Significant preoperative lagophthalmos
- Progressive cicatricial conjunctival disease.

## SURGICAL TECHNIQUE

A narrated video presentation describing this technique is available online (search term "live ptosis surgery"). White-line advancement involves advancement of the posterior surface of the levator aponeurosis via a transconjunctival posterior approach without resection of tarsus, conjunctiva, or Müller's muscle. The white line is best described as the distal free margin of the levator aponeurosis viewed from posteriorly and is continuous with the anterior surface of the aponeurosis.

In our practice, most patients first receive a bolus of intravenous sedation prior to administration of local anesthetic but remain alert for the remainder of the procedure. Local anesthesia is administered to all patients, regardless of whether the surgery is under general anesthesia. First, evert the eyelid and inject 0.5 mL of anesthetic (preferred choice is 0.5% bupivacaine with 1:200,000 epinephrine) subconjunctivally, just above the superior border of the tarsal plate (Fig. 64-1). Inject a further 1 mL subcutaneously, both along the skin crease and in the mid-pupillary pretarsal region. Prepare the patient in a sterile fashion, allowing time for the epinephrine to take effect. If a concurrent blepharoplasty is to be performed, excise skin and muscle first, at this stage.

Place a 4-0 silk traction suture through the gray line at the peak of the upper eyelid and evert the eyelid over a Desmarre's retractor (Fig. 64-2). Apply gentle diathermy at and also just above the superior border of the tarsus (Fig. 64-3). Create a conjunctival incision with a #15 Barde-Parker blade along this line (Fig. 64-4). Dissect Müller's muscle and conjunctiva off as a composite flap until the white line can be identified (Fig. 64-5). Place a double-armed 5-0 Vicryl suture centrally through the posterior belly of the white line (Fig. 64-6) in a forehand manner. Pass this through the conjunctival surface

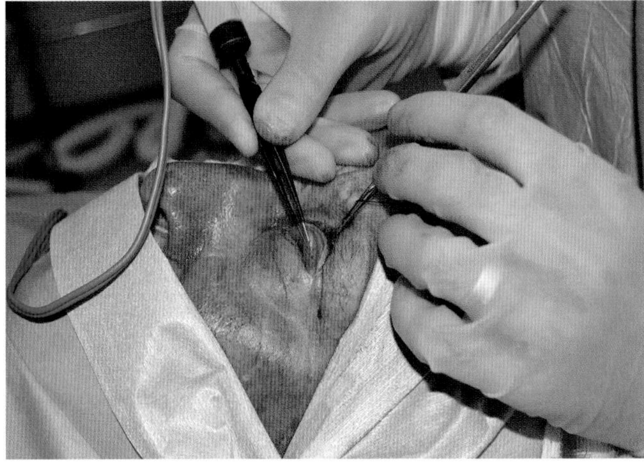

Figure 64-3 Apply a line of diathermy just above the superior border of the tarsus.

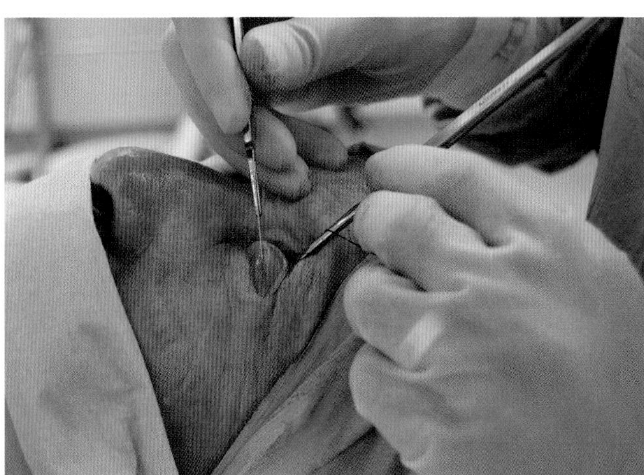

Figure 64-4 Carefully cut through only conjunctiva using a #15 Barde-Parker blade along the line of diathermy.

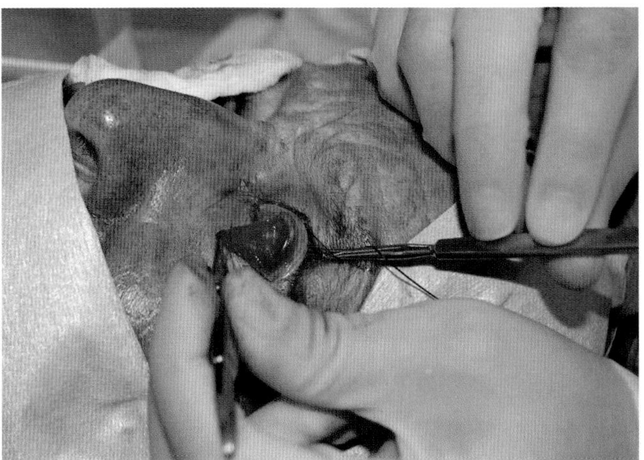

Figure 64-5 Dissect Müller's muscle and conjunctiva off as a composite flap until the white line is visualized.

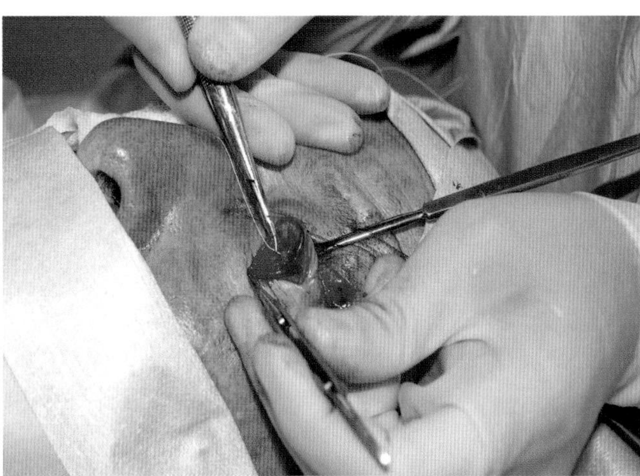

Figure 64-6 Place a double-armed 5-0 Vicryl suture centrally through the posterior belly of the white line in a forehand manner.

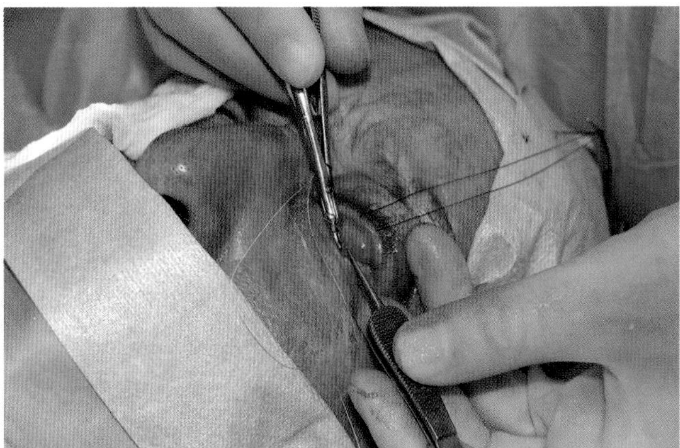

Figure 64-7 Pass this through the conjunctival surface of the tarsal plate, 1 mm below its superior border while ensuring there is no capture of orbital septum.

of the tarsal plate, 1 mm below its superior border (Fig. 64-7). Ensure there is no capture of orbital septum and pass the suture through to the skin and emerge in the region of the skin crease (Figs. 64-8A and B). Repeat with the second arm of the suture, passing through the tarsal plate in close proximity to the first bite while aiming to emerge through the same external exit point as the first suture to facilitate burying of the tied suture knot (Fig. 64-9).

Tighten the suture while ensuring there is no slippage and tie a slipknot to assess the eyelid height and contour (Fig. 64-10). If deemed satisfactory, surgery can then proceed to a similar stage on the contralateral side. If lid height is too low after the first suture, it can be relaxed and a second suture passed higher through the white line and again through the tarsal plate and skin, or the initial suture can be removed

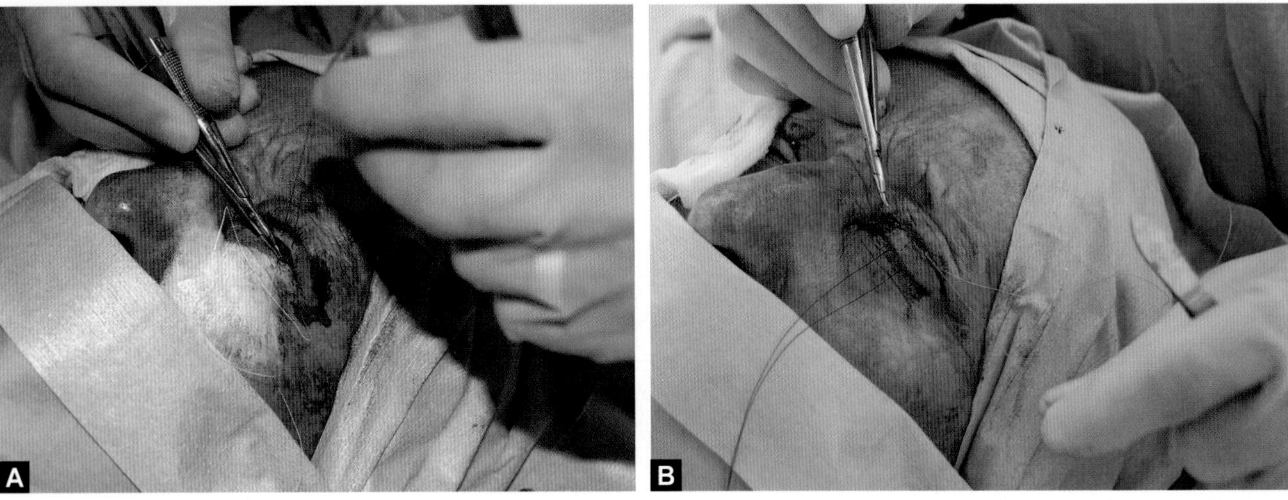


**Figures 64-8A and B** Rotate the eyelid (A) while holding the suture steady to safely pass the suture through to the skin, emerging in the region of the skin crease, (B) in this case a blepharoplasty has been performed.

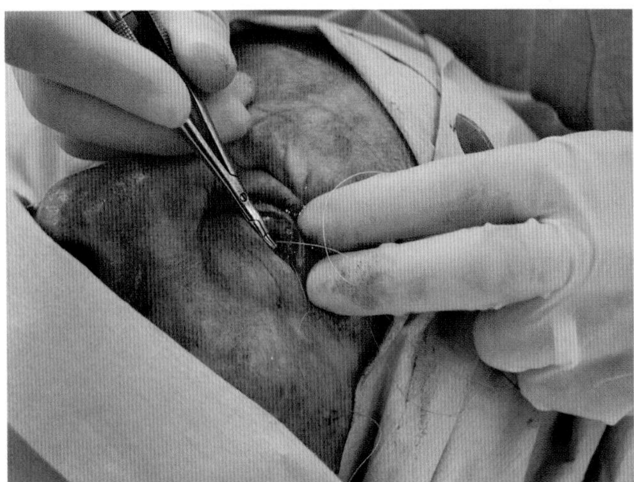

**Figure 64-9** Repeat with the second arm of the suture, passing through the tarsal plate in close proximity to the first bite while aiming to emerge through the same external exit point as the first suture to facilitate burying of the tied suture knot.

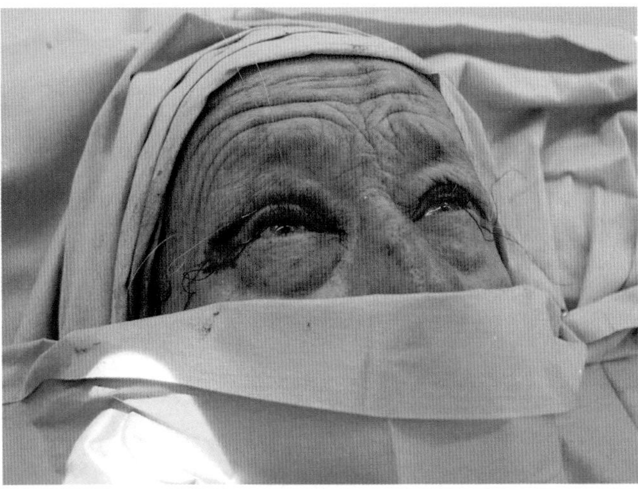

**Figure 64-10** Tighten the suture and tie a slipknot to assess the eyelid height and contour.

and repositioned. If the upper eyelid contour appears peaked after the first suture then untie and relax the suture before placing a second suture more central to the location of the peak. Altering the position of the second suture in this manner enables minor adjustments to eyelid height and contour without the undue delay of removing the first suture in the majority of cases. In such situations, the first suture was gently tied so as to act a "support" rather than a "cardinal" suture.

When the surgeon is happy with the eyelid height and contour, cut the bow of the slipknot and remove one end of the suture. Tie the other end and cut short. Müller's muscle and conjunctiva are left to heal spontaneously with no need for excision of these structures or for closure. If concurrent blepharoplasty has been performed, close the skin incision at this time.

## PEDIATRIC SURGICAL TECHNIQUE

Repeat the same steps as described above, but in cases where levator function was good (≥10 mm) and phenylephrine test had corrected upper eyelid height to within 1 mm of the contralateral upper eyelid, the first suture is passed through the junction of the superior edge of the white aponeurosis and levator. In severe ptosis with levator function <8 mm, pass the first suture through levator at a higher level (3–4 mm superior to the edge of the white aponeurosis). We have therefore coined the term "levatorpexy" for this technique as it effectively creates a pleat in levator when suturing to the tarsal plate.

We have often encountered a firm fibrous thin fat pad adherent between the distal levator and conjunctiva when dissecting into this postaponeurotic space. Before tying the first suture, a second suture was placed in the same manner through the levator muscle at the same vertical height but 2 mm medial to the first suture, then through the tarsus, 2 mm medial to the first and in the same way through to the skin. Sutures are tied on the skin aiming to exit each double-armed suture through the same exit site. Both Müller's muscle and conjunctiva are left to heal spontaneously with no excision or suturing of these structures.

## POSTOPERATIVE CARE

Prophylactic antibiotic ointment is prescribed four times daily to the operated eye(s) for 14 days if there is no contraindication. Sutures are left to absorb without removal. Patients are usually seen 1 week and 3 months after surgery. Ice packs during the first 5 days may reduce swelling and speed recovery.

## COMPLICATIONS

- Late "under correction" is more common than 'over correction' with this form of surgery.[18]
- If under corrected (as judged at the 3-month appointment), a further levator advancement can be performed and greater height achieved by placing the aponeurotic bites more proximally, toward the levator muscle.
- Over correction can be treated by removal of sutures at an early stage and by reseparating the layers. The benefit of white-line advancement is that no structures are removed, meaning release of the aponeurotic pleat should allow the patient to return to baseline.

## SURGICAL OUTCOMES: SCIENTIFIC EVIDENCE

White-line advancement results in a predictable outcome. Success rates approaching 90% have been reported and patients usually have a good eyelid contour.[18] Of those who require further surgery, the majority will be under corrected. The procedure can easily be combined with a blepharoplasty. A posterior approach is still justified in these cases as the orbital septum will remain unbreached.

Conventional anterior approach ptosis surgery in the presence of a functioning levator muscle also has success rates approaching 90% but varies depending upon the terms by which success is defined.[26-28] Concerns regarding unpredictability of lid height and eyelid contour remain, particularly residual medial under correction. Müller's muscle resection achieves similar success rates of 75–98%, with up to 90% achieving symmetry within 1.5 mm of the fellow eye.[14,20]

## PLACE OF THE TECHNIQUE IN SURGICAL ARMAMENTARIUM

- Newer techniques of posterior approach levator advancement are now an option in the majority of patients with ptosis and moderate to good levator function, even in phenylephrine negative cases.
- The technique is easy to teach and learn.
- A skin crease is reformed at the top of the tarsal plate as the sutures are externalized through the skin and tied.[19]
- Anatomy through this approach is easily identifiable, with minimal dissection. Respect for the normal physiology of the levator aponeurosis complex while maintaining tissue planes and tissues, means the technique is potentially reversible and reoperation easier.

## PEARLS AND PITFALLS

It is important that sutures are placed into healthy white aponeurotic sheet. Occasionally, after placement of sutures in what appears to be a white line, there can be an under correction of ptosis. We have found that this usually arises from erroneous placement of sutures into the orbital septum (anterior layer of levator) that can occasionally appear as a white line. In such cases, the levator aponeurosis is often significantly thin and can be found by further dissection closer to the conjunctiva beyond a thin Müller's muscle. As Müller's muscle disappears, a thin white line can be identified. Following this, further dissection between this white line and the conjunctiva can reveal a more healthy white sheet, that of the posterior surface of the levator aponeurosis. Placement of sutures into this white sheet, which is to say the healthier posterior surface of levator aponeurosis, will achieve the desired correction by a more effective advancement than simply plicating orbital septum to the tarsus.

## REFERENCES

1. Malhotra R, Salam A, Then SY, et al. Visible iris sign as a predictor of problems during and following anterior approach ptosis surgery. Eye. 2011;25:185-91.

2. Jones LT, Quickert MH, Wobig JL. The cure of ptosis by aponeurotic repair. Arch Ophthalmol. 1975;93:629-34.
3. Anderson RL, Beard C. The levator aponeurosis. Attachments and their clinical significance. Arch Ophthalmol. 1977;95:1437-41.
4. Anderson RL, Dixon RS. Aponeurotic ptosis surgery. Arch Ophthalmol. 1979;97:1123-8.
5. Anderson RL. Age of aponeurotic awareness. Ophthal Plast Reconstr Surg. 1985;1:77-9.
6. Bowman WP. Report of the chief operations performed at the Royal Ophthalmic Hospital for the quarter ending September 1857. R Lond Ophthalmol Hosp Rep. 1859;1:34.
7. Fasanella RM, Servat J. Levator resection for minimal ptosis: another simplified operation. Arch Ophthalmol. 1961;65:493-6.
8. De Blaskovics L. Treatment of ptosis: the formation of a fold in the eyelid and resection of the levator and tarsus. Arch Ophthalmol. 1929;1:672-80.
9. Agaston SA. Resection of levator palpebrae muscle by the conjunctival route for ptosis. Arch Ophthalmol. 1942;27:994.
10. Werb A. Ptosis. Trans Ophthalmol Soc N Z. 1976;28:29-32.
11. Putterman AM, Urist MJ. Müller muscle-conjunctiva resection. Technique for treatment of blepharoptosis. Arch Ophthalmol. 1975;93:619-23.
12. Collin R. A ptosis repair of aponeurotic defects by the posterior approach. Br J Ophthalmol. 1979;63:586-90.
13. Allen RC, Saylor MA, Nerad JA. The current state of ptosis repair: a comparison of internal and external approaches. Curr Opin Ophthalmol. 2011;22:394-9.
14. Dresner SC. Further modifications of the Müller's muscle-conjunctival resection procedure for blepharoptosis. Ophthal Plast Reconstr Surg. 1991;7:114-22.
15. Marcet MM, Setabutr P, Lemke BN, et al. Surgical microanatomy of the Müller muscle-conjunctival resection ptosis procedure. Ophthal Plast Reconstr Surg. 2010;26:360-4.
16. Berke RN. A simplified Blaskovics operation for blepharoptosis: results in 91 operations. Trans Am Ophthalmol Soc. 1951;49:297-350.
17. Ichinose A, Tahara S. Transconjunctival levator aponeurotic repair without resection of Mullers muscle. Aesthetic Plast Surg. 2007;31:279-84.
18. Patel V, Salam A, Malhotra R. Posterior approach white line advancement ptosis repair: the evolving posterior approach to ptosis surgery. Br J Ophthalmol. 2010;94:1513-8.
19. Goldberg RA. Cosmetic outcome of posterior approach ptosis surgery (an American Ophthalmological Society thesis). Trans Am Ophthalmol Soc. 2011;109:157-67.
20. Putterman AM, Fett DR. Muller's muscle in the treatment of upper eyelid ptosis: a ten-year study. Ophthalmic Surg. 1986;17:354-60.
21. Baldwin HC, Bhagey J, Khooshabeh R. Open sky Muller muscle-conjunctival resection in phenylephrine test-negative blepharoptosis patients. Ophthal Plast Reconstr Surg. 2005;21:276.
22. Kakizaki H, Malhotra R, Selva D. Upper eyelid anatomy: an update. Ann Plast Surg. 2009;63:336-43.
23. Marcet MM, Meyer DR, Greenwald MJ, et al. Proximal tarsal attachments of the levator aponeurosis: implications for blepharoptosis repair. Ophthalmology. 2013;120:1924-9.
24. Baldwin HC, Bhagey J, Khooshabeh R. Open sky Muller muscle-conjunctival resection in phenylephrine test-negative blepharoptosis patients. Ophthal Plast Reconstr Surg. 2005;21:276.
25. Anderson RL. Predictable ptosis procedures: do not go to the dark side. Ophthal Plast Reconstr Surg. 2012;28:239-41.
26. Jones LT, Quickert MH, Wobig JL. The cure of ptosis by aponeurotic repair. Arch Ophthalmol. 1975;93:629-34.
27. McCulley T, Kersten R, Kulwin D, et al. Outcome and influencing factors of external levator palpebrae superioris aponeurosis advancement for blepharoptosis. Ophthalmic Plast Reconst Surg. 2003;19:388-93.
28. Older J. Levator aponeurosis surgery for the correction of acquired ptosis. Ophthalmology. 1983;90:1056-9.

CHAPTER

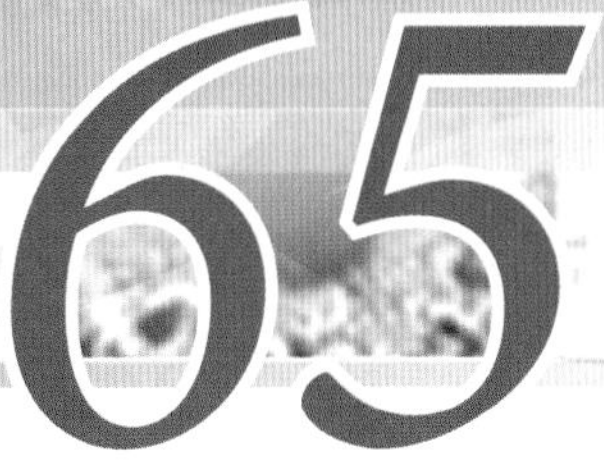

# Techniques in Frontalis Suspension

Louis Savar, Stuart R Seiff

## INTRODUCTION

Severe blepharoptosis resulting from minimal or absent levator function cannot be adequately repaired through surgery on the levator muscle or superior tarsal muscle (Müeller's muscle). The concept that the brow could be used to elevate a ptotic eyelid may date back as far 1801, with surgical refinements still being introduced today.[1,2] Frontalis suspension is most commonly used in cases of congenital ptosis; however, it is also used in patients with congenital fibrosis syndrome, cranial nerve III palsy, chronic external ophthalmoplegia, oculopharyngeal muscular dystrophy, myasthenia gravis and Marcus Gunn jaw winking. Urgent ptosis repair is indicated in children when developmental delay or amblyopia is suspected. Repair in the pediatric population may otherwise be delayed until school age.[3] Various suspension materials have been used and can be categorized as autologous, allograft, or synthetic. While each material has inherent advantages or disadvantages, it should be readily available, adjustable, well tolerated by surrounding tissues, and have long-lasting tensile strength.

## INDICATIONS

- Blepharoptosis resulting from minimal or absent levator function
  - Congenital ptosis
  - Congenital fibrosis syndrome
  - Cranial nerve III palsy
  - Chronic external ophthalmoplegia
  - Oculopharyngeal muscular dystrophy
  - Myasthenia gravis
  - Marcus Gunn jaw winking
- Repair should be performed urgently in children when amblyopia or developmental delay is suspected.

## CONTRAINDICATIONS

- Patients who will be unable to aggressively lubricate the ocular surface in the postoperative period
- Patients with poor frontalis function
- Patients with severe dry eye

## SURGICAL TECHNIQUE

### Selection of Suspension Material

#### *Autologous Tissues*

Autologous fascia lata, first described in the early 20th century for use in ptosis surgery, is the gold standard material for frontalis suspension.[4,5] More specifically, the tissue harvested comes from the iliotibial tract.[6] This fascia offers several advantages over other materials, including availability, no rejection and strong tensile strength with decreased risk of recurrent ptosis. Disadvantages include difficulty of postoperative adjustments, decreased availability of tissue in infants, and a second surgical site with possible complications of muscle herniation, hematoma, infection, or visible scar. Recently, Leibovitch[7] reported a series of infants all <3 years of age, who successfully underwent frontalis suspension procedures using autologous fascia lata. Alternative autologous materials used include temporalis fascia and palmaris longus tendon. The use of temporalis fascia has the additional advantages of not requiring a separate sterile field and minimal scarring since the incision is made behind the hairline.[8,9] The tissue tends to be more delicate and shorter than fascia lata.

*Autologous fascia lata:* Understanding of the anatomical landmarks of the thigh is key to harvesting adequate tissue.[10] The patient is positioned with the leg internally rotated and

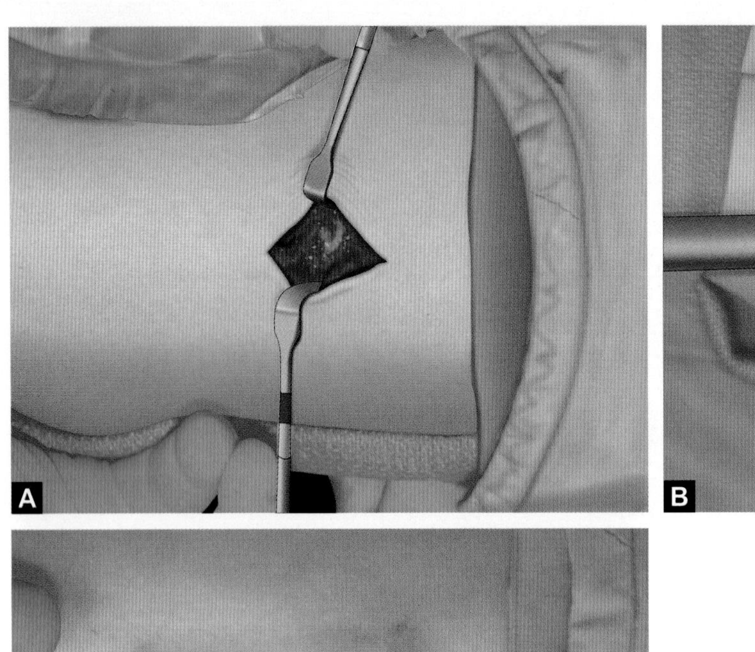

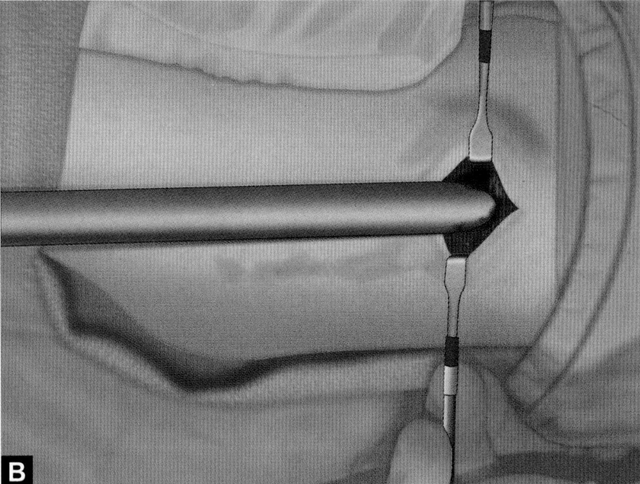

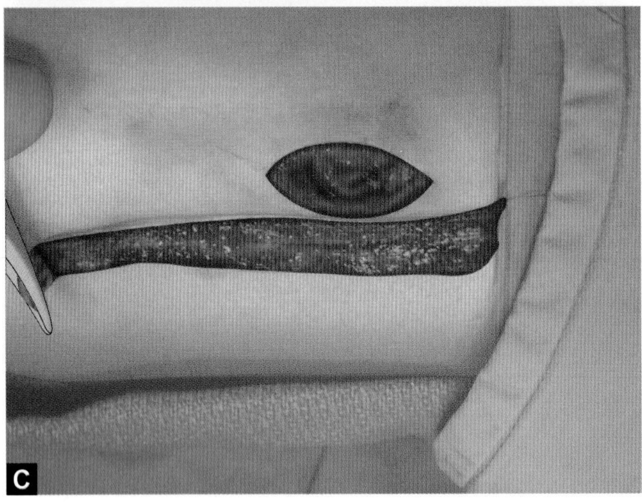

**Figures 65-1A to C** Harvesting autologous fascia lata. (A) Glistening fibers of the iliotibial tract visible after skin incision and dissection. (B) The fascia lata stripper is introduced through the incision around the fascia flap. (C) Representative fascia lata strip, which may then be cut into narrower strips.

partially flexed. A 3-cm vertical-skin incision is made on the lower lateral thigh approximately 5–10 cm above the lateral tibial condyle. Dissection is carried down to the glistening fibers of the iliotibial tract. The overlying soft tissues are cleared and two parallel incisions are made approximately 1 cm apart, in line with the fascial fibers, which course from the lateral tibial condyle superiorly and posteriorly toward the iliac crest. The inferior ends of the incisions are then joined by making a perpendicular incision in the fascia, thereby creating a flap of fascia. This flap is then introduced into the fascia lata stripper, which is then guided superiorly and posteriorly to fashion a 20-cm-long strip. This 1 × 20 cm strip is then cut into narrower strips 3–4 mm in width. The incision is closed in a layered fashion with 3-0 Vicryl suture in the deep subcutaneous tissue and a 5-0 fast absorbing gut interrupted suture for skin closure (Figs. 65-1A to C). Variations in fascia lata harvesting techniques have been described including a high leg incision and endoscopic approach, which may provide a less conspicuous scar and a lower risk of muscle herniation.[11,12]

*Autologous temporalis fascia:* A 3-cm skin incision is made vertically, approximately 4 cm behind the hairline and 2 cm above the ear. Blunt dissection is carried through the superficial temporal fascia down to the glistening deep temporal fascia. The temporalis fascia is incised horizontally and a 1-cm-wide strip is excised. The subcutaneous tissue is closed with 3-0 Vicryl and the skin is closed with staples or 5-0 fast absorbing gut suture.

*Autologous palmaris longus:* The palmaris longus tendon is present in approximately 80% of the population so it is necessary to check for its presence by having the patient oppose the tips of the thumb and little finger while flexing the wrist.[13] A bloodless surgical field is created by elevating the arm and placing a pressure bandage around the forearm.

A tourniquet is then placed above the elbow for 1 minute, prior to removal of the pressure bandage. The arm is situated in a supine position and 1-cm transverse incision is made along the wrist flexion crease. Dissection is carried through the superficial and deep fascia to the paratendon, which can be spread from the tendon using mosquito forceps. A second 1-cm incision is made approximately 10 cm proximal to the first in a transverse orientation, and again the tendon is isolated from the surrounding soft tissues. Traction on either end of the tendon confirms its course. The distal end is severed, externalized through the proximal incision. The tendon is then excised by severing the proximal end. The skin is closed with 6-0 nylon suture.

### *Allografts*

Preserved fascia lata was first promoted by Crawford for use in frontalis suspension with the benefit of not requiring a second surgical procedure, decreasing surgical time, and providing fascia for use in infants who may otherwise not have enough tissue available for harvesting.[10] Disadvantages compared to autogenous material include higher ptosis recurrence rates, increased granuloma and rejection rates, and the theoretical risk of disease transmission. Lyophilized banked fascia lata has been reported to have a recurrent ptosis rate approaching 50% 8 years after surgery.[14] Better results have been reported using irradiated, banked fascia lata, with failure rates of 21% up to 7 years after surgery.[15] Other preserved tissues, such as sclera and pericardium, tend to lose tensile strength and lead to high surgical failure rates.

### *Synthetic Materials*

Tillet and Tillet first described the use of silicone bands in frontalis suspension.[16] Subsequent improvements have led to the use of thinner 0.8–1.0-mm silicone rods. Silicone has several benefits over other materials, including availability, adjustability, elasticity, and being well tolerated by surrounding tissues.[17] Whereas many other materials become incorporated into surrounding tissues, silicone does not, allowing for adjustments or removal with ease even years after surgery. This is particularly important in patients with variable forms of ptosis such as chronic progressive external ophthalmoplegia or myasthenia gravis. Elasticity allows for easier lid closure, which is especially important in patients with poor Bell phenomenon and therefore at increased risk for exposure keratopathy, such as those with chronic progressive external ophthalmoplegia, myasthenia gravis, cranial nerve III palsy, and mechanical restriction of motility. Possible disadvantages include infection, exposure, and migration of the implant. Reported recurrent ptosis rates are low, 7–13%, and although initially described as a temporizing treatment until patients were old enough to undergo autologous fascia harvesting, some silicone suspensions have remained in place for over three decades.[17,18]

Other synthetic materials used in frontalis suspension include monofilament nylon, polypropylene, polyfilament cable-type suture, braided polyester, polyester fiber mesh, and expanded polytetrafluoroethylene (ePTFE). Smooth, nonporous, monofilament-like materials including nylon, polypropylene, and polyfilament cable-type suture are not integrated into the surrounding tissues and are more easily adjusted. Risks include cheese-wiring or slippage, granuloma formation, infection, and recurrence rates ranging from 28% to 69%.[19-21] Fragility of the material has led to post-traumatic recurrent ptosis. These materials are often used as temporizing measures due to their relative ease of placement and reversibility. Polyester fiber mesh and ePTFE provide scaffolding for fibrous ingrowth. While this characteristic may explain the long-term strength and lower ptosis recurrence rates compared to other synthetic materials, it also makes adjustment or removal more difficult. Infection or granuloma formation rates have been reported as high as 45%. Soaking the implants in antibiotic solution and meticulous wound closure may decrease these risks.[21,22]

## Placement of Suspension Material

Pediatric patients are usually able to tolerate a higher degree of lagophthalmos than adults, especially patients with poor Bell phenomenon. For this reason, in children that have otherwise normal corneal protective function, the lid margin height is usually set at the superior limbus during surgery. In those with higher risk for exposure keratopathy the lid height may be set at a lower level. A silicone sling should strongly be considered in these patients as it allows for a greater degree of passive lid closure and adjustability due to the lack of biointegration and elasticity. Several sling configurations have been described.

### *Double Triangle*

Crawford originally proposed the double triangle configuration for use with autogenous fascia but has since been used with other materials (Fig. 65-2A). Since there are two separate loops with three fixation points on the tarsus, this technique allows for good control of lid contour and long-term stability; however, it increases bulk and makes postoperative adjustments difficult. After anesthesia is administered a

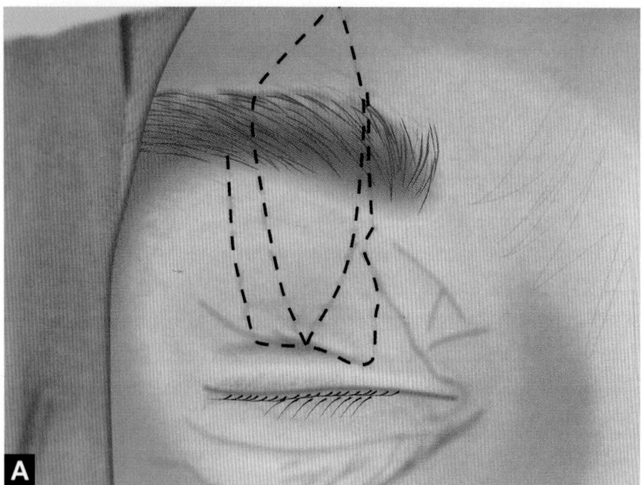


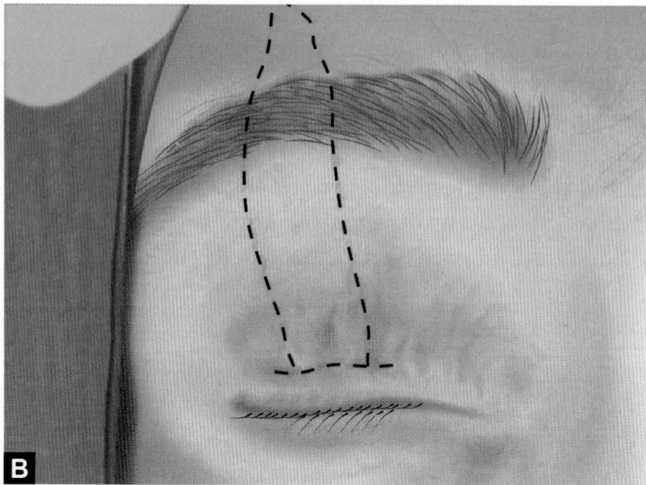


**Figures 65-2A and B** (A) Skin markings delineating the position of the six skin incisions and the planned course of the suspension material in the Crawford double triangle configuration. (B) Skin markings delineating the position of the five skin incisions and the planned course of the suspension material in the pentagonal configuration.

4-0 silk traction suture is placed in the upper lid margin. A Jaeger lid plate coated with ointment is then placed under the lid to protect the globe. A total of six skin incisions are made with the #15 blade, each 2–3 mm in length. Three eyelid skin incisions, carried down to the anterior tarsal surface, are made 2–3 mm above the lashes, one each above the lateral limbus, pupil, and medial limbus. Two skin incisions are made down to the periosteum just above the medial and lateral brow hairs in line with the previous supralash incisions. The final incision is made on the forehead, 10–15 mm above the midbrow in between the two brow incisions. This incision is carried through the frontalis muscle, and a pocket is created above the incision deep to the frontalis muscle using tenotomy scissors. A Wright needle is passed from the medial lid incision to the central lid incision. One end of the sling is threaded into the needle, which is then retracted back through the medial lid incision. The empty Wright needle is then passed from the medial brow incision to the medial lid incision, posterior to the orbital septum. Care must be taken not to pass the needle full thickness through the lid. The medial end of the sling is then threaded into the needle, which is retracted superiorly, externalizing the sling end from the medial brow incision. The empty Wright needle is then passed from the medial brow incision to the central lid incision, posterior to the orbital septum. The central end of the sling is threaded into the needle, which is retracted superiorly, so that both sling ends are now externalized at the medial brow incision. The same procedure is repeated at the lateral and central lid incisions with the two ends of a second strip of sling material externalized at the lateral brow incision. Each set of sling tails are adjusted to place the proper tension on the lid margin and create an appropriate contour. They are then tied forming two separate triangular loops based at the lid margin. One tail of each triangle is left long and the Wright needle is then used to pass the tails from the medial and lateral brow incisions out through the forehead incision. The ends of the two slings are tied with a square knot and secured with a nonabsorbable suture such as 6-0 nylon. The tails are trimmed to 10 mm in length and buried in the pocket deep to the frontalis muscle above the forehead incision. The forehead and brow incisions are then closed with subcutaneous 6-0 chromic gut suture, and the skin is closed with 6-0 fast absorbing gut suture. Some surgeons prefer to secure the sling material to the tarsal surface with a suture passed in the medial, central, and lateral lid incisions. This is also necessary if a single long lid crease incision is used for placement of the sling instead of the smaller stab incisions described above.

### *Rhomboid or Pentagonal*

Rhomboid[23] and pentagonal sling[24] configurations were popularized by Freidenwald and Fox (Fig. 65-2B). The advantages of this technique include using less graft material and easier adjustment. It is, thus, ideal for cases where postoperative adjustment is anticipated, and it is performed for most cases utilizing a silicone rod as the sling material. After anesthesia is administered a 4-0 silk traction suture is placed in the upper lid margin. A Jaeger lid plate coated with ointment is then placed under the lid to protect the globe. A total of five skin incisions are made with the #15 blade, each 2–3 mm in length (Fig. 65-3A). Two eyelid skin incisions carried down to the anterior tarsal surface are made 2–3 mm above the lashes in line with the medial and lateral limbus. Two skin incisions are made down to the periosteum just above the medial and lateral brow hairs in line with the previous supralash incisions. The final incision is made on the forehead, 10–15 mm above the midbrow in between the two brow incisions. This incision is carried through the frontalis muscle, and a pocket is created above the incision deep to the frontalis muscle using tenotomy scissors. The Wright needle is passed from the medial brow incision to the medial lid incision, posterior to the orbital septum. Care must be taken not to pass the needle full thickness through the lid. One end of the sling is then threaded into the needle, which is retracted superiorly, externalizing the sling end from the medial brow incision. Alternatively, a silicone rod with a long needle already attached may be used to pass the material without a Wright needle (Fig. 65-3B). The empty Wright needle is then used to pass the other sling end from the medial lid incision to the lateral lid incision, staying anterior to the tarsus, and from the lateral lid incision to the lateral brow incision in the same fashion performed on the medial side (Fig. 65-3C and D). The empty Wright needle is then passed from the forehead incision to the medial brow incision and used to pass the medial end of the sling along the needle track through the mid forehead incision (Fig. 65-3E). The lateral end of the sling is then passed through the forehead incision in the same fashion.

If using a silicone rod, the two tails are secured by placing a Watzke type silicone sleeve (Fig. 65-3F). Passing the tails in the same direction through the sleeve allows them to be more easily buried in the pocket created superior to the forehead incision. The sling is then adjusted to bring the lid to desired height and the sleeve is secured in place by passing a 5-0 nylon suture through the sleeve and around the sling tails. If using fascia or mesh material it is necessary to knot the tails together or suture them with nonabsorbable suture such as 5-0 nylon once the desired lid height is achieved. If other synthetic suture type material is used, the ends are knotted together. The tails are trimmed to 10 mm in length and buried in the pocket deep to the frontalis muscle above the forehead incision (Fig. 65-3G). The forehead and brow incisions are then closed with subcutaneous 6-0 chromic gut suture and the skin is closed with 6-0 fast absorbing gut suture (Fig. 65-3H). Some surgeons prefer to secure the sling material to the tarsal surface with a suture passed in the medial and lateral lid incisions. This is also necessary if a single long lid crease incision is used for placement of the sling instead of the smaller stab incisions described above.

### *Direct Fixation*

Spoor et al. described a broad, direct connection from the tarsal surface to the frontalis muscle without closed loops, a technique that has been modified with reasonable success.[25,26]

## MECHANISM OF ACTION

Frontalis suspension creates a link between the tarsus in the upper eyelid margin and the brow. This link allows for recruitment of the frontalis muscle to elevate the eyelid and clear the visual axis in the presence of a poorly functioning levator palpebrae superioris muscle.

## POSTOPERATIVE CARE

After the procedure, the eye and incisions are dressed with antibiotic ointment. Regardless of the type of material and technique chosen, a degree of lagophthalmos is expected in the postoperative phase and aggressive ocular lubrication is imperative (Fig. 65-4).

## SPECIFIC INSTRUMENTATION

*Crawford fascia stripper*: When harvesting autologous fascia lata, the fascia stripper may be utilized, as described earlier, to obtain an adequate length of tissue through a small incision

*Jaeger lid plate:* The lid plate, used to protect the globe, should be coated with ointment and placed between the eye and the eyelid when passing the fascia needle

*Wright fascia needle:* The fascia needle allows fascia to be passed subcutaneously and may also be used with synthetic materials that are not already attached to a needle.

## COMPLICATIONS

- Pain
- Infection
- Bleeding
- Granuloma formation
- Exposure of sling
- Keratopathy
- Ptosis recurrence

## PLACE OF THE TECHNIQUE IN SURGICAL ARMAMENTARIUM

Frontalis suspension is reserved for cases of blepharoptosis in which minimal or no levator function exists. It should be considered urgently in the pediatric population when

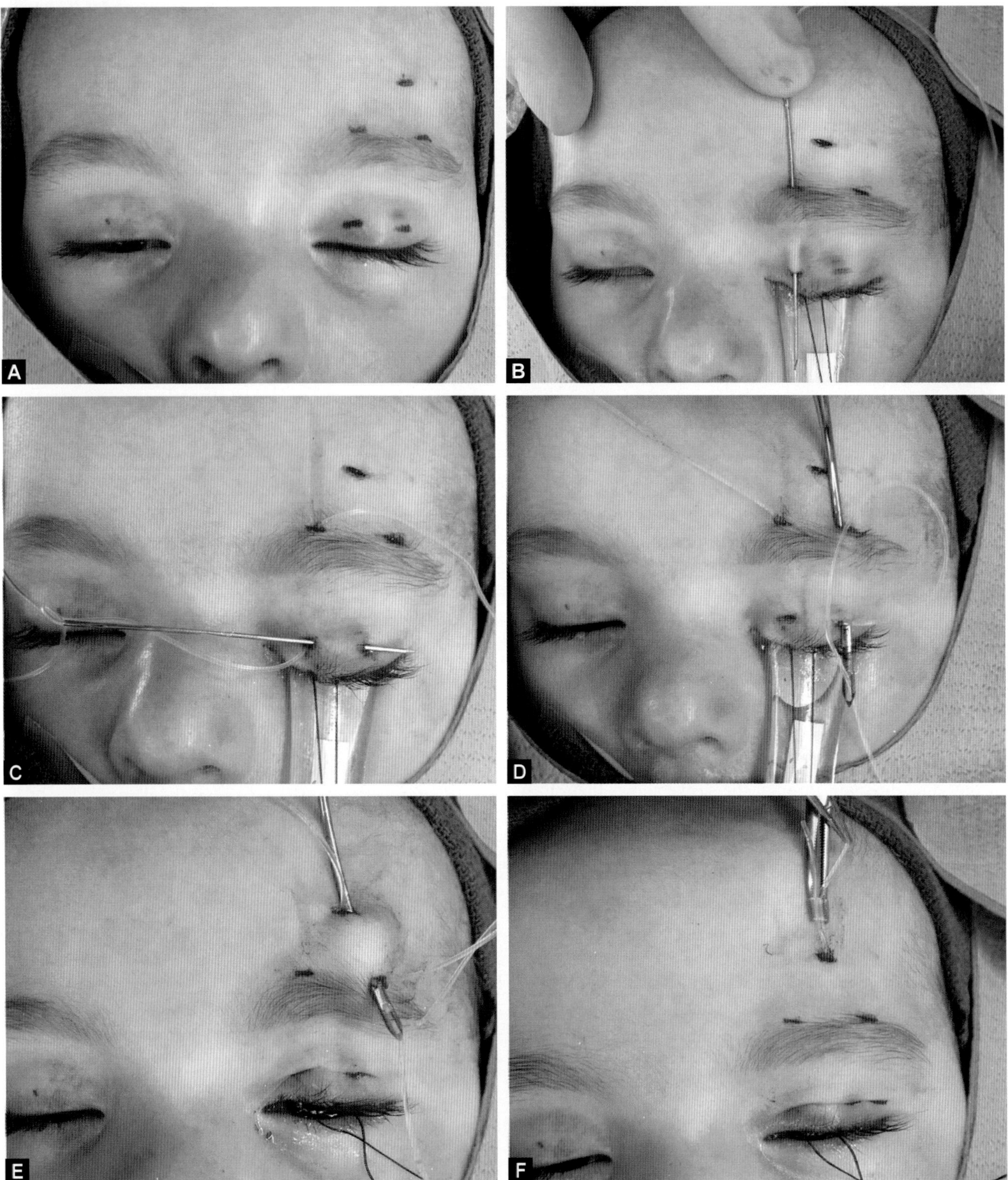


**Figures 65-3A to F** Frontalis suspension procedure. (A) Position of two eyelid skin incisions, two brow incisions, and single forehead incision. (B) The silicone sling is passed from the medial brow incision to the medial lid incision with Jaeger lid plate in place to protect the globe. (C) Passage of the sling from medial lid incision to lateral lid incision, anterior to tarsus. (D) Wright needle used to pass sling from lateral lid incision to lateral brow incision. (E) Wright needle used to pass sling from lateral brow incision to forehead incision. (F) After externalizing both ends of the sling from the forehead incision, the ends are trimmed and secured with a Watzke type silicone sleeve.

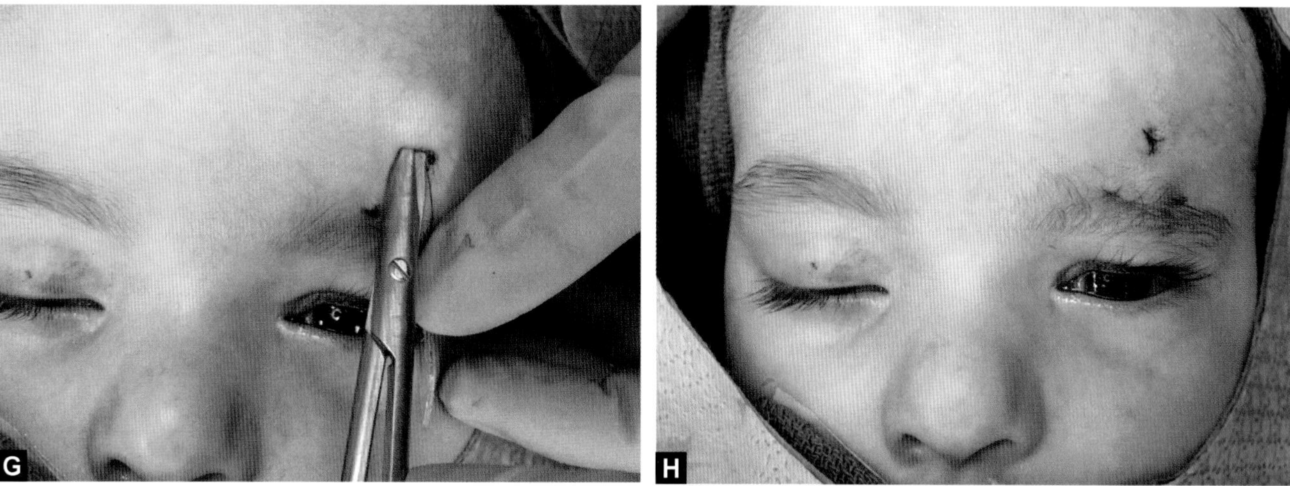

**Figures 65-3G and H** (G) A pocket is fashioned with blunt dissection deep to the frontalis muscle and superior to the forehead incision. (H) After burying the ends of the sling, all incisions are closed with absorbable suture.

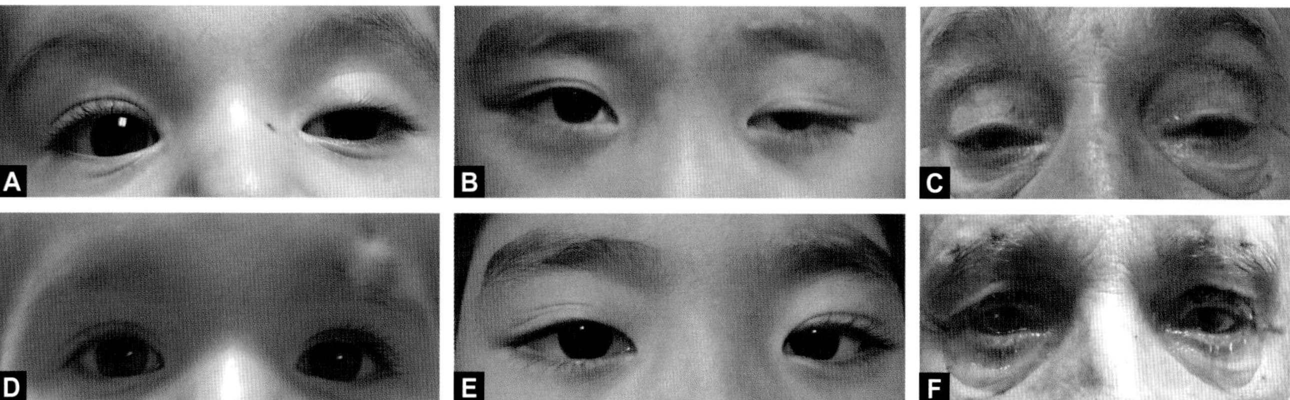

**Figures 65-4A to F** Representative preoperative (above) and postoperative (below) frontalis suspension photographs.

amblyopia or developmental delay is suspected. Caution must be taken in selection of suspension material and operative placement of lid height in patients with poor ability to protect the ocular surface.

## REFERENCES


1. Scarpa A. Saggio di osservazioni e d'esperienze sulle principali malattie degli occhi. Baldessare Comino Publisher. January 1, 1801.
2. Hunt RT. On the treatment of ptosis by operation. London Med Gaz. 1831;7:361.
3. Anderson RL, Baumgartner SA. Amblyopia in ptosis. Arch Ophthalmol. 1980;98(6):1068-9.
4. Payr E. Plastik mittels freier faszientransplantation bei ptosis. Dtsch Med Wochenschr. 1909;35:822.
5. Wright WW. The use of living sutures in the treatment of ptosis. Arch Ophthalmol. 1922;51:99-102.
6. Jordan DR, Anderson RL. Obtaining fascia lata. Arch Ophthalmol. 1987;105(8):1139-40.
7. Leibovitch I, Leibovitch L, Dray JP. Long-term results of frontalis suspension using autogenous fascia lata for congenital ptosis in children under 3 years of age. Am J Ophthalmol. 2003;136(5):866-71.
8. Neuhaus RW, Shorr N. Use of temporal fascia and muscle as an autograft. Arch Ophthalmol. 1983;101(2):262-4.
9. Tellioğlu AT, Saray A, Ergin A. Frontalis sling operation with deep temporal fascial graft in blepharoptosis repair. Plast Reconstr Surg. 2002;109(1):243-8.
10. Crawford JS. Repair of ptosis using frontalis muscle and fascia lata: a 20-year review. Ophthalmic Surg. 1977;8(4):31-40.
11. Naugle TC, Jr, Fry CL, Sabatier RE, et al. High leg incision fascia lata harvesting. Ophthalmology. 1997;104(9):1480-8.
12. Malhotra R, Selca D, Olver JM. Endoscopic harvesting of autogenous fascia lata. Ophthal Plast Reconstr Surg. 2007;23(5):372-5.
13. Lam DS, Ng JS, CHeng GP, et al. Autogenous palmaris longus tendon as frontalis suspension material for ptosis correction in children. Am J Ophthalmol. 1998;126(1):109-15.
14. Wilson ME, Johnson RW. Congenital ptosis. Long-term results of treatment using lyophilized fascia lata for frontalis suspensions. Ophthalmology. 1991;98(8):1234-7.

15. Esmaeli B, Chung H, Pashby RC. Long-term results of frontalis suspension using irradiated, banked fascia lata. Ophthal Plast Reconstr Surg. 1998;14(3):159-63.
16. Tillett CW, Tillett GM. Silicone sling in the correction of ptosis. Am J Ophthalmol 1966;62:521-3.
17. Carter SR, Meecham WJ, Seiff SR. Silicone frontalis slings for the correction of blepharoptosis: indications and efficacy. Ophthalmology. 1996;103(4):623-30.
18. Hersh D, Martin FJ, Rowe N. Comparison of silastic and banked fascia lata in pediatric frontalis suspension. J Pediatr Ophthalmol Strabismus. 2006;43(4):212-8.
19. Katowitz JA. Frontalis suspension in congenital ptosis using a polyfilament, cable-type suture. Arch Ophthalmol. 1979;97(9):1659-63.
20. Wagner RS, Mauriello JA, Jr, Nelson LB, et al. Treatment of congenital ptosis with frontalis suspension: a comparison of suspensory materials. Ophthalmology. 1984;91(3):245-8.
21. Wasserman BN, Sprunger DT, Helveston EM. Comparison of materials used in frontalis suspension. Arch Ophthalmol. 2001;119(5):687-91.
22. Mehta P, Patel P, Olver JM. Functional results and complications of Mersilene mesh use for frontalis suspension ptosis surgery. Br J Ophthalmol. 2004;88(3):361-4.
23. Friedenwald JS, Guyton JS. A simple ptosis operation; utilization of the frontalis by means of a single rhomboid-shaped suture. Am J Ophthalmol. 1948;31(4):411-4.
24. Fox SA. A new frontalis skin sling for ptosis. Am J Ophthalmol. 1968;65(3):359-62.
25. Spoor TC, Kwitko GM. Blepharoptosis repair by fascia lata suspension with direct tarsal and frontalis fixation. Am J Ophthalmol. 1990;109:314-7.
26. DeMartelaere SL, Blaydon SM, Cruz AA, et al. Broad fascia fixation enhances frontalis suspension. Ophthal Plast Reconstr Surg. 2007;23(4):279-84.

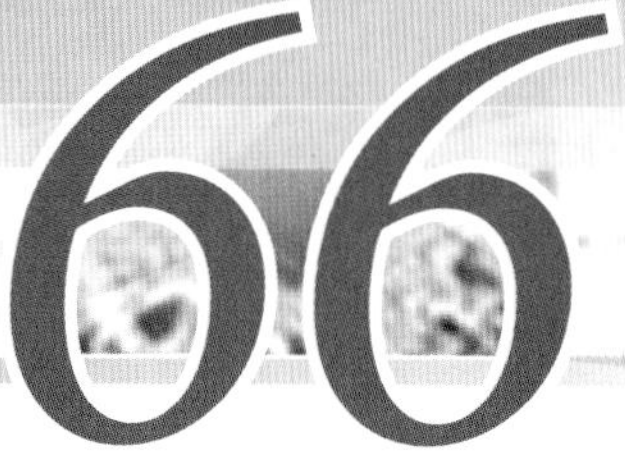


# Blepharoplasty

Shubhra Goel, Cat Nguyen Burkat

## INTRODUCTION

With aging, the periorbital tissues undergo histopathological changes that result in decreased tissue elasticity, tone, and volume. In the eyelid region, this may manifest as droopy eyelids that can lead to a tired appearance and even obscured vision. Blepharoplasty is one of the most popular cosmetic procedures for eyelid and facial rejuvenation.

Blepharoplasty, whether for aesthetic or functional purposes, is performed by removing redundant eyelid skin, excess herniated orbital fat, and hypertrophic orbicularis oculi muscle along the upper or lower eyelids. The primary goal of aesthetic blepharoplasty is the restoration of a youthful and natural eye. Enhanced superior and peripheral visual fields are the primary goal for those undergoing medically necessary blepharoplasty.

## INDICATIONS (FIGS. 66-1A TO D)

- Dermatochalasis (skin and/or fat) leading to obscured vision and heaviness over the upper eyelid margin.
- Dermatochalasis (skin and/or fat), due to age-related changes, for cosmetic improvement of the eyelid appearance
- Improvement of eyelid symmetry.
- Improvement of eyelid contour and crease definition, such as in Asian eyelids.
- Lower eyelid dermatochalasis (skin and/or fat) leading to eyelid bags or fullness.

## CONTRAINDICATIONS

- Upper or lower eyelid skin anterior lamellar shortening (secondary to previous surgery, burns, lasers, or trauma)
- Severe dry eyes (Fig. 66-2)
- Severe sulcus deformity (post-trauma, aging, previous surgery)
- Cicatricial entropion or ectropion of the eyelids
- Lower eyelid retraction
- Anticoagulation that cannot be discontinued for surgery
- Unrealistic expectations.

## SURGICAL TECHNIQUE

### Upper Lid Blepharoplasty

#### *Preoperative Evaluation (Fig. 66-3)*

- In addition to the routine general and ophthalmic examination, a detailed periocular and facial assessment is necessary. A Schirmer's test, or measurement of the tear lake meniscus should be performed in those with dry eyes. The cornea should be assessed for evidence of dry eyes, such as punctate surface keratopathy, scarring, and also evaluated for lagophthalmos and corneal hypoesthesia. In patients of Asian descent, the presence of an epicanthal fold should be documented, as well as the contour, low level, and definition of the desired eyelid crease. It is often helpful to assess old photographs together with the patient to better understand the patient's desired outcome and whether expectations are realistic.
- *Brow position*: The eyebrows and the eyelids should be considered a single unit to achieve optimal results. The male brow should typically rest at the level of the supraorbital rim, with a flat contour, in contrast to a female brow that is often much higher above the orbital rim and with a peaked or arched shape. Again, old photographs of the patient can better determine their natural brow contour. Aging leads to noticeable lateral brow ptosis and lateral

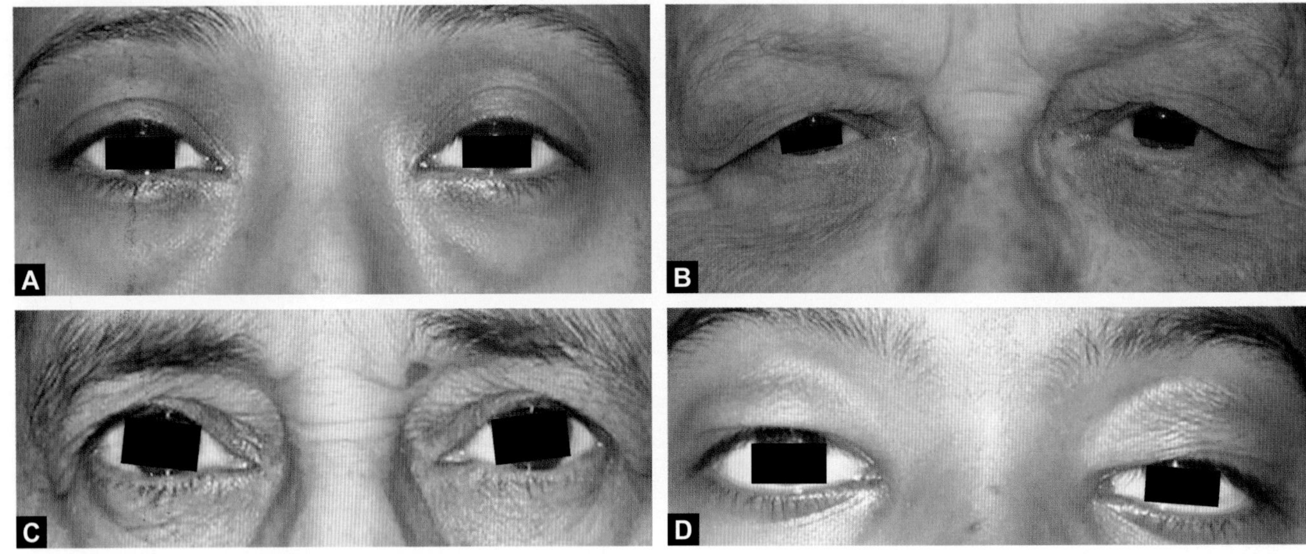


Figures 66-1A to D Common indications for blepharoplasty surgery.

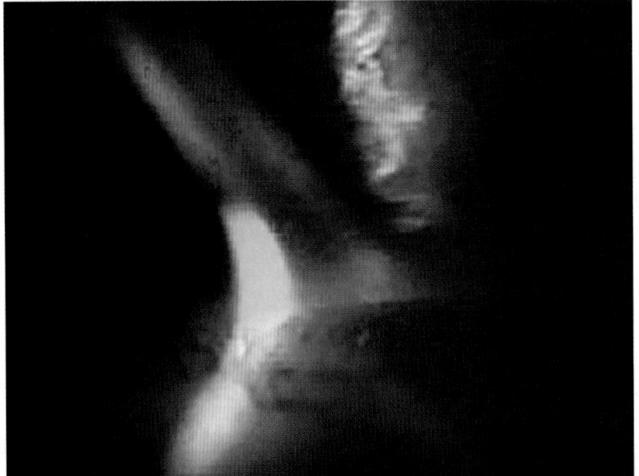

Figure 66-2 Relative contraindication for blepharoplasty. A tear meniscus measurement of < 0.2 mm using the slit-lamp beam may be suggestive of dry eyes.

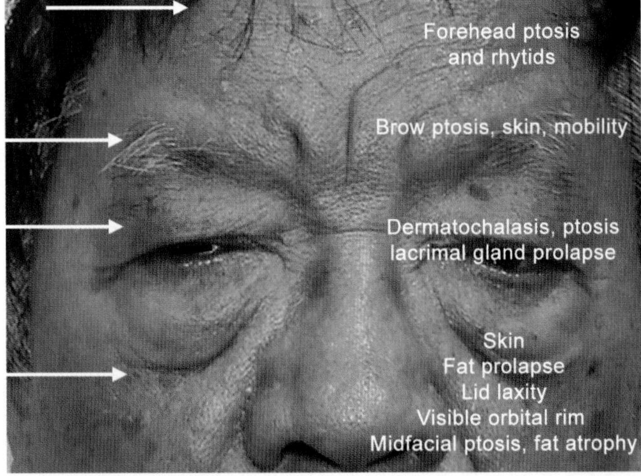


Figure 66-3 Preoperative evaluation. Facial parameters to be noted during evaluation of a patient for blepharoplasty surgery.

skin hooding first, due to the lack of frontalis muscle fibers attached to the lateral brow soft tissues. Significant brow ptosis leading to pseudodermatochalasis should be addressed via a brow elevation procedure, rather than blepharoplasty as this would further pull the eyebrows inferiorly into the orbital space (Figs. 66-4A and B). If true dermatochalasis is present in conjunction with brow ptosis, a combined brow lifting procedure and blepharoplasty can be performed through the same or different incisions.

- *Upper eyelid skin*: Assessment of the upper eyelid skin is of utmost importance and is measured in millimeters from the lash line to the thicker brow skin centrally, medially, and laterally (Fig. 66-5). Approximately, 20 mm of the upper eyelid should be retained for normal function and closure of the eyelids. However, each surgery should be individualized to the patient, and some may have smaller orbital spaces that only necessitate 16–18 mm of upper eyelid skin.[1-6] A conservative approach should first be taken, and the patient can be asked to open and close his or her eyes intraoperatively to assess whether more skin may safely be removed for a more pleasing outcome. It is also important to note the thickness, texture, and elasticity of the skin, as the patient may need to be counseled that the texture of the remaining skin may need ancillary procedures, such as

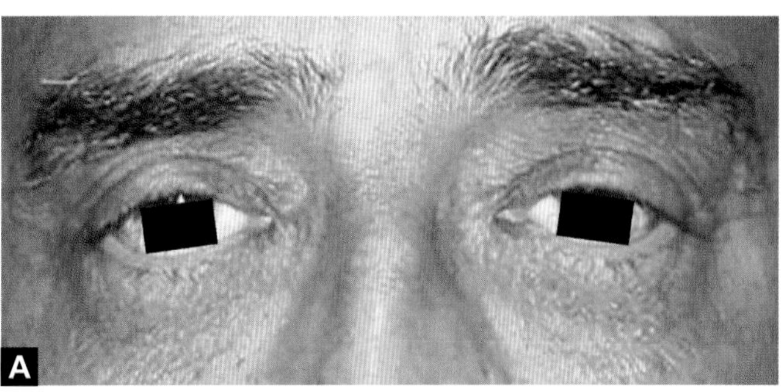


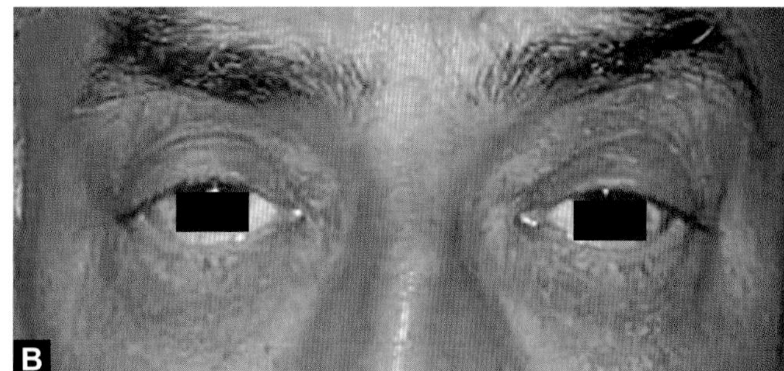


**Figures 66-4A and B** Brow position and its relation with the upper lid skin. A 60-year-old man with bilateral brow ptosis, involutional ptosis, and pseudodermatochalasis.

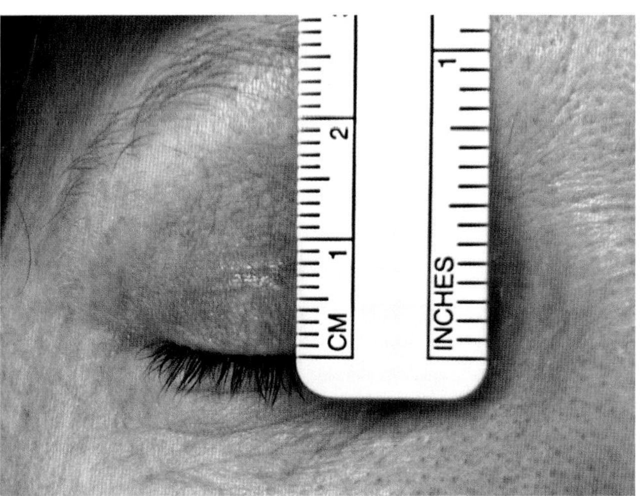


**Figure 66-5** Measurement of upper eyelid skin. The lid crease is measured on both sides. The amount of upper lid skin present is measured from the lid margin to the junction of the thin eyelid skin to the thicker brow skin. This junction is often inferior to the brow hairs and seen as a transition of skin thickness and color, with the brow skin lighter.

chemical peeling or laser resurfacing, to improve overall appearance. Gender considerations are important in assessing skin removal as well, as aggressive skin removal in men may lead to a feminized appearance, as opposed to retaining slightly more skin that will create a more natural skin fold and fullness that is typical for men. A conservative resection of the orbital fat will also minimize the appearance of a hollow and aged sulcus postoperatively.

- *Lid height*: The margin-to-reflex distance (MRD-1) should be documented for both sides. In some patients, the actual eyelid margin is in good position under the redundant overhanging skin, thus requiring only blepharoplasty surgery. In other patients, the lid margin clearly approaches the pupil, as opposed to the overhanging skin approaching the pupil and causing functional obstruction. Therefore ptosis correction, whether by internal or external approach, should be performed in conjunction with blepharoplasty surgery.
- *Lid contour and shape*: The eyelids should ideally have a positive canthal tilt, such that the lateral canthus is approximately 2 mm superior to the medial canthus. The lateral canthal angle should also demonstrate a sharp almond-shaped angle, in contrast to aging eyelids that may have a rounded and attenuated canthal angle.
- *Lid crease*: In most females, the upper lid crease should be 9–12 mm above the lash line. In males, it is typically lower at 7–9 mm above the lash line. In patients of Asian descent, the crease is sometimes less well defined, but located much lower at 4–6 mm. In case of multiple eyelid creases, the most prominent crease can be selected, keeping the crease level symmetric between the two upper eyelids. Redundant creases can be resected within the blepharoplasty skin flap.[1-6]
- *Orbital fat*: The degree of prolapsed orbital fat within the upper eyelids should be noted, and can be rated on the scale of 1+ to 4+. Fullness of the medial fat pad more than 2+ is often debulked as this results in a more aged appearance. Central preaponeurotic fat should be minimally contoured to maintain the natural fullness of youth. Excessive fullness of the lateral eyelid may be secondary to lacrimal gland prolapse that should be resuspended under the supraorbital rim during surgery (Figs. 66-6A and B).

## Surgical Technique (Figs. 66-7A to I)[1-6]

- A surgical marking pen and calipers are used to demarcate crescenteric upper eyelid blepharoplasty incisions with the lid crease placed at the desired height based on natural location, symmetry, gender, and ethnicity. Approximately, 18–20 mm of skin should be retained in both upper eyelids when measuring the superior incision line from the brow. The transition to eyebrow skin is often seen as thicker, lighter, and more porous skin and may be lower than the inferior edge of the eyebrow hairs, particularly in women due to brow plucking.

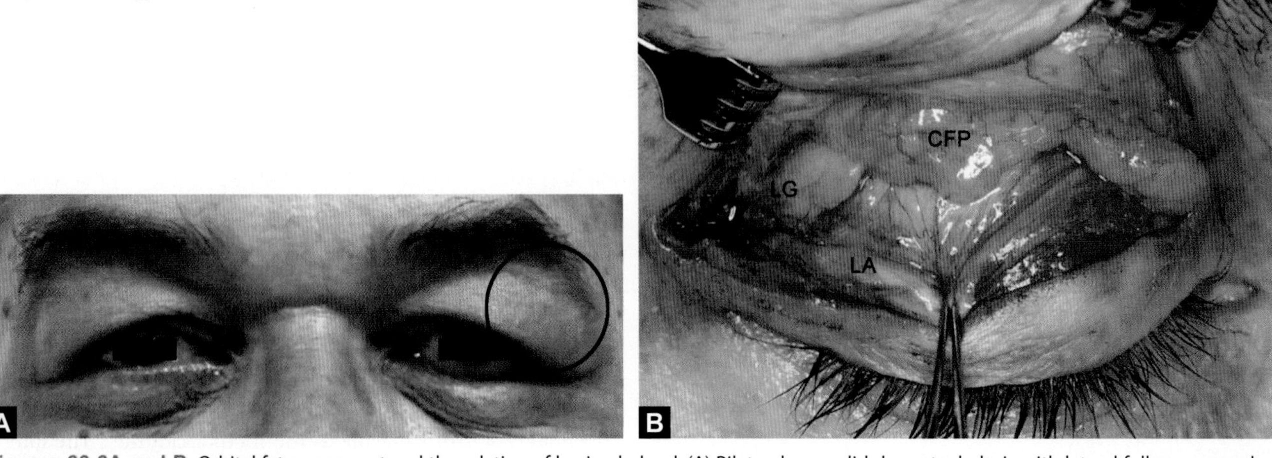


**Figures 66-6A and B** Orbital fat assessment and the relation of lacrimal gland. (A) Bilateral upper lid dermatochalasis with lateral fullness secondary to lacrimal gland prolapse. (B) Anatomical dissection demonstrating the upper lid medial and central fat pad (CFP), lacrimal gland (LG) prolapse laterally, and the underlying levator aponeurosis (LA).

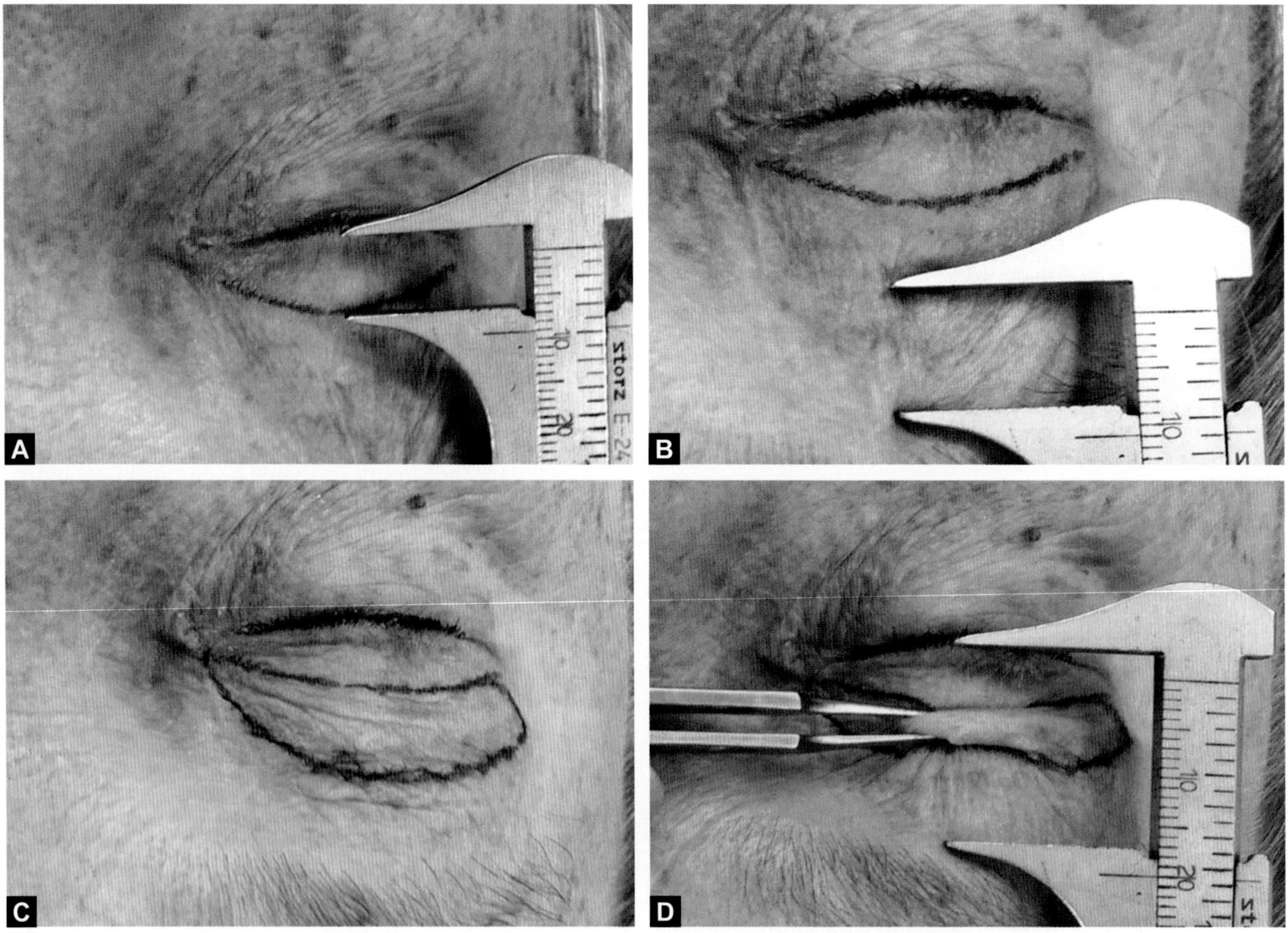

**Figures 66-7A to D** Skin Markings and basic surgical steps of upper lid blepharoplasty. (A) Marking the skin for upper lid blepharoplasty, surgeon's view. The lid crease is first measured and marked symmetrically. (B) The lid crease height is subtracted from 18–20 mm, and the remainder is measured from the junction of the lid to brow skin. (C) Typical upper lid skin markings for blepharoplasty surgery. (D) The skin pinch test between the inferior and superior markings confirms that 18–20 mm of upper lid skin have been maintained to preserve normal lid closure. Vertical tightening of the skin, or eversion of the lid margin with this test indicates excessive skin removal.

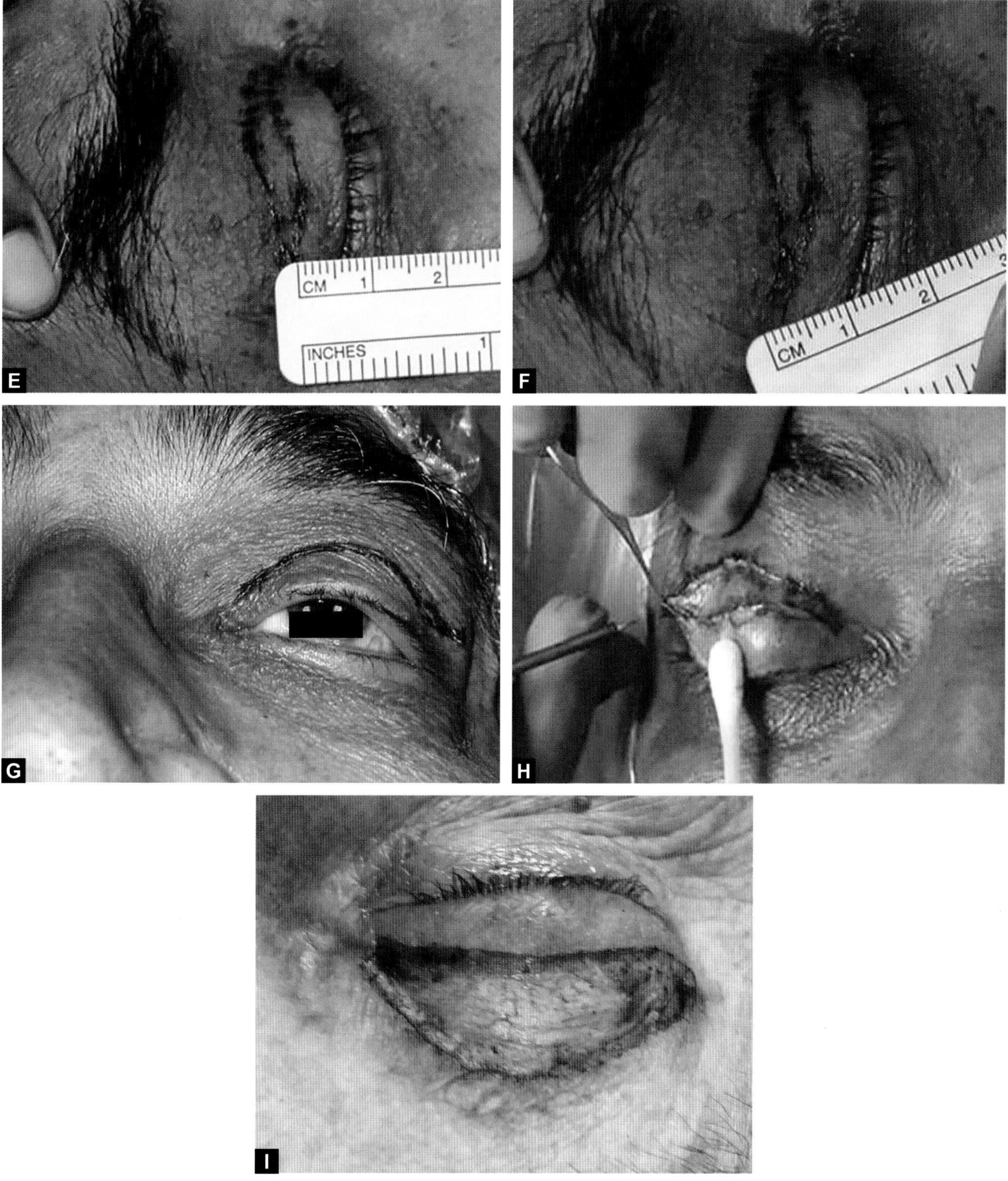


I

Figures 66-7E to I (E) The lateral skin marking and crease should taper down slightly, measure approximately 5 mm above the canthal angle and be symmetric on both sides. (F) In cases of concurrent brow ptosis, a lateral angled extension, which is blended into a crow's feet crease and approximately 10 mm from the canthus, can be useful for improving lateral skin hooding. (G) The medial extent of the skin marking typically should not extend past the upper punctum to avoid webbing. (H) An assistant can provide countertraction using a cotton-tip applicator or forceps to distract the skin edge away from the incision. This minimizes thermal injury to the skin edges during removal of the blepharoplasty flap and thus allows for optimal healing with less scarring. (I) Surgeon's view. A skin or skin–muscle flap is removed. The orbital septum is not opened yet, thus the levator muscle and aponeurosis are intact.

- Avoid incising medial to the upper punctum and lateral into the thicker temporal skin to avoid webbing of the skin. Likewise, the lateral incisions should not extend into or below the level of the lateral canthal raphe.
- The pinch technique is used to confirm the adequacy of retained skin. Eversion of the lashes or lid margin, or excessive vertical tightening of the remaining skin suggests overly aggressive skin excision.
- Brow ptosis may be measured by lifting the lateral brow up to the desired height above the superior orbital rim and measuring its excursion with a ruler. Brow ptosis should be corrected simultaneously to avoid the appearance postoperatively of residual skin redundancy laterally.
- Local infiltrative anesthesia using 2% lidocaine with 1:100,000 units epinephrine mixed in equal parts with 0.5% bupivacaine is given to both upper lids.
- The patient's face is prepped and draped in the usual sterile fashion.
- Corneal protectors lubricated with ophthalmic ointment are placed on both ocular surfaces.
- A 15 blade, $CO_2$ laser, or monopolar cautery tip is used to incise the eyelid skin along the previously placed markings. In patients with a predilection for hypertrophic or hyperpigmented scarring, such as pigmented skin, the 15-blade scalpel may be preferable to minimize tissue injury.
- The skin and orbicularis muscle are removed as single flaps generally, although a skin flap alone could be removed if there is preoperative concern for poor eyelid closure function. Such patients may include those with a history of Bell's palsy, dry eyes, decreased tear film or exposure signs, or elderly patients with no frank lagophthalmos but slow spontaneous blinking.
- The orbital septum is incised if there is significant fat prolapse preoperatively to isolate the underlying preaponeurotic fat pads. The fine attachments between the fat pads and the underlying levator complex are carefully lysed with the monopolar unit. If debulking is indicated based on the amount of preoperative fat prominence, the fat should be conservatively removed over a hemostat clamp or forceps, and the fat stump cauterized before release, to avoid orbital hemorrhage. Be certain that no vital structures, such as the levator aponeurosis or muscle, are included in the clamp prior to excision and cautery. The medial fat pad has a light yellow-white, creamy appearance, while the central fat pad is a darker yellow.
- The medial fat pads are carefully isolated and either thermally sculpted or debulked, taking care to cauterize the fat stump prior to release into the orbit. Avoid aggressively pulling or cauterization of the medial fat, as permanent injury to the trochlea and superior oblique tendon may occur.
- Fullness and prolapse laterally suggests lacrimal gland dystopia as there is no upper eyelid lateral fat pad anatomically. The lacrimal gland will exhibit a characteristic pink color, with a multilobulated shape. Failure to recognize this during surgery may lead to inadvertent lacrimal lobectomy and possible postoperative hemorrhage or chronic dry eye. On the other hand, if left uncorrected, this may result in eyelid asymmetry, persistent lateral fullness, and poor cosmesis.
- If preoperative evaluation demonstrated minimal to moderate fat prominence, the fat pads can often be thermally sculpted, with the Ellman round ball tip or the monopolar Colorado tip (held flat sideways), using a sweeping motion over an intact orbital septum. This approach limits the risk of orbital hemorrhage or injury to posterior lid structures, as well as requires much less operative time. Care should be taken to avoid aggressive thermal cautery of the septum, however, as eyelid retraction may occur.
- The upper eyelid incisions are closed with 7-0 Vicryl buried interrupted suture to close the orbicularis muscle layer, followed by 6-0 fast-absorbing plain gut suture to close the skin edges in a running or interrupted fashion. Alternatively, nonabsorbable Prolene or nylon suture may be used to close the incision to theoretically minimize hypertrophic scarring, although patients often appreciate the absorbable aspect. Absorbable sutures also save time in clinic without compromising the final appearance to the incisions and allow more flexibility for follow-up visits. Closure is performed from medial to lateral, as any dog-ear deformity, if present, is better addressed and camouflaged laterally (Figs. 66-8A and B).

## PEARLS

- Make the skin markings with a fine-tip marker prior to local anesthetic infiltration as this distorts the eyelid tissues
- Careful comparison of the eyelid creases on both sides helps obtain symmetry.
- Coexisting findings, such as levator dehiscence, lacrimal gland prolapse, and brow ptosis should be addressed concurrently to achieve the best results.
- Gender and ethnic variations are important to keep in mind when marking the skin flaps.
- The male brow is typically flatter and lower along the supraorbital rim.
- In Asian patients, the skin marking should blend medially with the epicanthal fold. A lower (4–5 mm)

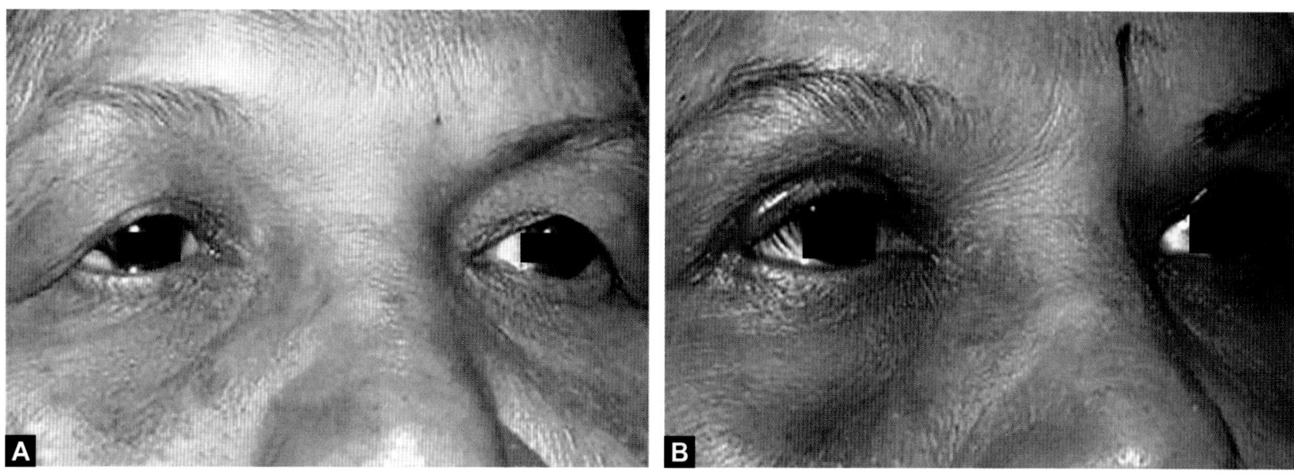

Figures 66-8A and B Postoperative photos of upper lid blepharoplasty performed in a 45-year old woman with temporal field limitation due to lateral hooding of redundant skin over the lid margin. Note the improvement of lateral hooding and temporal visual field following upper lid blepharoplasty.

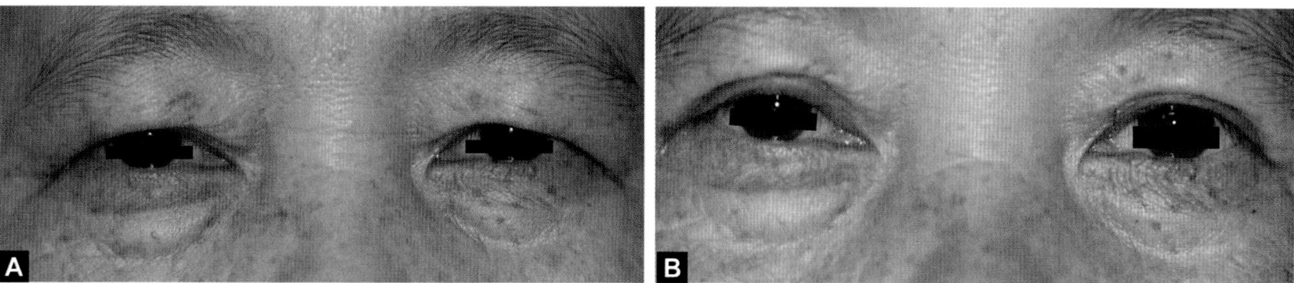

Figures 66-9A and B Preoperative and postoperative photos of conservative upper lid blepharoplasty in an Asian patient, taking care to maintain a low crease.

lid crease is natural and should be maintained to avoid Westernizing the eyelid appearance (Figs. 66-9A and B).

- Avoid excessive removal of the orbital fat pads in Asian eyelids, as a deep superior sulcus is less typical as compared the natural fullness of the entire lid sulcus in most Asian ethnicities.
- Upper eyelid skin should measure approximately 18–20 mm to avoid postoperative lagophthalmos.
- Conservative skin excision should be performed medially to avoid webbing and medial ectropion. A Burow's triangle should be excised, if necessary, to address excessive medial skin laxity.
- An additional 2–3 mm of skin may be removed laterally in cases of associated brow ptosis.
- Careful marking of the superior flap incision should be measured from the transition of the lid to brow skin. The transition to eyebrow skin is often seen as thicker, lighter, and more porous skin and may be lower than the inferior edge of the eyebrow hairs, particularly in women due to brow plucking.
- If the skin pinch leads to vertical striae, a tight upper lid, and/or eversion of the eyelid margin and lashes, the skin excision is too aggressive.
- The medial marking should not extend past the upper puncta to avoid webbing.
- The lateral markings should not extend into the thicker temporal skin or below the level of the lateral raphe.
- Aggressive skin and fat removal in men may lead to a hollow, feminized appearance. Retaining slightly more skin will create a more natural skin fold and fullness that is typical for men.
- Avoid aggressively pulling or cauterization of the medial fat, as permanent injury to the trochlea and superior oblique tendon may occur.
- Closure of the orbital septum is contraindicated.

## Lower Lid Blepharoplasty

### *Preoperative Evaluation (see Fig. 66-3)*

In general, the goal of lower lid blepharoplasty is to eliminate redundant skin, smooth the underlying musculature, tighten

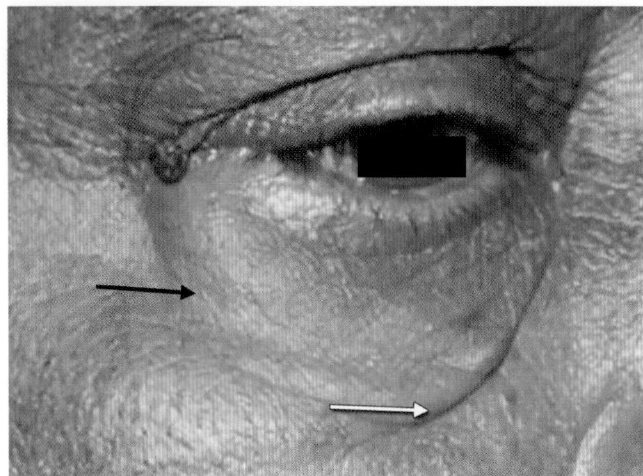

**Figure 66-10** Lower lid festoon and skin (fine arrow) with lateral fat prolapse (thick arrow).

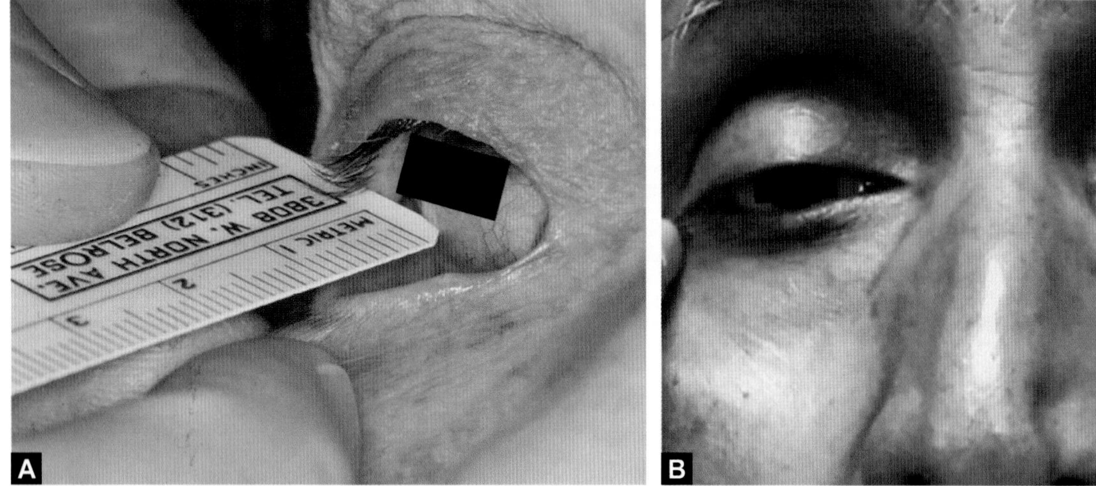


**Figures 66-11A and B** Tests for assessing the lid laxity. (A) Lower lid distraction test to quantify the degree of horizontal lid laxity. (B) Lower lid skin pinch to evaluate skin laxity and elasticity.

supporting structures, and sculpt or redrape excess orbital to blend the transition over the orbital rim between the lower eyelid and the cheek. In addition to the examination discussed in the upper lid blepharoplasty section, other important findings to evaluate include:

- *Skin*: The amount, depth, and location of rhytids are important to document. Skin turgor, texture, and tone, as well as dyschromias should also be considered. The presence of festoons or chronic eyelid edema may indicate chronic inflammation and may persist postoperatively (Fig. 66-10). The amount of redundant skin can be evaluated by asking the patient to look upward, or to open his or her mouth. This places the lower eyelid skin on stretch, and any excess skin with the lid in this position can be usually excised with less risk of postoperative cicatricial retraction or ectropion.
- *Lid position*: The lower lid should rest at the level of the inferior limbus or 1 mm below the limbus. Any amount of lower lid retraction should be documented and a lateral canthal tightening, with proper placement of the tarsal support suture higher along the orbital rim periosteum, should be considered.
- *Lid laxity*: The snapback test and distraction test are useful to determine the degree of horizontal laxity. On average, 4–5 mm of distraction, as the lid is gently pulled away from the globe surface, is considered normal (Figs. 66-11A and B). Likewise, if the lower lid is pulled down and released, and the lid margin does not quickly snap back to appose the ocular surface, this would suggest laxity, and a horizontal tightening procedure should be performed with blepharoplasty.

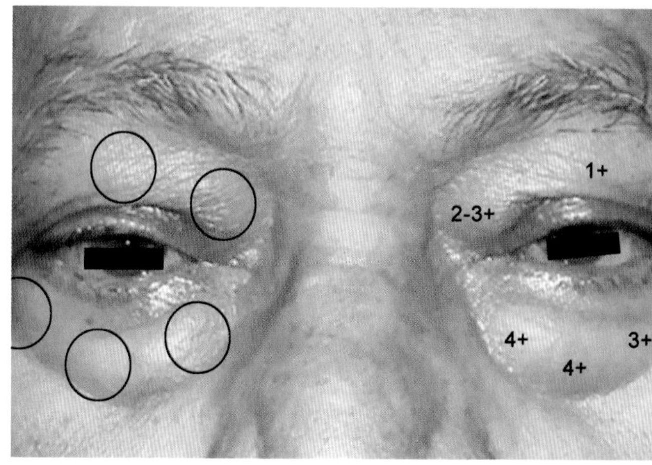


**Figure 66-12** Patient with upper and lower lid dermatochalasis and fat prolapse. Circles depict the location of upper lid (medial, central) and lower lid (medial, central, and lateral) orbital fat pads. Left side shows approximate grading of the prolapsed fat pads.

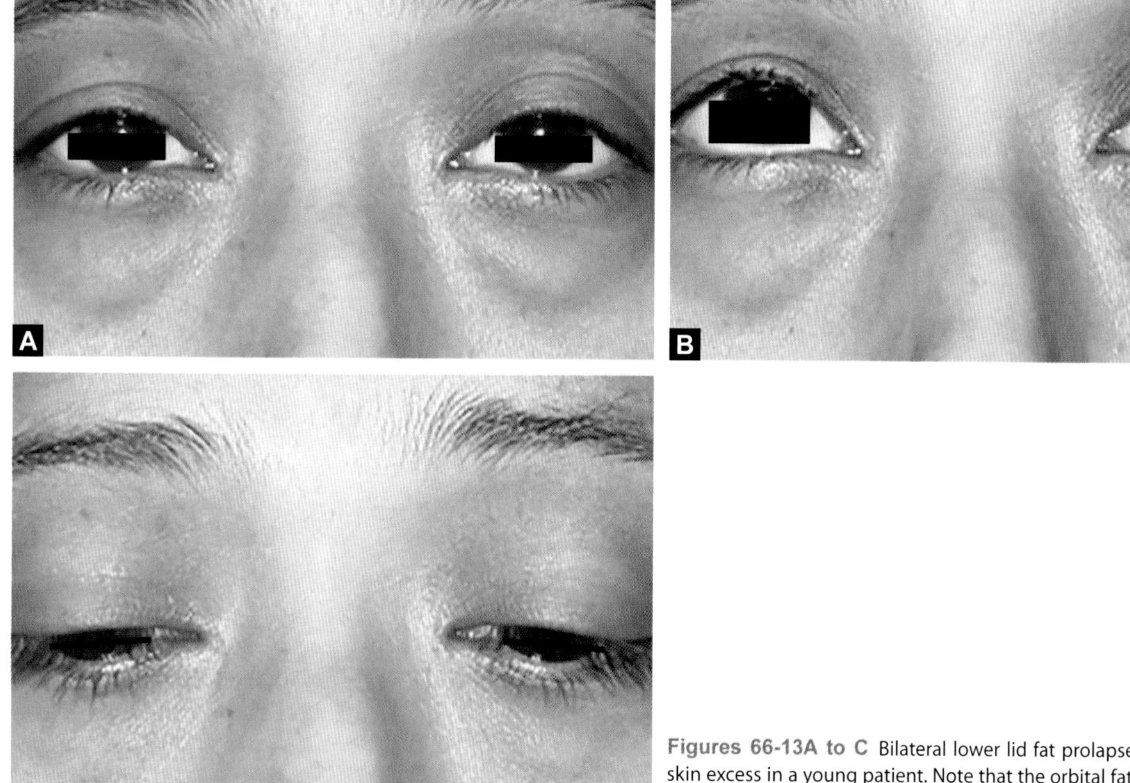


**Figures 66-13A to C** Bilateral lower lid fat prolapse without significant skin excess in a young patient. Note that the orbital fat pads become more prominent and full in upgaze and are less visible in primary and downgaze, in contrast to festoons, which do not change with gaze.

- *Fat prolapse or lack of fat*: The location and amount of prominence of each of the three lower lid fat pads is important to note in the upright position. If the patient is supine, the fat will fall back dependently and the degree of fat prominence can be difficult to see. Herniated orbital fat can also be noted by looking for areas of fullness in the lower eyelid that become more prominent as the patient looks up (Figs. 66-12 and 66-13). Excessive fat prolapse may require debulking. If the fat is moderate and the tear trough depressed then fat repositioning, rather than

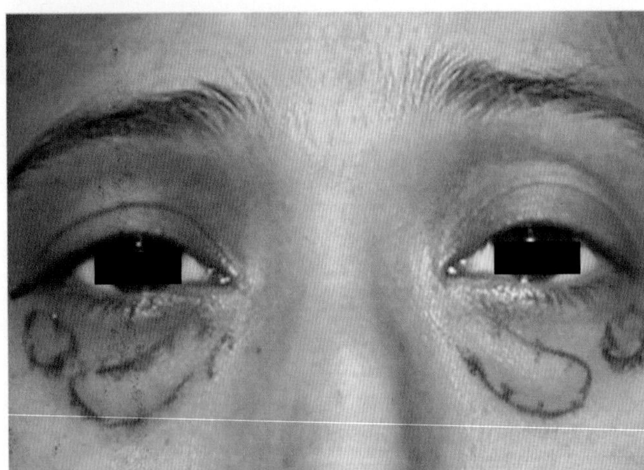

**Figure 66-14** Surgical steps in transcutaneous lower lid blepharoplasty. Preoperative markings in upright position delineating the areas of concern for the patient.

fat removal, should be considered to blend the lid–cheek junction. Lack of fat preoperatively should be discussed with the patient before surgery, as results would be suboptimal without concurrent volume augmentation to the lower lids and orbital rim sulcus. If there is significant lateral fat prolapse, this may be debulked first, as the lateral fat often retracts back behind the orbital rim once the other fat pads are addressed, making it more difficult to reach later.[1-4]

- *Other considerations*: A thorough evaluation should also note the shape and position of the canthal angles, orbicularis oculi muscle hypertrophy or corrugation, inferior scleral show and lid retraction, facial ptosis, tear trough deformity, thyroid proptosis presence of negative orbital vector.

## *Surgical Technique*

Lower lid blepharoplasty includes several approaches:

- Transcutaneous technique
- Transconjunctival technique
- Combined technique
- Adjunctive midface lifting.

1. Transcutaneous technique:
   a. Markings are made preoperatively in the upright position. The patient is asked to look up to assess the fat compartments to be addressed (Fig. 66-14).
   b. After infiltration with local anesthesia (same as in upper lid blepharoplasty), corneal eye shields are placed and the face is prepped and draped in usual sterile fashion.
   c. A subciliary incision is made 1–2 mm below the lash line and gently curved laterally for 1 cm into a crow's feet crease.
   d. Skin, with or without the orbicularis oculi muscle, is dissected.
   e. Strict hemostasis is important, and care is taken to preserve the eyelash follicles. Minimizing cautery at the subciliary incision may result in less scarring and lash loss.
   f. The orbital septum is button-holed over the prominent fat compartments and the fat isolated and completely freed circumferentially from the multilamellar orbital septum, cauterized at the base, and then excised with scissors or monopolar cautery. Fat pedicles can also be redraped, particularly medially and centrally, to add volume to significant tear trough sulci.
   g. Avoid excessive dissection and manipulation of the orbital septum layer, as this may predispose to cicatricial middle lamellar scarring and retraction complications.
   h. If any degree of lower lid laxity was present preoperatively, a lateral canthopexy or tarsal strip procedure should be performed to avoid postoperative retraction and ectropion. This can be combined with resuspension of the lateral orbital orbicularis muscle and/or suborbicularis oculi fat layer to the lateral orbital rim periosteum with additional 4-0 or 5-0 sutures.
   i. Excess lower lid skin and orbicularis muscle are redraped and carefully excised. The patient can be asked to open his or her mouth to see if the lower lid skin demonstrates vertical striae or downward movement of the lid that would suggest aggressive skin excision. A narrow pinch of skin and pretarsal orbicularis muscle may sometimes be sufficient if there is mild to moderate tissue excess (Figs. 66-15A and B). Aggressive orbicularis muscle removal may lead to destabilization of the eyelid margin, ectropion, weakened eyelid closure, or poor lacrimal pump mechanism.
   j. The lateral skin excision often angles downward and should blend into a natural relaxed skin tension crease.
   k. In cases of significant orbicularis muscle thickening or prominent dynamic corrugation, the lateral orbicularis muscle may be excised conservatively, and then redraped and secured to the maxillary bone lateral to the orbital rim to further smooth the lid contour while also providing additional horizontal support to the lid.

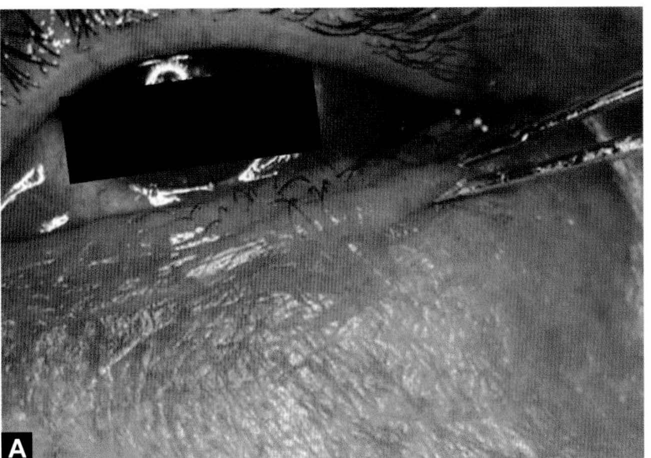


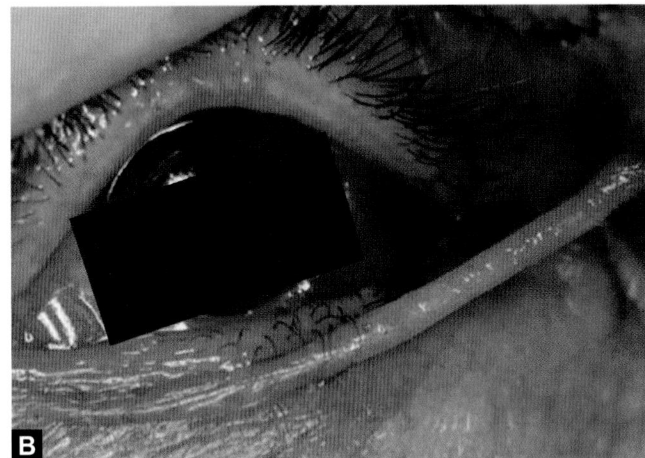


**Figures 66-15A and B** Surgical steps in transcutaneous lower lid blepharoplasty. In a patient with minimal skin redundancy, a small skin pinch (using forceps or a hemostat clamp) to remove a horizontal strip of subciliary skin can be performed. This minimizes dissection in the orbicularis and septal planes, thus decreasing the risk of postoperative retraction or ectropion.

l. The subciliary incision is closed with 6-0 fast-absorbing plain gut, nylon, or Prolene running or subcuticular suture.

2. Transconjunctival technique (Figs. 66.16A to D):
   a. Initial marking, anesthesia, and draping steps are similar to transcutaneous blepharoplasty above.
   b. This technique is ideal for patients with fat prominence but no significant skin redundancy. Alternatively, the transcutaneous incision and skin removal can be performed as above, and the fat debulking performed via a posterior approach.
   c. A Desmarres retractor is used to evert the lower eyelid and a Jaeger plate is used to protect the globe and provide gentle posterior pressure to prolapse the fat pads anteriorly toward the conjunctiva.
   d. Each of the three lower lid fat pads, the medial, central, and lateral, are accessed through a minimal 3–4 mm button-hole conjunctival incision over each fat pad. Through each button hole, the fat pad can be drawn forward with minimal tension. Fine attachments to the orbital septum can be felt and therefore, the base of the fat pad should be freed 360° circumferentially. An immediate release of more orbital fat can usually be seen once the septal attachments are fully released. This technique of freeing the base of the fat pad completely is particularly important when performing fat redraping, as incomplete release of the septal attachments will likely result in eyelid retraction or abnormal scarring within the septal layers.
   e. The fat pads can be clamped, if preferred, prior to excision. The stump of the resected fat should be controlled and cauterized prior to release to avoid orbital hemorrhage. Oxygen should be minimized at any time that electrocautery is used to avoid a spark fire.
   f. Fat should never be debulked posterior to the anterior orbital rim.
   g. The lateral fat is often undercorrected and therefore should be carefully addressed.
   h. When debulking the central fat pad, care is taken to neither instrument nor cauterize the inferior oblique muscle.

3. Combined technique:

   As mentioned previously, orbital fat is addressed through the transconjunctival approach while the skin–orbicularis complex is addressed transcutaneously. This theoretically avoids dissection in the plane of the orbital septum and thus may lead to less postoperative eyelid malposition (Figs. 66-17A and B). Alternatively, mild skin redundancy and laxity can be addressed with laser procedures rather than skin excision.

4. Adjunctive midface lifting:

   In patients with midfacial or facial descent, it may be optimal to elevate the suborbicularis oculi fat or superficial musculoaponeutic system to the periosteum lateral to the orbital rim. The orbitomalar ligament is typically released from the inferior orbital rim to fully mobilize the tissues. Midface lifting in conjunction with lower lid blepharoplasty decreases the mechanical weight of the ptotic midface, which can lead to retraction and/or ectropion after surgery. At the same time, it offers the benefits of restoring volume over the malar eminence and the inferior orbital rim, thus minimizing the tear trough deformity.

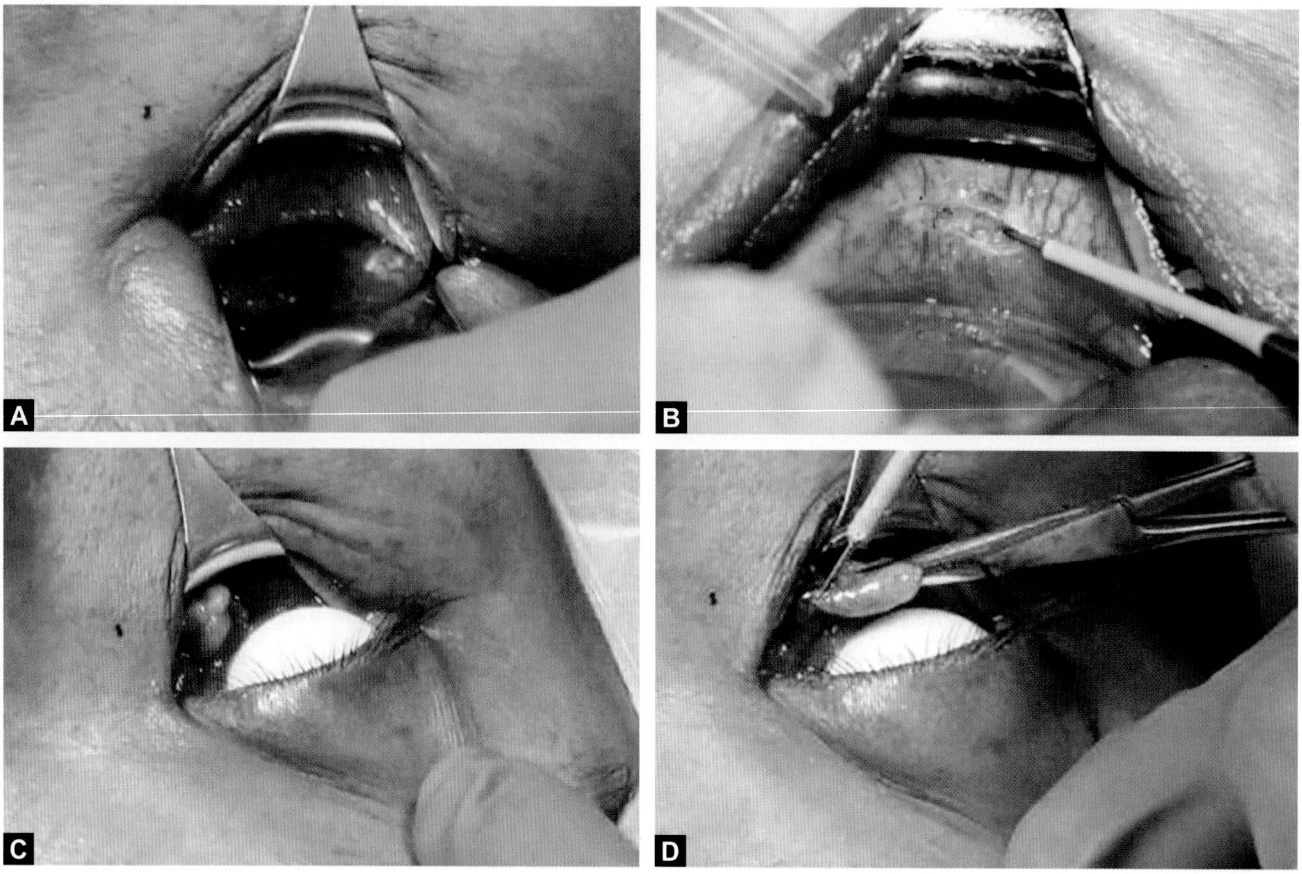

**Figures 66-16A to D** Surgical steps of transconjunctival lower lid blepharoplasty-fat debulking. (A) Desmarres retractor pulls the lower eyelid inferiorly while a Jaeger plate protects the globe. (B) Small 3-mm incisions, several millimeters inferior to the tarsus, can be made to access the individual fat pads. (C)Gentle posterior ballottement of the globe helps prolapse the fat pad anteriorly through the incision. (D) The fat is clamped with a hemostat and excised with cautery, or repositioned over the orbital rim if indicated.

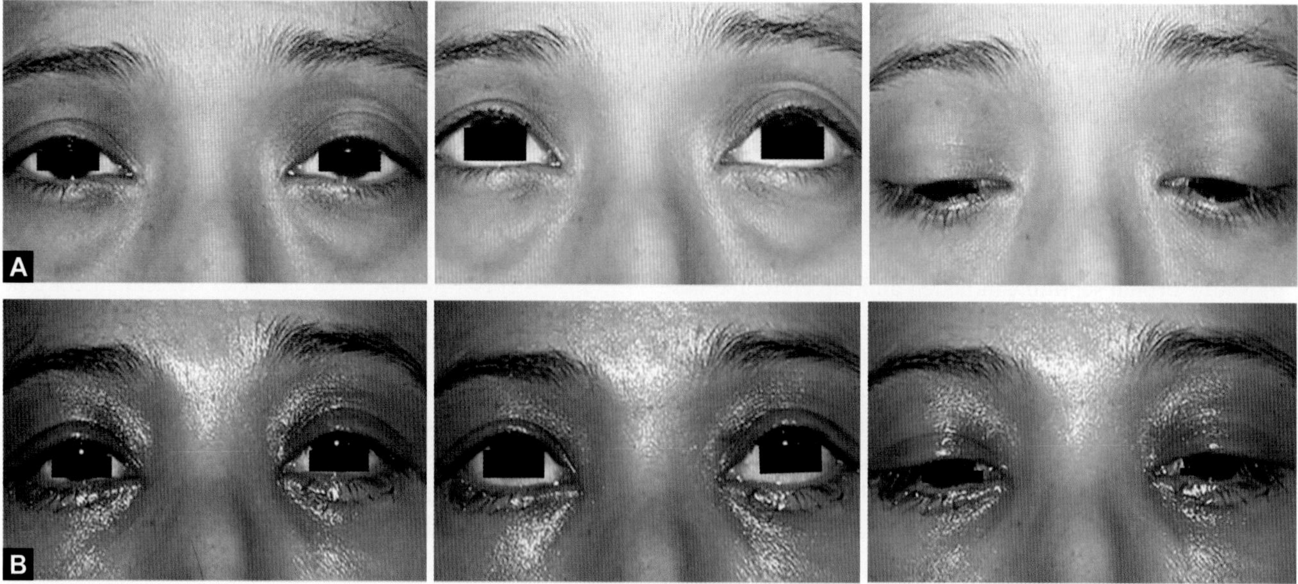


**Figures 66-17A and B** Postoperative photos 2 days after combined transconjuncival and skin pinch blepharoplasty demonstrates the improvement of the lower lid fullness.

## PEARLS

- It is important to be conservative when removing orbital fat. Draping or repositioning fat over the inferior orbital rim is often preferable to significant fat excision.
- Meticulous hemostasis is critical. It is a good practice to follow the clamp, cut, and cautery technique.
- Excessive skin removal laterally can lead to distortion, rounding, and ectropion of the lateral canthus, known as 'lateral canthal syndrome.'
- Always recreate a sharp lateral canthal angle to avoid rounding or web formation laterally.
- In the transconjunctival technique, the incisions should be placed 4–5 mm below the inferior tarsus, which corresponds to the inferior point of fusion between the lower lid retractors and the orbital septum. An incision too close to the tarsus may risk bleeding from the peripheral arcade arteries, but it is also above the level of the orbital fat such that dissection would travel through the joint fascia and approach the orbicularis muscle and skin, rather than the fat compartments.
- When possible, the transconjunctival approach is preferred as it leads to less lower lid retraction, scleral show, and postoperative ectropion. If excess skin is present, this can be removed through the subciliary approach or via a more conservative skin pinch that removes skin without muscle. Laser skin procedures can tighten mild skin laxity, and improve texture and color, without the need for surgery in select patients.
- The inferior oblique muscle between the medial and central fat pads should always be left undisturbed.

## COMPLICATIONS

- Retrobulbar hemorrhage with or without visual loss
- Infection
- Asymmetry
- Incomplete removal of redundant tissue, need for additional procedure
- Hypertrophic scarring or prolonged erythema of scar
- Aggressive skin resection leading to lagophthalmos (transient or permanent), cicatricial ectropion of the upper lid, web formation (incision placed too far medial)
- Blepharoptosis (levator muscle injury)
- Diplopia (superior or inferior oblique muscle damage)
- Hollowed out appearance (overly aggressive fat removal)
- Milia, suture granulomas.

## POSTOPERATIVE CARE

- Avoid strenuous activity, bending, or lifting heavy weights for 1 week
- Sleep with two pillows (approximately 45° elevation) for 1 week
- Start cold compresses immediately after surgery using washcloths soaked in a bowl of ice water, or a bag of frozen peas over a wet gauze. Cold compresses should be applied continuously as much as possible while awake for the first 48 hours
- Clean the operated area gently with warm water and a clean cotton-tip applicator if needed
- Avoid rubbing the eyelid area, forehead, or face to prevent dehiscence of the incisions
- Use topical lubricating eye drops frequently to prevent dry eye issues
- Avoid aspirin or ibuprofen for pain relief in the first several days after surgery
- Bruising typically resolves by 2 weeks
- May resume normal activities after 1 week
- Avoid makeup around the eyelids for at least 1 week; after that light makeup can be applied, but it should be carefully removed with a gentle cleanser to avoid incision dehiscence
- Contact lenses may be worn at 1–2 weeks after surgery, taking care to avoid pulling on the surgical eyelids during placement or removal of the lenses.

## CONCLUSION

Upper and lower eyelid blepharoplasty procedures can be very gratifying for both the surgeon and patient. It is important to identify the expectations of the patient preoperatively and determine pre-existing conditions that may lead to postoperative complications. A meticulous and individualized surgical approach, combined with appropriate postoperative care, can yield excellent results.

## REFERENCES


1. Spinelli HM. Atlas of aesthetic eyelid and periocular surgery. New York: Elsevier; 2004;Ch. 4:58-70.
2. Spinelli HM. Atlas of aesthetic eyelid and periocular surgery. New York: Elsevier; 2004;Ch. 5:72-89.
3. Hartstein ME, Holds JB, Massry GG. Pearls and pitfalls in cosmetic oculoplastic surgery. Berlin, Heidelberg: Springer; 2008;Part III:41-84.
4. Hartstein ME, Holds JB, Massry GG. Pearls and pitfalls in cosmetic oculoplastic surgery. Berlin, Heidelberg: Springer; 2008; Part IV:129-50.
5. Massry GG, Murphy MR, Azizzadeh B. Master techniques in blepharoplasty and periorbital rejuvenation. 2012;87-9.
6. Massry GG, Murphy MR, Azizzadeh B. Master techniques in blepharoplasty and periorbital rejuvenation. 2012;159-73.

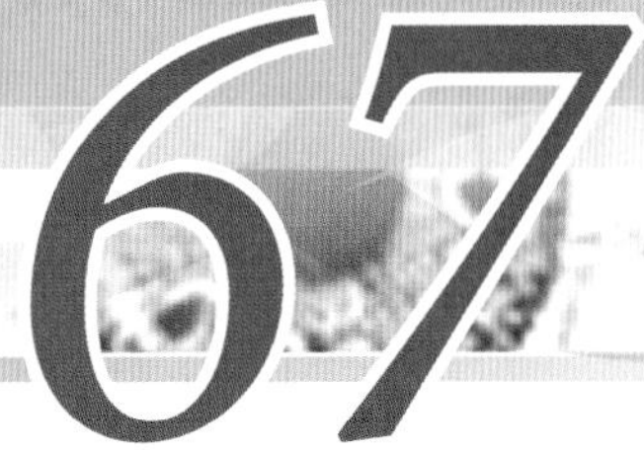

CHAPTER 67

# Brow Repair

Shubhra Goel, Cat Nguyen Burkat

## INTRODUCTION

The eyebrows play an important part in the face functionally and aesthetically. Brow repair is a general term describing the management of eyebrow ptosis. Eyebrow ptosis refers to drooping of the eyebrows and/or forehead, caused primarily by age-related degeneration of the muscles, skin, and forehead soft tissues. Gravitational forces and volume loss further contribute to these changes. Brow ptosis also leads to the appearance of redundant overhanging skin over the eyelids. Brow ptosis and secondary eyelid dermatochalasis not only result in a tired, sad, or angry look, but can also obstruct the field of vision.

## INDICATIONS

- Brow ptosis leading to secondary dermatochalasis and visual field restriction (Figs. 67-1A and B).
- Brow ptosis presenting in conjunction with significant upper lid dermatochalasis.
- Temporal brow ptosis causing lateral skin hooding over the lid margin and visual field restriction.
- Brow ptosis/loss of normal brow arch resulting in a cosmetic concern.
- Brow ptosis due to scarring (Fig. 67-2).
- Paralysis or weakness of the frontalis muscle due to facial nerve paralysis, myasthenia gravis, myotonic dystrophy, oculopharyngeal dystrophy, chronic progressive external ophthalmoplegia.
- Involuntary contraction of the orbital orbicularis oculi muscle that pulls the brow down in blepharospasm and facial dystonia.

### Anatomical Considerations

The eyebrows play an important role in facial expression, with their position dependent upon an interplay of elevators and

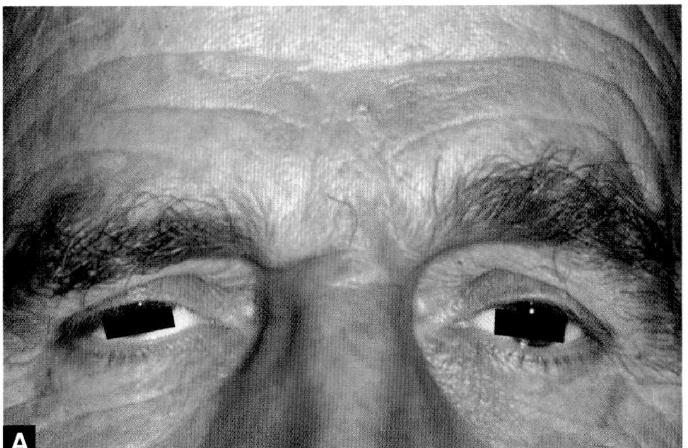

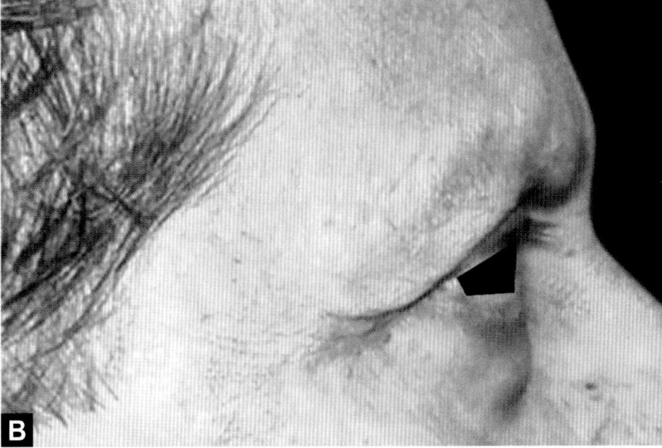

**Figures 67-1A and B** Functional indications for brow repair. (A) A 60-year-old man with asymmetric right brow ptosis causing mechanical eyelid ptosis and visual field obstruction. (B) A 40-year-old man with brow ptosis below the orbital rim causing pseudodermatochalasis.

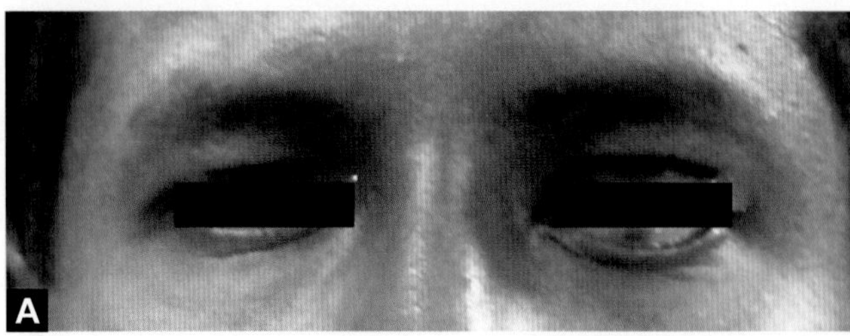
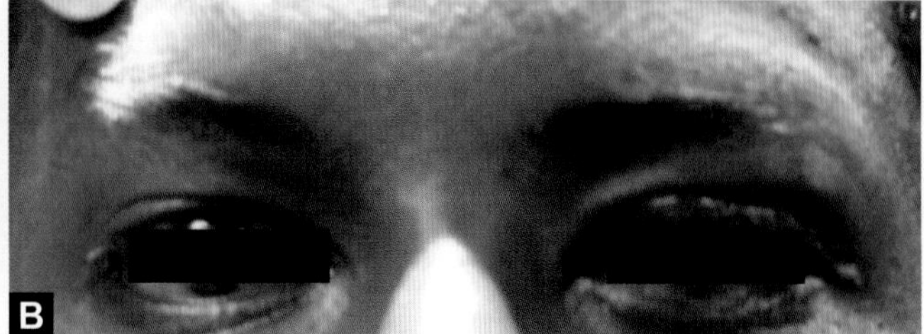

**Figures 67-2A and B** Functional indications for brow repair. (A) A 25-year-old man who presented with left eyelid retraction. Right brow ptosis and pseudodermatochalasis further contribute to asymmetry. (B) Asymmetry improves with left upper lid retraction repair and simulated right brow lift.

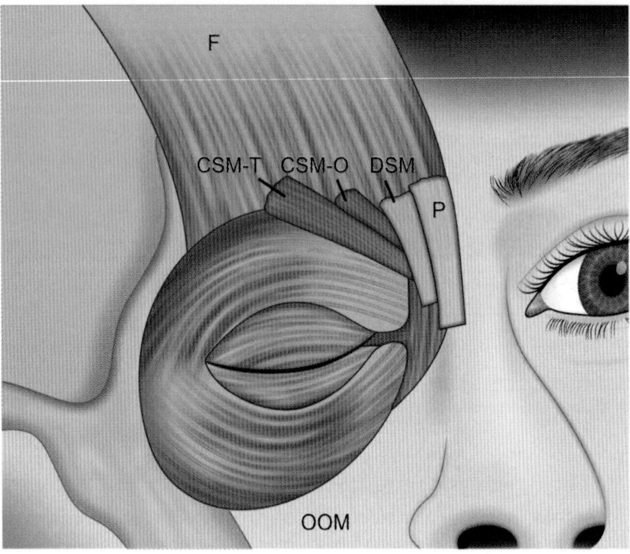


**Figures 67-3** Eyebrow musculature—brow elevator: frontalis muscle elevates the central and medial brow. Brow depressors: glabellar complex (corrugator supercilii—depresses the nasal eyebrow down and medially; procerus—depresses the medial eyebrow; depressor supercilii—depresses the medial eyebrow; orbital orbicularis oculi muscle—depresses entire brow, including lateral brow, toward eyelids).
(CSM-T: Corrugator supercilli muscle-Transverse; CSM-O: Corrugator supercilli muscle-Oblique; DSM: Depressor supercilli muscle; OOM: Orbicularis Oculi muscle; P: Procerus; F: Frontalis).

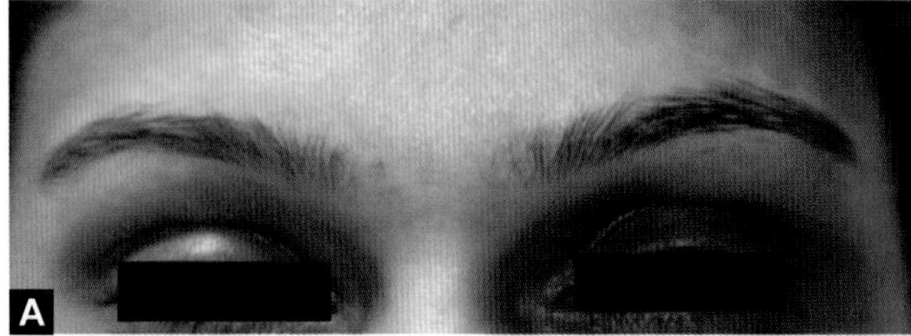
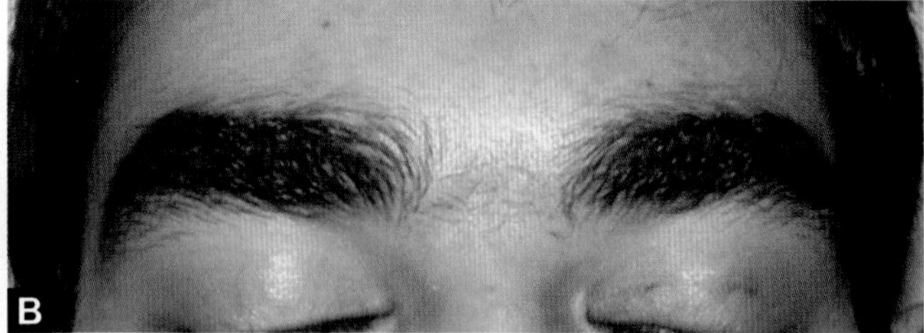

**Figures 67-4A and B** Typical brow configuration. (A) Typical arched, contoured, and higher female brow. (B) Typical flatter, lower, and fuller male brow.

depressors. The frontalis muscle is the sole elevator of the brow, whereas the eyebrow depressors include the glabellar muscle complex (corrugator supercilii, procerus, depressor supercilii) and the orbital portion of the orbicularis oculi muscles (Fig. 67-3).

## Topography

The head of the brow lies at the medial supraorbital ridge, the main body of the brow follows the supraorbital bony rim, and the tail overlies the lateral angular process of the frontal bone and extends to the zygomaticofrontal suture.[1-4] Topographically, an ideal female brow rests approximately 1 cm above the supraorbital rim with the maximum height of arch at the lateral canthus. In contrast, the male brow is typically flatter and lies lower along the supraorbital rim (Figs. 67-4A and B). Normal variations as well as ethnic differences in regard to the height and contour of the eyebrow should always be considered in the preoperative evaluation (Fig. 67-5).

# EVALUATION

The eyebrows and upper eyelids work together as integrated units in the upper face. Brow ptosis needs to be suspected in

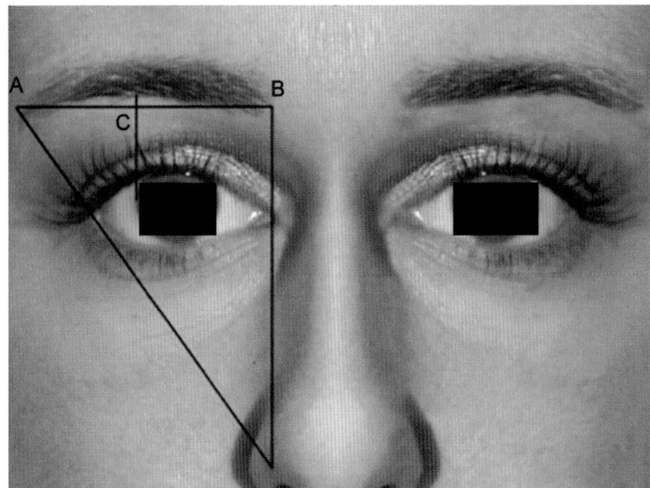


Figure 67-5 Brow topography – medially the brow begins at point B along a line drawn vertically with the medial canthal angle and the lateral nasal ala. The brow tail at point A lies along an oblique line drawn from the lateral canthal angle to the lateral nasal ala. The medial and lateral ends of the brow typically lie at the same horizontal level. The apex of the brow arch is located on a vertical line above the lateral limbus point C.

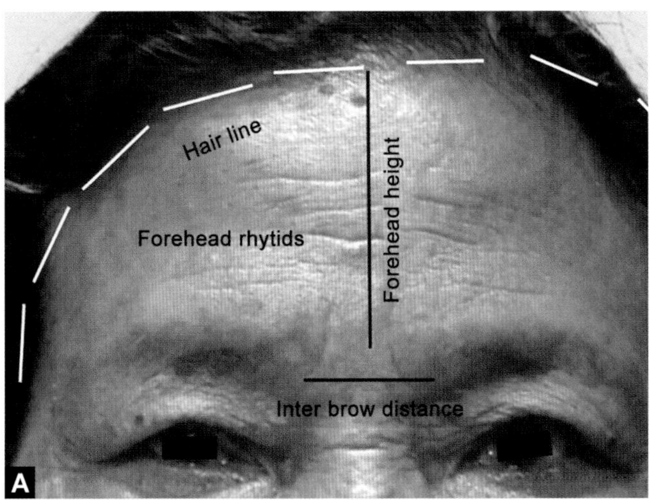


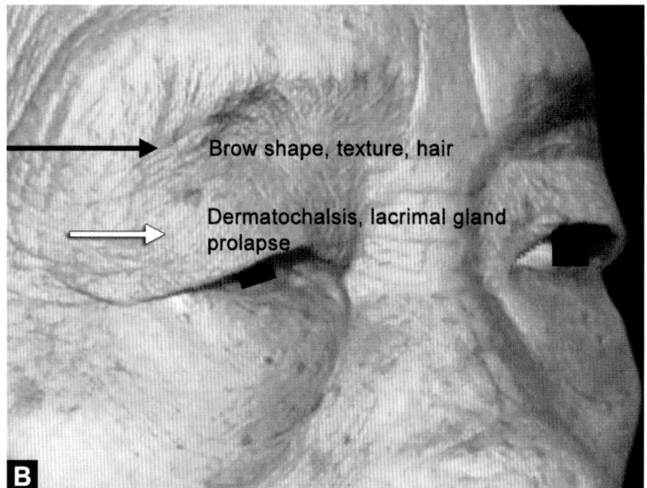


Figures 67-6A and B Brow assessment and measurements.

every patient with redundant upper eyelid skin, even if the brow position seems normal. Prominent transverse forehead creases due to chronic compensatory contraction of the frontalis muscles may indicate underlying brow ptosis. On examination, the frontalis muscle action should be negated by placing the hand over the forehead and asking the patient to close the eyes and relax. The actual brow position is then evident when the patient gently opens the eyes without using any forehead elevation.

In addition to a thorough ophthalmic examination, these additional parameters may help in determining the next appropriate surgical or nonsurgical management[1-4] (Figs. 67-6A and B).

- Hairline-high, low, alopecia, male-pattern baldness, hairstyle
- Forehead height
- Forehead transverse rhytids
- Frontalis muscle preference or asymmetry
- Eyebrow shape, contour, symmetry, and skin thickness
- Eyebrow hair distribution: plucking, thinning, tattoo
- Eyebrow mobility
- Concurrent dermatochalasis and/or eyelid ptosis
- Periocular fat prolapse/fullness
- Lacrimal gland proplapse
- Goldman visual fields (if functional indication).

## Brow Ptosis Measurement

Brow ptosis can be measured preoperatively to help determine the degree of descent, and thus the appropriate surgery that would most benefit the individual patient. The amount of brow ptosis can be measured by using a ruler held up to

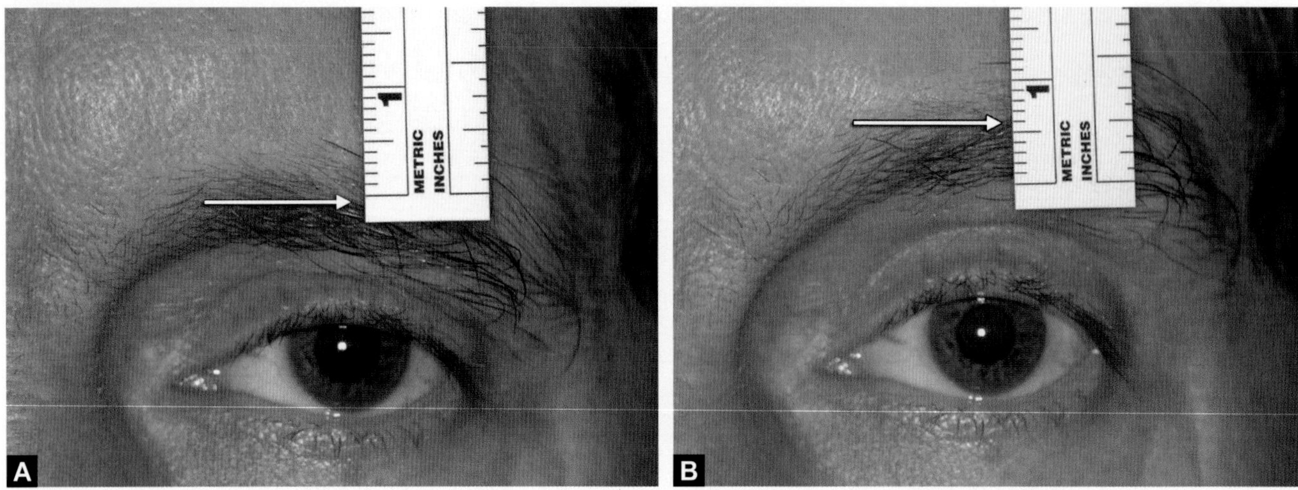


**Figures 67-7A and B** Measuring brow ptosis. (A) Ruler with the zero mark at the upper border of the brow when it is relaxed. (B) The brow is lifted until the desired position is achieved.

the brow, then lifting the brow to the desired height, and measuring this distance in millimeters (Figs. 67-7A and B).

While measuring brow descent, it is also important to note the degree of forehead compensation, and particularly whether there is asymmetry in frontalis muscle flexion. Often, there will be more prominent horizontal dynamic creases on one side, or the patient will noticeably elevate one forehead and brow higher. When the patient is asked to relax the forehead completely, the brows will typically look more symmetric. This clinical observation is crucial, as lifting the brows an equal amount on both sides during surgery would likely manifest as asymmetry postoperatively due to the pre-existing frontalis muscle preference. Therefore, the side on which the forehead prefers to elevate more should be surgically elevated to a lesser degree to result in more optimal postoperative symmetry.

## PREOPERATIVE PREPARATION

- Discontinuation of anticoagulants and anti-inflammatory drugs prior to surgery, unless medically contraindicated
- Counseling of the patient, including discussion of realistic expectations, risks, potential complications, postoperative care, and healing period
- Preoperative photographic documentation in primary, lateral, and three-forth profiles (Figs. 67-8A to C).

## SURGICAL TECHNIQUE

There are many different surgical and nonsurgical alternatives for brow elevation, including coronal, pretrichial, midforehead, temporal, supraciliary, internal (transblepharoplasty), endoscopic, and botulinum toxin techniques. The specific indications, advantages, disadvantages, and common complications for each have been summarized in Table 67-1. The basic surgical steps for some of the common approaches are highlighted below.[1-4]

- *Midforehead*: This procedure can be used to lift the entire brow rather than just laterally, by utilizing existing horizontal rhytids to camouflage the incisions. A horizontal strip of redundant skin and subcutaneous tissue are removed either as a long excision across the forehead, or divided into two separate excisions at different heights on each side of the forehead. If two crescents are removed, they should overlap centrally enough such that the medial eyebrows are sufficiently elevated. This is most useful for older male patients with thick, heavy sebaceous skin, or those with paralytic brow ptosis. It is less optimal for patients with minimal rhytids, or in whom a visible scar is not acceptable (Figs. 67-9 and 67-10)
- *Supraciliary*: This approach is best for patients with temporal brow droop and lateral skin hooding over the eyelid margin. The incision is typically placed over the lateral half to two thirds of the brow, depending on the extent of the lateral ptosis. A static or dynamic forehead rhytid just superior to the lateral brow may be used to camouflage the incision. The medial extent should end prior to the region of the supraorbital nerve to avoid postoperative numbness. Ideally, the medial aspect of the skin excision may be tapered slightly superiorly to blend into the forehead relaxed skin tension line, rather than curve downwards in a typical crescent that results in a more visible scar (Figs. 67-11 to 67-13). Women with very thin and tapered

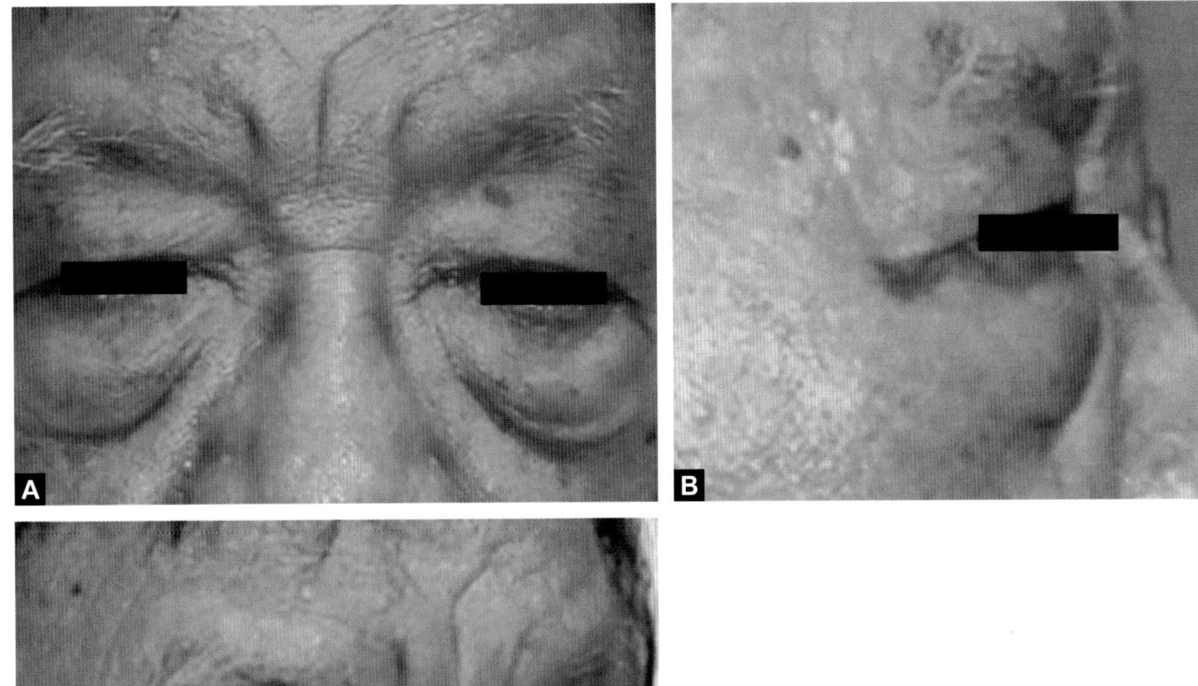


**Figures 67-8A to C** Photographic documentation show in (A) front view, (B) lateral view, and (C) three-fourth profile view.

TABLE 67-1 Synopsis of different brow lift techniques

| Brow lift approach | Specific indications | Advantages | Disadvantages | Complications |
|---|---|---|---|---|
| Coronal | • Moderate to severe brow ptosis and forehead rhytids<br>• Low or normal hairline<br>• Moderate to heavy forehead tissues | • Wide access for eyebrow muscle transection<br>• Direct excision of redundant skin | • Elevation of frontal hairline<br>• Long incision<br>• Forehead sensory changes | • Alopecia<br>• Asymmetry<br>• Skin necrosis<br>• Permanent overcorrection<br>• Facial nerve injury |
| Pretrichial | • Moderate to severe brow ptosis and forehead rhytids<br>• High hairline<br>• Heavy thick forehead tissues<br>• Paralytic forehead and brow ptosis | • Lowers a high hairline<br>• Direct access for eyebrow muscle transection<br>• Correction of medial and lateral brow ptosis<br>• Smoothing of forehead rhytids<br>• Direct excision of redundant skin | • Scar anterior to frontal hairline<br>• Not ideal with male pattern hair loss<br>• Less optimal if wears hair pulled back without bangs | • Hematoma<br>• Alopecia<br>• Visible scar<br>• Skin necrosis<br>• Damage to frontalis muscle and temporal branch of facial nerve<br>• Forehead sensory changes |

*Contd...*

*Contd...*

| Brow lift approach | Specific indications | Advantages | Disadvantages | Complications |
|---|---|---|---|---|
| Endoscopic | • Low to average hairline height<br>• Patients desiring minimal scars<br>• Mild to moderate brow ptosis<br>• Minimal to moderate forehead thickness | • Less alopecia risk<br>• Minimal injury to sensori-motor nerve units<br>• Small incisions<br>• Minimal scars<br>• Rapid recovery | • Expensive instrumentation<br>• Significant learning curve<br>• Less direct exposure<br>• Not ideal for paralytic forehead and brow ptosis | • Hematoma<br>• Forehead sensory changes<br>• Asymmetry<br>• Globe injury<br>• Facial nerve injury<br>• Elevation of hairline may create undesirable high forehead appearance |
| Midforehead | • Mainly in males with deep forehead furrows<br>• Patients with sparse frontal hairline | • Simple to perform<br>• No special instruments needed<br>• Reasonable camouflage of incisions within forehead rhytids<br>• Medial brow ptosis can be corrected | • Long scars may remain visible | • Hematoma<br>• Forehead sensory changes<br>• Asymmetry |
| Supraciliary | • Patients mainly desiring functional visual improvement of ptosis<br>• Patients with thick, bushy eyebrows or prominent supraciliary rhytids<br>• Paralytic brow ptosis | • Simple<br>• Significant degree of lift, especially if secured to higher frontal periosteum<br>• Easy access to brow<br>• Minimally invasive | • Visible scar above lateral brow<br>• Not ideal for thin eyebrows<br>• Does not correct medial brow ptosis | • Sensory changes if supraorbital neurovascular bundle is injured<br>• Alopecia<br>• Asymmetry<br>• Insufficient elevation |
| Internal (suture) | • Patients undergoing blepharoplasty<br>• Desire for minimally-invasive correction<br>• Mild to moderate lateral brow ptosis | • No visible scar<br>• Simple and fast<br>• Minimally-invasive<br>• No special instruments needed | • Moderate elevation<br>• No correction of forehead rhytids<br>• Does not correct medial brow ptosis<br>• Temporary discomfort at suture fixation point | • Insufficient elevation<br>• Possible brow dimpling |
| Internal (with absorbable implant) | • Patients undergoing blepharoplasty<br>• Desire for minimally-invasive correction<br>• Mild lateral brow ptosis | No visible scar<br>• Simple and fast<br>• Minimally-invasive | • Cost of implants<br>• Bone drilling required<br>• Palpable, tender implant in patients with thin skin<br>• May be less effective in patients with heavy thick brow tissues | • Infection<br>• Palpable implant<br>• Slow absorption may lead to chronic pain and inflammation at implant site<br>• Displacement of implant<br>• Inadequate elevation<br>• Erosion of overlying skin |
| Botulinum toxin | • For patients not interested in surgery<br>• Mild brow ptosis | • Quick results<br>• Noninvasive<br>• Lower cost | • Temporary results (months) | • Insufficient elevation<br>• Diffusion to adjacent tissues<br>• Eyelid ptosis |

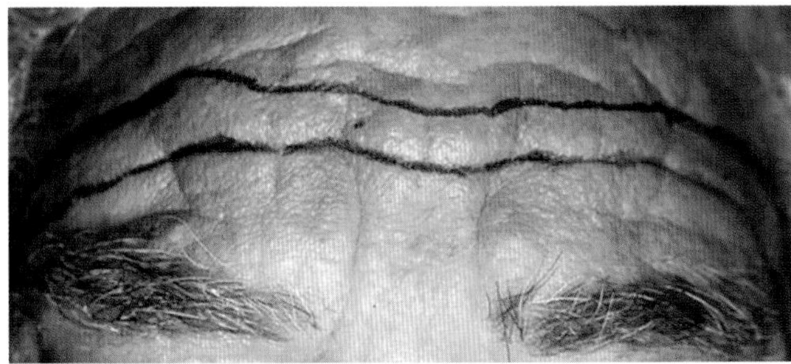

Figure 67-9 Midforehead brow lift markings within pre-existing rhytids.

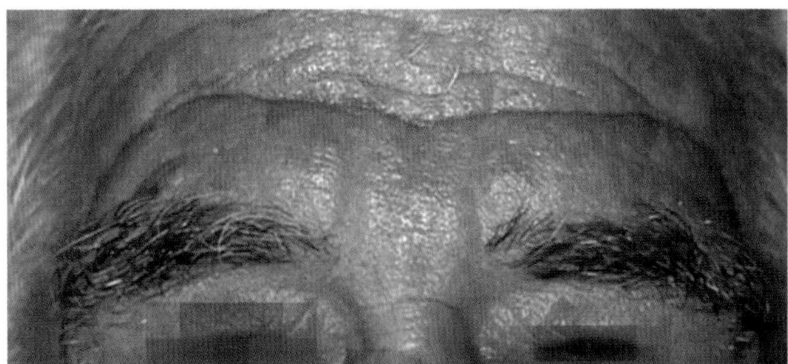

Figure 67-10 Midforehead brow lift, Postoperative, note the camouflaging of the scar within the normal rhytids.

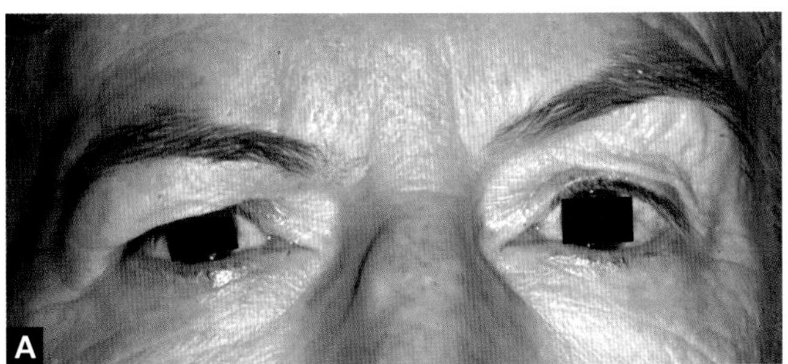


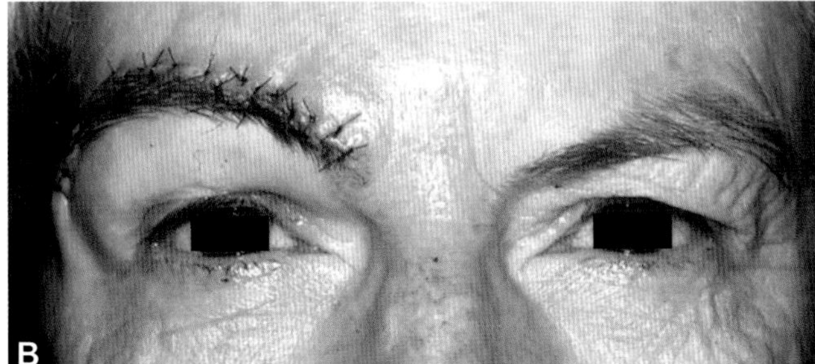


Figures 67-11A and B Patient with paralytic right brow ptosis underwent unilateral direct supraciliary lift.

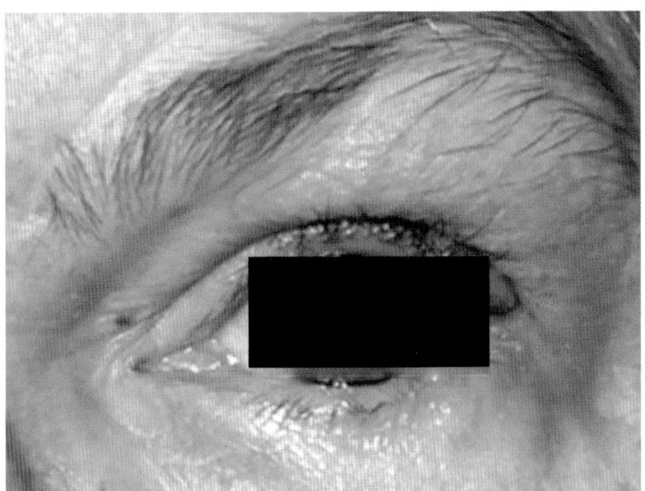

Figure 67-12 Poor scar following a full-length supraciliary incision.

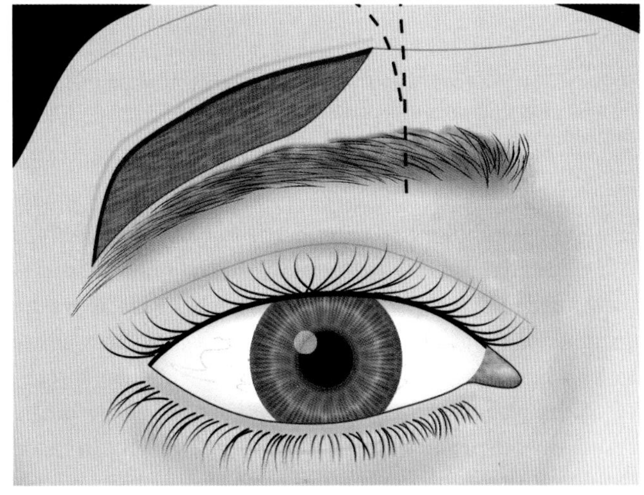

Figure 67-13 Modification of lateral supraciliary browlift with medial end tapered into a forehead crease.

eyebrows may not prefer this technique as the incisions cannot be easily covered with the brow hairs. The inferior edge of the incision can be further secured posteriorly to the underlying periosteum for more significant elevation

- *Internal*: The internal browpexy approach through the eyelid crease is minimally invasive and requires no additional incision when performed in conjunction with upper eyelid blepharoplasty. Preseptal dissection is performed to the superior orbital rim where the arcus marginalis is seen. Dissection then proceeds supraperiosteally over the frontal bone, posterior to the retro-orbicularis oculi fat pad to approximately 2 cm above the orbital rim (Fig. 67-14). This plane just over the periosteum is relatively avascular, as long as the brow fat is not entered. The entire lateral half of the brow should be dissected to create a sufficient dissection cavity over the lateral bone. Care should be taken to palpate the supraorbital notch to avoid dissection in this region. The lateral ligament that secures the tail of

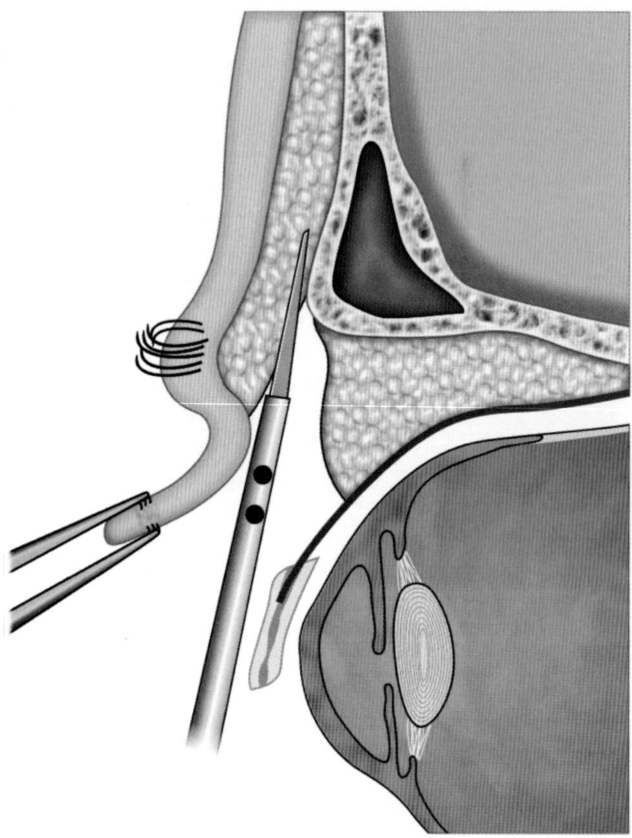

Figure 67-14 Schematic diagram of plane of dissection for internal browpexy. Dissection should proceed posterior to the brow fat and anterior to the periosteum.

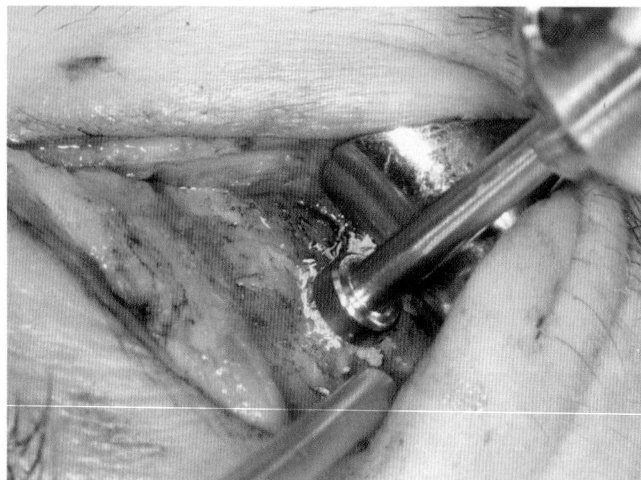

Figure 67-15 Drilling the frontal bone for placement of an absorbable implant device for internal browpexy lift.

the brow to the periosteum needs to be fully released to sufficiently mobilize the brow. Next, the brow fat pad is sutured to the periosteum approximately 1.5 cm above the superior orbital rim at the peak of the brow arch either by a nonabsorbable suture or by placement of an absorbable implant device (Fig. 67-15). The specific height can be adjusted depending on the desired brow height. In many older patients, the tail of the brow also requires an additional supporting suture to lift the brow as this lateral portion does not receive any compensatory frontalis muscle elevation. If the tail of the brow is not secured with a second suture in these patients, the brow may appear to have an unfavorable peaked or upside-down V shape to the contour.

- *Pretrichial*: This procedure is most beneficial for patients with significant forehead and brow ptosis, who have a relatively long forehead span, typically >6–6.5 cm. The incision is most crucial to the success and is placed just anterior to the hairline and placed in an irregularly irregular zigzag fashion to best camouflage the incisions. Long straight incisions are typically much more visible postoperatively. The incision is beveled to minimize scarring and avoid damage to the hair follicles. The plane of dissection is typically subcutaneous and therefore not as avascular as the coronal subperiosteal approach. However, as it is more superficial in dissection, the forehead rhytids are often more improved after surgery. Excess skin is removed superiorly as needed once the dissection is completed. Glabellar muscles can be weakened if preferred during this approach as well. Meticulous hemostasis is important in this dissection plane, and some surgeons may prefer utilizing a thrombin–fibrin glue sealant to help minimize potential space and bleeding. This technique is less ideal in patients with male pattern hair loss, or in females who wear the hair pulled back without bangs.
- *Botulinum toxin*: Chemical brow lifts using botulinum toxin A (Botox) can be an option in patients with minimal brow ptosis, or in those who wish to postpone surgery. Botox can be injected at precise locations to relax the corrugator and procerus muscles that pull the medial brow downwards and to the lateral orbital orbicularis oculi muscles that pull the lateral brow down. This is typically injected just below the lateral brow hairs approximately 0.5 cm above the orbital rim, to avoid eyelid ptosis. 2–4 units of Botox to target this lateral orbital orbicular is oculi muscle is an average dose (Figs. 67-16). The frontalis muscles that elevate the brow can then function unopposed. The desired effect can last ≥3 months.

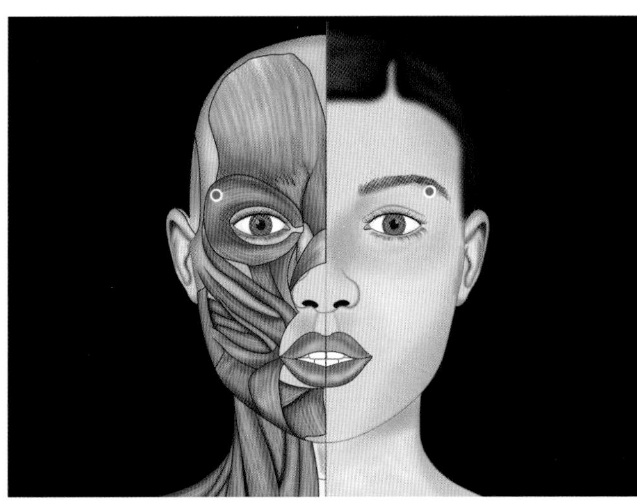

Figures 67-16 Schematic presentation to show the site for injecting Botox for chemical brow lift.

## POSTOPERATIVE CARE

- Apply cold compresses for 2 days continuously during waking hours.
- Avoid lifting, bending, strenuous activity, or exercise for ≥ 1 week.
- Keep the head elevated in the supine position for at least 1 week.
- Avoid rubbing the face or forehead area.
- Apply topical antibiotic ointment to the incisions if prescribed.
- Wash hair gently to avoid traction on the forehead and brow tissues.

## CONCLUSION

Performing a successful brow lift requires a thorough understanding of the integrated anatomy of the forehead, eyebrows, and eyelids. It is also important to understand the expectations of the patient before undertaking any surgical or nonsurgical correction. There are numerous surgical techniques available that can achieve excellent aesthetic results, and these continue to evolve with advancements in technology and a better understanding of senescent anatomical changes.

## REFERENCES

1. Albert DM, Lucarelli MJ. Oculofacial plastic, orbital, and lacrimal surgery. Clinical atlas of procedures in opthalmic and oculofacial surgery, 2nd edn. Oxford University press. 2012; Chap 70(7):716-32.
2. Fagien S. Putterman's cosmetic oculoplastic surgery, 4th edn. New York: Elsevier; 2008.
3. Nerad JA. Techniques in ophthalmic plastic surgery. New York: Elsevier; 2009:140-50, 177-87.
4. Dailey RA, Saulny SM. Current treatment for brow ptosis. Curr Opin Ophthalmol. 2003;14:260-6.

CHAPTER

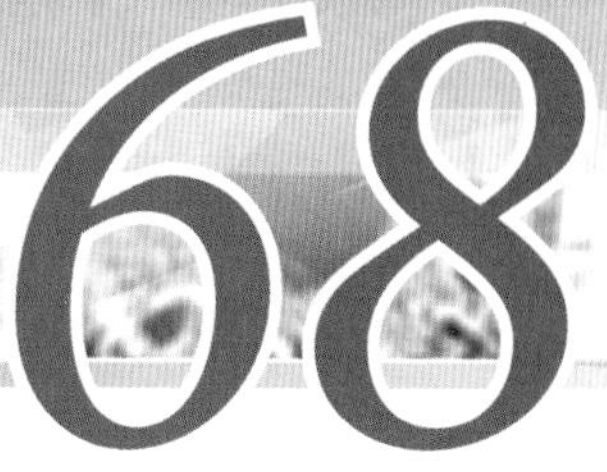


# Eyelid and Eyebrow Surgery in East Asians

Gangadhara Sundar

## ETHNIC CONSIDERATIONS IN OCULOFACIAL SURGERY—AN ASIAN PERSPECTIVE

Geographical Asia extends from Turkey in the west to Japan in the East, from Asian Russia and Mongolia in the North to the Malaysian Peninsula, and Indonesia to the South. Together with a total Asian population of 4.1 billion, which constitutes 57% of the world population,[1] the Asian diasporas are distributed globally as well. There are numerous cultural, social, economical variations between the various geographic regions with Asians being subdivided into the Middle Eastern Asians, South Asians, and East Asians. But from an oculofacial perspective, the East Asian population demonstrates a distinctive facial and periorbital anatomy compared with the South and West Asian populations, who are more similar to Caucasian anatomy that most surgeons are familiar with. Therefore, all oculofacial surgeons should familiarize themselves not only with traditional oculofacial anatomy, the spectrum of disorders, and their responses to various forms of external influences, but also with the more complex, little understood of the East Asian anatomy, pathology, and healing mechanisms.

We herewith highlight some of the distinct anatomical considerations of the East Asian eyelid, periorbital region, and the face. East Asians include the native ethnic populations of the following countries and its diaspora throughout the world. These include China and Hong Kong, Taiwan, North Korea, South Korea, Mongolia and Japan. They account for 37% of the Asian population. It is therefore imperative that the various terms such as Asian, East Asian, etc. be used in the appropriate context and perspective.

## GENERAL CONSIDERATIONS

In general, facial anthropometry and the ideals of beauty have common principles throughout the various ethnicities and geographic regions. The "Golden Ratio" of Divine Proportion (Φ, phi, 1:1.618) was first proposed and documented by the Ancient Greeks 2500 years ago and still forms one of the common foundations to ideal form and function in all living creatures. In addition, facial asymmetry and harmony of the various components of the face have been the hallmark of attractiveness and beauty.[2] The ideal human face has been proposed to be able to be equally divided into five portions horizontally and three portions vertically (Fig. 68-1). Evidence for this dates back to thousands of years with mentions made in the Indian Vedic Scripture of Samudrika Lakshana.[3]

## EAST ASIAN PERIORBITAL ANATOMY

There are several unique and special considerations to the form and structure of the East Asian face and the eyelids. These include distinct differences in anatomy and in tissue response to surgical trauma, resulting in an increase in postoperative complications and unpredictability[4] (Table 68-1).

## GENERAL FACIAL CONSIDERATIONS

In general, East Asians much like those of African descent have thicker skin, with an increased amount of pigmentation, regardless of complexion, compared to the Caucasians. It is possibly due to the same reason that it provides relative protection from ultraviolet damage with reduced and delayed age-related changes and skin malignancies as well. Moreover, because of relative lack of expression of emotion and

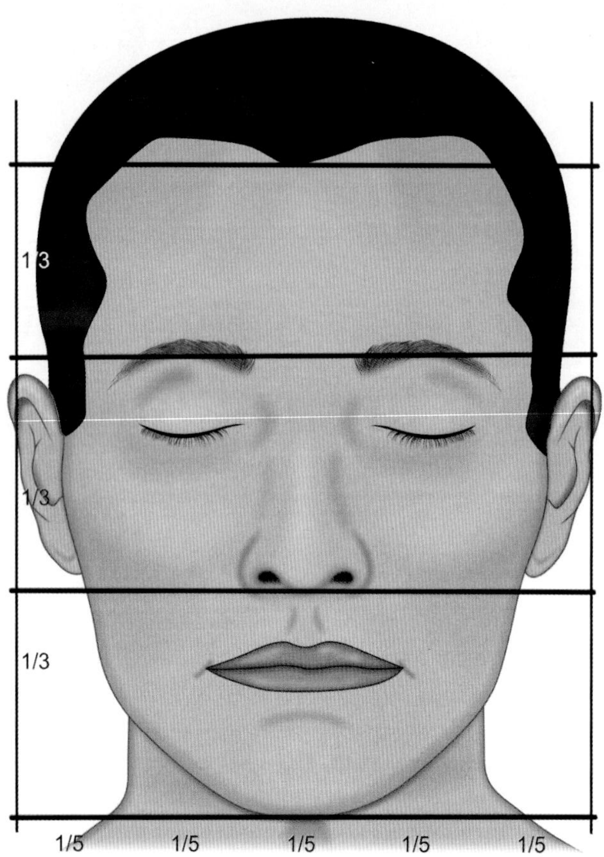


**Figure 68-1** Facial proportions: Rule of 1/3 and 1/5ths occidental vs East Asian.

subtle facial animation, the degree of dynamic rhytids and static rhytids are far less pronounced and less conspicuous as well. However, the combination of thicker skin and increased pigmentation predisposes them to increased inflammation, scarring, and hyperpigmentation to mechanical and thermal injury, natural, or iatrogenic. This in turn often results in undesirable hypertrophic scarring, hyper, and/or hypopigmentation with laser or surgical procedures.[5-7] It is therefore imperative to adequately assess and classify various skin types before embarking on various resurfacing procedures. Interestingly with global migration and ethnic admixture, these anatomical features may be subtle, and hence, biological origins of the individual be kept in mind when invasive and noninvasive procedures are being considered (Table 68-2).

## EYELID–PERIORBITAL CONSIDERATIONS

- *Eye brows*: In general, East Asians have a tendency to sparse eyebrow hair especially in females. Moreover, there is a natural tendency to low set eyebrows and flatter eyebrows in the rested and relaxed position (Fig. 68-2A). Due to the upper eyelid characteristics (absent lid crease, upper epiblepharon, and lash ptosis) constant frontalis overaction is common even in the young, resulting in severe brow ptosis in the elderly (Fig. 68-2B). The relatively sparse eye brows and the tendency to hypertrophic scarring of the thick and sebaceous forehead skin, especially with poor wound closure, makes it difficult to conceal incisions of the brow and midforehead, unless bushy eyebrows or deep rhytids are present
- *Upper eyelid*: Anatomical considerations in upper eyelid include an increased presence of fat in almost all layers of the upper eyelid.[11] These include the sub-brow, subcutaneous, and pretarsal planes often times with infiltration of the tarsus itself.[12] In addition, most experts believe that there is a much lower insertion of the orbital septum onto the levator aponeurosis, resulting in a lower projection of the preaponeurotic fat, onto the anterior surface of tarsus, and a generalized fullness of the upper eyelid[13] (Figs. 68-3A and B). While in occidental eyelids the upper eyelids generally have two fat pads: central and medial, not infrequently a lateral fat pad or presence is encountered in East Asians. The variable amount of levator aponeurotic slips to the overlying skin also contributes to the variability of the presence and prominence of the upper eyelid crease. In general, approximately 50% of the East Asians lack an obvious upper eyelid crease ("Double eyelid") and when present may be unilateral as well[14] (Fig. 68-4). When present the most common configuration is a nasally tapered crease ("Inner double eyelid"), which is buried within the medial epicanthal fold. An absent or weak upper eyelid crease results in an overhanging full upper eyelid with redundant skin, decreased "tarsal platform show". An exaggeration of the same results in the appearance of a narrow palpebral fissure, upper epiblepharon with lash ptosis and a sleepy, droopy eyelid appearance. As most of these are of developmental origin and thus long standing, this in turn results in eyelash ptosis, which when severe results in lash-corneal touch and keratopathy (Fig. 68-5). The overall height of the tarsus is also less (8 mm) compared with occidentals (10–12 mm), which may have implications in relation to the stability of the eyelid, availability of tarsus for resection, and reconstruction, etc
- *Lower eyelid*: The lower eyelid anatomy is similar to the upper eyelid with reduced tarsal height, absence of lower eyelid crease with increased tendency to a lower epiblepharon (Fig. 68-6A). In addition, there is the presence of

**TABLE 68-1** General characteristics of East Asian eyelid, periorbital, and facial region

| General facial considerations | Eyelid–periorbital considerations |
|---|---|
| Skin texture: thicker, more sebaceous | Eyebrows: less dense, low set, early browptosis<br>Smaller palpebral apertures, vertical and horizontal<br>Decreased margin-to-reflex distance, rounded eyelid margin, Sparser, straighter, thinner eyelashes |
| Increased skin pigmentation, Increased risk of postinflammatory hyperplasia | Upper eyelid: reduced tarsal height, absent, low or poorly formed eyelid crease, eyelash ptosis, epiblepharon, generalized increase in fat in all tissue planes |
| Decreased tendency to rhytids: static and dynamic | Lateral canthal angle considerations: higher, anterior |
| Increased inflammation and scarring | Medial canthal considerations: epicanthal fold, physiological telecanthus |
| Decreased incidence of skin cancers | Lower eyelid considerations: epiblepharon, eyelid ridge, rounding of eyelid margin |
| Short and shallow nasal bridge | Eyelash considerations: sparse, straight, thinner in young |

**TABLE 68-2** Various classifications of skin types and their response to photoexposure, iatrogenic injury, and relationship to ethnicity are in vogue[8-10]

| 2a. Fitzpatrick Classification (1975) | | |
|---|---|---|
| **Type** | **Complexion** | **Response to photoexposure** |
| Type I | Light, pale white | Always burns, never tans |
| Type II | White, fair | Usually burns, tans with difficulty |
| Type III | Medium, white to olive | Sometimes mildburn, gradually tans to olive |
| Type IV | Olive, moderate brown | Rarely burns, tans with ease to moderate brown |
| Type V | Brown, dark brown | Very rarely burns, tans very easily |
| Type VI | Black, very dark brown to black | Never burns, tans very easily, deeply pigmented |

| 2b. Lancer Ethnicity Grading (1998) | |
|---|---|
| **Geography** | **Skin type** |
| Asian Background | |
| Chinese, Korean, Japanese, Thai, Vietnamese, Filipino, Polynesian | LES Type 4 |
| African background | |
| Central, East, West African, Eritrean and Ethiopian North African, Middle Eastern Sephardic Jewish | LES Type 5/4 |
| European background | |
| Ashkenazy Jewish, Celtic, Central & Eastern European, Nordic, Northern European, Southern European, Mediterranean | LES Type 2, 3, 4 |
| North American background | |
| Native American (incl Inuit) | LES Type 3 |
| Latin/Central/South American background | |
| Central American, South American Indian | LES Type 4 |

LES (Lancer ethnicity scale) type risk factor
LES Type 1 – Very low risk
LES Type 2 – Low Risk
LES Type 3 – Moderate risk
LES Type 4 – Significant risk
LES Type 5 – High Risk

*Contd...*

*Contd...*

| 2c. Goldman's World Classification (2002) | | |
|---|---|---|
| 1. European / Caucasian | White | • Pale, cannot tan, burns easily, no post-inflammatory pigmentation<br>• B. Tan, rarely burns, rarely develops post-inflammatory pigmentation<br>• Deep tan, never burns, develops post-inflammatory pigmentation |
| 2. Arabic/Mediterranean/Hispanic | Light brown | • Pale, cannot tan, burns easily, no post-inflammatory pigmentation<br>• B. Tan, rarely burns, rarely develops post-inflammatory pigmentation<br>• Deep tan, never burns, develops post-inflammatory pigmentation |
| 3. Asian | Yellow | • Pale, cannot tan, burns easily, no post-inflammatory pigmentation<br>• B. Tan, rarely burns, rarely develops post-inflammatory pigmentation<br>• Deep tan, never burns, develops post-inflammatory pigmentation |
| 4. Indian | Brown | • Pale, cannot tan, burns easily, no post-inflammatory pigmentation<br>• B. Tan, rarely burns, rarely develops post-inflammatory pigmentation<br>• Deep tan, never burns, develops post-inflammatory pigmentation |
| 5. African | Black | • Pale, cannot tan, burns easily, no post-inflammatory pigmentation<br>• B. Tan, rarely burns, rarely develops post-inflammatory pigmentation<br>• Deep tan, never burns, develops post-inflammatory pigmentation |

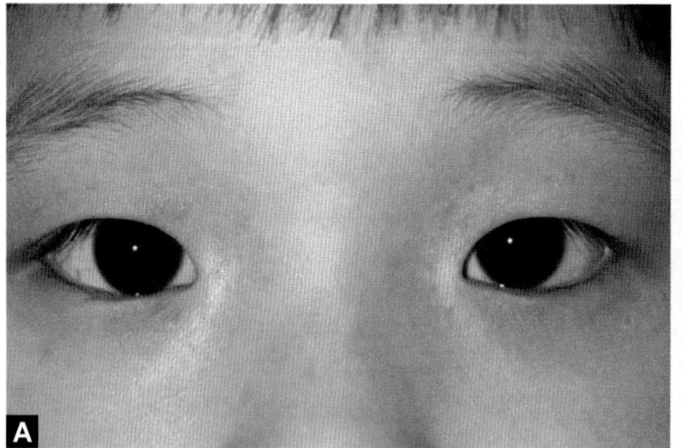


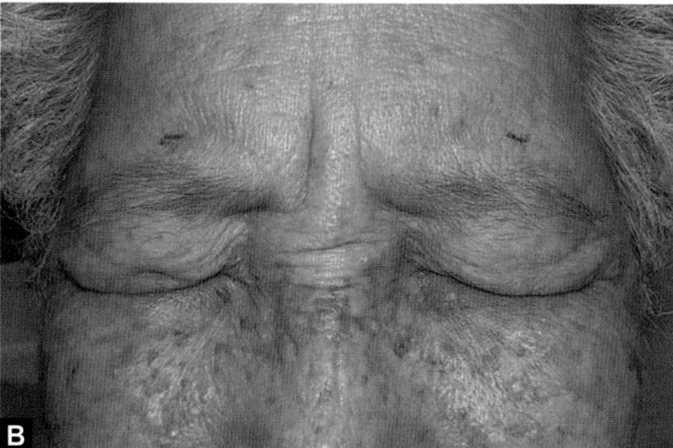


**Figures 68-2A and B** Periorbital surface anatomy in the young and the elderly. (A) Thin, sparse, slightly curved eyebrow, frontalis effort to clear visual axis. (B) Note position of superior orbital rim in relation to the eyebrow signifying severe brow ptosis.

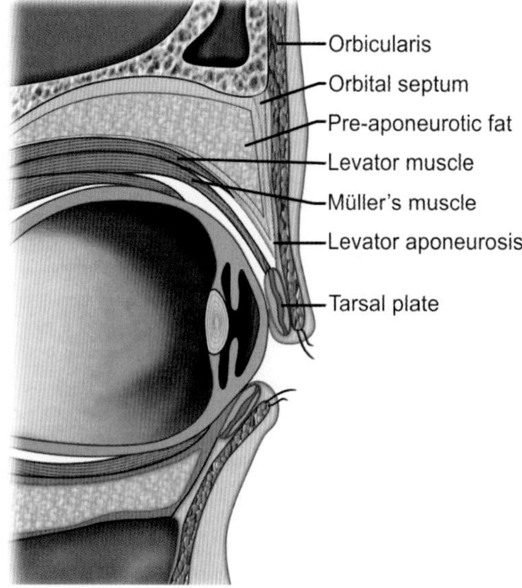


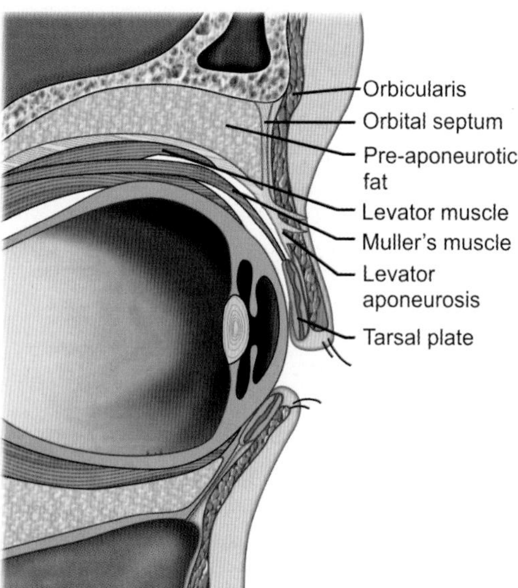


**Figures 68-3A and B** (A) East Asian upper eyelid. (B) Occidental upper eyelid.

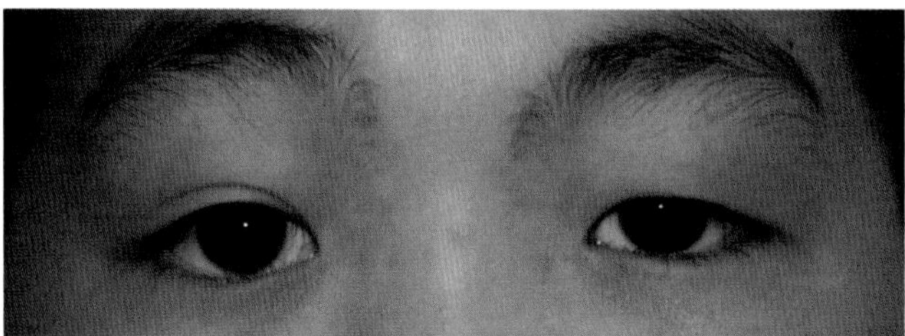

**Figure 68-4** Asymmetric eyelid creases in the same individual with variable tarsal platform show.

a fold of skin causing a "ridge" centrally and laterally in many children and young adults (Fig. 68-6B). The increased presence of upper and lower epiblepharon with lash ptosis, in addition to causing keratoconjunctivopathy (Fig. 68-6C), also results in deformed, distorted, and broken eyelashes (Fig. 68-6D), which may have clinical significance in the causation of corneal erosions

- *Lateral canthus*: Owing to the orbital rim—lateral canthal tendon relationship, the lateral canthal angle may be higher than in other ethnic groups, resulting in the classic Mongoloid slant, which in some individuals may be exaggerated. In such individuals, severe dermatochalasis often in combination with brow ptosis results in prominent lateral hooding (Fig. 68-7) often with visual field consequences and occasionally lateral canthal dermatitis as well.
- *Medial canthus*: A relatively common and characteristic variation is the presence of the epicanthal fold. The four common types include epicanthus supraciliaris, epicanthus palpebralis, epicanthus tarsalis, and epicanthus inversus[15] (Figs. 68-8A to D). In addition, the increased thickness of the skin and underlying soft tissue and tissue tension predispose incisions in this region to hypertrophic scarring and webbing and are thus best avoided. Common conditions where medial canthal incisions may be necessary include correction of telecanthus, blepharophimosis syndrome, external dacryocystorhinostomy, and medical epicanthoplasty. The presence of epicanthal folds and a shallow nasal bridge results in a distortion of midfacial horizontal proportions (rule of 5ths), resulting in physiological telecanthus (Fig. 68-9). For the same reason telecanthus from midfacial naso-orbital-ethmoidal fractures are also much less obvious in this population.
- *Lid margin—eyelash considerations*: The upper and lower posterior eyelid margins in cross section are generally more rounded than Caucasians resulting in relative marginal instability. This is one of the reasons that there is a continuum between epiblepharon and entropion and the increased incidence of entropion compared to ectropion. Just as East Asians have a propensity towards "sebaceous or oily" skin, likewise there is increased meibomian gland activity, often resulting in chronic inflammatory lid margin disease causing chalazia and trichiasis. East Asians also have finer and sparser eyelashes. As mentioned earlier, the presence of eyelash ptosis, upper and lower epiblepharon, eyelash imbrication upon eye closure is not uncommon, and there may be deformed, damaged eyelashes on lash–corneal touch.

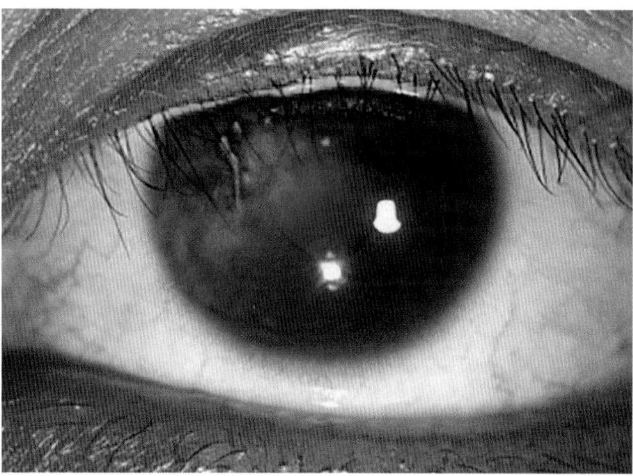

**Figure 68-5** Upper epiblepharon with lash–corneal touch and keratopathy.

## ASIAN EYELID SURGERY

Common eyelid surgeries include those for functional or esthetic indications with an overlap between the two in most situations. Moreover, owing to the intricate and complex eyelid–eyebrow interaction and consequences, brow ptosis is a commonly encountered condition, and thus, a brow lift is a common consideration as well. Common indications for eyelid surgery include congenital malformations and dysgenesis, e.g. simple and complex congenital ptosis, ethnic developmental conditions, e.g. epiblepharon, traumatic conditions, e.g. eyelid/canalicular lacerations, inflammations, e.g. chalazia, neoplasms: benign and malignant, and lastly involutional degenerative conditions, e.g. dermatochalsis, blepharoptosis, brow ptosis.

While the principles and concepts of eyelid surgeries in East Asians may be similar to other Asians and Caucasians,[16,17] there are special considerations, which shall be highlighted below. These include epiblepharon correction, medial epicanthoplasty, and East Asian blepharoplasty (double eyelid surgery). Esthetic indications for medial epicanthoplasty has dwindled over the years due to various factors: increased awareness and acceptance of medical epicanthal fold as a

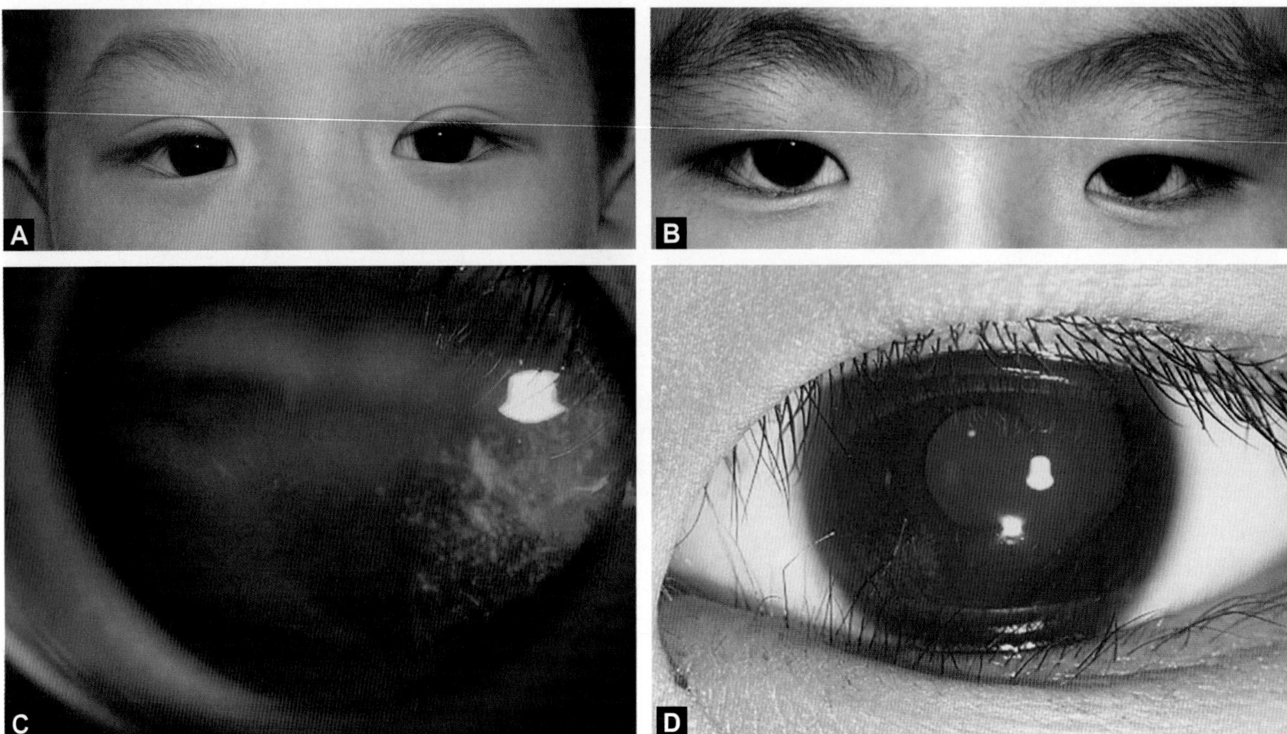

Figures 68-6A to D (A) Lower epiblepharon with visible skin fold. (B) Lower eyelid ridge. (C) Lash corneal touch with severe keratopathy. (D) Bent and broken eyelashes.

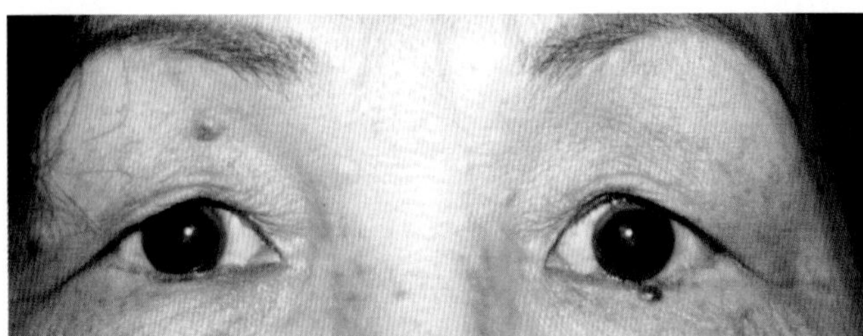

Figure 68.7 Prominent lateral hooding from upper dermatochalasis, absent lid crease, and brow ptosis resulting in frontalis overaction.

distinct feature of East Asians, greater unpredictability with increased scarring that is commonly associated with these open procedures.

## General Considerations

### Congenital Ptosis

Congenital ptosis may be classified into simple congenital ptosis (isolated levator dysgenesis) and complex congenital ptosis (Marcus Gunn jaw winking synkinetic ptosis, double elevator palsy, congenital III nerve palsy, Duane's eyelid retraction syndrome, blepharophimosis, etc.).[18] In each of the above, various implications include placement of surgical incision, especially when there are no pre-existing eyelid creases in the affected and the unaffected eyelid and the need or desire to create an eyelid crease, especially in cases of unilateral congenital ptosis. An overview of the evaluation, principles of management of simple congenital ptosis is shown below (Flowchart 68-1).

## Some General Guidelines in Congenital Ptosis Surgery in East Asians

Matching eyelid crease to contralateral side:

1. *If contralateral eyelid has no eyelid crease*: Options include either pure ptosis correction without forming an eyelid crease (incision above eyelid margin) or unilateral ptosis correction with bilateral upper eyelid crease formation
2. *If contralateral eyelid has well-developed eyelid crease*: Ptosis correction with symmetrical eyelid crease creation.

## East–Asian Blepharoplasty ("Double Eyelid Surgery")

This is a commonly desired and performed procedure in all patients of East Asian descent with functional, esthetic, and social goals. The goals of the procedure is to establish a natural appearing upper eyelid crease to enhance visibility of the upper eyelid (tarsal platform show), minimize hooding,

**Flowchart 68-1** Management of Simple Congenital Ptosis

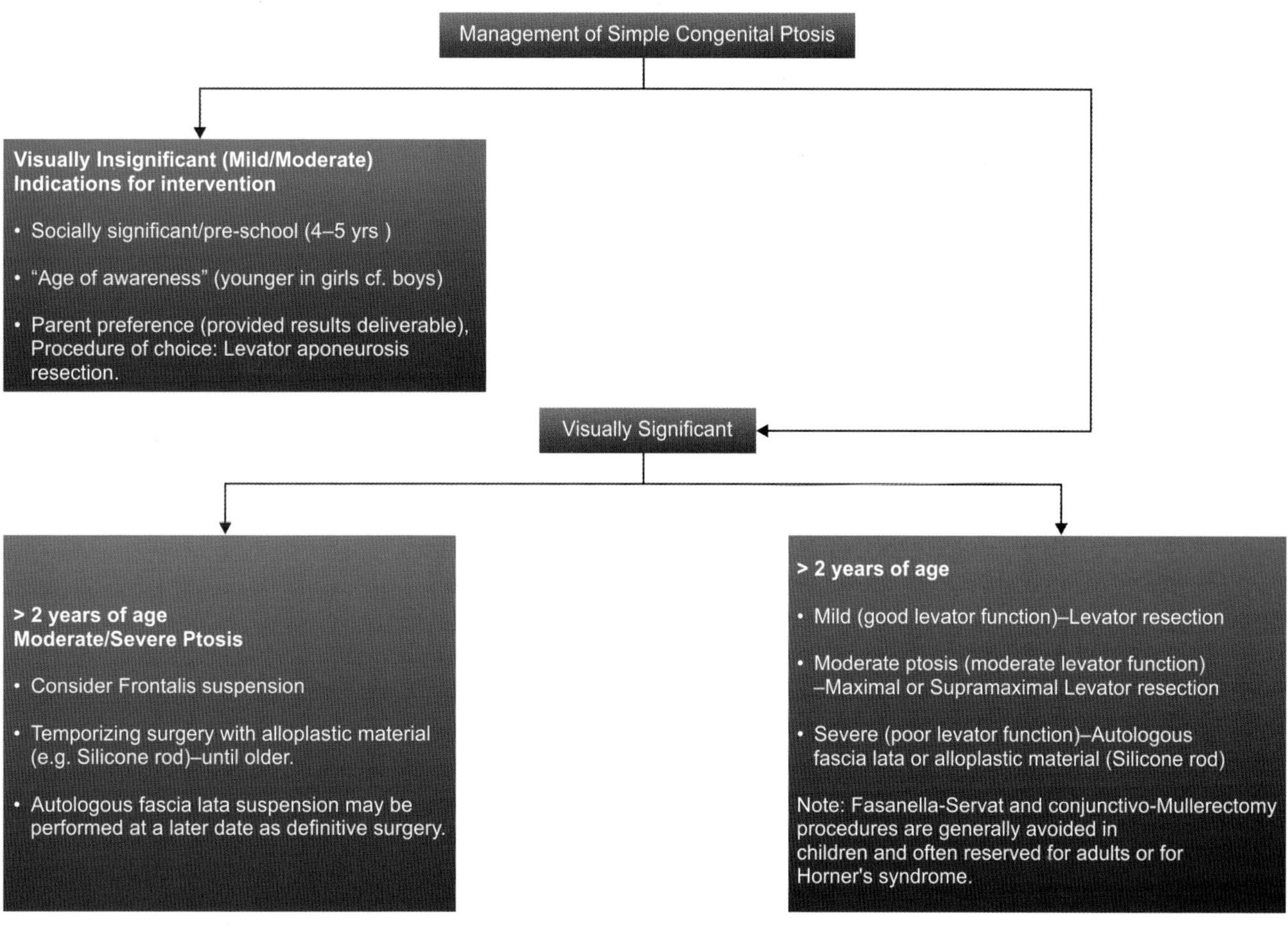


**Practical Tips**
- Differentiate visually significant from cosmetically significant congenital ptosis.
- *Remember:* Most common cause of visual loss in congenital ptosis is underlying refractive error or strabismus.
- Ensure proper informed consent from parents, including limitations of congenital ptosis correction
- Realistic expectation of parents/child re: eyelid height, contour, symmetry, lagopthalmos, need for additional revisions.
- Debate unilateral vs bilateral frontalis suspension in severe congenital ptosis with Marcus-Gunn jaw winking synkinetic ptosis.

with resultant eyelash ptosis correction, and finally not just with functional but esthetic benefits as well. Historically, it was described in the 1800s with periodic varied emphasis on open vs. closed techniques.[19] Challenges in East Asian blepharoplasty include predictability of height and symmetry of eyelid creases, permanency and depth of eyelid creases, and managing patient expectations. We shall herewith review some of the more commonly performed techniques including their pitfalls and advantages. All surgeries begin with good preoperative evaluation, patient desires and expectations, and a discussion of realistic expectations including potential adjustments for undesired outcomes.

- *Open technique*: This is performed by most oculofacial surgeons and has the following advantages: familiarity of surgical anatomy, more predictable outcomes with permanency of lid crease. Under local anesthesia, which could be performed either by a frontal nerve block or subcutaneous local infiltration, a lid crease incision is made as planned preoperatively with a conservative skin excision as desired. Dissection is performed to expose the superior tarsus and lower part of the levator aponeurosis by opening of the orbital septum. Fat in the inferiorly descended preaponeurotic space is cautiously trimmed maintaining hemostasis. Depending upon the eyelid crease desired (depth, dynamicity, etc.) delayed absorbable sutures (6-0 PDS) are placed anchoring the orbicularis along the inferior eyelid incision to the tarsus at a desired predetermined height or to the inferior edge of levator aponeurosis

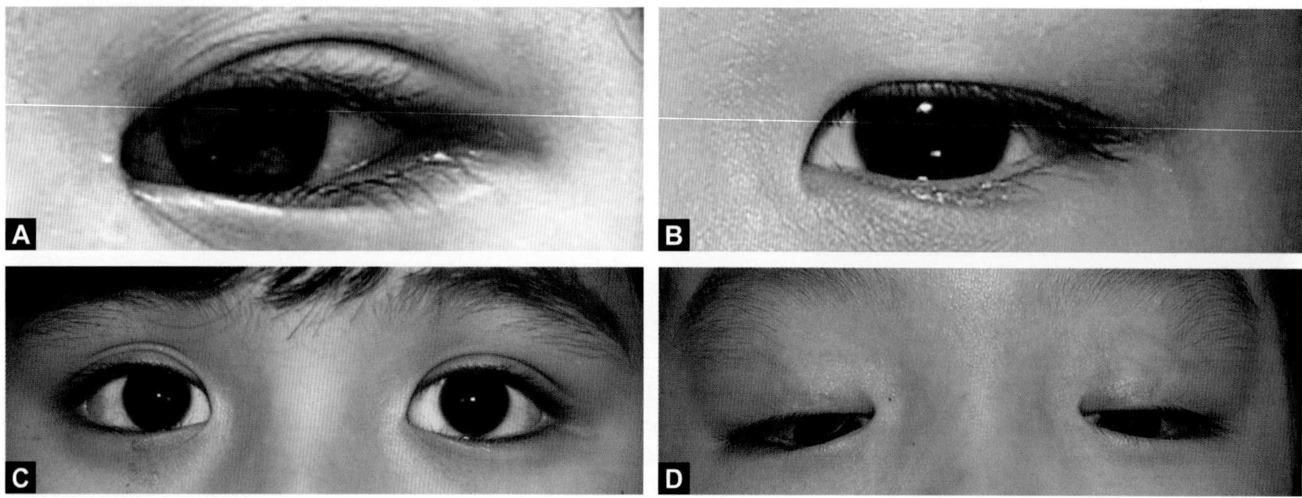

**Figures 68-8A to D** Epicanthal fold types.

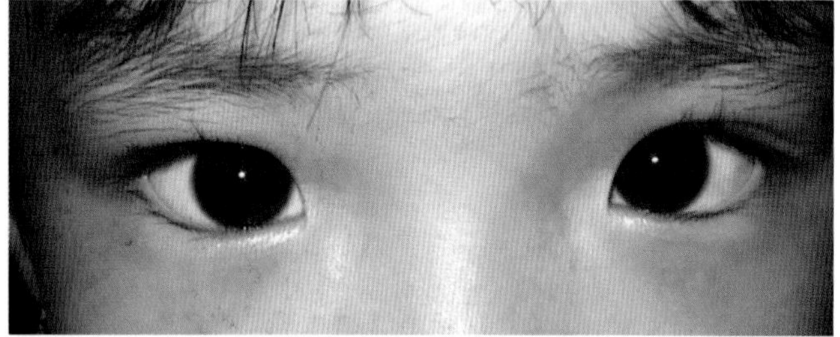

**Figure 68-9** Medial epicanthal fold with physiological telecanthus and pseudoesotropia.

or both, centrally, medially, and laterally. The skin incision is then closed as a running stitch (Figs. 68-10A to D). Variations of technique include anchoring of the orbicularis to the underlying tarsus or inferior edge of levator aponeurosis alone (Fig. 68-11A), and anchoring of the skin crease to the tarsus or levator aponeurosis (Fig. 68-11B). The goals of surgery are to create a natural, physiologically and ethnically appropriate dynamic eyelid crease, tarsal platform show, and correction of eyelash ptosis (Figs. 68-12A and B). While numerous techniques exist,[18,19] for the benefit of permanency and symmetry of eyelid creases an open technique is generally preferred, although the closed technique may have the advantage of simplicity, rapidity of procedure, and cost effectiveness.

Most patients achieve the desirable results with minimal complications.[20-22] Variations in outcomes include prolonged eyelid edema and/or inflammation, variability in depth and height of creases. These can be minimized with proper patient selection, symmetrical surgical technique with minimal iatrogenic trauma and dissection, use of noninflammatory sutures and avoiding early postoperative interventions unless gross over or undercorrection is present.

## Acquired Upper Eyelid Malpositions in Adults

These include dermatochalasis with lash ptosis, blepharoptosis: true (levator aponeurotic dehiscence—involutional or contact lens induced) or pseudoptosis (significant dermatochalasis, lateral hooding with brow ptosis), and increased tendency to entropion secondary to the above and also from chronic eyelid margin/postural lamellar inflammation. Also, owing to a reduced tarsal height, large resections of the tarsus/Müller's muscle, performed either as a component of tarsoconjunctivo-Müllerectomy (Fasanella-Servat procedure[23]) or conjunctivo-Müllerectomy (Putterman procedure[24]) may be difficult and hence avoided by some surgeons.

## Blepharoplasty for Dermatochalasis

The general principles of upper and lower blepharoplasty have a lot of similarities with those for the occidental patient. These include conservative skin and fat pad resection, meticulous hemostasis, addressing concomitant brow ptosis, and combining ptosis correction when appropriate. The differences however include addressing the "lateral fat pad", avoid excessive fat manipulation to prevent excessive scarring and lipogranulomata, determining and creating an appropriate eyelid crease (Figs. 68-13A and B) as discussed with the patient preoperatively and the reduced need for lower eyelid tightening in the middle aged patients Table 68-4.

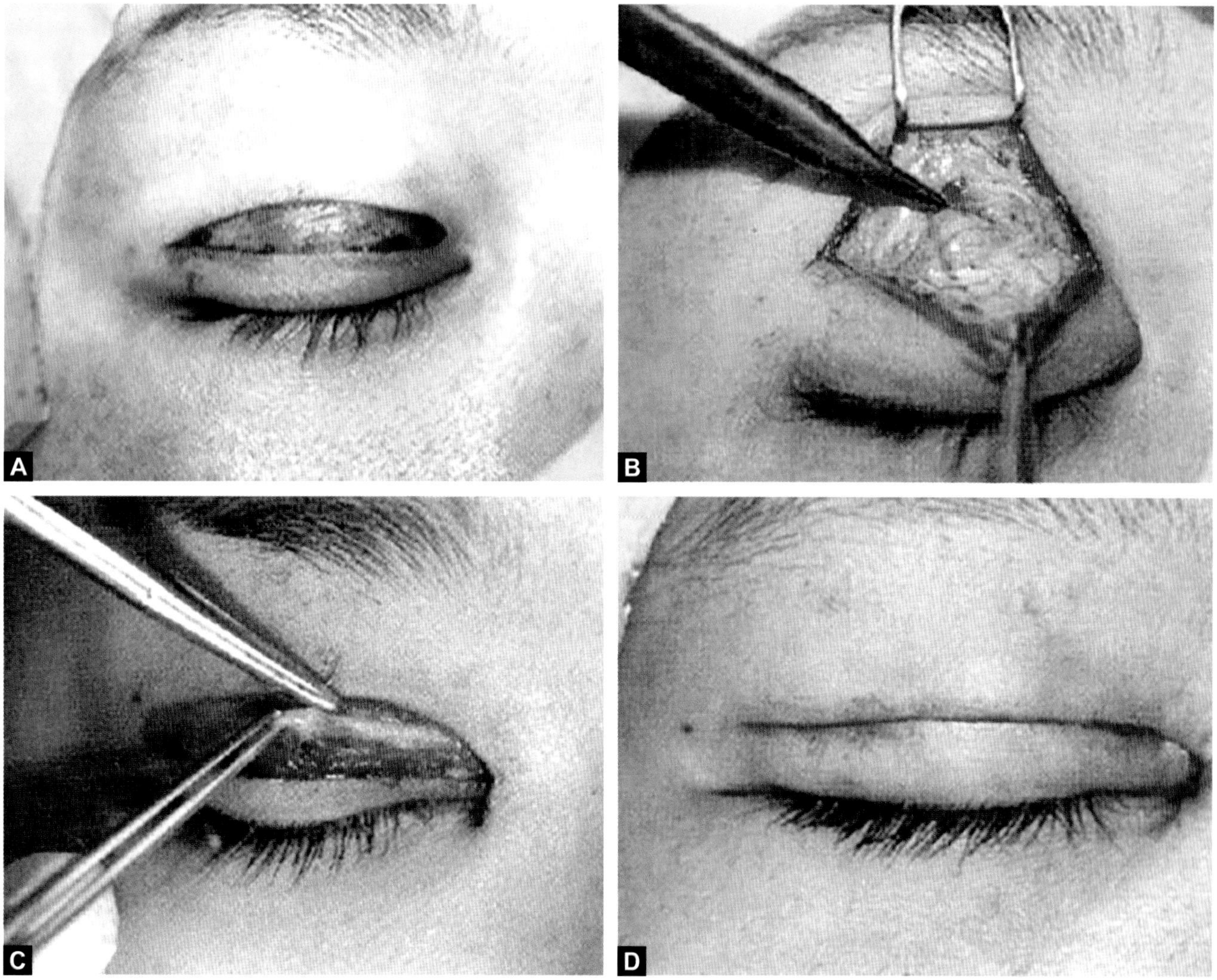

**Figures 68-10A to D** East Asian blepharoplasty.

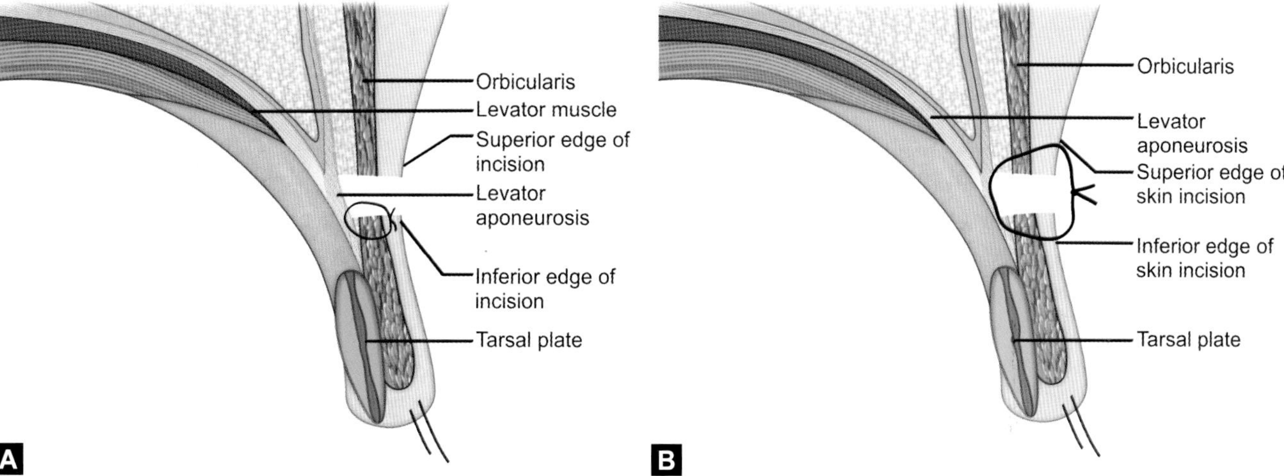


**Figures 68-11A and B** Demonstrating anchoring of the orbicularis or skin crease to the inferior edge of levator.

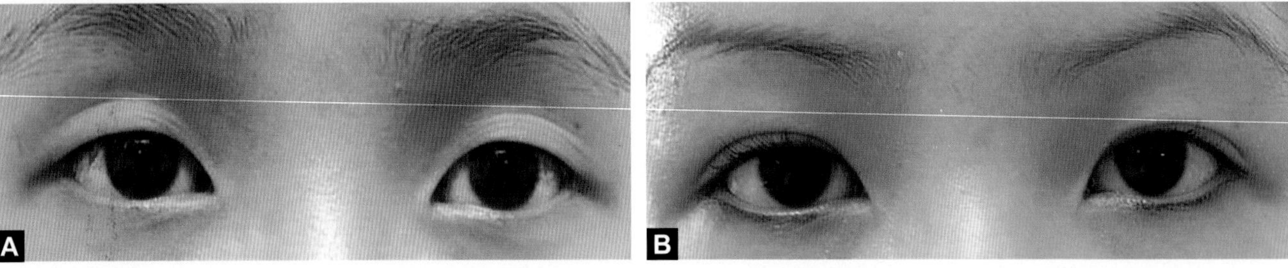

**Figures 68-12A and B** Preoperative and postoperative appearance of an ethnically compatible, natural looking eyelid crease.

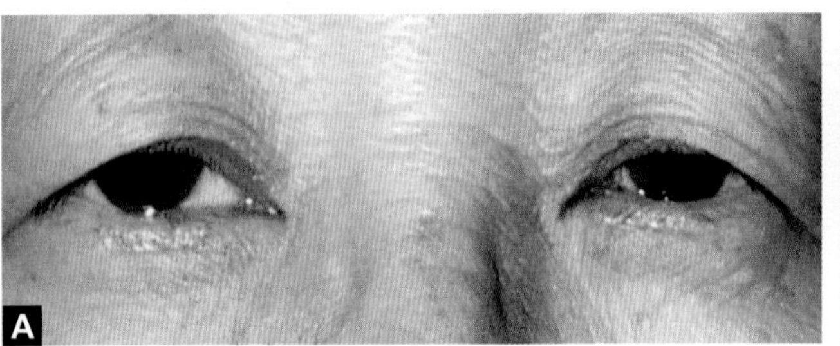

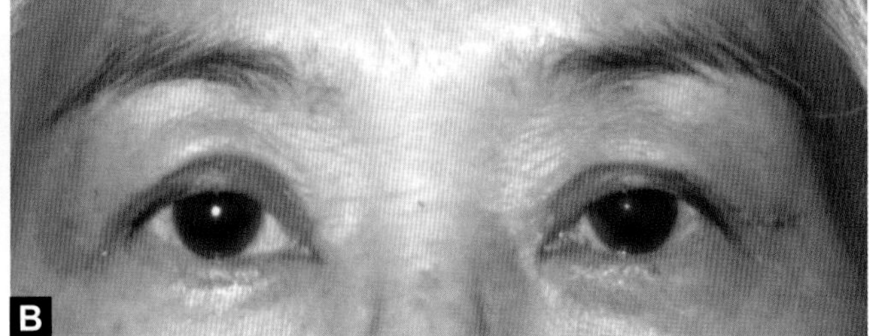

**Figures 68-13A and B** Upper blepharoplasty pre- and postoperative appearance.

**TABLE 68-4** Principles of adult ptosis corrections and blepharoplasty are similar to non-East Asians with some special considerations (listed below)

| |
|---|
| Increased incidence of pseudo/mechanical ptosis (Figs. 68-13A and B). |
| Development of new onset eyelid crease signifying levator disinsertion |
| Conservative skin excision recommended, especially in males. |
| Create a natural nasally tapered eyelid crease, lower in males compared to females. |
| Conservative or minimal postseptal, and sub-brow fat excision. |
| Minimize surgical trauma, cautery—to avoid postoperative unpredictable undesirable scarring. |
| Posterior approach ptosis might be more difficult owing to less horizontal laxity and relatively vertically short tarsus. |

*Lower eyelid considerations:* In general, Asians have a lower incidence of malignancies and less severe horizontal lid laxity especially in East Asians. These are significant factors to be taken into considerations in treating malpositions and eyelid reconstruction in adults. However, the increased eyelid margin instability from rounding of the eyelid margin predisposes East Asian patients to lower eyelid entropion, far more common than ectropion.[25] Absence of severe eyelid laxity in most patients facilitates minimally invasive techniques of lateral canthal manipulations, viz. lateral canthoplasty either through small lateral canthotomies or through the upper eyelid crease approach. A far more condition, especially in children and young adults is epiblepharon of eyelids, more commonly the lower eyelid.

## *Epiblepharon Correction*

Epiblepharon is a condition characterized by over-riding of the anterior lamella over the posterior lamella of the eyelids with resultant in-turning of eyelashes, abrading against the cornea and conjunctiva (Fig. 68-14). The lower eyelid is more involved than the upper eyelid. While in infants it may be asymptomatic because of the fine eyelashes and the gradual insidious onset of the condition, it is more symptomatic in school going children as the lashes grow longer and thicker, resulting in recurrent irritation, redness, discharge, tearing, or photophobia. Untreated epiblepharon with keratopathy may also result in corneal scarring (Figs. 68-15A to C ).

Most patients may be treated conservatively with lubricants and expectant management. However, in children who have persistent symptoms or keratopathy despite medical treatment, surgical treatment may be indicated and thus the most commonly performed oculoplastic surgery in this population. Although various techniques including nonsurgical and minimally invasive surgical techniques have been described the most common procedure is an open approach to the upper and lower eyelids. Lower epiblepharon correction is performed by the modified Hotz procedure.[26] After preoperative demarcation, a conservative spindle of redundant skin in the

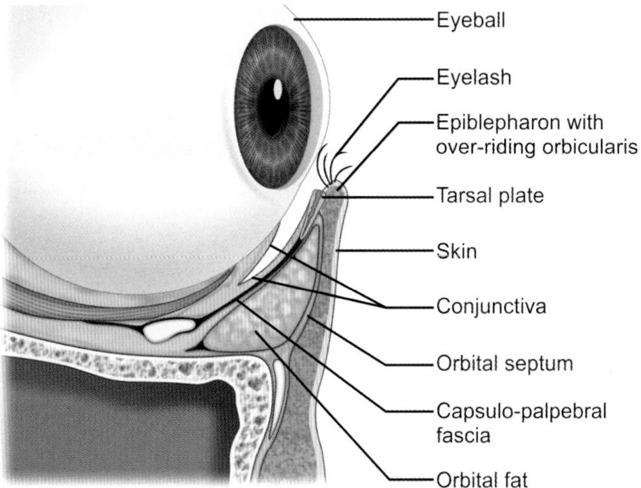


**Figure 68-14** Lower epiblepharon with lash cornea touch.

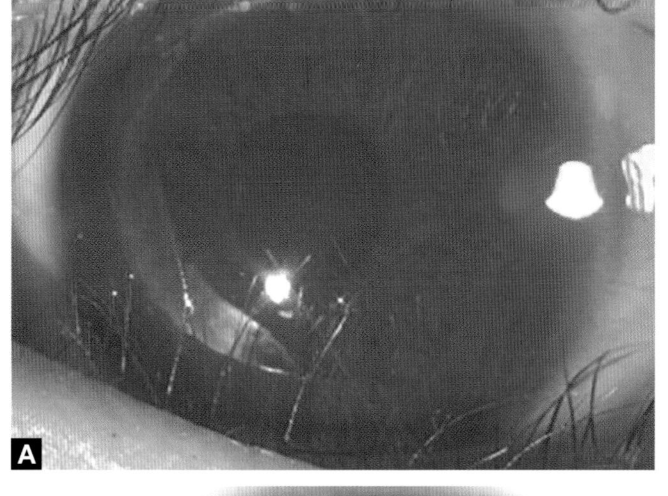


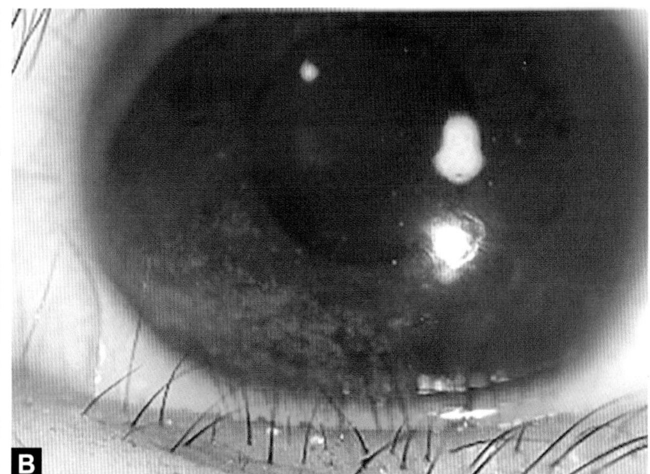


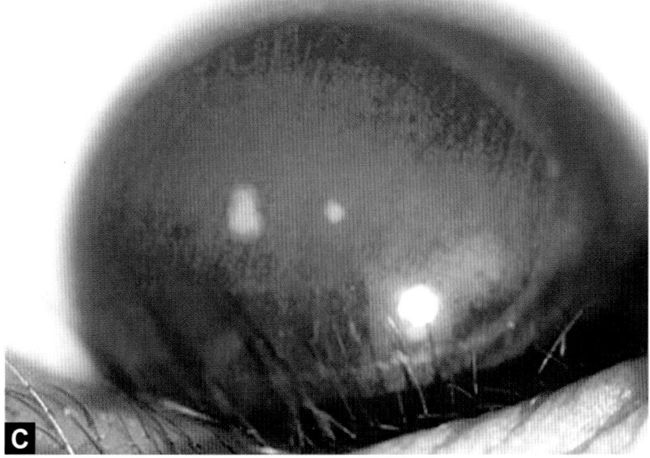


**Figures 68-15A to C** Epiblepharon with keratopathy (A) Mild, (B) moderate, (C) severe.

subciliary region is excised often with underlying infratarsal orbicularis especially medially to minimize undercorrection. Absorbable sutures (6-0 Vicryl) are used to anchor the orbicularis on either side of the incision to the anterior tarsus before closure of skin with a running nonabsorbable suture (6-0 Prolene) (Figs. 68-16A to E). Postoperative management is minimal with suture removal performed in 5–7 days and usually with good postoperative outcomes (Figs. 68-17A to D).

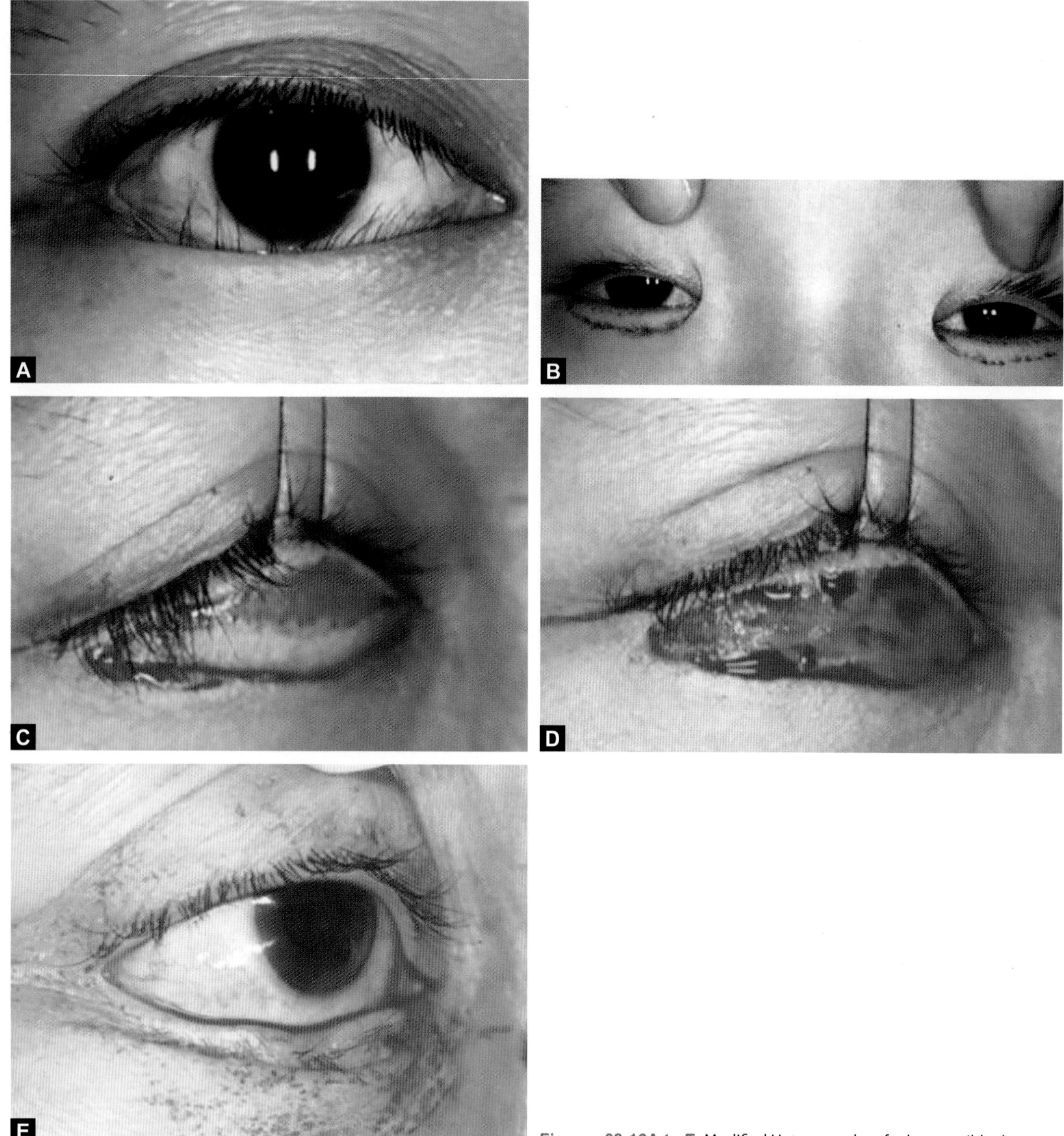

Figures 68-16A to E Modified Hotz procedure for lower epiblepharon.

Upper epiblepharon correction is very similar to the East Asian blepharoplasty and described above (*see* Fig. 68-10).

## *Brow Lift in East Asians*

Brow lifts are relatively common procedures performed in East Asians. A combination of heavy eyebrows and forehead with oily sebaceous skin, chronic exposure to bright sun in childhood resulting in chronic and sustained protractor contraction from squeezing, and chronic frontalis overaction to overcome lash ptosis and epiblepharon especially in individuals with poor, low, or absent eyelid creases predispose them to premature brow ptosis. In males, direct brow lift is the most

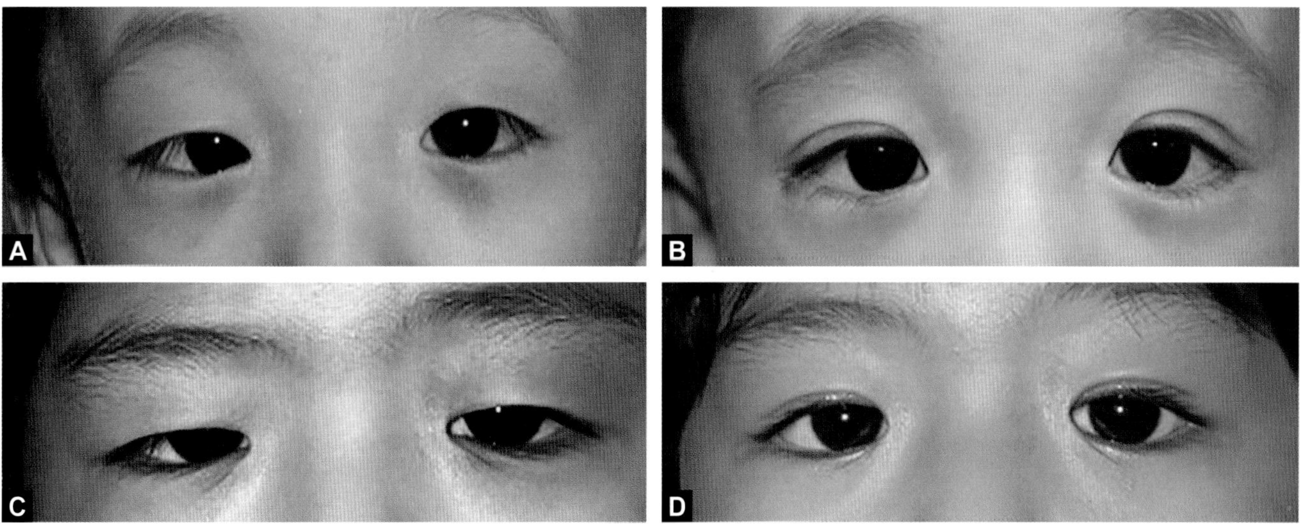


Figures 68-17 Pre- and postoperative appearance of four eyelid epiblepharon.

TABLE 68-5 Criteria to determine type of brow lift

| |
|---|
| Severity of brow ptosis |
| Gender |
| Eyebrow hair density |
| Height of forehead |
| Hairline: height, density |
| Balding pattern/predisposition |
| Midforehead rhytids: depth and location |
| Scalp hair density |
| Concomitant ptosis/dermatochalasis |
| Fitness for general vs local anesthesia |
| Patient's preference |

common procedure owing to the presence of a denser eyebrow, greater tolerance of a visible scar and inability to hide retrotrichial incisions from potentially receding hairlines. Females in contrast, are more conscious of potentially visible scar and thus more likely to have trichoplastic, endoscopic or nonendoscopic forehead lift and temporal lift. General guidelines, clinical considerations, and factors to be considered prior to offering browlift are highlighted in Table 68-5.

## Decision Making in Brow Lift Procedures (General Guidelines)

*Mild brow ptosis*: Chemical brow lift [botulinum toxin to brow depressors (orbicularis)], transblepharoplasty browpexy, transblepharoplasty endotine fixation, endoscopic (nonexcisional) brow lift.

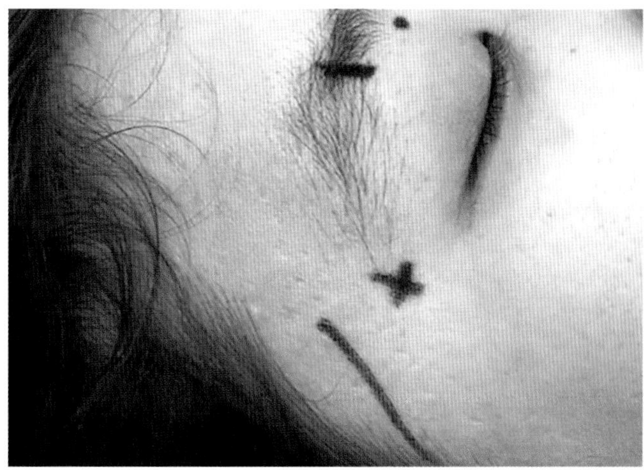

Figure 68-18 Danger zones of upper face showing supraorbital neurovascular bundle (short line), course of frontal branch of facial nerve (long line), and sentinel vein (X).

*Moderate to severe brow ptosis:* Short forehead with good scalp hair – choose retrotrichial (hairline) brow lift procedures (endoscopic brow lift, coronal brow lift).

Tall forehead—Choose eyebrow to pretrichial (hairline) procedures (pretrichial + temporal brow lift, midforehead brow lift (deep forehead creases), direct/supra brow lift). Avoid retrotrichial incisions that lengthen forehead.

Potential danger zones of the upper face[27] that should be kept in mind during dissections and patients appropriately counseled preoperatively are the supraorbital branch of the frontal nerve (V1) usually emerging from the supraorbital notch at the superomedial orbital rim, the frontal branch of the facial nerve innervating the frontalis muscle, and the sentinel vein (Fig. 68-18). Care should be taken to avoid damage to the nerves as damage to them may remain permanent resulting in patient dissatisfaction.[28,29]

Indications, contraindications, advantages, disadvantages, and complications of each technique is listed below Table 68.6.[28]

## SUMMARY

Eyelid and eyebrow surgery are common in East Asians, for both functional and cosmetic reasons. A meticulous understanding and knowledge of the anatomical variations,

TABLE 68-6 Brow lift procedures

| | Indications | Contraindications | Advantages | Disadvantages | Complications |
|---|---|---|---|---|---|
| Coronal (Fig. 68-19) | Dense scalp hair, no baldness expected, females, short forehead | Baldness – existing, expected, poor general health, broad forehead | Immediately hidden wound/scar | Large incision, requirement for GA, longer procedure | Alopecia, supraorbital paresthesia/anesthesia, frontal branch paresis/paralysis |
| Pretrichial/trichoplastic (Fig. 68-20) | Broad forehead, dense hairline | Receding hairline, short forehead | Well-hidden hairline with dense hair, faster procedure, direct visualization of "danger zones", GA/LA with MAC | Large wound, need for temporal incision for temporal lift | Supraorbital paresthesia/anesthesia, frontal branch paresis/paralysis |
| Midforehead lift (Fig. 68-21) | Deep midforehead static rhytids, tall forehead, male pattern baldness | Absent rhytids, unwilling patient | Simpler, faster, direct approach, LA with MAC, Direct visualization of danger zones | Potentially visible scar, need for temporal incision for temporal lift | Visible scar (poor patient choice, wound healing, supraorbital paresthesia/anesthesia, frontal branch paresis/paralysis |
| Direct/Suprabrow lift (Fig. 68-22) | Dense brow hair, unfit for GA, patient choice | Sparse eye brow | LA, simpler, faster, direct approach, No frontal branch of facial nerve damage | Potentially visible scar | Visible scar (poor patient choice, wound healing, supraorbital paresthesia/anesthesia, frontal branch paresis/paralysis |
| Internal browpexy | Patient unwilling for formal browlift procedure, minimal/impending brow ptosis | Moderate/severe brow ptosis | Blepharoplasty/ptosis incision only | No brow lift achieved | Recurrence, failure of procedure, transient puckering of temporal brow |
| Temporal brow lift | Lateral brow ptosis only | Unwilling patient, unfit for GA | Excellent temporal lift, hidden scar | None | Frontal branch of facial nerve paresis/paralysis, alopecia |

(LA: Local anesthesia; GA: General anesthesia; MAC: Monitored anesthetic care).

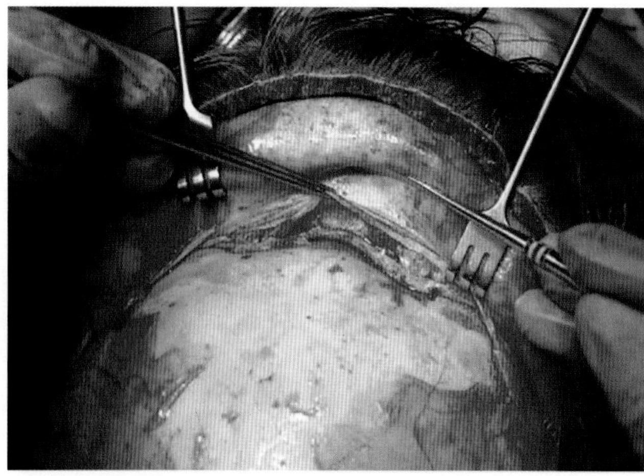

Figure 68-19 Arcus marginalis release in coronal brow lift.

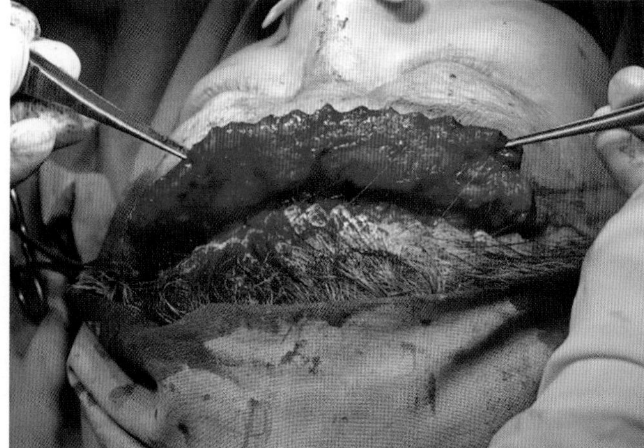

Figure 68-20 Pretrichial or Trichoplastic browlift.

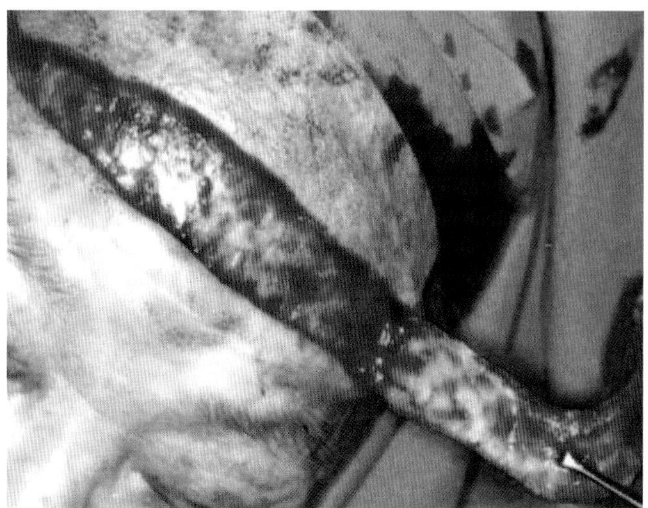

Figure 68-21 Midforehead lift.

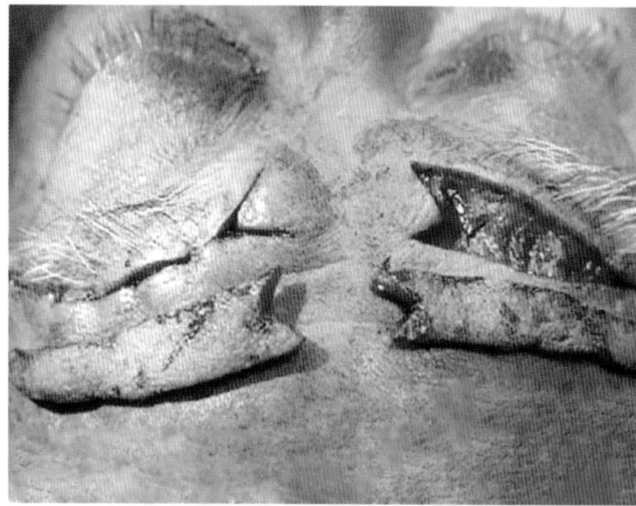

Figure 68-22 Direct brow lift.

response to pathological, mechanical and thermal trauma, controlled delivery of surgical techniques, and other therapeutic modalities, and realistic expectations go a long way in ensuring optimal functional, esthetic, and psychological outcomes.

## REFERENCES


1. www.en.wkipedia.org/wiki/world_population
2. Jefferson Y. Facial beauty: establishing a universal standard. Int J Orthodon. 2004;15:9-22.
3. www.tamilandvedas.wordpress.com/2012/05/26/scientific-proof-for-samudrika-lakshana/
4. McCurdy JA, Jr. Considerations in Asian cosmetic surgery. Facial Plast Surg Clin North Am. 2007;15(3):387-97.
5. Matory E, Jr. Ethnic considerations in Facial Esthetic Surgery. Philadelphia, PA: Lippincott-Raven 1998. ISBN 0-7817-0292-5.
6. Ranu H, Thng S, Goh BK, Burger A, Goh CL. Periorbital hyperpigmentation in Asians – an epidemiologic study and proposed classification. Dermatol Surg. 201137(9):1297-303.
7. Chan HH. Effective and safe use of lasers, light sources and radiofrequency devices in the clinical management of Asian patients with selected dermatoses. Lasers Surg Med. 2005;37(3):179-85.
8. Sachdeva S. Fitzpatrick skin typing – applications in dermatology. Indian J Dermatol Venerol Leprol. 2009;75(1):93-6.
9. Lancer HA. Lancer ethnicity scale (LES). Lasers Surg Med. 1998;22(1):9.
10. Goldman M. Universal classification of skin type. J Cosmet Dermatol. 2002:15:53-54.
11. Jeong S, Lemke BN, Dortzbach RK, et al. The Asian upper eyelid—an anatomical study with comparison to the Caucasian eyelid. Arch Ophthalmol. 1999;117(7):907-12.
12. Shen S. Medial pre-tarsal adipose tissue in the Asian upper eyelid. Ophthal Plast Reconstr Surg. 2008;24(1):40-2.
13. Amrith S. Oriental eyelids—anatomical and surgical considerations. Singapore Med J. 1991;32(5):316-8.
14. Seiff SF, Seiff BD. Anatomy of the Asian eyelid. Facial Plast Surg Clin N Am. 2007;15(3):309-14.
15. Chen WP. Asian blepharoplasty. Oxford, UK: Butterworth-Heinemann; 1995. ISBN 0-7506-9496-3.
16. McCord CD. Eyelid Surgery—principles and techniques. Philadelphia, PA: Lippincott-Raven; 1995. ISBN 0-7817—0293-3.
17. Fagien S. Putterman's cosmetic oculoplastic surgery, 4th edn. Philadelphia, PA: Saunders; 2008.
18. Sundar G. Pediatric oculoplastic surgery—a review. J Tamilnadu Ophthalm Assoc. 2009;47(3):13-19.
19. Nguyen MQ, Hsu PW, Dinh TA. Asian blepharoplasty. Sem Plast Surg. 2009;23(3):185-97.
20. Park JI. Asian facial cosmetic surgery. Philadelphia, PA: Saunders Elsevier; 2007. ISBN 1-4160-0290-1.
21. Chen WP. Upper blepharoplasty in the Asian patient 105-113. In: Fagien S (ed), Putterman's cosmetic oculoplastic surgery. Philadelphia, PA: Saunders Elsevier; 2008. ISBN 978-0-7216-0254-7.
22. Chee E, Choo CT. Asian blepharoplasty—an overview. Orbit. 2011;30(1):58-61.
23. Fasanella RM. Surgery for minimal ptosis: the Fasanella-Servat operation 1973. Trans Ophthalmol Soc UK. 1973;93:425-38.
24. Putterman AM, Urist MJ. Müller's muscle – conjunctival resection ptosis procedure. Ophthalmic Surg. 1978;9(3):27-32.
25. Carter SR, Chang J, Aguilar GL, et al. Involutional entropion and ectropion of the Asian lower eyelid. Ophthal Plast Reconstr Surg. 2000;16(1):45-9.
26. Sundar G, Young SM, Tara S, Tan AM, Amrith S. Epiblepharon in East Asian patients: the Singapore experience. Ophthalmol. 2010;117(1):184-9.
27. Seckel BR. Facial danger zones—avoiding nerve injury in facial plastic surgery. St. Louis, MO: Quality Medical Publishing; 1994. ISBN 0-942219-59-7.
28. Byun S, Mukovozov I, Farrokhyar F, Thoma A. Complications of browlift techniques: a systematic review. Aeshet Surg J. 2013;33(2):189-200.
29. Almousa R, Amrith S, Sundar G. Browlift – a South East Asian experience. Orbit. 2009;28(6):347-53.

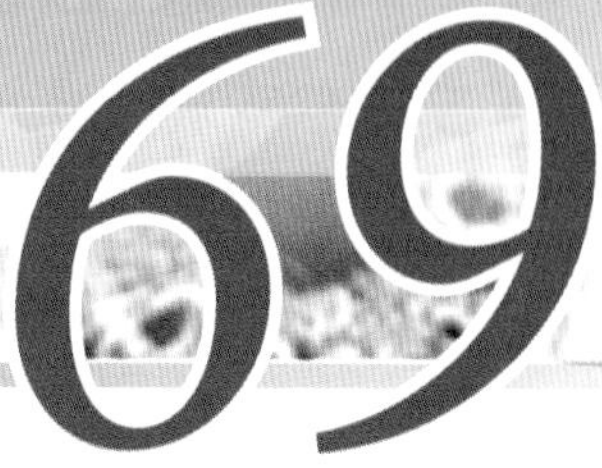


# Correction of Eyelid Retraction

Richard L Scawn, Jean-Paul Abboud, Don O Kikkawa, Bobby S Korn

## INTRODUCTION

Eyelid retraction may involve both upper and lower eyelids and is usually defined relative to the limbus in the vertical meridian of the pupil. A precise anatomical or numerical definition is difficult due to normal physiological variations especially with regard to ethnicity, myopia and age.[1-6] However, pathological lower lid retraction is usually considered when the lower eyelid extends below the lower limbus to expose sclera (Fig. 69-1). The normal upper eyelid position is approximately 0.5–1 mm beneath the upper limbus. Elevation above this position may be associated with disease, and any retraction above the limbus is likely to be pathological.[1-6]

Eyelid retraction may occur secondary to local, systemic, or central nervous system disease.[7,8] The most common causes of retraction are thyroid-related orbitopathy, an unintended consequence of cosmetic blepharoplasty or eyelid neoplasia excision. Other causes are listed in Table 69-1.

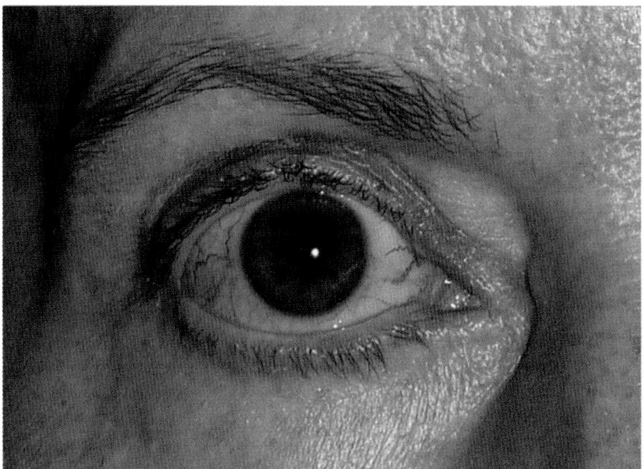

**Figure 69-1** Upper and lower eyelid retraction with scleral exposure superior and inferior to the limbus.

## INDICATIONS

- Exposure keratopathy in which conservative treatments, including topical lubrication and punctual occlusion, are inadequate or poorly tolerated
- Aesthetically unacceptable eyelid retraction.

## CONTRAINDICATIONS

- Medical contraindication to undergo local or general anesthesia
- Adverse reaction to specific spacer graft materials
- Donor-site morbidity for autologous grafts.

## SURGICAL TECHNIQUES

### Upper Eyelid Retraction

Upper eyelid retraction surgery is commonly carried out under local anesthesia (often with sedation) to enable titration of surgical dissection to upper lid position and contour.[9] Multiple techniques exist for upper eyelid lowering. A recent review of Graves upper eyelid retraction listed >50 published surgical technique manuscripts, with no conclusive opinion on the best surgical method.[6,10] Rather than dissect through the nuances of each technique, we summarize the principle methods.

### Retractor Overaction and Posterior Lamella Deficiency Predominates

#### *Levator–Müller Recession*

This involves recession of the levator palpebral superioris and Müller's muscles from their tarsal attachment.[6,10-16] An upper-lid skin-crease incision is made followed by dissection through

**TABLE 69-1** Etiology of upper and lower eyelid retraction

| | Upper eyelid retraction | Lower eyelid retraction |
|---|---|---|
| Neurogenic | • Dorsal midbrain syndrome<br>• Contralateral ptosis causing pseudoretraction (due to Hering's law)<br>• Aberrant regeneration of the oculomotor nerve<br>• Fracture of the orbital floor with associated inferior globe dystropia and increased innervation to eyelid retractors<br>• Sympathomimetic eyedrops (e.g. phenylephrine, apraclonidine) | • Orbicularis oculi weakness (e.g. facial nerve palsy) |
| Myogenic | • Thyroid-related orbitopathy<br>• Prior extraocular muscle surgery (e.g. superior rectus recession)<br>• Congenital fibrosis of the eyelid muscles | • Thyroid-related orbitopathy<br>• Flaccidity of lower eyelid muscles (e.g. botulinum toxin injection, orbicularis weakening)<br>• Postsurgical (e.g. inferior rectus recession) |
| Mechanical | • Eyelid malposition<br>• Globe prominence (e.g. severe myopia, exophthalmos, buphthalmos)<br>• Anterior lamellar shortening (e.g. contraction from neoplasms, burns, postsurgical, dermatoses)<br>• Postsurgical (e.g. upper eyelid blepharoplasty, ptosis repair, glaucoma filtration surgery with prominent bleb, scleral buckle)<br>• Contact lens wear | • Globe prominence (e.g. severe myopia, exophthalmos, buphthalmos)<br>• Anterior lamellar shortening (e.g. contraction from neoplasms, burns, postsurgical, dermatoses)<br>• Contact lens wear<br>• Postsurgical (e.g. lower eyelid blepharoplasty, scleral buckle) |

*Source*: Adapted and modified from Bartley GB. The differential diagnosis and classification of eyelid retraction.[4]

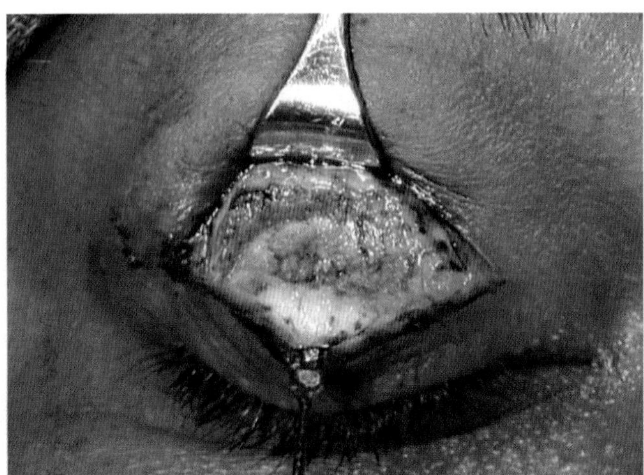

**Figure 69-2** Upper eyelid retraction repair with recession of levator palpebrae superioris and Müller's muscle.

orbicularis to the upper tarsal border. The levator and Müller's muscles are dissected free from the tarsus and the underlying palpebral conjunctiva either as separate structures or as a single-elevator complex using Westcott scissors, monopolar, or high-temperature cautery. The authors prefer a single elevator unit dissection beneath the orbital septum to minimize lid crease migration.[17] The dissection is continued superiorly until the desired lid height is achieved with care taken to keep the conjunctiva intact (Fig. 69-2). Frequent infiltration of local anesthetic aliquots on an insulin syringe between Müller's muscle and the conjunctiva facilitates dissection, hemostasis, and patient comfort in these vascularized inflamed tissues.[14] Asymmetric retraction correction, such as lateral flare, is managed using a more extensive dissection in that region.[6] Some authors routinely incise the lateral horn of the levator to aid lateral flare correction.[13]

The orbicularis is approximated with two or three 7-0 polyglactin 910 sutures (Ethicon Inc., Somerville, NJ, USA) and the skin is closed with either a running 6-0 fast absorbable gut or 6-0 polypropylene suture (Ethicon Inc., Somerville, NJ, USA). The addition of a "spacer", such as hard palate or donor sclera between the upper tarsal border and the recessed upper lid retractors has historically been advocated, but we rarely find this step necessary.[6]

The transconjunctival approach to upper lid lowering is well-established and yields good results. Müller's muscle can be recessed alone or in combination with the levator muscle and conjunctiva closure is not necessary.[6] Posterior approach proponents value avoiding a skin incision and leaving the anterior eyelid structures untouched should revisions be necessary.[18] The advantage of an anterior approach is ease of concurrent blepharoplasty and lid crease control.[15]

### Full-Thickness Upper Lid Recession (Blepharotomy)

This procedure involves an upper-lid skin-crease incision, dissection through orbicularis and the upper lid retractors to expose conjunctiva at the upper tarsal border. The conjunctiva is then excised medially and laterally creating a full-thickness blepharotomy.[19] This procedure requires less dissection and is potentially rapid. However, in the author's experience, the resultant lid contour is flatter compared with that of a Levator–Müller resection.

### Nonsurgical Methods

These include hyaluronic acid fillers, botulinum toxin, and triamcinolone, which are evaluated in conjunction with surgical techniques in the section "Scientific Evidence".

## Anterior Lamella Deficiency Predominates

Exposure symptoms due to anterior lamella deficiency may result from trauma, actinic damage, skin carcinoma excision, and after excessive skin excision in cosmetic blepharoplasty, which may sometimes be exacerbated by an excessive concurrent brow lift. Topical lubricants and punctal plugs are often adequate with symptoms often abating over 6 months; in cases exacerbated by recent surgery. However if these measures are unsuccessful, anterior lamella replacement is required. If the primary etiology is an excessive cosmetic brow elevation, a reversal could be considered.

### Full-Thickness Skin Graft

The ideal skin graft for the upper eyelid is contralateral eyelid skin, but this is often similarly afflicted. Alternatively, the posterior auricular or medial upper arm skin can be used.[20] A supraciliary incision[21] is made and any coexisting subcutaneous cicatrix undermined. The rationale for a supraciliary incision rather than lid crease incision advocated by other authors is twofold. The tarsus provides a stable platform to minimize contraction and the lid crease can be accurately placed since the crease will form at the upper graft border.[21,22] The required graft size is ascertained with upper eyelid on downward traction to assess the full extent of cicatrix. The donor skin is marked and excised using Westcott scissors. Excision with monopolar cautery is avoided to promote graft viability. Residual subcuticular fat or muscle is dissected off the graft to generate a thin graft and reduce its perfusion demands from the underlying tissue bed. The graft is secured with 6-0 polypropylene or 6-0 fast absorbing gut sutures. To minimize potential space for a hematoma or serosanguineous fluid, an anchoring 7-0 polyglactin suture is placed between the central graft and the underlying orbicularis (Fig. 69-3).

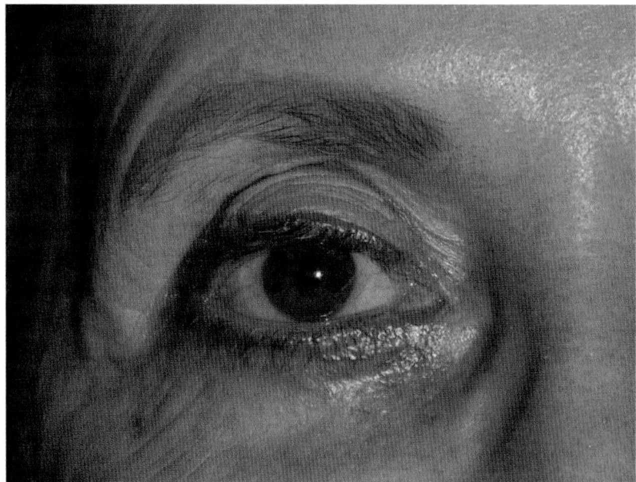

**Figure 69-3** Full-thickness skin graft to the upper eyelid to address anterior lamellar deficiency.

## Lower Eyelid Retraction

In the lower lids, retraction may be secondary to relative anterior or posterior lamella deficiency or middle lamella contracture. The choice of procedure is tailored to the etiology. A combination of procedures is often necessary with increasing lower lid retraction severity.

## Posterior or Middle Lamella Retraction

### Canthoplasty

A canthoplasty, as solitary procedure, is only able to address minor lower lid retraction. However, the lateral canthus is a critical aesthetic complex, and canthoplasty forms an important facet is in many lower lid retraction repair procedures. Multiple excellent techniques exist. A favored method of the authors is a variation of the "quick strip".[23] A small (3–4 mm) canthotomy and cantholysis is performed. A full-thickness triangle of lid tissue is excised proportional to the degree of horizontal laxity. Two 5-0 polyglactin sutures are used to reapproximate the shortened canthal angle to the superior crus of the lateral canthal tendon (LCT).[17] The addition of a 6-0 polyglactin canthal reformation suture through the upper and lower gray lines at the new lateral commissure is advocated by some to sharpen the canthal angle.[23]

### Lower Lid Retractor Recession

The lower eyelid is everted with a Desmarres retractor, and the conjunctiva is incised using a monopolar needle or Westcott scissors beneath the lower tarsal border. The dissection continues inferiorly to release the lower eyelid retractors from

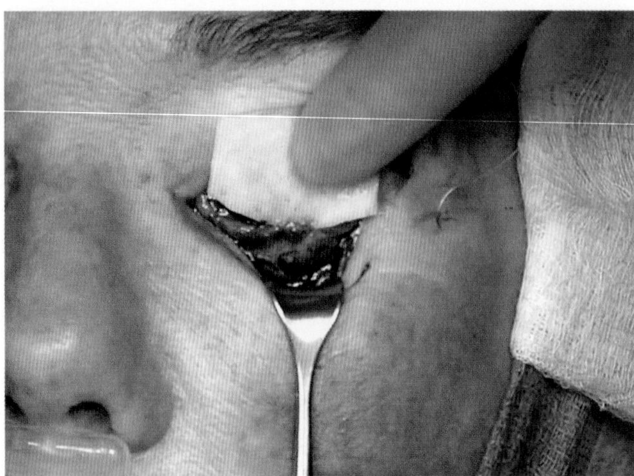

**Figure 69-4** Lower lid retraction repair with acellular dermal matrix spacer graft.

their insertion at the lower tarsal border. The dissection is continued into the fornix, releasing the orbicularis from the anterior surface of the retractors.[15,17,24] The retractors can be allowed to retract into the inferior fornix and the conjunctiva left to heal by secondary intention or sutured inferiorly to the orbicularis. Alternatively, a spacer can be sutured between the recessed retractors inferiorly and the lower tarsal border superiorly. A simple retractor release may be a useful adjunct in orbital decompression and orbital fracture repair.

### *Lower Lid Retraction with Acellular Dermis Matrix*

A lower lid retractor recession is performed as described in previous paragraph. Multiple types of alloplastic acellular dermis are available, such as Dermamatrix (Synthes, West Chester, PA, USA), Alloderm (Lifecell, Bridgewater, NJ, USA), and Enduragen (Stryker, MI, USA).[25-27] The acellular dermis is marked and cut from a sheet to the desired size and shape. In our experience, 1 mm of eyelid retraction correction requires 2.5–3 mm of Enduragen (data unpublished). The dermis spacer extendsthe length of the tarsus and is tapered at the medial and lateral ends to ensure a smooth soft tissue contour. The dermis spacer is secured superiorly to the inferior tarsal border and inferiorly the lower lid retractors with running 6-0 fast absorbing gut sutures (Fig. 69-4).

### *Alternative Posterior Lamella Spacers*

Other posterior lamella spacers include free tarsoconjunctival (TC) grafts, hard palate mucosa, and donor sclera.[28-31] Mucosal hard palate has been used a lower eyelid spacer for nearly 30 years. The mucosal lining facilitates rapid integration. As an autograft, the risk immunogenic inflammation or transmissible infections is avoided.[30] However, donor-site morbidity remains a concern. Dermis fat can be an effective posterior lamella spacer, particularly when eyelid retraction is accompanied by volume deficiency.[32] Complications include surface keratinization and hair growth, the latter occurring with inadequate hair follicle removal. We use a diamond burr or #10 Bard Parker blade to mechanically debride the epithelium and superficial dermis to ensure no residual hair follicles remain (Figs. 69.5A and B).

### *Orbitomalar and Suborbicularis Oculi Fat (SOOF) and Suspension with Single Drill Hole Fixation*

Multiple successful variations have been described in the elevation and fixation of the SOOF and midface.[33] We present one approach.[17,34] A canthotomy and cantholysis is performed. Dissection is continued inferiorly in the orbital septal plane to reach the inferior lateral orbital rim. The orbitomalar ligament is released using monopolar cutting cautery. A subperiosteal plane is created and dissection continued to ensure a freely mobile lateral midface. The periosteum of the lateral orbital rim is exposed and a high-speed drill is used to make a single hole 2 mm above the intended lateral canthal fixation position. One 4-0 polypropylene is passed twice through the cut LCT and the end temporarily secured with a bulldog clamp. Another 4-0 polypropylene suture is inserted in the SOOF in a locking fashion and the end again secured with a bulldog clamp. A crimped loop of 4-0 polypropylene is passed in an external-to-internal fashion though the osteotomy to engage the LCT suture, and then withdrawn externally thus drawing the LCT suture through the ostium. The SOOF suture is then tied to the LCT suture over the lateral orbital rim at the level of the frontozygomatic suture line.

### *Lower Lid Traction Sutures*

Temporary suspension (Frost) sutures from the lower lid to the brow are a useful adjunct to reduce traction on internal sutures in the early postoperative period when the tissues are most edematous. 5-0 Prolene sutures through the lower lid gray lines are secured firmly on the brow generating a vertical vector force.[17] These are usually removed within the first postoperative week. Skin bolsters should be used to prevent "cheese wiring" (Fig. 69-6).

## Anterior Lamella Retraction

### *Full-Thickness Skin Graft*

The lower lid is placed on upward traction with a 6-0 silk gray line suture, and a subciliary skin incision is made to

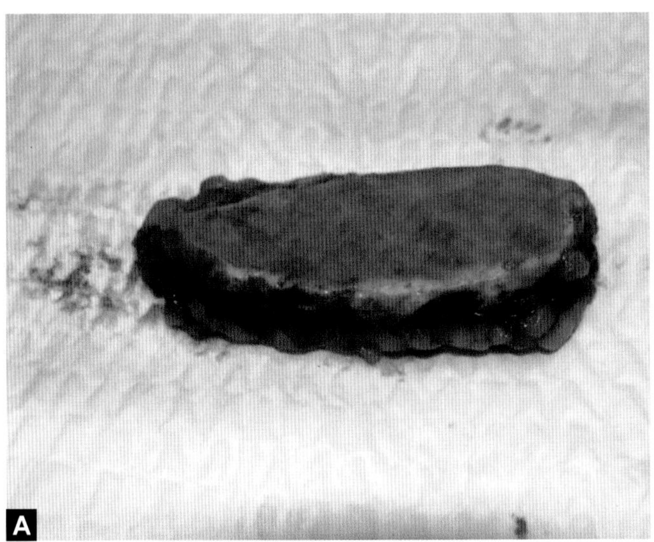


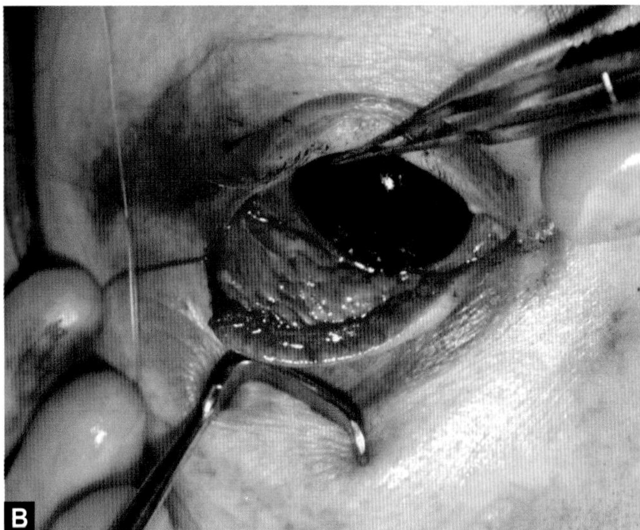


**Figures 69-5A and B** (A) Dermis fat graft after removal of epithelium. (B) Lower lid retraction repair with dermis fat graft

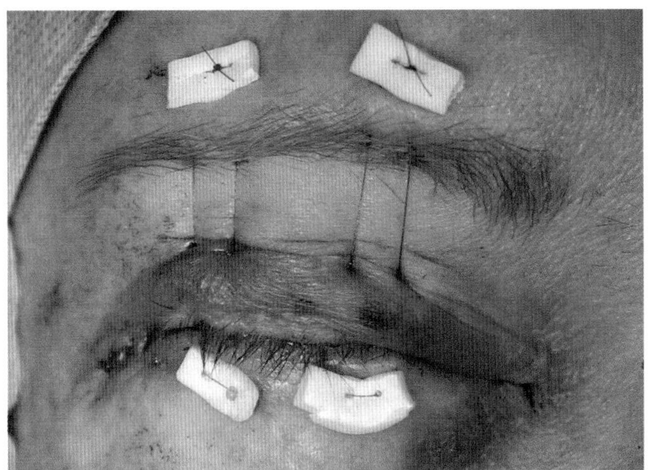

**Figure 69-6** Immobilization of lower lid with Frost suture after spacer graft placement and orbitomalar suspension.

the level of orbicularis muscle. A full-thickness skin graft is marked, sized, harvested, and thinned as described above in the section "Full-Thickness Skin Graft". "Oversizing" of a full-thickness skin graft is not necessary. The graft is secured with interrupted 6-0 fast absorbing gut or 6-0 polypropylene sutures. A canthoplasty is often necessary and a prophylactic SOOF suspension suture can be incorporated to minimize descent during the remodeling phase of wound healing. A 5-0 Vicryl suture is placed from the SOOF to the lateral orbital rim periosteum. Retraction in the early postoperative period is prevented by using lid margin traction sutures. A double- armed 6-0 Prolene (or silk) suture is placed over bolsters through the skin and gray line of the lower eyelid, passed through the upper lid gray line, and tied over bolsters to the brow. Alternatively, in cases where the postoperative retraction risk is low, a simple central tarsorrhaphy with 6-0 fast absorbing gut sutures can be used, which will absorb in about 5 days (Figs. 69-7A and B).

## POSTOPERATIVE CARE

An antibiotic/steroid ointment is placed in the eye and over the skin incisions in the operating room. This ointment is continued for approximately 2 weeks. An eye patch is used only if traction sutures have been placed, in which case the patch will be removed at the first postoperative visit and ointment omitted. An ice pack can be used to minimize ecchymosis in the first few days. However, if a skin graft has been used ice is avoided to promote graft perfusion. Some patients find the ice comforting and continue for a week or more. Oral antibiotics are used for patients undergoing spacer graft placement. Most patients do not require oral analgesia and a mild over the counter analgesic such acetaminophen/paracetamol will suffice. Moderate pain prescription analgesics (such as acetaminophen + hydrocodone) may be prescribed in the first week for patients undergoing drill hole fixation. Oral analgesic lozenges and antiseptic mouthwash are used postoperatively in hard palate graft (HPG) patients.[30] A hard palatal obturator for the first few weeks after HPG is also advocated by some.[30] A contact lens is often used to improve ocular surface irritation from posterior lamella grafts, particularly in HPG.[28] In HPG, the keratinized oral epithelium may undergo metaplasia to nonkeratinized epithelium in the recipient site although persistence of keratinization has also been demonstrated.[35,36]

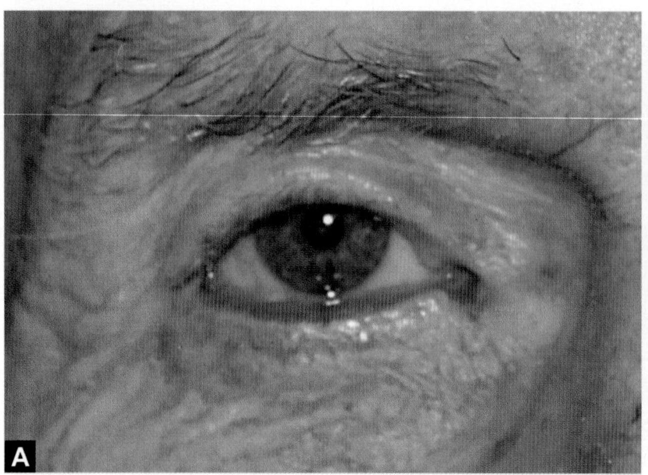

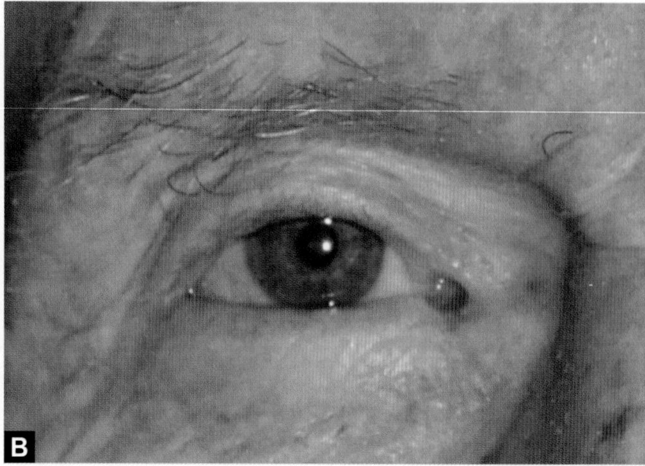

Figures 69-7A and B Before and after full-thickness skin graft to the lower eyelid.

## COMPLICATIONS

- Upper eyelid retraction surgery:
  - Ptosis (Over correction)
  - Under correction
  - Lid crease elevation
  - Asymmetry
  - Skin graft necrosis.
- Lower eyelid retraction surgery:
  - Ectropion
  - Dehiscence
  - Retraction
  - Graft donor-site morbidity
  - Chemosis
  - Posterior lamella graft extrusion
  - Skin graft necrosis.

## SURGICAL OUTCOMES: SCIENTIFIC EVIDENCE

Heterogenicity of pathology and surgical techniques make comparison of eyelid retraction surgery problematic. A paucity of level 1 evidence exists and most published literatures comprise uncontrolled case series. The techniques described herein for upper and lower lid retraction repair are well established with multiple series. Technical variations exist between authors, but the core principles remain.

In lower eyelid retraction repair, even the choice of spacer remains controversial.[30] The conclusion from the largest single surgeon series of lower eyelid retraction repair was that free TC, HPG, and sclera were effective in all retraction etiologies, although HPG was the favored material.[29] Acellular dermis is a relatively new eyelid spacer material.[25] Alloderm was prospectively compared with HPG in a series of 14 eyelids with equal success; however, Alloderm was associated with greater contraction and faired less well in reconstruction of contracted sockets.[26] Multiple acellular dermis material exists and as experience expands, improved evaluation against HPG will be possible.

Nonsurgical transient methods of reducing upper eyelid lid retraction extend back to the 1960s with adrenergic blockade using Guanethidine.[6] Botulinum toxin and hyaluronic acid filler have also been reported.[10,37] These techniques may represent a temporary alternative to surgical lid lowering in selected patients who wish to avoid surgery. The lid lowering effects of filler were modest. Although botulinum toxin is effective, variable outcomes, transient ptosis and diplopia were reported.[10,38] Improved predictability may be obtained using a transconjunctival approach and limiting use to patients with retraction of $\leq 2$ mm.[37] Subconjunctival triamcinolone can be used to improve eyelid retraction.[39] One randomized masked study of subconjunctival triamcinolone demonstrated mild to moderate improvement in recent onset thyroid-related upper eyelid retraction at the 24 week end point.[40] Limited evidence exists for a significant effect of triamcinolone in the quiescent, fibrotic phase. As eyelid surgery in thyroid-related retraction is usually deferred to the quiescent phase, triamcinolone's role in upper eyelid reconstruction is uncertain and traditional surgical techniques remain the mainstay.[40]

## REFERENCES

1. American Academy of Ophthalmology. Orbit eyelids and lacrimal system. San Francisco, CA: American Academy of Ophthalmology; 2007. Basic Clinical and Science Course; section 7.
2. Day RM. Ocular manifestations of thyroid disease: current concepts. Trans Am Ophthalmol Soc. 1959;57:572-601.

3. Small RG. Upper eyelid retraction in Graves' ophthalmopathy: a new surgical technique and a study of the abnormal levator muscle. Trans Am Ophthalmol Soc. 1988;86:725-93.
4. Bartley GB. The differential diagnosis and classification of eyelid retraction. Ophthalmology. 1996;103(1):168-76.
5. Harvey JT, Anderson RL. Lid lag and lagophthalmos: a clarification of terminology. Ophthalmic Surg. 1981;12:338-40.
6. Cruz AA, Ribeiro SF, Garcia DM, et al. Graves upper eyelid retraction. Surv Ophthalmol. 2013;58(1):63-76.
7. Bartley GB, Fatourechi V, Kadrmas EF, et al. Clinical features of Graves' ophthalmopathy in an incidence cohort. Am J Ophthalmol. 1996;121:284-90.
8. Bartley GB. The differential diagnosis and classification of eyelid retraction. Trans Am Ophthalmol Soc. 1995;93:371-87; discussion 387-9.
9. Putterman AM, Fett DR. Müller's muscle in the treatment of upper eyelid retraction: a 12-year study. Ophthalmic Surg. 1986; 17(6):361-7.
10. Kazim M, Gold KG. A review of surgical techniques to correct upper eyelid retraction associated with thyroid eye disease. Curr Opin Ophthalmol. 2011;22(5):391-3.
11. Ceisler EJ, Bilyk JR, Rubin PA, et al. Results of Müllerotomy and levator aponeurosis transposition for the correction of upper eyelid retraction in Graves disease. Ophthalmology. 1995; 102(3):483-92.
12. Baylis HI, Cies WA, Kamin DF. Correction of upper eyelid retraction. Am J Ophthalmol. 1976;82:790-4.
13. Harvey JT, Corin S, Nixon D, et al. Modified levator aponeurosis recession for upper eyelid retraction in Graves' disease. Ophthalmic Surg. 1991;22(6):313-7.
14. Mourits MP, Sasim IV. A single technique to correct various degrees of upper lid retraction in patients with Graves' orbitopathy. Br J Ophthalmol. 1999;83(1):81-4.
15. Tyers AG, Collin JRO. Colour atlas of ophthalmic plastic surgery, 3rd edn. Oxford, UK: Butterworth Heinemann Elsevier; 2008.
16. Kikkawa DO. Histopathologic analysis of palpebral conjunctiva in thyroid-related orbitopathy (an American Ophthalmological Society thesis). Trans Am Ophthalmol Soc. 2010;108:46-61.
17. Korn BS, Kikkawa DO. Video atlas of oculofacial plastic and reconstructive surgery. Philadelphia, PA: Elsevier Saunders; 2011.
18. Ben Simon GJ, Mansury AM, Schwarcz RM, et al. Transconjunctival Müller muscle recession with levator disinsertion for correction of eyelid retraction associated with thyroid-related orbitopathy. Am J Ophthalmol. 2005;140(1):94-9.
19. Elner VM, Hassan AS, Frueh BR. Graded full-thickness anterior blepharotomy for upper eyelid retraction. Trans Am Ophthalmol Soc. 2003;101:67-73; discussion 73-5.
20. Klapper SR, Patrinely JR. Management of cosmetic eyelid surgery complications. Semin Plast Surg. 2007;21(1):80-93. doi: 10.1055/s-2007-967753.
21. Shorr N, Goldberg RA, McCann JD, et al. Upper eyelid skin grafting: an effective treatment for lagophthalmos following blepharoplasty. Plast Reconstr Surg. 2003;112(5): 1444-8.
22. Verity DH, Collin JR. Eyelid reconstruction: the state of the art. Curr Opin Otolaryngol Head Neck Surg. 2004 Aug;12(4):344-8.
23. Barrett RV, Meyer DR. The modified Bick quick strip procedure for surgical treatment of eyelid malposition. Ophthal Plast Reconstr Surg. 2012;28(4):294-9.
24. Henderson JW, Relief of eyelid retraction—a surgical procedure. Arch Ophthalmol. 1965;74(2):205-16.
25. Cole PD, Stal D, Sharabi SE, et al. A comparative, long-term assessment of four soft tissue substitutes. Aesthet Surg J. 2011; 31(6):674-81.
26. Sullivan SA, Dailey RA. Graft contraction: a comparison of acellular dermis versus hard palate mucosa in lower eyelid surgery. Ophthal Plast Reconstr Surg. 2003;19(1):14-24.
27. McCord C, Nahai FR, Codner MA, et al. Use of porcine acellular dermal matrix (Enduragen) grafts in eyelids: a review of 69 patients and 129 eyelids. Plast Reconstr Surg. 2008; 122(4): 1206-13.
28. Patel BC, Patipa M, Anderson RL, et al. Management of post-blepharoplasty lower eyelid retraction with hard palate grafts and lateral tarsal strip. Plast Reconstr Surg. 1997;99(5):1251-60.
29. Oestreicher JH, Pang NK, Liao W. Treatment of lower eyelid retraction by retractor release and posterior lamellar grafting: an analysis of 659 eyelids in 400 patients. Ophthal Plast Reconstr Surg. 2008; 24(3):207-12. doi:10.1097/IOP.0b013e3181706840.
30. Wearne MJ, Sandy C, Rose GE, et al. Autogenous hard palate mucosa: the ideal lower eyelid spacer? Br J Ophthalmol. 2001; 85(10):1183-7.
31. Swamy BN, Benger R, Taylor S. Cicatricial entropion repair with hard palate mucous membrane graft: surgical technique and outcomes. Clin Experiment Ophthalmol. 2008;36(4):348-52.
32. Korn BS, Kikkawa DO, Cohen SR, et al. Treatment of lower eyelid malposition with dermis fat grafting. Ophthalmology. 2008; 115(4):744-51.
33. Ben Simon GJ, Lee S, Schwarcz RM, et al. Subperiosteal midface lift with or without a hard palate mucosal graft for correction of lower eyelid retraction. Ophthalmology. 2006;113(10):1869-73.
34. Oh SR, Korn BS, Kikkawa DO. Orbitomalar suspension with combined single drill hole canthoplasty [published online ahead of print Jun 27, 2013. Ophthal Plast Reconstr Surg.
35. Wobig JL, Loff HJ, Dailey RA. Vertical eyelid shortening. In: Levine MR (ed), Manual of oculoplastic surgery, 2nd edn. Boston: Butterworth Heinemann; 1996:143-4
36. Weinberg DA, Tham V, Hardin N, et al. Eyelid mucous membrane grafts: a histologic study of hard palate, nasal turbinate, and buccal mucosal grafts. Ophthalmic Plast Reconstr Surg. 2007;23:211-16.
37. Uddin JM, Davies PD. Treatment of upper eyelid retraction associated with thyroid eye disease with subconjunctival botulinum toxin injection. Ophthalmology. 2002;109:1183-7.
38. Costa PG, Saraiva FP, Pereira IC, et al. Comparative study of Botox injection treatment for upper eyelid retraction with 6-month follow-up in patients with thyroid eye disease in the congestive or fibrotic stage. Eye (Lond). 2009;23(4):767-73.
39. Chee E, Chee SP. Subconjunctival injection of triamcinolone in the treatment of lid retraction of patients with thyroid eye disease: a case series. Eye (Lond). 2008;22(2):311-5.
40. Lee SJ, Rim TH, Jang SY, et al. Treatment of upper eyelid retraction related to thyroid-associated ophthalmopathy using subconjunctival triamcinolone injections. Graefes Arch Clin Exp Ophthalmol. 2013;251(1):261-70.

CHAPTER

70

# Surgical Approaches and Techniques in Orbital Surgery

Geoffrey E Rose, David H Verity

## INTRODUCTION

Although orbital surgery was in the domain of neurosurgery in the past, with its higher morbidity of transcranial approaches, the management of orbital disease is now an ophthalmic specialty that employs more refined and aesthetic approaches with lower morbidity. However, the management of disease that extends outside the orbit (into cranium, pterygopalatine fossa, or paranasal sinuses) still requires comanagement with neurosurgeon, maxillofacial, or head-and-neck surgeons. One of six approaches can be used for almost all intraorbital surgery, the incisions tending to be placed in pre-existing skin rhytids or in the conjunctiva.

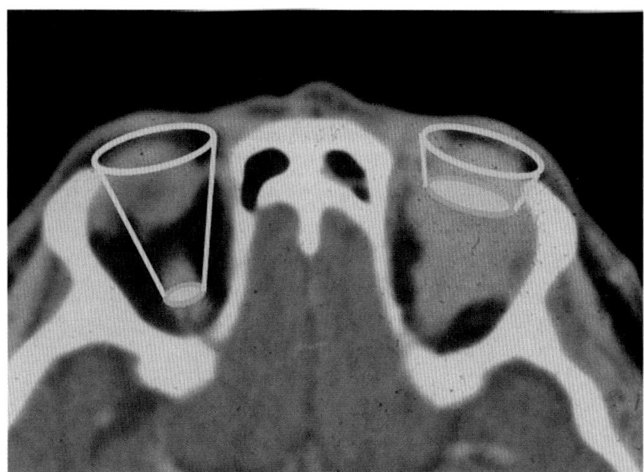

**Figure 70-1** The "conoid of view" in orbital surgery: from a surface incision that is spread open with retractors (yellow ellipses on scan), there will be a "conoid of view" into the depths with a finite area visible at the limit of exploration (turquoise ellipses). For a given-sized skin incision and resultant conoid, a shallow lesion will have a much greater visible area than that with a very deeply placed orbital lesion.

## KEY APPROACHES TO THE ORBIT

While a single approach will provide good access for most orbital surgery, the combination of two or more approaches may be considered with large or diffuse masses, for more extensive trauma, or with decompression of multiple walls. For any given approach, the size of the stretched skin incision, the ease of compression and displacement of intervening orbital tissues, and the depth of the lesion determine the extent of the "conoid of view" (COV), that is, a superficial lesion with a large skin incision will provide a wide and excellent COV, whereas the same incision being used to reach the deep retrobulbar space will have a long and narrow COV with only limited view of the lesion at its depth (Fig. 70-1).

### Upper-Eyelid Skin-Crease Approach

The upper-eyelid skin-crease incision, healing without visible external scar, provides ready access throughout the upper two thirds of the orbit and, if necessary and with some extra dexterity, down to the orbital floor. It is ideal for either incisional or excisional biopsies, with the skin incision being biased medially for superonasal masses and laterally for lacrimal gland masses and those abutting the lateral orbital wall (Fig. 70-2A). This incision, lying entirely within a line of relaxed skin tension in the upper lid, can be safely closed with a running 6-0 nylon (or 7-0 or 8-0 soluble sutures in children; Fig. 70-2B) and does not usually require any deep sutures.

Incision through the skin crease and underlying orbicularis muscle should be followed by an upward, preseptal dissection to avoid damage to the underlying levator muscle aponeurosis. Once alongside the extraconal preaponeurotic fat pad (and therefore clear of the levator aponeurosis), the

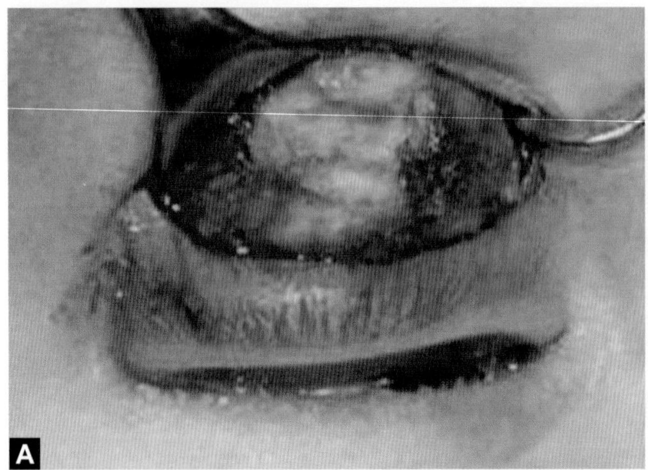

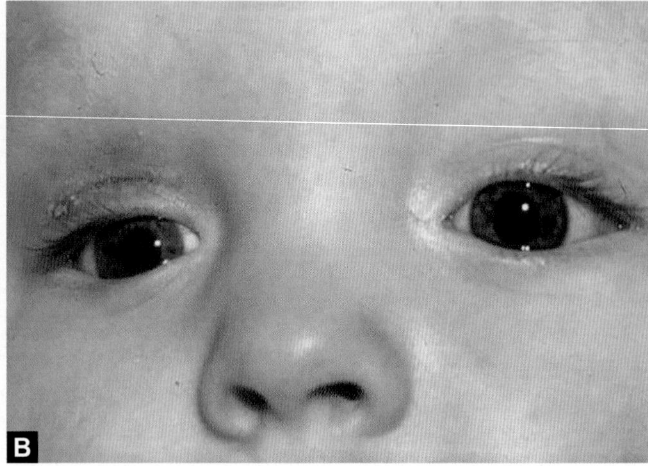

**Figures 70-2A and B** (A) The upper-lid skin-crease incision provides excellent access to lesions in the upper two thirds of the orbit and right back to the apex of the orbit. The inset shows a juvenile xanthogranuloma excised intact in an infant. (B) The incision naturally tends to close, rarely requires deep sutures, and heals extremely well, as shown in the same child at 2 weeks after surgery, where closure was performed with 7-0 absorbable sutures.

septum can be opened and the lesion sought within orbital fat. Most masses can be located by use of two "paddle retractors" to burrow, hand-on-hand, into the orbital depths until the lesion is seen—this directed burrowing being assisted by judicious palpation and a good knowledge of direction gained from study of imaging. Where orbital septa prevent onward spreading of the tissues, the septa can be "button holed" and opened by sharp dissection, after appropriate vascular diathermy. Masses along the orbital roof are best reached by downward displacement of the preaponeurotic fat pad, and masses involving the superior rectus or levator muscles reached by passage in the plane below the fat pad. The intraconal space is reached by either lateral or medial displacement of the superior rectus–levator complex and blunt dissection through the intraconal fat.

Lacrimal gland biopsies are best taken from the external surface of the orbital lobe and not from the palpebral lobe, the latter site often being spared the pathology and carrying a significant risk of true dry eye. Biopsy of the orbital lobe is achieved by following the preseptal plane out to the superolateral orbital rim and then dividing the arcus marginalis over about 2 cm to mobilize the whole gland inferomedially; removal of a good-sized specimen is relatively safe in this area and, with adequate hemostasis, has low morbidity.

A vacuum drain passed through the brow hairs is advisable where there has been surgery at the orbital apex, or after removal of a vascular lesion, and the drain removed after about 12 hours when it has stopped draining. Systemic prednisolone—with gastric protection—is typically used in a tailing dosage (starting at 1mg/kg/day) for about 10–12 days after surgery at the orbital apex, at the superior orbital fissure, or alongside the optic nerve. Nylon skin sutures can be removed at outpatient review 1–2 weeks after surgery, when the histology is often available and the definitive management discussed.

## Swinging Lower Eyelid Approach

Unless a subciliary blepharoplasty flap is required for resection of excessive skin or to allow correction of eyelid malpositions, the lower lid swinging flap—with its short outer canthal skin camouflaged in the inferolateral rhytid—has effectively superseded all direct transcutaneous approaches to the lower two thirds of the orbit. The scope of the lower lid swinging flap should be considered as equivalent to the upper-eyelid skin-crease incision, but with the horizontal incision placed on the internal surface of the eyelid—an approach not possible in the upper eyelid due to the importance of the levator apparatus. After division of the lower limb of the canthal tendon, the lower lid swinging flap has two variants, dependent on the position of the conjunctival incision within the lower fornix.

The "high flap"—where the internal incision is placed 1 mm below the tarsus (through the conjoined conjunctiva, lower lid retractors, and septum)—reaches the preseptal plane without disrupting orbital fat. Access to the preseptal plane is ideal for reaching the extraperiosteal space on the orbital floor and medial wall (Fig. 70-3A)—most usefully for repair of fractures, for bone decompressions (Fig. 70-3B), or to remove masses abutting or involving the periosteum. With the high flap, temporary fixation of the conjunctiva to the upper eyelid margin (using a 4-0 nylon suture) both protects the cornea

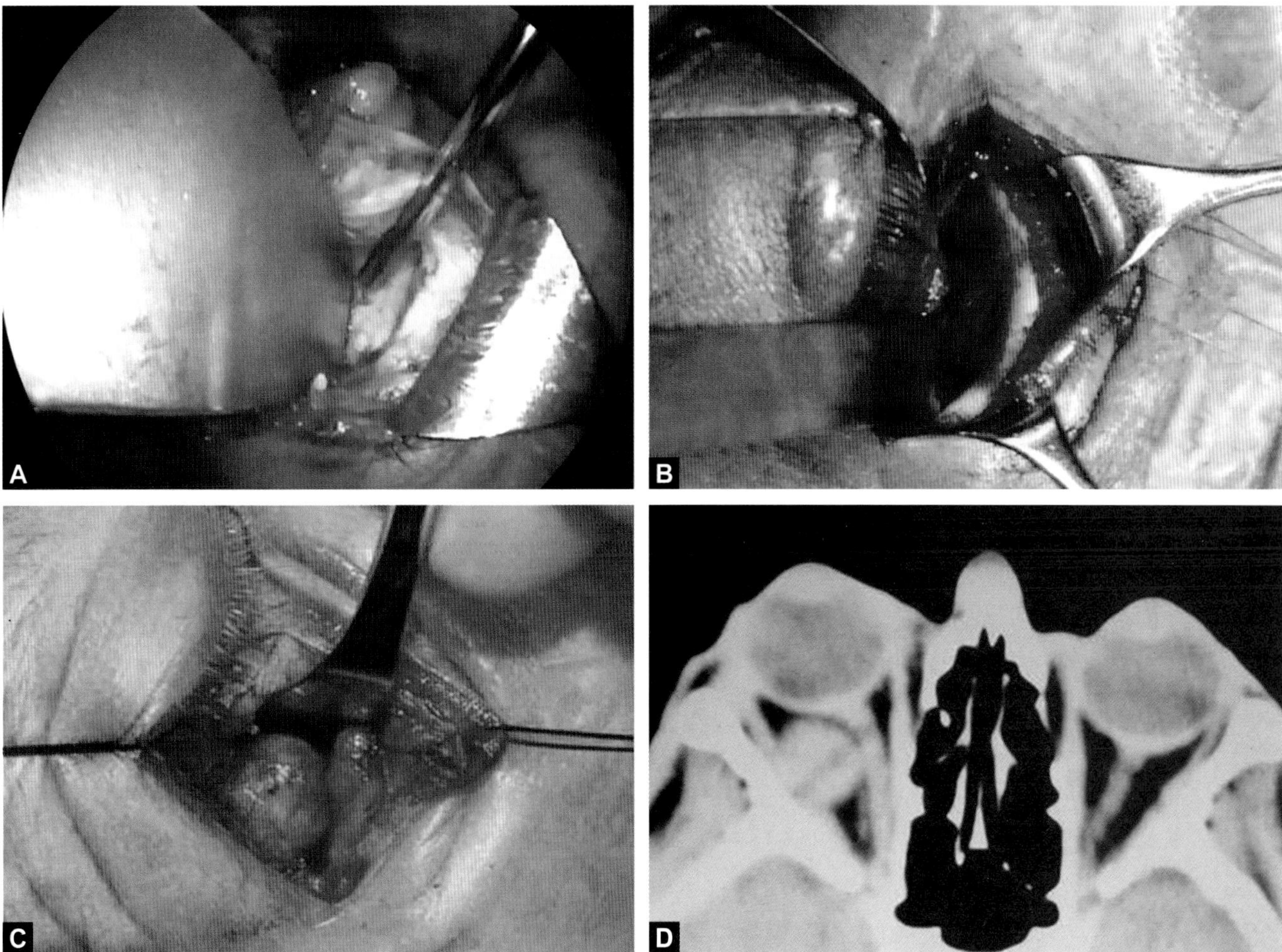

Figures 70-3A to D Two variants of the lower lid swinging flap: (A) The "high" variant, with incision just below the lower tarsal border, provides good access through the preseptal plane to the orbital floor and (B) good access for orbital floor and medial wall decompression. In contrast, the "low" variant – with internal incision placed low in the fornix— avoids the preseptal plane and gives access to (C) masses in the extraconal or (D) intraconal space.

and also eases dissection of the preseptal plane down to the orbital rim. If extensive access to the medial wall as well as the floor is required, the incision can be extended superomedially into a retrocaruncular incision and the inferior oblique origin divided, with the muscle held on a 5-0 absorbable suture for later refixation to its site of origin. When raising the periosteum across the orbital floor, it is important to seek out, diathermy and divide the perforating artery that passes from the medial edge of the infraorbital canal to the orbit; to fail to do so generally results in troublesome hemorrhage. Repair of the high flap is readily achieved by conjunctival closure with a 6-0 absorbable suture at the lateral end, at the medial end if the incision was extended into the retrocaruncular area, and then a layered repair of the lower limb canthotomy (tarsal plate and orbicularis to upper limb of tendon and orbicularis, skin-to-skin).

The internal incision for the "low flap" is placed along the lowest depths of the fornix and its length varied according to the required field of view; this incision through the conjunctiva and lower lid retractors enters the inferotemporal extraconal fat, and thereby gives access to the lower two- thirds of the orbit. Masses in the extraconal space can be resected back into the inferior orbital fissure (Fig. 70-3C) and the intraconal space accessed by division of the fibrous septa between the inferior and lateral recti (Fig. 70-3D).

## Lateral Canthotomy Approach

The lateral half of the orbit can be reached through a horizontal lateral canthotomy, with the benefits of rapid access and closure, and no loss of eyelid stability. It is particularly useful for biopsy of masses on the lateral orbital wall (Fig. 70-4A),

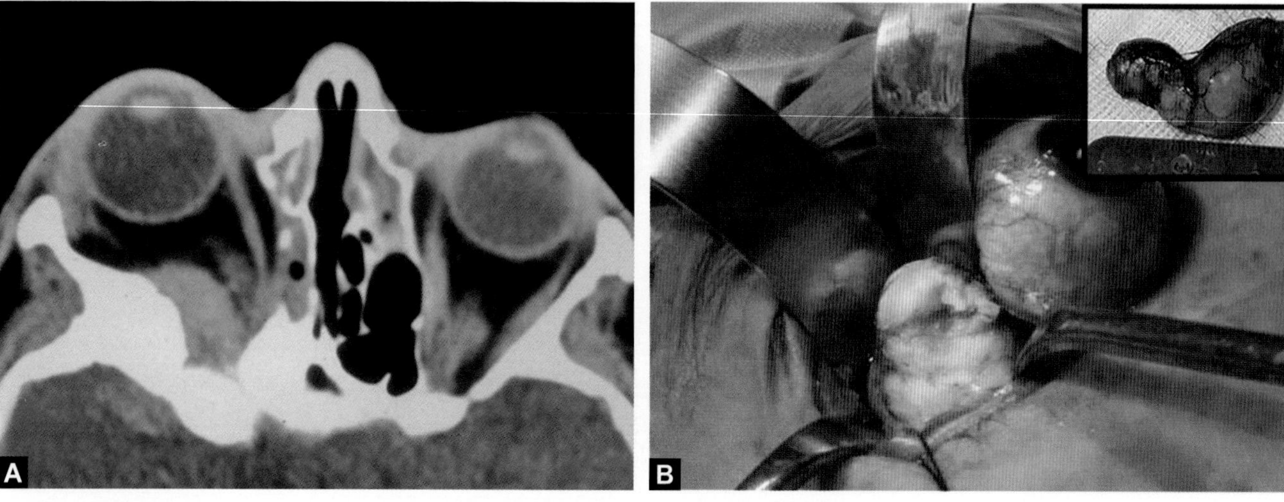

**Figures 70-4A and B** The canthotomy approach is ideal for access to masses along the lateral orbital wall, as with sphenoid wing meningioma (A), or for exploration of childhood orbits—as with excision of the intraorbital portion of the optic nerve (B).

for biopsy of diffuse masses (it being possible to biopsy muscle, fat, and lacrimal gland through this route), and also for removal of large masses from the relatively shallower orbits of children (Fig. 70-4B). The canthotomy alone provides a fair-sized rhomboid-shaped access, but this can be enhanced by division of the fascial connections to the lateral tubercle of the orbit, or by performing a partial conjunctival incision of the "low" swinging flap.

Closure of the canthotomy is readily achieved by alignment of the lid margins with a 6-0 soluble suture, then apposition of the upper and lower limbs of the tendon and skin closure.

## Lateral Orbitotomy with Bone Mobilization

The canthotomy approach to the deep orbit has only a very limited COV which, while adequate for incisional biopsy, might be too narrow for safe removal of orbital apex lesions; in such cases, outward swinging of the lateral orbital wall can markedly increase the COV by both widening the entrance incision and also shortening the path length (Fig. 70-5A). Bone-swinging lateral orbitotomy, now used considerably less with ascendancy of the "low" lower lid swinging flap, is still valuable for removal of pleomorphic adenomas of the lacrimal gland (the wider access aiding isolation of the posterior pole of the gland), and for removing lesions wedged into the orbital apex. Contemporary approaches utilize an extended upper-eyelid skin-crease incision (Fig. 70-5B), rather than the unsightly extended brow incision, and avoid removal (and devitalization) of the bone flap by hinging it laterally on the temporalis muscle (Fig. 70-5C). The extended lateral-half upper-eyelid incision also provides excellent access for lateral wall orbital decompression (Fig. 70-5D).

The upper-lid skin-crease incision is extended 1 cm toward the inferolateral rhytid, the orbital rim exposed, and the external periosteum incised widely at about 7 mm from the rim. The periosteum is then raised over the orbital rim and posteriorly across the lateral orbital wall, taking care to diathermy any perforating vessels. Parallel saw cuts are placed in the lateral wall, the upper being at the level of the superficial temporal line and the lower just above the zygomatic arch, and the temporalis muscle incised for 1 cm lateral to these two cuts to provide a "hinge" on which the bone can swing outward. Drill holes are placed in the rim either side of the osteotomies (to allow later suture fixation of the flap) and the internal face of the lateral wall weakened by "scoring" the bone about 1 cm behind the rim. While protecting the orbital contents with a malleable retractor, the bone is out fractured and the jagged bone edges trimmed, especially backward to enhance access to the orbital apex (Fig. 70-5E). The orbital contents can then be reached by opening the periosteum just behind the arcus marginalis (which is evident as an inflexion in the periosteum) and with backwards incision toward the apex of the orbit. After surgery, the bone flap is swung back into position and held with a 4-0 absorbable suture passed through the drill holes (Fig. 70-5F), the periosteum closed with the same suture, and the superficial tissues closed in layers. A vacuum drain is advisable after apical surgery and can be safely passed across the orbital rim, to exit through the lateral brow hairs.

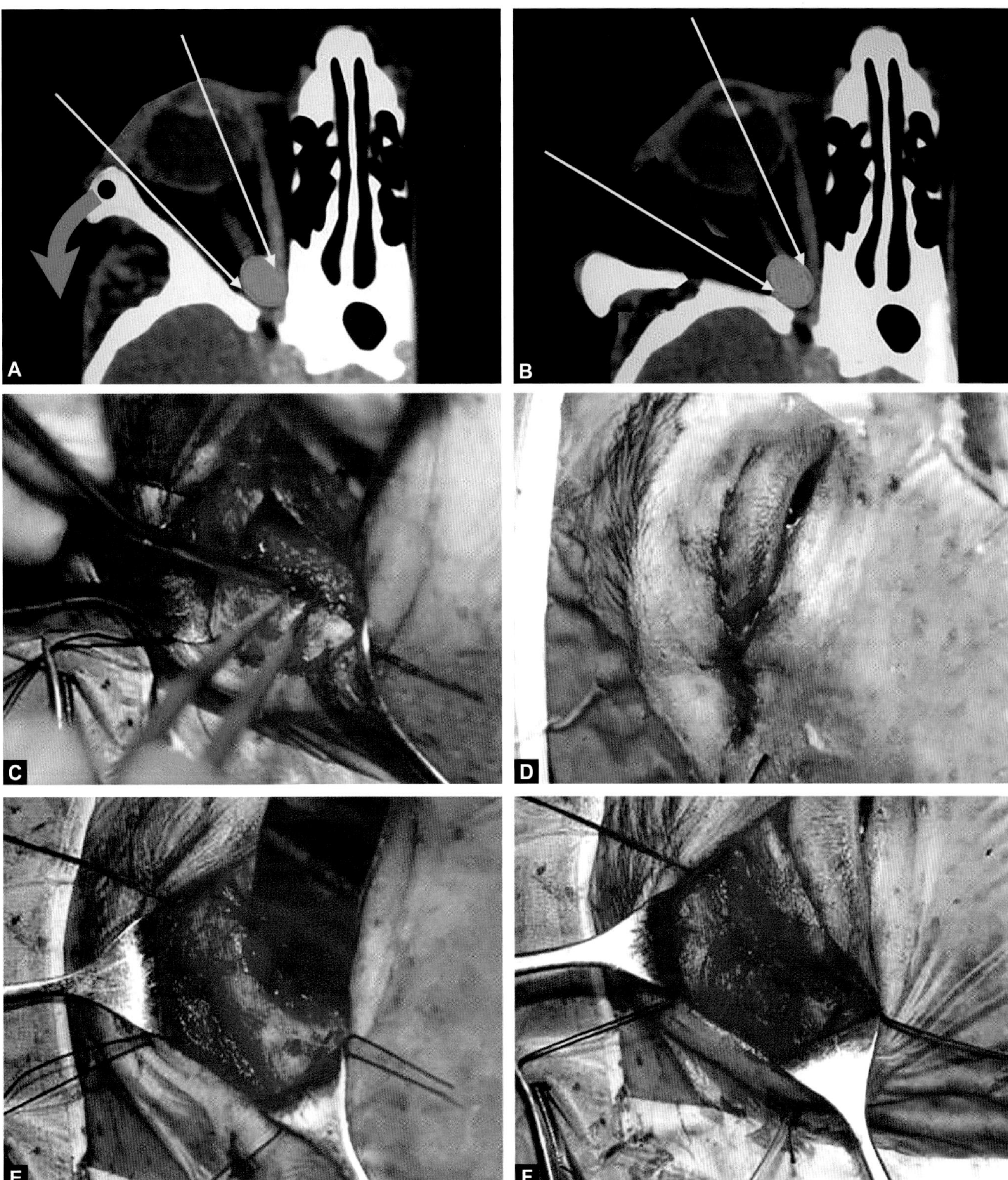


**Figures 70-5A to E** (A) Swinging out the lateral orbital wall in bone-swinging lateral orbitotomy leads to a greater "conoid of view" and also a shorter working distance to the orbital apex. (B) Contemporary lateral orbitotomy favors swinging the bone out on a hinge of intact temporalis muscle (thereby avoiding a devitalized orbital rim) and, likewise, placement of the cutaneous access into an extended upper-eyelid skin-crease incision. (C) Swinging the bone out on temporalis makes for easy reposition and fixation with 4-0 or 5-0 soluble sutures (D) and for ready closure of the periosteal flap to temporalis fascia with same suture (E and F).

### Transconjunctival Retrocaruncular Approach

The retrocaruncular approach to the orbit, passing behind the largely undisturbed lacrimal sac, provides excellent access to the medial orbital wall and medial half of the floor, together with the neighboring paranasal sinuses, and to masses biased medially within the orbit. Access to these areas is rapid, the closure very simple, and the incision leaves no visible scar. It is particularly valuable where decompression is required for compressive optic neuropathy (Fig. 70-6A).

The eyelids are parted using 2-0 traction sutures, the conjunctiva opened along the lateral border of the caruncle, and the tissues opened along the plane directed posteromedially behind the posterior lacrimal fascia. With the lacrimal sac protected by an 11-mm malleable retractor, the posterior lacrimal crest is exposed and the extraperiosteal plane entered anteriorly if needed—for example, if undertaking medial wall decompression; for intraorbital lesions it is unnecessary to disturb the periosteum. Placing a 16-mm-wide retractor within the extraperiosteal space is generally optimum for exposure of the orbital apex, and the medial half of the orbital floor is readily reached through the same incision (Fig. 70-6B). The conjunctival incision is closed with 7-0 absorbable sutures placed at the upper and lower edges of the caruncle.

### Conjunctival Peritomy

The conjunctival peritomy has a simple incision and standardized closure but, as compared to the larger incision of eyelid approaches, it tends to provide a limited and oblique view of deep orbital structures. Although the limited view may predispose to inadequate, crushed or nonrepresentative biopsies from the orbital depths, the peritomy is valuable for exploration of masses alongside the globe. Parabulbar masses can be reached by a neighboring peritomy of 120–180°, with radial relieving incisions, and the intraconal space reached by appropriate fenestration of the posterior Tenon's fascia.

## PRINCIPLES OF POSTOPERATIVE MANAGEMENT

Postoperative visual loss is, in most cases, almost certainly the result of arterial vasospasm in the posterior one third of the orbit, where the optic nerve has only a single and limited blood supply from perforating pial vessels; this arterial spasm is likely to be due to the vasospastic effect of several inflammatory mediators and free blood products, or due to direct contact with vessels on the surface of the optic nerve. Accumulation of fluid and inflammatory mediators can be reduced by placement of a vacuum drain (typically for 12 hours), by padding the operated orbit moderately firmly, and by nursing the patient in a semirecumbent position to reduce orbital venous pressure. Likewise, there should be good control of postoperative blood pressure and suppression of postoperative coughing, retching, or straining. For all but superficial orbital surgery, high-dose systemic glucocorticoids should be given during and after surgery to minimize vascular leakage and exudation of inflammatory mediators—with the steroids being continued in a tapering dosage for 10–14 days. Antibiotics should be given where there is a prolonged surgery, where there is disruption of the paranasal sinuses, or where an orbital implant has been placed.

As the only treatable cause of postoperative visual loss is a hemorrhage reaching arterial closing pressures, there is no actual rationale for leaving the orbit unpadded and monitoring pupillary signs. Arterial pressure hemorrhages are excruciatingly painful and cannot be ignored, and so our current regime is to monitor patients for severe or increasing pain after orbital surgery and then examine them if this arises; should the patient have a rock-hard orbit with gross proptosis, mechanical restriction of eye movements, and visual failure, the route for orbital exploration should be reopened as a matter of urgency, and any hematoma encouraged to drain prior to re-exploration under anesthesia to address the source of arterial hemorrhage.

With the exception of vigorous sports and heavy lifting or straining, the patient can pursue normal activities after orbital surgery, the restrictions applying for about 3 weeks. Nose-blowing and flying should be avoided for at least 2 weeks after repair of orbital fractures or after decompression of the medial orbital wall or floor.

## PREOPERATIVE CARE OF THE ORBITAL PATIENT

There are significant risks with orbital surgery some of which, such as loss of vision or persistent diplopia, will have a profound effect on their activities of daily living and their ability to work; indeed, for some professions the loss of vision in one eye, or debilitating diplopia, will be an absolute debarment. It is, therefore, imperative that the patient with orbital disease has the various treatment options clearly explained (including that of monitoring alone), and all the relevant complications and risks detailed before a final management is decided.

Although anterior, pre-equatorial orbital surgery has a low risk of major complication, there is still a small risk of complications such as periorbital sensory loss (rarely complete

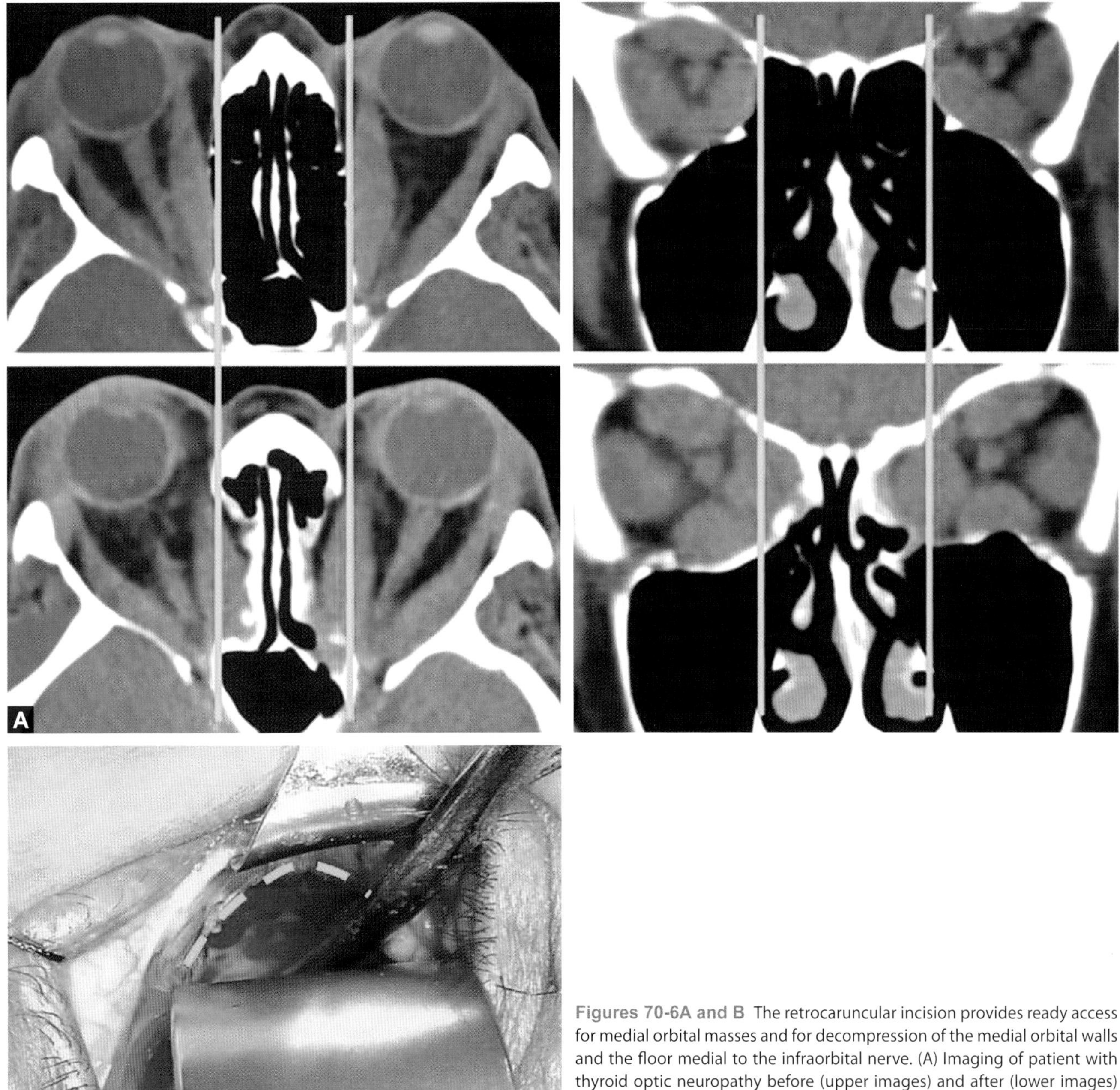


Figures 70-6A and B The retrocaruncular incision provides ready access for medial orbital masses and for decompression of the medial orbital walls and the floor medial to the infraorbital nerve. (A) Imaging of patient with thyroid optic neuropathy before (upper images) and after (lower images) medial wall and medial floor decompression. (B) The medial orbital wall is very rapidly reached through the retrocaruncular incision, the posterior lacrimal crest being indicated by the dotted line.

or permanent), mechanical restriction of globe movement, distortion of the eyelids or ptosis (with or without lagophthalmos), and ocular misalignment with restricted ductions. Surgery in the superonasal quadrant carries a small risk of motility disturbance due to trochlear damage, and care should be taken to avoid major disruption of the complex synovial sheaths around this structure and its tendon.

Operations within the retrobulbar intraconal space carry a somewhat greater risk of permanent visual loss (but still only a minority of cases), persistent motility disturbance requiring further corrective surgery, and persistent ptosis or mydriasis. Due to loss of lacrimal innervation entering the posterior pole of the lacrimal gland, resection of masses either within the orbital lobe (such as pleomorphic adenomas), or masses adherent to the posterior pole of the gland (such as deep orbital dermoid cysts) will often cause a loss of reflex tearing. Patients should be warned about this otherwise puzzling side effect of surgery in this particular area.

Because of the density of neurovascular structures at the apex, operations in the posterior one third of the orbit—despite all efforts to reduce inflammation due to tissue handling and thermal injury due to diathermy—are very often associated with an immediate postoperative "apex syndrome", with marked strabismus and global loss of eye movements, complete ptosis, mydriasis, and periorbital sensory loss. In most cases, these functions will return to normal over several months, but often with a dramatic improvement between weeks 8 and 12. Unfortunately, severe postoperative visual impairment, generally due to posterior ischemic optic neuropathy with no visible signs in the retina or optic nerve head, hardly ever improves and is associated with late diffuse optic atrophy.

Preoperative preparation of the patient should also include guidance about medications to be avoided before surgery—particularly any anticoagulants or antiplatelet agents; it should also be recognized that many foods—such as ginger, garlic, ginseng, and ginko—can influence hemostasis and should be avoided for some weeks prior to surgery. The type of anesthesia is dependent on the location of the lesion and the extent of surgery required: in many cases, local anesthesia is adequate for anterior biopsies; local anesthesia with deep sedation allows exploration of deeper lesions, but general anesthesia with systemic hypotension is usually required for surgery at the orbital apex and for procedures involving the orbital walls. Hypotensive anesthesia facilitates safer surgery by reducing the time of tissue handling and decreasing the accumulation of inflammatory blood products in the tissues; it may be achieved with either a volatile anesthetic agent (for example, isoflurane or sevoflurane) or with total intravenous anesthesia (TIVA) using a combination of propofol and remifentanil. TIVA is notable for allowing a smooth recovery from anesthesia (with less hypertensive rebound) and having a lower incidence of postoperative nausea and vomiting—these all being particularly desirable after orbital surgery.

## PEARLS AND PITFALLS

- Before embarking on Orbital Surgery a thorough knowledge of surgical anatomy of the orbit is necessary.
- Complications such as ptosis, diplopia, diminution of vision or rarely loss of vision must be explained to patient before surgery and proper consent should be obtained.
- Pre- and post-operative photographs of the patient and documentation of CT scan or MRI and ultrasonography are essential.
- A multidisciplinary approach is often required involving a team which consists of an oculoplastic surgeon, neurosurgeon, ENT surgeon, radiologist and pathologist.

## SUGGESTED READING

1. Davies BW, Hink EM, Durairaj VD. Transconjunctival inferior orbitotomy: indications, surgical technique, and complications. Craniomaxillofac Trauma Reconstr. 2014;7(3):169-74.
2. Sia DI, Chalmers A, Singh V, et al. General anaesthetic considerations for haemostasis in orbital surgery. Orbit. 2014;33(1): 5-12.
3. Markiewicz MR, Bell RB.Traditional and contemporary surgical approaches to the orbit. Oral Maxillofac Surg Clin North Am. 2012;24(4):573-607.
4. Marchal JC, Civit T. Neurosurgical concepts and approaches for orbital tumors. Adv Tech Stand Neurosurg. 2006;31:73-117.

CHAPTER

71

# Decompression Surgery

Robert A Goldberg, Daniel B Rootman

## BRIEF CONTEXTUAL HISTORY OF DECOMPRESSION

The idea of decompressing the orbit may be credited to the general surgeon Julius Dollinger in 1890 who accessed the lateral orbit via the lateral approach Kroenlein described a year earlier.[1] This surgery however was not widely adopted due to unsightly scars, and it was not until almost 40 years later that the issue was revisited.

In 1929, the Viennese otolaryngologist Oskar Hirsch described a removing of the orbital floor rather than the lateral wall and 2 years later the American Neurosurgeon Howard C. Naffziger described a superior decompression into the anterior cranial fossa. Completing the four walls of the orbit, the medial wall was first removed following an ethmoidectomy by Kistner in 1939. Walsh and Ogura later pioneered the combined medial and floor transantral approach in the late 1950s.[2,3]

In the 1980s, ophthalmic trained physicians began performing orbital decompression, first through the Ogura technique,[4] and then via transorbital approaches to the floor and medial wall.[5]

Transorbital decompression of the deep lateral wall was popularized by Goldberg et al. in the early 1990s.[6] This approach combined the transorbital approach developed earlier by Anderson and Linberg[5] with the sphenoid decompression techniques developed by MacCarty et al. in the 1970s,[7] without the need for a craniotomy. Orbital fat removal for decompression emerged around the same time, first by Olivari[8] and then Trokel et al.[9]

Over time, each wall and soft tissue compartment of the orbit has been decompressed together and separately through a range of incisions and approaches. However, these historical traditions continue to run through the specialties from where they began. Neurosurgeons tend toward cranial approaches, head and neck surgeons generally passing through the sinus cavities, and ophthalmic surgeons utilizing transorbital access.

## ANATOMIC REVIEW

The bony anatomy of the orbit can be conceptualized in terms of the four walls that comprise its barriers and the structures adjacent to each into which the orbital contents could potentially prolapse (Figs. 71-1A to D).

The frontal bone forms the vast majority of the orbital roof, with a small posterior contribution from the lesser wing of the sphenoid. Immediately adjacent to the thin frontal bone of the roof is the anterior cranial fossa. Extension into this space with orbital decompression is typically performed via a craniotomy; however, it can be accessed transorbitally or via frontal osteotomy.

The medial wall is a conceptual grouping of parts, or all, of four different bones: the maxillary, the lacrimal, the ethmoid, and the lesser wing of the sphenoid. The bones in this group are the thinnest in the orbit, measuring as thin as 0.2 mm. Overall, the length of the medial wall is 45–50 mm and the distance between the parallel medial walls is approximately 25 mm.

Immediately, adjacent to these bones are the ethmoid air cells, which extend in most cases to the level of the body of the sphenoid. However, the anterior wall of the sphenoid sinus can extend in some cases anterior to the orbital apex. In such configurations, it may be necessary to open the sphenoid sinus to completely decompress the orbital apex. In addition, the maxillary sinus will not infrequently extend superiorly to aerate part of the medial wall.

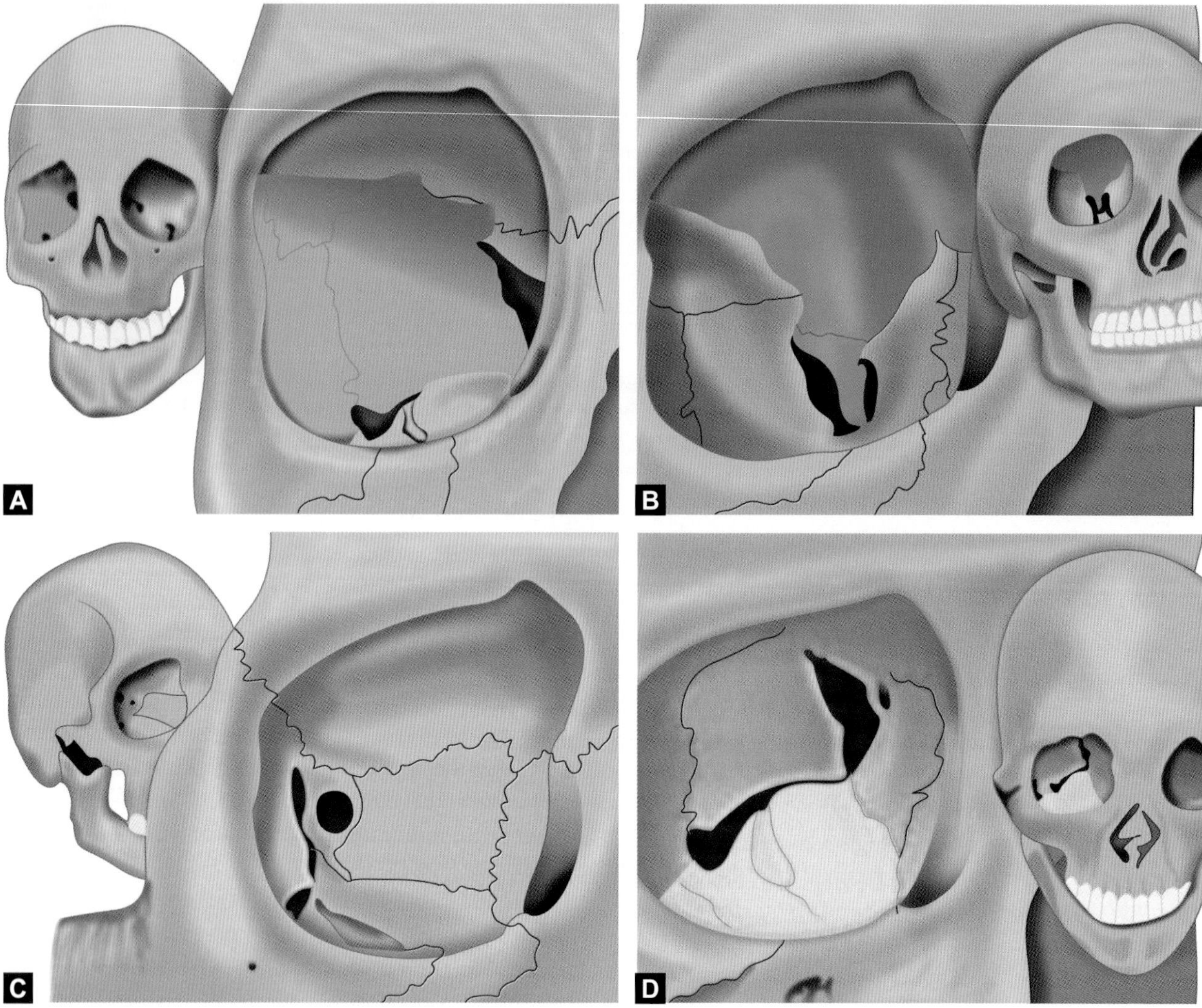

Figures 71-1A to D Four walls of the orbit.

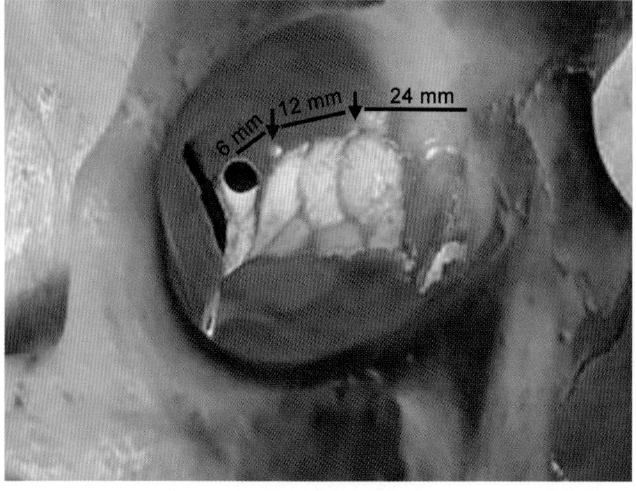


Figure 71-2 Medial wall with foramen indicated.

The frontoethmoidal suture is a critical landmark, delineating the medial wall from the roof of the orbit. Along this suture line the anterior and posterior ethmoidal foramen are found, with associated transmission of the anterior and posterior ethmoidal neurovascular bundles. The anterior foramen is located 24 mm from the anterior orbital rim. The posterior foramen is found roughly 12 mm posterior to the anterior foramen. The optic canal is generally located 6 mm posterior to posterior foramen. These structures must be identified and managed during medial wall decompression (Fig. 71-2).

The frontoethmoidal suture is of particular importance in identifying the superior extent the medial wall decompression. This suture is the medial fulcrum of the fovea ethmoidalis, and dissection above this point will lead to violation of the intracranial space.

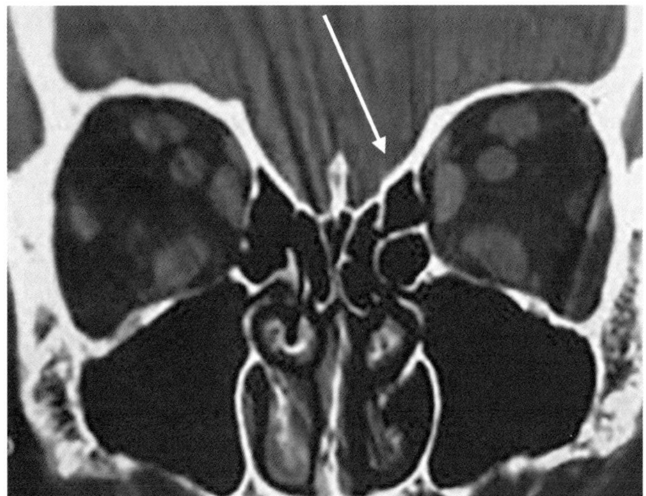

Figure 71-3 Fovea ethmoidalis.

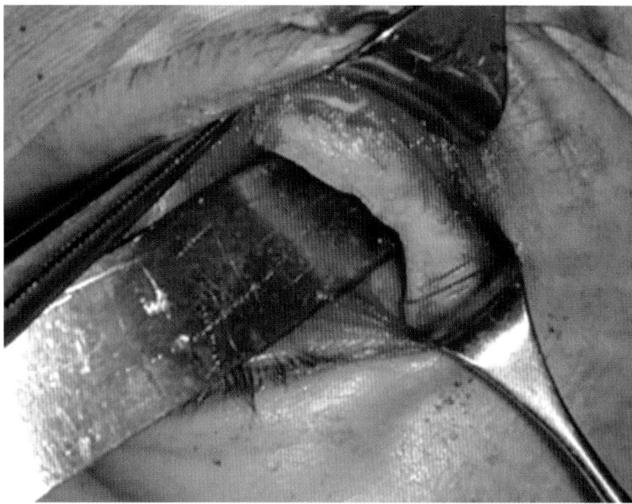

Figure 71-4 Lip of orbital rim.

It is also critical to understand the individualized conformation of the fovea ethmoidalis. This triangular invagination of the cribriform plate can be flat posteriorly, in which case it will extend perpendicular to the frontoethmoidal suture (Fig. 71-3). It could alternatively form an acute angle with the medial orbital wall anteriorly and extend deeply into the nasal cavity. In extreme cases, the fovea ethmoidalis may form the medial wall of the nasal cavity adjacent to the orbit posteriorly. Inadvertent entry into this space is possible if it is mistaken for additional ethmoid air cells.

The floor of the orbit is formed primarily by the maxillary bone, with smaller contributions from the zygoma laterally and the orbital process of the palatine bone posteriorly. The floor is triangular, slightly longer medially, and shorter laterally.

The lateral extent is delineated conceptually by a line running along the axis of the inferior orbital fissure. Although variability in the anterior extent of this fissure exists, it can often be encountered 15 mm posterior to the orbital rim. The floor is divided from the medial wall by the extent of the maxillary bone anteriorly and the palatine bone posteriorly. The lacrimal fossa is located anteromedially, with the insertion of the inferior oblique at its base.

The bony floor does not reach the posterior most extent of the orbit, it is a cone with the orbital process of the palatine bone at the apex. This point is still anterior to the optic canal by approximately 8–10 mm. The posterior border of the maxillary sinus is immediately anterior to this often found 35 mm from the orbital rim.

The implication of this anatomy is that decompression into the adjacent maxillary sinus will leave approximately 10 mm of orbit intact. Enlarging this space is critical for the management of dysthyroid optic neuropathy with a crowded apex. Thus, to complete an inferomedial decompression of the apex, the orbital process of the palatine bone should be removed.

The lateral wall is the most complex and possibly important of the four walls for the purposes of orbital decompression. It is formed primarily by the greater wing of the sphenoid, in addition to the zygoma anteriorly and the frontal bone superiorly. Again the shape of the lateral wall is triangular with the apex delineated by the superior and inferior orbital fissures, superiorly and inferiorly, respectively.

The lateral wall straddles the skull base and borders intracranial structures posteriorly and extracranial spaces anteriorly. In addition, the thickness of the bone is highly variable along the length of the wall. Anteriorly, the thick orbital rim is formed by the frontal and zygomatic bones.

Along the lateral and superior rim, there is a significant lip of bone extending into the mouth of the orbit. Unlike inferiorly and (to a lesser extent) medially, there is significant orbital volume lateral to, and beneath, the lip of the lateral wall. This is important when attempting to enter the orbit subperiosteally, as the surgeon must be careful to dissect at an acute angle to the rim rather than perpendicular to it (Fig. 71-4).

Posterior to the thick bone of the rim, the zygoma thins significantly leaving a virtual eggshell of bone centrally overlying the temporalis fossa. Inferiorly and superiorly at the level of the midorbit, the bone of the lateral wall thickens. Inferiorly in the body of the zygoma and superiorly in the frontal and zygomatic bones straddling the frontozygomatic suture.

The posterior portion of the lateral wall is formed by the sphenoid. This bone has a complex osteology and maintains relationships with the anterior cranial fossa superiorly, the middle cranial fossa posteriorly, the infratemporal/pterygopalatine fossae inferiorly, and the temporalis fossa anteriorly. There are two main areas of thick, cancellous bone within the greater wing of the sphenoid. First, superiorly extending from the tip of the superior orbital fissure connecting with the thicker bone segments of the frontal and zygomatic bones anteriorly. Inferiorly, the bone thickens again around the inferior orbital fissure extending back to the foramen ovale.

Approaching the lateral wall surgically requires an intimate knowledge of the anatomic relationships between orbit and surrounding structures, as well as the variation in bone thickness overlying these structures. Three-dimensional thinking is critical to lateral decompression surgery, to maintain safety and maximize volume expansion.

## AN INDIVIDUALIZED APPROACH TO SURGICAL REHABILITATION: THE "FIVE WALLS" OF DECOMPRESSION

In approaching the patient with congestive and disfiguring proptosis, it is beneficial to think outside of a defined "one size fits all" strategy. A graded and dynamic surgical decision-making process will benefit the patient by tailoring the congestive and proptosis needs of the individual patient while minimizing risk of surgical complications including consecutive strabismus.

Historically, there are five "walls" that can be decompressed: medial, floor, lateral, roof, and fat. Furthermore, elements of each approach can be tailored and/or combined to provide a graded amount of proptosis reduction while balancing the aggressiveness of the procedure.

In general, the order of decompression approaches at our institution follows the progression from fat to minimally invasive inferolateral wall, to deep lateral wall to medial/floor and finally roof in very extreme cases. These are generally progressively added as greater proptosis reduction is required.

Fatty decompression alone has been reported to provide between 3 and 6 mm of proptosis reduction, with postoperative incidence of new onset strabismus in the range of 7–8%.[10-13] The amount of fat removed can be graded, some suggesting as much as 6.5 cc can be excised.[11,12] This variable and modest amount of proptosis reduction can provide an initial, minimally invasive option for patients that require only a small amount of proptosis reduction and can additionally be effective to reduce congestion.

Combining fat removal with hand-carved boney removal over the inferolateral zygomatic and maxillary bones can augment this procedure.[14] Fat decompression can also be combined with boney decompression along any wall and will increase proptosis reduction in such cases.[15-21]

The choice of the first wall for boney decompression is controversial. At our institution, we approach the deep lateral wall as initial and often the only therapy. Primarily, this is for conceptual reasons. By enlarging the orbital space in a posterior axial plane, the deep lateral wall decompression anatomically corrects proptosis in an anatomically appropriate way. Thus, allowing the orbital contents to prolapse posteriorly while maintaining the horizontal and vertical relationships between the muscles and fat septae. In additional, the eggshell drilling of the orbital cavity maintains the normal boney distinction between the orbit and each of the adjacent anatomic compartments, thus avoiding complications caused by abnormal communication between the orbit and surrounding spaces (pulsation, oscillopsia, temporal wasting, frontal sinus obstruction, etc). Empirically, there is suggestion that the proptosis reduction is comparable to other approaches and the incidence of consecutive motility deficits and diplopia may be reduced.[22]

The second wall to be decompressed is typically the medial wall, often including the posterior portion of the floor. This is a particularly useful approach for dysthyroid optic neuropathy, where the decompression can involve the posterior floor and extend to the annulus of zinn, thus decompressing the crowded orbital apex.[23-28] Often, the medial wall is combined with lateral in what has been termed a "balanced decompression".[21,29-34]

The third wall to be decompressed is often the anterior floor, which alone can lead to high rates of diplopia.[35,36] This three-wall decompression technique is typically reserved for the most severe cases of malignant exophthalmos with exposure, congestion, and globe subluxation.[16,37-41]

Finally, decompressing the roof, although a primary access point for neurosurgical purposes, is rarely necessary and likely does not add significantly to the proptosis reduction achieved with three wall plus fat decompression. However, in extreme cases this four-wall approach can provide further proptosis reduction.[42]

Overall, the choice of what to decompress should be individualized based on the patients' clinical picture, cosmetic and functional needs, boney and soft tissue anatomy, and surgeon's experience and preference. Flexibility and adaptability are highly desirable features in approaching this surgery.

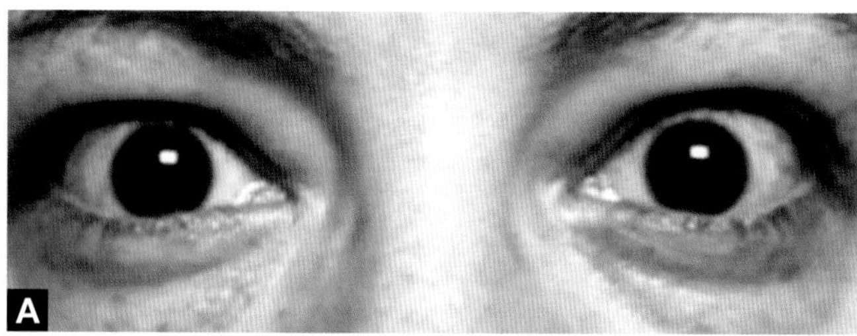


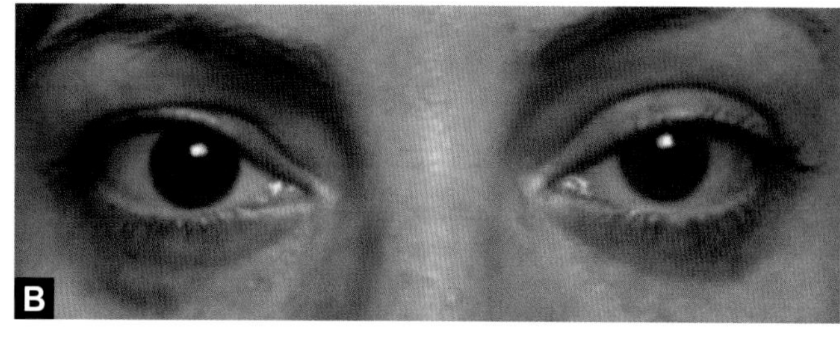


Figures 71-5A and B Pre- and postminimally invasive decompression.

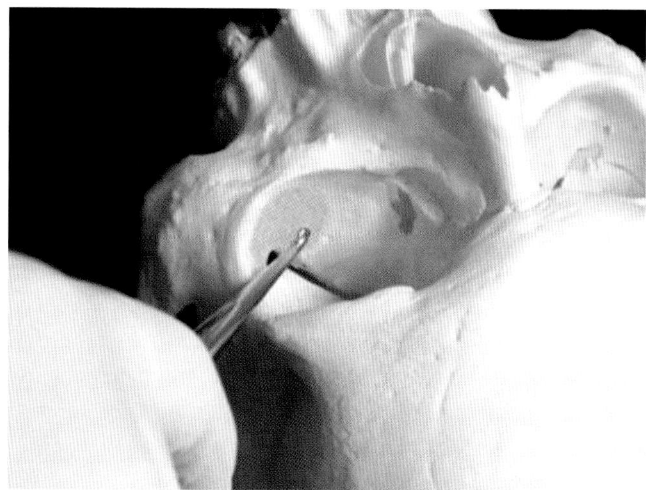

Figure 71-6 Minimally invasive curette of basin.

## TECHNIQUES: MINIMALLY INVASIVE, STANDARD DEEP LATERAL WALL AND EXTENDED MEDIAL/POSTERIOR FLOOR DECOMPRESSION

### Minimally Invasive Transconjunctival Decompression

In cases of mild proptosis, minimal congestion and/or an individual with a naturally prominent orbital rim configuration (Figs. 71-5A and B), it may be reasonable to perform a minimally invasive decompression. We prefer to use a transconjunctival approach to the floor with conservative removal of the thick bone within the body of the zygoma with and associated small anterolateral maxillary sinus osteotomy.[14]

For this technique, a transconjunctival incision is made 4 mm below the inferior tarsus extending from the caruncle to the lateral fornix. Dissection in the preseptal plane is continued to expose the inferior orbital rim. A periosteotomy is made immediately posterior to the arcus marginalis. The entire floor is exposed subperiosteally extending laterally to reveal the body of the zygoma anterior and lateral to the inferior orbital fissure.

The thick bone of the lateral maxilla and zygomatic body (the "basin")[43] are then carved utilizing a sharp 2–4 mm curette. The boney removal should include the marrow space of the inferior zygoma and a small portion of the floor overlying the maxillary sinus (Fig. 71-6). This small decompression will open the anterolateral orbit and may increase volume by 1.0–1.5 cc.[43]

The periosteum is then opened widely along the lateral floor and a fatty decompression is performed. Fat resection is primarily performed in the space between the inferior and lateral rectus. Extensive blunt dissection with a blunt tip scissors in this fat space will break up septae and allow the fat to prolapse. A #10 French Frazier tip suction is then used to engage the fat, drawing it forward. In some cases, simple suction alone may be sufficient for removal; however, a small amount of cutting at the base of the suction tip is often required. Bleeding in the small vessels within the fat space is not typically a problem and will usually resolve with irrigation and/or instillation of epinephrine containing local anesthetic and/or some gentle pressure on the globe. Bipolar cautery should always be available, used with suction and irrigation when necessary.

Approximately, 2.5 mm of proptosis reduction can be achieved with this combined method.[14] There is minimal risk of new onset diplopia and/or motility restriction. Thus, it is an excellent approach for patients who require only minimal decompression, and it can be combined with lower eyelid retraction or lower blepharoplasty surgery utilizing the same incision.

### Transcaruncular Deep Medial Wall Decompression

The medial wall decompression is particularly useful as a primary approach in cases of dysthyroid optic neuropathy and as an adjunct to deep lateral wall decompression in cases requiring large amounts of proptosis reduction.

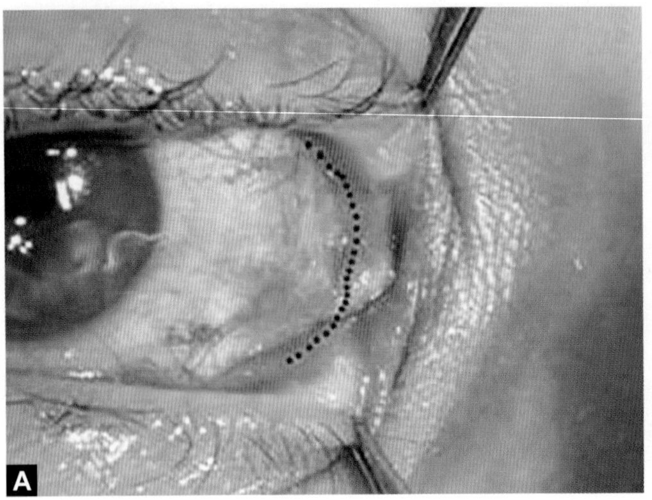

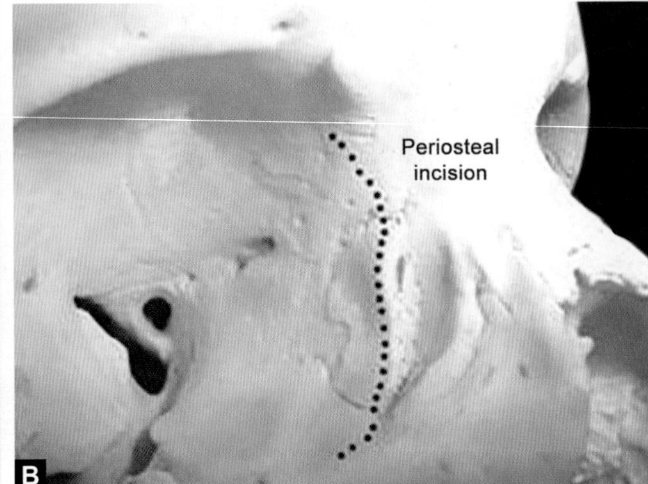


Figures 71-7A and B Transcaruncular incision.

The incision is designed to split the caruncle horizontally (Figs. 71-7A and B). It is then extended along the upper and lower fornices to create a wide opening extending 180° around the medial conjunctival surface. The Stevens scissors are then placed into the crux of the subcaruncular tissue and advanced to the medial wall. The posterior lacrimal crest is palpated. It is critical to stay posterior to the posterior lacrimal crest to avoid damage to the nasolacrimal system. The scissors are then opened widely (preceded by a small amount of cutting) and a malleable retractor is advanced into this space. Creating this passage from the conjunctival surface to the medial wall should be performed in a deliberate manner to maintain a single plane for further dissection.

The periosteum is then incised with cutting cautery and a subperiosteal plane is created. This opening should be extended to mirror the wide conjunctival opening, extending from the roof to the floor. This wide opening will prevent tearing the periosteum during later posterior dissection.

The anterior ethmoidal neurovascular bundle can then be identified, cauterized, and divided. It is easiest to identify the artery by starting the subperiosteal dissection on the roof, approaching the vessel from above. The line of the anterior and posterior ethmoid artery marks the frontoethmoid suture and will serve as the superior extent of the boney dissection, to avoid entry into the cranial vault. In addition, care should be taken when dissecting medially in the nasal cavity as the fovea ethmoidalis can extend inferiorly in this position and appear similar to an ethmoid air cell. The configuration of the fovea ethmoidalis should be assessed preoperatively on coronal imaging.

The initial boney opening can be created with any blunt-tipped instrument such as a suction tip or a curved snap. Once an opening into the sinus is created, a series of Takahashi forceps and rongeurs are used to expand the osteum. The lamina propecia osteotomy is extended anteriorly to approximately the level of the anterior ethmoidal foramen or slightly anterior to this landmark. Extension substantially anterior to this may increase the risk of globe dystopia and strabismus, without providing significant axial proptosis reduction.

Posteriorly, the anterior wall of the sphenoid sinus is identified by feel, as this bone will be firmer than the walls of the ethmoid sinuses. This landmark provides a general guide to the posterior extent of the dissection. It is rare that one will be required to extend the decompression posterior to the anterior wall of the sphenoid sinus; however, it is critical to remove the deep lamina papyracea over the posterior ethmoid cells until it is flush with the anterior wall of the sphenoid sinus.

The floor can then be removed up to the anterior border of the medial wall osteotomy. The medial wall of the maxillary sinus should also be shaved down to the floor of the sinus. This is particularly important posteriorly, where the maxillary sinus ends and the orbital process of the palatine bone is found (Figs. 71-8A and B). This bone should be removed to create a 180° continuity in the decompressed space and allow for complete prolapse of the apical contents into the ethmoid sinus—maxillary sinus—pterygopalatine fossa.

The periosteum is then opened to the posterior extent of the osteotomy, and blunt dissection is used to break up any fibrous septae and allow for free orbital prolapse. Fatty decompression of the inferomedial and inferolateral spaces can augment the procedure at this point. Closure is with a single-buried suture reapproximating the caruncle.

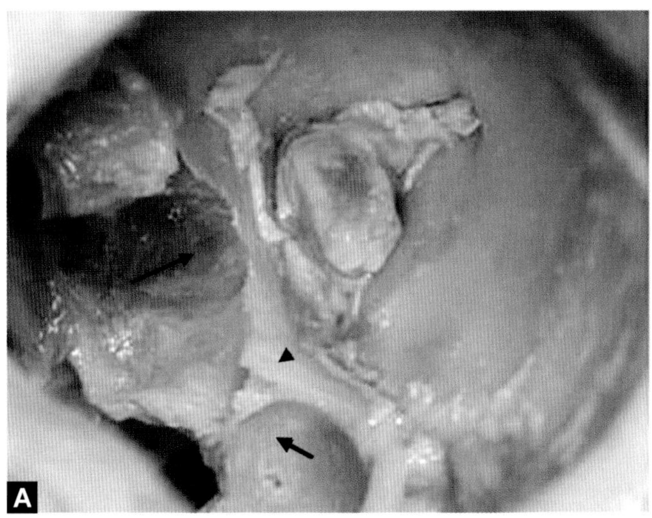

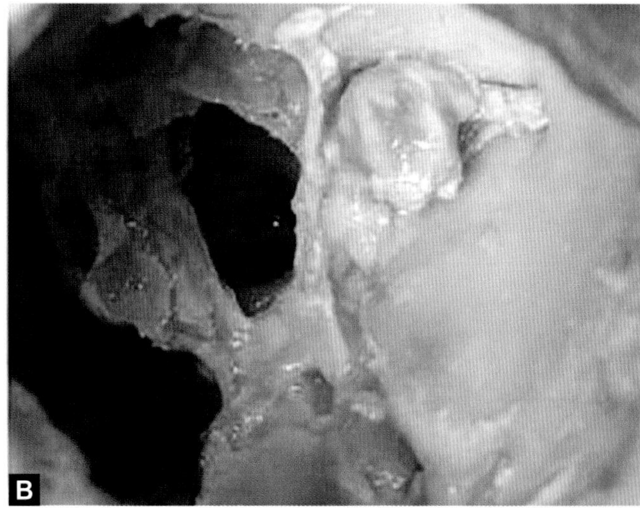

Figures 71-8A and B (A) Posteromedial strut. Arrowhead: orbital process of palatine bone; long arrow: posterior ethmoid; short arrow: posterior wall of maxillary sinus. (B) Posteromedial strut removed with continuity between the pterygopalatine fossa, posterior ethmoid, and orbit (note: posterior wall of ethmoid is removed with continuity into sphenoid sinus).

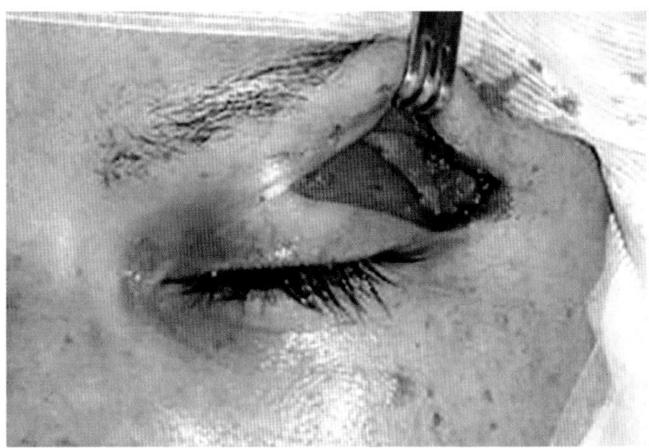

Figure 71-9 Modified lid crease incision.

## Transorbital Transcranial Deep Lateral Wall Decompression

For cases where 2–5 mm of proptosis reduction is the goal, the deep lateral wall decompression is ideal. The approach into the orbit is through a modified lid crease incision (Fig. 71-9). After opening the skin and subcutaneous tissue, blunt vertical dissection onto the superior rim will spread the fibers of the orbicularis. This motion will minimize bleeding and is less traumatic to the orbicularis as a whole.

Sharp and blunt dissection through the exposed retro-orbicularis oculus fat will reveal the orbital rim, which can then be further cleaned bluntly with cotton tip applicators. A wide exposure of the rim is critical, from the midorbit superiorly to below Whitnall's tubercle laterally.

A #15 Bard Parker blade or cutting cautery can then be used to create an incision through the periosteum 3 mm anterior to the arcus marginalis. Care is taken to follow the curvature of the rim along the entire extent of the exposure.

A sharp Freer elevator is then used to elevate the periosteal flap. It is critical to follow the acute curvature of the orbital rim to avoid spilling fat as one enters the orbit. Additional elevation of the periosteum heading toward the temporalis fossa will be required to drill out the lacrimal gland fossa later.

The tire iron technique is then used to lift the periosteum of the orbital rim in an en glove fashion extending down to the midorbit inferiorly and superiorly. This will release tension on the periosteal flap during the apical dissection.

Dissection is then carried posteriorly to expose the tip of the inferior and superior orbital fissures. In a possibly half of cases there may be a small fossa transmitting a recurrent branch of the middle meningeal artery just anterior to the tip of the superior orbital fissure. If this vessel is evident it can be cauterized and cut in cases requiring maximal lateral decompression, which will extend to the superior orbital fissure.

The lacrimal keyhole is then created.[43] Using a high-speed burr the orbital rim around the lacrimal fossa is then thinned. The region of boney reduction is variable but typically will extend from Whitnall's tubercle to the ¼ point of the orbital roof, with tapered edges at both ends. The rim is narrowed, and the thick bone of the lacrimal fossa can be thinned out (Fig. 71-10). This bone shaving allows for straight access to the posterior orbit for visualization and instrumentation during deep orbital drilling. It also will allow the lacrimal gland to prolapse, adding to the decompression effect.

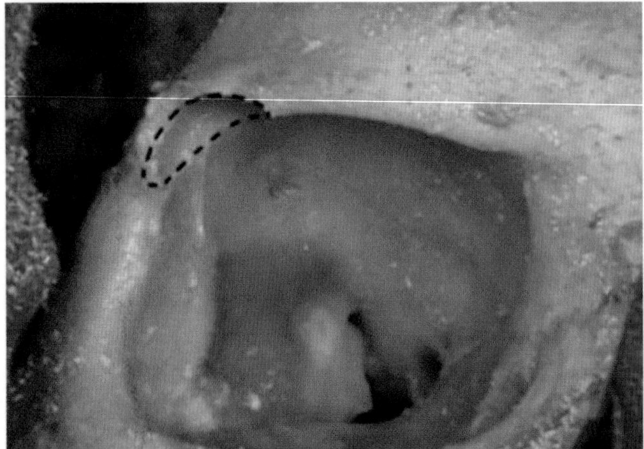

**Figure 71-10** Lacrimal "keyhole".

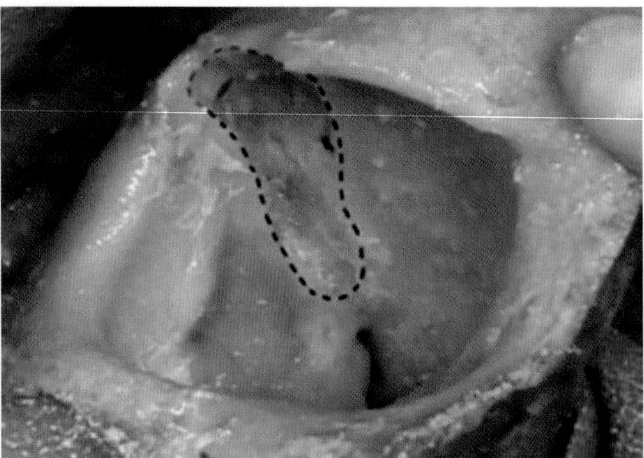

**Figure 71-11** The river of the superior orbital fissure.

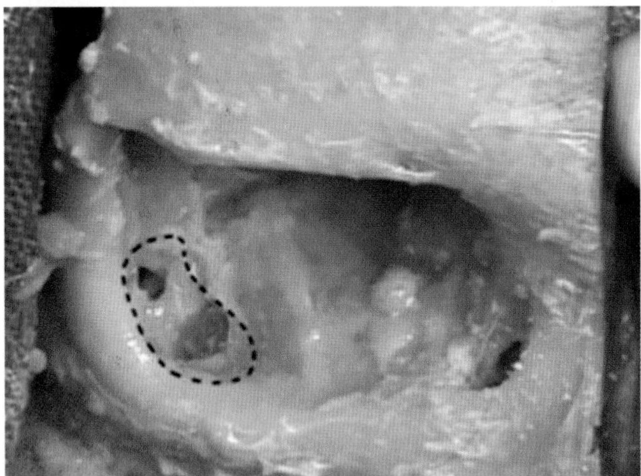

**Figure 71-12** The basin of the inferior orbital fissure.

The next area of boney removal is the lake of diploe found within the greater wing of the sphenoid immediately superior to the inferior orbital fissure. Drilling anterior and superior to the tip of the inferior orbital fissure will enter this space. Boney removal can proceed until the inferior orbital fissure is completely skeletonized. A curette can also be used to smooth out this diploic space.

Opening the lake of diploe around the inferior orbital fissure will reveal in cross section the river of diploe extending from this position to a point approximately 5 mm anterior to the superior orbital fissure. Drilling along this line leads into the second pocket of diploe within the greater wing of the sphenoid extending anterior from the tip of the superior orbital fissure up to the frontozygomatic suture. Part of this space may involve thick sections of the zygomatic and/or frontal bone (Fig. 71-11). After drilling out this river of diploe, there may be a cliff of bone along the posterior edge of the boney dissection. Removal of this ledge is important to allow the tissues to prolapse into the space created by bone work.

Lastly, depending on the amount of decompression desirable, the basin of the inferior orbital fissure can be removed. This area of thick cortical bone is safe and the deep lateral wall drilling can start in this position depending on surgeon's preference. The bone extends around the anterior tip of the inferior orbital fissure within the body of the zygoma. It can be drilled out to the point of exposing the buccal fat pad and may extend partially into the lateral edge of the maxillary sinus (Fig. 71-12). Extending too far into the anterior maxillary sinus should be avoided as this can lead to hypoglobus and strabismus, without providing significant proptosis reduction.

Finally, the periosteum should be opened back into the areas of boney dissection. A wide opening is desirable. Further blunt dissection of the orbital fat will break up adhesions and allow free movement of soft tissue into the boney cavities posteriorly. Additional fatty decompression in the inferolateral compartment can be performed utilizing the suction method outlined earlier.

Hemostasis is assured and then the periosteum and soft tissues overlying the orbital rim can be approximated if so desired. The skin is then closed.

## Managing Intraoperative and Early Postoperative Complications in Decompression Surgery

Perioperative complications are rare overall in deep lateral decompression; however, they can and do occur. Intraoperatively, one should be prepared to manage small venous bleeds from vessels in the bone or fat. If the source of the bleeding can be identified directly with standard suction and irrigation techniques, gentle bipolar cautery can be applied. If it is more diffuse or difficult to find in the fat, irrigation with epinephrine containing local anesthetic and then packing with gentle pressure can usually resolve the oozing. Bone wax is effective for bleeding of diploic vessels, but it should be used sparingly, as excessive wax can lead to late granulomas. A pressure patch can be applied after surgery if some diffuse ozzing is still present at the end of the case. Periodically checking the patient in postoperative care is important to monitor for a compartment syndrome. Any elevation in the orbital pressure should be managed with standard orbital hemorrhage techniques including cantholysis and in extremely rare circumstances, embolization.

Should a small amount of dura be exposed in the deep lateral orbit, this can usually be managed conservatively, especially if no cerebrospinal fluid is expressed. Should the dura be opened, small leaks in young patients typically respond well to packing with orbital fat. Extensive or persistent leaks may require neurosurgical management and we typically will close the wound, awaken from anesthesia and transfer care to complementary services. This allows for neurosurgical evaluation, planning and care in specialized neurosurgical operating suites.

## REFERENCES


1. Alper MG. Pioneers in the history of orbital decompression for Graves 'ophthalmopathy. Documeta Ophthalmologica. 1995; 89:163-71.
2. Ogura JH, Walsh TE. The transantral orbital decompression operation for progressive exophthalmos. Laryngoscope. 1962; 72:1078-97.
3. Walsh TE, Ogura JH. Transantral orbital decompression for malignant exophthalmos. Laryngoscope. 1957;67:544-68.
4. Baylis HI, Call NB, Shibata CS. The transantral orbital decompression (Ogura technique) as performed by the ophthalmologist: a series of 24 patients. Ophthalmology. 1980;87:1005-12.
5. Anderson RL, Linberg JV. Transorbital approach to decompression in Graves' disease. Arch Ophthalmol. 1981;99:120-4.
6. Shorr N, Baylis HI, Goldberg Ra, et al. Transcaruncular approach to the medial orbit and orbital apex. Ophthalmology. 2000;107:1459-63.
7. MacCarty CS, Kenefick TP, McConahey WM, et al. Ophthalmopathy of Graves' disease treated by removal of roof, lateral walls, and lateral sphenoid ridge: review of 46 cases. Mayo Clin Proc. 1970;45:488-93.
8. Olivari N. Transpalpebral decompression of endocrine ophthalmopathy (Graves' disease) by removal of intraorbital fat: experience with 147 operations over 5 years. Plastic and reconstructive surgery. 1991;87:627-41; discussion 42-3.
9. Trokel S, Kazim M, Moore S. Orbital fat removal. Decompression for Graves orbitopathy. Ophthalmology. 1993;100:674-82.
10. Chang M, Baek S, Lee TS. Long-term outcomes of unilateral orbital fat decompression for thyroid eye disease. Graefe's archive for clinical and experimental ophthalmology = Albrecht von Graefes Archiv fur klinische und experimentelle. Ophthalmologie. 2013;251:935-9.
11. Richter DF, Stoff A, Olivari N. Transpalpebral decompression of endocrine ophthalmopathy by intraorbital fat removal (Olivari technique): experience and progression after more than 3000 operations over 20 years. Plastic and reconstructive surgery. 2007;120:109-23.
12. Robert P-YR, Rivas M, Camezind P, et al. Decrease of intraocular pressure after fat-removal orbital decompression in Graves disease. Ophthalmic Plast Reconstr Surg. 2006;22:92-5.
13. Wu C-H, Chang T-C, Liao S-L. Results and predictability of fat-removal orbital decompression for disfiguring graves exophthalmos in an Asian patient population. Am J Ophthalmol. 2008;145:755-9.
14. Ben Simon GJ, Schwarcz RM, Mansury AM, et al. Minimally invasive orbital decompression: local anesthesia and hand-carved bone. Arch Ophthalmol. 2005;123:1671-5.
15. Chiarelli AGM, De Min V, Saetti R, et al. Surgical management of thyroid orbitopathy. J Plast Reconstr Aesthet Surg: JPRAS. 2010;63:240-6.
16. Chu Ea, Miller NR, Grant MP, et al. Surgical treatment of dysthyroid orbitopathy. Otolaryngol Head Neck Surg: official journal of American Academy of Otolaryngology-Head and Neck Surgery. 2009;141:39-45.
17. Goldberg Ra. Advances in surgical rehabilitation in thyroid eye disease. Thyroid: official journal of the American Thyroid Association. 2008;18:989-95.
18. O'Malley MR, Meyer DR. Transconjunctival fat removal combined with conservative medial wall/floor orbital decompression for Graves orbitopathy. Ophthalmic Plast Reconstr Surg. 2008;25:206-10.
19. Tieghi R, Consorti G, Franco F, et al. Endocrine orbitopathy (Graves disease): transpalpebral fat decompression in combination with 3-wall bony expansion. J Craniofacial Surg. 2010; 21:1199-201.
20. Unal M, Leri F, Konuk O, et al. Balanced orbital decompression combined with fat removal in Graves ophthalmopathy: do we really need to remove the third wall? Ophthalmic Plast Reconstr Surg. 2003;19:112-8.
21. van der Wal KG, de Visscher JG, Boukes RJ, et al. Surgical treatment of Graves orbitopathy: a modified balanced technique. Int J Oral Maxillofacial Surg. 2001;30:254-8.
22. Goldberg Ra, Perry JD, Hortaleza V, et al. Strabismus after balanced medial plus lateral wall versus lateral wall only orbital decompression for dysthyroid orbitopathy. Ophthalmic Plast Reconstr Surg. 2000;16:271-7.
23. Girod Da, Orcutt JC, Cummings CW. Orbital decompression for preservation of vision in Graves' ophthalmopathy. Arch Otolaryngol Head Neck Surg. 1993;119:229-33.
24. Hallin ES, Feldon SE, Luttrell J. Graves' ophthalmopathy: III. Effect of transantral orbital decompression on optic neuropathy. Br J Ophthalmol. 1988;72:683-7.
25. Jeon C, Shin JH, Woo KI, et al. Clinical profile and visual outcomes after treatment in patients with dysthyroid optic neuropathy. Korean J Ophthalmol: KJO. 2012;26:73-9.

26. Perry JD, Kadakia A, Foster Ja. Transcaruncular orbital decompression for dysthyroid optic neuropathy. Ophthalmic Plast Reconstr Surg. 2003;19:353-8.
27. Schaefer SD, Merritt JH, Close LG. Orbital decompression for optic neuropathy secondary to thyroid eye disease. The Laryngoscope; 1988:712-6.
28. Soares-Welch CV, Fatourechi V, Bartley GB, et al. Optic neuropathy of Graves disease: results of transantral orbital decompression and long-term follow-up in 215 patients. Am J Ophthalmol. 2003;136:433-41.
29. Alsuhaibani AH, Carter KD, Policeni B, et al. Orbital volume and eye position changes after balanced orbital decompression. Ophthalmic Plast Reconstr Surg. 2011;27:158-63.
30. Graham SM, Brown CL, Carter KD, et al. Medial and lateral orbital wall surgery for balanced decompression in thyroid eye disease. Laryngoscope. 2003;113:1206-9.
31. Kacker A, Kazim M, Murphy M, et al. "Balanced" orbital decompression for severe Graves' orbitopathy: technique with treatment algorithm. Otolaryngol Head Neck Surg: official journal of American Academy of Otolaryngology-Head and Neck Surgery. 2003;128:228-35.
32. Sellari-Franceschini S, Berrettini S, Santoro A, et al. Orbital decompression in graves' ophthalmopathy by medial and lateral wall removal. Otolaryngol Head Neck Surg: official journal of American Academy of Otolaryngology-Head and Neck Surgery. 2005;133:185-9.
33. Takahashi Y, Kakizaki H, Shiraki K, et al. Improved ocular motility after balanced orbital decompression for dysthyroid orbitopathy. Canad J Ophthalmol J Canadien d'ophtalmologie. 2008; 43:722-3.
34. Unal M, Ileri F, Konuk O, et al. Balanced orbital decompression in Graves' orbitopathy: Upper eyelid crease incision for extended lateral wall decompression. Orbit (Amsterdam, Netherlands). 2000;19:109-17.
35. Garrity JA, Fatourechi V, Bergstralh EJ, et al. Results of transantral orbital decompression in 428 patients with severe Graves' ophthalmopathy. Am J Ophthalmol. 1993;116:533-47.
36. Tallstedt L, Papatziamos G, Lundblad L, et al Results of transantral orbital decompression in patients with thyroid-associated ophthalmopathy. Acta Ophthalmol Scand 2000;78(2): 206-10.
37. Barkhuysen R, Nielsen CCM, Klevering BJ, et al. The transconjunctival approach with lateral canthal extension for three-wall orbital decompression in thyroid orbitopathy. J Cranio-maxillo-facial Surgery: official publication of the European Association for Cranio-Maxillo-Facial Surgery. 2009;37:127-31.
38. Cansiz H, Yilmaz S, Karaman E, et al. Three-wall orbital decompression superiority to 2-wall orbital decompression in thyroid-associated ophthalmopathy. J Oral Maxillofacial Surg: official journal of the American Association of Oral and Maxillofacial Surgeons. 2006;64:763-9.
39. Lee TJ, Kang MH, Hong JP. Three-wall orbital decompression in Graves ophthalmopathy for improvement of vision. J Craniofacial Surg. 2003;14:500-3.
40. McNab AA. Extracranial orbital decompression for optic neuropathy in Graves' eye disease. J Clin Neurosci: official journal of the Neurosurgical Society of Australasia. 1998;5:186-92.
41. Pezato R, Pereira MD, Manso PG, et al. Three-wall decompression technique using transpalpebral and endonasal approach in patients with Graves' ophthalmopathy. Rhinology. 2003;41: 231-4.
42. West M, Stranc M. Long-term results of four-wall orbital decompression for Graves' ophthalmopathy. Br J Plast Surg. 1997; 50:507-16.
43. Goldberg RA, Kim AJ, Kerivan KM. The lacrimal keyhole, orbital door jamb, and basin of the inferior orbital fissure. Arch Ophthalmol. 1998;116:1618-24.

CHAPTER

72

# Endoscopic Orbital Surgery

Kelvin KL Chong, Nicole C Tsim

## INTRODUCTION

Endoscopic surgery utilizes fiberoptic scopes through small incisions or natural body orifice to diagnose and treat disease. Another closely related term is minimally invasive surgery (MIS), emphasizing the advantage of reduced body cavity invasion.

Endoscopic surgery utilizes fiberoptic illumination, magnification, and real-time image capturing. This allows "keyhole" incisions with better cosmesis (shorter or absent skin wound), reduced tissue dissection (less surgical trauma), and thus quicker recovery.[1] Endoscopic/laparoscopic surgery is now widely practiced by general surgeons, gynecologists, and ear nose throat surgeons.

The MIS is a key focus in ophthalmic research and development. However, endoscopic orbital surgery was initially adopted by sinus surgeons and is yet to catch up with the rest of ophthalmic subspecialties. Inherent limitations for endoscope use in the orbit include an anatomically confined bony compartment and thus possibility of compressive collateral damage during the creation of an optical cavity (compared to that within the abdominal and pelvic cavity), the absence of fluid-filled cavities (compared with ventricles and vitreous space), and the presence of freely mobile orbital fat obscuring the endoscopic view.

To date, endoscopic approaches to the orbits are primarily performed through paranasal sinuses to the medial (ethmoid), inferior orbit (maxilla), and optic nerve (ethmoid, sphenoid) or through the subperiosteal potential space to reach all quadrants of the orbit during endoscope-assisted orbitotomies.[2,3]

## INDICATIONS

### Orbital Decompression: Thyroid-Associated Orbitopathy

Indications for orbital decompression include dysthyroid optic neuropathy (DON), globe subluxation, congestive orbitopathy, malignant exophthalmos (exposure keratopathy, uncontrolled intraocular pressure), and proptosis. During endoscopic decompression, the ethmoidal sinuses are removed before the medial and/or the medial part of inferior wall of the orbit, whereas the lateral part of the floor can be accessed via the transantral or endoscope-assisted transconjunctival/subciliary approach.[3,4] Medial wall is often decompressed for DON while combinations of other bone (floor, lateral wall) and/or fat removal decompression via transantral, transconjunctival, or transcutaneous approaches were used for the remaining indications above.

### Biopsy or Drainage of Orbital Lesions

Endoscopic transethmoidal, transantral, or trans-sphenoidal approach can be considered when lesions are located primarily in the medial, inferomedial, and apical orbit, respectively, where they lie close to the adjacent sinus cavities.[5] Intraoperative neuronavigation allows quicker lesion localization, confining operative field and limiting collateral damage.

Medially or inferiorly based subperiosteal orbital abscesses, developed as infective complication of rhinosinusitis, can be managed with concomitant functional endoscopic sinus surgery (FESS), removal of lamina papyracea, and opening of periorbita for abscess drainage.[6]

Intraorbital or periorbital foreign body, when located in medial and inferior orbit, may also be removed through the paranasal sinuses, often with the use of navigation system or fluoroscopic guidance.

### Orbital Fracture Repair

Repair of orbital wall fracture is indicated in cases with significant enophthalmos, persistent diplopia due to entrapment of orbital tissues, or large fracture size (> 2 $cm^2$). While transcaruncle approach allows direct and quick access to the medial wall, visualization may be improved by the use of an endoscope in fractures extending near to the apex. Both transethmoidal and transantral approach have been reported for repair of fractures of the medial and inferior walls while orbital access is required for subsequent implant placement.

### Traumatic Optic Neuropathy (TON)

The TON is a clinical diagnosis made with evidence of acute optic neuropathy attributable to recent history of trauma. Imaging studies may show fractures of the optic canal, sphenoid sinus, and orbital apex with or without bony fragments impinging on the nerve.

Patients with secondary nerve injury from edema, hematoma, or bony impingement of the optic nerve may benefit from optic canal decompression surgery. Endoscopic decompression of the optic nerve may be used alone or in combination with high-dose corticosteroids. Early surgery within 7 days after initial insult was found to be associated with better prognosis. The largest clinical trial to date (IONTS, International Optic Nerve Trauma Study), however, did not show any benefit of optic canal decompression compared with conservative treatment or systemic corticosteroid therapy alone.[7] In the authors' institute, patients are offered the options of high-dose intravenous methylprednisolone when there is no medical contraindication and are assessed on a case-by-case basis for surgery if the following are evident. The risks of potential life-threatening and intracranial complications such as carotid artery injury, stroke, cerebrospinal fluid leak, or postoperative bleeding, however, must be balanced with the potential gain in useful vision.

#### *Indications for Surgical Decompression in TON*

- Failure for vision to improve after 72 hours of high-dose steroid therapy.
- Progressive visual loss during steroid therapy.
- Contraindication to steroids with progressive visual loss.
- Loss of vision with computer tomography (CT) scan evidence of fracture or hematoma impinging on optic nerve.

## CONTRAINDICATIONS TO ENDOSCOPIC SURGERY

- Relative:
  - Insufficient instrumentation or working knowledge with endoscopes.
  - Patients with altered periorbital anatomies (congenital, traumatic, iatrogenic) without relevant imaging studies available.
- Absolute:
  - Uncontrolled bleeding tendencies.

## SURGICAL TECHNIQUE

Patients are prepared and draped as for endoscopic sinus or orbital surgery, typically under general anesthesia and endotracheal intubation. Local anesthetic is infiltrated around the surgical field. Transcaruncular ethmoidal, submucosal over the superior buccal gingiva, subconjunctival, or subcutaneous infiltration is given with 2% Lignocaine and 1:200,000 epinephrine solutions for hemostasis. Ribbon gauzes, cotton buds, or neuropatties soaked in topical vasoconstrictants, e.g. 5% cocaine solution is placed into the nasal cavity for mucosal decongestion and vasoconstriction.

### Medial Wall Orbital Decompression[4]

Surgery starts with uncinectomy and middle meatotomy (Figs. 72.1 to 72.3), followed by removal of anterior, middle, and posterior ethmoid air cells using cutting forceps and/or powered instruments (debrider). Middle meatotomy prevents obliteration of the maxillary sinus drainage by subsequently prolapsing orbital tissues (Fig. 72-4). The frontal recess should be preserved during removal of the most anterosuperior ethmoid air cells (agger nasi). Skull base is recognized by the presence of fovea ethmoidalis and the thickness of the overlying bone (Fig. 72-5). A complete ethmoidectomy until the sphenoid sinus entry leaving only the lamina papyracea is thus made. The medial wall can then be removed by cracking through using a seeker probe or a periosteal elevator then continued with Blakesley forceps (Fig. 72-6). Depending on the size and location of the lesion and/or extent of decompression required, the lamina papyracea may be removed up to the sphenoethmoidal junction. The periorbita should be kept intact at this stage (Fig. 72-7). The anterior and posterior ethmoidal vessels are useful landmarks of the superior limit at frontoethmoidal suture (Fig. 72-8).

Medial part of the floor may be removed, but the anterior ethmoidomaxillary strut should be preserved to support the

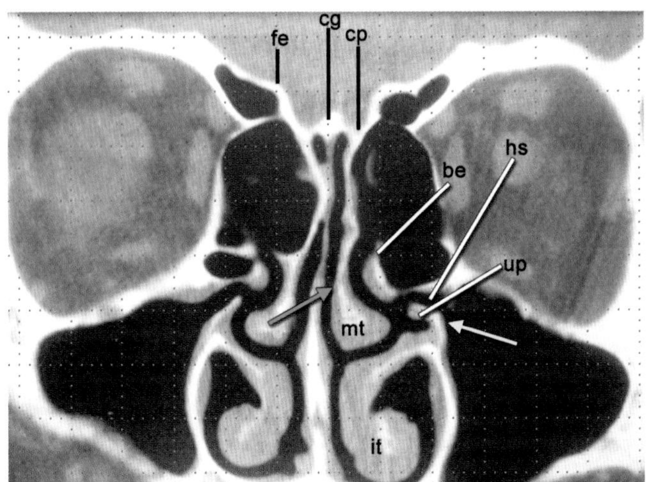


Figure 72-1 Coronal computed tomography of normal orbits and paranasal sinuses. Middle turbinate (blue arrow) and uncinated process (yellow arrow) are important endoscopic landmarks during transethmoidal medial wall decompression. (be: Bulla ethmoidalis; up: uncinated process; cg: crista galli; cp: cribriform plate; hs: hiatus semilunaris; fe: fovea ethmoidalis; mt: middle turbinate; it: inferior turbinate).

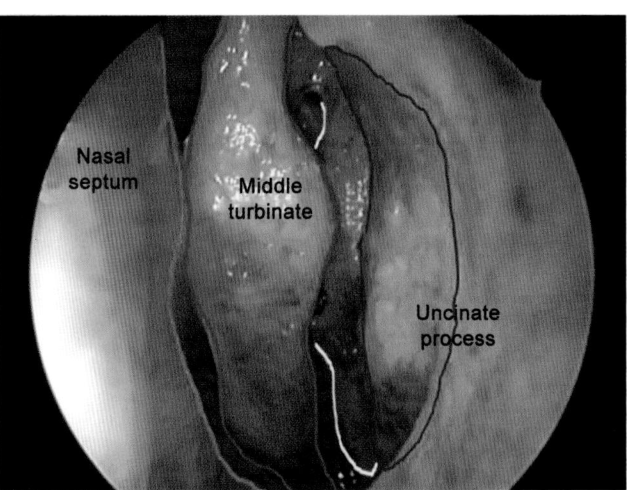


Figure 72-2 Endoscopic view of left nostril. Important endonasal landmarks at the start of endoscopic orbital decompression.

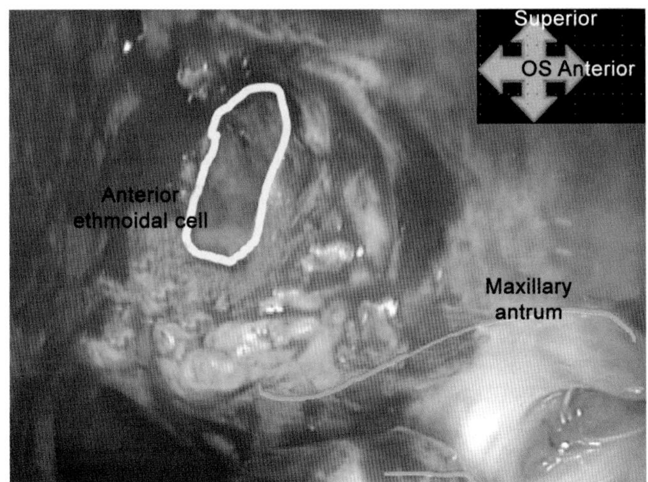


Figure 72-3 Endoscopic view of left nostril during anterior ethmoidal cell removal.

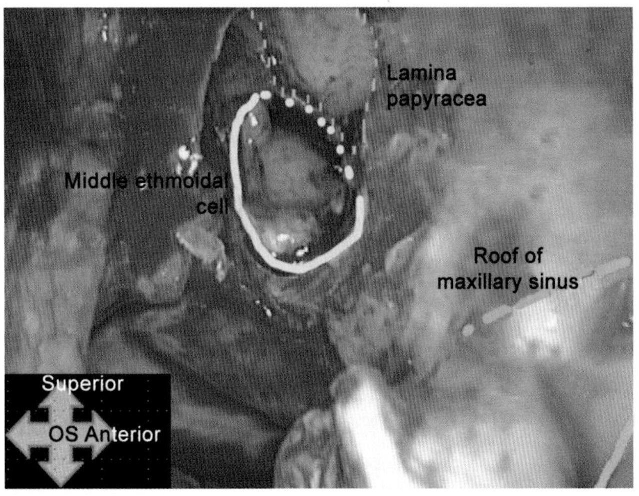


Figure 72-4 Endoscopic view of left nostril during middle ethmoidal cell removal, part of the medial wall (lamina papyracea), and the roof of the maxillary sinus seen through the antrum.

globe and to avoid postoperative hypoglobus and diplopia (Fig. 72-9). The medial bony floor of the orbit is removed as far laterally as the infraorbital nerve (ION).

Exposed periorbita is then slit opened posteroanteriorly with a curved sickle, a bent 18-gauge needle or crescent knife (Fig. 72-10). A periosteal sling parallel to the medial rectus muscle may help decrease postoperative esotropia (Fig. 72-11). The degree of proptosis reduction is reassessed to decide on further periosteal release, bony and/or fat removal (Fig. 72-12).

Endoscopic transethmoidal orbital decompression can be combined with lateral (transcutaneous), inferior (transantral, subconjunctival, swinging eyelid) bony and/or fat removal decompression for different indications (DON versus proptosis or both), and degree of proptosis reduction (Figs. 72-13A and B).

## Optic Canal Decompression — Transethmoidal or Trans-sphenoidal Approach

For cases of TON indicated for surgical intervention, the medial aspect of the optic canal may be decompressed

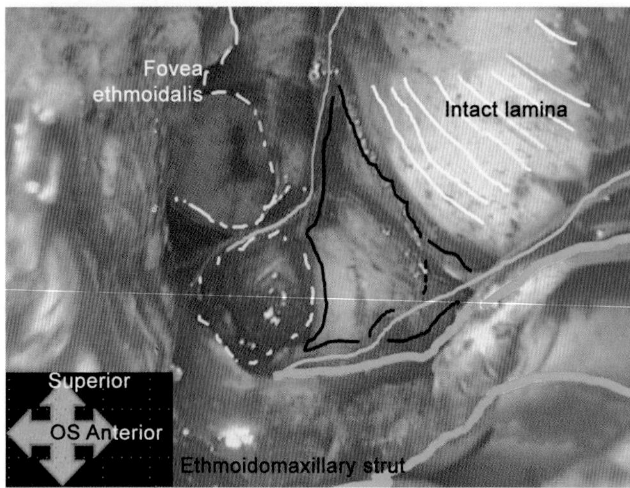


Figure 72-5 Endoscopic view of left nostril showing intact medial wall (right), skull base represented by fovea ethmoidalis (above left), and ethmoidomaxillary strut (below right).

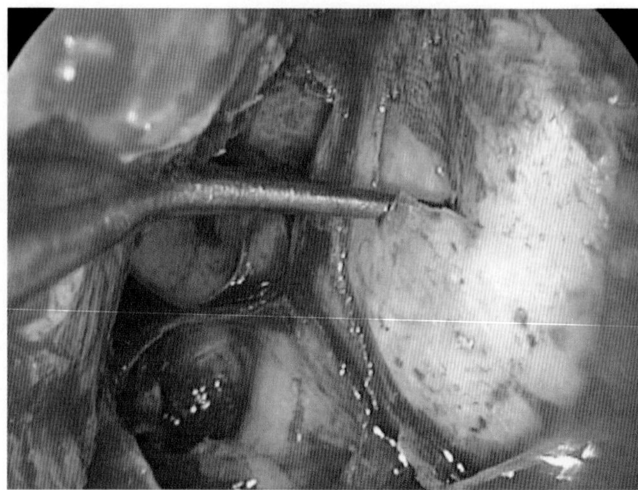

Figure 72-6 Endoscopic view of left nostril showing seeker probe initiating the removal of lamina papyracea.

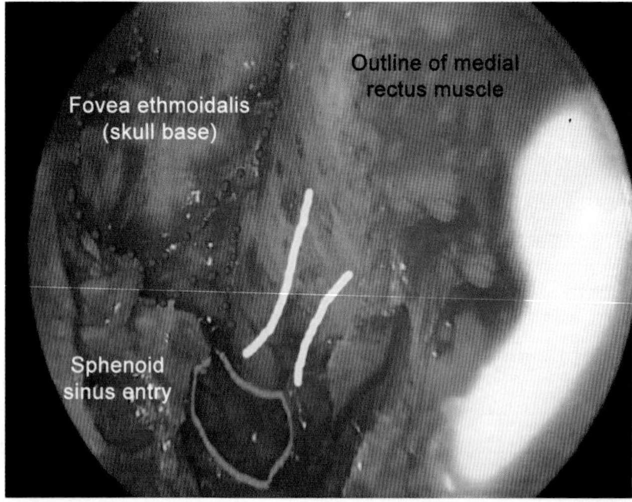


Figure 72-7 Endoscopic view of left nostril showing medial periorbital with a silhouette of medial rectus muscle.

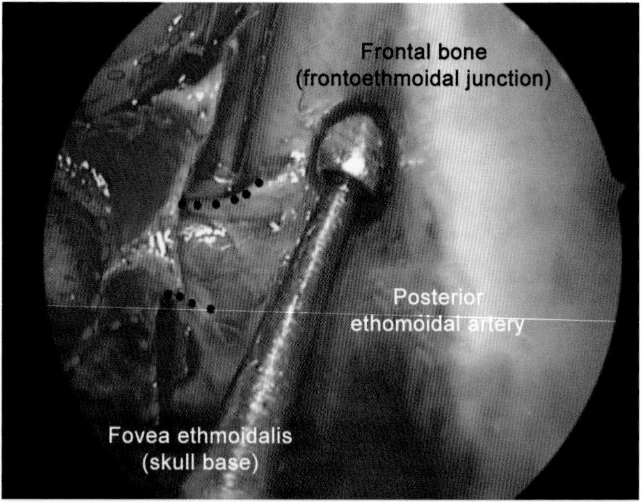


Figure 72-8 Endoscopic view of left nostril showing posterior ethmoidal artery marking the frontoethmoidal junction.

endoscopically through the ethmoid or sphenoid sinus. During transethmoidal approach, complete ethmoidectomy is performed until sphenoid sinus entry; while the sphenoid while the sphenoid ostium may be identified through the superior turbinate with or without a midline posterior bony septoplasty during trans-sphenoidal approach[4] (Fig. 72-14). Once the sphenoid sinus is reached, the medial and lateral optocarotid recesses should be identified, and the location of the optic canal and carotid artery identified and confirmed with navigation system if available (Fig. 72-15). Under endoscopic view, a long-handled diamond burr is used to drill open one segment, typically the middle part of the bony optic canal, with constant irrigation to prevent heat damage to the underlying optic nerve (Fig. 72-16). Once the canal bone is drilled thin, a periosteal elevator is used to peel or elevate the remaining bone away from the optic nerve and sheath. The rest of the bony canal is readily removed with a 1-mm sphenoid rongeur mechanically from the apex toward the chiasm (Fig. 72-17). The optic nerve sheath should be examined for any laceration, particular when there is associated canal fracture (Figs. 72-18 and 72-19). If indicated, the entire length of the optic nerve sheath and the annulus of Zinn are incised with a sickle, crescent knife or a bent 18-gauge needle, exposing the underlying pia matter. Incisions should be shallow, as the

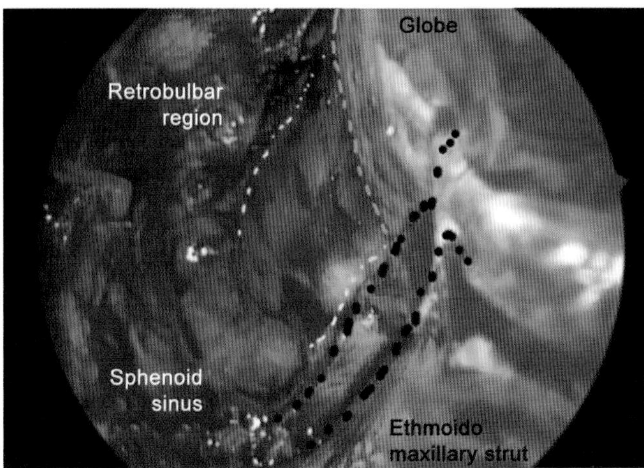


Figure 72-9 Endoscopic view of left nostril showing the intact medial periorbita (yellow) and the outline of the globe (blue) after complete ethmoidectomy, bounded posterior by sphenoid sinus entry (green), and inferiorly by ethmoidomaxillary strut (black).

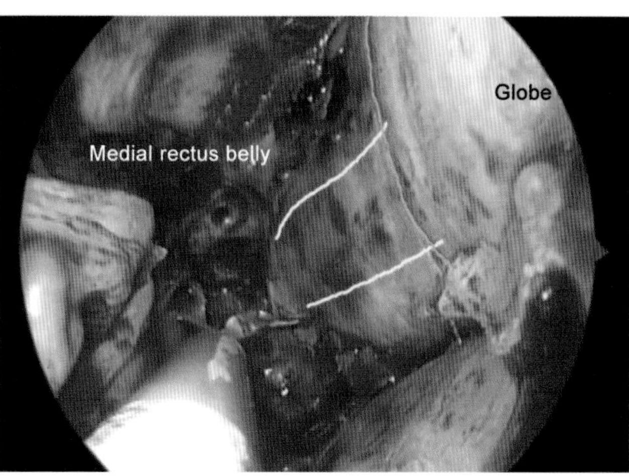


Figure 72-10 Endoscopic view of left nostril showing incision of the medial periorbita along the medially rectus belly silhouette (yellow) with a bent crescent blade.

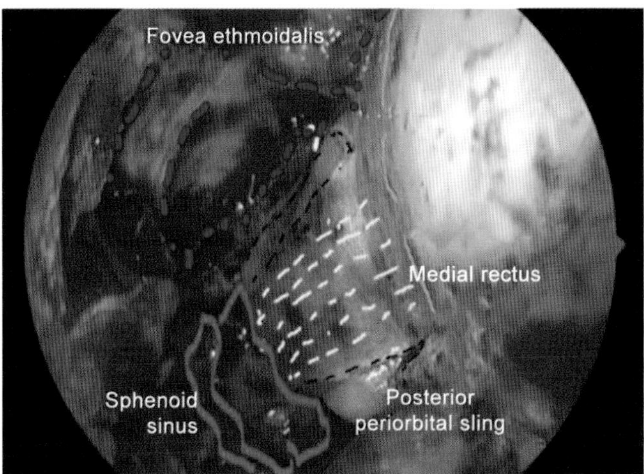


Figure 72-11 Endoscopic view of left nostril showing the periosteal sling (yellow dotted lines) and prolapse of orbital fat (black outline) after initial incisions.

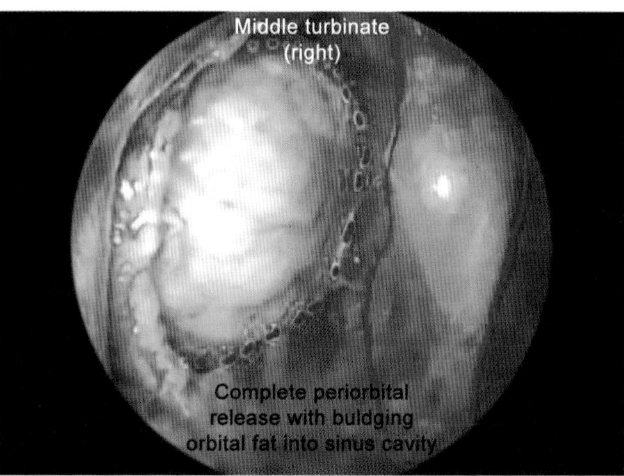


Figure 72-12 Endoscopic view of right nostril showing complete periosteal release the orbital fat prolapsed in the sinus cavity (blue dotted lines). Middle turbinate outlined in red.

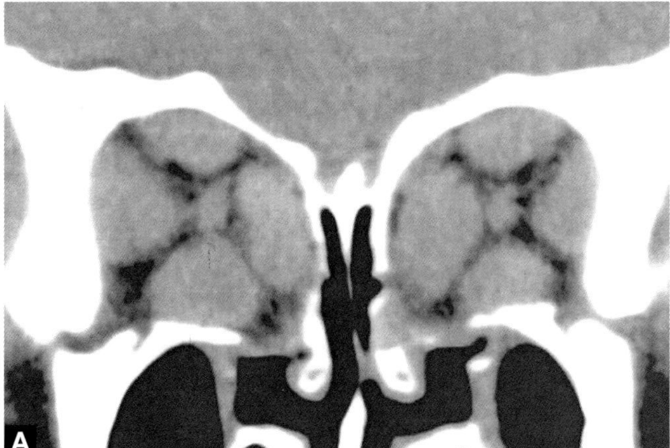


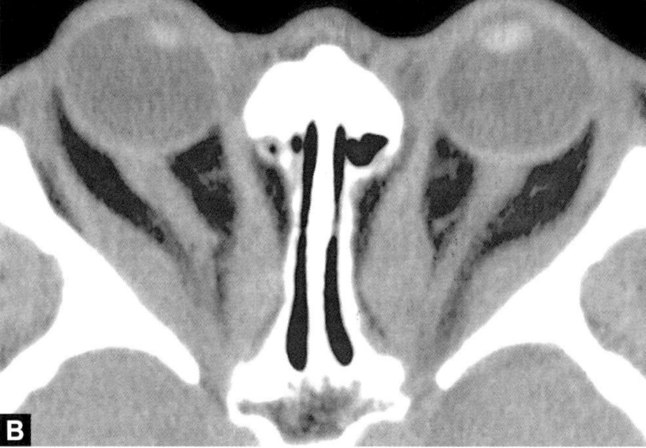


Figures 72-13A and B Postoperative computed tomographic scan of a patient after bilateral endoscopic medial wall decompression for dysthyriod optic neuropathy. Coronal (A) and axial (B) showing complete ethmoidectomy and prolapse of orbital tissues into the sinus cavities.

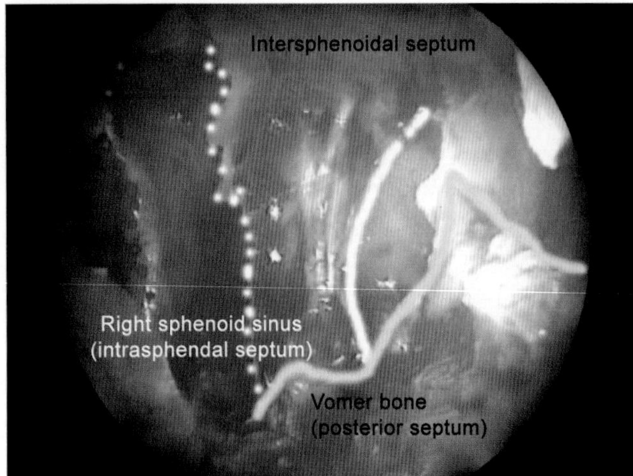


**Figure 72-14** Endoscopic view of right nostril during trans-sphenoidal optic canal decompression. The intrasphenoidal septum within the right sphenoid sinus is highlighted by blue dotted line, whereas the intersphenoidal septum (midline) is highlighted by white line. Part of the posterior nasal septum (vomer bone) has been removed and outlined in yellow.

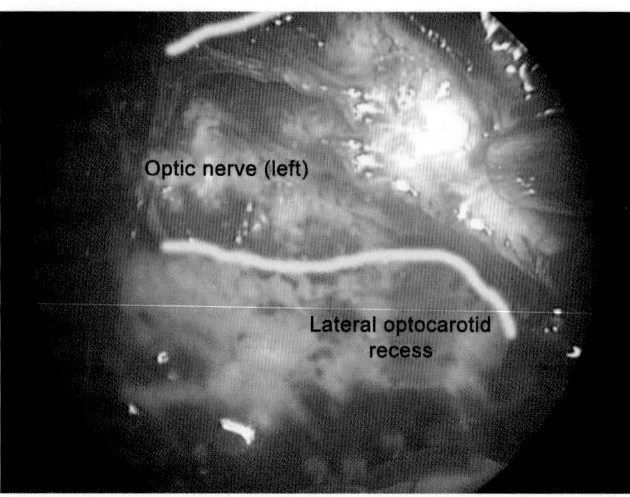


**Figure 72-15** Endoscopic view of left nostril during trans-sphenoidal optic canal decompression. Left optic nerve is outline in yellow and the lateral optocarotid recess is shown. Carotid prominence is at the right lower corner of the figure.

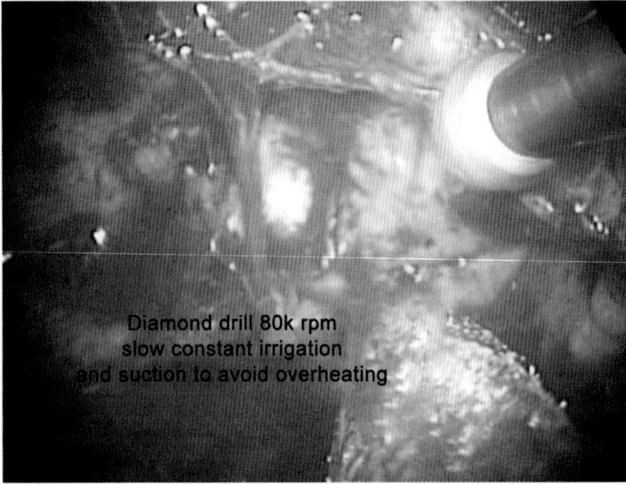


**Figure 72-16** Endoscopic view of left nostril during trans-sphenoidal optic canal decompression showing diamond drill at 80 krpm with constant irrigation to avoid overheating the underlying optic nerve.

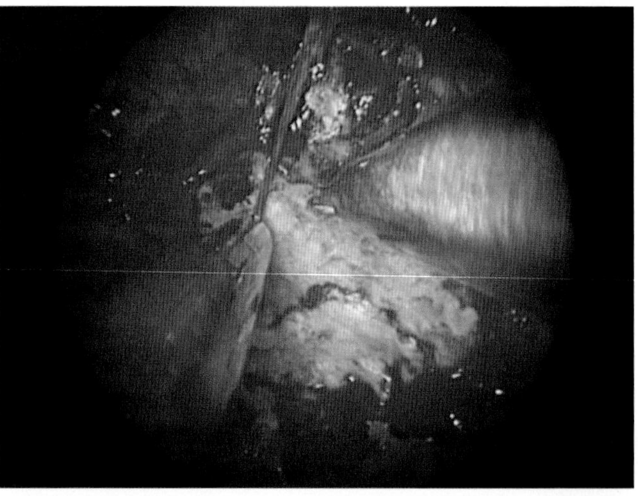

**Figure 72-17** Endoscopic view of left nostril during trans-sphenoidal optic canal decompression. Once a keyhole is made over the middle of the optic canal, the medial aspect of the bony canal can be deskeletonized with 1-mm ronguer mechanically.

superomedial quadrant of the cone is where damage to the inferiorly positioned ophthalmic artery can occur (Figs. 72-20 and 72-21).

## Endonasal Transethmoidal or Endoscope-Assisted Transcaruncular Approach for Medial Wall Fracture Repair[8,9]

Forced-duction test is performed and degree of restriction of medial rectus recorded. An ethmoidectomy is performed as above using transethmoidal approach. Frequent irrigation and gentle pressure on the globe will help differentiating blood clot, bone fragments from prolapsing orbital tissue, the latter should be preserved. Dissection continues posteriorly until the whole fracture is completely exposed. An implant is then inserted through a separate caruncular incision as below.

If the endoscope-assisted, conjunctival approach is contemplated, a curvilinear incision is made either between the skin and caruncle (precaruncle), at the junction of posterior one third of caruncle (transcaruncle) or between the plica and caruncle (retrocaruncle) with scissors and extended into the fornices. A pair of blunt-tipped, Stevens' tenotomy scissors are

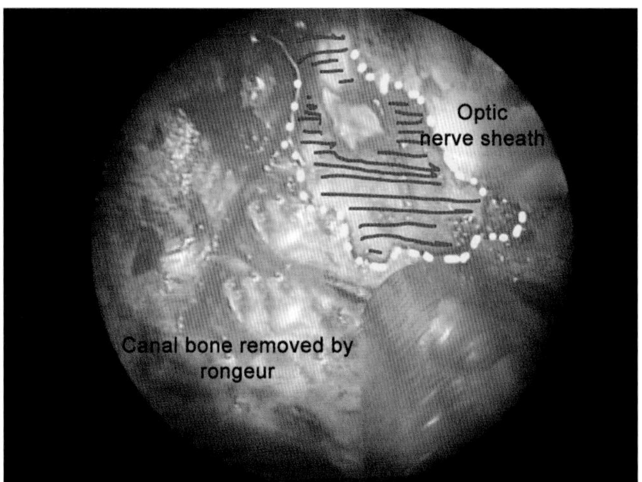


Figure 72-18 Endoscopic view of left nostril during trans-sphenoidal optic canal decompression. A closer look at a segment of the optic canal deskeletonized (yellow dot) showing the underlying optic nerve sheath (blue lines).

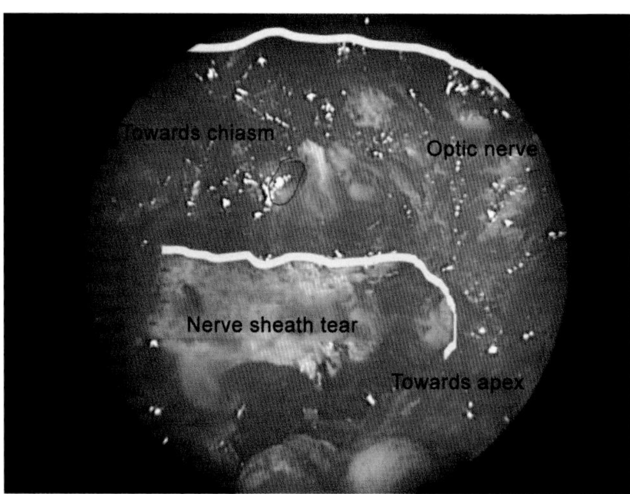


Figure 72-19 Endoscopic view of left nostril during trans-sphenoidal optic canal decompression. At the end of the procedure, the medial aspect of the optic canal is completely deskeletonized from orbital apex toward the chiasm. In this case there is a nerve sheath tear due to the fracture of overlying optic canal bone.

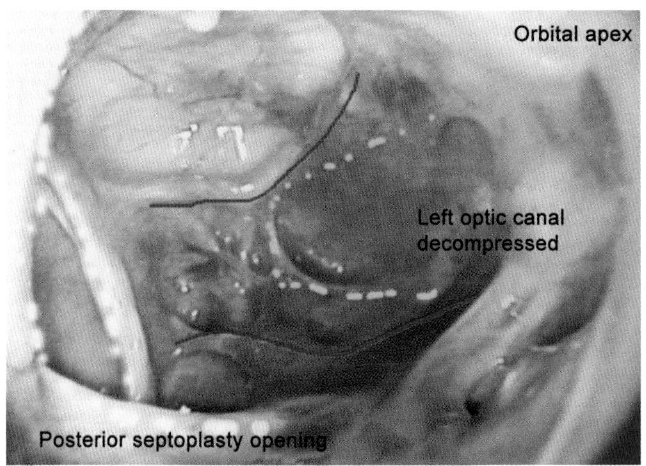


Figure 72-20 Endoscopic view of right nostril after trans-sphenoidal optic canal decompression. Looking through the posterior septoplasty opening the area of decompressed optic canal was mucosalized at post-operative 1 month.

used to palpate the posterior lacrimal crest where the blades are opened and a malleable retractor is inserted posteriorly. Blunt dissection exposes the medial periosteum, which is incised with a cutting monopolar cautery. Subperiosteal cavity is prepared by lifting the periosteum off the medial orbital wall. A 4.0 mm, 0° endoscope is then introduced into the prepared site for manipulation under direct visualization. The dissection is extended to expose the boundaries of the fracture. The assistant retracts gently and laterally the orbital contents using a malleable retractor and wet neuropatties with frequent monitoring of mydriasis (sign of iatrogenic apical compression). Unstable bony fragments should be removed and prolapsed orbital tissues repositioned. The anterior and posterior ethmoidal vessels can be cauterized.

For either approach, surgeons decide on the implant (permanent versus absorbable, smooth versus porous, synthetic versus autologous/allogenic) e.g. thin porous polyethylene sheet can be cut into appropriate size and contoured to fit into the bony defect. Forced-duction test should be repeated before the conjunctival incision is closed with 6-0 absorbable sutures.

## Removal of Orbital Tumor[1-3,10]

### *Extraconal Lesions*

Extraconal lesions located primarily over the medial orbit can be approached via the transethmoidal approach as described above. The amount of lamina papyracea removal or periosteal opening depends on the location of the lesion. Navigational device is helpful to locate the lesion endonasally and limit the amount of dissection. Well circumscribed lesion, e.g. cavernoma can often be bluntly dissected away from the prolapsing orbital fat and the medial rectus.

### *Intraconal Lesions[10]*

Small, purely intraconal lesions may require temporary disinsertion of the medial rectus. Disinsertion may be considered if there is inadequate endonasal retraction of the rectus when the lesion is lateral to the medial rectus. A blunt retractor is inserted endonasally under the inferior border of the posterior medial rectus muscle to retract it superomedially to expose the orbital apex. Alternatively, retraction of the detached muscle is

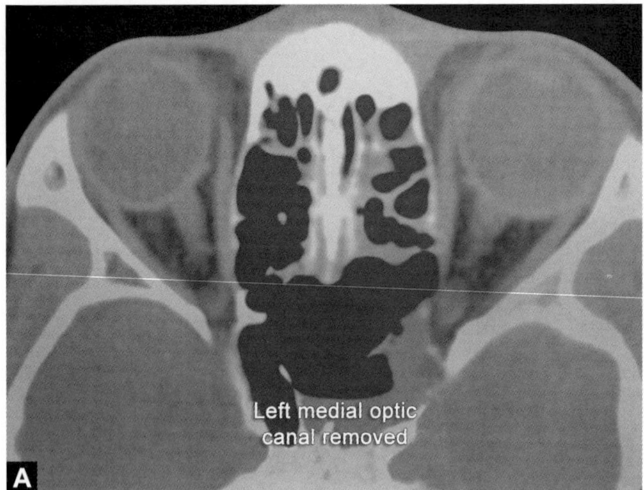


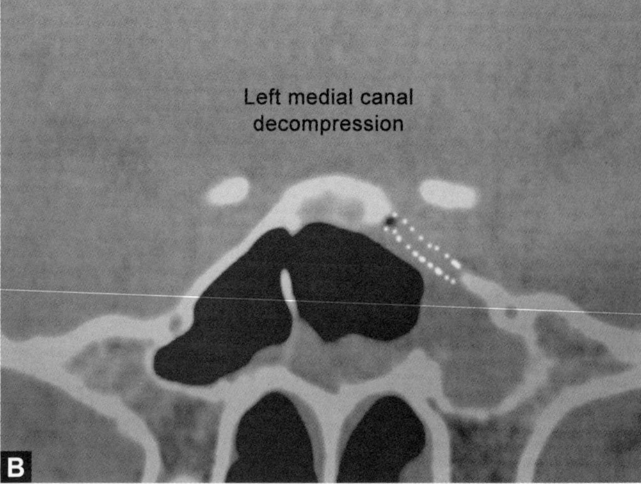


**Figures 72-21A and B** Postoperative computed tomographic orbit scan after left trans-sphenoidal optic canal decompression. Axial (A) and coronal (B) scan showing the removal of medial optic canal (white dotted line).

achieved through a transcaruncular incision using thin malleable retractors or squint hooks, and a 3- or 4-hand surgical technique is used to bluntly dissect out the lesion. After the tumor is removed, the detached medial rectus is sutured back onto the globe. The medial wall can be reconstructed by thin sheet of medpor implant similar to a fracture repair.

### Inferior Orbitotomy—Transantral Approach[11]

An upper gingivobuccal sulcus incision is made on the lesion side. Subperiosteal plane is entered and the ION should be identified and preserved while an antrostomy window is created through the anterior wall of maxillary sinus, using a cutting drill then enlarge using rongeur. Both 0° and 30° endoscopes are used to examine the fracture and the posterior edge of the fracture will be readily visualized, as with the intraorbital portion of the ION and the inferior orbital fissure (Fig. 72-22). Mucosal and bony fragments are removed similar to medial wall fracture repair. An implant of choice can then be inserted through a transconjunctival or swinging eyelid approach (Figs. 72-23 and 72-24). The gingivobuccal incision is closed with interrupted 4-0 Vicryl (absorbable) sutures.

The above approach can be adopted for additional inferior wall orbital decompression (lateral to the ION) or removal of lesions located in the posterior part of inferior orbit.

## MECHANISM OF ACTION

Endoscopic orbital surgery has the advantage of an illuminated, magnified view through paranasal sinuses or subperiosteal cavities. When dissecting from outside the orbit (i.e. through sinuses), it also avoids pressure on the orbital apex during deep retraction, which may be beneficial in cases with compromised optic nerve function (e.g. DON).

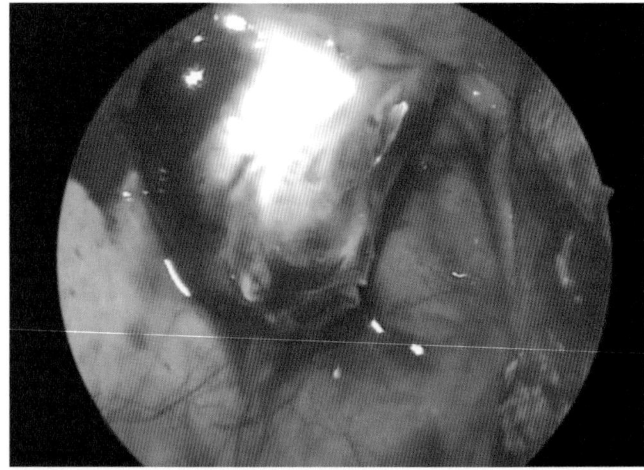

**Figure 72-22** Transantral endoscopic view of the right blowout fracture (day 7 post-injury). Evidence of orbital tissue prolapse, bony fragments, resolving hematoma and mucosal healing.

## POSTOPERATIVE CARE

Patients are nursed in reverse Trendelenburg position to minimize venous congestion. They should be offered frequent ice packs over the eyes and are instructed to avoid nose blowing to prevent surgical emphysema when sinuses are entered. Gentle saline douching may be started when epistaxis stops with topical nasal steroid spray similar to post-FESS care. Air travel should be avoided within 6 weeks. Postoperative antibiotics and systemic steroid may be given according

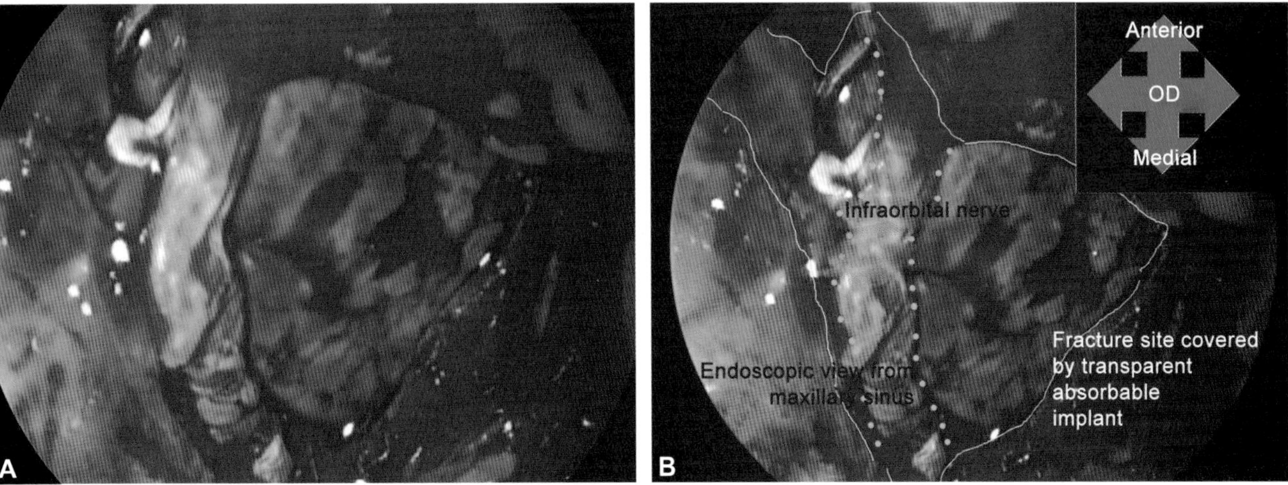


**Figures 72-23A and B** (A) Transantral endoscopic view of the right blowout fracture post-reduction and absorbable (transparent) implant insertion. (B) The fracture is outlined in yellow while the infraorbital nerve in blue dotted line. The prolapsed orbital tissue was reduced, and the defect was covered by a thin sheet of transparent absorbable implant.

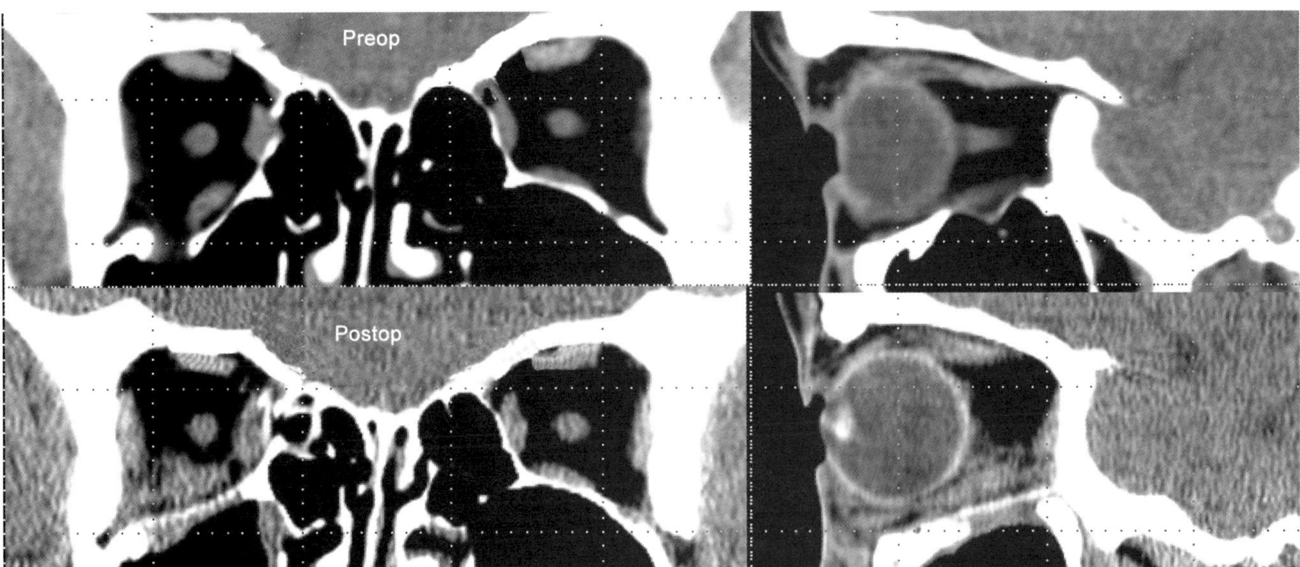


**Figure 72-24** Preoperative (above) and postoperative (below) computed tomographic scan of the same patient of Figures 72.21 and 72.22 showing reduction of orbital fracture, repositioning of prolapsed orbital tissue and replacement of orbital defect with implant in coronal (left) and axial (right) scans.

to the operative indications (e.g. dysthyriod optic neuropathy), as well as the amount of swelling anticipated. Visual acuity and pupillary reaction should be monitored as in standard orbital surgeries.

## SPECIFIC INSTRUMENTATION

In the authors' institute, the operating surgeon holds the endoscope and stands on the right side of the patient. In transsphenoidal approach, surgeon may operate bimanually through both nostrils and a lens holder is used. Video screen should be positioned along the visual axis of the operating surgeon while navigation device is positioned over the head side of the patient.

Most surgeries are performed with a 0°, 4-mm endoscope. Oblique-viewing (30°, 45°, 75°) endoscopes are helpful in visualizing the lateral aspect, anterior floor (transantral), or frontal region during superior orbitotomy. Endonasal instruments (e.g. monopolar/bipolar cautery, burr, ronguer) are long handled, with sheath cover to avoid mucosal damage. Thin malleable or long-blade retractors are also important during deep orbital retraction.

## COMPLICATIONS

General complications include bleeding (epistaxis, retrobulbar hemorrhage), infection (sinusitis, orbital cellulitis), nasolacrimal injury, cerebrospinal fluid leak, injury to the extraocular muscles, vessels, oculomotor, ciliary, and optic nerves. Below are complications specific to each indication.

- Orbital decompression:
  - Diplopia
    - Commonest with isolated floor > combined medial and floor with anterior strut removal > anterior strut-sparing medial and floor decompression > combined medial and lateral wall > isolated lateral wall > fat removal decompression.
  - Infraorbital hypoesthesia (floor decompression).
- Orbital fracture repair:
  - Persistent enophthalmos, diplopia, implant-related complications (migration, infection, peri-implant hemorrhage and fibrosis).
- Traumatic optic neuropathy:
  - Carotid artery injury—stroke and uncontrolled bleeding.

## SURGICAL OUTCOMES: SCIENTIFIC EVIDENCE/ META-ANALYSIS

The Cochrane review of surgical orbital decompression for thyroid eye disease demonstrated that there was limited conclusion to be drawn from only two randomized controlled trials that were studied.[12] The reviewers could not recommend any particular intervention for orbital decompression in thyroid eye disease due to the diversity of methodology used. Techniques to reduce proptosis were comparable. Comparing surgical three-wall decompression versus methylprednisolone pulsed therapy for DON, current uncontrolled studies suggest that balance decompression by removing medial and lateral wall with or without fat removal may be the most effective surgical method and is associated with fewer side effects.

## PLACE OF THE TECHNIQUE IN SURGICAL ARMAMENTARIUM

Endoscopic and combined open and endoscopic (endoscopic-assisted) techniques for decompression, fracture repair, removal of orbital lesions, and foreign bodies have been increasingly reported in the literature. However, orbital surgeons should be aware of the distinct advantages and inherent limitations of endoscope use in the orbit. On the other hand, contemporary oculofacial surgeons should be comfortable operating with endoscope, often built on prior experience in endoscopic dacryocystorhinostomies and forehead lifts. Finally, orbital surgeons should be familiar with sinonasal sinonasal, and to an extent, intracranial anatomies, in a way similar to sinus or neurosurgeons that operate in the orbits.

## REFERENCES


1. Murchison AP, Rosen MR, Evans JJ, et al. Endoscopic approach to the orbital apex and periorbital skull base. Laryngoscope. 2011; 121:463-7.
2. Tsirbas A, Kazim M, Close L. Endoscopic approach to orbital apex lesions. Ophthal Plast Reconstr Surg. 2005;21(4):271-5.
3. Prabhakaran VC, Selva D. Orbital endoscopic surgery. Indian J Ophthalmol. 2008;56(1): 5-8.
4. Pletcher SD, Sindwani R, Metson R. Endoscopic orbital and optic nerve decompression. Otolaryngol Clin North Am. 2006; 39(5):943-58.
5. Karaki M, Akiyama K, Kagawa M, et al. Indications and limitations of endoscopic endonasal orbitotomy for orbital lesion. J Craniofac Surg. 2012;23(4):1093-6.
6. Bhargava D, Sankhla D, Ganesan A, et al. Endoscopic sinus surgery for orbital subperiosteal abscess secondary to sinusitis. Rhinology. 2001;39(3):151-5.
7. Levin LA, Beck RW, Joseph MP, et al. The treatment of traumatic optic neuropathy: the International Optic Nerve Trauma Study. Ophthalmology. 1999;106(7):1268-77.
8. Wu W, Jing W, Selva D, et al. Endoscopic transcaruncular repair of large medial orbital wall fractures near the orbital apex. Ophthalmology. 2013;120(2):404-9.
9. Han K, Choi JH, Choi TH, et al. Comparison of endoscopic endonasal reduction and transcaruncular reduction for the treatment of medial orbital wall fractures. Ann Plast Surg. 2009; 62(3):258-64.
10. Wu W, Selva D, Jiang F, et al. Endoscopic transethmoidal approach with or without medial rectus detachment for orbital apical cavernous hemangiomas. Am J Ophthalmol. 2013;156(3): 593-9.
11. Ducic Y, Verret DJ. Endoscopic transantral repair of orbital floor fractures. Otolaryngol Head Neck Surg. 2009;140(6): 849-54.
12. Boboridis KG, Bunce C. Surgical orbital decompression for thyroid eye disease. Cochrane Database Syst Rev. 2011;(12): CD007630.

CHAPTER

73

# Orbital Blowout Fractures

Rakesh M Patel, Allen M Putterman

## INTRODUCTION

Orbital fractures are due to blunt force trauma applied to the orbit. Frequently, there is concern for a concurrent globe injury as well, and therefore, ophthalmology is oftentimes the initial service consulted for evaluation of these patients. It is essential the ophthalmic surgeon understand the key principles that determine if the patient needs surgical repair or if observation is in order for the patient.

## EVALUATION

The first step in examining a patient that has suffered orbital trauma is to evaluate the globe for injury. This includes performing a complete ophthalmic examination including a dilated fundoscopic examination. In particular, one must carefully assess the globe for rupture or retinal tears/detachments as these require urgent treatment and take precedence over the fractures. Critical elements of the examination to evaluate for an orbital fracture include assessing diplopia, extraocular motility, enophthalmos, hypo-ophthalmus, infraorbital nerve sensation, and palpable orbital rim step-off. In addition, dental malocclusion or pain with opening of the jaw should be assessed as this may be indicative of a zygomaticomaxillary complex fracture.

Restricted extraocular movements after blunt trauma may be secondary to hemorrhage and edema of the orbital soft tissues, entrapment of orbital soft tissue or extraocular muscle in a fracture site, or paresis of an extraocular muscle. Decreased sensation to the midface, upper lip, and gums on the side of injury is consistent with injury to the infraorbital nerve. Hypo-ophthalmus may result from the globe sinking inferiorly into the maxillary sinus from an orbital floor fracture.

In patients suspected of orbital fracture, computed tomographic (CT) scan is valuable in assessment of the bony architecture of the orbit. Both coronal and axial cuts of the orbit should be evaluated to define the extent of the orbital fracture. Occasionally, magnetic resonance imaging (MRI) may be obtained to evaluate for soft tissue entrapment in a fracture defect that may not have been well visualized on CT scan.

## PATHOPHYSIOLOGY

An orbital blowout fracture is by definition a fracture of the orbital walls with the orbital rims remaining intact. There are two prominent theories to explain why an orbital blowout fracture occurs. In the hydraulic theory, the traumatic force is transmitted to the orbital contents increasing the intraorbital pressure. The weakest portions of the orbit, the orbital floor and the medial wall, will then fracture.[1] The maxillary and ethmoid sinuses act like a pressure valve, ultimately absorbing the force of trauma. In the buckling theory, traumatic force is applied directly to the orbital rims, which is transmitted through the bone to the thinner orbital walls resulting in a fracture of these walls.[2] It has been shown that both mechanisms likely play a role in blowout fractures.[3]

## INDICATIONS

Indications for surgical repair of an orbital blowout fracture have been historically controversial. Many advocated early repair of fractures due to concerns of the patient developing enophthalmos and diplopia.[4,5] Others prefer a more conservative approach as there is often spontaneous improvement without intervention.[6-9] While the decision to decide whether to repair the fracture early has become easier with improved

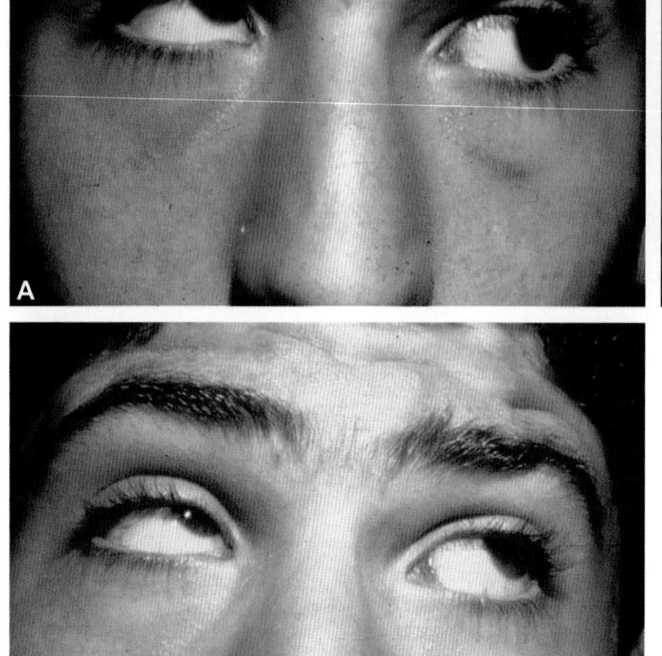

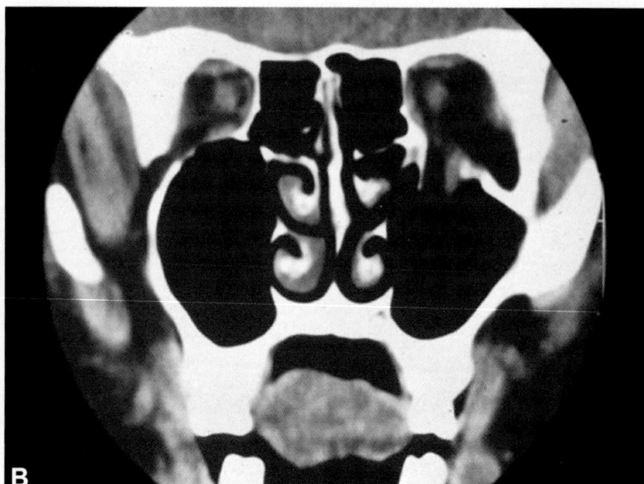

**Figures 73-1A to C** Orbital floor fracture. (A) Inability to elevate the left eye after blunt trauma. (B) Computed tomographic scan reveals herniated inferior rectus muscle into the orbital floor fracture defect. (C) After floor fracture repair with supramid implant. Note improved elevation of left eye.

imaging modalities, there certainly are a segment of patients where the decision is not so straightforward. We describe our practice pattern in managing patients with orbital blowout fractures below.

## Early Treatment

In patients who present with an orbital fracture, there are clinical signs that would indicate surgery is in order. Two primary indications that surgery should be performed early include: (1) The patient has severe enophthalmos or hypo-ophthalmos that is cosmetically unacceptable or (2) the patient has severe diplopia that is visually intolerable and does not improve over time, has a positive forced duction test, and imaging evidence of extraocular muscle entrapment exists (Figs. 73.1A to C).[6] For this patient population, surgery should be performed as soon as possible, waiting no > 2–3 weeks. If the aforementioned findings are not present then one should observe these patients over the next few months.[6-9] Many patients may present with a large orbital blowout fracture without the above findings on initial examination. Although aware that some physicians will advise surgical repair in this setting due to concerns of the patient developing subsequent enophthalmos, we believe one cannot accurately predict whether a patient will develop this complication based upon the fracture size alone. Therefore, we still advocate observing patients with such large fractures that have minimal enophthalmos and hypo-ophthalmos.

A white-eyed blowout fracture with entrapment of the inferior rectus muscle in the pediatric population is an entirely different entity that requires a different management strategy.[10] Please refer to section "White-Eyed Blowout Fracture" for further discussion.

### *Enophthalmos/Hypo-Ophthalmos*

Enophthalmos is a rare finding in the acute setting of trauma as the orbital tissues are typically edematous preventing retrograde movement of the globe. Therefore, the patient needs to be followed closely over the subsequent weeks to determine if the patient is developing severe enophthalmos, which is an indication for surgery. The amount of enophthalmos present in a patient can be formally measured using a Hertel exophthalmometer.

Hypo-ophthalmos may occur with a large orbital floor fracture where the globe descends into the maxillary sinus. As with enophthalmos, this finding may not be evident in the acute setting due to swollen orbital tissues although a severe case of acute hypo-ophthalmos after trauma has been reported that required urgent repair.[11,12] Again, we follow these patients over the next few weeks to determine if the patient is developing significant globe descent. To measure hypo-ophthalmos, we align the long edge of a ruler with the medial canthi of both eyes and note where the ruler bisects the globe. The physician can then assess if one globe is inferiorly displaced relative to the other.

If enophthalmos or hypo-ophthalmus present early and is unacceptable to the patient, early surgical repair of the fracture is advised. To make the assessment in a timely fashion, we prescribe steroids to the patient if no contraindication is present. This will speed up the resolution of the orbital edema and therefore narrow the window to determine if the patient needs surgery.[13]

## *Diplopia*

The other primary indication for early surgical repair is intolerable diplopia. Many patients in the acute setting of an orbital fracture have diplopia. Putterman et al. hypothesized this frequently occurs due to the edematous or hemorrhagic orbital fat being entrapped into the fracture site.[9] Whitnall previously noted there are vertical fibrous bands that connect the inferior extraocular muscles to the posterior–inferior orbital fat and periosteum.[14] Koornneef elaborated further stating the entire orbital connective tissue and adipose tissue complex play a vital role in extraocular motility.[15,16] It is this inferior tissue that may be "stuck" in the fracture defect of the floor preventing adequate movement of the globe and causing diplopia in the acute setting. Putterman et al. showed this diplopia frequently improved over time to a point where it was no longer visually disturbing to the patient.[9] Potential reasons for why this improvement occurs is resolution of the orbital fat edema and hemorrhage or stretching of the orbital fat. To this end, we again prescribe steroids in the acute setting to help speed up the resolution of the edema and/or hemorrhage in hopes of resolving the double vision.[13] However, if diplopia is truly secondary to an entrapped extraocular muscle, the steroids are unlikely to work in which case surgery is warranted.

A great tool in assessing diplopia is forced ductions and forced generations. These tests help determine if the diplopia is paretic versus restrictive in nature. After instillation of topical anesthetic drops, a cotton-tipped applicator soaked in 4% lidocaine is applied to the inferior limbus for 1 minute. A toothed forceps then grasps the episcleral limbus at this position and attempts to move the eye up and down. If there is difficulty in movement, this may be indicative of entrapped orbital tissue or extraocular muscle and therefore considered a positive forced duction test. A forced generation test is performed by asking the patient to look up or down while holding the episcleral limbus with toothed forceps. If there is significant tension on the forceps, this is considered a negative test. However, if there is minimal pull to the forceps, the test is considered positive and the patient may have a paretic muscle. For a medial wall fracture that is concerning for entrapment, 4% lidocaine may instead be applied to the nasal limbus and forced ductions/generations are once again performed in a similar fashion.

Another essential tool is the CT scan. Coronal cuts of the orbit are particularly valuable to assess if the extraocular muscle is entrapped in the fracture defect. If an entrapped extraocular muscle is not evident on CT scan yet the suspicion remains for entrapment, MRI is occasionally useful as it may better delineate the soft tissue herniating into the fracture defect (Figs. 73.2A to C).

## *Management*

It is the findings from the above examination tools that best determine the course of management. If the patient has disabling diplopia that is not improving on steroids over a 2- to 3-week period or unacceptable enophthalmos or hypo-ophthalmos develops, early surgical repair of the fracture is advocated.[6] This is further supported by positive forced duction testing with a negative forced generation and radiographic evidence of extraocular muscle entrapment. Meanwhile, if the diplopia does improve or resolve without objectionable enophthalmos and hypo-ophthalmos, observation is warranted. This is further supported by negative forced ductions, positive forced generations, and no radiographic evidence of muscle entrapment.[6]

## *Surgical Technique*

If surgery is pursued, our preference is to repair the orbital floor fracture with a lateral canthotomy/cantholysis and a

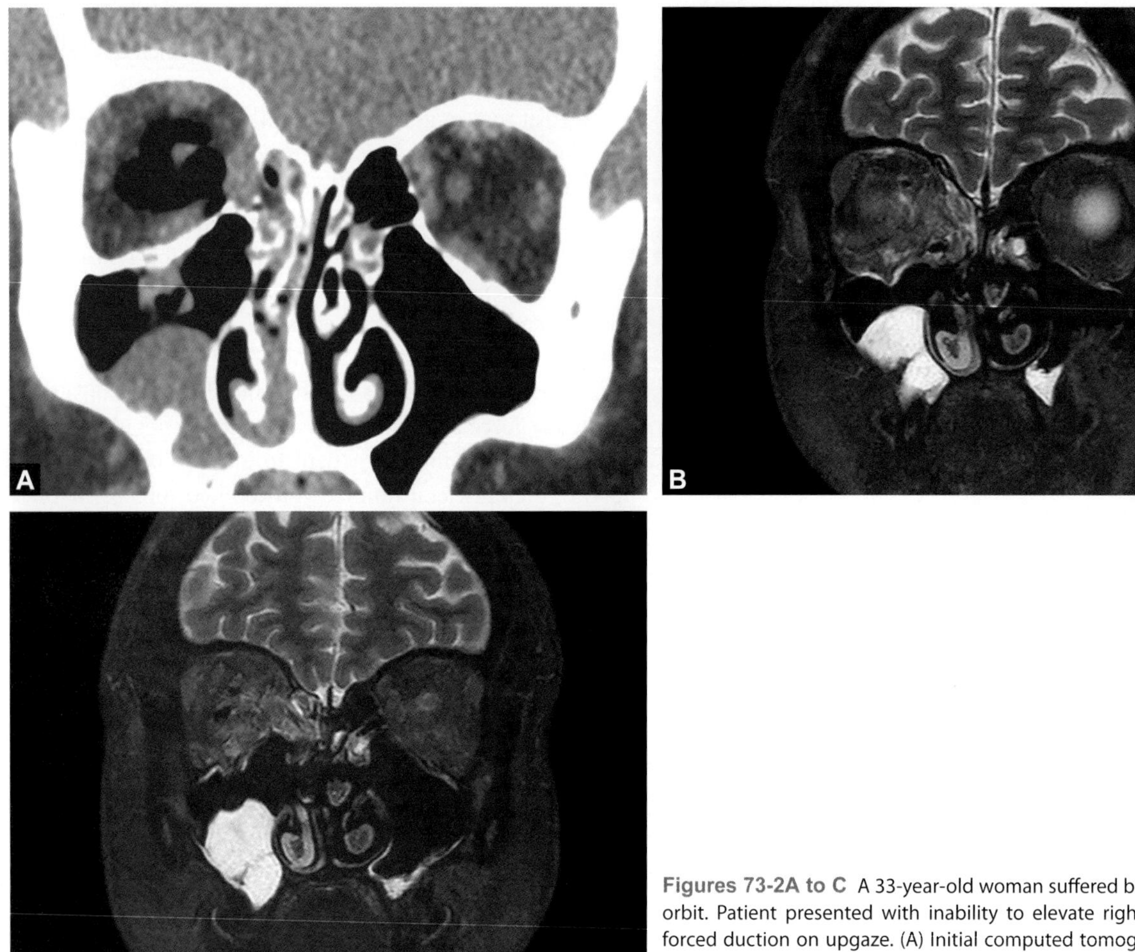

**Figures 73-2A to C** A 33-year-old woman suffered blunt trauma to right orbit. Patient presented with inability to elevate right eye with positive forced duction on upgaze. (A) Initial computed tomographic scan read as medial wall fracture only. (B and C) Magnetic resonance imaging revealed orbital soft tissue herniated into the orbital floor fracture defect.

transconjunctival dissection to the orbital rim under general anesthesia.[6] After a subperiosteal dissection into the orbital floor, the entire rim of the fracture defect is identified and the orbital contents are released from the fracture defect. An orbital floor implant, such as a silastic implant, is then placed and fixated in a previously described technique where the anterior tongue of the implant is inserted into the fracture site.[17,18] If the fracture defect is much larger, a titanium implant covered with silastic is frequently used, which may be fixated to the inferior orbital rim with drill holes and a 4-0 Prolene suture.

If a medial wall fracture requires repair, two primary surgical approaches are utilized. The transcaruncular approach provides adequate exposure of the medial orbital wall without leaving a scar.[18,19] The Lynch incision may also be utilized to access the medial wall providing even greater exposure[20]; however, it frequently leaves unsightly scars. Our implant material of choice is typically either silastic or titanium.

## Late Treatment

Late treatment of orbital fractures is indicated in patients with diplopia that, although improved initially, did not entirely resolve and remain visually handicapping or objectionable enophthalmos or hypo-ophthalmos developed. After 5–6 weeks from the initial date of trauma, we find orbital fracture surgery to have less than desirable outcomes.[6] Therefore, in these patients, we prefer alternative modalities of treatment to improve functional and/or aesthetic outcome.

### *Enophthalmos/Hypo-Ophthalmos*

If there is significant hypo-ophthalmos, a custom made silastic orbital floor implant is placed using a similar technique to the orbital fracture repair (Figs. 73.3A and B).[21] The implant thickness will be determined by the degree of preoperative hypo-ophthalmos. Typically, the implant will be 2–3-mm

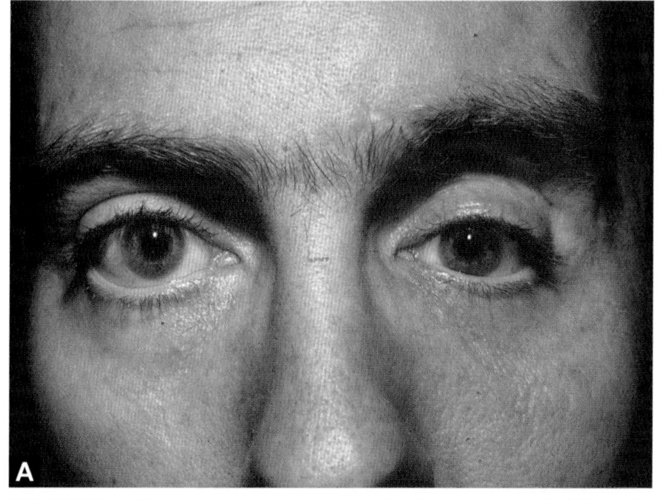


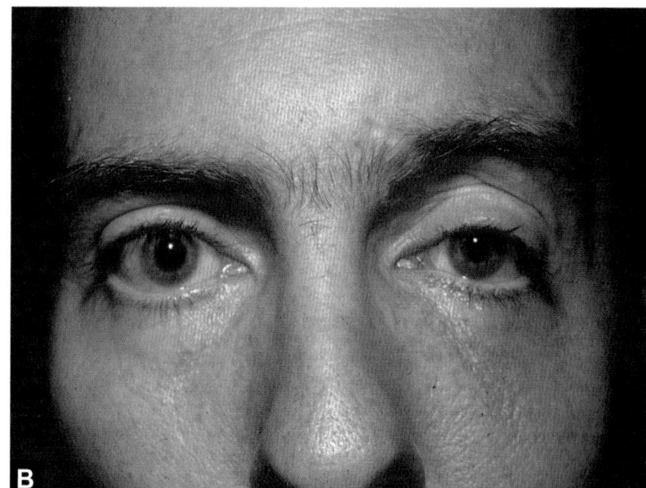


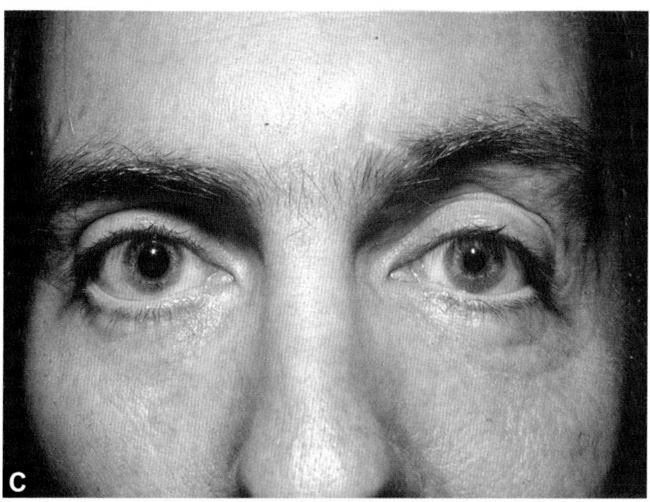


**Figures 73-3A to C** Orbital floor fracture. (A) Note the hypo-ophthalmos and ptosis on the left. (B) After late repair of fracture with custom silastic orbital floor implant; hypo-ophthalmos is improved but ptosis remains. (C) After conjunctival Mueller's muscle resection on the left.

thick anteriorly transitioning to 6–10-mm thick posteriorly. The implant will be fixated to the orbital rim as previously described.

If enophthalmos is associated with a narrow palpebral fissure and a decreased margin-to-reflex distance-1 (MRD-1), we advocate performing a Mueller's muscle-conjunctival resection ptosis procedure (MMCR, Figure 73.3C).[22,23] Briefly, one drop of 10% phenylephrine is instilled into the upper fornix with the patient in a supine position. After approximately 5 minutes, if the patient's eyelid elevates to a suitable level that the patient likes, an MMCR is performed. This will create an illusion that both eyes appear symmetric and therefore mask the enophthalmos.

If enophthalmos is present with a normal palpebral fissure, but the patient has a deep supratarsal sulcus of the upper eyelid or hollowing of the lower eyelid, a contralateral blepharoplasty may be performed with the goal again being to achieve a symmetric appearance of the eyes (Figs. 73.4A and B). For the upper eyelid, this may be performed by removing the skin, orbicularis, and fat while creating a higher eyelid crease. For the lower lid, this may be completed through a transconjunctival blepharoplasty with debulking of the lower eyelid fat pads. These techniques will mask the enophthalmos, creating a more pleasing aesthetic appearance for the patient.

## Diplopia

Diplopia is most bothersome in primary gaze and in the reading position of downgaze. For a patient with an orbital fracture and bothersome diplopia that although initially improving but did not completely resolve, strabismus surgery is preferred. In our experience, we have primarily encountered the need to perform such surgeries in orbital floor fractures. The type of surgery will depend on the type of strabismus and is not to be performed until the diplopia measurements stabilize. For patients with difficulty looking down but who have a

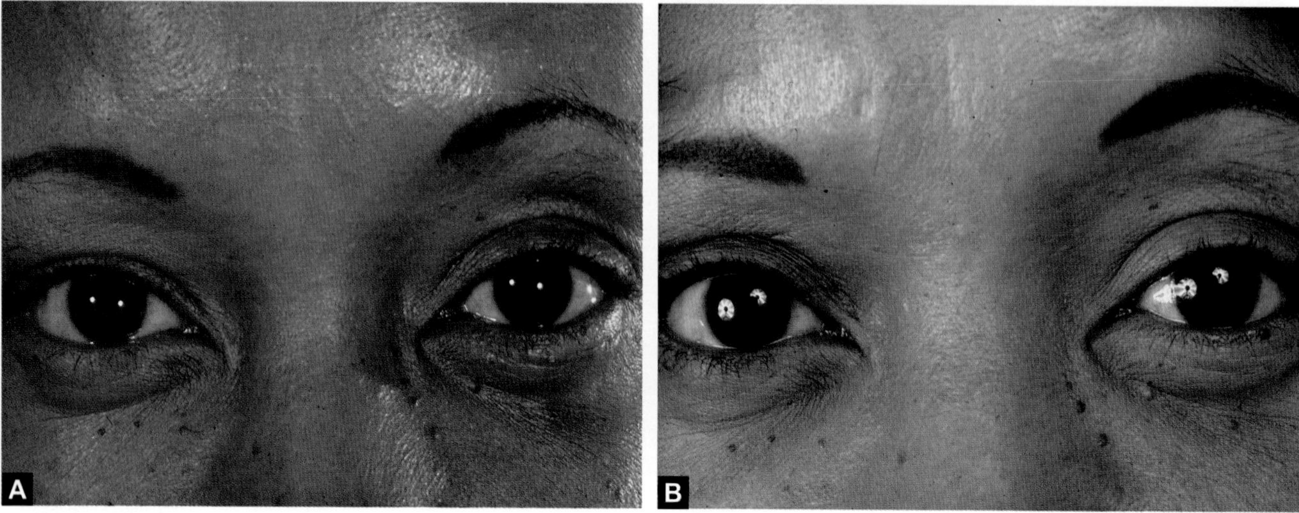


**Figures 73-4A and B** (A) Left orbital floor fracture – note enophthalmos and deepened supratarsal sulcus of the left upper eyelid. (B) After right upper eyelid blepharoplasty – note improved symmetry of the upper eyelids.

negative forced duction on upgaze, a modified reverse Knapp procedure is performed by transposing the medial and lateral rectus muscles posterior to the inferior rectus muscle insertion. If the forced duction is positive on upgaze, an inferior rectus muscle recession on an adjustable suture is performed. After several months, this is followed by a modified reverse Knapp procedure.[6] We find this to be more successful in resolving the diplopia as opposed to performing a late repair of the orbital floor fracture.

## WHITE-EYED BLOWOUT FRACTURE

Pediatric patients with a white-eyed blowout fracture require an entirely different management strategy altogether. These patients are typically young with minimal external signs of trauma that developed a severe motility deficit after injury. Jordan et al. eloquently described the criteria to diagnose a white-eyed blowout fracture after blunt trauma: (1) patients < 18 years of age, (2) minimal soft-tissue signs of injury, (3) significant motility restriction, (4) no enophthalmos, and (5) minimal to no fracture on radiographic scan.[10] For these patients, it is advocated that surgical repair should be performed urgently within 1–2 days (Figs. 73.5A to D). If the patient also has severe nausea and vomiting or symptomatic bradycardia, this may indicate an oculocardiac reflex secondary to extraocular muscle entrapment and could require emergent treatment.[24] Intraoperatively, a trapdoor fracture may be visualized where the fractured bone snapped back into near-normal anatomic position with incarcerated tissue.[25] If the repair is not performed in a timely manner, muscle ischemia may result leading to permanent motility deficits.[26]

## CONCLUSION

Orbital blowout fractures are a common entity that presents to the ophthalmologist. Frequently, it is obvious when surgery is necessary and when it is not. For patients with evidence of entrapment on imaging, diplopia that is not improving, and positive forced duction testing, early surgical repair of the fracture is advocated within 2–3 weeks or sooner. Similarly, early surgical intervention is advised for patients with unacceptable enophthalmos or hypo-ophthalmos. For patients without diplopia and those who exhibit no signs of enophthalmos or hypo-ophthalmos, observation is warranted.

However, there is a subset of patients where the decision to operate or not is much more challenging. For patients with diplopia acutely after trauma that is improving, further observation is warranted for up to 1–3 months. However, if the diplopia fails to completely resolve after this time frame and remains visually disturbing, strabismus surgery is offered to the patient. For patients who develop late hypo-ophthalmos, a silastic orbital floor implant may be placed to elevate the globe. If the patient develops late enophthalmos with a decreased MRD-1, an MMCR may be performed on the affected side. Instead, if the enophthalmos is associated with a deep supratarsal sulcus or lower eyelid hollowing, a contralateral blepharoplasty may be performed. Finally, a white-eyed blowout fracture is an entirely different entity that requires urgent treatment to prevent permanent motility deficits.

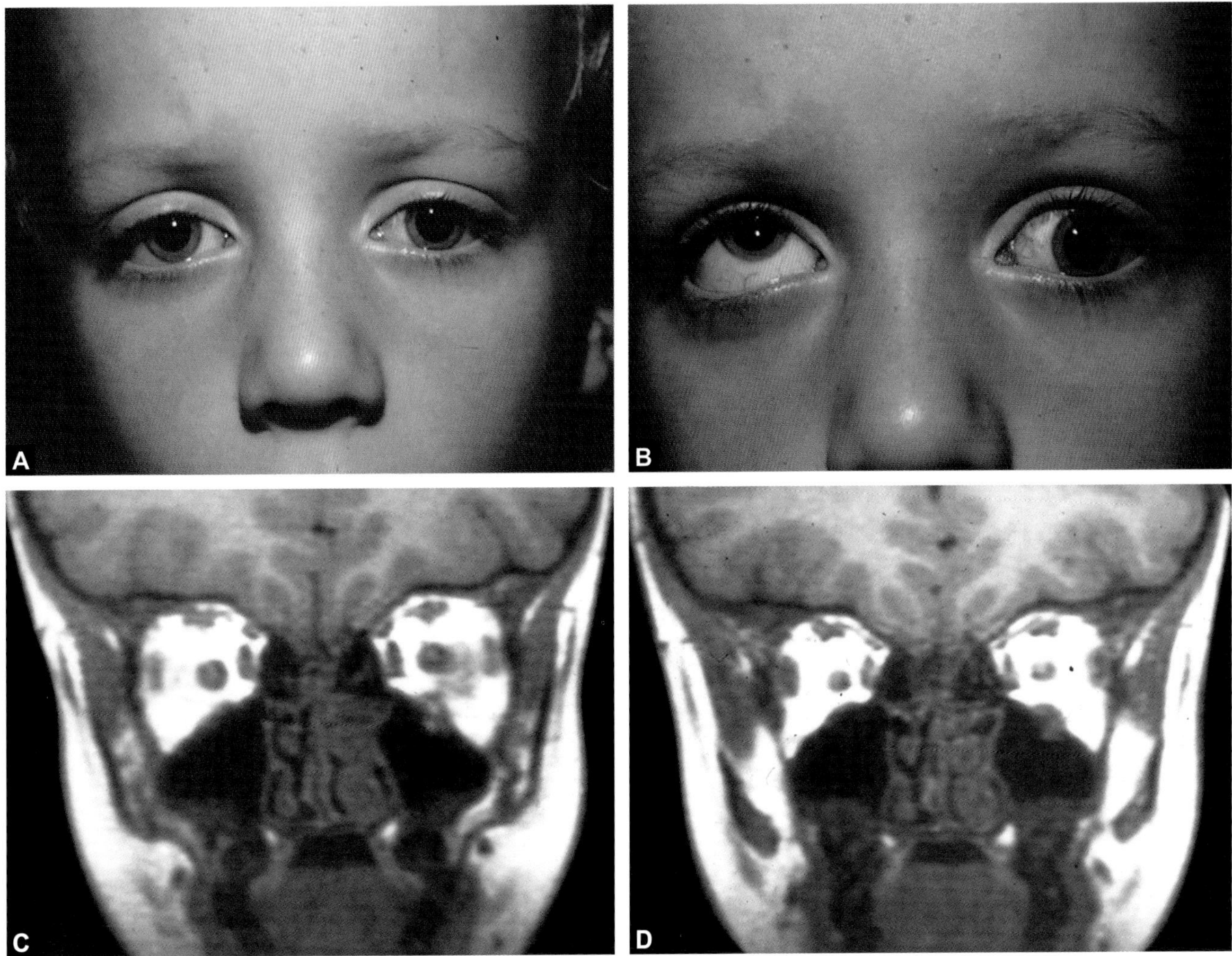


**Figures 73-5A to D** White-eyed blowout fracture. (A) Patient is orthophoric in primary gaze. (B) Patient is unable to elevate the left eye. (C and D) Magnetic resonance imaging of the same patient. Note herniation of the inferior rectus muscle into the fracture defect of the left orbital floor.

## REFERENCES


1. Smith B, Regan WR. Blow-out fractures of the orbit. Am J Ophthalmol. 1957;44(6):733-9.
2. Fujino T, Makino K. Entrapment mechanisms and ocular injury in orbital blowout fracture. Plast Reconstr Surg. 1980;65(5):571-6.
3. Warwar RE, Bullock JD, Ballal DR, et al. Mechanisms of orbital floor fractures: a clinical, experimental, and theoretical study. Ophthal Plast Reconstr Surg. 2000;16(3):188-200.
4. Smith B, Converse JM. Early treatment of orbital floor fractures. Trans Am Acad Ophthalmol Otolaryngol. 1957;61(5):602-8.
5. Converse JM, Smith B, Obear MF, et al. Orbital blow-out fractures: a ten-year survey. Plast Reconstr Surg. 1967;39(1):20-36.
6. Putterman AM. Management of blow-out fracture of the orbital floor: a conservative approach. Surv Ophthalmol. 1991;35(4):292-8.
7. Putterman AM. Late management of blowout fractures of the orbital floor. Trans Sect Ophthalmol Am Acad Ophthalmol Otolaryngol. 1977;83(4 Pt 1):650-9.
8. Putterman AM. Dr. Allen M. Putterman on the subject of blowout fractures of the orbital floor. Ophthal Plast Reconstr Surg. 1985;1(1):73-4.
9. Putterman AM, Stevens T, Urist MJ. Nonsurgical management of blow-out fractures of the orbital floor. Amer J Ophthalmol. 1974;77(2):232-9.
10. Jordan DR, Allen LH, White J, et al. Intervention within days for some orbital floor fractures: the white-eyed blowout. Ophthal Plast Reconstr Surg. 1998;14(6):377-90.
11. Berkowitz RA, Putterman AM, Patel DB. Prolapse of the globe into the maxillary sinus after orbital floor fracture. Amer J Ophthalmol. 1981;91(2):253-7.
12. Abrishami M, Aletaha M, Baheri A, et al. Traumatic subluxation of the globe into the maxillary sinus. Ophthal Plast Reconstr Surg. 2007;23(2):156-8.

13. Millman AL, Della Rocca RC, Spector S, et al. Steroids and orbital blowout fractures – a new systematic in medical management and surgical decision-making. Adv Ophthalmic Plast Reconstr Surg. 1987;6:291-300.
14. Whitnall SG. The anatomy of the human orbit and accessory organs of vision, 2nd edn. London, United Kingdom: Oxford University Press; 1932: 300-16.
15. Koornneef L. Current concepts on the management of orbital blow-out fractures. Ann Plast Surg. 1982;9(3):185-200.
16. Koornneef L. Details of the orbital connective tissue system in the adult. Acta Morphol Neerl Scand. 1977;15(1):1-34.
17. Smith B, Putterman AM. Fixation of orbital floor implants: description of a simple technique. Arch Ophthalmol. 1970;83:598.
18. Garcia GH, Goldberg RA, Shorr N. The Transcaruncular approach in repair of orbital fractures: a retrospective study. J Craniomaxillofac Trauma. 1988;4(1):7-12.
19. Shorr N, Baylis HI, Goldberg RA, et al. Transcaruncular approach to the medial orbit and orbital apex. Ophthalmology. 2000;107(8):1459-63.
20. Lynch RC. The technique of a radical frontal sinus operation which has given me the best results. Laryngoscope. 1921;31: 1-5.
21. Putterman AM, Millman AL. Custom orbital implant in the repair of late posttraumatic enophthalmos. Am J Ophthalmol. 1989;108(2):153-9.
22. Putterman AM, Urist MJ. Muller's muscle-conjunctiva resection. Technique for treatment of blepharoptosis. Arch Ophthalmol. 1975;93(8):619-23.
23. Putterman AM, Urist MJ. Treatment of enophthalmic narrow palpebral fissure after blow-out fracture. Ophthalmic Surg. 1975; 6(3):45-9.
24. Sires, Bryan S. Orbital trapdoor fracture and oculocardiac reflex. Ophthal Plast Reconstr Surg. 1999;15(4):301.
25. Soll DB, Poley BJ. Trapdoor variety of blowout fracture of the orbital floor. Am J Ophthalmol. 1965;60:269-72.
26. Smith B, Lisman RD, Simontan J, et al. Volkmann's contracture of the extraocular muscles following blow-out fracture. Plast Reconstr Surg. 1984;74(2):200-16.

CHAPTER

74

# Optic Nerve Sheath Fenestration

Nathan Abraham, Christopher I Zoumalan

## INTRODUCTION

Optic nerve sheath fenestration (ONSF) has long been used as a surgical treatment option for conditions in which there is an elevated intracranial pressure. First described by De Wecker in 1872, ONSF has traditionally been considered an effective surgical strategy in idiopathic intracranial hypertension (IIH).[1-3] Among the benefits of ONSF in IIH, improvement of vision is among the most dramatic, noted primarily in the ipsilateral eye. Reductions in headaches and disc edema have also been noted. In addition, benefits have been reported in the contralateral eye by a filtration effect propagated throughout the cerebrospinal fluid (CSF) circulatory system.

## INDICATIONS

The primary indication for ONSF has been for use in IIH, yet several cases have documented its efficacy in successful stabilization or reversal of vision loss due to optic nerve sheath hemorrhage, cryptococcal meningitis with papilledema, and intracranial breast cancer metastases with papilledema.[4-6] ONSF has not been shown to be an effective measure for improving vision loss due to anterior ischemic optic neuropathy.[7,8] A recent study showed ONSF to be equally effective in the pediatric population compared to adults.[9]

The IIH, also known as pseudotumorcerebri, is primarily seen in obese females, ages 20–45 years old, has no known etiology, and requires the following for diagnosis (Dandi criteria):

- Signs and symptoms of increased intracranial pressure (headache, nausea, transient visual obscurations lasting seconds, double vision, dizziness, emesis).
- Elevated CSF pressure (> 200 mm Hg in nonobese adults and > 250 mm Hg in obese adults).
- Normal neuroimaging studies.
- Normal neurologic examination (with the exception of papilledema and/or cranial nerve palsies).
- No other identifiable cause such as medications (including vitamin A, tetracycline, oral contraceptive pills, nalidixic acid, lithium, steroid use, or withdrawal).

Common symptoms of IIH are headache, transient visual obscurations, intracranial noises (pulsatile tinnitus), photopsia, retrobulbar pain, diplopia, and sustained visual loss.[10-15]

## PREOPERATIVE EXAMINATION

Evaluation for ONSF should begin with a thorough ophthalmic history and physical examination including visual acuity, color vision, pupillary assessment, motility, visual field testing, and funduscopic examination to determine the existence and extent of papilledema (swelling of optic nerve). A full neurological examination is also warranted to search for signs of focal neurological deficits common in IIH, paying close attention for cranial nerve deficits. Emergent head imaging (computed tomography and magnetic resonance imaging) is necessary and critical for ruling out intracranial lesions including dural venous thrombosis and neoplasms, both of which can cause papilledema. Lumbar puncture is needed to evaluate CSF composition and opening pressure. Blood pressure should also be monitored.

The treatment of IIH begins with medical management, starting with weight loss, acetazolamide or furosemide, and systemic steroids if needed. If visual loss persists despite the above measures, ONSF should be considered. Preoperative discussion should include the risk of complications, as ONSF is performed in close proximity to the optic nerve and other

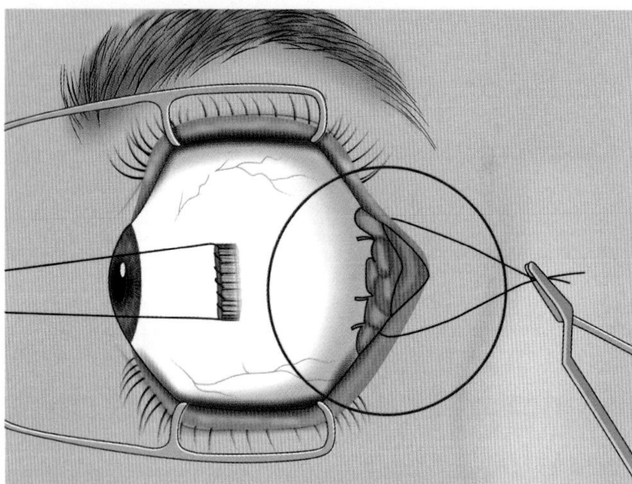

**Figure 74-1** A 4-0 silk suture is passed in a running stitch fashion through the muscle stump to be used as a traction suture.

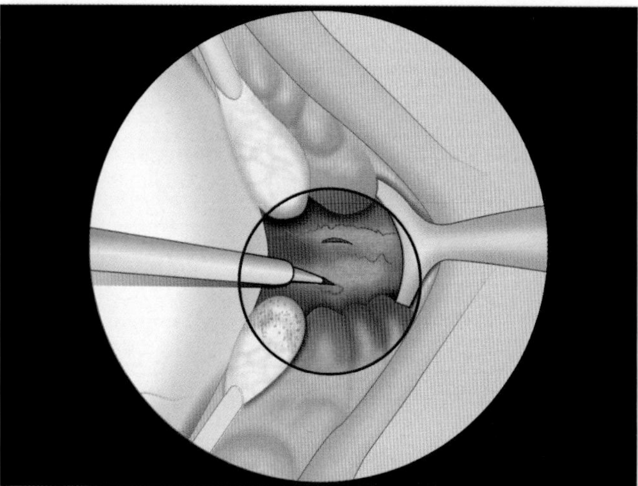

**Figure 74-2** During exposure, prolapsing orbital fat can often obscure the field and may be retracted using a Schepens orbital retractor and cotton-tipped applicators.

vital visual structures within the orbital cavity. Continued medical management is warranted postoperatively, as ONSF is not curative. IIH patients with bilateral visual disturbance should first have ONSF performed on the more severely affected eye.

## SURGICAL TECHNIQUE

General anesthesia is recommended for this procedure. Local anesthesia may be an appropriate option based on the overall health of the patient and experience of the surgeon.

Equipment:

- Bipolar cautery
- Wire lid speculum
- Westcott scissors
- Ophthalmic fine-toothed forceps
- Jameson muscle hook (× 2)
- Double-armed 5-0 Vicryl suture with spatulated needle
- 4-0 silk suture
- Malleable retractor
- Schepens orbital retractor
- Cotton tip applicators
- Long neurobayonet-toothed forceps and scissors
- Long-handled 15° blade or Supersharp blade
- Trans-sphenoidal or Bellucci scissors.

The patient should be placed in the supine position. Patients should avoid anticoagulants perioperatively and should notify their surgeon of any outpatient anticoagulation.

There are a variety of approaches and techniques for performing ONSF. This chapter focuses on a transconjuctival medial orbitotomy approach. One advantage of this approach is the possibility of obtaining an optic nerve sheath biopsy after sheath decompression.

Following general anesthesia, the eye, and eyelid are prepared and draped in a standard ophthalmic surgical fashion. An eyelid speculum is then fastened. Peritomy at the nasal limbus is performed with relaxing incisions allowing for dissection down to bare sclera. The medial rectus muscle is identified and isolated using a muscle hook. Next a double-armed 5-0 Vicryl suture is passed through the insertion of the medial rectus with locking bites at the inferior and superior aspects of the muscle. The muscle is then disinserted with Westcott scissors. A 4-0 silk suture is passed in a running stitch fashion through the muscle stump to be used as a traction suture (Fig. 74-1).

If hemostasis becomes necessary, bipolar or needle-point cautery may be used. The globe is rotated laterally using 4-0 silk traction suture. Care must be given to rotate the globe periodically, thereby releasing tension and avoiding ischemia. Proper exposure of the optic nerve sheath is aided by careful retraction of the orbital soft tissue using a malleable retractor. During exposure, prolapsing orbital fat can often obscure the field and may be retracted using a Schepens orbital retractor and cotton-tipped applicators (Fig. 74-2).

After adequate exposure is achieved, the planned incision point can be outlined with a marking pen. The incision point should be in the distal aspect of the nerve sheath, thereby avoiding damage to the nerve itself. Making the incision 2–3 mm from the globe ensures avoidance of damage to the

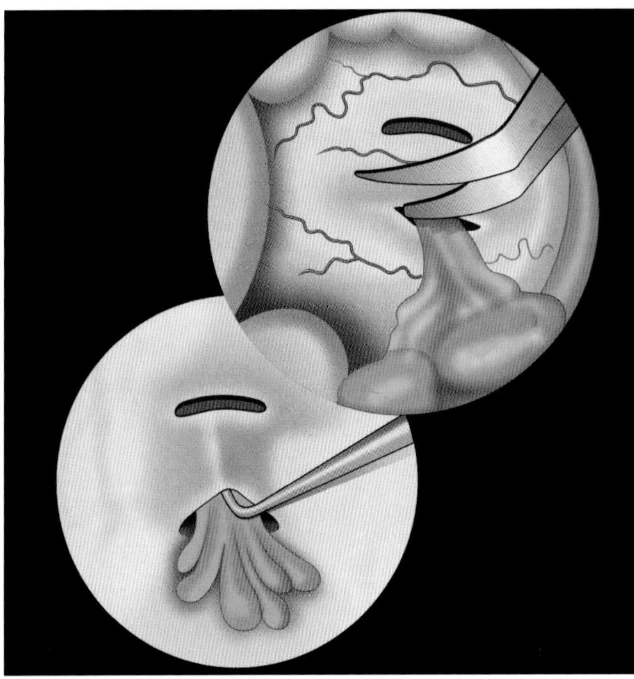

Figure 74-3 The edge of the incision should be everted with fine-toothed neurosurgical forceps and Bellucci scissors introduced to extend the incision to a length of 5–7 mm.

vascular supply, primarily through a plexus of short ciliary vessels. The longitudinal incision along the nerve sheath can be made using a long 15° blade or a Supersharp blade, similar to the one used for paracentesis formation in cataract surgery. The path of the incision should be an upward and away manner to avoid injury to the nerve itself.

Once the incision into the optic nerve sheath is made, an egress of fluid may be observed, which indicates release of the CSF under high pressure. The edge of the incision should be everted with fine-toothed neurosurgical forceps and Bellucci scissors introduced to extend the incision to a length of 5–7 mm (Fig. 74-3). Again, care should be taken to stay superficial, with the inferior blade tenting the dura and arachnoid layer to avoid contact with deeper tissue. A second incision, parallel to the first may be created in the same fashion. A superior oblique hook may be used to elevate the dura and arachnoid through the initial incision to assist in subsequent incisions. The introduction of the hook will also release any adhesions.

Another option may be to excise this entire window of tissue between the incisions. Occasionally, this may be indicated for biopsy purposes if the etiology is in question. Hemostasis in the orbit is performed with Cottonoids and cotton-tipped applicators, as well as light bipolar cautery if needed. The traction suture is then removed. The medial rectus muscle is reattached to its insertion point using the 5-0 Vicryl suture. The conjunctiva is then reapproximated with an absorbable suture.

## POSTOPERATIVE CARE

Anticoagulation should be avoided in the immediate postoperative period. Systemic antibiotics should be administered intraoperatively and continued overnight. If need be, intravenous steroids may be given perioperatively and overnight. Monitoring visual acuity and pupil checks a few hours postoperatively is critical. The patient may be admitted overnight for observation. One week of antibiotic-steroid eye drop is standard. If needed, a tapered oral steroid regimen may be given on a case-by-case basis. Recovery is relatively pain free and rarely necessitates narcotic use. Optic nerve function should be assessed 1–2 weeks postoperatively to ensure proper healing. Recovery of vision and optic nerve function often occur in parallel and happens rapidly over the first several weeks postoperatively.

## COMPLICATIONS

Temporary diplopia, sudden loss of vision (either from a vascular occlusive event, direct injury to nerve, or a hemorrhage), orbital or intrasheath hemorrhage resulting in vision loss, and pupillary abnormality from damage to parasympathetic nerve fibers.

## REFERENCES


1. De Wecker L. On incision of the optic nerve in cases of neuroretinitis. Int Ophthalmol Cong Reps. 1872;4:11-4.
2. Moskowitz B. Optic nerve sheath fenestration. In: Della Rocca RC, Bedrossian EH, Arthurs BP. Ophthalmic plastic Surgery: decision making and techniques. 1. New York: McGraw-Hill; 2002:291-4.
3. Alsuhaibani AH, Carter KD, Nerad JA, et al. Effect of optic nerve sheath fenestration on papilledema of the operated and the contralateral nonoperated eyes in idiopathic intracranial hypertension. Ophthalmology. 2011;118(2):412-4.
4. Muthukumar N. Taumatichaemorrhagic optic neuropathy: case report. Br J Neurosurg. 1997;11:166-7.
5. Milman T, Mirani N, Turbin RE. Optic nerve sheath fenestration in cryptococcal meningitis. Clin Ophthalmol. 2008;2:637-9.
6. Gasperini J, Black E, Van Stavern G. Perineural metastasis of breast cancer treated with optic nerve sheath fenestration. Ophthal Plast Reconstr Surg. 2007;23:331-3.
7. Jablons MM, Glaser JS, Schatz NJ, et al. Optic nerve sheath fenestration for treatment of progressive ischemic optic neuropathy. Results in 26 patients. Arch Ophthalmol. 1993;111:84-7.

8. Glaser JS, Teimory M, Schatz NJ. Optic nerve sheath fenestration for progressive ischemic opticneuropathy. Results in second series consisting of 21 eyes. Arch Ophthalmol. 1994;112:1047-50.
9. Thuente DD, Buckley EG. Pediatric optic nerve sheath decompression. Ophthalmology. 2005;112:724-7.
10. Berman D, Miller NR. New concepts in the management of optic nerve sheath meningiomas. Ann Acad Med Singapore. 2006; 35:168-74.
11. Goh KY, Schatz NJ, Glaser JS. Optic nerve sheath fenestration for pseudotumorcerebri. J Neuroophthalmol. 1997;17:86-91.
12. Mauriello JA, Jr, Shaderowfsky P, Gizzi M, et al. Management of visual loss after optic nerve sheath decompression in patients with pseudotumorcerebri. Ophthalmology. 1995;102:441-5.
13. Vanderveen DK, Nihalani BR, Barron P, et al. Optic nerve sheath fenestration for an isolated optic nerve glioma. J AAPOS. 2009;13:88-90.
14. Wilkes BN, Siatkowski RM. Progressive optic neuropathy in idiopathic intracranial hypertension after optic nerve sheath fenestration. J Neuroophthalmol. 2009;29:281-3.
15. Wall et al. Brain 1991, PMID 1998880.

CHAPTER

75

# Orbital Implants

Sima Das, Santosh G Honavar

## INTRODUCTION

A wide variety of materials have been used as orbital implants for restoring the orbital volume following loss of an eye. Orbital implants also impart motility to the prosthesis and maintain cosmetic symmetry with the fellow eye. The history of orbital implant dates back to 1885, when Mules decided to implant "artificial vitreous" in the form of a glass sphere after an evisceration.[1] A similar implant was introduced by Frost in the following year who put it in Tenons' capsule following enucleation. A wide variety of implants have been tried since then ranging from gold, paraffin, glass as well as "natural" approaches like ox bone, acrylic, fat, rubber, wire, silk, and rabbit eye. Based on the type of material used, the design of the implant and the technique of implantation, orbital implants can be divided into the following major categories:[2]

- Nonintegrated (nonporous) and integrated (porous) implants.
- Nonintegrated, semi-integrated, integrated, biointegrated, and biogenic implants.
- Buried and exposed implants.

The choice of implant varies from patient to patient as well as depends on the surgeons' preference and the availability of pegging facilities. All implants have their own advantages and limitations and there is no clear implant of choice for all patients. However, an ideal implant should fulfill the following criteria:[3]

- It should get incorporated with orbital tissues.
- It should be biocompatible and should not cause any rejection, allergic, or inflammatory reactions.
- It should not be biodegradable.
- It should compensate for the volume loss of the eye.
- There should not be any complications associated with the implant like infection, extrusion, and migration.
- It should allow maximum motility of the prosthesis.
- It should provide stimulus for orbital growth.
- It should be readily available, inexpensive, and easy to use.

None of the currently available orbital implants fulfill all these criteria and the search for the ideal implant is far from over. The classic spherical orbital implants have persisted as the most effective orbital implant with minimal complications and still remain the most commonly used orbital implant. This chapter will provide an overview of the commonly used orbital implants and salient features of the implantation techniques.

## NONINTEGRATED IMPLANTS

Nonintegrated implants have a smooth, nonporous surface that does not allow fibrovascular ingrowth into their inorganic body. The extraocular muscles are either tied over the implant or sutured to the wrapping material used to cover some of these implants (Figs. 75-1A and B). They have no direct connection with the ocular prosthesis and they provide motility by surface tension at the conjunctivoprosthesis interface. They provide good volume replacement. Some amount of ocular motility is also imparted when the extraocular muscles are imbricated in front of the implant. Silicone, acrylic, and polymethyl methacrylate (PMMA) are the most commonly used nonintegrated spherical implants.[4] The spherical implants can be placed in the orbit either unwrapped or wrapped in material such as autogenous sclera, banked sclera, autogenous fascia lata, polyglactin/polyglycolic mesh, and Gore-Tex sheet.[5,6] Wrapping material helps to decrease the postoperative exposure rate of the implant. Modification of the surgical

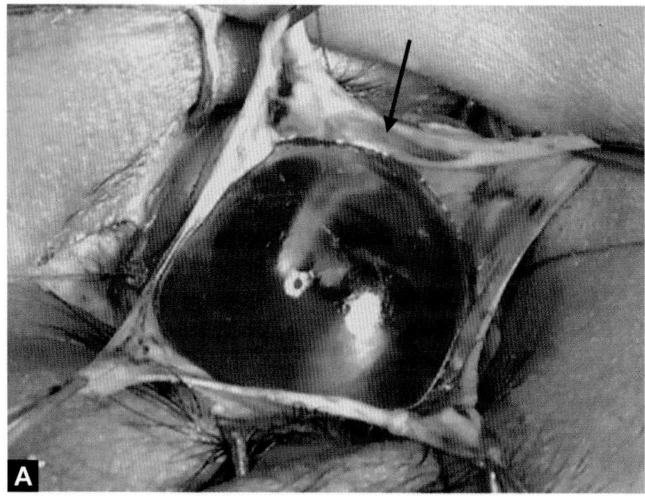


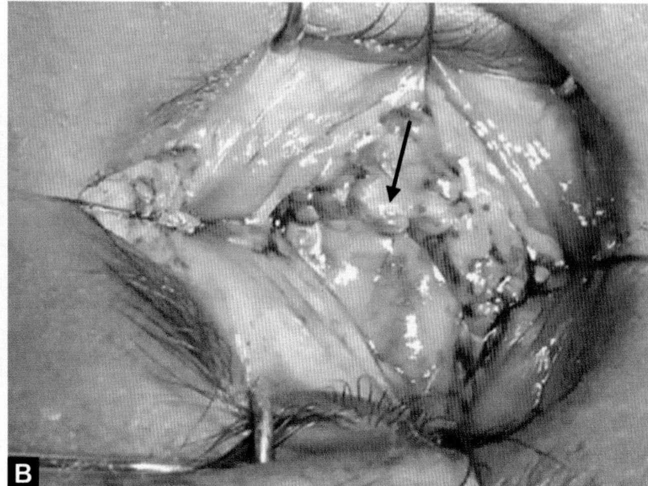


**Figures 75-1A and B** Polymethyl methacrylate implant insertion within the posterior tenons after myoconjunctival enucleation (A) Posterior tenons closed over the implant. (B) muscles sutured to respective fornices.

implantation technique has also helped to reduce the exposure rates of these implants. One limitation reported with these implants is their migration because of overlying rectus muscle contraction.

## INTEGRATED IMPLANTS

Integrated implants have a rough, porous surface that allows for ingrowth of fibrovascular tissue from the anophthalmic socket, thus allowing for true integration of the implant into orbital tissues. The integration makes these implants more resistant to migration and extrusion. They may also have provisions for drilling "pegs" or "posts" that connect them to the ocular prosthesis for added motility. Hydroxyapatite and porous polyethylene are the most commonly used porous implants and are described below.

### Hydroxyapatite

The hydroxyapatite implant was first introduced by Dr Perry in 1985. The implant material is formed from a salt of calcium phosphate that is normally present in the human mineralized bone and is derived from living corals found in deep sea waters. Hydroxyapatite is nontoxic, nonallergenic, and biocompatible and nonbiodegradable. The porous hydroxyapatite matrix is infiltrated by the host fibrovascular tissue when it is implanted into orbital soft tissues.[7,8] Vascularization of a porous implant can be assessed radiographically with contrast-enhanced magnetic resonance imaging (MRI). Implants with a grade 3 or 4 vascularization (equal to or greater than orbital rim) are believed to be adequately vascularized. This assessment is essential prior to drilling a hole for pegging as it is important to identify central avascular zone and also because it has been shown than implants with >75% vascularization tend to bleed during drilling.[9,10] The pore structure and orientation of the pores determine the extent of the vascularization, and poor vascularization of the implant can lead to extrusion.[11] Higher surface exposure rate is also associated with the use of unwrapped hydroxyapatite implants. Rough surface of the implant causes it to erode through the thin conjunctiva and Tenon's layers. Wrapping the implant with appropriate material reduces the exposure rate. Extraocular muscles can be attached directly to the wrapping material of the implant causing better implant motility. The various wrapping materials that have been used for this purpose are donor sclera, autologous tissue like fascia lata or synthetic materials like Vicryl mesh.

Exposure and infection are the most common complications reported with hydroxyapatite implant, although exposure maybe more related to the surgical implantation technique and the wrapping material used rather than the implant material itself[11-13] (Figs. 75-2A to C). An exposure rate between 3% and 7.6% has been reported in various series.[14,15] Other reported complications associated with hydroxyapatite implant include conjunctival thinning and erosion causing late exposure, orbital hemorrhage, socket discharge, pyogenic granuloma formation, and persistent socket pain. Other potential drawbacks include brittle and speculated nature of the implant material that precludes direct suturing of the extraocular muscles and makes insertion of the implant difficult.

Hydroxyapatite represents a significant advancement in cosmetic rehabilitation of anophthalmic socket. However,

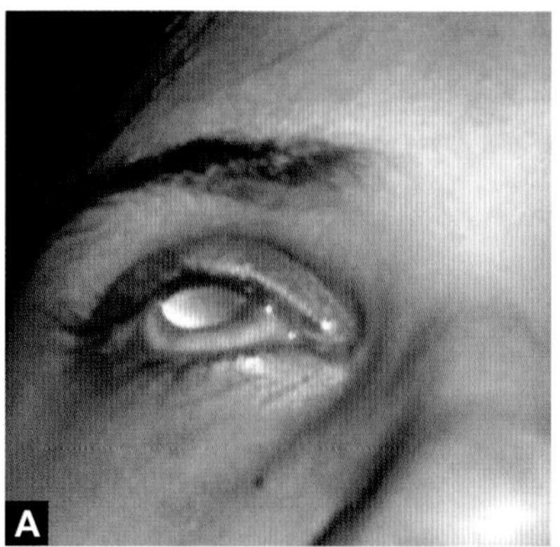

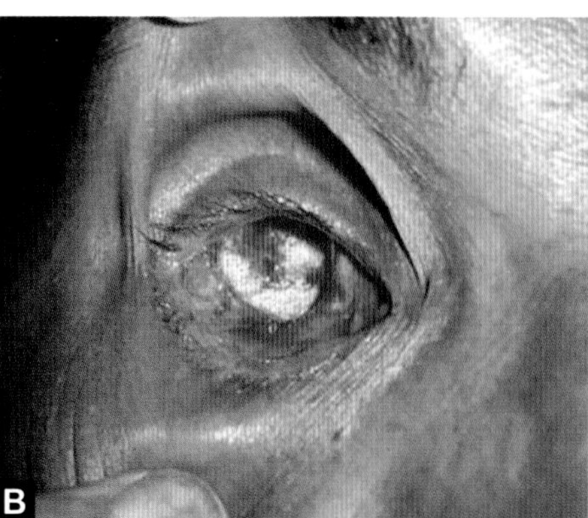

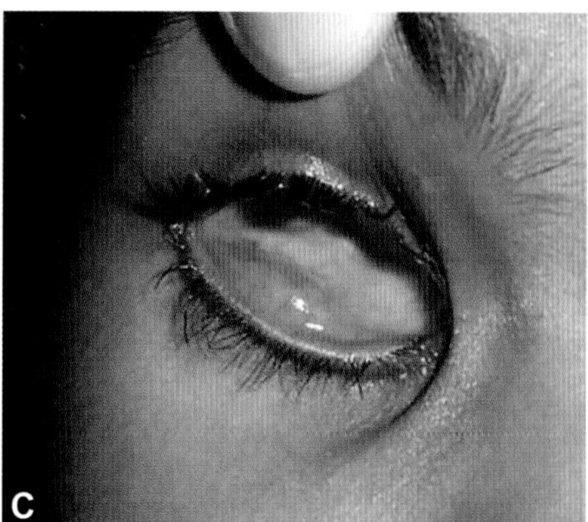


**Figures 75-2A to C** Implant exposure and migration: (A) Exposure of polymethyl methacrylate (PMMA) implant, (B) exposure of hydroxyapatite implant, (C) migration of PMMA implant inferiorly following enucleation.

better understanding of the limitations associated with use of hydroxyapatite has decreased its popularity considerably. The high cost of the implant as well as the additional cost of the wrapping material, drilling procedure, and peg placement has led to the search for porous implants of reduced cost and complication profile. Synthetic hydroxyapatite implant costs almost half that of coralline hydroxyapatite and can be an alternate to the above when cost is a concern. It is currently available in its third-generation form. However, the complications and the problems associated with synthetic hydroxyapatite implant remain similar to that of the coralline implant.

### Porous Polyethylene

Introduced as an orbital implant in 1991, this is another type of integrated implant material and is similar to hydroxyapatite in that it allows fibrovascular ingrowth. However, the surface of porous polyethylene implant is smooth in contrast to hydroxyapatite implants. The advantage conferred by this property is that they do not require additional wrapping material and it is easier to implant them with minimal tissue drag. Also, the muscles can be directly sutured to their surface and they are less expensive as compared to hydroxyapatite implants. The smother surface also causes less irritation of the overlying conjunctiva thus reducing the chances of late exposure. Porous polyethylene implants are available in spherical, egg, conical, and mounded shapes.[16,17] To reduce conjunctival abrasion, the anterior surface can be made of smooth nonporous surface and retaining the porous surface posteriorly to allow for fibrovascular ingrowth.

With the introduction of porous polyethylene implant, there has been a trend shift from hydroxyapatite to the use of porous polyethylene as evidenced by the ASOPRS survey done in 1995 and 2002.[18,19] This shift may be explained by the easier availability, low cost, and ease of implantation of porous polyethylene implants. In the 2002 survey, it was also observed that most surgeons did not wrap the implants (59.8%) or use a motility peg (91.8%).

Various complications like infection, exposure, and extrusion have been reported with these implants as well. The reported rates of exposure vary from 3.7% to 21.6%. Limited literature is available comparing the exposure rates of hydroxyapatite and porous polyethylene implants. Tabatabaee et al. compared 198 wrapped hydroxyapatite implants with 53 unwrapped porous polyethylene implants after primary enucleation, and concluded that the rates of extrusion were significantly higher (Odds ratio: 7.97) in the latter group.[20]

### Bioceramic

Chemically, this material is aluminium oxide and is similar to other porous implants. It is strong, easy to manufacture, and less expensive when compared to other synthetic implants. It was approved for use by the FDA in 2000. Jordan et al. reported positive results in their series, with an exposure rate of 9.1%.[21]

## WRAPPING OF POROUS IMPLANTS

Various materials like donor sclera and bovine pericardium, autologous tissues like fascia lata, and synthetic materials like polyglactin mesh have been used for wrapping the orbital implant prior to its placement into the orbit.

### Donor Sclera

Freshly frozen donor sclera has been the most popular and successful wrapping material for orbital implants over the years.[18] It is readily available and easy to use, and can be

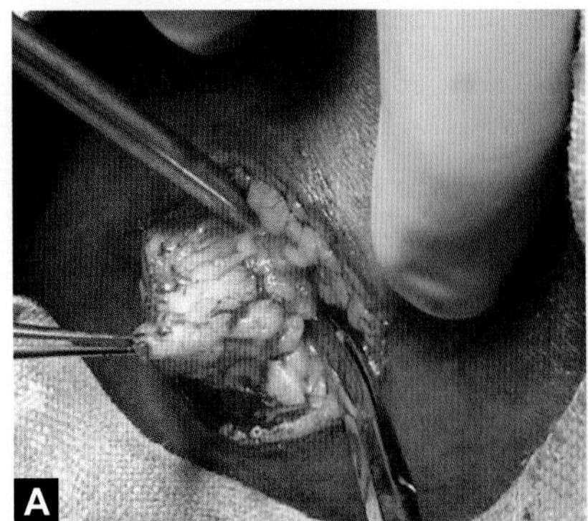
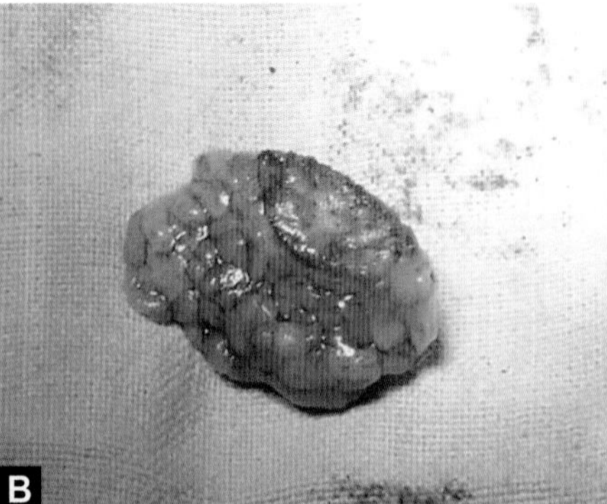
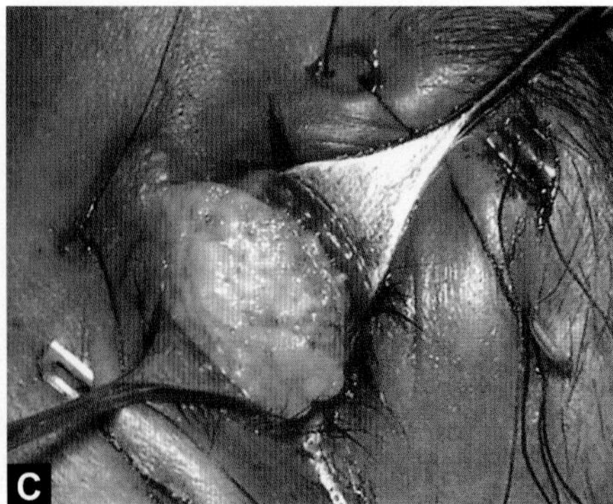

**Figures 75-3A to C** Technique of dermis fat graft implantation. Dermis fat graft harvested from the gluteal region (A), trimmed to appropriate size (B), and inserted into the socket and (C) sutured to the conjunctival edges.

sutured to the implant with 4-0 or 5-0 nonabsorbable sutures. However, its use has reduced in recent years due to the possibility of disease transmission.[22] Other processed donor tissues like human pericardium, fascia lata, dura mater, and bovine pericardium have also fallen into dispute for similar reason and due to the high cost.

## Autologous Tissue

Autologous tissues include fascia lata, temporalis fascia, auricularis muscle complex, pericardium, and pericranium.[23,24] The main advantage is that they vascularize rapidly and there is no risk of a foreign body response. However, they require an additional surgical procedure at another site, prolonging the surgical and recovery times. Scarring at the donor site is another concern, especially in cases with fascia lata.

## Synthetic Mesh

Vicryl (polyglactin 910) is the most common synthetic material used for wrapping implants. The advantages of synthetic mesh lie in the ease of insertion and attachment of extraocular muscles. It has a multitude of holes to allow good vascularization. Also, it eliminates the risk of disease transmission and the need for a second surgical procedure for donor tissue, thus bringing down postoperative morbidity. It is easily available, nonantigenic, and inexpensive. Jordan et al. reported good results with Vicryl mesh in their series with only four cases of conjunctival dehiscence.[25] Another material that has been explored for wrapping implants is Gore-Tex (polytetrafluoroethylene), although no added advantage over unwrapped silicone implants was demonstrated by Morax et al.[26]

Wrapping materials make the insertion of implants with rough surfaces easier by reducing the tissue drag and provide volume augmentation; it provides a barrier over the speculated surface of the implant though the role of wrapping in reducing implant exposure is debated.[27] It allows for precise fixation of the extraocular muscles over the implant surface and thus theoretically improves the implant motility and allows smooth movement of the prosthesis. However, wrapping increases the cost of the procedure and there is a theoretical risk of disease transmission when donor tissue is used. Current evidence suggests a deceasing trend toward the use of wrapping material.[19]

## Dermis Fat Grafting

Though dermis fat grafting is not considered often as a conventional orbital implant, it is an excellent material for implantation of pediatric anophthalmic sockets and fulfills most of the criteria of an ideal implant. It is a composite implant providing volume augmentation as well as causes expansion of the socket surface (Figs. 75-3A to C). The extraocular muscles can be sutured to the graft providing some amount of motility. It is specifically advantageous in children as it can grow with the age of the child thus allowing for bony socket expansion.[28] Since it an autologous material, chances of infection and exposure are minimal. However, fat atrophy can cause late volume loss in adults implanted with dermis fat graft. Socket discharge and hair growth on the surface of the graft are other problems sometimes associated with dermis fat grafts.

# PEGGING OF POROUS IMPLANTS

Pegging allows for coupling of the orbital implant with the prosthesis, thereby increasing the motility of the artificial eye and hence the overall cosmetic appearance of the patient. Though pegging provides definite improvement in prosthesis motility, it is not widely practiced by many surgeons due to the satisfactory results obtained without pegging. Pegging is done after adequate vascularization of the porous implant that can be confirmed on contrast-enhanced MRI. Fibrovascular ingrowth may occur at different rates in different individuals and an avascular area of the implant may predispose to implant extrusion. Titanium peg systems are currently preferred as they are biocompatible and better tolerated by soft tissues than the polycarbonate pegs used earlier.[29]

Though pegging is thought to provide better prosthesis motility, there is not much evidence comparing the motility of pegged versus nonpegged prosthesis. This coupled with the fact that pegging increases the cost of the procedure considerably, there is need for repeat surgical procedure and the complications associated with peg like extrusion, infection, and granuloma formation are the reasons why some surgeons do not prefer pegging of the implant. Also not every patient is a suitable candidate for peg placement. Small children and adults over 65 years or patients with chronic debilitating illness or collagen vascular disease who might be noncompliant with follow-up and might not take adequate care of the peg are not suitable candidates for peg placement.[30]

## IMPLANT SELECTION

The search for an ideal orbital implant is still ongoing and there is little consensus regarding orbital implant material and design among surgeons. Most surgeons have their own preference about spherical versus shaped implant, integrated versus nonintegrated, and wrapping or unwrapped implant; the implant selection is also determined by the cost and whether pegging is planned or not.

In the author's practice, following enucleation, porous implant is used only in patients where future pegging is planned. Porous polyethylene remains the porous implant of choice and a spherical implant is used with anterior surface covered with scleral cap to which the extraocular muscles are sutured. Vascularity of the implant is checked radiographically with MRI before planning the pegging procedure. In cases where pegging is not planned, spherical PMMA implant is inserted within muscle cone following myoconjunctival technique of enucleation. Appropriate-sized spherical PMMA implant is also the preferred implant following evisceration. Dermis fat graft is preferred in children with anophthalmic socket with both volume loss and conjunctival shortening. It is also preferred in reconstruction of irradiated socket where the vascularity is compromised and there is higher possibility of extrusion of alloplastic implant.

## REFERENCES


1. Sami D, Young S, Petersen R. Perspective on orbital enucleation implants. Surv Ophthalmol. 2007; 52(3):244-65.
2. Moshfeghi DM. Enucleation. Survey Ophthal. 2000;44(4): 277-301.
3. Piest KL, Welsh MG. Pediatric enucleation, evisceration and exenteration techniques. In Katowitz JA (ed.), Pediatric Oculoplastic Surgery. New York: Springer; 2002. pp. 617-27, Chap 32.
4. Beard C. Remarks on historical and newer approaches to orbital implants. Ophthalmic Plast Reconstr Surg. 1995;11: 89-90.
5. Custer PL, Kennedy RH, Woog JJ, et al. Orbital implants in enucleation surgery: a report by the American Academy of Ophthalmology. Ophthalmology. 2003; 110:2054-61
6. Nunnery WR, John DNg, Kathy JH. Enucleation and evisceration. In: Spaeth G (ed.), Ophthalmic Surgery: Principles and Practice, 3rd edition. Philadelphia, PA: Elsevier; 2003. pp. 485–507.
7. Shields CL, Shields JA, De Potter P. Hydroxyapatite orbital implant after enucleation: experience with initial 100 consecutive cases. Arch Ophthalmol. 1992;110(3):333-8.
8. Shields CL, Shields JA, Eagle RC Jr, et al. Histopathologic evidence of fibrovascular ingrowth four weeks after placement of the hydroxyapatite orbital implant. Am J Ophthalmol. 1991; 111(3):363-6..
9. De Potter P, Shields CL, Shields JA, et al. Role of magnetic resonance imaging in the evaluation of the hydroxyapatite orbital implant. Ophthalmology. 1992;99(5):824-30.
10. Jamell GA, Hollsten DA, Hawes MJ, et al. Magnetic resonance imaging versus bone scan for assessment of vascularization of the hydroxyapatite orbital implant. Ophthalmic Plast Reconst Surg. 1996;12(2):127-30.
11. Nunery WR, Heinz GW, Bonnin JM, et al. Exposure rate of hydroxyapatite spheres in the anophthalmic socket: histopathologic co relation and comparison with silicone sphere implants. Ophthal Plast Reconst Surg. 1993;9(2):96-104.
12. Goldberg RA, Holds JB, Ebrahimpour J. Exposed hydroxyapatite orbital implants: report of six cases. Ophthalmology. 1992; 99(5):831-6.
13. Shields CL, Shields JA, De Potter P, et al. Problems with the hydroxyapatite orbital implant: experience with 250 consecutive cases.Br J Ophthalmol. 1994;78(9):702-6.
14. Oestreicher JH, Liu E, Berkowitz M. Complications of hydroxyapatite orbital implants. A review of 100 consecutive cases and a comparison of dexon mesh (polyglycolic acid) with scleral wrapping. Ophthalmology. 1997;104(2):324-9.
15. Jordon DR, Gilberg s, Mawn L, et al. The synthetic hydroxyapatite implant: a report on 65 patients. Opthal Plast Reconstr Surg. 1998;14(4):250-5.
16. Karesh JW, Dresner SC. High density porous polyethylene (Medpor) as a successful anophthalmic implant. Ophthalmology. 1994;101(10):1688-95; discussion 1695-6.
17. Rubin PA,Popham J, Rumeldt S. et al. Enhancement of the cosmetic and functional outcome of enucleation with the conical orbital implant. Ophthalomology. 1998;105(5):919-25..

18. Hornblass A, Biesman BS, Eviatar JA. Current techniques of enucleation: a survey of 5,439 intraorbital implants and a review of the literature. Ophthal Plast Reconstr Surg. 1995;11(2): 77-86; discussion 87-8.
19. Su GW, Yen MT. Current trends in managing the anophthalmic socket after primary enucleation and evisceration. Ophthal Plast Reconstr Surg. 2004;20(4):274-80.
20. Tabatabaee Z, Mazloumi M, Rajabi MT et al. Comparison of the exposure rate of wrapped hydroxyapatite (Bio-Eye) versus unwrapped porous polyethylene (Medpor) orbital implants in enucleated patients. Ophthal Plast Reconstr Surg. 2011;27(2): 114-8.
21. Jordan DR, Klap per SR, Gilberg SM et al. The bioceramic implant: evaluation of implant exposures in 419 implants. Ophthal Plast Reconstr Surg. 2010;26(2):80-2.
22. Tullo AB, Buckley RJ, Kelly T et al. Transplantation of ocular tissue from a donor with sporadic Creutzfeldt-Jakob disease. Clin Experiment Ophthalmol. 2006;34(7):645-9.
23. Gayre GS, Debacker C, Lipham W et al. Bovine pericardium as a wrapping for orbital implants. Ophthal Plast Reconstr Surg. 2001;17(5):381-7.
24. Lee SY, Kim HY, Kim SJ, et al. Human dura mater as a wrapping material for hydroxyapatite implantation in the anophthalmic socket. Ophthalmic Surg Lasers. 1997;28(5):428-31.
25. Jordan DR, Klapper SR, Gilberg SM. The use of vicryl mesh in 200 porous orbital implants: a technique with few exposures. Ophthal Plast Reconstr Surg. 2003;19(1):53-61.
26. Morax S. Use of GORE-TEX (polytetrafluoroethylene) in the anophthalmic socket. Adv Ophthalmic Plast Reconstr Surg. 1990;8:82-7.
27. Li T, Shen J, Duffy MT. Exposure rates of wrapped and unwrapped orbital implants following enucleation. Ophthal Plast Reconstr Surg. 2001;17(6):431-5.
28. Tarantini A, Hintschich C. Primary dermis-fat grafting in children. Orbit. 2008;27(5):363-9.
29. Salour H, Eshaghi M, Abrishami M et al. Complications of hydroxyapatite pegging: comparison between polycarbonate and titanium peg system. Eur J Ophthalmol. 2007;17(3):408-12.
30. Jordan DR, Klapper SR. Surgical techniques in enucleation: the role of various types of implants and the efficacy of pegged and nonpegged approaches. Int Ophthalmol Clin. 2006;46(1): 109-32.

CHAPTER

76

# Contracted Socket

Fairooz P Manjanadavida, Santosh G Honavar

## INTRODUCTION

Contracted socket is defined as a socket where a reasonably sized prosthesis cannot be placed or maintained. It can be soft tissue contraction leading to fornix shortening and or bony contraction. Mustarde has classified it into true acquired contracted socket and congenital underdeveloped socket.[1] The contributing factors in acquired type include inappropriate surgical techniques, failure of volume replacement with orbital implant, ill-fitting prosthesis, postoperative socket infection, exposure to radiation, and severe injury with excessive loss of soft tissue. However, it varies in degree of severity.

According to Krishna, soft tissue socket contraction is graded from 0 to V, depending on the severity of surface loss[2] (Figs. 76-1A to E). Apart from the surface contraction in acquired socket, there are other essential features that predict the outcome of treatment. These include volume loss and degree of socket dryness. Therefore, the Krishna classification is modified including these essential parameters (Table 76-1) Tawfik et al. classified contracted socket as Grade I to V, depending upon the severity.[3] Grading of the socket is essential in planning appropriate surgical management. The recommended nomogram in the management of contracted socket takes into consideration volume and surface loss. Both the aspects have to be addressed for an optimal cosmetic outcome (Table 76-2). Apart from the orbital soft tissue and/or bony contraction, restoration of periocular deformity including superior sulcus deformity, upper eyelid ptosis, lower eyelid malposition, and bony hypotrophy mandates attention.

## ACQUIRED CONTRACTED SOCKET

Clinical features:

- Displacement of ocular prosthesis
- Narrow palpebral fissure
- Lower lid malposition
- Conjunctival scarring
- Absent fornices.

### Preoperative Clinical Evaluation

It is essential to perform a preliminary clinical evaluation of the socket to plan appropriate management. The steps include includes external evaluation, slit lamp biomicroscopy, and photographic documentation. Assessment is done with and without prosthesis.

- With prosthesis
  - Eyelid position
  - Presence of ptosis
  - Lower lid ectropion or entropion
  - Horizontal eyelid laxity
  - Superior sulcus deformity
  - Prosthetic position (undersized/oversized)
  - Prosthetic motility
  - Hertel's exophthalmometry (to assess grade of enophthalmos)
  - Cosmesis.
- Without prosthesis
  - Conjunctival surface and fornices
  - Implant location (central/migrated)
  - Implant exposure/extrusion
  - Implant motility
  - Presence of discharge
  - Schirmer's test.

## INDICATIONS AND GOAL OF SURGERY

The major indication for surgery in contracted socket is inability to retain an ocular prosthesis with frequent displacement.

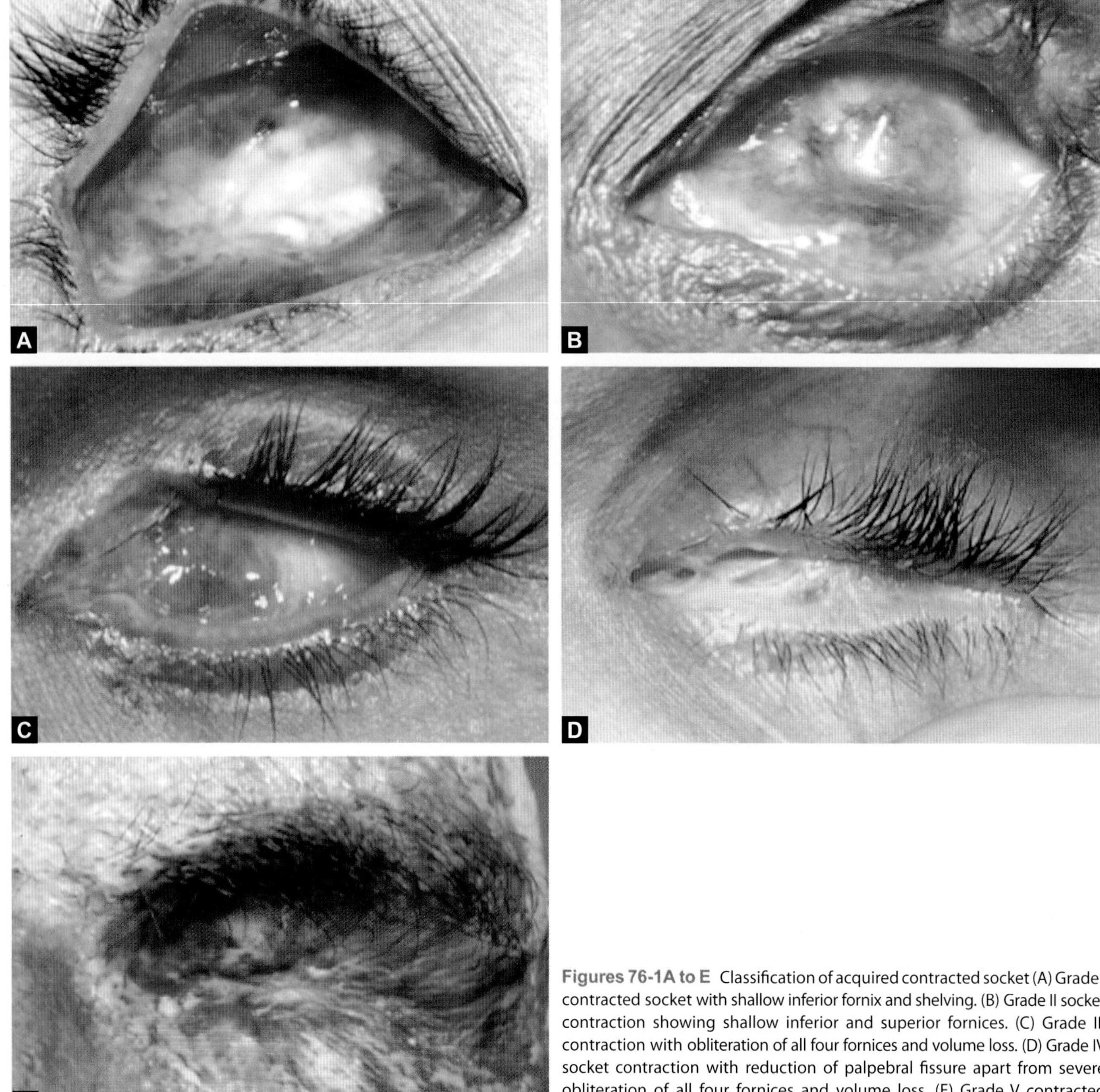

Figures 76-1A to E Classification of acquired contracted socket (A) Grade I contracted socket with shallow inferior fornix and shelving. (B) Grade II socket contraction showing shallow inferior and superior fornices. (C) Grade III contraction with obliteration of all four fornices and volume loss. (D) Grade IV socket contraction with reduction of palpebral fissure apart from severe obliteration of all four fornices and volume loss. (E) Grade V contracted socket, refractory socket with recurrence after multiple failed procedure.

TABLE 76-1 Modified Krishna classification for acquired contracted socket

| Grade | Severity | Surface loss | Volume loss | Schirmer's test (mm) |
|---|---|---|---|---|
| Grade 0 | None | Normal socket with deep and well-formed fornices. No contraction | Absent | >15 |
| Grade I | Minimal | Shallow inferior fornix or shelving of the inferior fornix | Absent | >10–15 |
| Grade II | Mild | Loss of both inferior and superior fornices | Absent | >5–10 |
| Grade III | Moderate | Loss of inferior, superior, medial, and lateral fornices | Present | >2–5 |
| Grade IV | Severe | Loss of all the fornices and reduction of palpebral aperture | Present | 0–2 |
| Grade V | Very severe | Recurrence of contraction of socket after multiple failed procedures | Present | 0 |

TABLE 76-2 Contracted socket—management algorithm

| Shallow fornix | Surface loss | Volume loss | Management |
|---|---|---|---|
| Yes | No | No | Prosthetic revision<br>FFS |
| Yes | + (mild) | No | FFS with conjunctival incision/sieving |
| | ++ (moderate) | No | FFS with AMG |
| | +++ (severe) | No | FFS with MMG |
| Yes | No | Yes | Secondary implant |
| Yes | Yes | Yes | DFG |
| Yes | Yes/dry | Yes (severe) | Vascular pedicle graft<br>Exenteration prosthesis |

(AMG: Amniotic membrane graft; DFG: Dermis fat graft; FFS: Fornix formation sutures; MMG: Mucous membrane graft).

The primary goal is to create the fornix with adequate surface and restore the volume of the socket to necessitate the placement of cosmetically optimal custom ocular prosthesis.[3-7] Secondary goal is restoring periocular anatomy that enhances the cosmesis.

## SURGICAL TECHNIQUES

There are wide varieties of surgical procedures available in socket restoration. Several graft materials have been used in socket reconstruction including, amniotic membrane graft (AMG), mucous membrane graft (MMG), split-thickness skin graft, autologous dermis-fat graft, and vascularized muscle pedicle flaps.[7-13] The choice of surgery solely depends on the grade of contraction and type of contraction.

### Fornix Formation Sutures

The main principle of socket reconstruction is creation of a deep fornix to retain the custom ocular prosthesis. Sutures are passed through respective fornices, lower and upper. Nonabsorbable sutures are passed through the intended part of the fornix transconjunctivally. The needle is passed through the periosteal layer at the orbital rim, to exit at the skin surface corresponding to the inferior orbital rim. Bolsters are placed for adequate fixation. Similar sutures are passed central, medial, and lateral along the inferior and the superior orbital rim. Inferomedial and superolateral sutures are passed superficially to prevent damage to the lacrimal apparatus and lacrimal gland, respectively. Figs. 76-2A to F illustrates the technique. The sutures are removed approximately after 2 weeks postoperatively.

### Grade I Contracted Socket

In the presence of minimal contraction with inferior forniceal shortening without volume loss, surface restoration alone provides good outcome. In certain situations, lower fornix appears absent or shallow due to implant migration. This can be addressed by replacing the migrated implant, preferably by an integrated implant to minimize the risk of recurrence.

The various techniques and surgical procedures performed are as follows.

### Conjunctival Incision/Sieving Technique

It is a simple and effective method in restoring surface as well as inferior fornix. Major advantage is rapid healing and prevents donor-site morbidity. But the indications are limited.

- Technique:
  - *Conjunctival incision*: Horizontal incision extending from lateral and medial fornices 3-mm short of the canthi is performed. Conjunctiva is released from the underlying scar tissue and mobilized through the central linear incision. Inferior fornix formation sutures are passed central, medial, and lateral. Adequate-sized conformer is placed ensuring well centration.
  - *Conjunctival sieve/mesh*: Similar to the conjunctival incision technique, surface is expanded by creating multiple horizontal incisions. Vertical incision is made at the lateral fornix, through which the conjunctiva is released from the underlying scar tissue. The dissection is continued until the entire surface is freed from the scar tissue ensuring mobility of the overlying conjunctiva. This is followed by multiple stab incision over the conjunctiva 3–4 mm apart.[14] The inferior fornix is mobilized and fornix formation sutures are placed in a similar fashion as mentioned earlier.

### Grade II Contracted Socket

The socket where both inferior and superior fornices are shallow is calssified as GradeII/ mild contracted socket. Surface restoration requires expansion of surface with suitable allogenic or autologous grafts. The most commonly used grafts include amniotic membrane and mucous membrane.

### Amniotic Membrane Graft

The AMG is widely used in ocular surface reconstruction after trauma or chemical injury and surgical excision of conjunctival mass. Similarly, AMG is an accepted useful technique in restoring surface in mild to moderate socket contraction.[8,12] It has the ability to promote the growth and migration

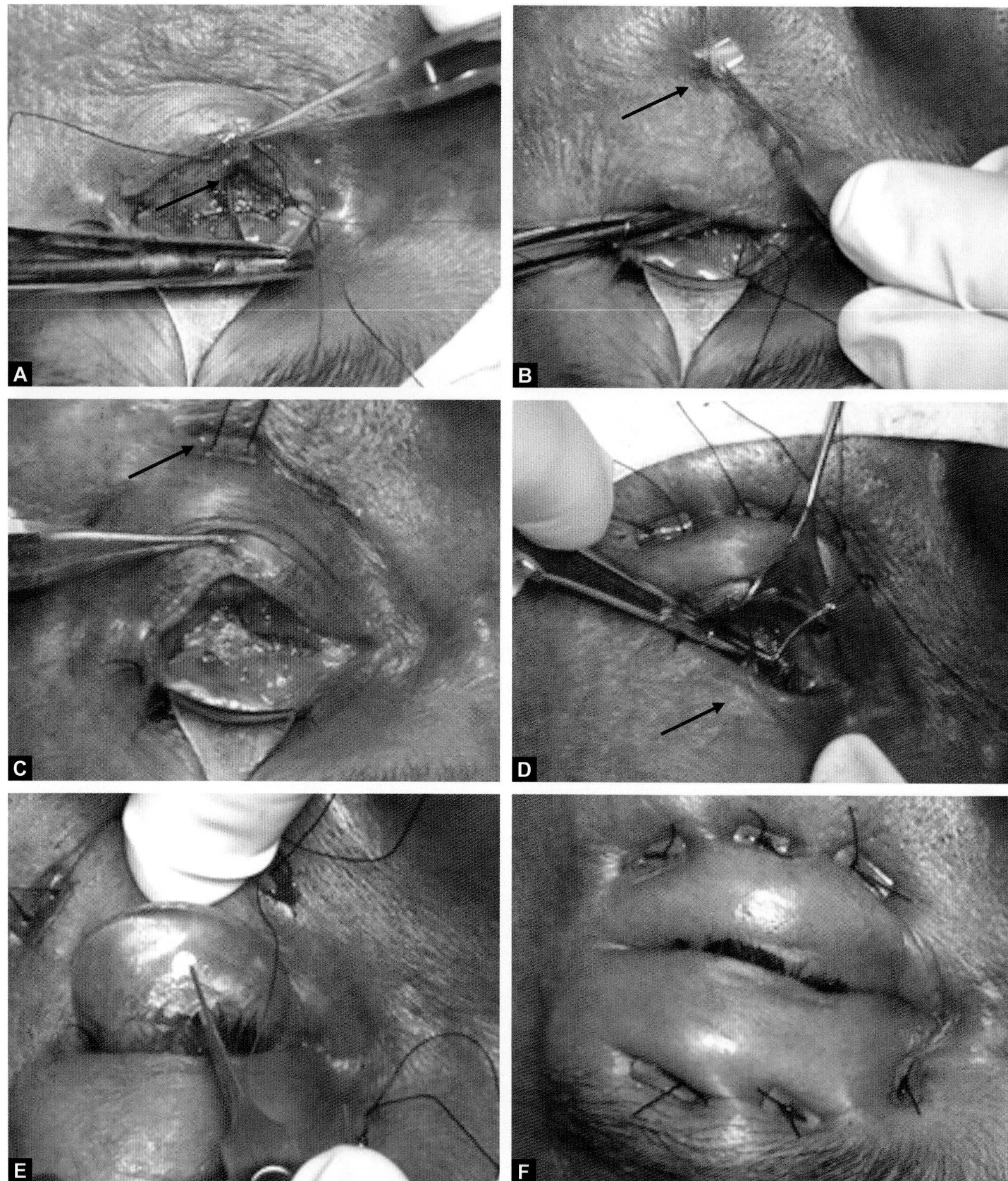


Figures 76-2A to F Illustrates the technique of fornix formation in contracted socket. (A) Intended fornix is marked below the tarsal edge and needle with 4-0 silk suture is passed centrally transconjunctivally. (B) The needle exits at the inferior orbital rim passing through the periostium and secured with a bolster. (C) The other end of the suture is passed with a free needle in a similar fashion, fixed by a bolster. (D) After passing the central, medial, and lateral sutures, superior fornix is fixed similarly passing through the periostium and securing the suture at the superior orbital margin. (E) Conformer of appropriate size is placed. (F) Sutures of both upper and lower lids are tied tight in an alternate manner.

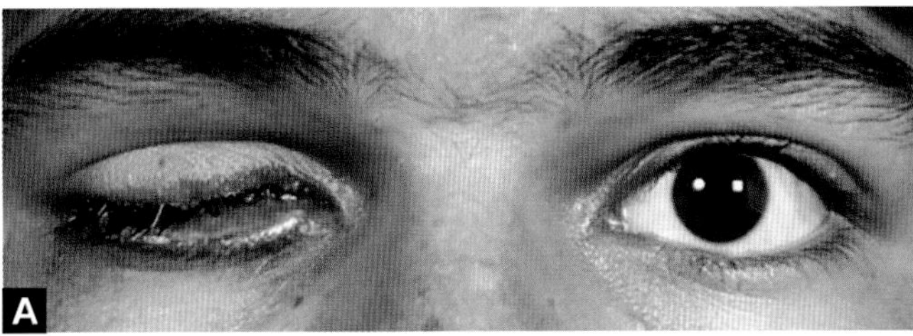
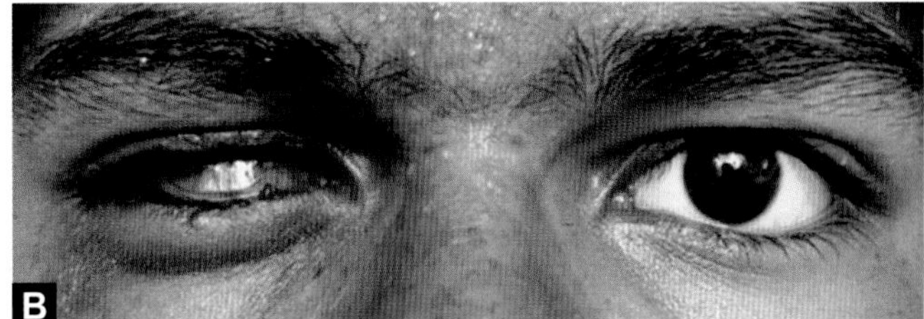

**Figures 76-3A and B** Grade I contracted socket surgically corrected with amniotic membrane graft and inferior fornix fixation.

of normal conjunctival epithelium and to a greater extent prevents fibrosis and scar formation.

*Technique:* The surface or recipient bed is prepared for the placement of AMG. Socket is horizontally incised from lateral to medial canthi, and healthy conjunctiva is dissected from the underlying scar tissue with blunt dissection. After release of the conjunctiva, inferior and superior fornix formation sutures are passed as per the requirement and tied tight. Following which further assessment of the donor bed is performed and appropriate sized AMG is placed over the surface. After drying the surface, fibrin glue is applied and graft held in position (Figs. 76-3A and B). Conformer is placed, and tarsorrhaphy performed to be removed a week later. After complete epithelialization of the surface, custom ocular prosthesis is placed.

## Mucous Membrane Graft

Mucous membrane is harvested from the oral, buccal, or nasal mucosa and serves as an ideal graft for moderate socket contraction with surface loss.[9] Major drawback is the limited success rate in dry, irradiated socket. Vascularity of the recipient bed plays a major role in the survival of the graft making it unsuitable for severe dry contracted socket. MMG lacks goblet cells with reduced success in dry socket.

*Technique:* As mentioned above, the recipient bed of the socket is prepared by releasing the healthy conjunctiva from the underlying scar tissue. Meticulous dissection should be carried out avoiding cauterization of the bed. Fornix formation sutures are placed superiorly and inferiorly as appropriate. The recipient bed is assessed and measurement taken. Donor tissue can be harvested from labial, buccal, or nasal mucous membrane. Adequate-sized tissue is harvested in excess, approximately 30%, as the graft may shrink in size. The donor site is closed directly with interrupted absorbable sutures with smaller grafts and, alternatively amniotic membrane can be placed with tissue glue, to cover the donor area. This will reduce the morbidity, increase comfort, and enhance rapid healing. Harvested graft is placed in the recipient bed, and the edges are sutured with interrupted 6-0 Vicryl sutures, followed by quilt sutures to anchor the graft to the bed (Figs. 76-4A to D). Appropriate sized conformer is placed and tarsorrhaphy performed to be removed after 1 week, to receive a custom-made ocular prosthesis after complete healing.

## Grade III Contracted Socket

The contraction of all four fornices with volume loss is considered as grade III or moderate socket contraction. The goal remains both surface and volume restoration. The options include MMG and dermis fat graft. The former achieves only surface restoration but fails to provide volume. In that case orbitotomy and buried orbital implant placement is recommended along with mucous membrane. Fat transfer into the orbit may also be considered to augment the volume. Dermis fat graft is ideal in such situation as it restores surface along with augmentation of volume.[7,10,15]

## Dermis Fat Graft

It is a biogenic autologous fat graft with overlying dermis, carefully separated from the epidermis. The main advantage is the restoration of both volume and surface loss. The fat replaces volume and the overlying dermis provides the surface for conjunctiva to epithelialize over the dermis and expand the surface. The most ideal site for harvesting the graft is the nonhair baring area of the buttocks, junction of anterior superior iliac spine, and greater trochanter. The major risk factor for graft failure is irradiated sockets and, severe contraction with reduced vascularity making it unsuitable in selected cases.[16]

*Technique:* The socket is prepared in a similar manner as mentioned earlier and, the fornix formation sutures are placed. After measuring the recipient bed (socket) with calipers, the donor site is marked with an extra 30% to ward against graft contraction. Epidermis is separated from the dermis by subepidermal injection of anesthetic agent achieving a peu-de-orange appearance. The epidermis is carefully dissected and removed with a #15 Bard Parker knife or diamond dusted

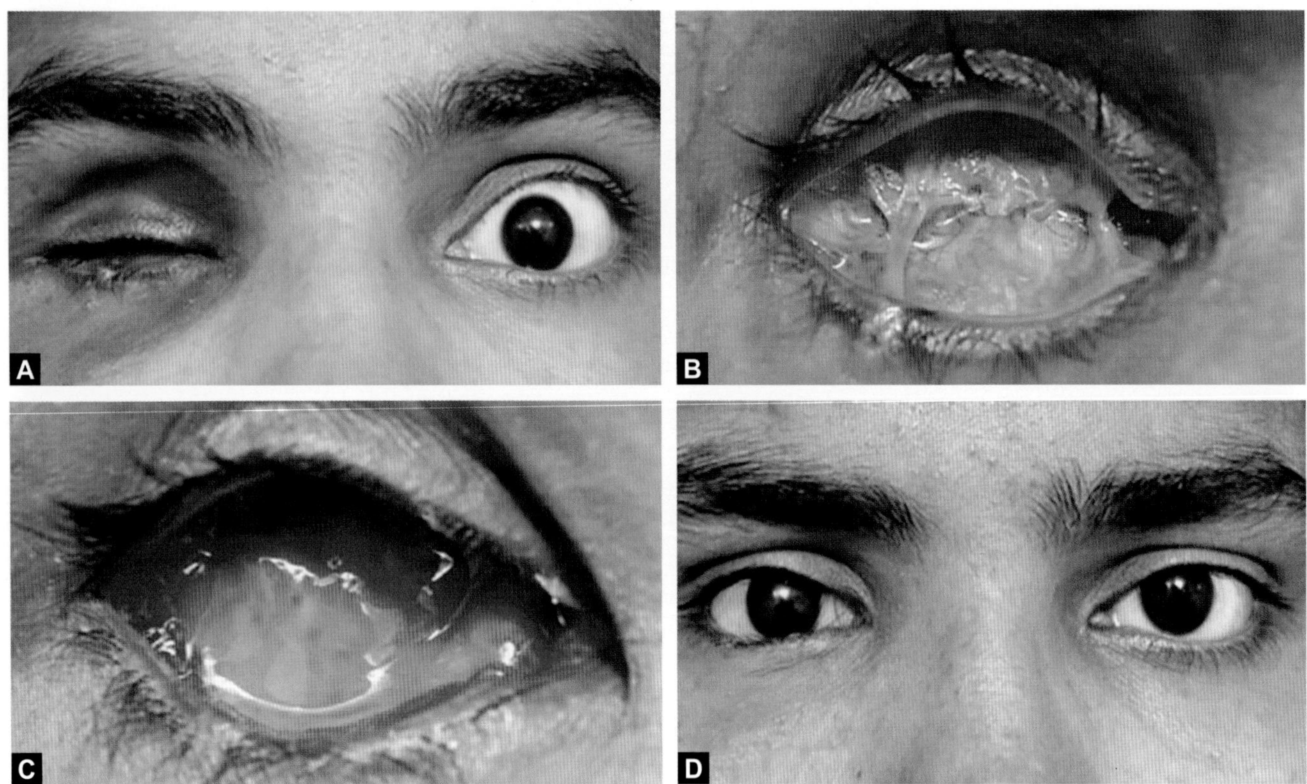


**Figures 76-4A to D** (A) and (B) showing moderate socket contraction with shallow fornix and fibrous bands. (C) Shows the appearance of the socket after 3 weeks postoperative. (D) Custom ocular prosthesis is placed at 6 weeks after ensuring complete healing of the socket.

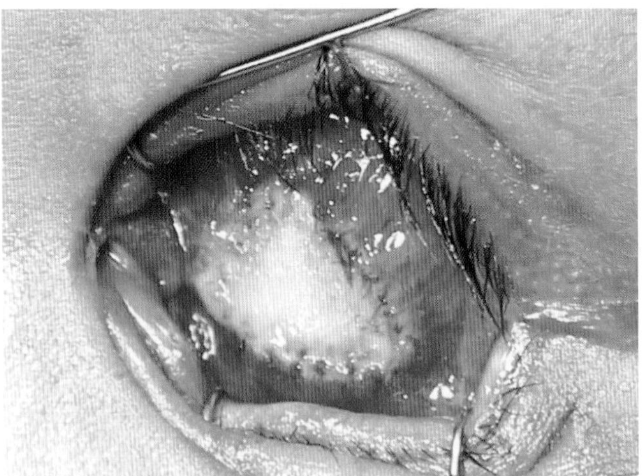

**Figure 76-5** Dermis fat graft placed in the recipient bed in a 6-year-old child. The edges of dermis are approximated to the conjunctival edge with 6-0 Vicryl sutures 360°.

burr. Deep incisions are placed to harvest the graft with a #11 Bard Parker knife. The donor area is closed in layers with vertical mattress sutures. The harvested graft is placed in the recipient bed and held in place with interrupted 6-0 Vicryl sutures 360° (Fig. 76-5). Care must be taken not to oversize the graft, as it may affect graft conjunctivalization leading to central necrosis and graft failure. The graft is assessed for complete conjunctivalization, occurring 8–10 weeks postoperatively. Thereafter ocular prosthesis is placed (Figs. 76-6A and B).

## Grade IV Contracted Socket

This category of socket includes those with absent fornices and reduction of palpebral fissure to a narrow slit. There is severe contraction with both surface and volume loss. Most often these sockets are dry with extensive scarring due to irradiation or repeated surgeries. Restoration of surface with MMG followed by additional surface and volume augmentation with dermis fat graft can be attempted in a stepwise manner (Figs. 76-7A to D). Variety of other grafts has been used, including split thickness skin graft, transposition grafts, and pedicle graft requiring multidisciplinary team approach of oculoplastic, maxillofacial, and craniofacial surgeons. The goal is to provide a vascular graft to overcome the compromised vascularity of the socket. If the microenvironment of the socket bed has adequate vascular supply, split-thickness skin graft has favorable outcome. With the advent of microsurgical

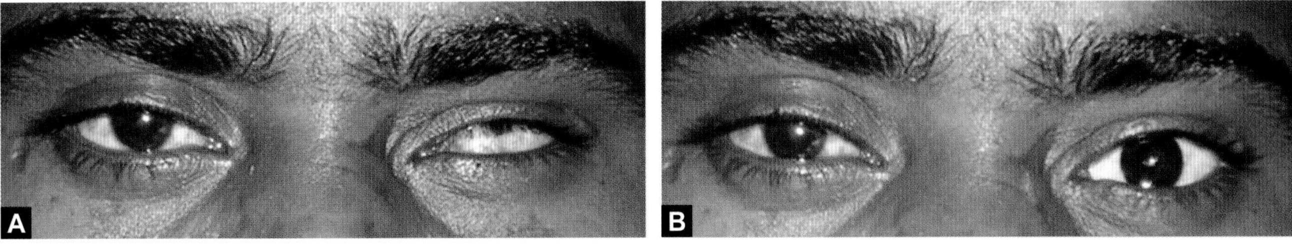

Figures 76-6A and B Conjunctivalized dermis fat graft at 8 weeks fitted with custom ocular prosthesis.

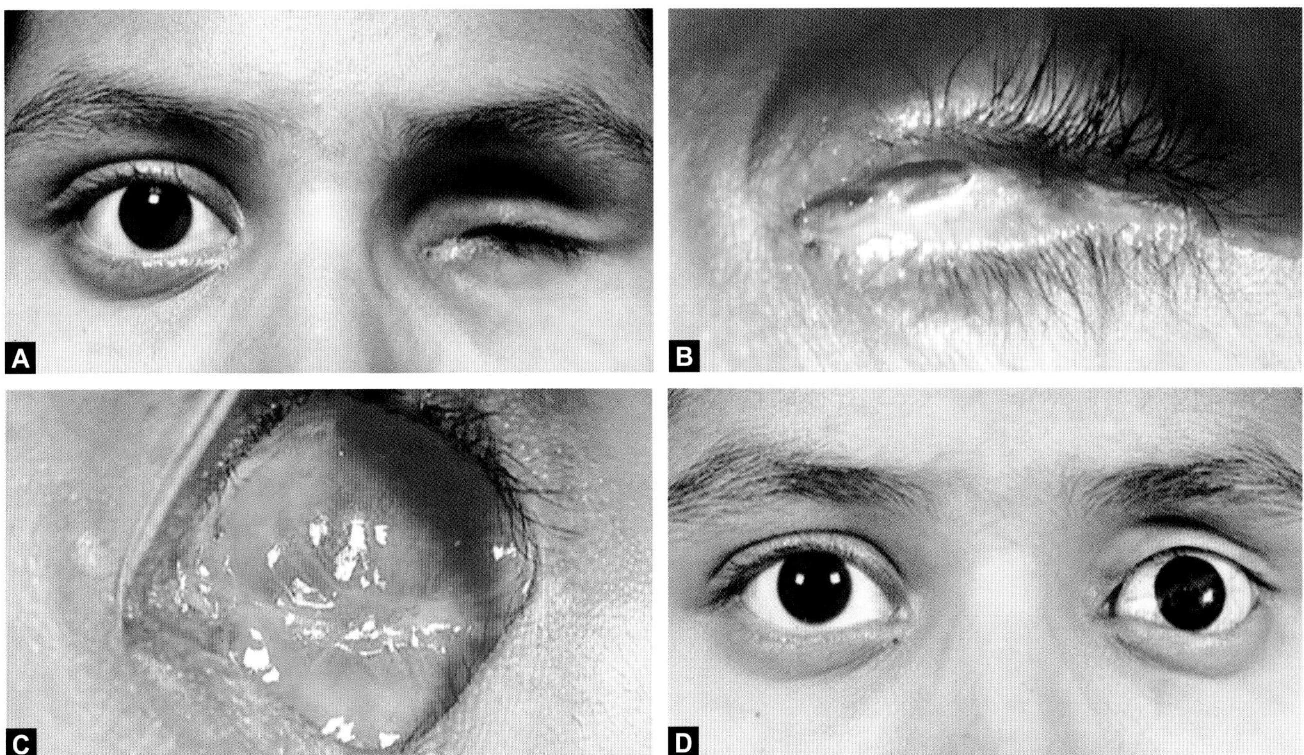

Figures 76-7A to D (A) and (B) showing severe socket contraction with obliterated fornices and narrow palpebral fissure following previous ocular surface reconstruction for chemical injury. (C) Surface and volume expanded in staged procedure with mucous membrane graft followed by dermis fat graft with satisfactory cosmesis.

procedures, severe contraction with compromised vascularity is reconstructed with vascular pedicle graft, such as temporal artery pedicle graft, radial forearm flap, thoracodorsal artery perforator adipose tissue grafts.[13,17] The vascular anastomosis is achieved through the superficial temporal artery and or facial artery where pedicle is tunneled subcutaneously. The additional advantage of thoracodorsal artery perforator adipose tissue grafts includes volume augmentation.[17]

## Grade V Contracted Socket

These are the sockets that have failed multiple surgeries with very severe soft tissue contraction. Apart from the socket deformity, there is complete obliteration of the palpebral fissure with deformed eyelids. It becomes surgically challenging to provide adequate surface and volume. Custom-made exenteration prosthesis can improve cosmesis (Figs. 76-8A to C).

Following socket reconstruction, attention may be required for periocular cosmetic reformation. Surgical rehabilitation of sulcus deformity and lid deformities may be required additionally to have favorable outcome. Most commonly, superior sulcus deformity is seen in anophthalmic sockets as a part of postenucleation socket syndrome. Sulcus deformities are addressed with hyaluronic acid fillers or fat transfer and can restore normal anatomical contour to a greater extent.[18] Lower eyelid deformities such as retraction or entropion can be corrected with spacer grafts. Patients own auricular, palatal

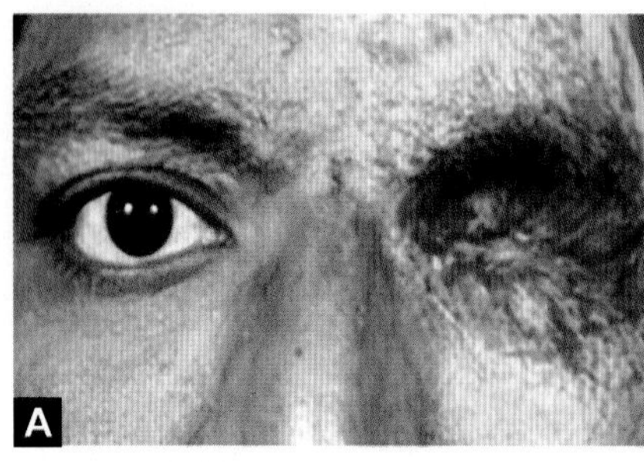
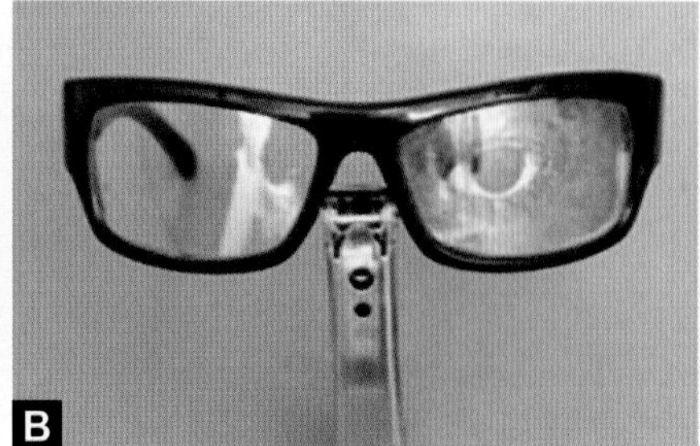
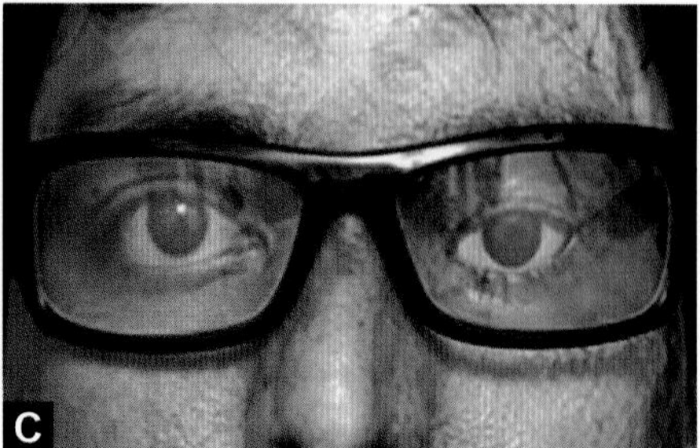

**Figures 76-8A to C** Very severe contracted socket following vitreolage and, refractory to multiple procedures, fitted with spectacle mounted custom-made exenteration prosthesis.

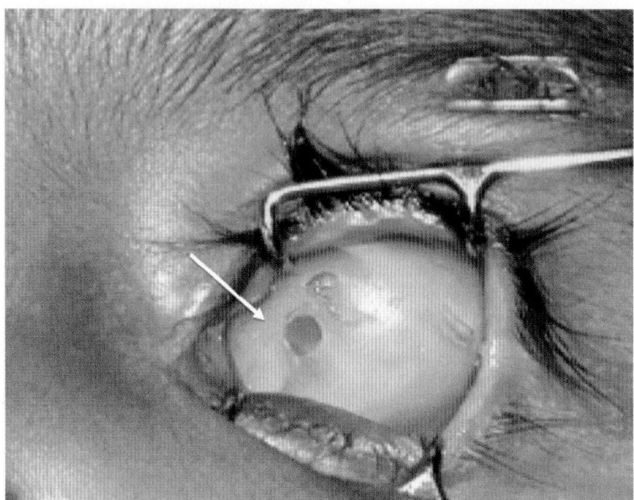

**Figure 76-9** Showing custom-made hydrogel socket expander placed in a 1-year-old child for soft tissue expansion. It is kept in position preventing rotation with external suture fixation.

or nasal septal cartilege, or preserved human acellular dermis can be used for this purpose.[19]

Bony contraction may require expansion of the orbit for improved cosmesis. It can be achieved by osteotomies and expansion of orbit vertically and horizontally as in congenital anophthalmia. The defect in the orbital bone is replaced by split-skull bone grafts.[20,21]

## CONGENITAL CONTRACTED SOCKET

This entity falls into the category of bony contraction and soft tissue contraction due to maldeveloped eyeball. It can be anophthalmia or microphthalmia because of which there is no stimulation for orbital growth. Genetics and environmental factors play a pivotal role in the embryonic maldevelopment.[22] Presence of an eyeball is essential for normal orbital growth and, absence of which lead to severe facial deformity. The main principle in the management is to stimulate normal growth of orbit and soft tissue at the earliest as possible. The aim is to attain orbital growth, expand the conjunctival space and eyelid palpebral length.[23,24]

Management requires a stepwise progressive expansion of the soft tissue followed by stimulation of orbital growth and expansion. Attempts are made to expand the soft tissue with serial acrylic conformers of increasing size until custom-made conformers are fitted.[23] After placing the custom-made conformers tarsorrhaphy is performed to hold it in place for appropriate duration. To avoid repeated anesthesia, cyanoacrylate glue can also be used for closure of eyelid. The results with serial acrylic conformers are gratifying. Hydrogel osmotic expanders have been used by various authors to achieve socket expansion with encouraging results (Fig. 76-9). After ensuring adequate surface expansion, orbital hydrogel expanders are placed into the orbit. This can be achieved through conjunctival incision and implant placement. It is reported that the implant can expand 30 times its original volume.[22-24] Injectable pellet expanders have been used for socket expansion. The pellets are introduced transcutaneously through the inferior orbital rim.[25] However, inferior migration of the expanders has been observed making it a less favorable technique.[26] A preliminary result of inflatable silicone globe expanders with titanium T-plate in congenital anophthalmia was recently published with satisfactory results.[27]

Dermis fat graft is an ideal autologous implant in anophthalmic and microphthalmic eyes. It has an additional benefit, especially for socket reconstruction in children following soft tissue expansion (Figs. 76-10A to D). The advantage is the reported growth of dermis fat graft in children that leads to normal development of the bony orbit.[7,10,23,28-30] Apart from donor-site morbidity, associated limitations include graft atrophy and hypertrophy that may require augmentation and debulking, respectively. Implantation of dermis fat graft of appropriate size is still considered rewarding in pediatric anophthalmic and microphthalmic eyes, ideally performed

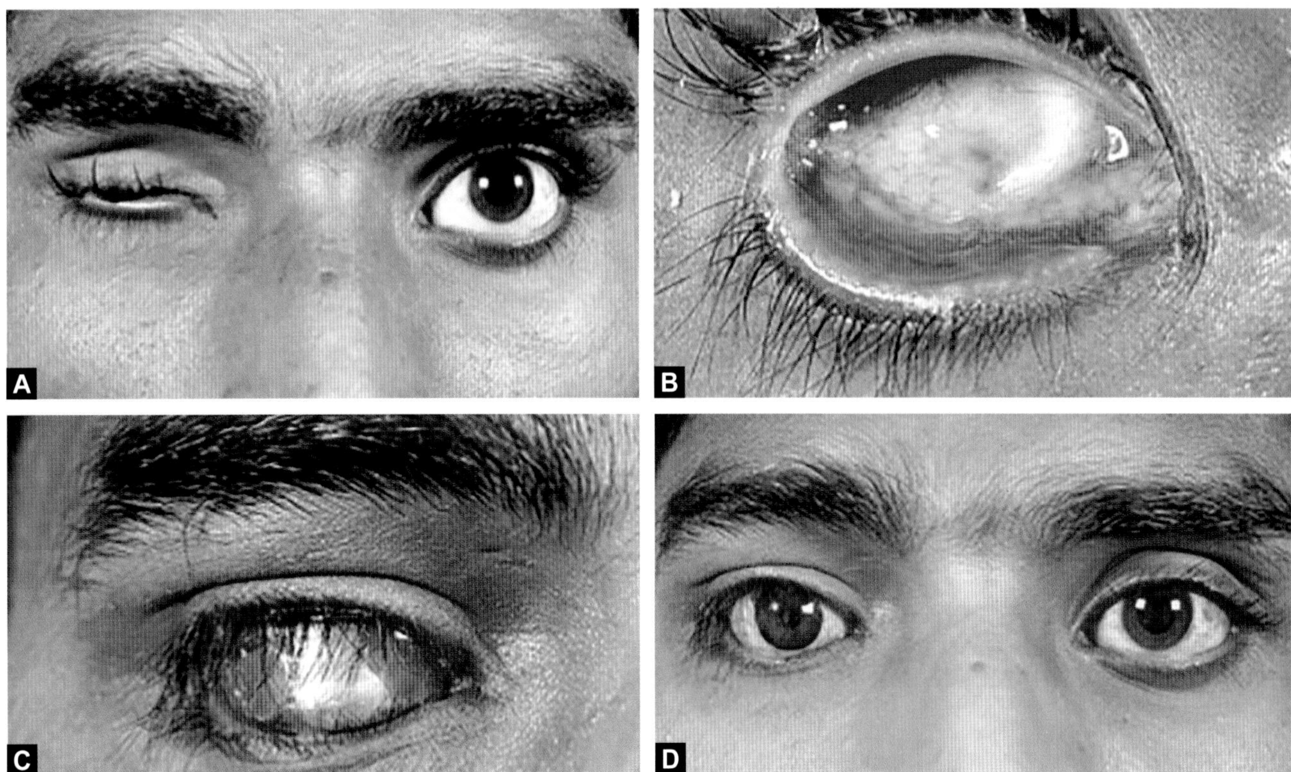


**Figures 76-10A to D** (A) and (B) Showing congenital anophthalmia in a teenager. (C) Conjunctivalized dermis fat graft seen behind the conformer 6 weeks after surgery. (D) Custom ocular prosthesis was fitted 10 weeks postoperative after complete conjunctivalization.

before 3 years of age. Orbital volume can also be restored with lateral orbitotomy and implant placement. In severe bony contraction, bony expansion is achieved by osteotomy and cranial bone grafts.

## CONCLUSION

Contracted socket and its management are extremely challenging and parallel the severity of contraction. It is essential to undertake meticulous preoperative evaluation and, classification for appropriate surgical planning. Nevertheless, surgical techniques have evolved since recent years using various substrate grafts for augmenting the surface and volume. The key factor is to develop deep fornices that can stabilize the prosthesis by fixation of fornices to the periostium. It is not difficult to attain satisfactory cosmesis in mild to moderate contracted socket, whereas severe contraction requires a highly skilled multidisciplinary team approach. Congenital anophthalmos and microphthalmos mandates socket rehabilitation earliest as possible to prevent severe ocular and facial deformity. More conservative approach should be devised and executed in congenital socket reconstruction.

## PEARLS

- Clinical history and meticulous examination aids in planning of management
- Grading includes surface loss and volume loss
- Principle of socket surgery is fornix fixation
- Restore and retain the available conjunctiva
- High rate of graft failure in socket with compromised vascularity
- Periocular cosmetic reformation is considered for overall better cosmesis
- Eyelid deformities can be corrected to a great extent with prosthetic revision
- An expert ocularist can help optimize cosmesis

## REFERENCES

1. Mustarde JC. General principles and management of contracted socket. Orbit. 1986;5(2):77-80.
2. Krishna G. Contracted sockets (aetiology and types). Indian J Ophthalmol. 1980;28:117-20.
3. Tawfik HA, Raslan AO, Talib N. Surgical management of acquired socket contracture. Curr Opin Ophthalmol. 2009; 20(5): 406-11.

4. Collin JR, Moriarty PA. Management of the contracted socket. Trans Ophthalmol Soc U K. 1982;102(Pt 1):93-7.
5. Putterman AM, Scott R. Deep ocular socket reconstruction. Arch Ophthalmol. 1977;95(7):1221-8.
6. Quaranta-Leoni FM. Treatment of the anophthalmic socket. Curr Opin Ophthalmol. 2008;19(5):422-7.
7. Betharia SM, Patil ND. Dermis fat grafting in contracted socket. Indian J Ophthalmol. 1988;36(3):110-2.
8. Bajaj MS, Pushker N, Singh KK, et al. Evaluation of amniotic membrane grafting in the reconstruction of contracted socket. Ophthal Plast Reconstr Surg. 2006;22:116-20.
9. Nasser QJ, Gombos DS, Williams MD, et al. Management of radiation-induced severe anophthalmic socket contracture in patients with uveal melanoma. Ophthal Plast Reconstr Surg. 2012;28(3):208-12.
10. Smith B, Bosniak SL, Nesi F, et al. Dermis-fat orbital implantation: 118 cases. Ophthalmic Surg. 1983;14(11):941-3.
11. Björnsson A, Einarsson O. Repair of the contracted eye socket using a flap from the upper eyelid. Plast Reconstr Surg. 1984; 74(2):287-91.
12. Poonyathalang A, Preechawat P, Pomsathit J, et al. Reconstruction of contracted eye socket with amniotic membrane graft. Ophthal Plast Reconstr Surg. 2005;21(5):359-62.
13. Li D, Jie Y, Liu H, et al. Reconstruction of anophthalmic orbits and contracted eye sockets with microvascular radial forearm free flaps. Ophthal Plast Reconstr Surg. 2008;24:94-7.
14. Xin W, Wei X, Yun-Ping L, et al. Meshed conjunctival incision technique: an efficient technique for contracted eye socket. J Plast Reconstr Aesthet Surg. 2013;66(5):688-92.
15. Guberina C, Hornblass A, Meltzer MA, et al. Autogenous dermis-fat orbital implantation. Arch Ophthalmol. 1983;101(10): 1586-90.
16. Raizada K, Shome D, Honavar SG. Management of an irradiated anophthalmic socket following dermis-fat graft rejection: a case report. Indian J Ophthalmol. 2008;56:147-8.
17. Koshima I, Narushima M, Mihara M, et al. Short pedicle thoracodorsal artery perforator (TAP) adiposal flap for three-dimensional reconstruction of contracted orbital cavity. J Plast Reconstr Aesthet Surg. 2008;61(12):e13.
18. Anderson OA, Tumuluri K, Francis ND, et al. Periocular autologous Coleman fat graft survival and histopathology. Ophtahl Plastic Reconstr Surg. 2008;24(3):213-7.
19. Lee EW, Berbos Z, Zaldivar RA, et al. Use of DermaMatrix graft in oculoplastic surgery. Ophthal Plast Reconstr Surg. 2010;26(3): 153-4.
20. Zhang R. Reconstruction of the anophthalmic orbit by orbital osteotomy and free flap transfer. J Plast Reconstr Aesthet Surg. 2007;60(3):232-40.
21. Arvanitis P, Stratoudakis A, Alexandrou C. Secondary orbital implant insertion in an anophthalmic patient after orbital reconstruction. Orbit. 2007;26(4):275-7.
22. Gonzalez-Rodriguez J, Pelcastre EL, Tovilla-Canales JL, et al. Mutational screening of CHX10, GDF6, OTX2, RAX and SOX2 genes in 50 unrelated microphthalmia-anophthalmia-coloboma (MAC) spectrum cases. Br J Ophthalmol 2010;94: 1100–1104
23. Quaranta-Leoni FM. Congenital anophthalmia: current concepts in management. Curr Opin Ophthalmol. 2011;22(5):380-4.
24. Gundlach KK, Guthoff RF, Hingst VH, et al. Expansion of the socket and orbit for congenital clinical anophthalmia. Plast Reconstr Surg. 2005;116:1214-22.
25. Schittkowski MP, Guthoff RF. Injectable self inflating hydrogel pellet expanders for the treatment of orbital volume deficiency in congenital micro- phthalmos: preliminary results with a new therapeutic approach. Br J Ophthalmol. 2006;90:1173-7.
26. Tao JP, LeBoyer RM, Hetzler K, et al. Inferolateral migration of hydrogel orbital implants in microphthalmia. Ophthal Plast Reconstr Surg 2010;26:14 – 17.
27. Tse DT, Abdulhafez M, Orozco MA, et al. Evaluation of an FAIROOZ Page 17/5/2014 clinical experience. Am J Ophthalmol. 2011;151(3):470-82.
28. Heher KL, Katowitz JA, Low JE. Unilateral dermis-fat graft implantation in the pediatric orbit. Ophthal Plast Reconstr Surg. 1998;14(2):81-8.
29. Tarantini A, Hintschich C. Primary dermis-fat grafting in children. Orbit. 2008;27(5):363-9.
30. Mitchell KT, Hollsten DA, White WL, et al. The autogenous dermis-fat orbital implant in children. J AAPOS. 2001;5(6):367-9.

CHAPTER

77

# Enucleation

Sima Das, Santosh G Honavar

## INTRODUCTION

Enucleation is one of the commonly performed surgeries in ophthalmology and involves the removal of the entire globe along with a portion of the optic nerve from the orbit. Enucleation may be considered the oldest operation of ophthalmology; in 1841, O'Ferrel and Bonnet separately described their technique of enucleation, which involved separation of the tenons and extraocular muscles and removal of the globe.[1] The idea of orbital implants was first introduced by Mules and Frost who suggested use of a hollow glass sphere as implant.[2] The modern day enucleation techniques are based on the foundation laid down by these pioneers.

Enucleation surgery as a treatment modality is primarily indicated for intraocular tumor and end-stage ocular disease. The goal of the surgery is to remove the affected eye safely and effectively, remove the underlying disease pathology, and provide excellent long-term cosmetic outcome. Various modifications of the surgical technique have been done over the years to achieve these goals. This chapter discusses the indications, technique, complications of standard enucleation procedure.

## INDICATIONS

Enucleation is the treatment of choice for primary intraocular malignancy, which is not amenable to any other form of therapy, has potential for metastasis, or has created a blind painful eye. Following are the situations where enucleation is indicated[3] (Figs. 77-1A to C).

### *Intraocular Malignancy*

Retinoblastoma and choroidal malignant melanoma are the two most common tumors, which need enucleation. With improvement in technology eye sparing techniques have proven more and more effective for management of these tumors. However, certain subset of these patients still need removal of the eye by enucleation. For retinoblastoma enucleation, it is imperative to remove a long optic nerve stump of at least 15 mm along with the eyeball to be able to remove the disease completely. Several modifications of the standard technique have been described to achieve this goal, including cutting the optic nerve from medial aspect and using straight scissors for cutting the nerve.

### *Trauma*

The decision to enucleate an eye after severe ocular trauma remains controversial. However, enucleation of a severely traumatized globe with no visual prognosis may be justified in certain cases to prevent the possible risk of sympathetic ophthalmia to the other eye. Although the exact incidence of sympathetic ophthalmia is not known, it has been estimated to be as high as 3–5% in some series.[4] Although attempt should always be made to do a primary globe repair after severe ocular trauma, in some situations such as severely traumatized eye with no visual prognosis and where repair is not possible, a primary enucleation is indicated provided the patient is conscious to understand the implication of the surgery and provide consent for the same.[5] Enucleation for prevention of sympathetic ophthalmia can also be done as secondary procedure within 2 weeks of the trauma.[6-8] In case of onset of sympathetic ophthalmia in the fellow eye, enucleation of the damaged eye at the earliest have been found to provide a better final vision in the sympathizing eye.[3,8]

### *Painful Blind Eye*

Painful blind eye after trauma or any end-stage ocular disease like neovascular glaucoma, uveitis, and chronic retinal

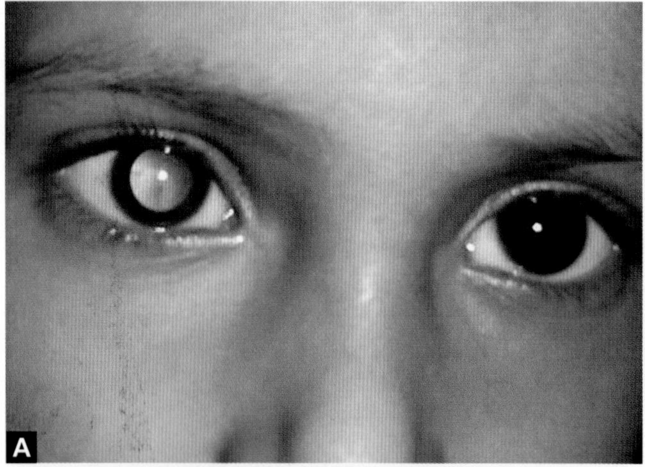


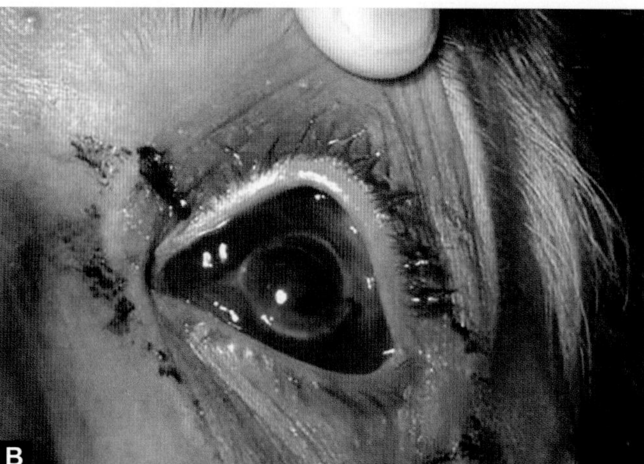


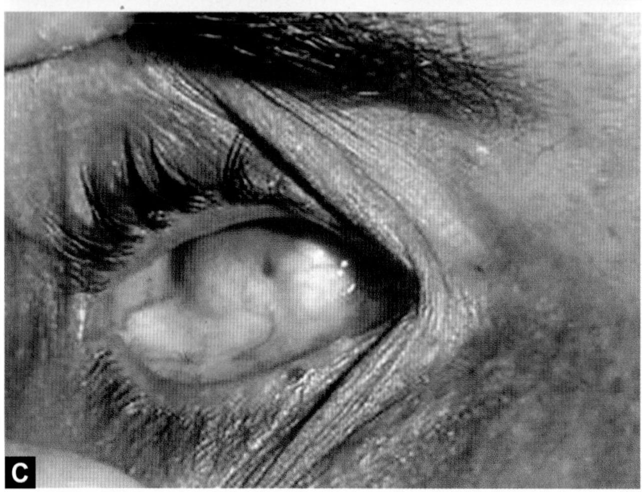


**Figures 77-1A to C** Indications of enucleation. (A) Advanced intraocular retinoblastoma. (B) Globe rupture after trauma with nil visual prognosis. Enucleation is indicated to prevent development of sympathetic ophthalmia. (C) Blind painful phthisical eyeball with volume loss in the socket.

detachment is another indication for enucleation. Enucleation is reserved for those cases where conservative treatment modalities for pain relief like medications and cyclocryotherapy is ineffective.[3]

### *Blind Disfigured Eye*

Enucleation is also indicated for cosmetically disfiguring blind eye to restore the overall appearance and preserve the self-image of the patient. Blind disfigured phthisis or atrophic bulbi can harbor underlying malignancy like melanoma.[9,10] Such eyes with suspicion of intraocular malignancy where detailed evaluation is not possible due to media opacity and the periodic follow-up with ultrasound or magnetic resonance imaging is not feasible should preferably be enucleated.

### *Congenital Microphthalmos*

Congenital severe microphthalmos with extremely shrunken eyeball can hamper the growth of the orbital bone and cause orbital hypoplasia.[11] Early enucleation and placement of a large sized orbital implant in these cases can stimulate the bony orbital growth and restore orbital symmetry.

## Enucleation Surgery

### *Preoperative Evaluation*

In addition to a detailed ophthalmic evaluation, preoperative evaluation should consist of documentation of the indication for enucleation and visual potential of the fellow eye. A detailed discussion has to be held with the patient about the need for the surgery and the alternative treatment available, and the patient must be counseled regarding the realistic surgical and cosmetic outcome. A written informed consent should be obtained from the patient or from the legal guardians in case of minors prior to the surgery. In cases, where enucleation is done for an intraocular malignancy, a metastatic workup should be done prior to surgery. Any systemic disease such as hypertension and diabetes needs to be controlled before surgery. Blood thinners like aspirin are discontinued prior to surgery in consultation with physician.

Removing the wrong eye is the most devastating complication in ophthalmology. Hence, it is absolutely essential for the surgeon to personally identify the correct eye on the operating table by doing chart review and ophthalmoscopic evaluation before starting the surgery.

## *Anesthesia*

Enucleation is preferably done under general anesthesia with a retrobulbar injection of lignocaine and epinephrine to reduce bleeding and provide postoperative comfort. Although retrobulbar anesthesia can provide adequate analgesia, handling of the extraocular muscles can stimulate oculocardiac reflex and transection of the optic nerve can cause Augenblink phenomenon with distressing visual sensations.[3,12] Hence, in patients where the surgery has to be done under local anesthesia due to medical contraindications for general anesthesia, adequate sedation should be ensured.

## *Surgical Technique*

The conventional technique of enucleation involves dissection of the conjunctiva and tenons, disinsertion of the extraocular muscles, transection of the optic nerve, removal of the globe, and placement of an orbital implant in the intraconal space. The extraocular muscles are either left loose or tied over the implant conventionally. Several modifications of this technique have been done, primarily to increase the implant and prosthesis motility. Authors currently follow the myoconjunctival technique of enucleation where the extraocular muscles are attached to the respective fornices instead of imbricating over the implant.[13,14] This technique has been found to impart better implant and prosthetic motility. Following are the steps of the myoconjunctival technique of enucleation:

*Peritomy and disinsertion of extraocular muscles*: Eyelids are retracted with speculum and 360° limbal peritomy performed. A small lateral canthotomy can be done in cases of retinoblastoma to facilitate insertion of the enucleation scissors to obtain a long optic nerve stump. Small radial incision can be given at the edge of the conjunctival peritomy in inferolateral quadrant to facilitate prolapse of the globe. The posterior Tenon's capsule is bluntly dissected off the globe by spreading a blunt tip tenotomy scissor between the sclera and the tenons in the quadrants between the extraocular muscles. The extraocular muscles are hooked, separated from surrounding tenons by blunt dissection and tagged with 4-0 silk suture just posterior to the insertion (Fig. 77-2A). A 6-0 Vicryl tag suture is passed through the muscle belly about 5–6 mm from the insertion. The muscle is transected between the two sutures. The medial rectus is transected first, followed by the inferior, lateral, and superior rectus in that sequence. The oblique muscle are hooked, dissected from the tenons and transected. The inferior oblique is clamped and cut using bipolar cautery to prevent bleeding from the muscle.

*Optic nerve transection:* A gentle traction is applied with the silk sutures to cause luxation of the globe out of the orbital rim. Gentle downward traction on the fornices with eye speculum facilitates this. This maneuver straightens the optic nerve and helps in obtaining a long optic nerve stump. Inability to luxate the globe freely could be due to a small conjunctival opening or residual extraocular muscle fibers or anterior tenons adhesions on the globe. Conjunctival opening is expanded with radial cuts if needed. The globe is inspected carefully again to dissect out all remaining tenons attachment. Vortex veins can be identified and cauterized if required. Authors prefer to use a blunt tip 15° curved tenotomy scissors from the lateral aspect to transect the nerve. The nerve can also be transected from the medial aspect using a straight enucleation scissors. The closed enucleation scissors is introduced between the lateral rectus and globe, strumming the optic nerve, and reaching the orbital apex. The scissors is then lifted up by about 2-mm from the apex to prevent damage to the structures that pass through the superior orbital fissure. The blades of the scissors are opened, the nerve is gripped firmly between the blades, and transected with single bold cut while maintaining a gentle traction on the globe. Remaining Tenon's capsule adhesion can be dissected bluntly and the globe removed. Hemostasis is obtained by firm digital pressure over the socket with dry gauze for several minutes.

In cases where the muscle traction sutures are not applied, a curved hemostat can be used to grasp the remnant of the lateral rectus insertion and provide traction on the globe. In the "no touch" technique of enucleation, instead of the muscle traction sutures, a cryoprobe is applied to the sclera and helps to provide traction.[15] In this technique, no direct pressure is applied to the globe while doing enucleation for intraocular malignancy. Metastatic spread of the tumor by embolization has been postulated to happen due to pressure on the globe during enucleation.[16] Though no studies have proven the efficacy of the no touch technique in preventing metastasis of intraocular melanoma, it is imperative that traction on the globe should be kept to a minimum while enucleating an eye harboring a malignancy.

*Implant placement and closure:* A spherical polymethylmethacrylate (PMMA) implant is preferred by the authors for volume replacement after enucleation. The size of the implant is decided based on the age of the patient and the axial length. In adults, a 20–21-mm implant could be easily inserted without causing any undue tension on the wound closure. The edges of the posterior Tenon's are identified (Fig. 77-2B). In cases where the posterior Tenon's capsule is thin and friable or disrupted accidentally during the dissection, it can be identified by following the extraocular muscle tunnels. The posterior layer of the muscle tunnel is formed by the posterior Tenon's. Location of the intraconal fat also helps in identifying the posterior Tenon's. The edges of the posterior Tenon's are held with forceps, and the implant is pushed into the intraconal space as far back in the orbit as possible (Fig. 77.2C). The posterior Tenon's are next closed with 6-0 Vicryl interrupted sutures (Fig. 77-2D). The extraocular muscles are sutured just short of the respective fornices by passing the preplaced muscle suture through the Tenon's–conjunctiva complex (Fig. 77-2E). The anterior Tenon's are closed with 6-0 Vicryl interrupted sutures and conjunctiva closed with 6-0 Vicryl running suture (Figs. 77-2F and G). Care should be taken while suturing the conjunctiva to avoid any invagination of the conjunctival edges, which might cause implantation cyst formation later and preclude prosthesis wear. The exteriorized muscle sutures are tied on the conjunctival surface and the knot left exposed (Fig. 77-2H). Appropriate sized PMMA conformer is inserted into conjunctival cul de sac, suture tarsorrhaphy done, antibiotic ointment applied, and the pressure patch is left overnight.

In cases where enucleation is done for intraocular tumor, the enucleated eyeball should be inspected for any gross extraocular extension of the tumor; scleral thinning; irregular contour; induration or vascularity; dilatation of the vortex veins; and the optic nerve for thickening, adherence or nodularity of its sheath, and its length. All the suspicious scleral areas are marked for the pathologist to obtain sections from. The eyeball is sent for histopathological evaluation in 10% formalin.

### Advantage of the Myoconjunctival Technique of Enucleation

- Better implant centration and reduced chances of migration.
- Increased prosthetic motility due to deepening of the fornices with muscle contraction.
- Inexpensive procedure as PMMA implant is used.
- Decreased chances of implant exposure due to secure three layer closure of the Tenon's and conjunctiva over the implant.

## POSTOPERATIVE CARE

Postoperatively the patient receives systemic antibiotics, analgesics and topical antibiotic, and steroid eyedrops. If there is no contraindication, a short course of systemic steroid can be given for excessive postoperative swelling. Tarsorrhaphy suture is removed after 1 week and prosthesis fitting can be done after 6–8 weeks.

## COMPLICATIONS

### Intraoperative and Early Postoperative Complications

- *Hemorrhage*: Although minimal periorbital ecchymoses and hemorrhage is common postoperatively, excessive intraoperative bleeding is unusual during enucleation. Retrobulbar injection of lignocaine with adrenaline preoperatively can help in intraoperative hemostasis. The bleeding from the central retinal vessels following optic nerve transection can usually be controlled by firm digital pressure. Use of cautery is rarely required and should be done with caution near the orbital apex to prevent damage to the extraocular muscles and oculomotor nerves.
- *Loss of extraocular muscles*: This can be prevented by placing the muscle tag sutures meticulously. Lost muscle can be traced by identifying the muscle tunnel between the anterior and posterior Tenon's and grasping the muscle within the tunnel.
- Removal of the wrong eye is the most devastating complication in ophthalmology and can be prevented by careful review of the patient charts, marking the eye and confirmation of the eye to be operated on table by the surgeon before starting the surgery.
- *Orbital infection*: Postoperative orbital infection is uncommon following enucleation. Orbital infection is reported to be more common with the use of porous implants and might require removal of the implant.[17-19]
- *Orbital apex injury*: Injury to the delicate structures of the orbital apex can occur while dissection is done in the posterior orbit in an attempt to remove long optic nerve stump or excessive cautery is done to the posterior orbital tissue to control intraoperative bleeding. Injury to the oculomotor nerve can cause postoperative ptosis.
- Excessive traction on the optic nerve can cause chiasmal traction and postoperative visual field defects in the fellow eye.[20]

## Late Complications

- Late complications are usually in the form of postenucleation socket syndrome and are due to inadequate orbital volume replacement with a small implant[21,22] (Figs. 77-3A to C). Missed orbital fracture in an anophthalmic socket can also cause postenucleation socket syndrome.[23] The features of postenucleation socket syndrome include

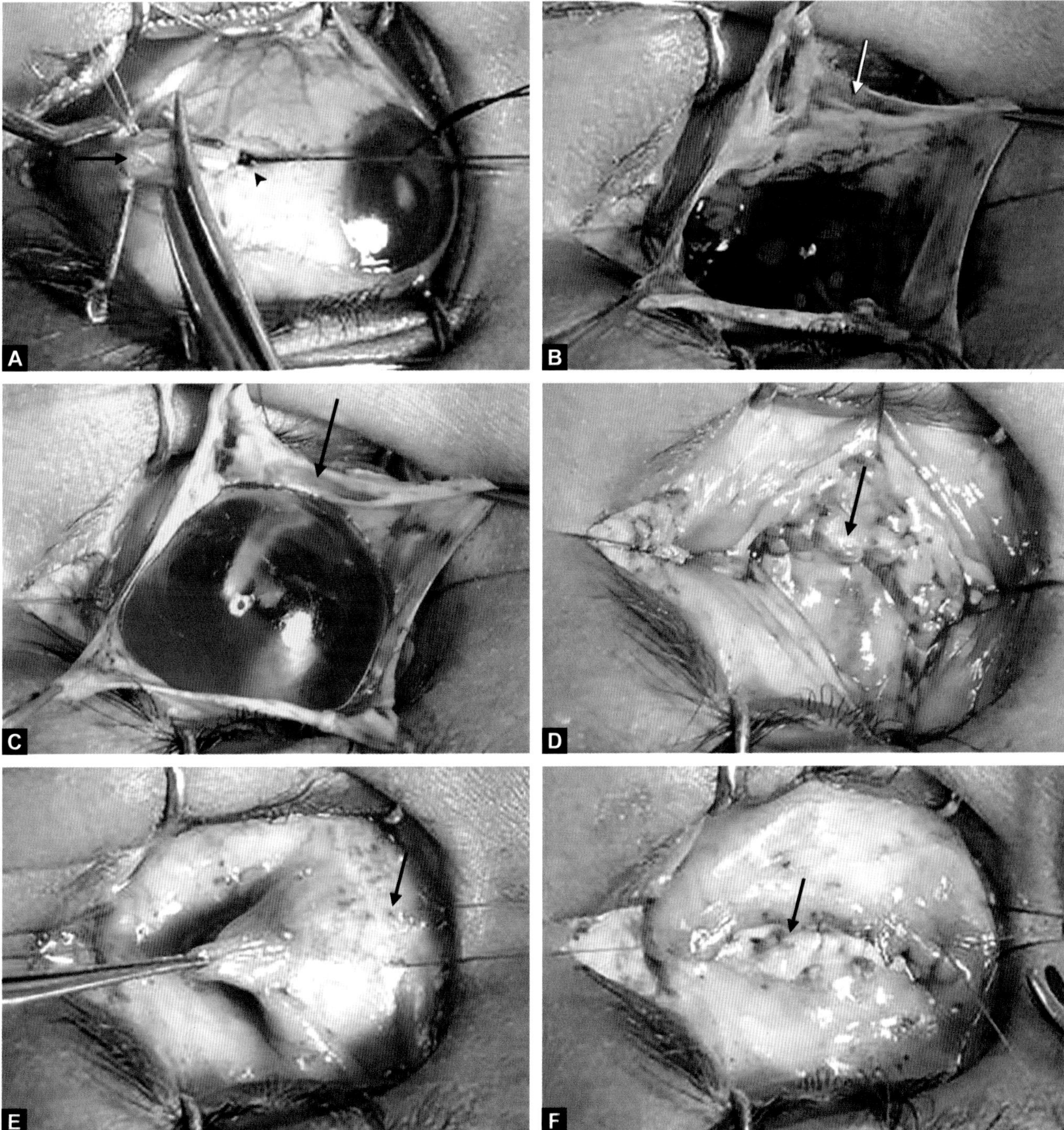

**Figures 77-2A to F** Technique of myoconjunctival enucleation. (A) Extraocular muscles are isolated, tagged with 4-0 silk and 6-0 Vicryl sutures and cut in between the sutures. (B) Posterior Tenon's and intraconal space identified after removing the globe. (C) Appropriate sized spherical polymethylmethacrylate implant placed within the intraconal space behind the posterior Tenon's. (D) Posterior Tenon's closed with 6-0 Vicryl interrupted sutures. (E) Recti muscle sutured just short of the respective fornices using preplaced 6-0 Vicryl sutures. (F) Anterior Tenon's closed with 6-0 Vicryl interrupted sutures.

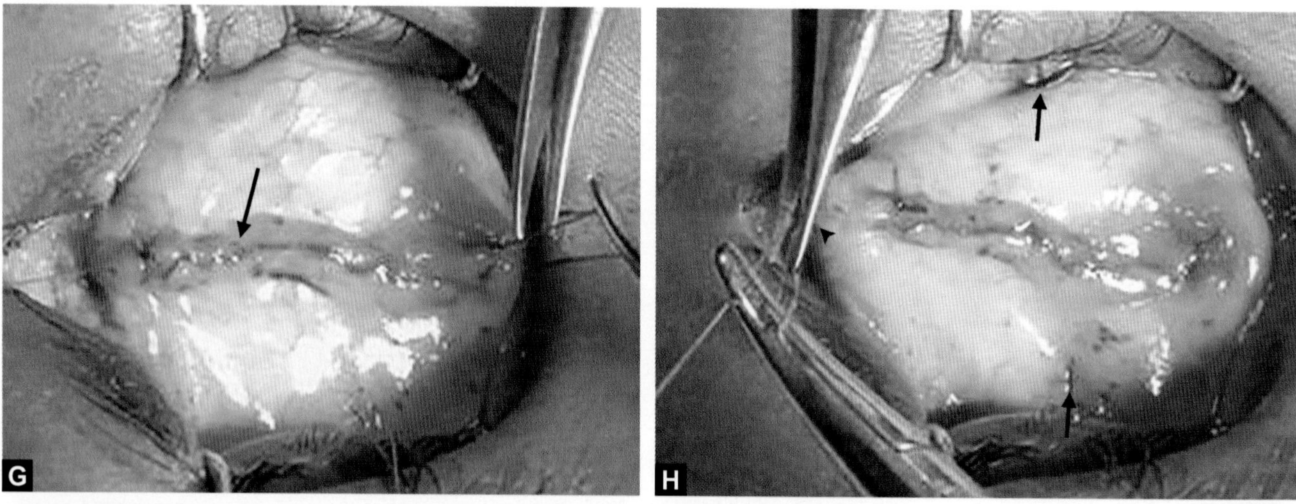


**Figures 77-2G and H** Technique of myoconjunctival enucleation. (G) Conjunctiva closed with 6-0 Vicryl running suture. (H) Exteriorized muscle sutures are tied and cut.

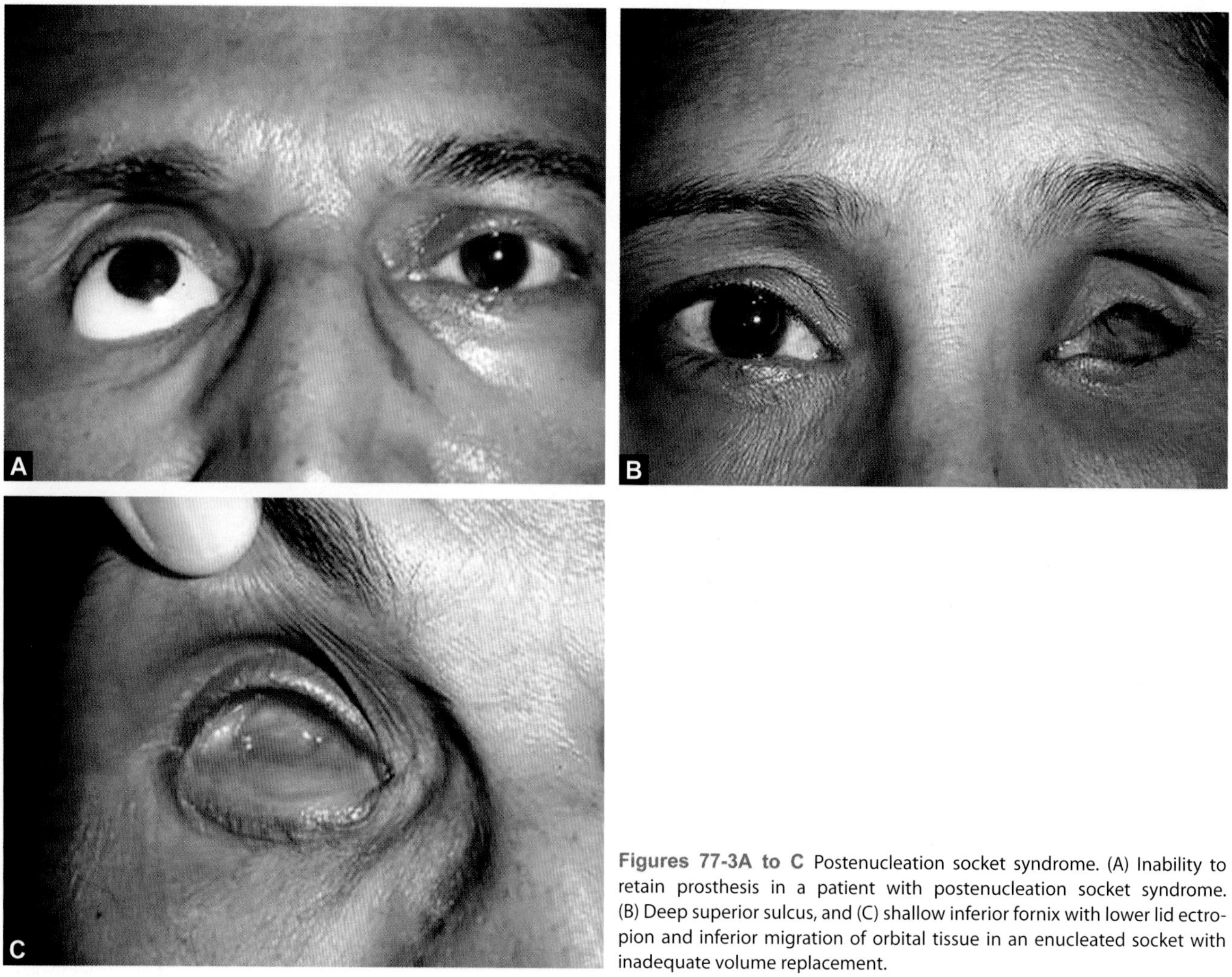

**Figures 77-3A to C** Postenucleation socket syndrome. (A) Inability to retain prosthesis in a patient with postenucleation socket syndrome. (B) Deep superior sulcus, and (C) shallow inferior fornix with lower lid ectropion and inferior migration of orbital tissue in an enucleated socket with inadequate volume replacement.

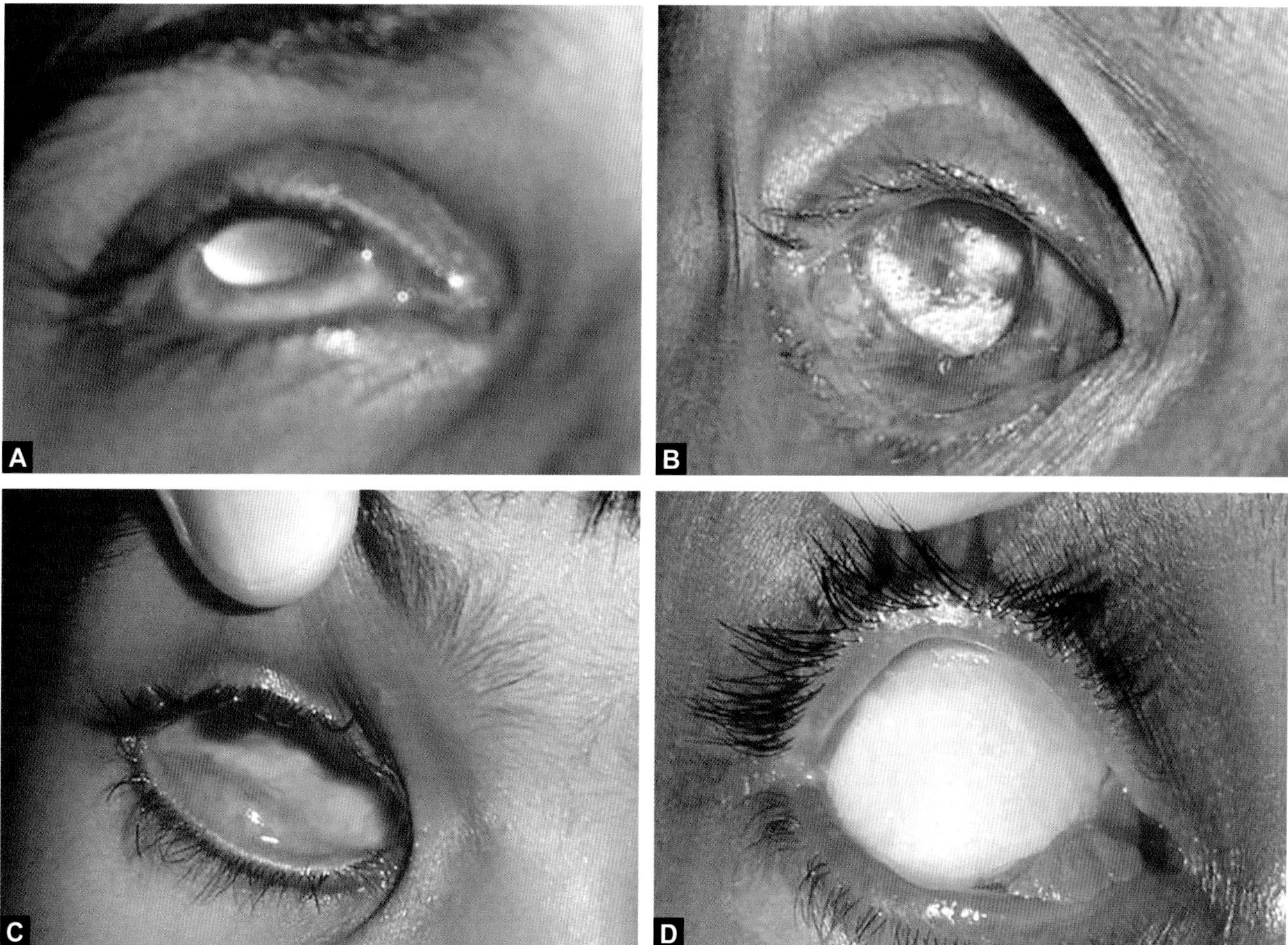


**Figures 77.4A to D** Complications of enucleation. (A) Exposure of an oversized polymethylmethacrylate implant. (B) Hydroxyapatite implant exposure with chronic socket infection and discharge. (C) Inferior implant migration causing shallowing of inferior fornix after enucleation for retinoblastoma. Enucleation was done by the conventional technique with imbrication of the extraocular muscles over the implant. (D) Exposure of an oversized porous polyethylene implant requiring removal of the implant.

superior sulcus deformity, lower lid ectropion, stretching and shallowing of the inferior fornix, and inferior migration of orbital tissues.

- Implant exposure and migration and socket contracture are the other late complications of enucleation (Figs. 77-4A to D). Migration of the implant can occur due to placement in locations other than the intraconal space or due to imbrications of the muscles over the implant as in conventional technique of enucleation.[24] Superotemporal migration can cause ptosis due to pressure over the levator aponeurosis. Inferior migration of the implant can cause shallow inferior fornix and nonretention of the prosthesis.
- Exposure of the implant can occur after infection or due to dehiscence of the wound or due to placement of an oversized implant. Early exposure needs immediate revision of the socket and covering the area of the exposure with patch graft. Implant exposure after placement of an integrated implant could be due to slow vascularization of the implant and erosion of the overlying tenons and conjunctiva by the porous implant. Using a wrapping material with porous implants can reduce this complication.[19] Spontaneous healing of an exposed porous implant is rare.[25] Exposure of a porous implant might require removal of the nonvascularized part of the implant with a drill and covering the exposure with a patch graft.

## PROSTHESIS FITTING

A custom-made prosthesis can be fitted in the socket about 6–8 weeks after the surgery. Till that time an acrylic conformer is kept inside the socket to prevent any surface contracture. The conformer should be large enough to apply gentle pressure and stretching of the fornices while allowing closure of the eyelids comfortably. A conformer with a central opening is preferable as it allows for the discharge and secretions from behind the conformer to drain out. A slight vaulting of the conformer prevents undue pressure over the conjunctival sutures and promotes faster healing. Along with prosthesis, patients are also advised to use protective eyewear to prevent any accidental trauma to the fellow sighted eye. Patients are also advised to refrain from participating in contact sports, which carries risk of ocular injury.

## CONCLUSION

Enucleation as a management modality is indicated for intraocular tumors not amenable to other forms of treatment and for pain relief and cosmetic rehabilitation of blind painful and disfigured eyes. The decision to enucleate the eye should be taken after a detailed discussion with the patients about the realistic surgical and cosmetic outcome. A meticulous surgical technique with attention to minimal tissue manipulation, gentle handling of the conjunctiva, identification and preservation of extraocular muscles, placing an appropriate sized implant in central intraconal space are essential for creating an adequate socket with optimal volume and surface suitable for fitting prosthesis.

## REFERENCES


1. Jordan DR, Klapper SR. Surgical techniques in enucleation: the role of various types of implants and the efficacy of pegged and nonpegged approaches. Int Ophthalmol Clin. 2006;46:109-32.
2. Mules PH. Evisceration of the globe, with artificial vitreous. Trans ophthalmol Soc U K. 1885;5:200-6.
3. Moshfeghi DM. Enucleation. Survey Ophthalmol. 2000;44(4): 277-301.
4. Hogan MJ, Zimmerman LE. Ophthalmic pathology: an atlas and textbook. Philadelphia, PA: WB Saunders; 1962.
5. Esmaeli B, Elner SG, Schork MA, et al. Visual outcome and ocular survival after penetrating trauma: a clinicopathologic study. Ophthalmology. 1995;102:393-400.
6. Green WR. Uveal tract. In: Spencer WH (ed), Ophthalmic pathology: an atlas and textbook, vol. 3, 4th edn, Philadelphia, PA: WB Saunders Company; 1996:1997-2039.
7. Jennings T, Tessler HH. Twenty cases of sympathetic ophthalmia. Br J Ophthalmol. 1989;73:140-5.
8. Lubin JR, Albert DM, Weinstein M. Sixty-five years of sympathetic ophthalmia: a clinicopathologic review of 105 cases (1913–1978). Ophthalmology. 1980;87:109-21
9. Duke-Elder S, ed. Cysts and tumors of the uveal tract: diagnosis of malignant melanoma. In: System of ophthalmology, vol. 9, Chapter 6, St. Louis: CV Mosby; 1966: 896.
10. Yanoff M, Fine B. Ocular pathology. Hagerstown, MD: Harper & Row; 1975.
11. Kennedy RE. Effects of early enucleation on the orbit in animals and humans. Trans Am Ophthalmol Soc. 1964;62:459.
12. Munden PM, Carter KD, Nerad JA. The oculocardiac reflex during enucleation. Am J Ophthalmol. 1991;111(3):378-9.
13. Shome D, Honavar SG, Raizada K, et al. Implant and prosthesis movement after enucleation: a randomized controlled trial. Ophthalmology. 2010;117(8):1638-44.
14. Yadava U, Sachdeva P, Arora V. Myoconjunctival enucleation for enhanced implant motility. Result of a randomised prospective study. Indian J Ophthalmol. 2004;52(3):221-6.
15. Fraunfelder FT, Wilson RS. A new approach for intraocular malignancy: the "no touch" technique. In: Jakobiec FA (ed), Ocular and adnexal tumors. Birmingham, UK: Aesculapius; 1978: 39-45.
16. Zimmerman LE, McLean IW, Foster WD. Does enucleation of the eye containing malignant melanoma prevent or accelerate the dissemination of tumour cells? An unanswered question! In: Jakobiec FA (ed), Ocular and adnexal tumors. Birmingham, UK: Aesculapius; 1978.
17. Jordan DR, Brownstein S, Rawlings N, et al. An infected porous polyethylene orbital implant. Ophthal Plast Reconstr Surg. 2007;23(5):413-5.
18. Hong SW, Paik JS, Kim SY, et al. A case of orbital abscess following porous orbital implant infection. Korean J Ophthalmol. 2006;20(4):234-7.
19. Tabatabaee Z, Mazloumi M, Rajabi MT, et al. Comparison of the exposure rate of wrapped hydroxyapatite (Bio-Eye) versus unwrapped porous polyethylene (Medpor) orbital implants in enucleated patients. Ophthal Plast Reconstr Surg. 2011;27(2): 114-8.
20. Tabatabaei SA, Soleimani M, Khodabandeh A. A case of auto nucleation associated with a contralateral field defect. Orbit. 2011;30(3):165-8.
21. Steinkogler FJ. The treatment of the post-enucleation socket syndrome. J Craniomaxillofac Surg. 1987;15(1):31-3.
22. Tyers AG, Collin JR. Orbital implants and post enucleation socket syndrome. Trans Ophthalmol Soc U K. 1982;102 (Pt 1): 90-2.
23. Ataullah S, Whitehouse RW, Stelmach M, et al. Missed orbital wall blow-out fracture as a cause of post-enucleation socket syndrome. Eye (Lond). 1999;13( Pt 4):541-4.
24. Allen L. The argument against imbricating the rectus muscles over spherical orbital implants after enucleation. Ophthalmology. 1983; 90(9):1116-20.
25. Custer PL, Trinkaus KM. Porous implant exposure: Incidence, management, and morbidity. Ophthal Plast Reconstr Surg. 2007; 23(1):1-7. Review.

CHAPTER

78

# Evisceration

Vikas Menon

## INTRODUCTION

History of evisceration surgery goes back to about 200 years when it was performed by Bears in 1817 in a surgery complicated by expulsive hemorrhage. Noyes reported the use of evisceration as a treatment of bad intraocular infections. Subsequently, the procedure started gaining ophthalmologists interest as a useful procedure for a variety of conditions. Mules introduced the glass sphere in 1884 as a primary implant to be inserted in the scleral shell after evisceration.[1]

Evisceration has certain advantages over enucleation as it is less time consuming, requires no orbital tissue or muscle dissection, causes less disturbance of normal orbital anatomy, and causes a lesser incidence of late onset fat atrophy or socket contraction, leading to an overall better orbital volume and better prosthesis motility.

## INDICATIONS

The primary indication for evisceration is a painful or a disfigured nonseeing eye where the goal of treatment is to provide relief from pain or adequate cosmesis. Clinical situations requiring evisceration include endophthalmitis, phthisis bulbi, staphylomatous globes, traumatic injury, and end-stage glaucoma. Many of these patients have prior history of cataract surgery, penetrating keratoplasty, glaucoma surgery, or retina surgery[2] (Figs. 78-1 and 78-2).

## CONTRAINDICATIONS

Possibility of an intraocular malignancy is the most important contraindication to evisceration, as there is risk of dissemination of the tumor upon opening such a globe. Hence, it

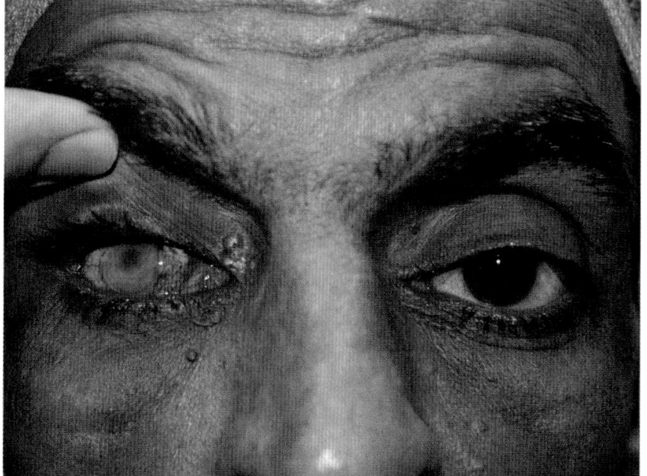

**Figure 78-1** Right atrophic bulbi following multiple surgeries for retinal detachment.

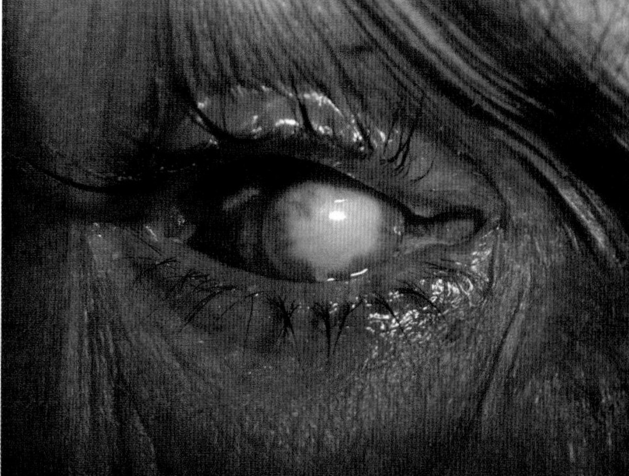

**Figure 78-2** Severe endophthalmitis requiring evisceration.

is mandatory to do a thorough clinical evaluation, aided by appropriate imaging like ultrasonography, CT, or MRI scan in every patient to rule out malignancy.

Even though with some modifications to the standard technique, like relaxing sclerotomies or four petal technique[3] it is possible to place an adequate-sized implant after evisceration in many hypoplastic or phthisical globes, extremely shrunken or small eyeballs are better treated with enucleation to avoid compromizing volume replacement.

Cases where there is requirement of a thorough histologic examination of the tissues should be subjected to enucleation, as it provides the pathologist with an intact globe and properly maintained anatomy. Even though sympathetic ophthalmia has been reported to be extremely rare after evisceration, it is preferable to do enucleation in cases of penetrating trauma where the globe is very badly disrupted. Patients having preexisting nystagmus and requiring removal of eye can have bizarre movements of prosthesis after evisceration, and are better subject to enucleation.

## SURGICAL TECHNIQUE

Before the surgery is undertaken, a choice has to be made about the type of implant to be used and size of the implant. Both porous and nonporous implants can be used in evisceration and there is no clear-cut consensus about superiority of one over the other.[4] The author prefers to use nonporous polymethyl methacrylate (PMMA) spherical implant because of its overall low complication rate, ease of availability, and cost.

Implant size is another important factor that needs to be taken into consideration as part of surgical planning. Ideally, the prosthesis should contribute 2.0 mL to the overall volume replacement in a socket. Prosthetic volumes >3.0 mL are bulky and can lead to secondary eyelid problems such as ectropion and lower lid laxity over a period of time.[5] Kaltreider and Lucarelli have provided a useful and simple formula for calculating the implant size. They suggest an implant with diameter AL-3 mm for evisceration, where AL is axial length of the normal eye. With this formula they were able to eliminate clinically unacceptable superior sulcus deformity and enophthalmos in 85% of their patients.[6]

So far, there is no consensus about placing the implant in an infected eye. Many avoid placing the implant at the time of evisceration;[7,8] others prefer to place the implant at the time of surgery even though there may be small risk of extrusion.[9] Delayed primary placement of implant has also been described with good results.[10]

### Anesthesia

Evisceration can be performed under local anesthesia in most patients unless there is an obvious indication for general anesthesia. Local anesthesia is in the form of a retrobulbar injection of lidocaine with 1:100,000 epinephrine and bupivacaine.

### Technique

The lids are kept retracted with a wire speculum. 360° conjunctival peritomy is done with Westcott scissors (Fig. 78-3). Conjunctiva and Tenon's are separated posteriorly upto insertion of recti or even slightly beyond. A limbal incision is then made with a no 11 scalpel blade, which is then extended all around with scissors for removal of the corneal button (Fig. 78-4). Cornea needs to be removed completely. After removal of cornea, the uveal tissue is separated from the sclera with the help of an evisceration spoon and an attempt is made to remove all the uveal tissue adherent to the scleral shell (Fig. 78-5). The inner side of the empty scleral cup is then cleaned with a sponge soaked in absolute alcohol to eliminate any infective material and to denature any remnants of the uveal tissue. A PMMA spherical implant is placed inside the scleral shell after enlarging the scleral opening as required (Fig. 78-6). Relaxing posterior sclerotomies can be made to allow placement of a larger sized implant. Sclera, Tenon's, and conjunctiva are closed separately with 6-0 polyglactin sutures (Fig. 78-7). A conformer is placed in the socket at the end and a temporary suture tarsorrhaphy is done to prevent extrusion of the conformer in the early postoperative period due to edema (Fig. 78-8).

In case a porous implant is used, all the steps of surgery are similar except that the implant needs to be soaked in saline for some time before implantation to remove all the air from the pores and it is mandatory to do posterior sclerotomies to allow the fibrovascular ingrowth to take place.

### Postoperative Care

Systemic antibiotics and analgesics are given for 5–7 days. A pressure dressing is kept in place and removed after 24 hours. Some surgeons prefer to keep the pressure bandage on for 3–5 days. Topical antibiotic-steroid drops are started subsequently except in grossly infected eyes where steroids are withheld in the early postoperative period. Tarsorrhaphy can be opened at 1 week, and the socket is generally ready for prosthesis after 6 weeks (Fig. 78-9).

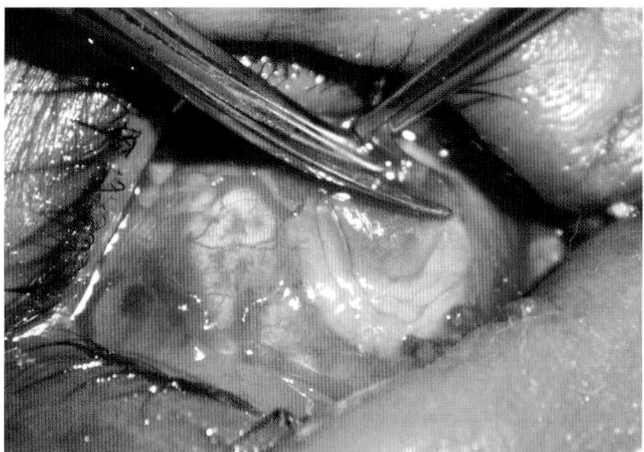

Figure 78-3 Conjunctival peritomy.

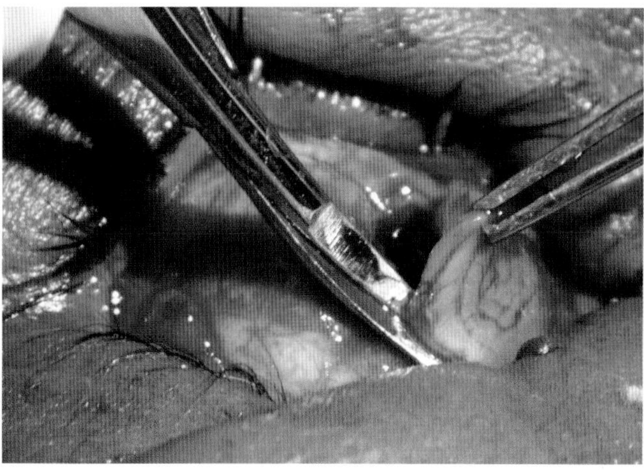

Figure 78-4 Removal of cornea.

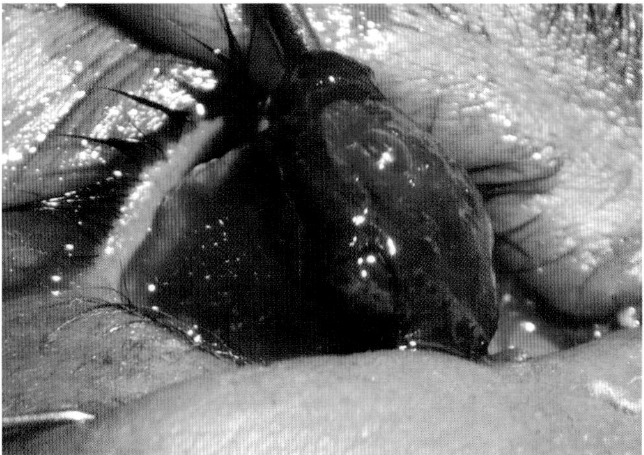

Figure 78-5 Removal of intraocular contents.

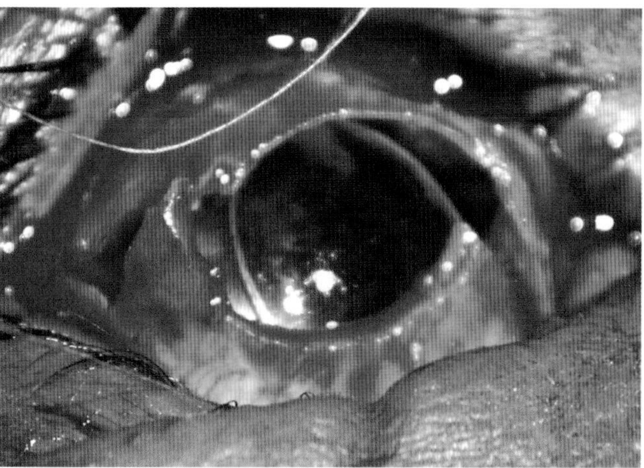

Figure 78-6 Sclera being sutured after implantation of nonporous polymethyl methacrylate spherical implant.

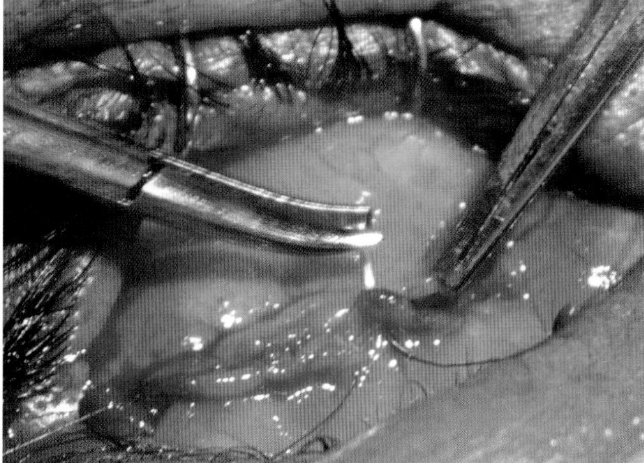

Figure 78-7 Conjunctiva being closed by running absorbable suture after closure of scleral and Tenon's in separate layers.

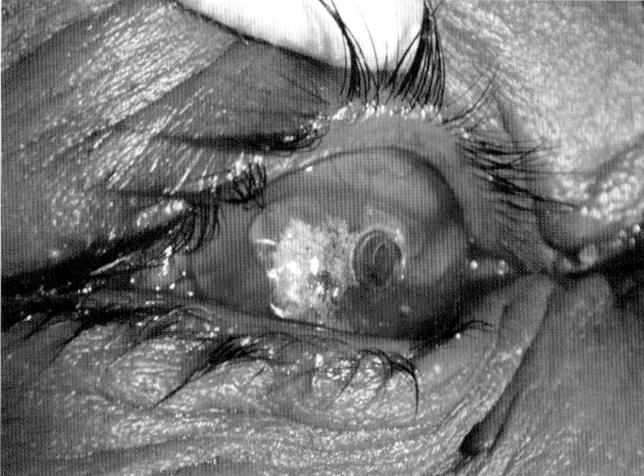

Figure 78-8 Conformer in place at the end of surgery.

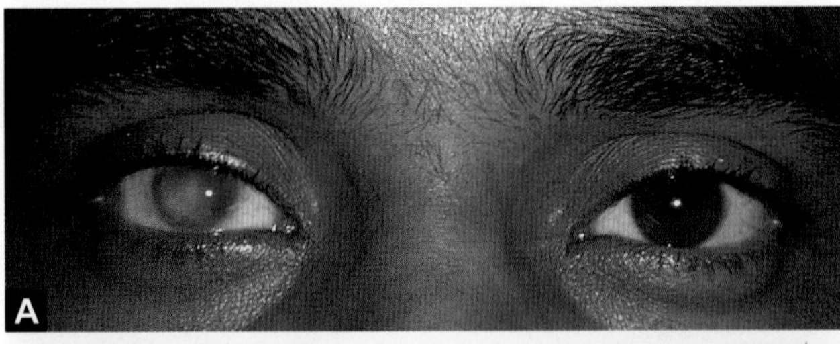


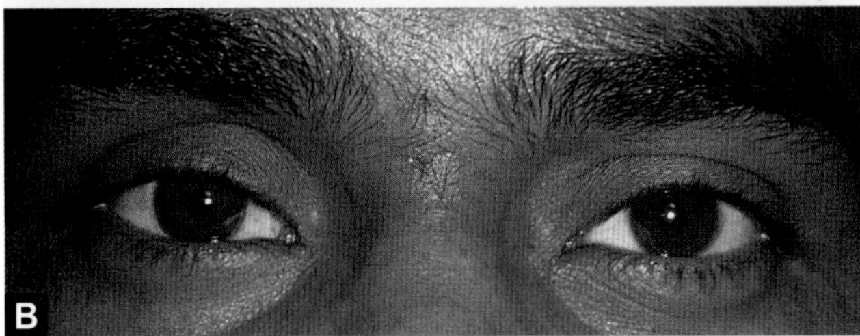


**Figures 78-9A and B** Pre- and post-evisceration with a well-fitted prosthesis.

## COMPLICATIONS

- *Bleeding*: Usually occurs from vortex veins or retained uveal tissue.
- *Implant exposure*: Incidence of this complication is higher with porous implants than with nonporous ones. In a recent publication, it has been reported as 7.7% without pegging and 34.5% with pegging for porous implants.[11] Exposure requires covering the exposed area with a dermis fat or a scleral graft. In case the area of exposure is very large, the implant can be removed and a secondary implant inserted.
- *Implant extrusion*: More commonly seen in infected eyes and cases where a disproportionately large implant size is used. A secondary implant is usually required.
- *Sympathetic ophthalmia*: Complete removal of uveal tissue is recommended at the time of evisceration to prevent sympathetic ophthalmia. Fortunately this complication is extremely uncommon. Only one case of sympathetic ophthalmia has been reported after evisceration in the last 25 years reflecting the rarity and improvement in treatment.[12]
- *Deep supratarsal sulcus*: Most often occurs due to inadequate volume replacement or fat atrophy.
- *Lax lower eyelid*: It occurs due prolonged use of a heavy prosthesis.
- *Contracted socket*: It is less common nowadays where a proper primary surgery was done, but can still occur as a result of excessive fibrosis in the socket in cases of bad trauma, chemical, or thermal injury.
- *Miscellaneous*: Persistent pain, pyogenic granuloma, and infection.

## PEARLS AND PITFALLS

- Evisceration is a safe and effective procedure for most blind eyes requiring relief from pain or better cosmesis.
- Intraocular malignancy is an absolute contraindication for evisceration. All necessary investigations must be done prior to surgery to rule out malignancy and routine histopathology must be done for intraocular tissues removed in all cases.
- Implant should be able to provide adequate volume replacement in the socket and chosen according to the surgeon's experience and comfort.

## REFERENCES


1. Meltzer MA, Schaefer DP, Della Rocca RC. Evisceration. In: Della Rocca RC, Nesi FA, Lishman RD (eds), Smith's ophthalmic plastic and reconstructive surgery, Vol 2. St.Louis: CV Mosby; 1987. pp. 1300-7.
2. Chaudhry IA, AlKuraya HS, Shamsi FA, et al. Current indications and resultant complications of evisceration. Ophthalmic Epidemiol. 2007;14(2):93-7.
3. Sales-Sanz M, Sanz-Lopez A. Four-petal evisceration: a new technique. Ophthal Plast Reconstr Surg. 2007;23(5):389-92.
4. Beard C. Remarks on historical and newer approaches to orbital implants. Ophthal Plast Reconstr Surg. 1995;11:89-90.
5. Kaltreider SA. The ideal ocular prosthesis: analysis of prosthetic volume. Ophthal Plast Reconstr Surg. 2000;16:388-92.
6. Kaltreider SA, Lucarelli MJ. A simple algorithm for selection of implant size for enucleation and evisceration: a prospective study. Ophthal Plast Reconstr Surg. 2002;18: 336-41.
7. Hughes WL. Evisceration. Arch Ophthalmol. 1960;63:60-4.
8. Smith BC, ed. Ophthalmic Plastic and Reconstructive Surgery. Vol 2. St. Louis: CV Mosby; 1987. pp. 1300-7.
9. Dresner SC, Karesh JW. Primary implant placement with evisceration in patients with endophthalmitis. Ophthalmology. 2000;107:1661-5.
10. Shore J, Dieckert P, Levine M. Delayed primary wound closure: use to prevent implant extrusion following evisceration for endophthalmitis. Arch Ophthalmol. 1988;106:1303-8.
11. Jordan DR. Problems after evisceration surgery with porous orbital implants. Ophthal Plast Reconstr Surg. 2004;20:374-80.
12. Griepentrog GJ, Lucarelli MJ, Albert DM, et al. Sympathetic ophthalmia following evisceration: a rare case. Ophthal Plast Reconstr Surg. 2005;21:316-8.

CHAPTER

79

# Orbital Exenteration

Sima Das, Santosh G Honavar

## INTRODUCTION

Orbital exenteration involves removal of the eyeball along with the orbital soft tissue structures.[1-3] The resulting deformity is often severe, and cosmetic rehabilitation is difficult. Hence, this procedure should be reserved for life-threatening malignancies or infections. The resulting deformity caused by the surgery is also socially and psychologically distressing for the patient; therefore, reconstruction and cosmetic rehabilitation should be part of the surgical planning.

Orbital exenteration is one of the oldest described surgeries. With advances in technology for early diagnosis and availability of globe sparing aggressive management modalities for orbital and periocular tumors, exenteration is rarely performed currently except as a last resort.[4,5]

## INDICATIONS

Orbital exenteration is usually reserved for management of orbital tumors, infections, and deformities, which are not amenable to other forms of therapy (Figs. 79-1 and 79-2).[2,3,6-14] Following are the main indications for orbital exenteration:

- Life-threatening primary orbital malignancies like adenoid cystic carcinoma of the lacrimal gland.
- Intraocular malignancies with orbital extension like retinoblastoma, choroidal malignant melanoma.
- Orbital extension of periocular malignancies like:
  - Carcinoma paranasal sinuses.
  - Conjunctival squamous cell carcinoma.
  - Eyelid malignancies like sebaceous gland carcinoma, basal cell carcinoma, and squamous cell carcinoma.
  - Skin malignancies.
- Life-threatening sino-orbital mucormycosis and other fungal infections with vascular thrombosis causing tissue necrosis. Exenteration is needed for debridement of the necrosed tissues and allows penetration of the antifungal medications.
- Recalcitrant diffuse orbital inflammations causing intractable pain not responding to conservative management.
- Severe orbital contracture with inability to wear a prosthesis.
- Benign conditions like:
  - Neurofibromatosis with orbital deformity.
  - Orbital meningioma and lymphangioma causing disfiguring proptosis.

## TYPES OF ORBITAL EXENTERATION

Depending upon the amount of structures removed, orbital exenteration can be divided into various types (Table 79-1).[3,15] The procedure is tailored to the individual patient and the particular type of the procedure chosen depends on the extent of the disease as determined from the examination of the orbit and surrounding structures and results of imaging findings like computed tomographic scan and magnetic resonance imaging. Exenteration can be divided into the following types.

### Anterior Exenteration

Anterior exenteration is an extended form of enucleation where, in addition to globe, variable amount of bulbar conjunctiva, palpebral conjunctiva, and posterior eyelid lamina is removed. A shallow socket lined with anterior lamella of the lids is left behind. Anterior exenteration is indicated for advanced conjunctival malignancies not amenable to complete surgical excision.

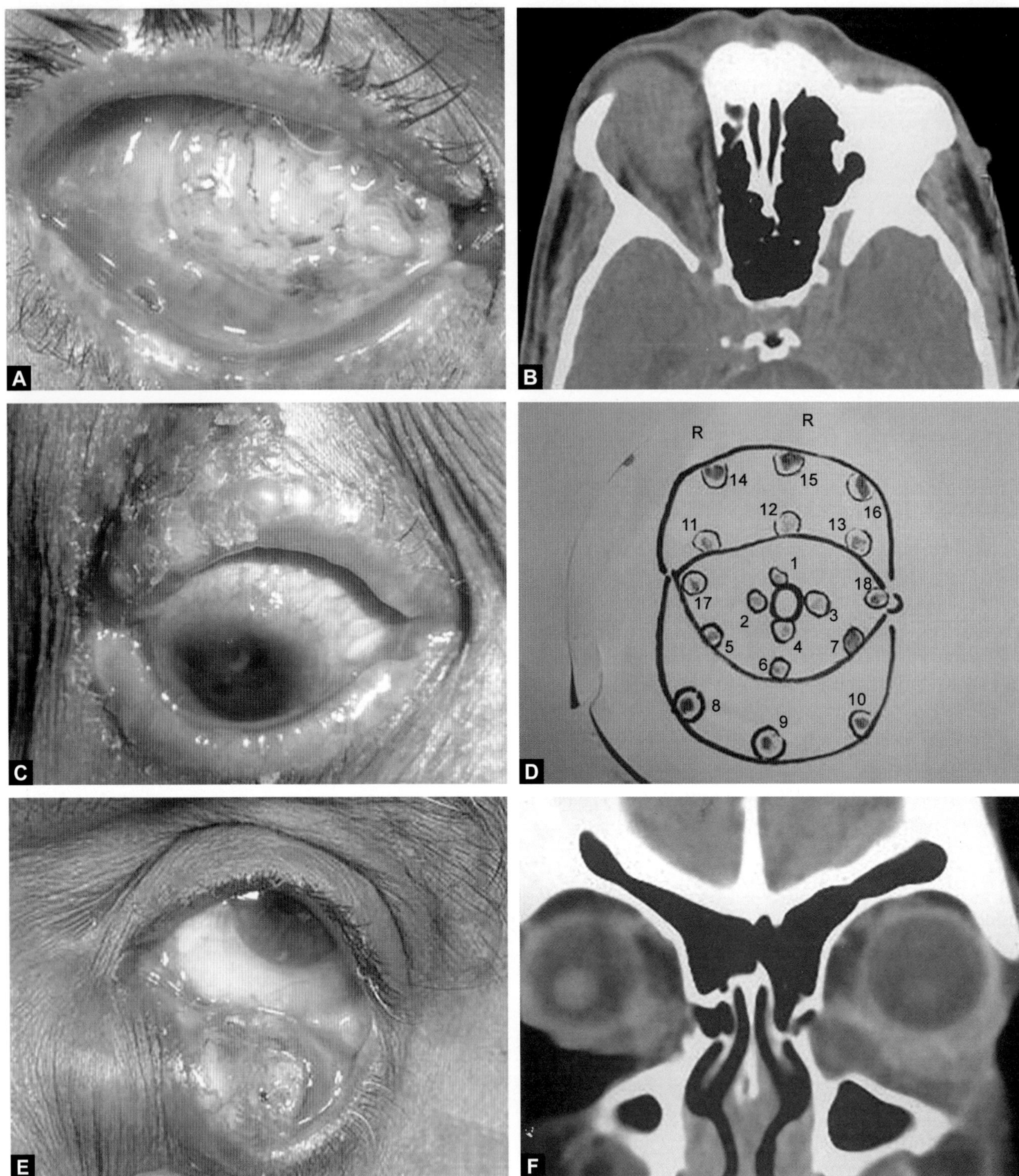


Figures 79-1A to F Indications of orbital exenteration for ocular malignancies. (A) Advanced conjunctival squamous cell carcinoma. (B) Computed tomographic (CT) scan showing orbital extension of the tumor. (C) Pagetoid sebaceous gland carcinoma presenting as unilateral diffuse blepharoconjunctivitis. (D) Conjunctival map biopsy revealed diffuse involvement of the upper and lower bulbar and palpebral conjunctiva by the tumor with all 18 biopsy sites positive. Anterior orbital exenteration was done for this patient. (E) Lower eyelid sebaceous gland carcinoma. (F) CT scan shows extension of the tumor to the inferior orbit.

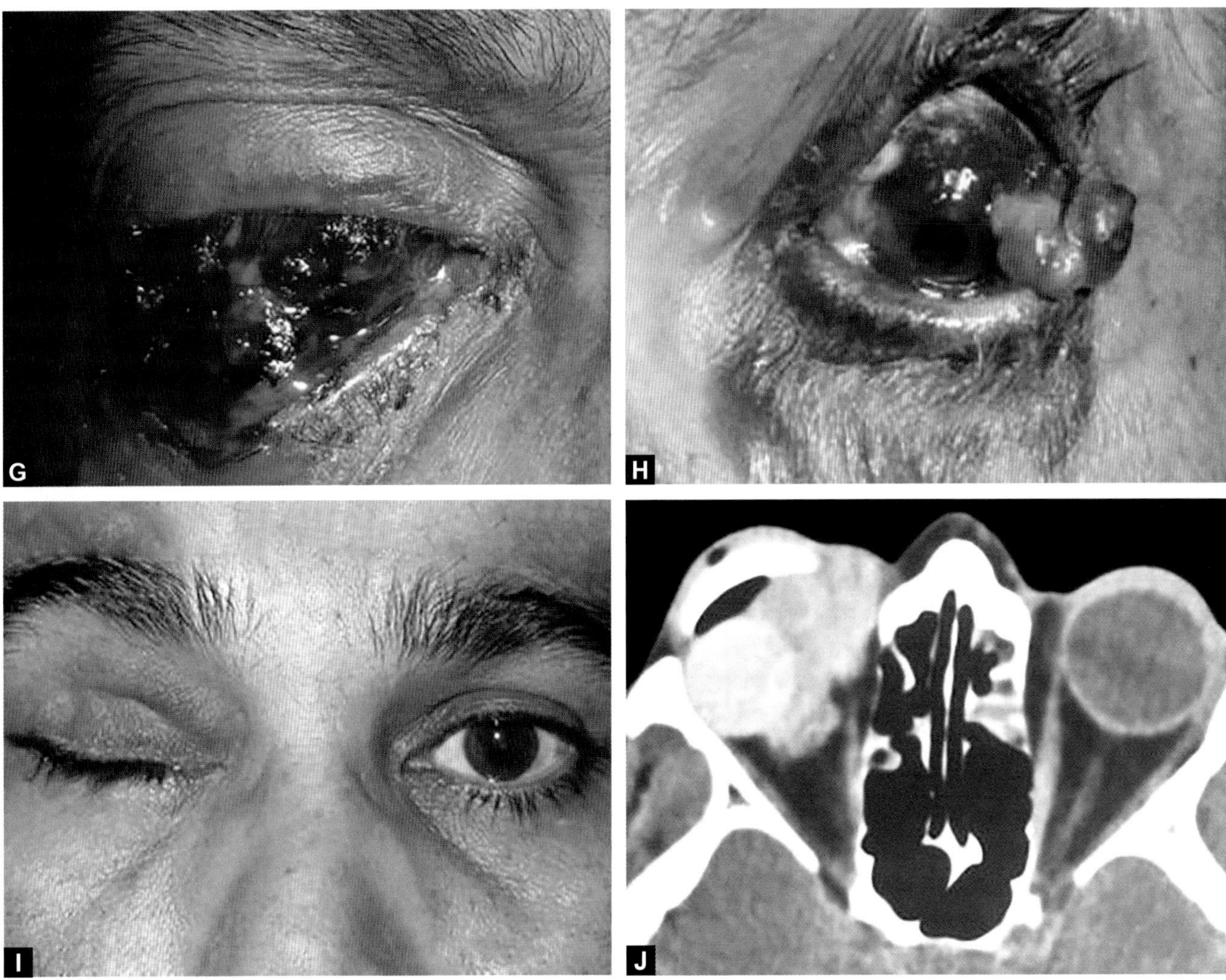

Figures 79-1G to J (G) Conjunctival malignant melanoma with orbital involvement requiring exenteration for tumor debulking. (H) Diffuse conjunctival melanoma arising from primary acquired melanosis (PAM) with atypia. Note involvement of the eyelid skin by PAM requiring eyelid sacrificing orbital exenteration. (I) Orbital recurrence of uveal melanoma following enucleation. (J) CT scan showing recurrent tumor in the medial orbit with lateral displacement of the implant.

## Subtotal or Eyelid Sparing Exenteration

Eyelid sparing orbital exenteration is indicated for intraocular tumors with extrascleral extension, orbital tumors, eyelid and ocular surface tumors with involvement of only the conjunctiva or subconjunctival tissue, and no full-thickness involvement of the eyelids. Here full thickness of the eyelid margins and rest of the posterior lamina are removed leaving behind rest of the anterior lamina of the eyelid with skin and variable amount of orbicularis. Primary closure of the exenteration cavity is done by apposing the residual eyelid margins. This technique was first popularized by Coston and Small.[1,3] This is the most commonly performed technique in the author's practice.

### *Advantages*

- Faster healing time.
- Excellent cosmetic result.
- Smooth skin-lined orbital cavity.
- Postoperative radiation tolerated well because of a skin-lined cavity.

### *Drawback*

- Tumor recurrence might not be detected early.

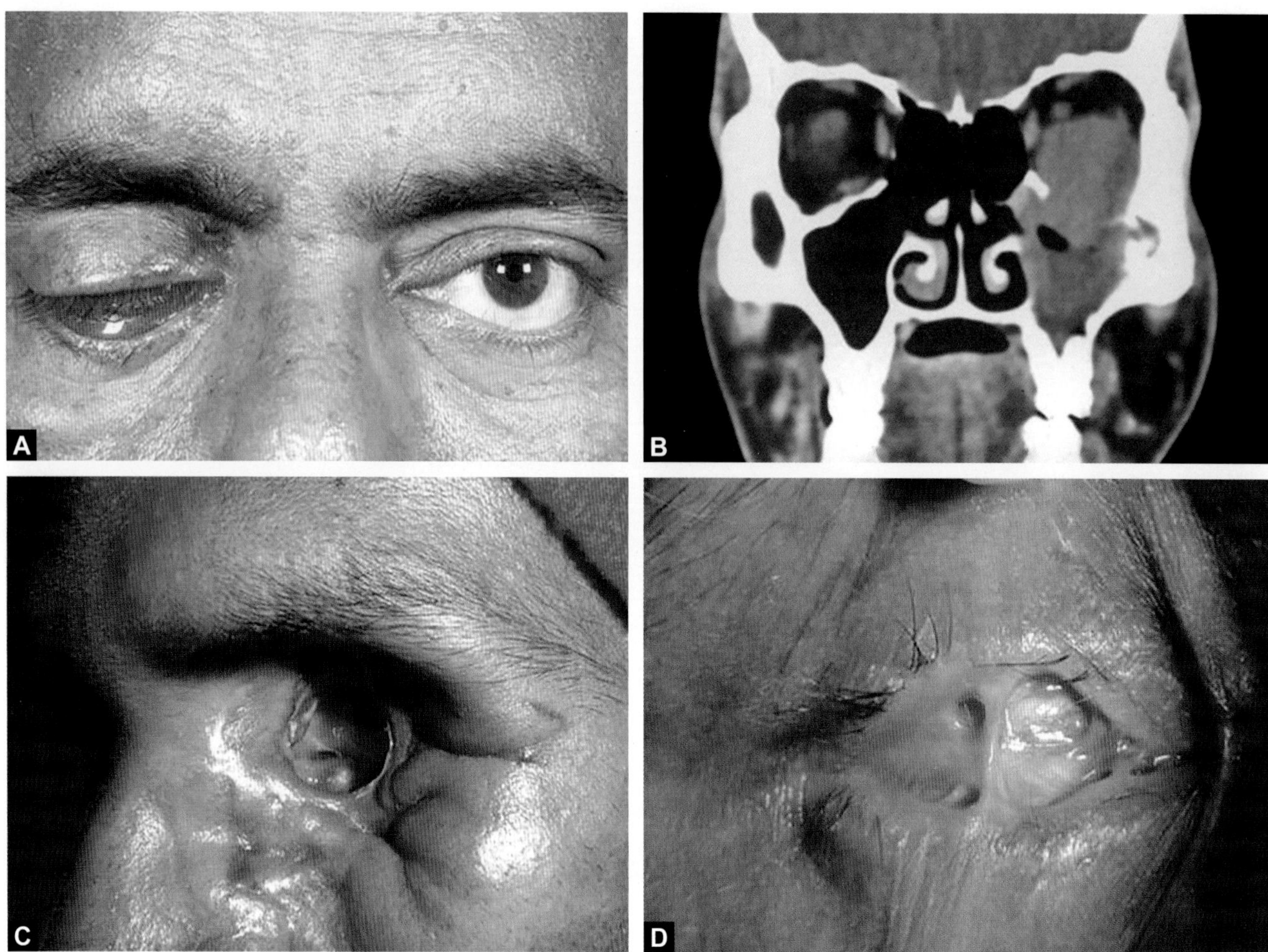

Figures 79.2A to D Indication of orbital exenteration for nontumorous causes. (A) Sino-orbital mucormycosis not responsive to conservative treatment in an immunocompromised patient. (B) Computed tomographic appearance of recurrent sino-orbital fungal granuloma following debulking caused by Aspergillus fumigatus. (C) Extended orbital exenteration with partial maxillectomy was done for this patient. (D) Severely contracted socket with inability to retain ocular prosthesis in a young patient following chemical injury. Anterior exenteration was followed by orbital prosthesis fitting for cosmetic rehabilitation of this patient.

TABLE 79-1 Types of orbital exenteration

| Type | Contents removed | Contents preserved | Final appearance |
|---|---|---|---|
| Anterior exenteration/ extended enucleation | Globe, posterior lamella of eyelid, conjunctival sac | Periorbita, posterior orbital contents | Shallow socket, immobile eyelids present |
| Lid sparing exenteration/subtotal exenteration | Orbital contents including periosteum of orbital walls. Eyelid margins | Anterior lamina of the eyelid including skin and some orbicularis muscle | Deep orbit. Residual skin and orbicularis edges sutured together forming a smooth lining |
| Total exenteration/ eyelid sacrificing | Orbital contents, periorbita and lids | Bare orbital bones with or without a skin graft | Spectacle mount or glued prosthesis can be fitted after the healing is complete |
| Radical/extended exenteration | Dissection involves paranasal sinuses, face, jaw, palate, skull base | Frontal bone if removed is replaced, cavity covered with myocutaneous vascular flap with vascular anastomosis | Cavity can be filled with myocutaneous vascular flaps or a maxillofacial prosthesis can be used to close the palatal defect along with split skin graft |

### Total Orbital Exenteration or Eyelid Sacrificing Orbital Exenteration

This procedure is done mainly for eyelid malignancies extending to the orbit or primary orbital or paranasal sinus malignancies with orbital extension and involving the eyelid skin. The orbital contents including the periorbita and the eyelids are removed. The procedure can be sometimes combined with radical craniofacial surgery or radical sinus surgery. The bare orbital cavity can be allowed to heal by spontaneous granulation or covered using a temporalis muscle flap, dermis fat graft, or split-thickness skin graft.[16,17]

#### *Advantages*

- Healing by granulation tissue usually gives rise to shallower and much smoother socket, which is cosmetically better.
- The socket is open for examination for any signs of local recurrence.

#### *Disadvantages*

- Open socket requires a closure follow-up and regular dressing with Vaseline gauze till the cavity is epithelized completely.
- Prolonged healing time, especially if healing is allowed by spontaneous granulation.
- Incomplete healing.
- Sino-orbital fistula formation leading to orbital discharge.
- Malodorous socket especially if skin graft is used to cover the socket.
- Infection.

### Extended Orbital Exenteration

When primary or secondary malignancies of the orbit involve the adjacent bones and surrounding structures like paranasal sinus, temporal fossa, etc. an extended orbital exenteration is indicated. It is a multidisciplinary procedure involving orbital surgeon, neurosurgeon, and faciomaxillary reconstructive surgeon. The morbidity and mortality are much higher than the other types of exenteration. In addition to the complications associated with the other types of exenteration, exposure of the intracranial contents is associated with a high risk of mortality and morbidity. The final cosmetic appearance is also extremely poor.

## PREOPERATIVE EVALUATION

Preoperative evaluation of a patient for exenteration includes evaluation for metastatic disease and regional lymph node assessment. The extent of the disease determines the extent of the exenteration; hence, this should be determined and documented appropriately. For extensive disease with distance metastasis where treatment is palliative, alternative management options like radiotherapy or limited resection might be more appropriate and should be discussed with the patient. Preoperative surgical planning should also include consideration for reconstruction options like use of regional flaps or free grafts. In case of extensive disease with high risk of local recurrence, it might be preferable to do total exenteration leaving the cavity open to detect any recurrence at the earliest. Since orbital exenteration causes considerable facial disfigurement and psychological distress, counseling the patient and setting up realistic goals to rehabilitation is extremely important. A written informed consent is obtained prior to surgery with patient fully informed of the postoperative facial deformity and loss of vision in the eye. Exenteration does not guarantee a complete cure from the disease, hence patient needs to be emphasized the need for close follow-up postoperatively to detect any tumor recurrence and metastasis.[18,19] Exenteration is usually done under general anesthesia. As blood loss is expected during surgery, one or two units of blood should be kept ready for transfusion if required.

## SURGICAL TECHNIQUE

The eyelid margins are sutured with 4-0 silk and the suture ends are left long. This helps in giving traction and allows for the mobilization of the orbital tissues during dissection. The incision for the surgery depends on the type of the exenteration being done. In case of eyelid sparing technique, an upper eyelid crease and subciliary incision is given and joined at the medial and lateral canthus about 4 mm from the lid margin (Figs. 79-3A and 79-4A). In eyelid sacrificing method, skin incision is given over the orbital rim all around the eyeball, and dissection is done to reach the periosteum over the orbital rim (Figs. 79-3B and 79-4B). Dissection is done in the suborbicularis plane to reach the orbital rim periosteum (Fig. 79-5). The rest of the surgical steps are similar in both techniques.

The periosteum is incised 360° around the orbital rim and separated from the bone with periosteal elevator (Fig. 79-6). The periorbita is separated from the bone of all four orbital walls up to the orbital apex. Transection of the nasolacrimal duct in the medial orbital wall and the inferior orbital fissure structures inferolaterally is required for complete separation of the periorbita from orbital bones. The superior and inferior orbital blood vessels are cauterized with bipolar cautery while separating the periorbita to avoid bothersome bleeding.

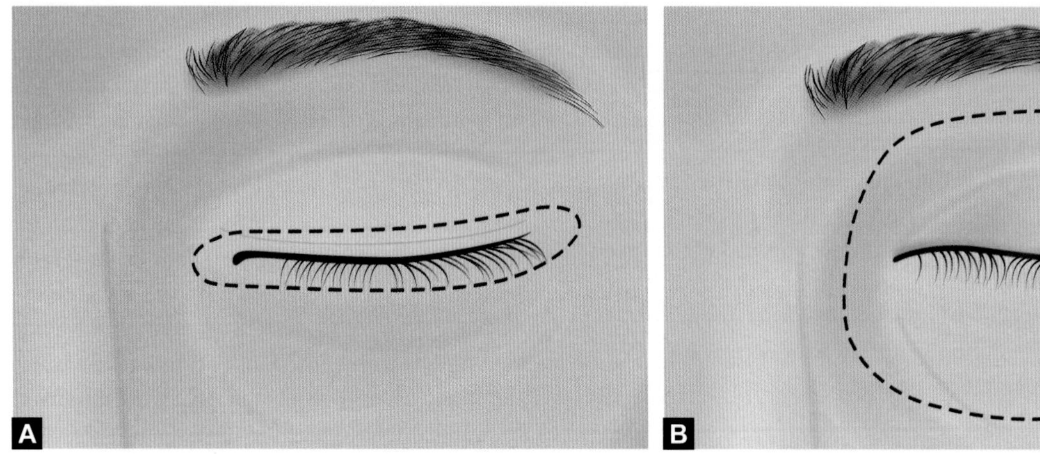


**Figures 79-3A and B** Incisions for orbital exenteration. (A) In eyelid sparing technique, the incision is given in upper and lower lid crease and anterior lamina of the eyelid is preserved. (B) In eyelid sacrificing technique, the incision is given along the orbital rim.

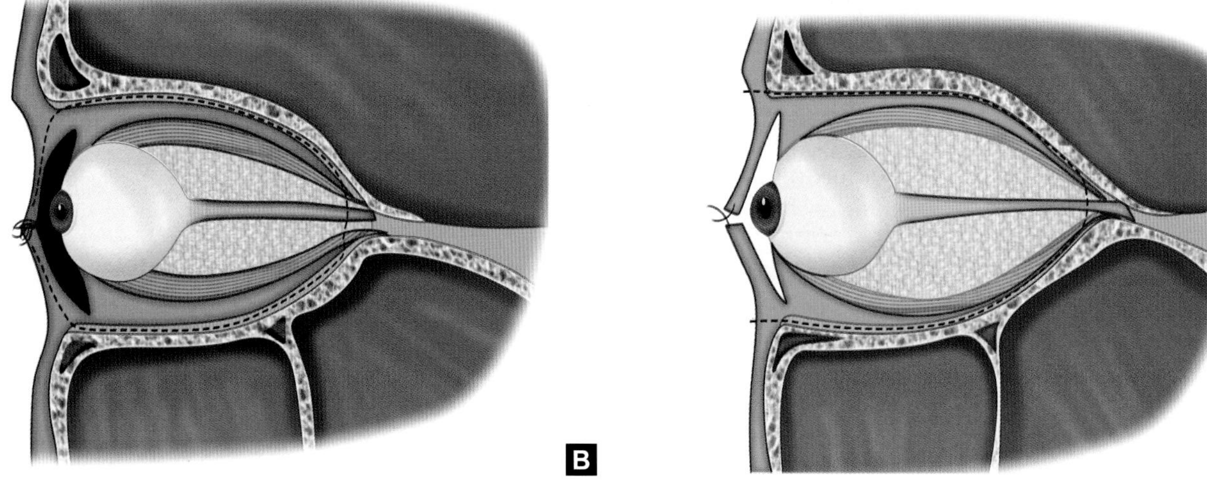


**Figures 79-4A and B** Incision line and plane of dissection showing the extent of tissue removal in exenteration. Dotted line indicates the plane of dissection. (A) Dissection plane in eyelid sparing technique. (B) Dissection plane in eyelid sacrificing exenteration.

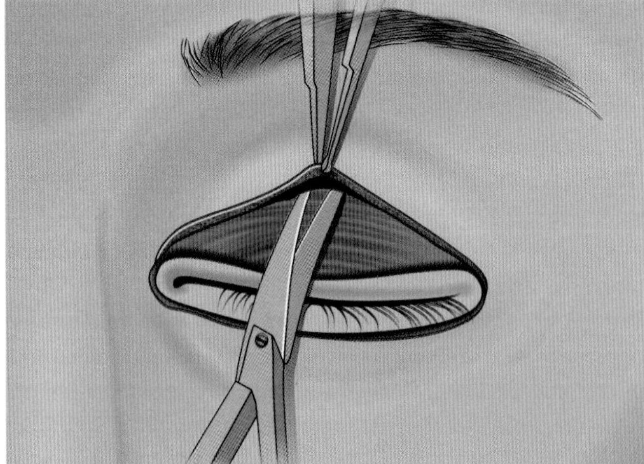

**Figure 79-5** Dissection done in the suborbicularis plane in eyelid sparing orbital exenteration.

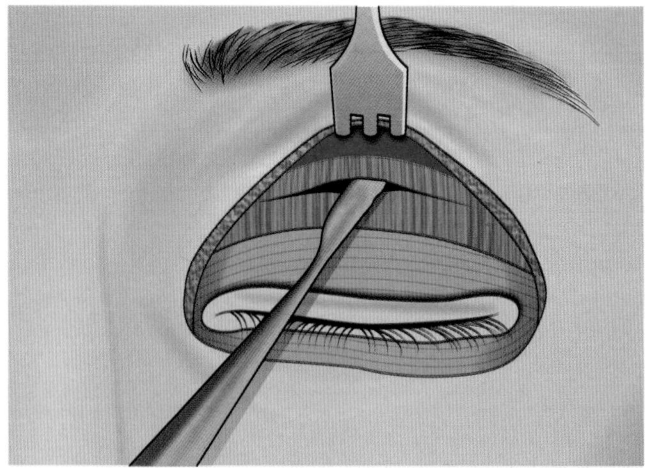

**Figure 79-6** The periosteum is incised just outside the orbital rim and periorbita separated from the orbital walls.

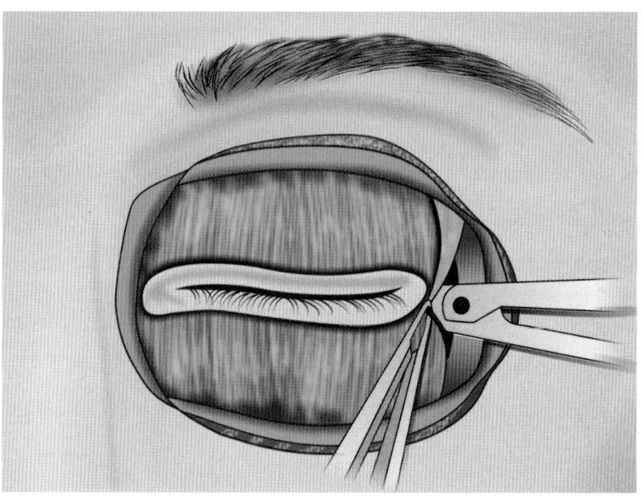

**Figure 79-7** Tissues at the orbital apex are cut with curved scissors after separating the periorbita from all the orbital walls.

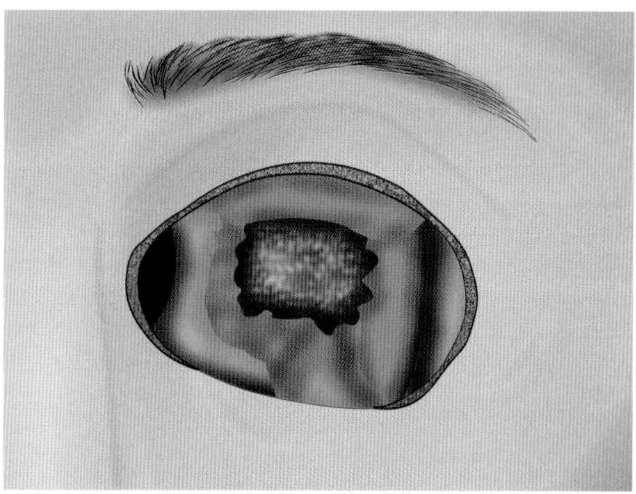

**Figure 79-8** Appearance of the bony orbital cavity after exenteration. Residual soft tissue at the posterior orbit provides vascular supply if a split thickness skin graft is used to cover the cavity.

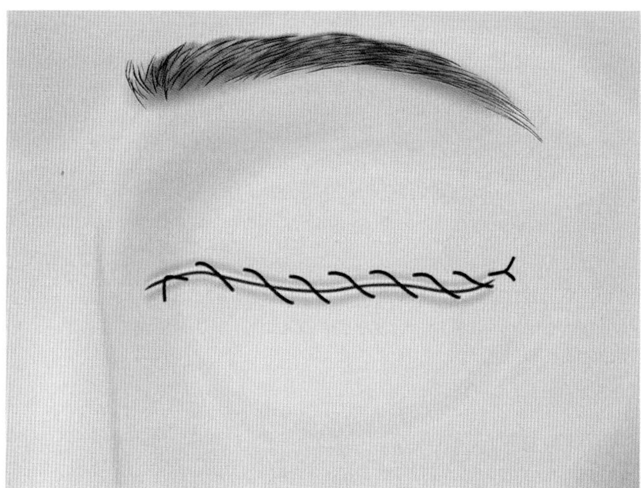

**Figure 79-9** Direct closure of the eyelid margins after eyelid sparing exenteration forming a skin lined cavity.

It is important not to breach the periorbita while separating it from orbital bones. After dissecting the orbital contents free, a clamp is applied across the tissues at the orbital apex. The apical tissues are cut with enucleation scissors and the orbital contents removed with an intact periorbital lining (Fig. 79-7). Brisk bleeding is encountered at this stage. The cavity is packed immediately with gauze and firm digital pressure applied for several minutes. The bleeding blood vessels can be directly visualized, clamped, and cauterized. Gelfoam can also be left over the apical tissues to control ooze from the tissues. The cavity is inspected for bony destruction and extension of the disease to surrounding structures which might necessitate further excision (Fig. 79-8).

Once hemostasis is achieved the reconstruction option is decided upon. In eyelid sparing technique, the eyelid margins are sutured together to form a skin-lined cavity (Fig. 79-9). In eyelid sacrificing technique, the cavity can be packed with petroleum gauze and left to heal by granulation or can be covered with a split skin graft. Other reconstructive options like temporalis muscle flap or local or distant skin muscle flaps might be required especially in cases where the bony walls are violated, and re-establishment of the orbital barriers become functionally and cosmetically important. The reconstruction can be done during the primary surgery, but it is preferable to do it at a second sitting allowing for an observation period to detect tumor recurrence.

## POSTOPERATIVE TREATMENT

The patient is prescribed systemic antibiotics and anti-inflammatory drugs postoperatively. Wound is cleaned with disinfectant solution, and antibiotic ointment is applied. Strict wound hygiene is maintained to prevent any wound gape or infection. In eyelid sparing technique, the socket collection is aspirated regularly till the aspirate reduces to 2–5 mL.[3] This allows for the cavity to collapse and promotes faster healing (Figs. 79-10 and 79-11).

In eyelid sacrificing method where the cavity is left to heal by granulation, daily dressing needs to be done with petroleum gauze till the cavity heals. Note has to be made of any possible tumor recurrence. Healing takes about 6–8 weeks time, and a prosthesis fitting can be considered once the cavity has a smooth epithelial lining (Fig. 79-12).

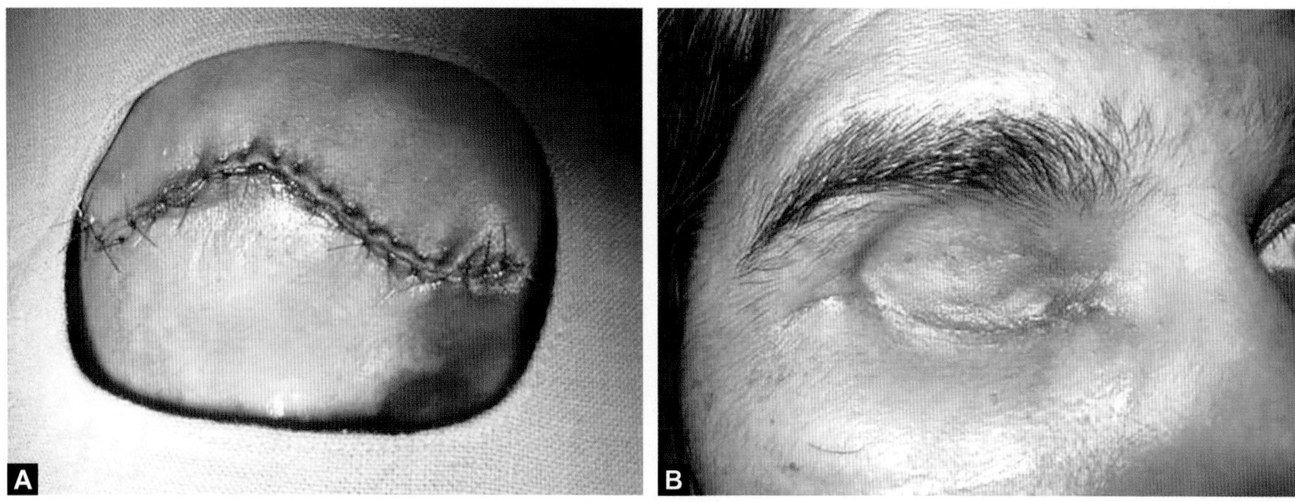

**Figures 79-10A and B** Appearance of the exenterated cavity. (A) immediately after skin closure in eyelid sparing exenteration. (B) Appearance 3 months postoperatively.

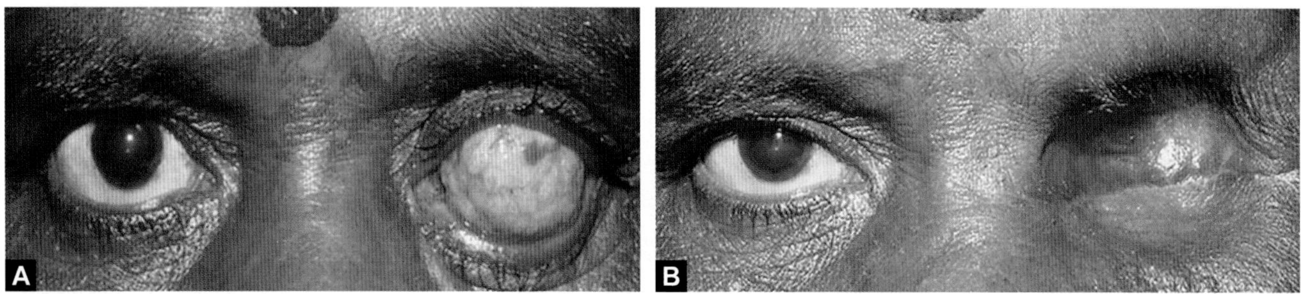

**Figures 79-11A and B** (A) A patient with squamous cell carcinoma of the conjunctiva with anterior orbital extension. (B) Smooth and concave skin cover over the exenterated cavity 3 months following eyelid-sparing orbital exenteration.

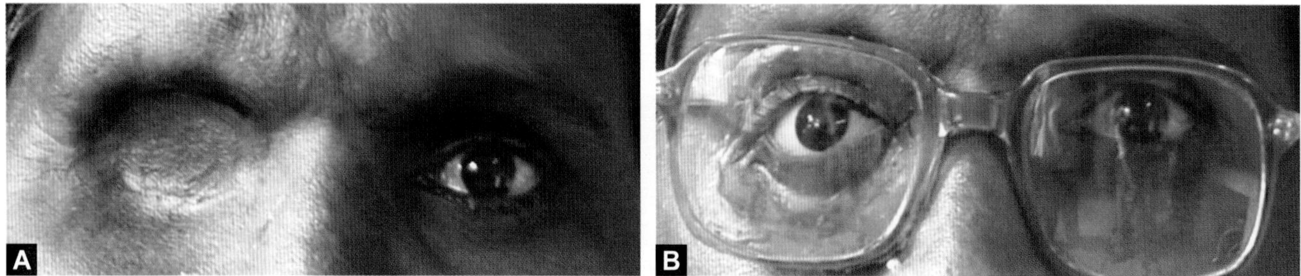

**Figures 79-12A and B** (A) Six-month postoperative appearance of a patient with sebaceous gland carcinoma who underwent partial eyelid-sparing orbital exenteration. (B) Acceptable consmesis with an exenteration prosthesis.

## COMPLICATIONS OF EXENTERATION

Intraoperative complications include excessive bleeding or cerebrospinal fluid leak if the dura is breached in cases of extended exenteration. A neurosurgical team is required in cases of extended exenteration where such complication is anticipated. Early complications include wound dehiscence due to infection, hemorrhage or due to compromised blood flow to the flap or skin graft. Skin breakdown can also occur after radiation treatment to the exenterated socket (Fig. 79-13A). Sino-orbital fistulae can form early or in late postoperative period and can be functionally and cosmetically disabling to the patient. Temporalis muscle flap can be used in these cases as a secondary reconstructive option. Numbness over the

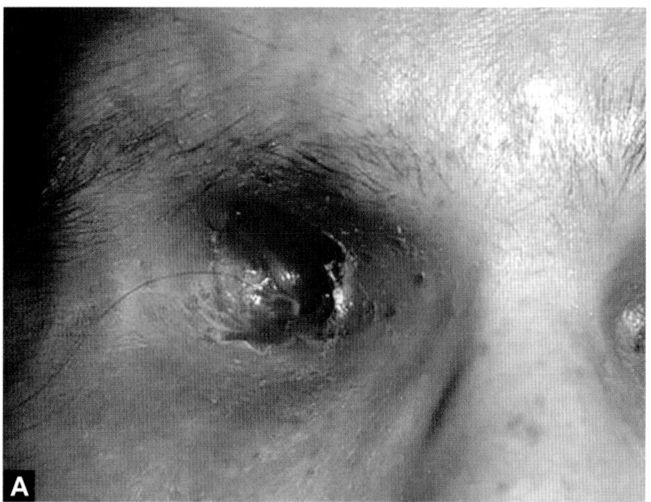


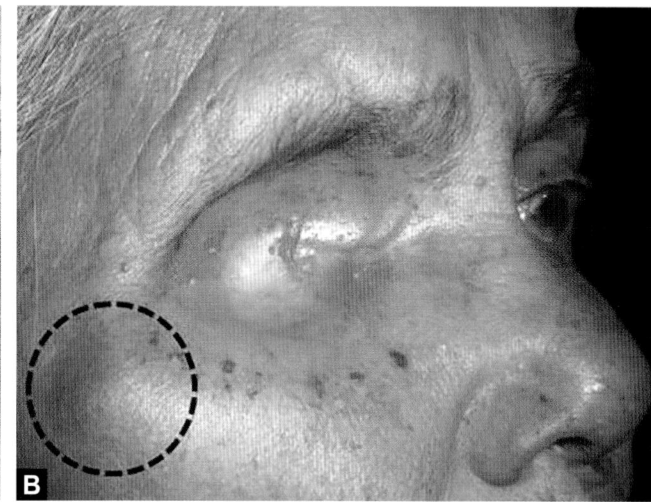


**Figures 79-13A and B** Complications of exenteration. (A) Skin breakdown and fistulae formation following radiotherapy to socket exenterated for orbital extension of uveal melanoma. (B) Tumor recurrence (indicated by dotted line) following exenteration for conjunctival melanoma.

forehead and cheek area is common after exenteration due to injury to branches of fifth cranial nerve. It tends to diminish with time, and patient needs to be informed about this complication preoperatively.

Tumor recurrence following exenteration is more common during the first year after surgery (Fig. 79-13B). All orbital tissues obtained during exenteration should be routinely sent for histopathological examination to assess for tumor-free margins. This helps in planning adjunctive treatments like chemotherapy or radiotherapy. Even tumor-free margins might not guarantee complete remission and recurrence rates of 7–10% have been reported in cases of locally invasive tumors like basal cell or squamous cell carcinoma when all the involved tissue was removed and clear margins were seen on histopathology.[9,17]

Orbital exenteration per say does not increase the survival rate. Especially, in the setting of malignant melanoma, exenteration might help in local tumor control but might not improve survival.[19]

## Prosthesis Fitting

Orbital prosthesis fitting after exenteration can be done after the cavity has completely healed. A good bony support and epithelized soft tissue covering are a must for providing support for the prosthesis and for planning an osseointegrated implant. An orbital prosthesis is custom made and can be either mounted on the spectacles or can be retained using adhesive or osseointegrated implants (Fig. 79-12). Spectacle mounted prosthesis can slip and has to be removed everytime the spectacle needs to be cleaned. Adhesive or osseointegrated implant retention eliminates this problem and might be preferred by the patients. Although pupil dilating orbital prosthesis is available, problems like high cost, inability to move the eye or blink, irritation of the skin, and need for frequent socket cleaning needs to be discussed with the patient before planning prosthetic rehabilitation.

## CONCLUSION

Orbital exenteration is a radical and disfiguring surgery with very specific indications. The rate of orbital exenteration has shown a decreasing trend in the recent years because of the early diagnosis of tumors and availability of alternative treatment modalities like plaque brachytherapy, chemotherapy, and radiotherapy.

Recent reports also suggest that exenteration of the orbit does not guarantee a complete remission of the disease and might not prevent metastasis. Hence, the surgery should be reserved for life-threatening tumors or infections, and postoperative long-term follow-up is mandatory to detect local recurrence and metastasis. Rehabilitation of the exenterated socket is very important as the surgery is psychologically distressing. Proper preoperative counseling to set realistic goals and an individualized approach for socket reconstruction goes a long way in providing satisfactory cosmetic outcome.

## REFERENCES

1. Coston TO, Small RG. Orbital exenteration-simplified. Trans Am Ophthalmol Soc. 1981;79:136-52.

2. Shields JA, Shields CL. Orbital exenteration. In: Shields JA, Shields CL (eds), Intraocular tumors. A text and atlas. Philadelphia, PA: WB Saunders; 1992:40-2.
3. Shields JA, Shields CL, Demirci H, et al. Experience with eyelid-sparing orbital exenteration: the 2000 Tullos O. Coston Lecture. Ophthal Plast Reconstr Surg. 2001;17(5):355-61.
4. Shields JA, Shields CL, Freire JE, et al. Plaque radiotherapy for selected orbital malignancies: preliminary observations: the 2002 Montgomery Lecture, part 2. Ophthal Plast Reconstr Surg. 2003;19:91-5.
5. Meldrum ML, Tse DT, Benedetto P. Neoadjuvant intracarotid chemotherapy for the treatment of advanced adenoid cystic carcinoma of the lacrimal gland. Arch Ophthalmol. 1998;1163: 315-21.
6. Kennedy RE. Indications and surgical techniques for orbital exenteration. Ophthalmology. 1979;86:967-73.
7. Pushker N, Kashyap S, Balasubramanya R, et al. Pattern of orbital exenteration in a tertiary eye care centre in India. Clin Exp Ophthalmol. 2004;32(1):51-4.
8. Maheshwari R, Review of orbital exenteration from an eye care centre in Western India. Orbit. 2010;29(1) 35-8.
9. Nemet AY, Martin P, Benger R, et al. Orbital exenteration: a 15-year study of 38 cases. Opthal plast Reconstr Surg. 2007;23(6): 468-72.
10. Hargrove RN. Indications for orbital exenteration in mucormycosis. Ophthal Plast Reconstr Surg. 2006;22:286-91.
11. Nithyanandam S. Rhino-orbito-cerebral mucormycosis. A retrospective analysis of clinical features and treatment outcomes. Indian J Ophthalmol. 2003;51:231-6.
12. Viestenz A, Colombo F, Holbach LM. Orbital exenteration in therapy-resistant painful scleritis-associated inflammation of orbital soft tissues. Klin Monbl Augenheilkd. 2002;219(6):462-4.
13. Jackson IT, Laws ER, Jr, Martin RD. The surgical management of orbital neurofibromatosis. Plast Reconstr Surg. 1983;71(6): 751-8.
14. Kwiat DM, Bersani TA, Hodge C, et al. Surgical technique: two-step orbital reconstruction in neurofibromatosis type 1 with a matched implant and exenteration. Ophthal Plast Reconstr Surg. 2004;20(2):158-61.
15. Yeatts RP. The esthetics of orbital exenteration. Am J ophthalmol. 2005;139:152-3.
16. Mauriello JA Jr, Han KH, Wolfe R et al. Use of autogenous split-thickness dermal graft for reconstruction of the lining of the exenterated orbit. Am J Ophthalmol. 1985;100:465-7.
17. Ben Simon GJ, Schwarcz RM, Douglas R, et al. Orbital exenteration: one size does not fit all. Am J Ophthalmol. 2005;139(1): 11-7.
18. Esmaeli B, Ahmadi MA, Youssef A, et al. Outcomes in patients with adenoid cystic carcinoma of the lacrimal gland. Ophthal Plast Reconstr Surg. 2004;20:22-6.
19. Blanco G. Diagnosis and treatment of orbital invasion in uveal melanoma. Can J Ophthalmol. 2004;39:388-96.

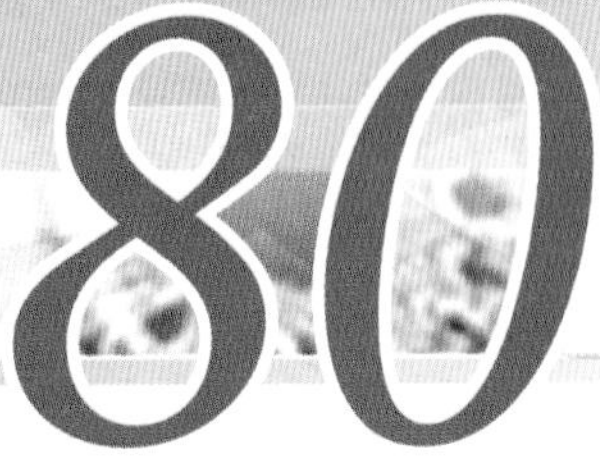

CHAPTER 80

# Nasolacrimal Duct Probing and Irrigation

Ashley Lundin, Cat Nguyen Burkat, Shubhra Goel

## INTRODUCTION

Congenital dacryostenosis is one of the most common lacrimal system problems in children and may lead to epiphora with or without mucopurulent discharge. The most common etiology of congenital dacryostenosis is the complete or partial failure of canalization of the Valve of Hasner. Other less common causes include osseous obstruction due anomalous passages, deviated nasal septum, or impaction of the inferior turbinate.[1-3] Idiopathic or primary acquired nasolacrimal duct obstruction accounts for the majority of lacrimal system problems in adults. It is postulated that inflammation of unknown cause results in occlusive fibrosis of the nasolacrimal system causing obstruction and subsequent epiphora.[4-8] Probing and syringing remain the gold standard in the management and diagnosis of congenital and acquired dacryostenosis and are used to assess the anatomy and functional status of the lacrimal drainage system.

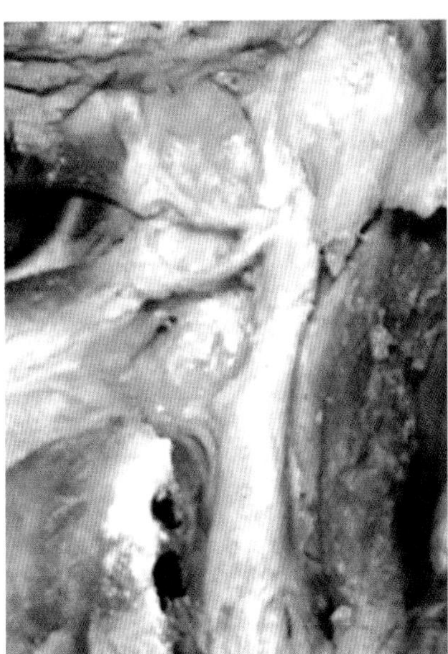

**Figure 80-1** Cadaver dissection of the lacrimal excretory system, right side.

## ANATOMY

The anatomy of the lacrimal system can be divided into three components:

- Secretory:
  - Lacrimal gland—reflex and emotional tear secretion.
  - Accessory lacrimal glands of Wolfring and Krause—basal tear production.
- Distributory:
  - Eyelids—blinking motion distributes tears across ocular surface.
  - Tear film—complex composition of tear film (mucous, aqueous, lipid layers) assists in maintaining tears on ocular surface.
- Excretory (Fig. 80-1):
  - Puncta:
    - The puncta measure 0.2–0.3 mm in diameter and sit on a small elevation called the lacrimal papillae.
    - The superior punctum rests ~ 0.5–1.0 mm more medial than the inferior punctum.
  - Canaliculi:
    - The proximal canaliculus is short (2 mm) and perpendicular to the lid margin. The distal canaliculus travels horizontally for 8–10 mm and curves posterior and medially toward the lacrimal sac. In 90% of people, the superior and inferior canaliculi join to form a common canaliculus that is 0–5 mm

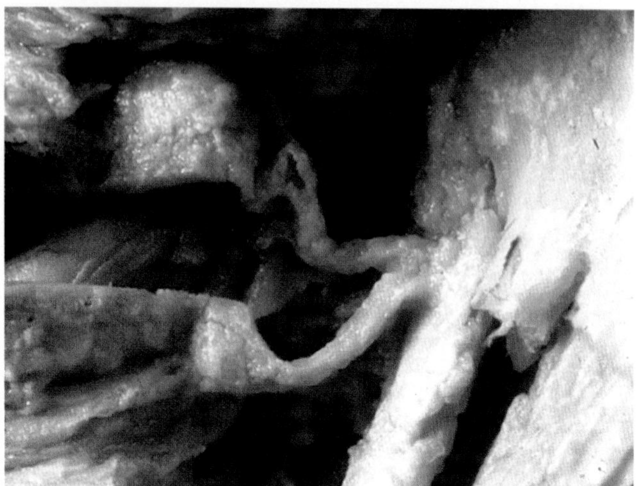

Figure 80-2 Closer view of the cavaderic dissection, demonstrating the longer inferior canaliculus, and the combined common canaliculus entering the superior lacrimal sac.

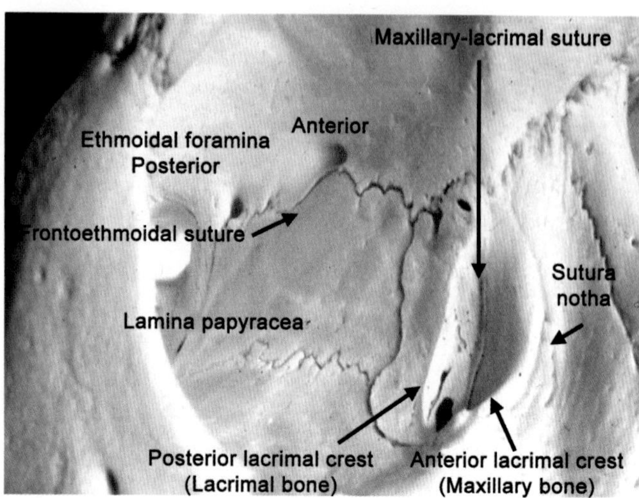


Figure 80-3 Bony orbital structures of the lacrimal sac fossa.

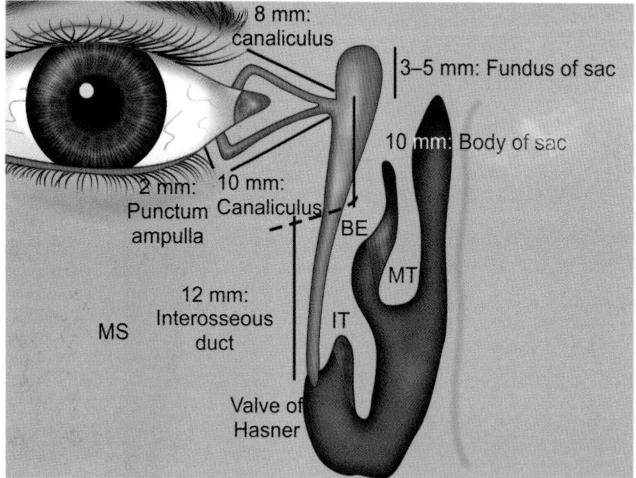


Figure 80-4 Schematic diagram of the approximate dimensions of the lacrimal excretory system.
(BE: Bulla ethmoidalis; IT: Inferior turbinate; MS: Maxillary sinus; MT: Middle turbinate).

in length (Fig. 80-2). The common canaliculus then enters the lacrimal sac at an abrupt angle of >45°. A potential mucosal flap is created by the abrupt angle of the common canaliculus as it enters the lacrimal sac, termed the Valve of Rosenmuller.

- Nasolacrimal sac:
  - The sac rests within the lacrimal sac fossa of the anteromedial orbit (Fig. 80-3).
  - The body and apex of the sac together measure 12–15 mm in length (anteroposterior diameter of 4–8 mm, 3–5 mm in width). The entrance of the common canaliculus is typically 3–5 mm below the fundus apex.
- Nasolacrimal duct:
  - The nasolacrimal duct extends inferiorly from the nasolacrimal sac as a proximal interosseous (12–15 mm) and intermeatal portion (5 mm) (Fig. 80-4). There is a lateral and posterior slope to the nasolacrimal duct as it travels inferiorly, which follows the shape of the lateral nasal wall (Fig. 80-5).
  - The distal duct exits into the inferior meatus of the nose below the anterior aspect of the inferior turbinate.
  - The valve of Hasner, located at the distal duct, represents a mucosal flap that prevents reflux of tears and nasal mucosal secretions back into the lacrimal system.[9,10]

## INDICATIONS

Tearing is a common, but nonspecific complaint of lacrimal system dysfunction. It may occur as a result of several processes including hypersecretion, often from reflexive tearing due to irritation from blepharitis, dry eye, corneal abrasion, conjunctivitis, keratitis, ectropion or entropion, and trichiasis. Epiphora, or an overflow of tears onto the cheek, is frequently secondary to obstruction, partial or total, of the lacrimal outflow system.

Congenital nasolacrimal obstruction is the most common cause of tearing within the first 2 years of life, often secondary to an imperforate valve of Hasner or less commonly due to osseous obstruction of anomalous passages, or a deviated nasal septum.

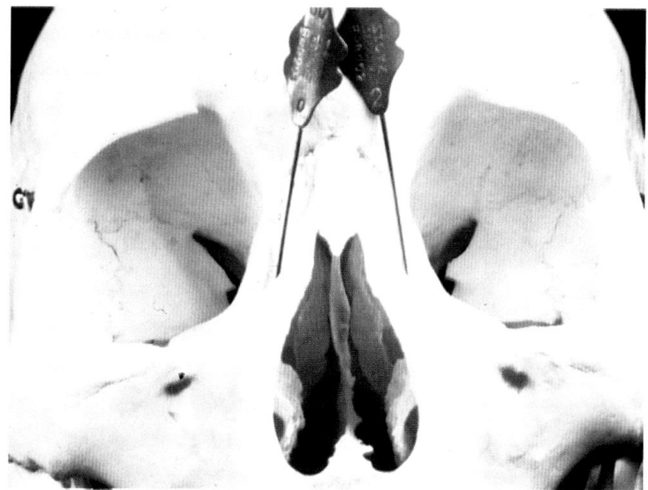

**Figure 80-5** Probes within the lacrimal system demonstrate a lateral and posterior slope to the nasolacrimal duct as it travels inferiorly along the lateral nasal wall.

**TABLE 80-1** Therapeutic and diagnostic indications

| Therapeutic indications | Diagnostic indications |
|---|---|
| Primary congenital dacryostenosis | Primary congenital dacryostenosis |
| Failed primary probing | Secondary congenital dacryostenosis |
| Chronic dacryocystitis | Failed primary probing |
| Neonatal acute dacryocystitis | Partial acquired dacryostenosis |
| Congenital dacryocele | Tearing in adults |

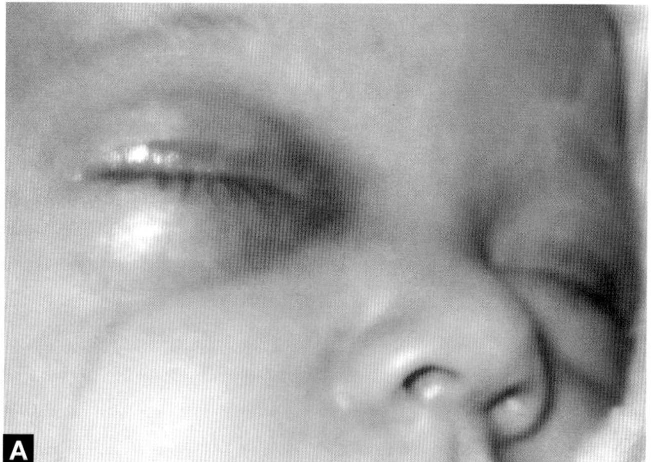

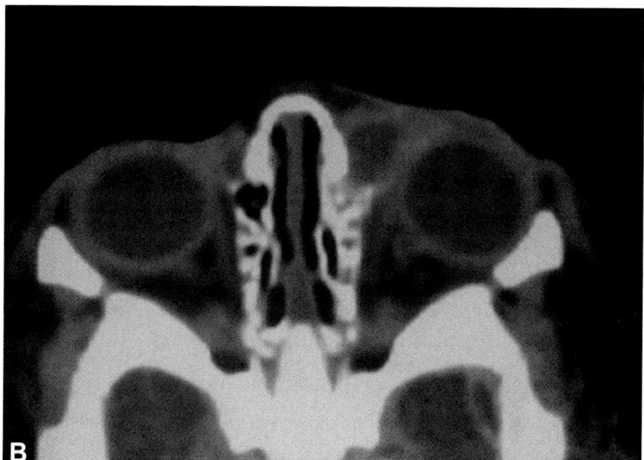

**Figures 80-6A and B** Congenital dacryocystocele, bilateral sides. (A) Clinical photo, (B) Computed tomographic image demonstrating bilateral lacrimal sac and ductal cysts.

In contrast, nasolacrimal obstruction in adults has a wide range of possible etiologies:

- Conjunctivochalasis obstructing the punctum
- Megalocaruncle
- Punctal stenosis or malposition
- Canalicular stenosis (from trauma, iatrogenic, or drugs)
- Lacrimal sac tumors or trauma
- Idiopathic acquired nasolacrimal duct stenosis (most common cause of tearing in adults).
- Mechanical obstruction from retained foreign body (i.e. punctal plug)

If nasolacrimal dacryostenosis is suspected, nasolacrimal duct probing and irrigation is indicated to determine the etiology of tearing.

## Therapeutic Indications: (Table 80-1)

- Primary congenital dacryostenosis
- Failed primary probing
- Chronic dacryocystitis in children
- Neonatal acute dacryocystitis
- Congenital dacryocystocele (Figs. 80-6A and B).

## Diagnostic Indications

- Primary congenital dacryostenosis
- Secondary congenital dacryostenosis
- Failed primary probing
- Partial acquired dacryostenosis
- Tearing in adults.

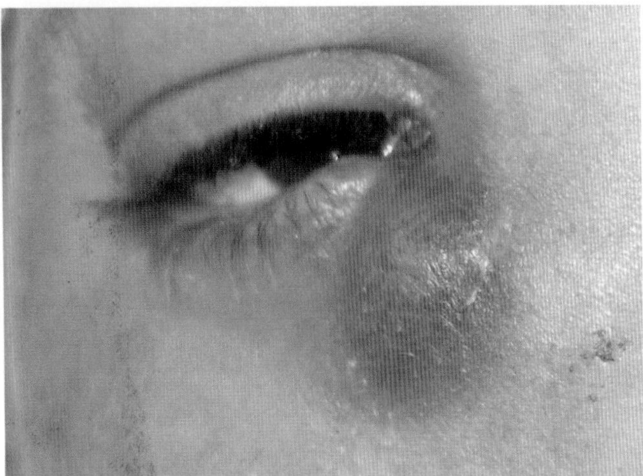

**Figure 80-7** Acute dacryocystitis, right side.

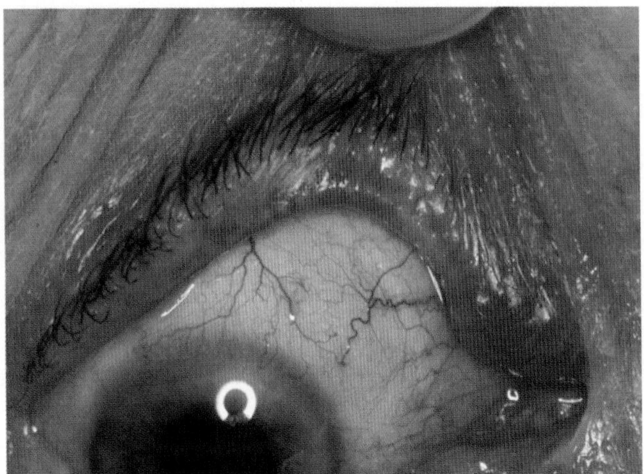

**Figure 80-8** Acute canaliculitis, with erythema, edema, and tenderness of the right upper eyelid margin medial to the punctum.

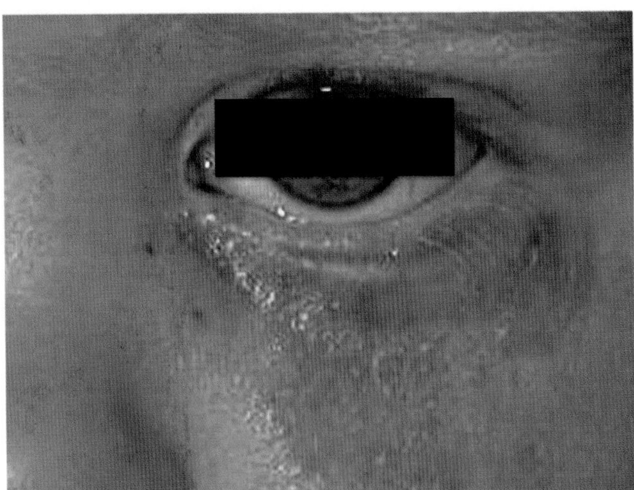

**Figure 80-9** Clinical photograph of congenital dacryostenosis, manifesting as mattering, discharge, and skin irritation of the left side.

## CONTRAINDICATIONS

- Acute dacryocystitis (Fig. 80-7)
- Acute canaliculitis (Fig. 80-8).

## TIMING OF NASOLACRIMAL DUCT PROBING AND IRRIGATION

There has been significant controversy regarding the proper timing for nasolacrimal duct probing and irrigation in congenital nasolacrimal duct obstruction (Fig. 80-9):

- 96.4% success rate was reported in a study by Katowitz and Welsh[7] when probing was done prior to 13 months of age. A gradual decrease in the success rate was noted with increasing age.
- 92.6% success rate in children >36 months of age was reported by Robb.[11]
- Kushner[3] reported a 100% success rate in patients with simple congenital nasolacrimal duct obstruction (obstruction involving the valve of Hasner) irrespective of the patient's age. This dropped to 36% in children with complicated nasolacrimal duct obstruction between the ages of 18 and 48 months.
- 97% success rate noted in children between 24 and 36 months, 75% for 37–48 months, and 42% beyond 48 months of age by Honavar et al.[12]
- Baggio et al.[13] reported a success rate of 91.3% when the probing was performed between birth and 7 months of age.
- A general consensus regarding the timing of nasolacrimal duct probing and irrigation can be summarized as:
- Conservative management (massage) of congenital nasolacrimal duct obstruction until 12 months of age.
- Consider nasolacrimal duct probing between 12 and 18 months if conservative treatment fails.
- Probing prior to 12 months of age may be beneficial in special cases (mucocele, child awaiting intraocular surgery, repeated episodes of dacryocystitis, and amniotocele).

## INSTRUMENTATION

- Setting:
  - Office for most adults.
    - Operating room if additional procedure is planned, i.e. silicone intubation, dacryocystorhinostomy.
  - Operating room for children (office may be considered if <9 months old).

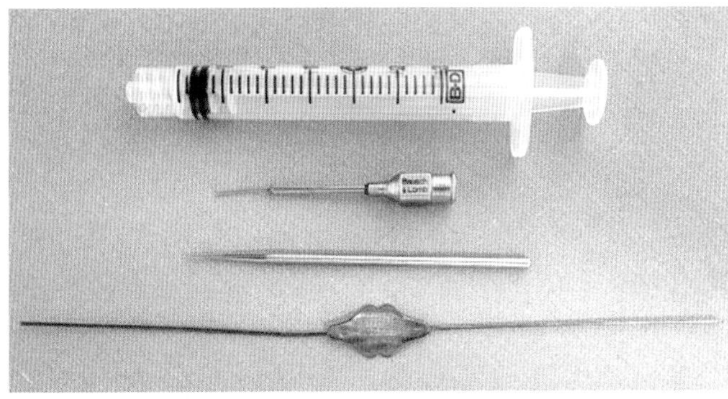

Figure 80-10 Basic instrumentation for probing and irrigation in the office.

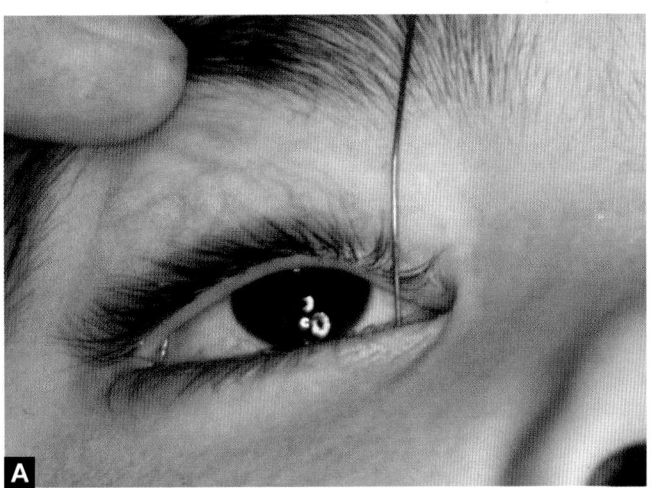

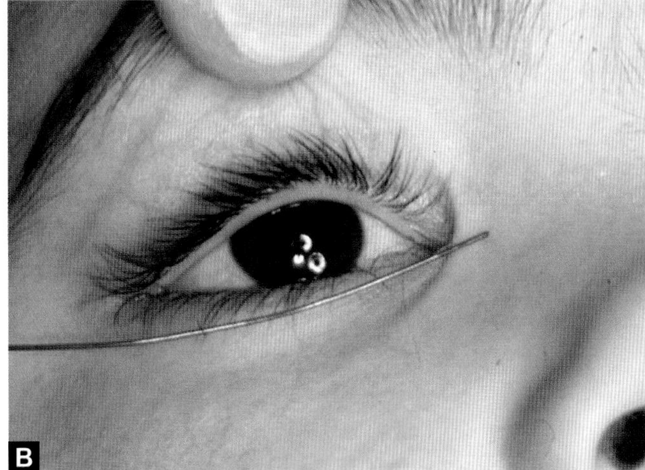

Figures 80-11A and B Probe first perpendicular to the margin for 2 mm (A), then horizontal to the eyelid margin slightly upward or downward toward the medial canthal angle in respect of the proximal anatomy (B).

- Anesthesia:
  - Topical.
    - Adults.
    - Proparacaine 0.5% or tetracaine 0.5% ophthalmic solution.
  - General.
    - Children.
    - Laryngeal mask airway or endotracheal tube.
- Instrumentation (Fig. 80-10):
  - Punctal dilator.
  - 1- or 3-cc syringe.
  - Saline, distilled, or tap water.
  - Silver or gold tipped blunt cannula, 21- or 23-gauge.
  - Double-ended Bowman probe, size #0-00.

## TECHNIQUE

- Instructions—diagnostic:
  - Stand on the side of the patient that is being probed and irrigated.
  - Place one drop of topical anesthetic on the ocular surface (proparacaine 0.5% or tetracaine 0.5% ophthalmic solution).
  - Digital pressure over the lacrimal sac is performed to check for mucopurulent regurgitation. If positive, stenosis and blockage of the nasolacrimal duct is confirmed.
  - A #0-00 Bowman probe can be lubricated with ophthalmic ointment for easy passage.
  - Dilate the superior and inferior puncta with a punctal dilator.
  - The Bowman probe is first entered perpendicular to the margin for 2 mm (Figs. 80-11A and B), then advanced parallel to the lid margin toward the nasolacrimal sac while applying gentle counter traction to avoid "accordion folding" of the canaliculi that could result in false passages (Fig. 80-12).
    - A "hard stop" as the probe reaches the medial wall of the lacrimal sac indicates patency of the system up to the nasolacrimal sac.

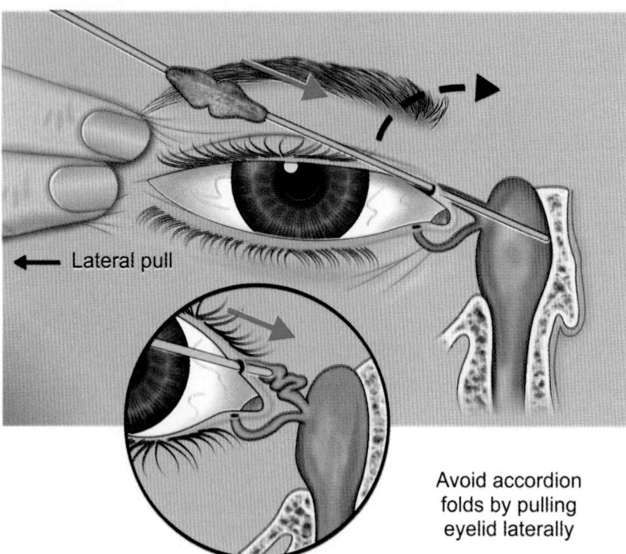


Figure 80-12 Pull the eyelid laterally to avoid accordion folds of the canaliculus that could result in false passages.

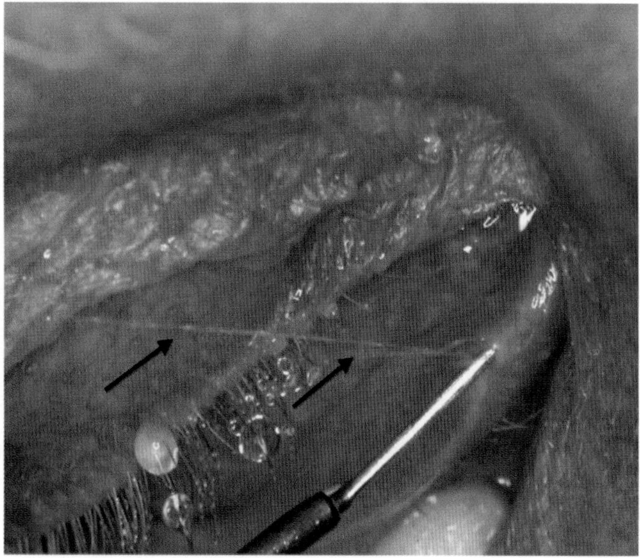

Figure 80-13 Reflux through the same punctum being irrigated suggests obstruction of the irrigated canaliculus (inferior).

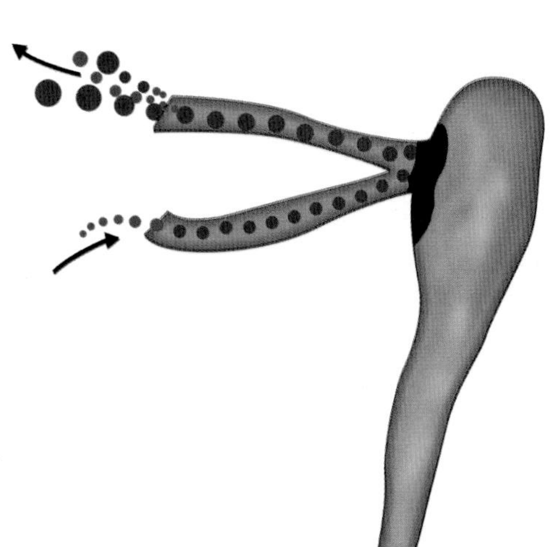

Figure 80-14 Schematic diagram. Reflux through the opposite punctum only suggests obstruction at the common canaliculus.

- A "soft stop" suggests that there is stenosis or obstruction of the canaliculi, and the location of any focal stenoses or obstructions can be documented by measuring the Bowman probe from the punctum to the level of the soft stop.

- A blunt 21- or 23-gauge cannula, attached to a 1- or 3-cc syringe filled with sterile saline or tap water, is then advanced into the inferior punctum and proximal canaliculus. A 1–2 cc of fluid is flushed into the system, and attention is directed toward the medial canthal area to observe for signs of possible obstruction. See below for possible outcomes.[14]
  - Reflux through the irrigated punctum indicates obstruction of the same irrigated canaliculus (Fig. 80-13).
  - Reflux through the opposite punctum suggests obstruction at the common canaliculus or more distal structures (Fig. 80-14).
  - Distension of the lacrimal sac indicates obstruction of the nasolacrimal duct.
  - Irrigation into the nose indicates an anatomically, but not necessarily functional, patent system.
  - Partial irrigation into the nose accompanied by some amount of reflux indicates a partial nasolacrimal duct obstruction (Fig. 80-15).
  - *Note*: care should be taken when interpreting the results of this test. It may appear normal anatomically in the presence of functional obstruction. In addition, irrigation of the lacrimal system is done with a hydrostatic pressure that is far above the normal tear flow, and may demonstrate a normal result when, in fact, a partial functional obstruction is present.

- Instructions—therapeutic (i.e. congenital obstruction):
  - Performed in the office or operating room.
  - Intranasal application of a vasoconstrictor such as oxymetazoline HCL 1% may be used to limit bleeding.
  - The steps are performed as for diagnostic probing above, until a "hard stop" is felt along the medial wall of the nasolacrimal sac.

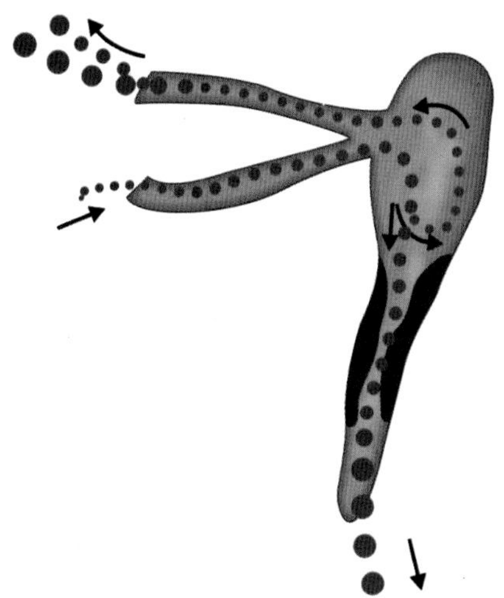

Figure 80-15 Schematic diagram. Partial irrigation into the nose accompanied by some amount of reflux from the opposite punctum indicates a partial lacrimal duct obstruction.

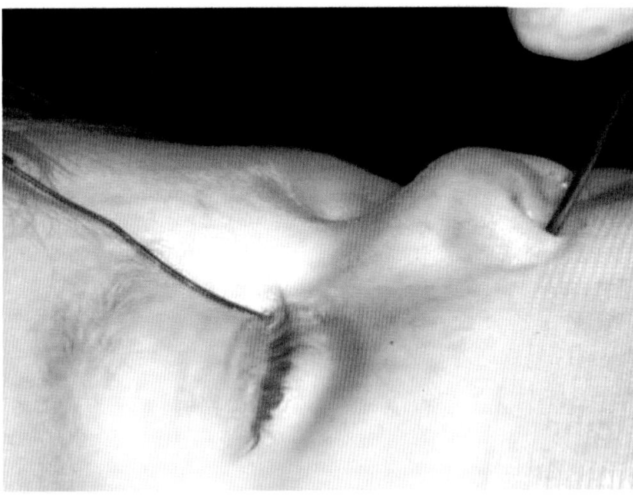

Figure 80-16 Probe should be parallel to the nose and resting flat along the brow rim to help locate the correct angle of the duct.

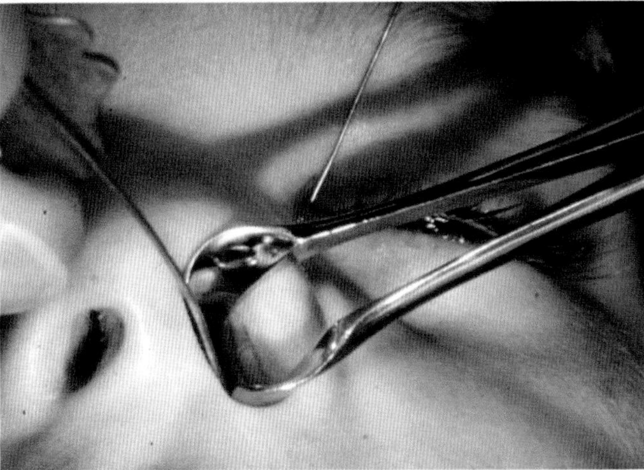

Figure 80-17 A second Bowman probe can be gently passed into the nostril and directed posterolaterally until it touches the first, to confirm the entrance of the first probe into the nose.

- The probe is then rotated vertically so that the external end lies flat against the patient's brow, and the probe is parallel with the nasolacrimal duct. It is then directed inferiorly and slightly posterolaterally down the nasolacrimal duct (Fig. 80-16). If resistance is met, do not force the probe as this may create a false passage.
- For congenital dacryostenosis, the Bowman probe is advanced into the nasolacrimal duct until a "pop" is felt as the probe passes through the membrane of the imperforate valve of Hasner.
- To confirm the presence of the Bowman probe in the nose, a second Bowman probe is passed into the nose and directed posterolaterally until it touches the first (Fig. 80-17).
- A silicone tube may be placed through the dilated system if indicated.

## POSTOPERATIVE CARE

Patients should be educated about the possibility of minor epistaxis or blood-tinged tears for 1–2 days after any nasolacrimal system procedure and therefore should avoid exercise and strenuous activity for several days. A topical vasoconstrictor, such as oxymetazoline HCL 1%, may be used BID X 1 week to reduce bleeding if needed. Rapid epistaxis that does not abate with nasal pressure should be seen urgently to evaluate for intranasal arterial bleeding that may require packing or cauterization. Patients should also be advised regarding signs of postoperative infection including fever, medial canthal erythema, increasing medial canthal pain, and mucopurulent discharge from the nasal vestibule or medial canthus. Antimicrobial prophylaxis with a topical antibiotic is not routinely indicated, but it may be started if there is any concern for postoperative infection. Parents may also be instructed to continue Criggler massage for 1 month after probing and irrigation for children with congenital nasolacrimal duct obstruction.

## COMPLICATIONS

- Bleeding.
- Infection.
  - Postoperative preseptal cellulitis, acute dacryocystitis.
- Creation of false passage—be sure to angle the probe in the direction of the canaliculi and duct at all times.

- Scarring in the inferior meatus, canaliculus.
- Inability to pass the probe down the nasolacrimal duct.
- Continued tearing, need for additional surgery.

## CONCLUSION

It is important to understand lacrimal system anatomy prior to performing any lacrimal system procedure. Nasolacrimal duct stenosis and obstruction are common problems for both children and adults. Nasolacrimal duct probing and irrigation are a beneficial diagnostic and therapeutic tool. Controversy exists regarding the correct timing of probing and irrigation in congenital obstruction.

## REFERENCES


1. Jones LT, Wobig JL. The Wendell L. Hughes Lecture. Newer concepts of tear duct and eyelid anatomy and treatment. Trans Sec Ophthalmol Am Acad Ophthalmol Otolaryngol. 1977;83:603-16.
2. Petersen RA, Robb RM. The natural course of congenital obstruction of the nasolacrimal duct. J Pediatr Ophthalmol Strabismus. 1978;15(4):246-50.
3. Kushner BJ. Congenital nasolacrimal system obstruction. Arch Ophthalmol. 1982;100(4):597-600.
4. Shermeatro C, Gladstone GJ. Adult nasolacrimal duct obstruction (Review). J Am Osteopathic Assoc. 1994;3:229-32.
5. Hurwitz JJ, Cooper PR, McRae DJ, Chemoweith DR. The investigation of epiphora. Can J Ophthalmol. 1977;12:196-8.
6. Joseph JM, Zoumalan CI. Lacrimal System Probing and Irrigation. Updated July 25, 2011. Available at: http://emedicine.medscape.com/article/1844121-overview.
7. Katowitz JA, Welsh MG. Timing and initial probing and irrigation in congenital nasolacrimal duct obstruction. Ophthalmology. 1987;94(6):698-705.
8. Hurwitz JJ. The lacrimal syst, 1st edn. Philadelphia, PA: Lippincott-Raven. 1996
9. Olver J. Colour atlas of lacrimal surgery. 1st edn. Woburn, MA: Butterworth-Heinemann; 2002.
10. Linberg JV. Contemporary issues in ophthalmology-lacrimal surgery, 1st edn. New York, NY: Churchill Livingstone, Inc. 1988.
11. Robb RMS. Success rates of nasolacrimal duct probing at time intervals after 1 year of age. Ophthalmology. 1998;105(7):1307-10.
12. Honavar SB, Prakash VE, Rao GN. Outcome of probing for congenital nasolacrimal duct obstruction in older children. Am J Ophthalmol. 2000;130(1):42-8.
13. Baggio E, Ruban JM, Sandon, K. Analysis of the efficacy of early probing in the treatment of symptomatic congenital lacrimal duct obstruction in infants. Apropos of 92 cases. J Fr Ophthalmol. 2000;23(7):655-62.
14. Nesi FA, Lisman RD, Levine MR. Smith's ophthalmic plastic and reconstructive surgery, 2nd edn. St Louis, MO: Mosby-Year Book Inc.; 1998.

CHAPTER

81

# External Dacryocystorhinostomy

Sima Das

## INTRODUCTION

Surgery for lacrimal drainage problems had existed in the middle ages in the form of either drainage of an abscess or sac extirpation. Dacryocystectomy was considered the treatment of choice for nasolacrimal duct (NLD) obstruction until the introduction of external dacryocystorhinostomy (DCR) procedure by Toti in 1904.[1] Toti's procedure involved creation of a communication between the lacrimal sac and nasal cavity by resecting part of lacrimal sac, bone and nasal mucosa. Modification of this technique was made by Dupuy-Dutemps and Bourguet by approximating the mucosal flaps to create an epithelium lined tract.[2] Modern-day external DCR is essentially the same technique originally described by Toti with minor modifications.

Though DCR currently is performed by both external and endonasal approach, external approach still remains the gold standard against which the results of other drainage procedures are compared. The goal of the surgery is to make an adequate sized bony ostium that remains so after allowing for shrinkage and to ensure a mucosa lined anastomosis.[3] Both these goals can be met adequately through an external approach DCR, thus ensuring a high success rate.

## SURGICAL ANATOMY

Knowledge of the relevant surgical anatomy is essential before planning any surgical intervention in the lacrimal outflow pathway[4] (Fig. 81-1). The lacrimal punctum in the upper and lower lid courses vertically for about 2 mm and then horizontally parallel to the eyelid margin before joining together for 1–2 mm to form the common canaliculus. The common canaliculus opens into the nasolacrimal sac at the level of medial canthal tendon about 2–5 mm below the fundus of the sac. Rarely, the lacrimal canaliculi may open separately into the sac. The nasolacrimal sac is about 10 mm in vertical dimension. It lies in the lacrimal fossa between the anterior and the posterior lacrimal crest. The anterior lacrimal crest is formed by the nasal process of maxilla and is a continuation of the inferior orbital rim. This forms an important surgical landmark for identifying the lacrimal sac and defining the boundary of the bony ostium. The lacrimal fossa is bounded posteriorly by the posterior lacrimal crest that is the posterior limit of the lacrimal bone and abuts the lamina papyracea of the ethmoid bone. This is also an important surgical landmark as the infracture of the bone for creating the bony osteum is started from this site. The lacrimal sac continues inferiorly to enter the maxillary bone and form the NLD that opens in the inferior meatus of the nose about 2–2.5 mm posterior to the vestibule. The lacrimal fossa lies lateral to the middle meatus of the nose and hence the bony ostium opens into the middle meatus of the nose.

## INDICATIONS OF DCR

DCR is indicated for the treatment of disorders of the lacrimal outflow pathway.[5] Following are the common situations where DCR is the treatment of choice (Figs. 81-2A to F):

- Primary acquired NLD obstruction causing symptomatic epiphora.
- Chronic dacryocystitis causing symptomatic epiphora, discharge and repeated acute attack of dacryocystitis. It is preferable to wait for about 4–6 weeks after an acute attack of dacryocystitis before proceeding with external DCR.
- Secondary acquired NLD obstruction following trauma, nasal tumor excision, etc.

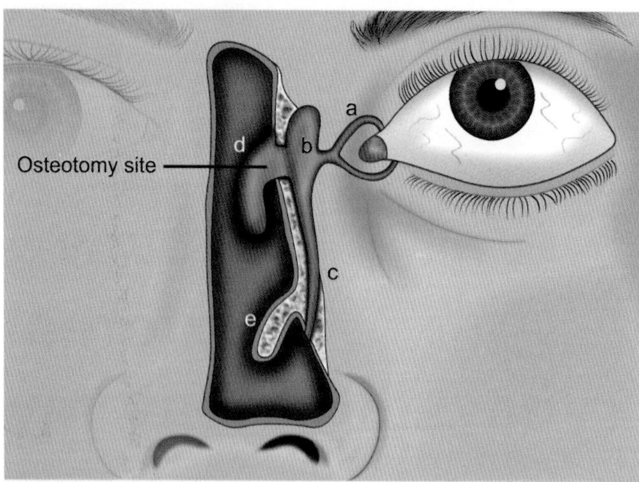


**Figure 81-1** Schematic diagram of the anatomy of the lacrimal outflow pathway, nasal cavity, and position of the osteotomy in dacryocystorhinostomy surgery. (A) Canaliculi, (B) Lacrimal sac, (C) Nasolacrimal duct, (D) Middle turbinate, (E) Inferior turbinate.

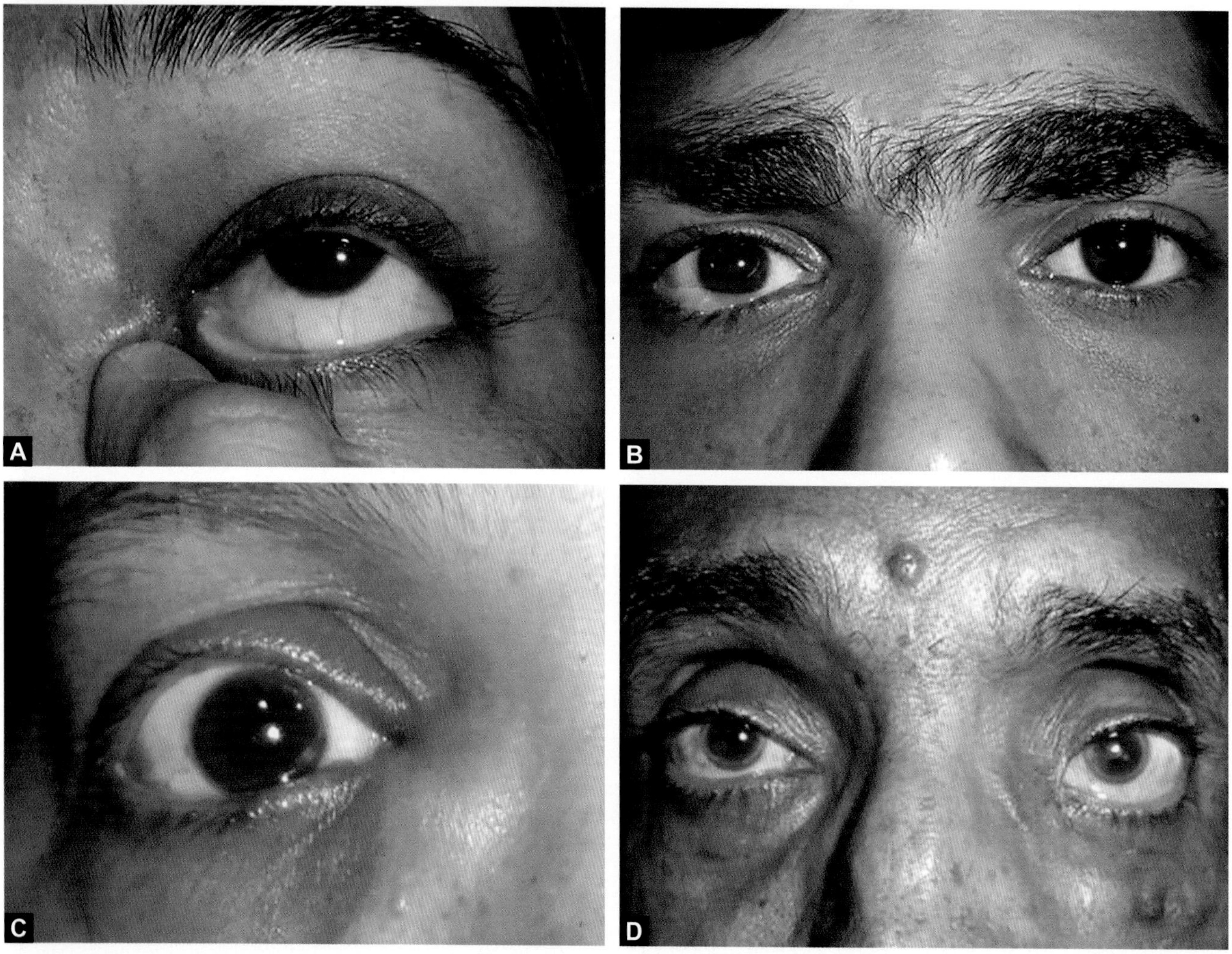

A B C D

**Figures 81-2A to D** Indications of dacryocystorhinostomy. (A) Chronic dacryocystitis with a positive ROPLAS test. (B) primary acquired nasolacrimal duct obstruction in an adult, note the positive dye disappearance test. (C) lacrimal mucocele. (D) left nasolacrimal duct obstruction following facial trauma, note the rounding of the medial canthus and sac distension on left side.

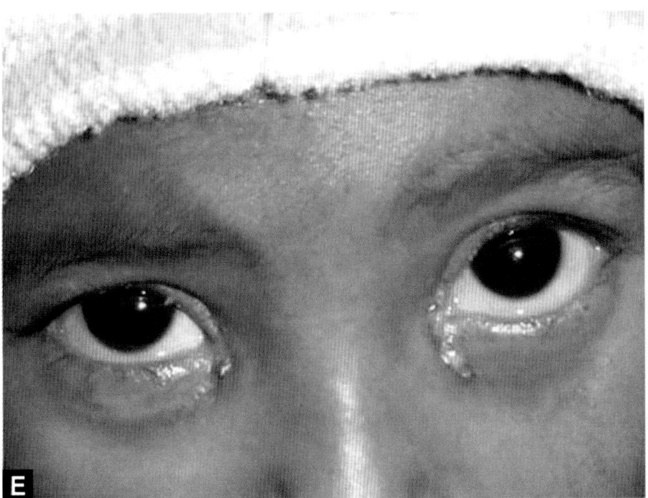

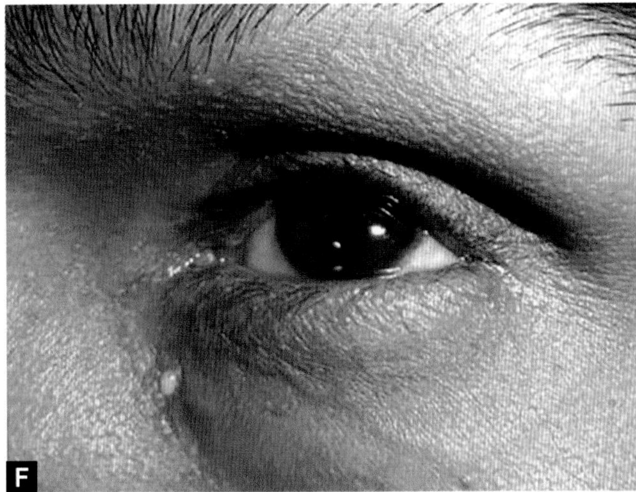

**Figures 81-2E and F** (E) congenital nasolacrimal duct obstruction in a child not resolving with probing with history of repeated acute dacryocystitis (F) congenital lacrimal fistula associated with nasolacrimal duct obstruction.

- Congenital NLD obstruction not amenable to other treatment like probing and intubation.
- As an adjunct to other procedures like canaliculodacryocystorhinostomy or conjunctivodacryocystorhinostomy and Jones tube placement.
- Dacryolithiasis.
- Partial NLD obstruction or atonic sac causing symptomatic epiphora.

## PREOPERATIVE PREPARATIONS

Preoperative evaluation of patients for DCR should include a detailed history about systemic conditions like hypertension, diabetes, and use of any medications that alter the coagulation profile. Good control of blood pressure is essential before taking up the patient for surgery to minimize intraoperative and postoperative bleeding. Bleeding and clotting time is tested preoperatively to rule out any bleeding diathesis. Medications like aspirin and warfarin can be discontinued temporarily before the surgery in consultation with the physician. Any history of nasal pathology or previous nasal or lacrimal surgery should be elicited as it has a bearing on the surgical plan. Nasal examination with endoscope is required in patients suggestive of intranasal pathology. Preoperative imaging with computed tomography (CT) scan is indicated in patients with secondary acquired NLD block following facial trauma, tumor excision, or in cases with suspected sinonasal mass lesion. Dacryocystography might be required in patients with failed lacrimal surgery to look for remnant of the sac.[6]

## ANESTHESIA

Most cases of DCR can be done as an office procedure (Fig. 81-3) under local anesthesia.[7,8] Sedation might be needed in patients who are apprehensive. In authors practice, general anesthesia (GA) is advocated for pediatric cases in few cases of post-traumatic NLD block where concurrent removal of bony callus might be needed or in adult patients who refuse surgery under local anesthesia. The nasal mucosa is anesthetized first using 10% lignocaine nasal spray. Local anesthesia is given with a mixture of 2% Xylocaine with adrenaline and 0.5% bupivacaine. Adrenaline helps in vasoconstriction and minimizes blood loss during surgery. Waiting for 10–15 minutes after giving the block helps in effective vasoconstriction. In patients where use of adrenaline is contraindicated, anesthesia is given with a combination of 2% Xylocaine and 0.5% bupivacaine. The anesthesia is given at three sites using 16 mm 26G needle, approximately 1.5–2 mL at each site.[8]

- The infratrochlear nerve that supplies the lacrimal sac is infiltrated by passing the needle just below the trochlea and entering the extraconal space along the superomedial orbital wall.
- Infraorbital nerve block is given by injecting over the orbital floor periosteum at the level of infraorbital foramen at the maximum depth allowed by the needle.
- Local infiltration at the site of incision injecting deeper till the level of the periosteum over the anterior lacrimal crest.

Intravenous sedation is injected in selected patients to allay anxiety. General anesthesia with cuffed endotracheal

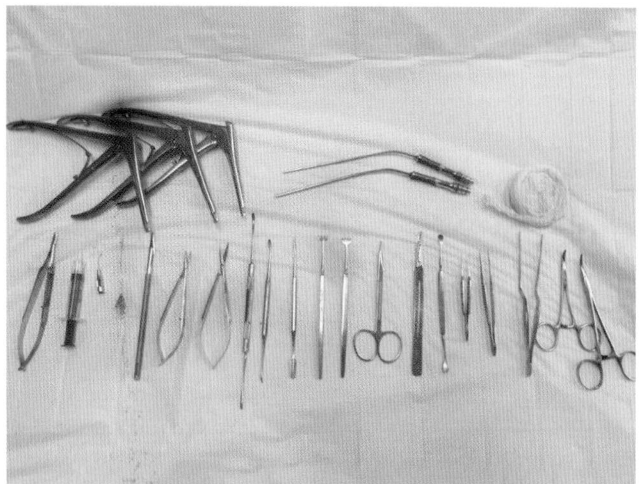

Figure 81-3 Instruments used during dacryocystorhinostomy surgery.

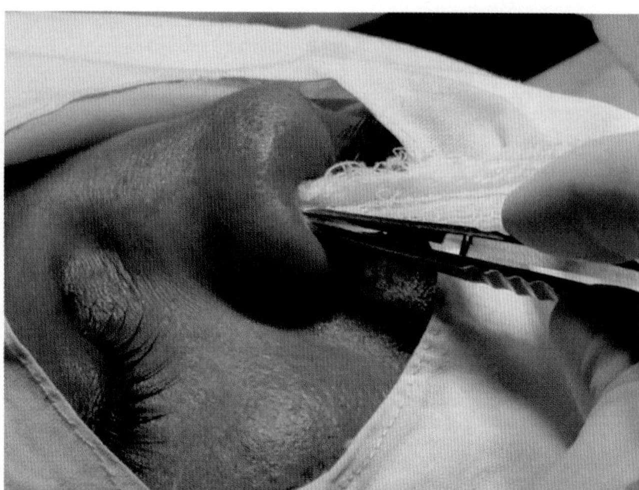

Figure 81-4 Preoperative nasal packing being done with gauze soaked in 4% lignocaine.

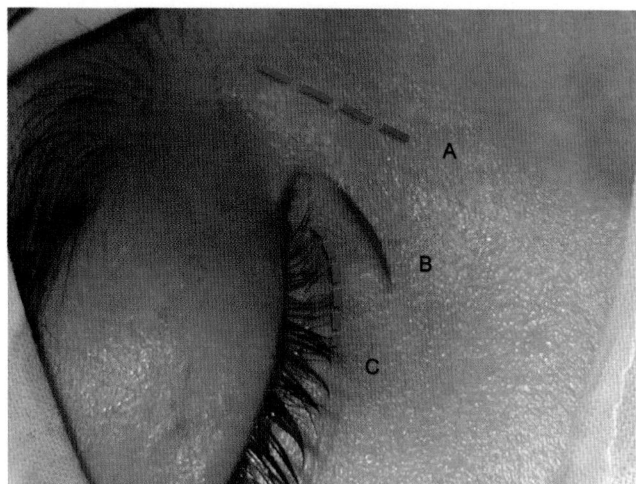


Figure 81-5 Various incision used for dacryocystorhinostomy. (A) Straight incision along the root of the nose about 10 mm from medial canthus, (B) tear trough incision, and (C) lower eyelid subciliary incision.

tube is advocated in children. Local infiltration with Xylocaine with adrenaline is given along the site of the incision even in patients under GA to minimize blood loss during surgery. Nasal packing of the middle turbinate area is done with gauze piece soaked in 4% lignocaine and 0.1% oxymetazoline for anesthesia and decongestion of the nasal mucosa (Fig. 81-4).

## SURGICAL PROCEDURE

### Incision for External DCR

A straight incision at the site of the midpoint of the medial canthus and nasal bridge or a curvilinear incision 3 mm medial to the medial canthus are the most commonly used DCR incisions that give adequate exposure for creation of a bony ostium (Fig. 81-5). Curvilinear incision placed along the tear trough can give excellent exposure and has excellent cosmetic appearance postoperatively. The author's current approach is to use a tear trough incision placed along the inferior orbital rim extending from below the level of MCT (medial canthal tendon) for about 10–15 mm. Subciliary incision can also give adequate exposure of the surgical site and have good aesthetic outcome.[9]

### Lacrimal Sac Dissection

The orbicularis is separated through the skin incision by blunt dissection by spreading a straight tenotomy scissor along the length of the incision. The periosteum over the anterior lacrimal crest is dissected using periosteal elevator or a blunt tip suction cannula. Bleeding noted at this stage can be controlled by using cautery. The lacrimal sac is separated from the anterior crest using a periosteal elevator, and the lacrimal fossa is exposed (Fig. 81.6). Disinsertion of the medial canthal tendon is not necessary in most cases, and adequate exposure can be obtained by giving traction on the wound edges using retractors.

### Bony Ostium Formation

The bony osteotomy is initiated at the junction of the lacrimal bone and lamina papyracea by infracturing the bone at this site. A 1 or 1.5 mm Kerrison punch is introduced between the lacrimal bone and nasal mucosa and the osteotomy is initiated (Fig. 81-7). The osteotomy is continued vertically upwards for 3–4 mm above the anterior crest till it is possible to insinuate the punch easily between the bone and mucosa. The osteotomy is then mushroomed out superiorly and inferiorly

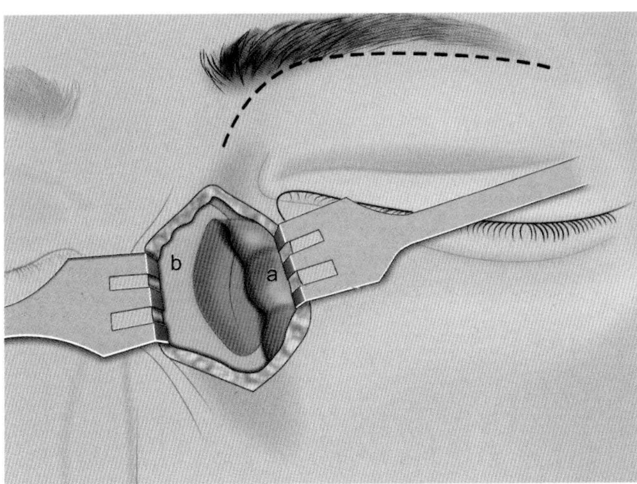


Figures 81-6 Exposure of the lacrimal sac, anterior lacrimal crest and lacrimal fossa through a tear trough incision. (a) Lacrimal sac and anterior (b) lacrimal crest.

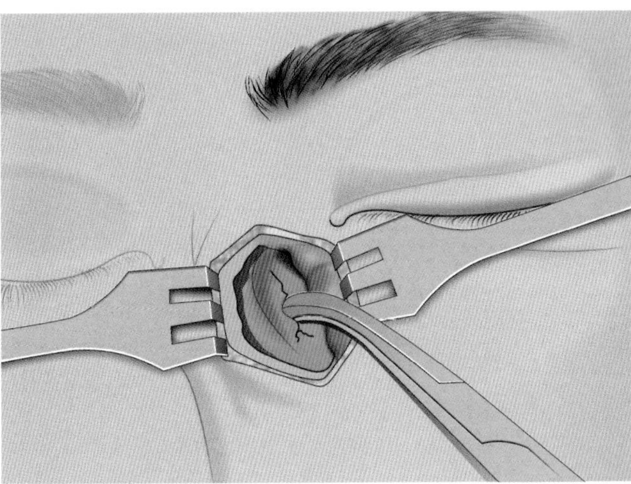

Figure 81-7 Infracture of the thin bone of lamina papyracea with a curved hemostat. Osteotomy is started from this site.

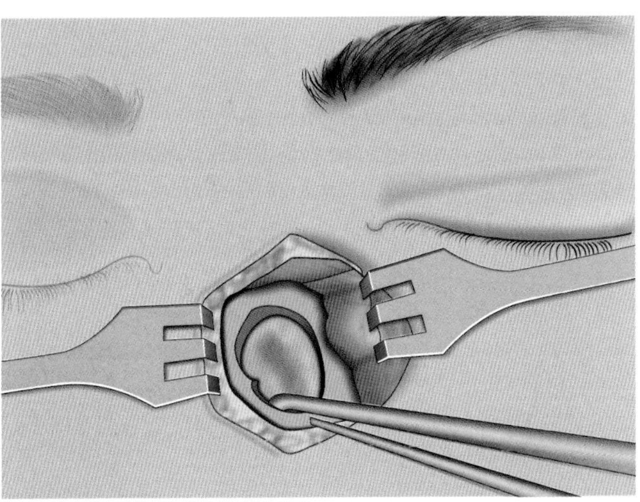

Figure 81-8 Osteotomy being done using bone punches and extended till about 3–4 mm above the level of anterior lacrimal crest.

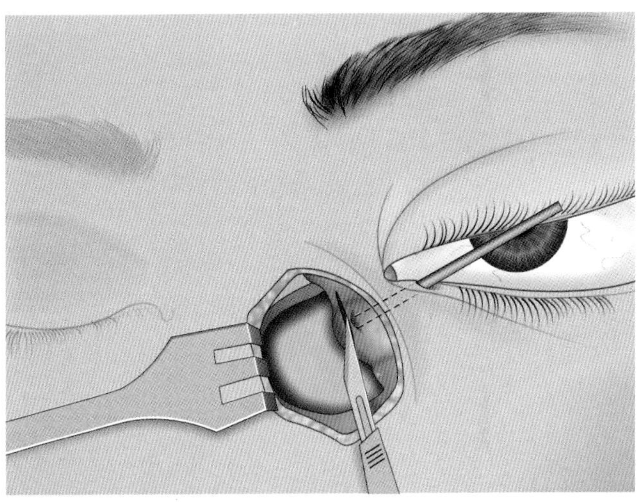

Figure 81-9 Opening of the lacrimal sac by a straight horizontal incision. Note the tenting of the sac using a lacrimal probe to prevent cutting the medial wall of the sac accidentally.

from the edges of the groove (Fig. 81-8). The punch should be held perpendicular to the bone and pressure should be applied near the tip of the punch handle away from the fulcrum for effective punching. The superior edge of the bone underlying the MCT is best removed by holding the punch in a reverse grip or by using a Citelli reverse cutting punch. The extent of the completed ostium are superiorly about 2 mm above the MCT, inferiorly till the upper edge of NLD, posteriorly including the lamina papyracea, and anteriorly till 3–4 mm above the level of anterior crest. Ultrasonic surgical aspirator (Sonopet Omni, Synergetic, Inc, O'Fallon, MO) can also be used for removal of bone during DCR with minimal collateral soft tissue damge.[10]

## Mucosal Flaps Creation and Anastomosis

The mucosal flaps are made next. The lacrimal sac flaps are made by inserting a no. 1 Bowman probe into the sac, though one of the canaliculi and tenting the sac as posterior as possible. Using the probe as the guide, a vertical incision is given in the medial wall of the sac from the fundus till sac-NLD junction to slit open the sac lumen (Fig. 81-9). The incision should be given over the probe to make a large anterior sac flap. Mucopurulent discharge from the sac can come out at this stage confirming a full thickness opening of the sac mucosa. The incision is extended superiorly and inferiorly with curved Castroviejo scissors till the fundus of sac and the upper end

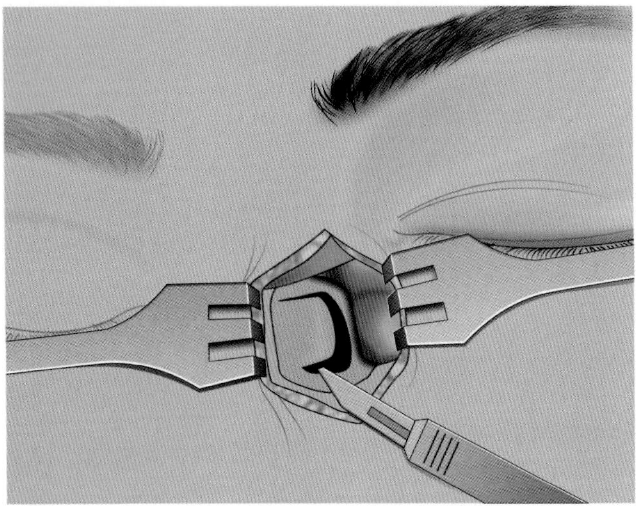

**Figure 81-10** Rectangular nasal mucosal flap being made.

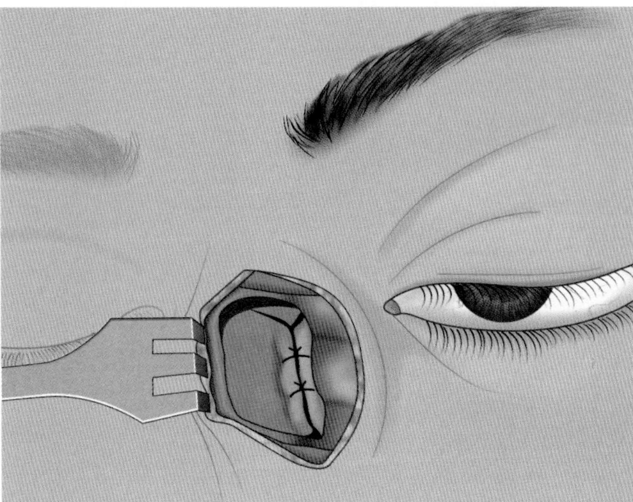

**Figure 81-11** Suturing of the anterior flaps of lacrimal sac and nasal mucosa.

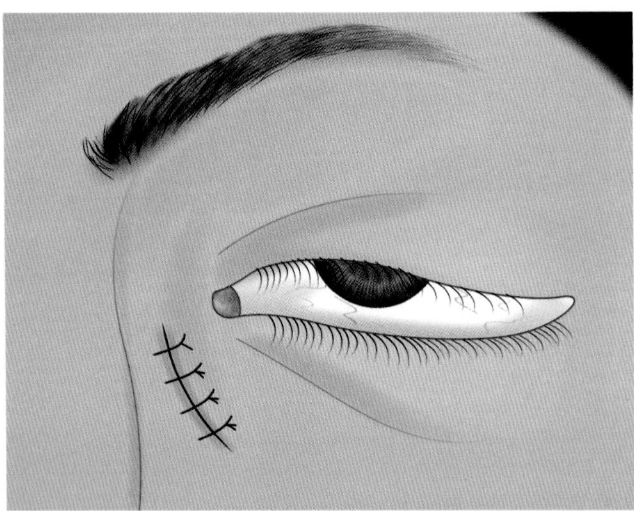

**Figure 81-12** Skin closure with interrupted sutures.

of NLD and relaxing cuts are given at the edges of the incision to create anterior and posterior flaps. The posterior flap can be excised if only anterior flap suturing is planned.

The nasal mucosa is opened by giving two vertical full thickness mucosal cuts along the superior and the inferior bony edges of the osteotomy margin. The two vertical cuts are joined inferiorly to raise a rectangular flap hinged superiorly along the anterior crest (Fig. 81-10). The residual posterior edge of the flap is trimmed. The anterior flap is also trimmed off before suturing to prevent any sagging of the flaps at the site of the anastomosis. Prominent middle turbinate occluding the site of the osteum can be trimmed by doing partial turbinectomy at this stage. The nasal mucosal and anterior lacrimal flaps are sutured with 6-0 absorbable suture (Fig. 81-11). The apposition of the flaps should be edge to edge to prevent any sagging of the flaps at the site of the anastomosis. Tenting of the sutured flaps to the periosteum or orbicularis can also be done to prevent sagging of the flaps over the passage.

### Closure

The skin orbicularis is sutured with interrupted sutures, the nasal mucosal packing removed and syringing done to confirm free passage of fluid (Fig. 81-12). Nasal cavity is repacked and eye is patched.

## POSTOPERATIVE TREATMENT

Postoperatively, the patient is started on oral antibiotics and analgesics for 5 days. The eye patch is removed next day, the nasal pack is removed gently and note is made of any nasal bleed. Patient is started on topical antibiotic eye drops. Wound cleaning is done with Betadine 5% solution, antibiotic ointment is applied over sutures; nasal decongestant drops and steroid nasal spray are prescribed for 2–3 weeks. Sutures are removed after 1 week and establishment of patency checked by doing syringing. Patient is followed up at 1 week, 6 weeks, 6 months, and yearly thereafter.

## INDICATION OF INTUBATION

Use of intubation in routine uncomplicated DCR patients is controversial as tube induced granulation tissue formation can itself be a cause of closure of the anastomosis. In author's practice it is indicated in cases with canalicular stenosis, fibrosed sac with inadequate mucosal flaps, repeat DCR or in case of loss of mucosal flaps during surgery. If indicated, a bicanalicular Silastic tube is commonly used. The lacrimal probe with the attached tube is passed through the upper and lower canaliculi through the osteotomy to the nasal cavity and taken out through the nose with the help of a hemostat. The probes are removed, multiple surgical knots are tied to secure the tube in the nose and excess tube is cutoff just inside the nostril. The mucosal flaps are then sutured and rest of the surgery is completed.

## INDICATION OF ANTIMETABOLITES

Use of adjunctive antimetabolites like mitomycin C during routine external DCR is controversial. Antimetabolites act by their antifibrotic effect thereby reducing the scarring and closure of the anastomosis site. Larger final ostium size and increased success rate has been reported with the intraoperative use of adjunctive antimetabolites at various concentrations.[11,12] However, their use during uncomplicated routine external DCR is controversial. Author's use of Intraoperative mitomycin C is limited to repeat DCR with extensive soft tissue scarring.[13] Mitomycin C is used at concentration of 0.02% and cottonoids soaked in the injection is placed at the site of the anastomosis for 3 minutes after creating the mucosal flaps. Care is taken to avoid the cottonoid touching the skin edges of the incision that can predispose to cutaneous fistulae formation at the incision site postoperatively. At the end of 3 minutes, the cottonoids are removed and the anastomosis site irrigated thoroughly with sterile ringer solution before proceeding with closure of the flaps and the incision.

## COMPLICATIONS OF DCR

Complications of DCR can be divided into intraoperative and postoperative complications. Excessive bleeding is the most common intraoperative complication. The following precautions can help in minimizing the bleeding during surgery:

- Bleeding can be minimized by good preoperative blood pressure control and giving anxiolytics and sedation if the patient seems to be apprehensive.
- Anesthesia using local infiltration of lignocaine along with adrenaline wherever permissible.
- Careful placement of the incision avoiding the angular vein
- Use of preoperative nasal decongestant and tight nasal packing during surgery. Excessive bleeding intraoperatively can be controlled at times by changing the nasal packing.
- Availability of a good electrocautery or a radiofrequency cautery during surgery.
- Use of a suction cannula during surgery.
- Availability of bone wax to stop any excessive periosteal ooze or bleed from the bone.
- Raising the head end of the operating table if required.

These steps will minimize the bleeding during surgery in most cases. Rarely, accidental injury to the anterior ethmoidal vessels can happen. This might need a posterior nasal packing to stop the bothersome bleeding. To avoid this complication, the superior edge of the osteum should not be extended posteriorly behind the anterior edge of lamina papyracea.

Injury to the cribriform plate and cerebrospinal fluid leak is a rare complication. It is more likely to occur during pediatric DCR as children have a low lying cribriform plate compared to adults and are more prone to accidental injury while punching the bone superiorly. Hence in children, the superior edge of the ostium is limited till the level of the medial canthal tendon. Rarely, meningitis has been reported after DCR surgery.[14,15]

Loss of the mucosal flaps can occur at times during surgery either due to damage to the nasal mucosa while creating the ostium or injury to the sac while dissecting. In case of loss of the nasal mucosal flap, the lacrimal sac flap can be sutured to the edge of the periosteum or to the orbicularis muscle. Loss of both the flaps will need an anastomosis between the orbicularis and soft tissues. A bicanalicular intubation is preferred in these cases to maintain the patency of the ostium.

Early postoperative complications include secondary nasal bleeding, wound infection, wound dehiscence, excessive nasal crusting. Secondary bleeding usually occurs between day 4 and 10, is seen in about 3.8% cases and can usually be managed conservatively.[16] Excessive nasal crusting might need endoscopic cleaning to prevent blockage at the site of the osteum.

## DCR IN SPECIAL SITUATIONS

### DCR with Fistulectomy

Lacrimal fistulae can be congenital or acquired following episode of acute dacryocystitis and burst lacrimal abscess. Acquired fistulous tract closes spontaneously after reestablishment of patency after a DCR and does not require separate dissection of the fistulous tract. Since most fistulous opening are present inferolateral to the sac, the surgical incision for DCR can be placed such that the fistulae is included in the incision and the tract closes along with closure of the skin incision. Congenital fistula, in contrast, is an epithelium lined

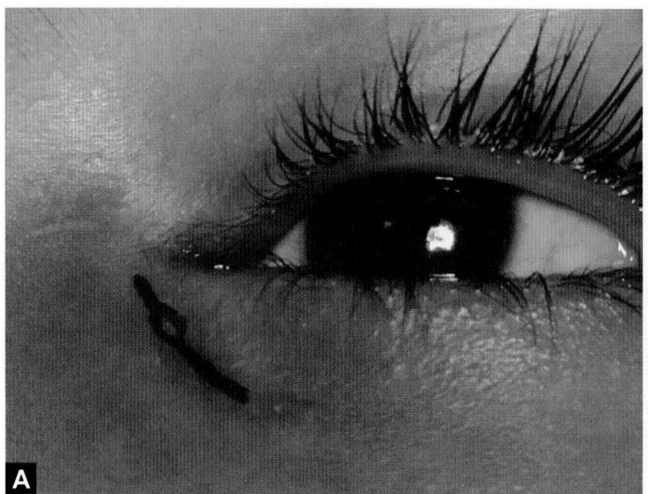

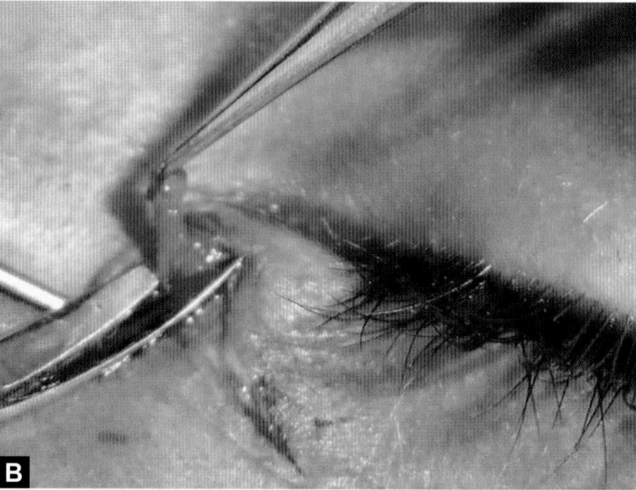

**Figures 81-13A and B** Dacryocystorhinostomy (DCR) incision including the congenital fistulous tract in cases of DCR with fistulectomy surgery (A). The fistulous tract is dissected and excised before proceeding with DCR (B).

tract and needs dissection and excision of the tract to prevent recurrence of the fistulae. The incision for DCR in these cases are placed such to include the fistulous opening (Figs. 81-13A and B). A lacrimal probe is inserted into the fistula that is used as a guide to dissect and trace the tract till its entry into the sac or canalicular system. The dissected tract is excised and the mucosal edges closed with 8-0 Vicryl sutures. A routine DCR is then performed though the skin incision. In cases where the fistulous tract is communicating with the canaliculi, a bicanalicular Silastic intubation is done along with DCR to prevent canalicular scarring and stenosis later.

### Concerns in Pediatric DCR

There are certain anatomical differences that should be kept in mind and technique of external DCR in children needs to be modified accordingly.[17,18] The lacrimal fossa and anterior lacrimal crest is not very well defined in children. Hence there might be some difficulty in defining the boundaries of the osteotomy. The superior edge of the osteotomy should not extend beyond the level of medial canthal tendon as the cribriform plate is low lying in children and can be damaged accidentally while creating the osteotomy. In children, the blood loss during surgery should be kept to minimum as they have a lower blood volume compared to adults. Though wound healing is faster in children, the incision length should be kept minimum, not more than 2 cm to avoid any visible scar. If concurrent canthoplasty is planned for epicanthal fold or telecanthus repair, DCR can be done through the same canthoplasty incision. In children with NLD block associated with craniofacial anomalies, a CT scan should preferably be done preoperatively to rule out underlying bony anatomical anomaly and plan the surgery accordingly. Irrespective of the age of the child, probing should be done for all children before starting the surgery if it has not been done earlier. Though probing has the highest success rate in younger children less than 1 year, about 75% success rate has been reported for children between 3 and 10 years, hence a trial of probing on table before proceeding with DCR is worthwhile.[19]

## RESULTS OF EXTERNAL DCR

External DCR is considered the gold standard in the treatment of NLD obstruction. A high surgical success rate of about 95% is reported in many studies. However, when functional success as defined by dye test is also included in the criteria for success the success rate declines to about 70%.[20-22] The surgical success also depends on the type and etiology of obstruction with postsaccal obstructions having a higher success rate than presaccal obstruction.[21] Higher failure rate has been reported in post-traumatic cases.

Inappropriate size and location of the ostium, common canalicular scarring, shrinkage of the rhinostomy site due to granulation tissue formation, and fibrosis remain the most common cause of failure of the surgery.[23,24] Failure can be prevented by making an adequate sized bony ostium, appropriately placed adjacent to the middle meatus, and lined by mucosal flaps. Failure can also occur due to "sump syndrome". Here the ostium is present with patent syringing but small remnant of the sac inferiorly causes mucopurulent discharge to collect and spill back to conjunctival cul-de-sac. In cases where reoperation is required for failed external DCR, revision of the osteotomy site can be done endonasally, excessive granulation and scar tissue excised and a bicanalicular intubation is done.[25,26]

## SUMMARY

External DCR is one of the most commonly performed oculoplastic surgery. The currently performed surgical technique remains essentially the same as described about a century ago with only minor modifications. If done appropriately, this technique has a high success rate of over 95%. Many surgeons now prefer an endonasal approach DCR over external DCR with comparable success rate reported in experienced hands. Though the primary advantage of endonasal approach remains avoidance of skin incision, the cutaneous scar in external DCR is not persistent and is not perceived as cosmetic blemish by most patients.[27,28] With the use of small incisions, hidden lid crease and tear trough incision along the natural skin tension lines, the risk of a visible scar is considerably reduced. Also, other advantages like requirement of simple and inexpensive equipments, short operative time, high success rate, and ability to obtain tissue biopsy make external DCR the gold standard and preferred surgical option for NLD obstruction and dacryocystitis.

## REFERENCES


1. Toti A. Nuovo metodo conservatore di cura radicalle delle suppurazioni cronicle del sacco lacrimale. Clin Mod Firenze. 1904; 10:385-9.
2. Dupuy-Dutemps B. Note preliminaire sur un procede de dacryocystorhinostomie. Ann Ocul Par. 1920;27:445.
3. Ali MJ, Naik MN, Honavar SG. External dacryocystorhinostomy: tips and tricks. Oman J Ophthalmol. 2012;5(3):191-5.
4. Yeatts RP. Lacrimal laceration. In: Roy FH (ed.), Master Techniques in Ophthalmic Surgery. Media, PA: Williams & Wilkins; 1995.
5. Dortzbach RK: Dacryocystorhinostomy. Ophthalmology. 1978; 85:1267-70.
6. Francisco FC, Carvalho AC, Francisco VF, et al. Evaluation of 1000 lacrimal ducts by dacryocystography. Br J Ophthalmol. 2007;91(1):43-6.
7. Knežević MM, Stojković MŽ, Vlajković GP, et al. Pain during external dacryocystorhinostomy with local anaesthesia. Med Sci Monit. 2011;17(6):CR341-6
8. Ciftci F, Pocan S, Karadayi K, et al. Local versus general anaesthesia for external dacryocystorhinostomy in young patients. Ophthal Plast Reconstr Surg. 2005;21(3):201-6.
9. Dave TV, Javed Ali M, Sravani P, et al. Subciliary incision for external dacryocystorhinostomy. Ophthal Plast Reconstr Surg. 2012;28(5):341-5.
10. Sivak-Callcott JA, Linberg JV, Patel S. Ultrasonic bone removal with the Sonopet Omni: a new instrument for orbital and lacrimal surgery. Arch Ophthalmol. 2005;123:1595-7.
11. Kao SCS, Liao CL, Jason HS, et al. Dacryocystorhinostomy with intraoperative mitomycin C. Ophthalmology. 1997;104:86-91.
12. You YA, Fang CT. Intraoperative mitomycin C in dacryocystorhinostomy. Ophthal Plast Reconstr Surg. 2001;17(2):115-9
13. Yeatts RP, Neves RB. Use of mitomycin C in repeat dacryocystorhinostomy. Ophthal Plast Surg. 1999;15:19-2.
14. Usul H, Kuzeyli K, Cakir E, et al. Meningitis and Pneumocephalus. A rare complication of external dacryocystorhinostomy. J Clin Neurosci. 2004;11(8):901-2.
15. Seider N, Kaplan N, Gilboa M, et al. Effect of timing of external dacryocystorhinostomy on surgical outcome. Ophthal Plast Reconstr Surg. 2007;23(3):183-6.
16. Tsirbas A, McNab AA. Secondary haemorrhage after dacryocystorhinostomy. Clin Experiment Ophthalmol. 2000;28(1): 22-5.
17. Nowinski TS, Flanagan JC, Mauriello J. Pediatric dacryocystorhinostomy. Arch Ophthalmol. 1985;103(8):1226-8.
18. Kropp TM, Goldstein JB, Katowitz WR. Management of pediatric lower system problems: dacryocystorhinostomy. Pediatr Oculoplast Surg. New York:Springer, 2002:325-36.
19. Thongthong K, Singha P, Liabsuetrakul T. Success of probing for congenital nasolacrimal duct obstruction in children under 10 years of age. J Med Assoc Thai. 2009;92(12):1646-50.
20. Fayers T, Laverde T, Tay E, et al. Lacrimal surgery success after external dacryocystorhinostomy: functional and anatomical results using strict outcome criteria. Ophthal Plast Reconstr Surg. 2009;25(6):472-5.
21. Delaney YM, Khooshabeh R. External dacryocystorhinostomy for the treatment of acquired partial nasolacrimal obstruction in adults. Br J Ophthalmol. 2002;86(5):533-5.
23. Ben Simon GJ, Joseph J, Lee S, et al. External versus endoscopic dacryocystorhinostomy for acquired nasolacrimal duct obstruction in a tertiary referral center. Ophthalmology. 2005; 112:1463-8.
24. Konuk O, Kurtulmusoglu M, Knatova Z, et al. Unsuccessful lacrimal surgery: causative factors and results of surgical management in a tertiary referral center. Ophthalmologica. 2010;224(6): 361-6.
25. Welham RA, Wulc AE. Management of unsuccessful lacrimal surgery. Br J Ophthalmol. 1987;71(2):152-7
26. Orcutt JC, Hillel A, Weymuller EA Jr. Endoscopic repair of failed dacryocystorhinostomy. Ophthal Plast Reconstr Surg. 1990;6(3):197-202.
27. Sharma V, Martin PA, Benger R, et al. Evaluation of the cosmetic significance of external dacryocystorhinostomy scars. Am J Ophthalmol. 2005;140:359-62.
28. Olver JM. Tips on how to avoid the DCR scar. Orbit. 2005; 24(2):63-6. Review.

CHAPTER

# 82

# Dacryocystorhinostomy: Endonasal

Jane Olver

## INTRODUCTION

Transnasal dacryocystorhinostomy (DCR) was first described by Caldwell in 1893 to open the lacrimal sac and drain the tears into the nose for the relief of epiphora from nasolacrimal duct obstruction. In 1913, Western countries made a nasal window resection of the upper nasolacrimal duct and further developed endonasal DCR. Toti advocated the external approach DCR and Dupuy-Dutemps developed this with sutured mucosal flaps in the early 19th century, which became the foundation for mid and late 20th century external DCR. In the 1990s with the advent of the Hopkins rigid endoscope, endonasal DCR again emerged, called endonasal endoscopic (EE) DCR.

External approach DCR and EE-DCR are virtually the same operation with similar aims but have a different surgical approach to the lacrimal sac, from outside and inside the nose. The aim of DCR surgery, whether by the external skin incision approach or by the EE approach, is to create a large bony and corresponding lacrimal sac opening along the entire vertical height of the lacrimal sac into the lateral nasal wall, through which the tears can drain unimpeded. There should be no mucosal, bony fragments or close middle turbinate or septum with which the ostium could form a synechiae and an obstruction.

External DCR has a proven track record and is quick and effective. It has been regarded as the gold standard of lacrimal surgery. Endonasal endoscopic dacryocystorhinostomy is now the first choice of DCR surgery for patients with epiphora from a blocked nasolacrimal duct. It is being actively taught worldwide to ophthalmologists in training.

## DEFINITION

*Definition of DCR Surgery*: Creation of a new opening between the tear lake, the lacrimal sac and the inside of the nose via which the tears will flow unimpeded into the nose with resultant relief of a watering eye.

There are several different types of DCR:

- External via skin incision
- Endonasal with microscope or headlight
- Endonasal endoscopic (4 mm rigid endoscope)
- *COEXEN-DCR*: Combined External and Endoscopic endonasal DCR where there is a narrow nasal space and septal prominence or synechiae, particularly for a complicated redo DCR, usually under local anesthesia but can be under general anesthesia. Gives all options and allows to check three dimensionally, both from the outside and inside the nose simultaneously.
- Transcanalicular endoscopic (approximately 1 mm microendoscope)

All of the above can be with silicone bicanalicular intubation.

There are also two other types of DCR:

- Conjunctivo-DCR with Jones type glass bypass tube
- Canalicular-DCR with silicone intubation

In this chapter, EE-DCR is described.

## INDICATIONS

The clinical aims of EE-DCR are the relief of:

- A watering eye from nasolacrimal duct obstruction.
- Mucous discharge and reflux from nasolacrimal duct obstruction with a mucocele.

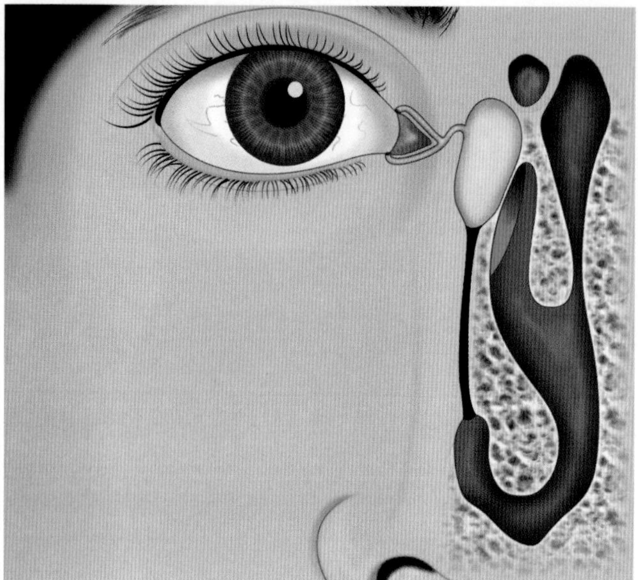

Figure 82-1 Blocked nasolacrimal duct and mucocele.

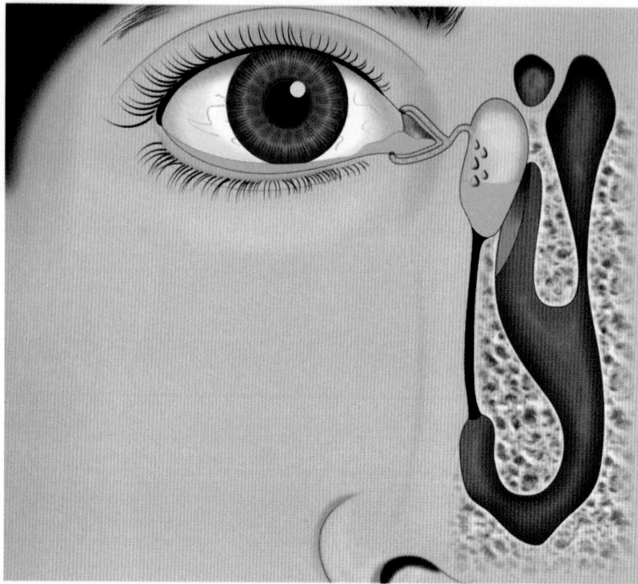

Figure 82-2 Tears wash back over eye from large lacrimal sac.

- Acute dacryocystitis from a stagnant, nonregurgitating infected mucocele and nasolacrimal duct obstruction.

The main advantage of EE-DCR over the external DCR is avoidance of a scar on the side of the nose. It is also precise, minimally invasive intranasal surgery as new functional endoscopic sinus surgery (FESS) instruments ensure accuracy inside the nose. The surgeon can see the actual wound site–the one inside the nose–during surgery and monitor its healing after surgery using endoscopic visualization (Figs. 82-1 and 82-2).

## CONTRAINDICATIONS

Patients with significant canalicular obstruction or loss in whom a CDCR or canalicular-DCR are indicated.

Patients with other causes of a watering eye, which are as follows:

- Hypersecretion
- Functional watering secondary to abnormal eyelid position or laxity.

## SURGICAL AIMS, SUCCESS, AND FAILURE

### Surgical Aims

The surgical aim is to create a bony osteotomy or rhinostomy in the maxilla and lacrimal bone and open the entire length of the lacrimal sac into lateral nasal wall. This large opening is to allow for free tear flow into nose. There should be no intervening bony or mucosal remnants or ethmoid air cell or middle turbinate blocking the opening. If necessary, an anterior ethmoidectomy of the agger nasi air cell and a partial anterior turbinectomy should also be performed (Figs. 82-3 to 82-5).

If the opening made is too small, the tears may drain only intermittently and not cope with an additional load of tears such as in cold weather or crying. If the opening made is too high in relation to the lacrimal sac base, then a sump syndrome may occur with intermittent mucous and tears wash back over the eye (Figs. 82-6 and 82-7).

### Surgical Failure

Surgical failure is mainly from scar tissue formation at various locations, most commonly the ostium. It is more likely to occur if there is:

- Local mucosal inflammation
- Untreated or recurrent intranasal disease
- Small ostium
- Tight silicone tubes
- Residual mucosal/tiny bony fragments
- Adjacent obstructing turbinate.

Intraostium mucosal granulomas occur from the silicone tubes rubbing on the ostium mucosa healing edge as they move with each blink. This can cause a blocked ostium with symptoms of mucous discharge and watering, with a subsequent scarred ostium and failure. Although granulomas can be treated medically with topical steroid drops, they may require cauterization with silver nitrate and extirpation surgically. Pre-existing polyps or recurrent polyps or other nasal disease can also obstruct the ostium and predispose to poor function or resultant failure (Figs. 82-8 and 82-9).

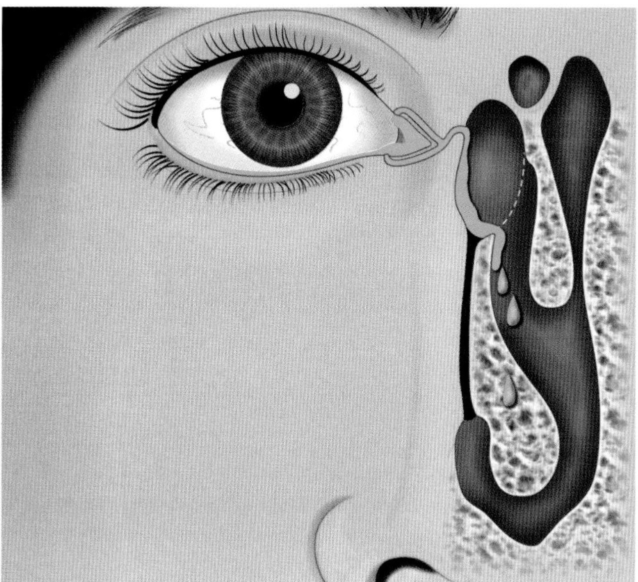
Figure 82-3 Post dacryocystorhinostomy open ostium.

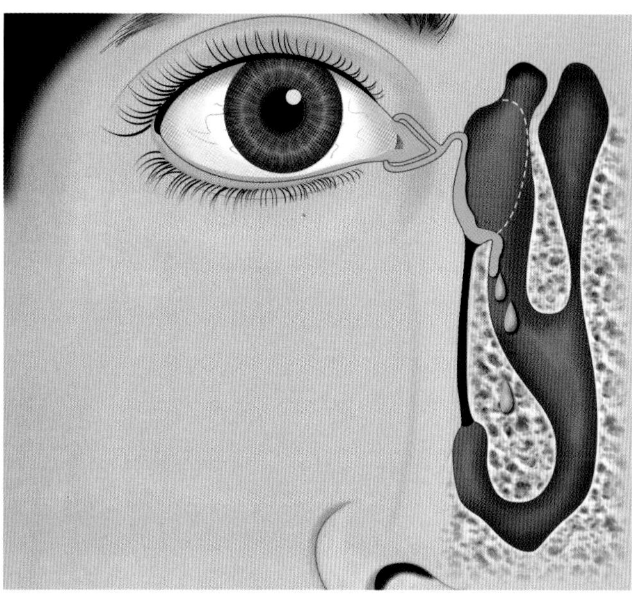
Figure 82-4 Post dacryocystorhinostomy open ostium and anterior ethmoid.

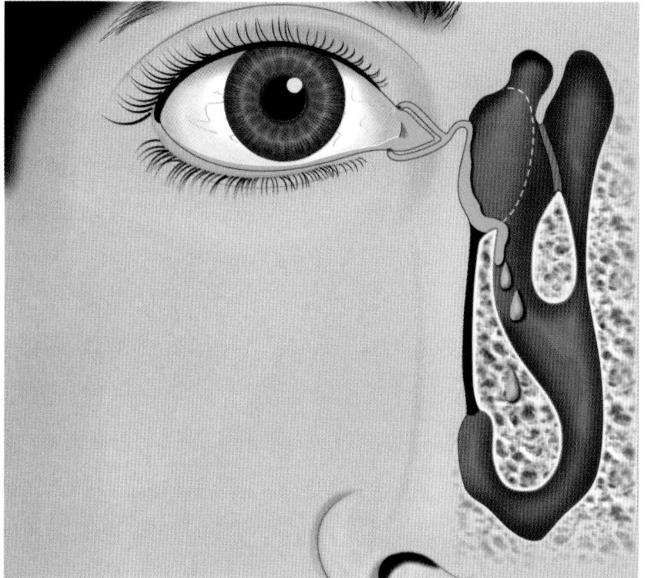
Figure 82-5 Post dacryocystorhinostomy open ostium and anterior ethmoid and anterior turbinectomy.

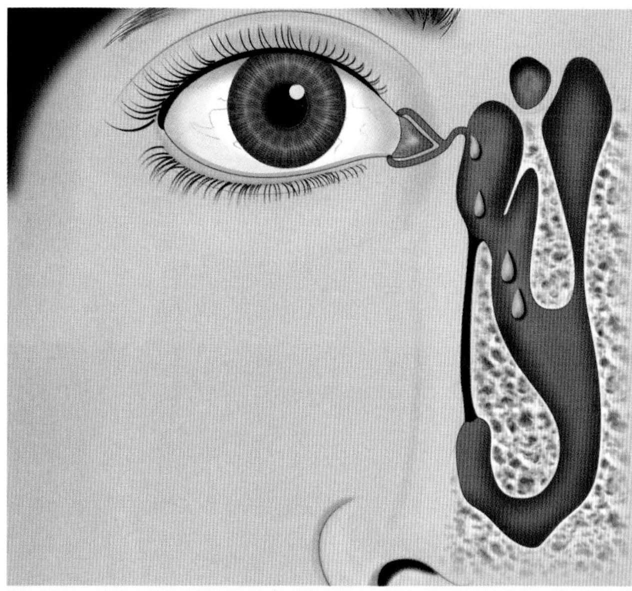
Figure 82-6 Post dacryocystorhinostomy small low opening that risks failure.

Mucosal adhesions caused by local inflammation, infection, undue trauma, and mucosal loss can lead to failure from scar tissue over the common canalicular opening, at the ostium, and within the lacrimal sac remnant (Figs. 82-10 to 82-12).

If small remnants of thin bone such as the uncinate process or lacrimal bone are left, there may be irregular healing and a convoluted tear drainage through the ostium, causing intermittent watering (Fig. 82-13).

Scar tissue can form between a paradoxically curved middle turbinate and the ostium where the turbinate mucosal is very close to the surgical ostium. Postoperative swelling causes adhesion and scarring between the turbinate and ostium. Similarly, if there is a septal deviation that is not addressed by septoplasty, scarring between the septum and turbinate and ostium can occur that is difficult to address (Figs. 82-14 and 82-15).

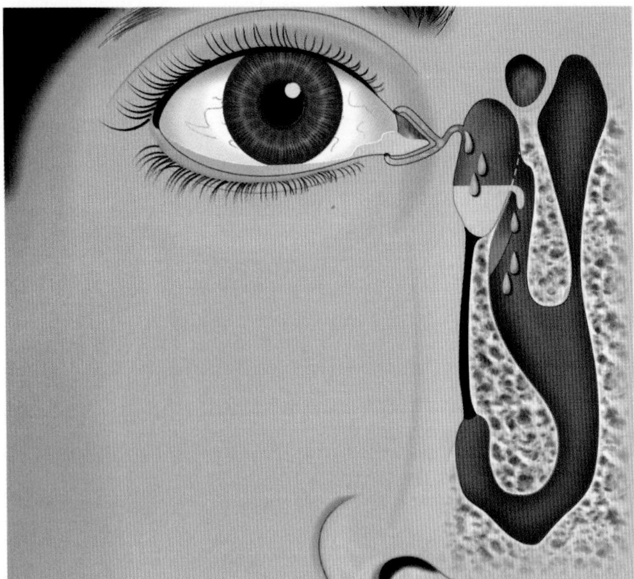

**Figure 82-7** Post dacryocystorhinostomy small high opening and sump syndrome cause watering and wash back of tears and mucous over eye.

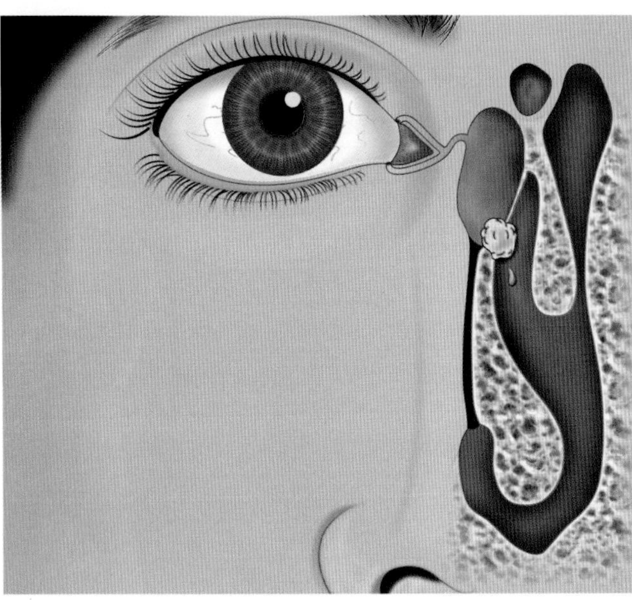

**Figure 82-8** Ostium granuloma causes intermittent watering and mucous discharge from eye and nose.

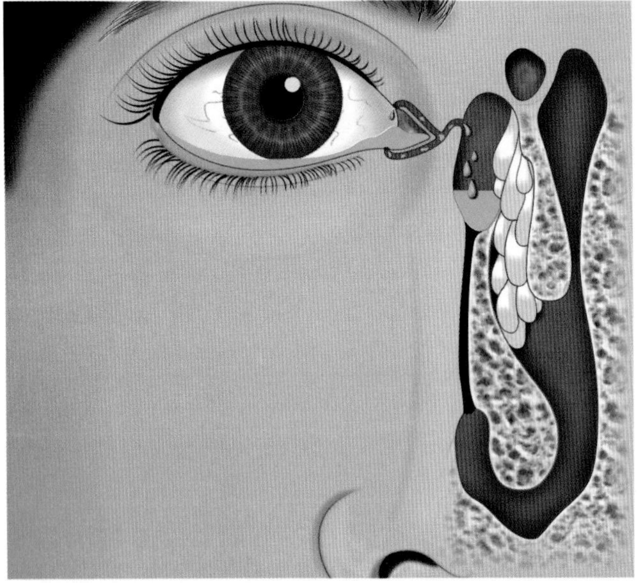

**Figure 82-9** Post dacryocystorhinostomy good sized ostium blocked by recurrent polyps.

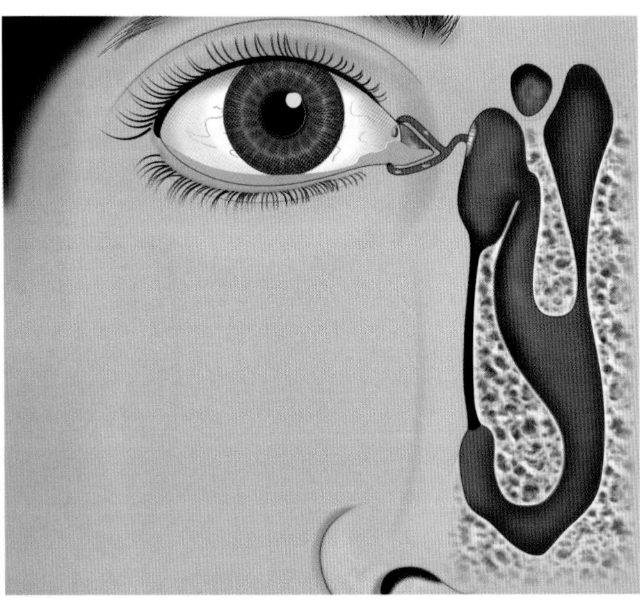

**Figure 82-10** Fine scar membrane over distal end common canaliculus into sac.

## Surgical Success

Surgical success is measured subjectively and objectively, at least 3 months after the silicone tubes have been removed (if inserted). The patients' opinion of the watering and the surgeons' assessment on syringing and nasal endoscopy are used to gauge success. It should be in the range of 90–95% success. A positive functional endoscopic dye test where a drop of fluorescein 1% is instilled in the conjunctival fornix appears at the ostium within seconds and drains down the lateral nasal wall, which indicates a functioning ostium (Fig. 82-16).

## Surgical Steps

### *Preparation: Anesthesia and Decongestant*

Surgery can be carried out under local anesthetic if only rongeurs are used for removal of the maxillary bone, and

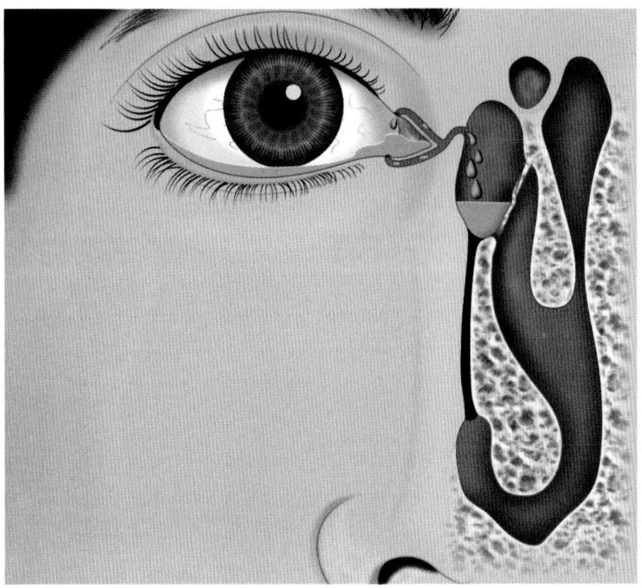
Figure 82-11 Thin membrane over ostium opening.

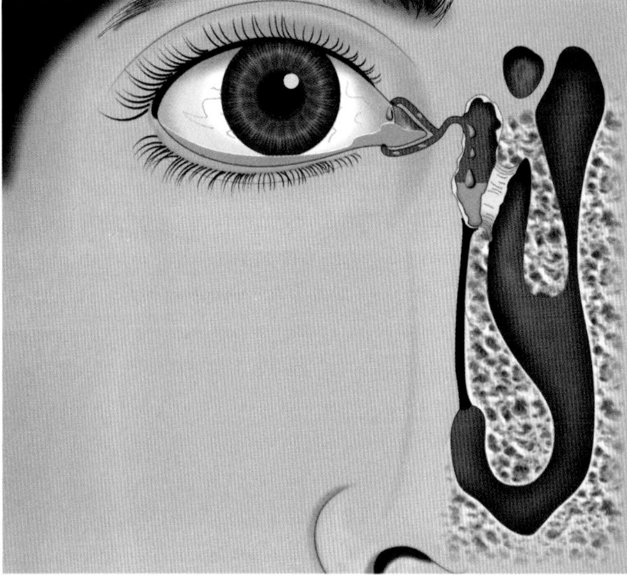
Figure 82-12 Small sac with intraluminal scarring and thick ostium scar.

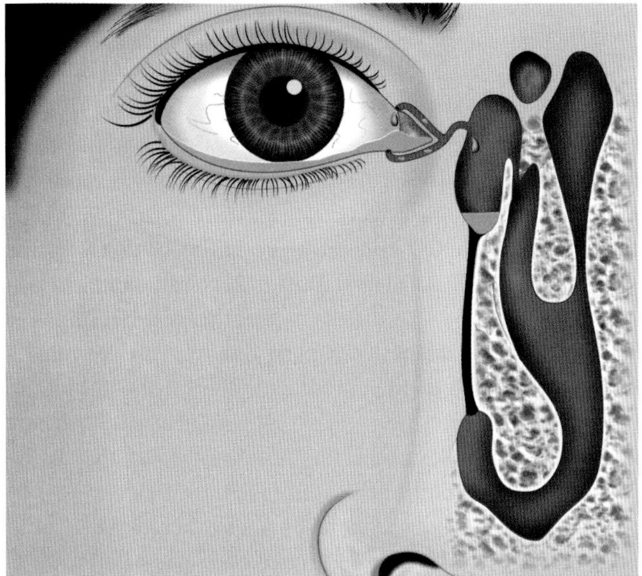
Figure 82-13 Very small high opening ostium with convoluted exit due to residual mucosal or small bony fragments.

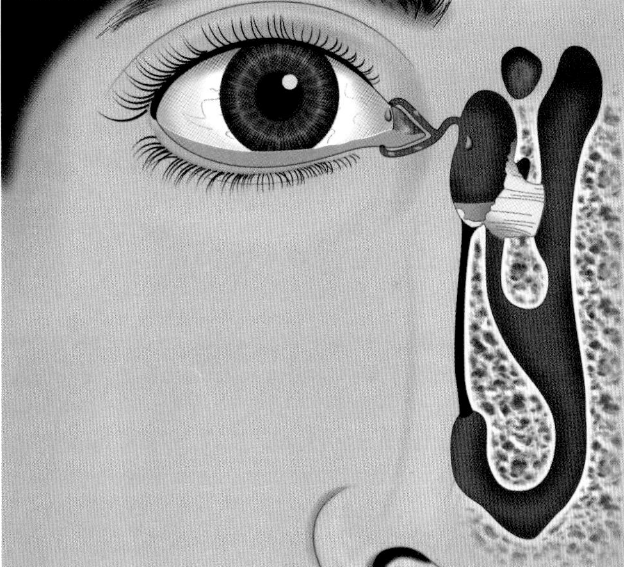
Figure 82-14 Thick scar (synechiae) between ostium and middle turbinate.

under general anesthesia only if mechanical instruments such as the diamond bur for bone and the microdebrider oscillating blade for mucosa are used, due to the large amount of irrigation required. Even if the patient is under general anesthetic condition, local anesthesia is also used. A combined external and EE-DCR can be done under local anesthesia if irrigation is not required.

Nasal mucosa:

- Vasoconstricted with co-phenylcaine nasal spray.
- Topical adrenaline 1 in 10,000 soaked patties.
- Local anesthetic injection 2 mL of lignocaine and adrenaline 1 in 80,000.

Subcutaneous tissue over lacrimal sac:

- 2–3 mL of a mixture of 4 mL of bupivacaine 0.5%, 4 mL of xylocaine with adrenaline 1 in 200,000 and 2 mL of dexamethasone.

Ocular surface:

- Topical proxymethacaine and tetracaine.

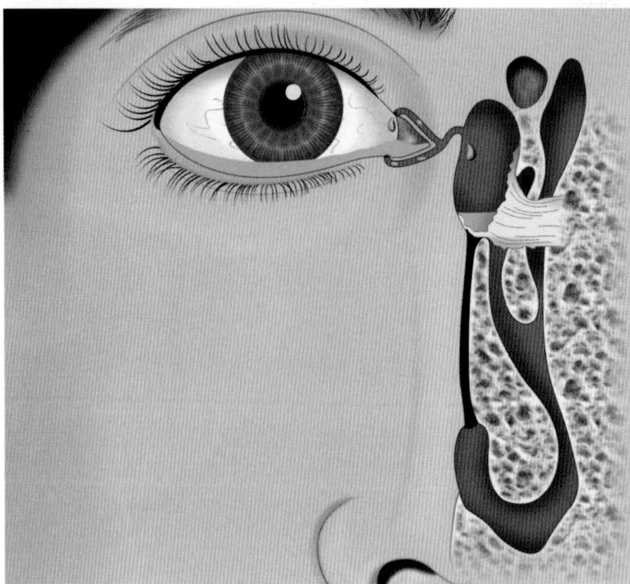

Figure 82-15 Thick scar (synechiae) between ostium, middle turbinate, and septum.

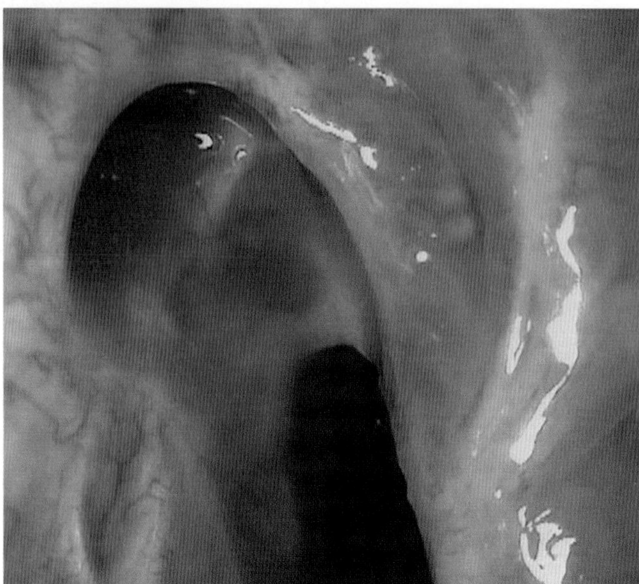

Figure 82-16 Right positive functional endoscopic dye test.

## Surgery: Instrumentation

*Ophthalmic instruments*: Ophthalmic instruments such as curved Westcott scissors are used for anterior partial middle turbinectomy to help complete the nasal flaps. The angled keratome blade is also invaluable for opening the lacrimal sac. HPMC gel mixed with fluorescein 2% irrigated into the lacrimal sac helps visualize the inside when cutting into the sac and making the sac flaps.

*FESS instruments:* The most important is the Freer's elevator and micro-Blakesley forceps. Also used are Medtronic 25° diamond bur, a 3.5 mm oscillating bur, long-handled Barde Parker number 15 blade, nasal aspiration, Lusk seeker, adrenaline 1 in 1000 on small neurosurgical patties, endoscope demister solution, O´Donoghue bicanalicular silicone intubation, and Nasopore internal dressing.

## Endoscopic Endonasal Surgical Steps

*Photos from a right-sided primary endonasal endoscopic DCR*

Once the nasal mucosa is well decongested, focus the endoscope light onto the middle turbinate and its shoulder where it has its lateral wall anterior attachment (Fig. 82-17). Use a long-handled size 15 Barde Parker blade to make a nasal mucosal flat 10–12 mm long from 4 mm above the middle turbinate shoulder, to at least half way down the middle turbinate. A microendoscopic transcanalicular light source with its tip placed in the lacrimal sac is not necessary and its insertion can damage the canaliculus (Fig. 82-18).

Bleeding should be small and can be aspirated or an adrenaline pattie placed for a few seconds that both absorbs blood and vasoconstricts the nasal mucosa (Fig. 82-19). After elevating the flap with the Freer's elevator, fold the nasal mucosal flap back over the middle turbinate to expose the maxillary bone and lacrimal crest (Fig. 82-20).

Use the 20° DCR burr to make the rhinostomy in the maxillary bone. This has irrigation and aspiration attached to it (Fig. 82-21). One the outer surface of the entire lacrimal sac has been exposed when the maxillary ostium is large enough, inflate the sac with HPMC mixed with fluorescein 2% Minims. In the picture below, the sac is clearly seen (Fig. 82-22). There is also a small hole toward the apex of the sac that is the partially opened anterior ethmoid agger nasi cell.

Start to open the sac with the angled keratome 1.7 mm knife quite anteriorly in order to make a large posterior lacrimal sac flap and expose the inside of the sac with the common canalicular opening (Fig. 82-23). As the sac is opened, the inside of the lumen and the fluorescein in HPMC starts to be seen (Fig. 82-24).

Gently push the posterior lacrimal sac mucosal flap back so that its edge sits right next to the edge of the posterior nasal flap. The inside of this sac looks edematous and the fluorescein stained lining of the inside of the lacrimal sac is seen (Fig. 82-25). If necessary reduce the nasal lacrimal flap with a 3.5 mm diamond oscillating bur at 3000–5000 revs per minute (Fig. 82-26). If required, use the Kerrison rongeur to augment the bony ostium (Fig. 82-27).

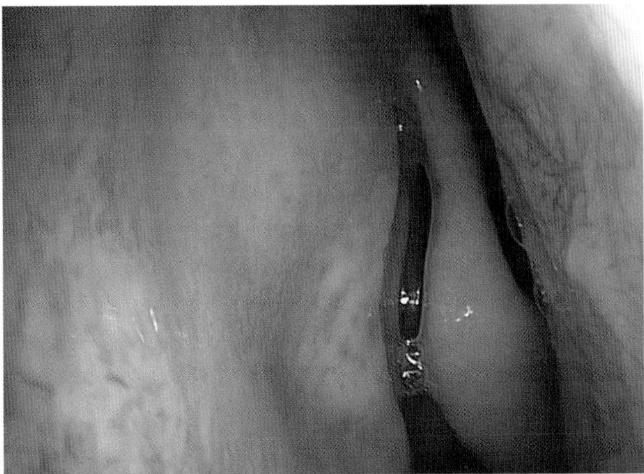

Figure 82-17 Right nasal space showing lateral wall and middle turbinate.

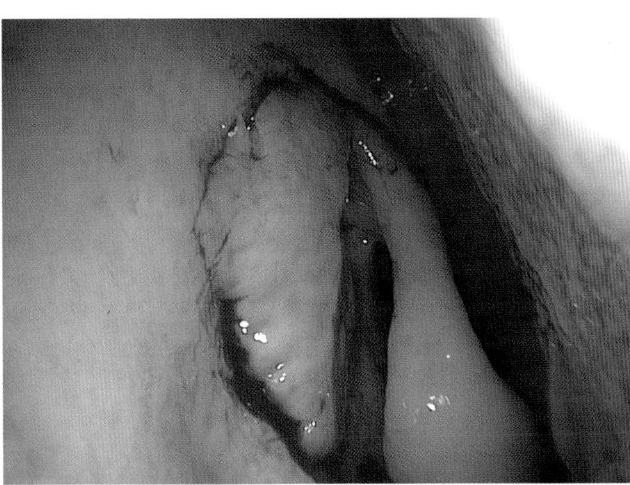

Figure 82-18 Nasal mucosal incision.

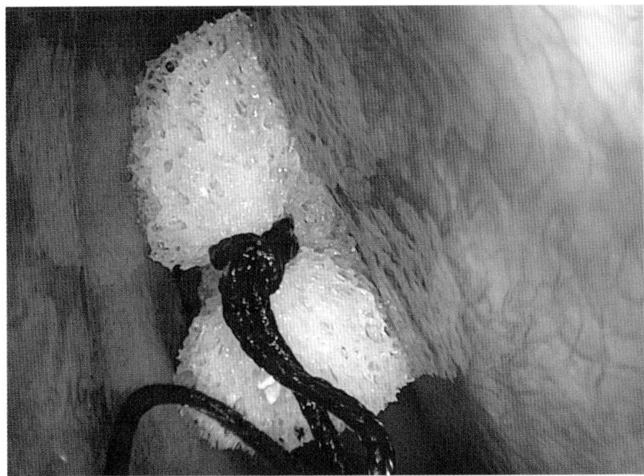

Figure 82-19 Adrenaline patty to vasoconstrict and absorb small amount of blood.

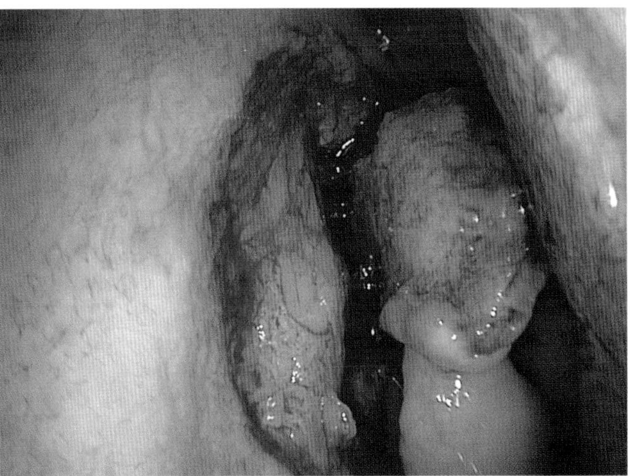

Figure 82-20 Nasal mucosal flap reflected over middle turbinate to protect turbinate.

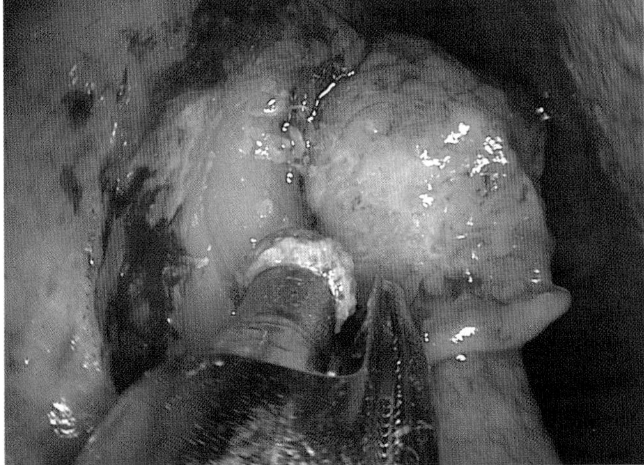

Figure 82-21 Diamond bur to remove thick maxilla bone.

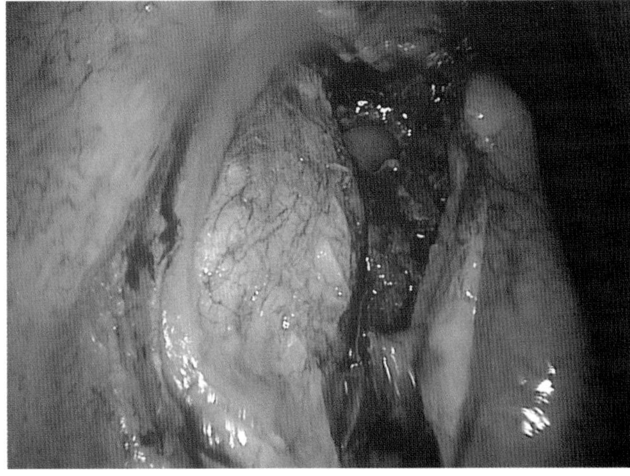

Figure 82-22 Maxillary ostium. The lacrimal sac of outer mucosal surface is seen. The sac is inflated with HPMC and fluorescein.

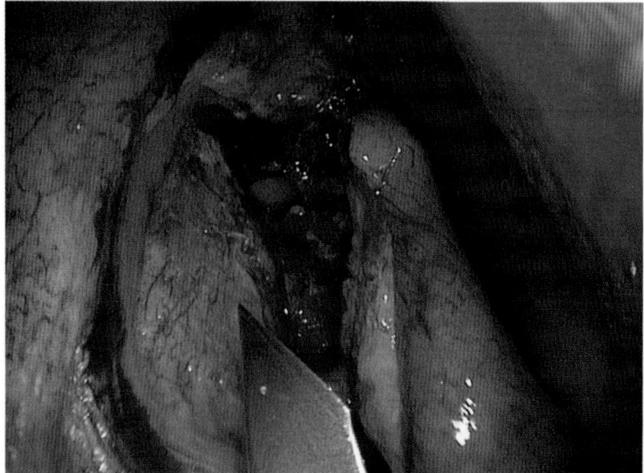

**Figure 82-23** Keratome poised to open sac vertically.

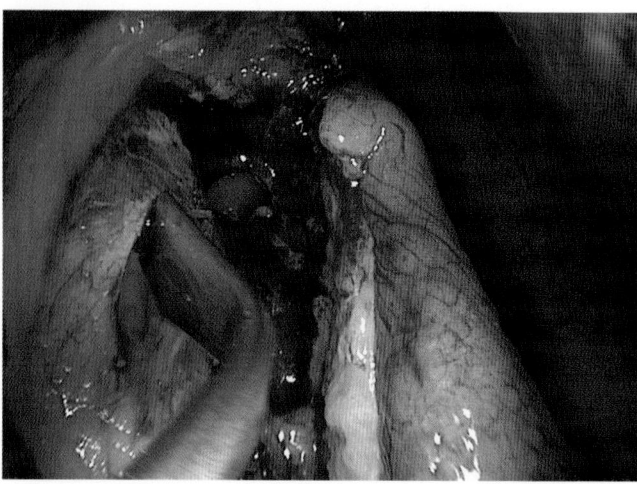

**Figure 82-24** Keratome partially opened sac and lumen with fluorescein visible.

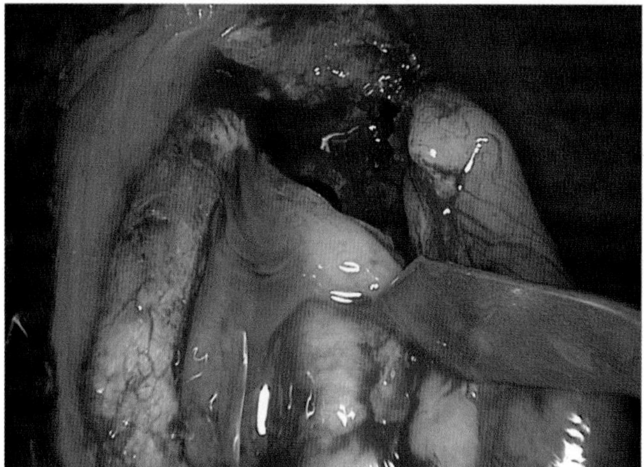

**Figure 82-25** Keratome reflecting lacrimal sac mucosal flap toward the nasal mucosal flap that has been trimmed to fit and give mucosa-to-mucosa apposition without sutures.

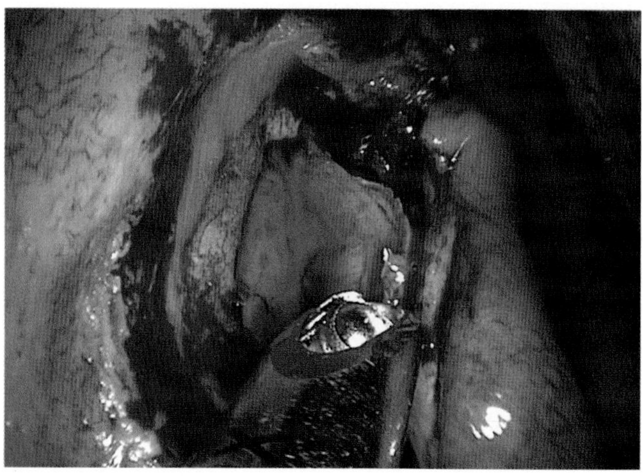

**Figure 82-26** Microdebrider oscillating blade to delicately trim tiny amounts of mucosa and improve edges smoothness and fit.

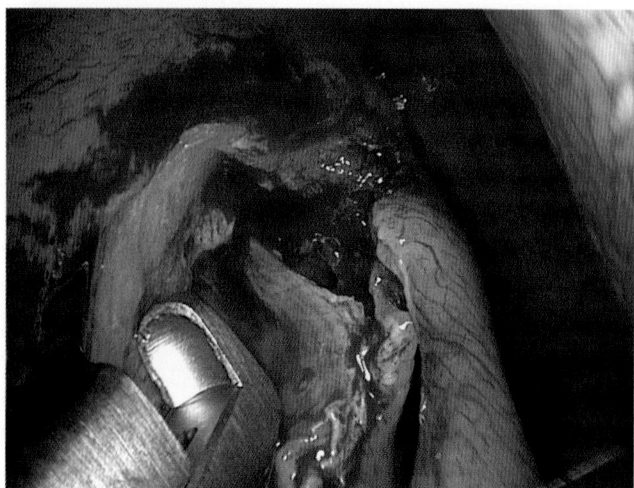

**Figure 82-27** Kerrison rongeurs to remove maxilla bone anterior.

Approximate the mucosal flaps and pass silicone O´Donoghue tubes and knot these. Before cutting the tubes, place a half-sized Nasopore absorbable dressing in the ostium. This serves to tamponade the ostium open and also reduces postoperative bleeding. The tubes are then trimmed to fit snuggly inside the nose (Fig. 82-28).

## ADJUNCTIVE PROCEDURES

Anterior partial turbinectomy if there is marked paradoxical curvature, anterior displaced or marked concha bullosa of the middle turbinate, or partial anterior ethmoidectomy if there is a large agger nasi air cell, both of which can be done during the EE-DCR surgery. Septoplasty may be sometimes required either prior to or at the same time as EE-DCR.

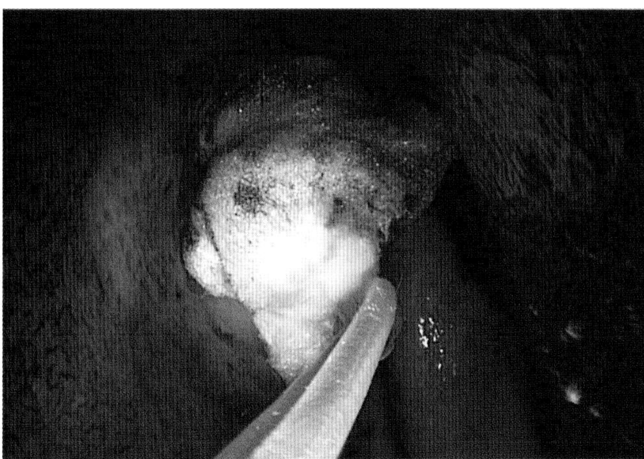

**Figure 82-28** Nasopore packing in ostium, wrapped around O´Donoghue silicone tubing emerging from common canaliculus.

## CONTROVERSIES

### Silicone Bicanalicular Intubation

Tubes are commonly used and are left in for between 4 and 6 weeks. They do keep the common canalicular opening open but can predispose to periosteal granuloma where they rub on the ostium edge with each blink if left in too long. It is a good prognostic sign if the tubes are seen to be moving with each blink.

### Mitomycin C

Topical periostium applied mitomycin C can influence healing and hence scarring and may have a role in more difficult cases with a strong tendency to scar, e.g. in Afro-Caribbean and trauma. However, the peer-reviewed literature is undecided.

### Mechanical Instrumentation

Mechanical instrumentation means power tools inside the nose and these do get high enough and through the thickest part of the maxillary bone; however, they are expensive and the patient has to be under general anesthetic because of the irrigation used to wash and cool the tissue and aspiration required. Kerrison rongeurs of different sizes and angles can achieve almost the same exposure as powered tools, but can sometimes fail to open the upper part of the lacrimal sac where the maxillary bone is thickest.

### Cost

Powered tools are more expensive than simple bone rongeurs. Overall endonasal DCR is more expensive to do than external DCR.

### General Anesthesia

This has been mentioned above in relation to endonasal DCR.

### Postoperative Care

Commitment by the surgeon and patient is essential:

- NeilMed nasal douche twice daily 6 weeks, Flixanase nasal spray twice daily, g chloramphenicol qds.
- No vigorous nose blowing for 5 days. No swimming for 2 weeks.
- See at 1 week and aspirate the remaining Nasopore dressing, any crusts, and clots out. Irrigate.
- See at 3 weeks and repeat nasal endoscopy and decide when will be ready for removal of tubes.
- Removal of tubes around 5 weeks.

### Complications

- Bleeding
- Surgical emphysema if breach the lamina cribosa and they blow nose
- Watering while Nasopore pack in situ
- Granuloma
- Scarring.

## SURGICAL OUTCOMES

Surgical success depends on a large ostium and tidy surgery without undue postoperative inflammation. The main cause of failure is granuloma and scar tissue. Surgical success is measured by subjective improvement and objective patent syringing and a positive functional endoscopic dye test. Success range is from 84% to 96%. Outcomes of EE-DCR and external DCR are now very similar. Most studies have not shown significant improvement in surgical outcome with antimetabolites. Patient satisfaction is high, equal with that of external approach DCR.

## REDO-DCR

Good results are achieved with endoscopic DCR to redo of both primary failed external and endoscopic DCR. Some have preparation for Jones tubes if there is a long slit canaliculus, functional failure (lid pump), and marked canalicular obstruction.

## PEARLS AND PITFALLS

- *Pearls*: Big opening, no small fragments of bone or mucosa. Low threshold to do combined external and endonasal endoscopic DCR.
- *Pitfalls*: Damaging nasal mucosa by frequent instrumentation entry especially to septum and causing synechiae. Operating within a nose that is too narrow.

## SUGGESTED READING

1. Ben Simon GJ, Joseph J, Lee S, et al. External vs Endoscopic DCR for acquired nasolacrimal duct obstruction in a tertiary referral centre. Ophthalmology. 2005;112:1463-8.
2. Hii BW, McNab AA, Friebel JD. A comparison of external and endonasal DCR in regard to patient satisfaction. Orbit. 2012; 31:67-76.
3. Hull S, Lalchan SA, Olver JM. Success rates in powered endonasal revision surgery for failed dacryocystorhinostomy in a tertiary referral center. Ophthal Plast Reconstr Surg. 2013;29: 267-71.
4. Jutley G, Karim R, Joharatnam N, et al. Patient satisfaction following endoscopic endonasal dacryocystorhinostomy: a quality of life study. Eye (Lond). 2013;27:1084-9.
5. Karim R, Ghabrial R, Lynch T, et al. A comparison of external and endoscopic endonasal dacryocystorhinostomy for acquired nasolacrimal duct obstruction. Clin Ophthalmol. 2011;5:979-89.
6. Leong SC, Macewen CJ, White PS. A systematic review of outcomes after dacryocystorhinostomy in adults. Am J Rhinol Allergy. 2010;24:81-90.
7. Minasian M, Olver J. The value of nasal endoscopy after dacryocystorhinostomy Orbit. 1999;18(3):167-76.
8. Moore WM, Bentley CR, Olver JM. Functional and anatomical results after two types of endoscopic endonasal dacryocystorhinostomy Ophthalmology. 2002;109:1575-82.
9. Olver JM. The success rates for endonasal dacryocystorhinostomy Br J Ophthalmol. 2003;87:1431.
10. Zaidi FH, Symanski S, Olver JM. A clinical trial of endoscopic vs external dacryocystorhinostomy for partial nasolacrimal duct obstruction. Eye (Lond). 2011;25:1219-24.

CHAPTER 83

# Punctal and Canalicular Surgery

David H Verity, Geoffrey E Rose

## INTRODUCTION

Punctal and canalicular occlusion has diverse etiologies (Tables 83-1 to 83-3), and surgery for canalicular block carries a guarded prognosis even in the most experienced hands. Lacrimal pump function, being dynamic, depends both on anatomical patency and normal lacrimal pump physiology; thus, restoration of anatomical conductance is not always followed by improved lacrimal outflow. The prime example is noted in patients who appear to have recovered fully after idiopathic facial nerve palsy: despite normal canalicular structure, incomplete stimulation of the orbicularis fibers surrounding the canaliculus and lacrimal sac can still cause troublesome lacrimal flow symptoms, this in the absence of lid atony or corneal exposure. The purpose of this chapter is to outline the surgical approaches to managing punctal and canalicular occlusion, with the caveat that surgery is not predictably followed by symptomatic relief—this being due to the prerequisite for both structural and physiological integrity of the lacrimal outflow apparatus. Although the management of canalicular injury is comprehensively reviewed elsewhere, the principles that underscore canalicular surgery following a primary repair are similar, irrespective of the original cause for the occlusion.

**TABLE 83-1** Causes of punctal obstruction.

| |
|---|
| Congenital punctal atresia |
| Iatrogenic causes (see causes for canalicular obstruction) |
| Inflammatory causes: |
| • Stagnant tear lake with distal lacrimal outflow obstruction |
| ▪ Ocular surface inflammatory disorders |
| ◦ Drug eruptions (such as Stevens–Johnson syndrome) |
| ◦ Ocular mucus membrane pemphigoid |

**TABLE 83-2** Causes of canalicular obstruction

| |
|---|
| Congenital canalicular atresia |
| Infection |
| • Chronic staphylococcal lid disease |
| • Periocular herpes simplex infection |
| • Microbial canaliculitis |
| Systemic inflammatory diseases |
| • Ocular mucus membrane pemphigoid[a] |
| • Drug eruptions (Stevens–Johnson syndrome) |
| • Lichen planus |
| Iatrogenic causes |
| • Topical treatment |
| ◦ Drop preservatives |
| ◦ Mitomycin C[b] |
| • Lacrimal stents and plugs (in particular intracanalicular plugs) |
| • Probing in children with injury to the posterior wall of the common canaliculus |
| • Chemotherapeutic agents |
| ◦ 5-fluorouracil (including S1 chemotherapy)[c] |
| ◦ Taxanes: Docetaxel (Taxotere) and paclitaxel |
| • Local radiotherapy[d] |

[a]Canalicular occlusion in mucus membrane pemphigoid results from distal spill-over of conjunctival inflammation and causes proximal canalicular obstruction. However, in these patients (and those with SJS) primary tearing is uncommon due to the effect of conjunctival fibrosis on goblet cell function and aqueous tear delivery via the lacrimal ductules.

[b]Some authors advocate temporary punctal occlusion to reduce canalicular toxicity whilst using MMC drops. This carries the additional advantage of increasing bioavailability of the drug to the ocular surface.

[c]5 FU is a potent inhibitor of DNA synthesis. S-1 is an oral fluoropyrimidine agent consisting of 5-fluorouracil and two modulators of 5-FU metabolism. Canalicular epithelial complications occur in about 6% of patients, and include punctal narrowing and focal or diffuse canalicular stenosis. A quarter of such patients will require DCR with placement of a bypass tube.

[d]Radiotherapy to the medial canthal region for tumour control is nearly always complicated by canalicular occlusion.

**TABLE 83-3** Noncanalicular obstruction: causes and approximate incidence

| Cause | Annual incidence (%)* |
|---|---|
| Herpes simplex infection | 8/23 (35%) |
| Iatrogenic causes (e.g. syringing) | 6/23 (26%) |
| Cicatricial conjunctival disease† | 6/23 (26%) |
| Chemotherapy: 5-fluorouracil | 2/23 (9 %) |
| Lichen planus | 1/23 (5%) |

*Authors' experience of caseload at Moorfields Eye Hospital over an 8-year period.

†Including risk factors for conjunctival fibrosis (for example, topical glaucoma therapy or severe chronic blepharitis).

## PUNCTAL SURGERY

The contribution of apparent punctal stenosis (Fig. 83-1) to lacrimal symptoms can be difficult to determine, and is probably overestimated given the guarded prognosis following punctoplasty in the absence of other coexistent causes for lacrimation. In these authors' opinion, punctal enlargement is only considered once other treatable causes for lacrimation are addressed, including causes of evaporative dry eye and lid malposition. Furthermore, since punctal stenosis often occurs in the presence of nasolacrimal duct stenosis or occlusion, lacrimal syringing should be performed after punctal dilation and before considering formal punctoplasty. This, and the observation that punctal stenosis occurs only rarely after dacryocystorhinostomy (DCR), suggests that a stagnant and toxic tear lake (due to distal outflow impedance) contributes to fibrous contracture of the punctal annulus and, in such cases, distal outflow obstruction should logically be the first addressed.

### Punctal Enlargement

Where it is desirable to enlarge the punctum, this can be achieved by performing a "three snip" excision of the posterior wall of the ampulla, being as vertical as it is longitudinal and so avoiding an unnecessarily long—or slit-like—punctal and canalicular enlargement. Where there is a closed punctum with an overlying conjunctival membrane, the aperture can often be retrieved with an incision using the oblique edge a 19G needle over the punctal 'hill.' Note, however, that a flat lid contour overlying the anticipated position of the punctum suggests congenital atresia and, in such rare cases, punctal retrieval is unlikely to be successful. In all cases, failure to identify the mucosal-lined lumen indicates a more extensive canalicular block, and the patient should be offered open lacrimal drainage surgery with retrograde intubation (v.i.).

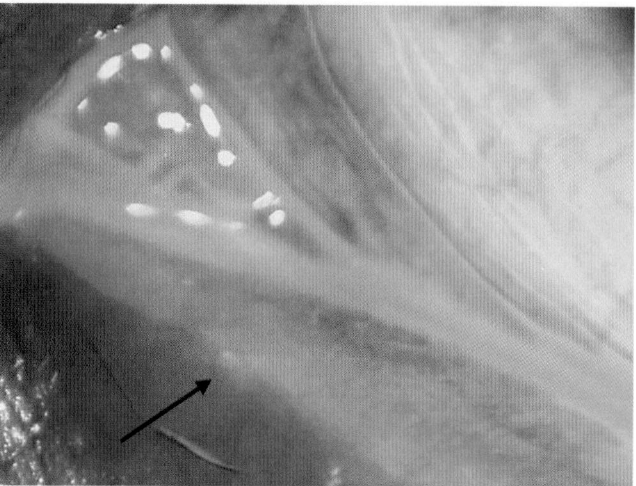

**Figure 83-1** Punctal stenosis (arrow) with fluorescein dye retention.

### Punctal Closure

For true ocular sicca syndromes (for example, with Sjögren's syndrome, or after high-dose radiotherapy for lacrimal gland malignancies), permanent canalicular closure should be considered; where complete tear deficiency is certain—as in the latter example—closure can be performed at the time of orbital surgery. In other cases, and where there is no evidence for pre-existing canalicular obstruction, a trial with a retrievable silicone punctal plug should be performed prior to considering permanent closure. Note that permanent intracanalicularplugs should never be used, as these can lead both to canalicular inflammations and injury to the common canaliculus (Figs. 83-2A and B). Maximal topical therapy should always precede surgical closure, both because of the irreversible nature of surgery and the unpredictable effect of occlusion. Where permanent closure is indicated, the inferior punctum is usually occluded first. This can be achieved either by thermal cautery inside the horizontal portion of the canaliculus or by selective excision of the membranous wall of the ampulla with a tissue punch or feather blade. With the latter technique, a 7/0 absorbable mattress suture is passed through the peripunctal tissues and tied over the skin to reduce the risk of spontaneous recanalization. Whichever approach is favored, the patient should be warned of the risk of subsequent lacrimal flow symptoms and, conversely, that of possible reopening of the canaliculus: the less destructive the method of closure, the greater the risk of spontaneous reopening.

A further, reversible approach (termed the "punctal patch" procedure) has been advocated, with better long-term closure rates claimed than some traditional techniques. This procedure involves excision of a 2 mm by 2 mm superficial block

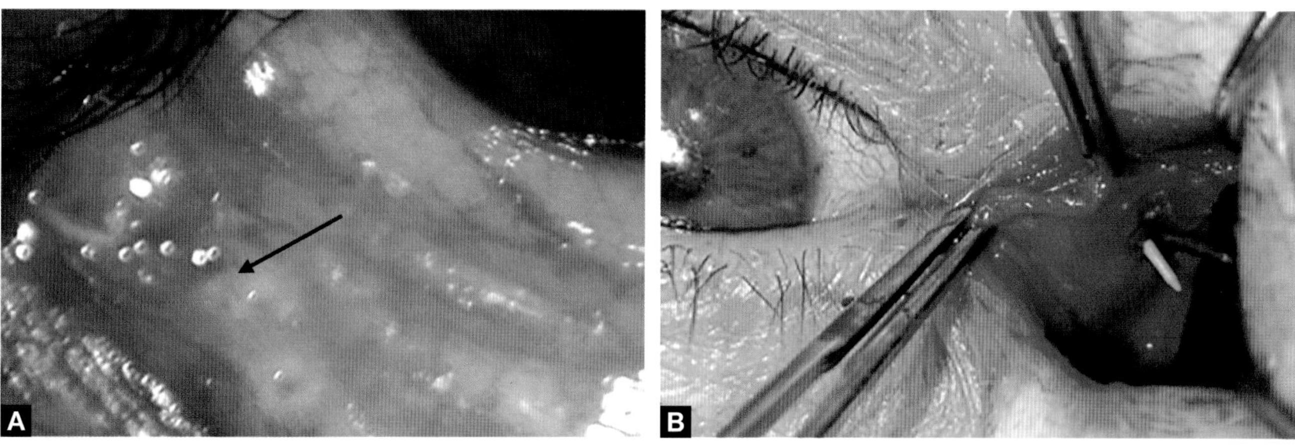

**Figures 83-2A and B** Intracanalicular plugs: Part (A) shows plug lodged in the midcanaliculus and part (B) shows a different plug that has eroded through the back of the common canaliculus into the sac posterior to the common canalicular opening.

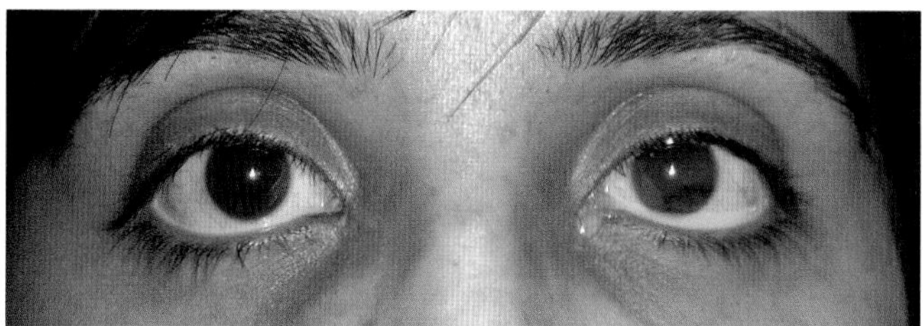

**Figure 83-3** Left fluorescein dye retention and lacrimal "flow" symptoms due to canalicular stenosis.

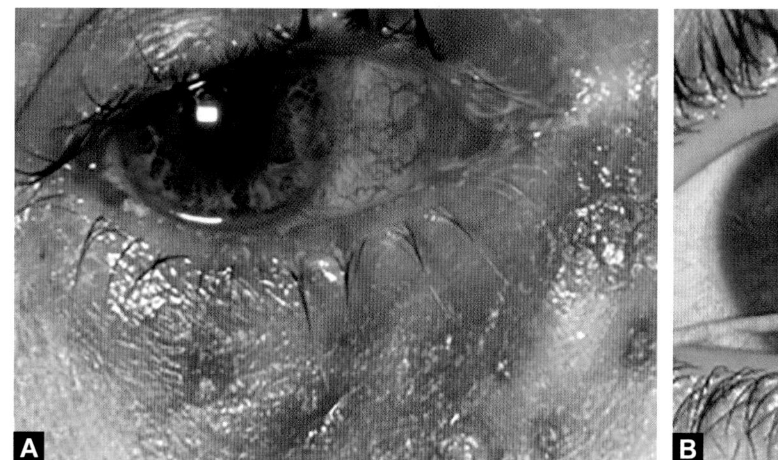

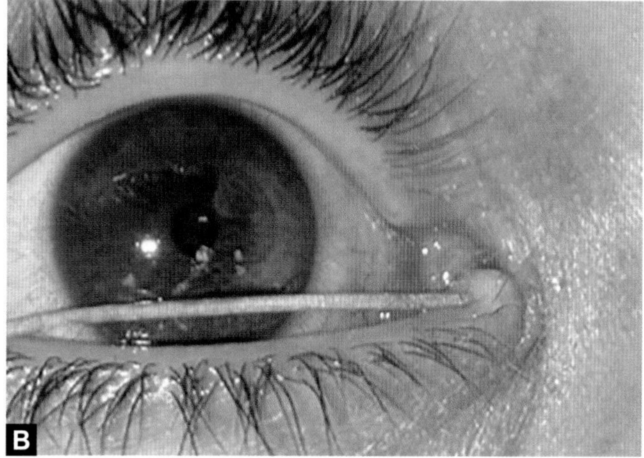

**Figures 83-4A and B** Herpes simplex: Part (A) shows primary herpetic infection of the eyelids and part (B) shows inferior canalicular occlusion at 2 mm (different case).

of the membranous surface overlying the punctum (and including the superficial part of the annulus) and placing a bulbar conjunctival patch graft over the defect. Other authors, citing both the risk of graft necrosis and the loss of even the smallest amount of bulbar conjunctiva in severe sicca syndromes, have proposed a 180° rotational graft of a block of marginal tissue containing the punctum (termed the "punctum switch graft")—although the results of larger studies to determine its long-term efficacy are awaited.

## CANALICULAR SURGERY

All chronic canaliculitis will lead to secondary fibrosis, reduced canalicular conductance, and increased risk of lacrimal flow symptoms (Fig. 83-3), although the degree of functional loss depends on the cause, with mild epithelial inflammation (as seen with Herpes Simplex, Figs. 83-4A and B) causing less severe and widespread contracture than deeper, subepithelial inflammation (as seen with canalicular involvement in lichen

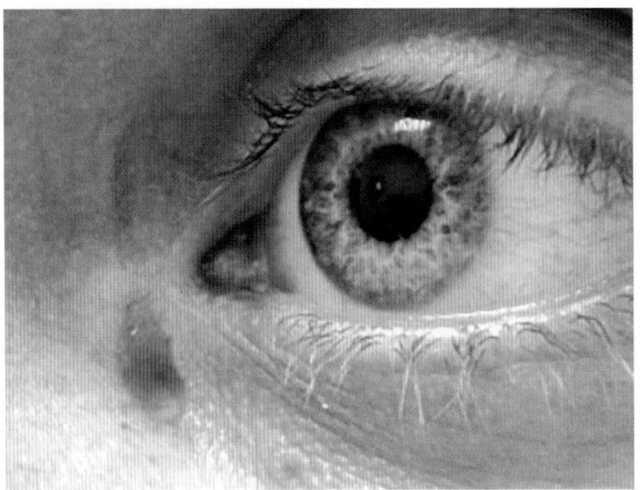

Figure 83-5 Congenital lacrimal fistula.

planus). Paradoxically, although microbial canaliculitis often presents with many months of chronic inflammation, such patients are rarely troubled by symptoms after treatment—this probably being due to expansion of the canalicular lumen by stones and debris, with no significant reduction in canalicular cross-sectional area after resolution of the condition.

## Surgery for Congenital Accessory Canaliculi (Congenital Fistulae)

The congenital lacrimal fistula is rare and often missed, with failure to recognize that tear spillage is from the ostium below the medial canthal tendon, rather than over the medial end of the eyelid *per se* (Fig. 83-5). Although some advocate fistulectomy alone, backwash of tears from an accessory canaliculus is indicative of distal outflow impedance. For this reason, fistulae are best dealt with by performing a standard DCR and excising the fistula intact as far as its communication with the common canaliculus is concerned. Excision of the fistula (as a "sock" of tissue) is performed with a feather blade either directly or by approaching it perpendicularly from a DCR skin incision (Figs. 83-6A to C). The tissues overlying the excised fistula (orbicularis and skin) are closed in layers to prevent its reopening, although this should not occur when satisfactory DCR is also performed.

## Canaliculotomy for Infective Canaliculitis

Swelling over the affected canaliculus with a chronic, creamy and mucoid discharge are the hallmarks of microbial canaliculitis (Figs. 83-7 and 83-8), but unfortunately such symptoms are often missed for very long periods, being misdiagnosed as chronic conjunctivitis, chalazion, or nasolacrimal duct obstruction, with consequent inappropriate and ineffective treatment. Microbial canaliculitis is effectively cured by performing a 5–6 mm canaliculotomy with fine scissors, and the intracanalicular debris massaged out of the lumen—passing from medially to laterally—using two cotton buds placed either side of the eyelid (Fig. 83-9). Some authors advocate midcanalicular canaliculostomy, to preserve the punctal annulus, and others have suggested expression of debris on the slit lamp microscope without opening the canaliculus; the latter technique is likely to fail in all but the mildest of cases, due to sequestration of large "stones" in the expanded canaliculus, or anterograde displacement of debris into the lacrimal sac.

It is essential that all debris is removed at surgery, and that material is not washed distally by inappropriate syringing or probing, as this carries a risk of anterograde dissemination of infection. A short course of postoperative topical chloramphenicol suffices, as the majority of organisms are sensitive to this antibiotic; topical pre- or post-operative penicillin treatment is not required. The longitudinal incision usually heals without significant defect and—with the rare exception of primary lacrimal sac infection—recurrent symptoms generally indicate the inadequate evacuation of canalicular debris at primary surgery. One caveat exists however: the clinician should check for a history of placement of canalicular plugs or stents; these carry a worse prognosis and should, if possible, be retrieved at surgery.

## The Injured Canaliculus

Surgery for canalicular injury is covered in depth elsewhere, but the key principles of repair are summarized as follows. First, canalicular injuries should not be considered in isolation, and injury to other local structures should also be suspected. Knowledge of the mechanism of injury—if available—will alert the clinician to the presence of retained foreign bodies or to collateral damage to the medial canthus, the paranasal sinuses, or the cranial cavity. Where there is doubt, imaging should be obtained: careful inspection of the soft tissue windows on CT will often reveal retained organic material, these usually having subtle enhancement at the edge of the foreign body. In the absence of more serious injuries (for example, globe or intracranial trauma), a patient with a canalicular laceration—whether inferior, superior, or both—can be safely repaired on the next available routine operating list, although preferably within 48 hours. Examination under general anesthesia tends to be easier and allows assessment of the medial canthal tendon (MCT), and the extent of

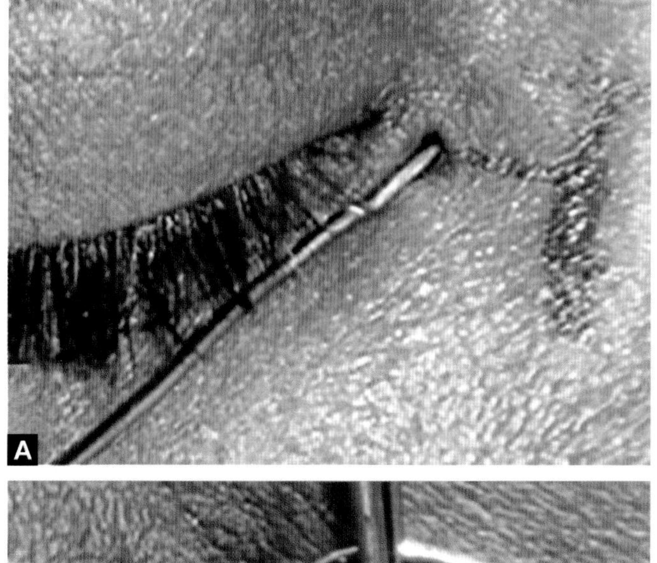


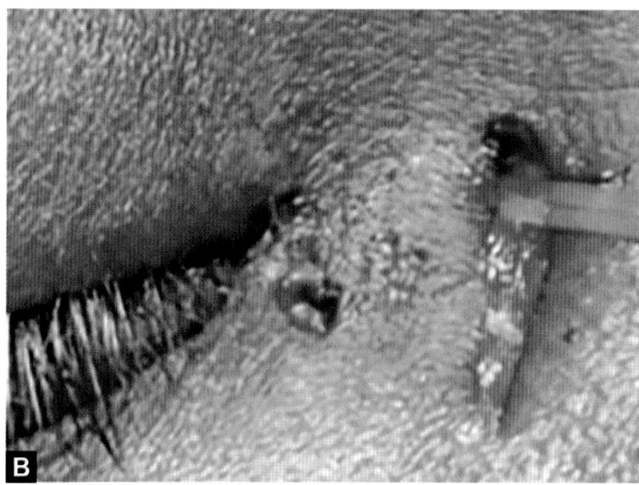


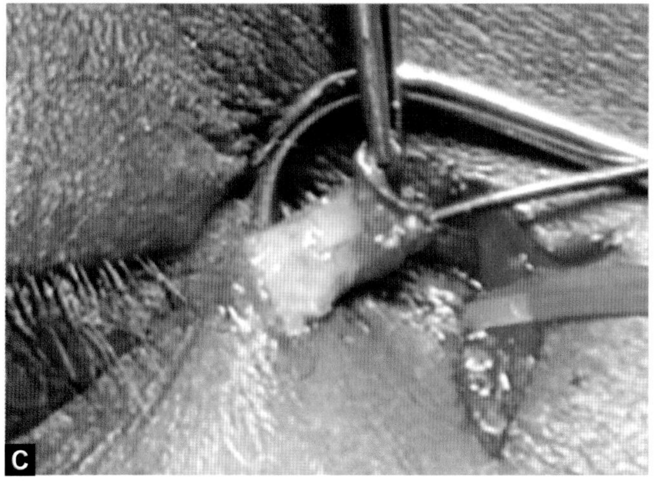


**Figures 83-6A to C** Surgery for symptomatic congenital lacrimal fistula: Part (A) showing marking for dacryocystorhinostomy (DCR) and right-angle incision to fistula; (B and C) different case showing DCR (completed) and separate intact excision of the accessory canaliculus.

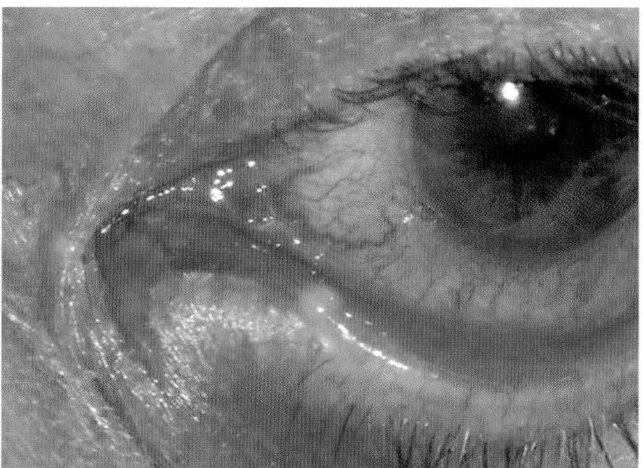

**Figure 83-7** Chronic canaliculitis with typical creamy white discharge.

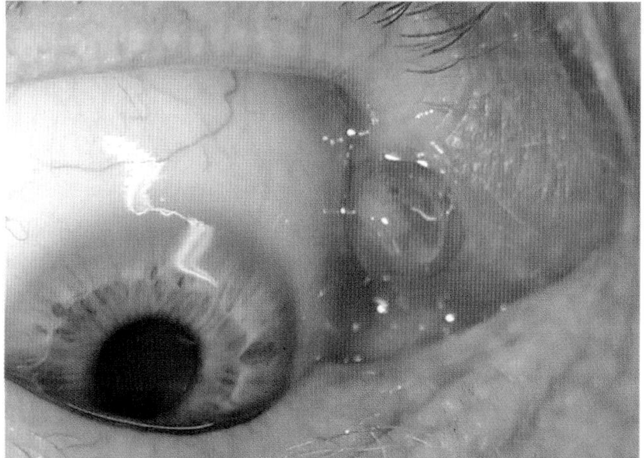

**Figure 83-8** Granuloma associated with chronic canaliculitis of the upper eyelid.

canalicular injury, although early closure of soft tissue lacerations by fibrinous exudate can mask quite extensive injuries. Where dehiscence of the posterior limb of the MCT has occurred, repair is indicated to minimize subsequent anterior displacement of the medial canthus (a secondary "Centurion syndrome"), as this tends to cause residual

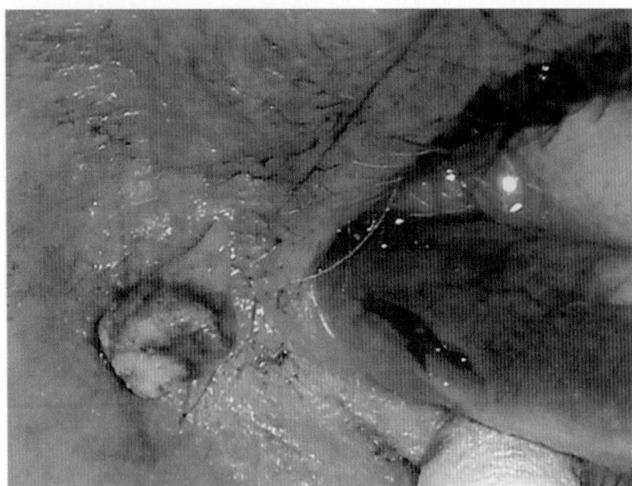

**Figure 83-9** Canaliculotomy with expression of debris and associated "stone".

lacrimal symptoms, even with canalicular patency. Using a transconjunctival retrocaruncular approach, a 5/0 absorbable or 4/0 polypropylene suture is placed through the periosteum overlying the posterior lacrimal crest and the corresponding medial aspect of the eyelid tarsus or residual tendinous tissue; such sutures should be placed before repair of any canalicular laceration.

The best technique for identifying the distal cut end of a canaliculus remains controversial, and techniques include the use of an eyed pigtail probe, canalicular syringing with a viscoelastic material, fluorescein or air through an uninjured fellow canaliculus, and constriction of the adjacent vascularized tissue by local application of phenylephrine or epinephrine—this latter method revealing the distal canaliculus as a pale "ring" (Figs. 83-10A to D). In practice, the latter maneuver is the most useful, although the pigtail probe has recently attracted renewed interest. In the authors' experience, timely surgery using the operating microscope, hemostasis and careful observation of the deep medial canthal region, together with local vasoconstriction, are generally sufficient to reveal the distal surface of the canaliculus in the vast majority of cases. A silicone stent—be it a shortened monocanalicular or a self-retaining bicanalicular variant—is inserted before the tissues are closed. Deep 5/0 absorbable sutures are placed to repair the posterior limb of the MCT, and a 7/0 absorbable suture is used for the pericanalicular tissues. The distal end of the stent is first advanced into the cut end of the distal canaliculus before these sutures are drawn tight and tied, thereby both reuniting the cut ends of the canalicular surfaces over the silicone stent (which acts as a guide), and restoring the posterior vector of the medial eyelid(s). The stent(s) are left in position for 3–6 weeks when they are readily removed, with the long-term outlook reflecting the severity of the original injury.

## Proximal and Midcanalicular Occlusion

The prognosis for lacrimal surgery depends on the location and extent of the canalicular block, with extensive or distal canalicular occlusion carrying the worst prognosis—as, for example, with the long and severe occlusions of lichen planus. The success of primary lacrimal intervention is related to the distal length of residual healthy canaliculus: with a lengthy proximal and midcanalicular occlusion, retrograde canaliculostomy of the very limited residual distal canaliculus (if present at all) results in a medially placed and static inner canthal pseudopunctum that is likely to be nonfunctional, even if anatomically patent. Where there is only a short proximal block, the residual healthy canaliculus remains an active part of the lacrimal pump mechanism and symptomatic control tends to be better.

Although clinical examination identifies complete proximal or midcanalicular obstruction, the treatment of choice is external DCR with retrograde canaliculostomy: primary placement of a canalicular bypass tube should be avoided for three reasons. First, the extent of occlusion cannot be determined before surgery, and may be limited to a short proximal length with significant residual healthy canaliculus. Second, DCR bypasses the normal physiological resistance within the nasolacrimal duct, thereby reducing the overall outflow impedance —irrespective of the state of the residual canalicular system. Third, even when a patient is likely to require a secondary bypass tube, the optimum stability of the tube is achieved after prior open DCR once the primary carunculectomy site and medial canthal tissues have healed.

# SURGICAL TECHNIQUE

## Dacryocystorhinostomy with Retrograde Canaliculostomy

Obstruction sited in the first 7 mm of a canaliculus should be treated by DCR with retrograde canaliculostomy. The extent of the block is determined by retrograde probing of the canaliculus through the open sac, and the patient should therefore be warned of the possible need for primary placement of a glass canalicular bypass tube in the event that no common canaliculus is found.

Surgery entails creating a large osteotomy, this aiding formation of the largest possible soft tissue window (with minimal impedance to tear flow) and unobstructed

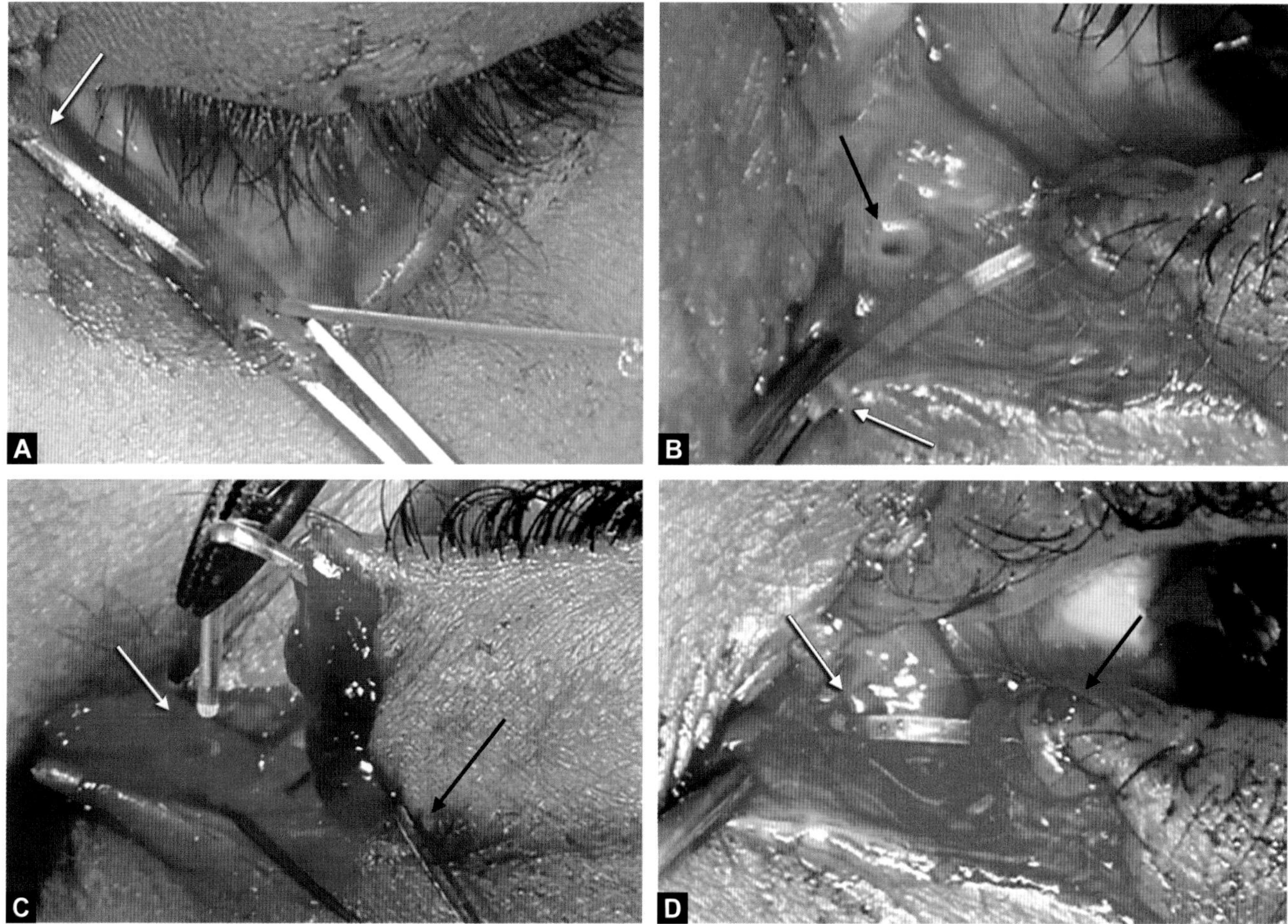


**Figures 83-10A to D** Canalicular repair: (A) Placement of the monocanalicular silicone stent (arrow showing uncut end), (B) identification of the distal canaliculus (closed arrow) and shortened silicone stent, (open arrow), (C) insertion of the stent into the distal canaliculus (open arrow, with closed arrow showing pre-placed sutures), and (D) silicone stent maintained in collagen annulus by the stnet "heel" (closed arrow) with distal stent in the distal canaliculus (open arrow).

movement for a canalicular bypass tube, should one become necessary. Likewise, primary carunculectomy should be performed in all such cases, as later placement of a bypass tube is more successful where the carunculectomy bed has healed.

Once the posterior mucosal flaps have been sutured, the internal common canalicular opening is probed in a retrograde fashion using a '1' gauge Bowman probe with an 80° bend at about 8 mm from its end. The end of this angulated probe is directed gently into the common opening, maintaining minimal traction on the anterior sac flap to avoid unnecessary tissue distortion. Passing the probe as far laterally as possible along each canaliculus in turn, a 1–2 mm square fenestration (or "pseudopunctum") is created in the canalicular wall overlying the tip of the probe (Figs. 83-11A and B). The bodkin on a silicone stent is similarly bent to allow retrograde intubation of the most accessible canaliculus, passing from the internal opening towards the new "pseudopunctum", and the bodkin retrieved and straightened. The fellow canaliculus is then intubated in an anterograde fashion through its corresponding real punctum or "pseudopunctum", and the tubes tied in the nose.

In severe obstructions where only the common canaliculus is present, its lateral end is opened into the carunculectomy bed and—as in cases where only a single canaliculus is retrievable—the returning end is passed through the fibrous annulus of the fellow punctum and into the nasal space; this "blind" return to the nasal space is facilitated by passing a 19-gauge needle through the tissue first, thereby creating a track which enters the opened sac away from the common canalicular opening. Note that monocanalicular stent(s) cannot be used in this scenario because the new "pseudopunctum" has no retaining annulus.

The skin sutures are removed 7–10 days after surgery and the silicone stent 3–4 weeks later. Although a "blind return"

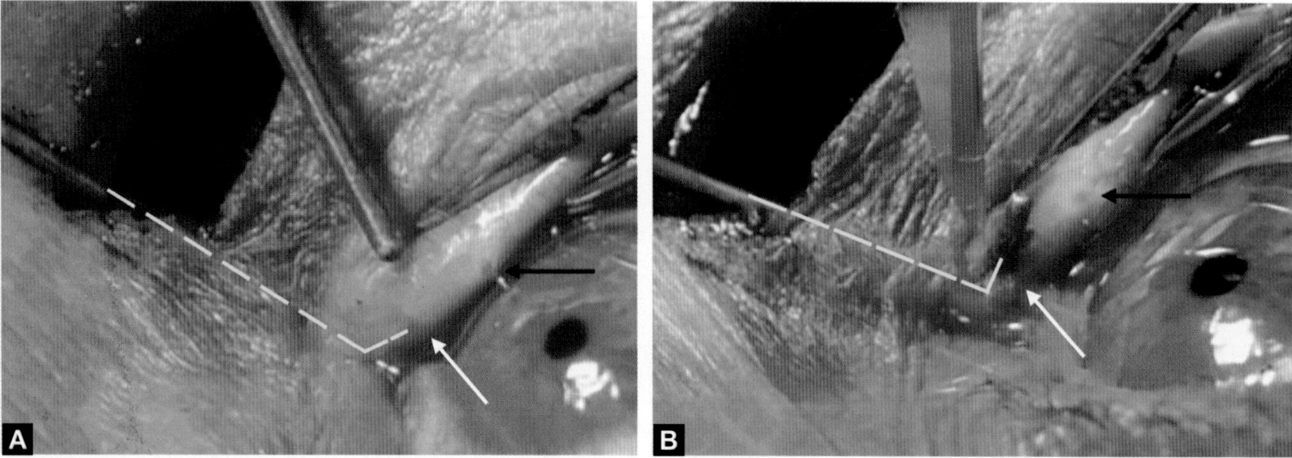


**Figures 83-11A and B** Retrocanaliculostomy for midcanalicular obstruction: Part (A) shows the '1' Bowman probe being placed ab interno into the proximal upper canaliculus (dotted line showing path of the probe, with open arrow and second probe identifying the probe tip in the canaliculus, and the closed arrow identifying the natural punctum). Creation of the pseudopunctum is shown in part (B), in which an E11 blade is used to create a fenestration over the probe end (open arrow).

has been performed in the absence of a healthy punctal annulus, the stent should be removed early to avoid pressure erosion through the canaliculi (so-called "cheesewiring").

## Surgical Technique: Placement of a Canalicular Bypass Tube

Also referred to as conjunctivodacryocystorhinostomy, placement of a Jones' canalicular bypass tube is required in the absence of any functional canaliculus. Whilst some surgeons favor primary placement of bypass tubes, and some advocating placement without prior DCR (the tube being passed directly into the nasal space through the anterior ethmoid sinuses), the current authors only very rarely perform primary placement of such tubes and never without prior DCR. Although primary placement is occasionally indicated, secondary placement is generally preferable due to improved tube positioning and stability in a medial canthal bed that has healed after prior DCR and carunculectomy.

A lacrimal bypass tube acts as an aqueduct, or lacrimal "bridge", between the medial canthal tear lake and the nasal space and it replaces one dynamic component of the lacrimal pump—the canaliculus—with an alternative, albeit truncated, dynamic system.[e] For this reason, placement of a bypass tube without prior DCR (resulting in a rigid immobile conduit) should be avoided.

In primary Jones' tube placement, a large rhinostomy is performed and the posterior mucosal flaps are sutured.[f] After carunculectomy, diathermy is applied to the caruncular bed, and the point of Nettleship dilator or punctal seeker is used to define a track between the medial canthus and the nasal space, the track then being expanded with a double-ended ("bullhorn") dilator (Figs. 83-12A and B); this approach permits precise placement of the canthal and nasal ends of the tube, with greater control than that afforded by sole use of the wider-tipped "bullhorn" dilator.

An appropriate tube is selected, being long enough to lie in the midnasal space but without touching the septum, and is inserted into the track over a '1' Bowman probe. Due to the subtle flange at the nasal end, tube placement requires firm pressure with both thumbnails, with an assistant gently supporting the end of the Bowman probe.[g] For optimum drainage, the tube should enter the medial canthus immediately behind the mucocutaneous junction of lower lid margin, and be orientated 30–40° downward with the far end lying freely within the nasal space in front of the middle turbinate (Fig. 83-13). The ostium should neither lie too deeply—this risking episcleral erosion and inflammation—nor too anteriorly, where it will rest proud of the tear lake. With primary placement of a tube, an encircling 6/0 nylon suture should be placed to keep the ostium out of the healing caruncular bed; such a suture is passed through the medial lower lid,

---

[e] Lid movement, with a sweep of tears medially into the canthal region, corresponding medial canthal mobility, air passage over the tube ostium in the nose (creating a relative vacuum within the tube), and the slight sub-atmospheric nasal pressure occurring during inhalation are all dynamic processes.

[f] Surgery is performed under general anaesthesia; nasal vasoconstriction with local anaesthesia creates an atypically capacious nasal space and can result in misguided nasal positioning of the bypass tube.

[g] Note, use of any other device to exert pressure on the tube end tends to shatter it.

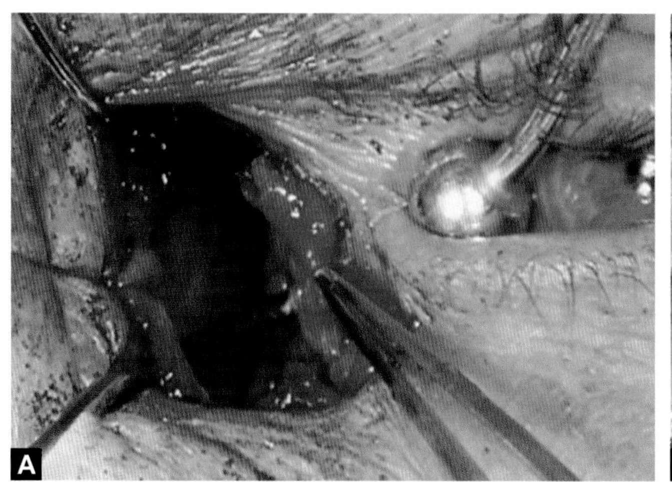


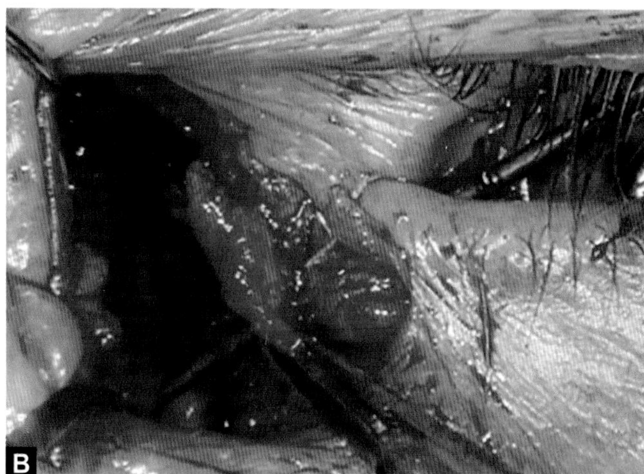


**Figures 83-12A and B** Insertion of a primary Lester Jones lacrimal bypass tube: Part (A) shows the use of the bullhorn dilator to create a track before passing the glass bypass tube over a '1' Bowman probe (B).

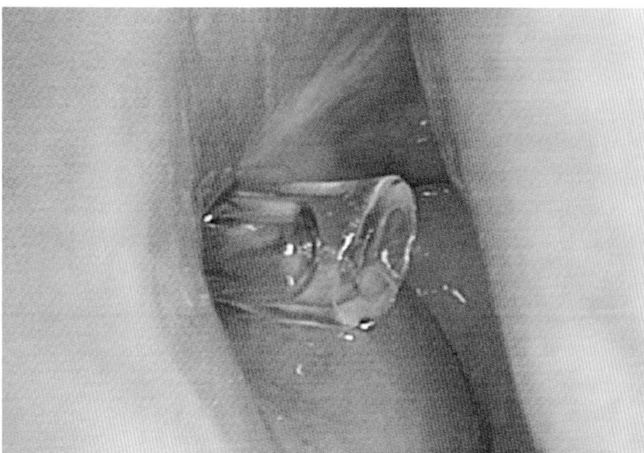

**Figure 83-13** Endoscopic view of the lacrimal bypass tube, with the distal end being in the mid-nasal space.

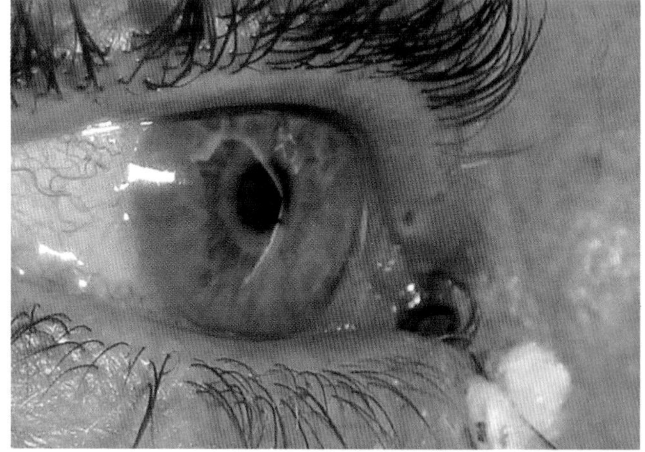

**Figure 83-14** First placement of bypass tube showing encirclement suture tied over a cotton wool bolster.

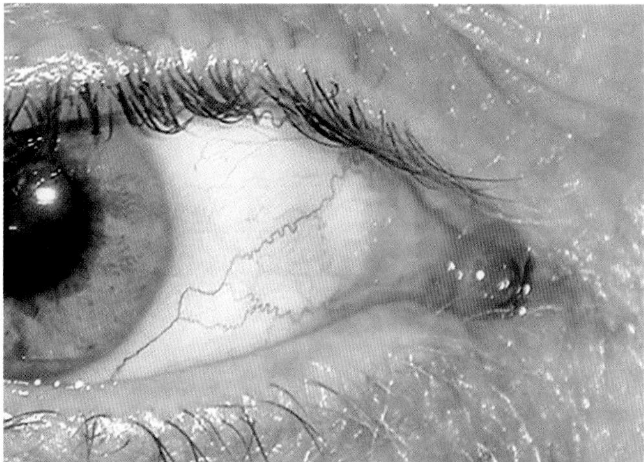

**Figure 83-15** Optimal bypass tube placement, being partly below the lower lid margin with the tube opening lying in the lacrimal "sump" created by prior carunculectomy.

three times around the tube neck, and then back out to the surface of the lid—where it is tied over a bolster and removed 7–10 days later (Fig. 83-14). The patient is prescribed a 2-week course of a topical steroid-antibiotic combination, and a nasal decongestant if required. The tube should permit free passage of saline from the conjunctival sac into the nose (Fig. 83-15).

Secondary placement of a Jones' bypass tube (Fig. 83-16) is performed in a similar manner, but an encircling suture is not required unless further caruncular debulking has been performed and a nasal endoscope used to confirm the position of the tube end.

## Surgical Technique: DCR and Annular Encirclement for Lacrimal Agenesis

The extremely rare cases of complete lacrimal agenesis, generally only identified at the time of attempted DCR in a child,

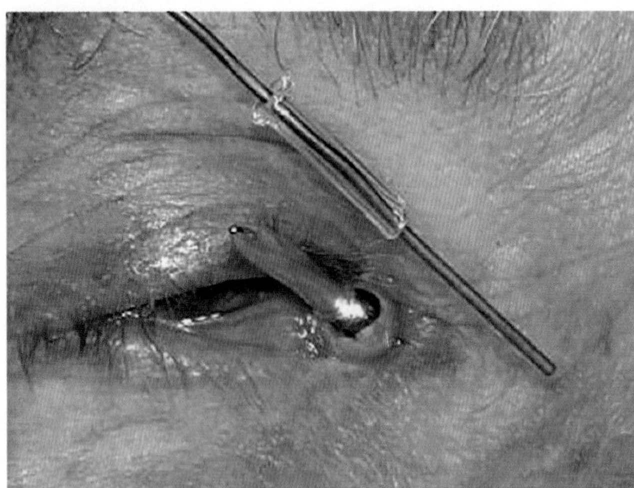

Figure 83-16 Secondary placement of Lester Jones tube, with bullhorn dilator in place and a suitable length tube positioned over a '1' probe for insertion.

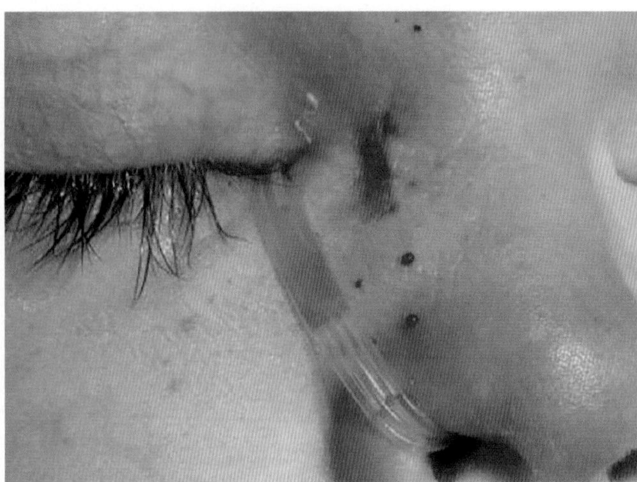

Figure 83-17 Surgery for congenital lacrimal agenesis showing multiple "rings" of silicone intubation.

can be managed by creation of a large fistula between the carunculectomy site and the nasal space. The fistula is maintained by placement of multiple "rings" of silicone intubation (Fig. 83-17), this encircalage being removed at about 4 weeks after surgery; the silicone stenting must not be too tight, so as to avoid pressure ischemia of the nasal rim. The parents should be advised of the likelihood of requiring later placement of a bypass tube if symptoms persist beyond the age of 9 or 10 years.

## KEY POINTS

- All canalicular inflammations lead—to varying degrees—to a reduced canalicular conductance.
- Canalicular patency does not imply normal dynamic function.
- Infective canaliculitis, being frequently misdiagnosed and resulting in chronic discharge at the inner canthus, requires canaliculotomy and evacuation of all infected material and debris.
- Periocular primary herpes simplex infection can cause canalicular and common canalicular epithelial inflammation, with secondary stenosis or occlusion.
- Lichen planus, in contrast, causes extensive canalicular occlusion due to subepithelial fibrosis.
- Other causes of canalicular stenosis include chemotherapeutic agents (e.g. radioiodine, 5-fluorouracil, S1 chemotherapy, mitomycin C, and the Taxane group).
- Symptomatic congenital accessory canaliculi are best managed with fistula excision and formal lacrimal drainage surgery.
- Complete congenital lacrimal agenesis may be managed with dacryocystorhinostomy and ring intubation, with a high likelihood of requiring later placement of a canalicular bypass tube in early adulthood.
- Punctal stenosis per se is best managed by removing the posterior wall of the ampulla (in contrast to the standard longitudinal "three snip" punctoplasty).
- Occlusion of the proximal and mid canaliculus should be managed with dacryocystorhinostomy, retrograde canaliculostomy, and silicone intubation.
- Management of a membranous obstruction of the common canaliculus includes dacryocystorhinostomy, membranectomy, and anterograde intubation.
- The only indication for primary placement of a canalicular bypass tube is the total absence of all distal canalicular and common canalicular structures.
- In patients undergoing dacryocystorhinostomy with retrograde canaliculostomy for proximal or midcanalicular block, a carunculectomy should be considered at the time of primary lacrimal drainage surgery.
- When a canalicular bypass tube is placed for the first time, a temporary encirclement suture should be placed around the neck of the tube, as this keeps the flange of the tube proud of the surface during healing of the raw epithelial bed.

## SUGGESTED READING

1. Ali MJ, Honavar SG, Naik M. Endoscopically guided minimally invasive bypass tube intubation without DCR: evaluation of drainage and objective outcomes assessment. Minim Invasive Ther Allied Technol. 2013;22:104-9.

2. Bourkiza R, Lee V. A review of the complications of lacrimal occlusion with punctal and canalicular plugs. Orbit. 2012;31: 86-93.
3. Chak M, Irvine F. Rectangular 3-snip punctoplasty outcomes: preservation of the lacrimal pump in punctoplasty surgery. Ophthal Plast Reconstr Surg. 2009;25:134-5.
4. Chalvatzis NT, Tzamalis AK, Mavrikakis I, et al. Self-retaining bicanaliculus stents as an adjunct to 3-snip punctoplasty in management of upper lacrimal duct stenosis: a comparison to standard 3-snip procedure. Ophthal Plast Reconstr Surg. 2013; 29:123-7.
5. Chatterjee S, Rath S, Roy A, et al. 20G silicone rod as mono-canalicular stent in repair of canalicular lacerations: experience from a tertiary eye care centre. Indian J Ophthalmol. 2013;61: 585-6.
6. Durrani OM, Verity DH, Meligonis G, et al. Bicanalicular obstruction in lichen planus: a characteristic pattern of disease. Ophthalmology. 2008;115:386-9.
7. Eiseman AS, Flanagan JC, Brooks AB, et al. Ocular surface, ocular adnexal, and lacrimal complications associated with the use of systemic 5-fluorouracil. Ophthal Plast Reconstr Surg. 2003; 19:216-24.
8. Esmaeli B, Golio D, Lubecki L, et al. Canalicular and nasolacrimal duct blockage: an ocular side effect associated with the antineoplastic drug S-1. Am J Ophthalmol. 2005;140:325-7.
9. Esmaeli B, Hidaji L, Adinin RB, et al. Blockage of the lacrimal drainage apparatus as a side effect of docetaxel therapy. Cancer. 2003;98:504-7.
10. Gogandy M, Al-Sheikh O, Chaudhry I. Clinical features and bacteriology of lacrimal canaliculitis in patients presenting to a tertiary eye care center in the Middle East. Saudi J Ophthalmol. 2014;28:31-5.
11. Hussain RN, Kanani H, McMullan T. Use of mini-monoka stents for punctal/canalicular stenosis. Br J Ophthalmol. 2012; 96:671-3.
12. Joganathan V, Mehta P, Murray A, et al. Complications of intra-canalicular plugs: a case series. Orbit. 2010;29:271-3.
13. Khu J, Mancini R. Punctum-sparing canaliculotomy for the treatment of canaliculitis. Ophthal Plast Reconstr Surg. 2012;28: 63-5.
14. Kintzel PE, Michaud LB, Lange MK. Docetaxel-associated epiphora. Pharmacotherapy. 2006;26:853-67.
15. Kopp ED, Seregard S. Epiphora as a side effect of topical mitomycin C. Br J Ophthalmol. 2004;88:1422-4.
16. Liang X, Lin Y, Wang Z, Lin L, et al. A modified bicanalicular intubation procedure to repair canalicular lacerations using silicone tubes. Eye. 2012;26:1542-7.
17. Liu B, Li Y, Long C, et al. Novel air-injection technique to locate the medial cut end of lacerated canaliculus. Br J Ophthalmol. 2013;97:1508-9.
18. Madge SN, Malhotra R, Desousa J, et al. The lacrimal bypass tube for lacrimal pump failure attributable to facial palsy. Am J Ophthalmol. 2010;149:155-9.
19. Naik MN, Kelapure A, Rath S, et al. Management of canalicular lacerations: epidemiological aspects and experience with Mini-Monoka monocanalicular stent. Am J Ophthalmol. 2008; 145:375-80.
20. Nam SM. Microscope-assisted reconstruction of canalicular laceration using Mini-Monoka. J Craniofac Surg. 2013;24: 2056-8.
21. Port AD, Chen YT, Lelli GJ Jr. Histopathologic changes in punctal stenosis. Ophthal Plast Reconstr Surg. 2013;29:201-4.
22. Shahid H, Sandhu A, Keenan T, et al. Factors affecting outcome of punctoplasty surgery: a review of 205 cases. Br J Ophthalmol. 2008;92:1689-92.
23. SmartPlug Study Group. Management of complications after insertion of the SmartPlug punctal plug: a study of 28 patients. Ophthalmology. 2006;113:1859.
24. Soiberman U, Kakizaki H, Selva D, et al. Punctal stenosis: definition, diagnosis, and treatment. Clin Ophthalmol. 2012; 6:1011-8.

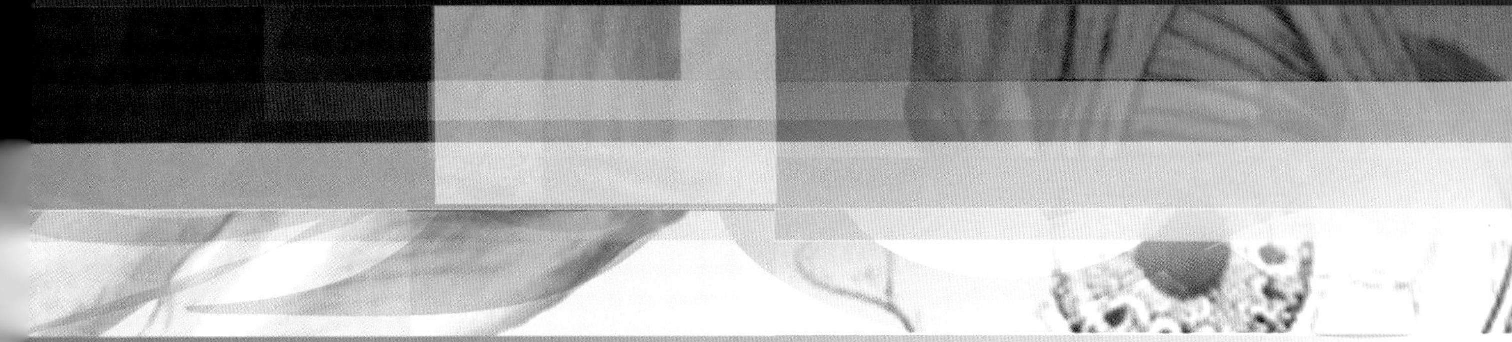

# Section 7

# Oncology Surgeries

*Section Editor* Bertil Damato

CHAPTER

# 84

# Introduction to Oncology Section

Bertil Damato

## INTRODUCTION

In addition to surgical tumor removal, expert techniques in ocular oncology include various forms of phototherapy, radiotherapy and pharmacotherapy, some of which involve surgical procedures, which are mentioned in this section.

## SURGICAL EXCISION

Tumor excision has always been the principal form of treatment for tumors (Figs. 84-1A and B). The main aim of primary tumor excision is to prolong life, although with some diseases, such as choroidal melanoma, it is not known whether or not it actually does so in a particular patient (Figs. 84-2A and B).[1] Other objectives include the prevention of a painful and unsightly eye, if possible conserving the eye and vision.

In some patients, the tumor may already have been sterilized by radiotherapy so that the objective of surgical resection would be to treat or prevent local morbidity arising as a result of the toxic irradiated tumor.[2,3]

## RADIOTHERAPY

Radiotherapy can be administered prior to surgery, to prevent tumor seeding (i.e. "neoadjuvant radiotherapy").[4] Radiotherapy can also be applied after surgical resection, to prevent local tumor recurrence (i.e. "adjunctive radiotherapy").[5,6] Radiotherapy is also useful as a means of controlling any local tumor recurrences after local resection.

Radiotherapy is often the sole form of treatment. In such cases, surgical procedures include plaque insertion and removal as well as insertion of tantalum markers for proton beam radiotherapy (Fig. 84-3).

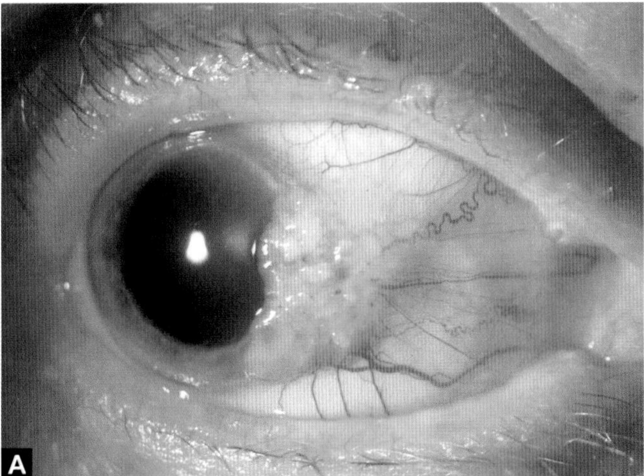


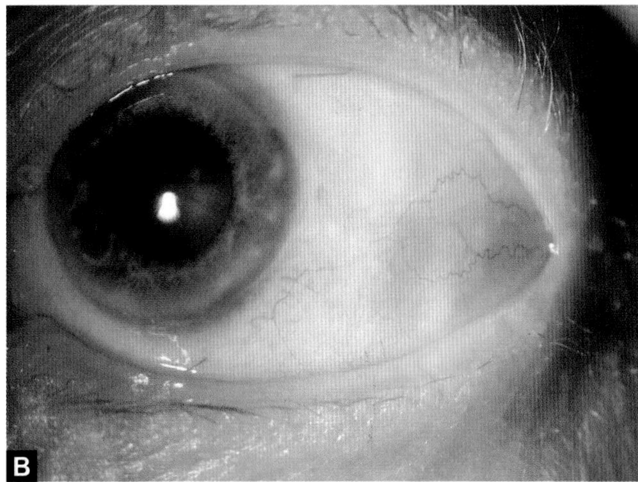


**Figures 84-1A and B** (A) Conjunctival squamous cell carcinoma before treatment and (B) after surgical excision with adjunctive ruthenium plaque brachytherapy and topical chemotherapy with 5-fluorouracil drops.

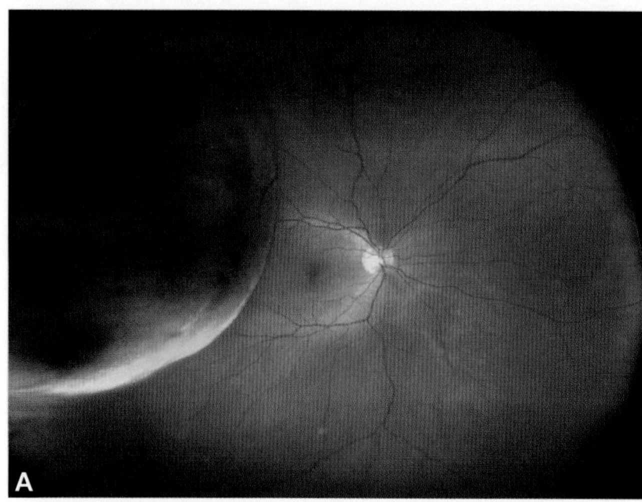

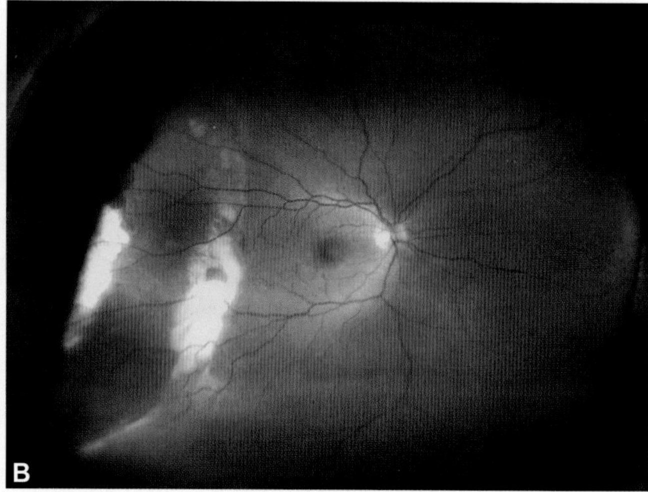

Figures 84-2A and B Right fundus of a 37-year-old woman with a temporal choroidal melanoma measuring 16.4 mm basally and 8.4 mm in thickness (A) Fundus appearance a few days after exoresection with adjunctive ruthenium plaque brachytherapy (B) Despite the good surgical result, the prognosis for survival was poor because the tumor showed epithelioid cells and chromosome 3 loss, which indicate a high mortality as a result of metastatic spread before ocular diagnosis and treatment.

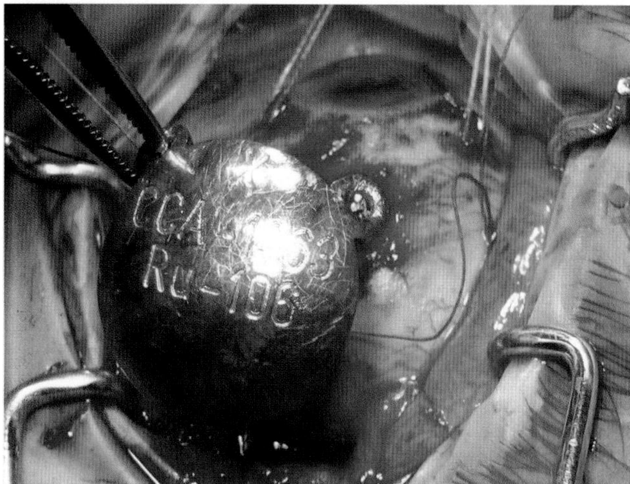

Figure 84-3 Ruthenium plaque. The success of therapeutic modalities such as brachytherapy and proton beam radiotherapy depends on the surgical skill with which the plaque and markers are inserted.

## PHOTOTHERAPY

Phototherapy plays a major role in the treatment of retinoblastoma, administered alone or in combination with chemotherapy.

Phototherapy can also be administered to destroy any tumor remnants after surgical resection (e.g. after endoresection).[7] It is also used for retinopexy after endoresection or biopsy.

Transpupillary thermotherapy can be administered as primary treatment. Alternatively, it can be used to reduce exudation from an irradiated choroidal melanoma.[8]

Photodynamic therapy is mostly deployed for vascular tumors. It is sometimes administered for other tumors, such as uveal melanoma, either as primary treatment or for exudation after radiotherapy. Photodynamic therapy is also useful in patients with recurrent hyphema from an irradiated iris melanoma.[9]

Some forms of pharmacotherapy involve surgery and these include intra-arterial chemotherapy and intraocular injections, which are described in this section.

## CRYOSURGERY

Cryosurgery is useful in the treatment of intraocular tumors, such as retinoblastoma, vasoproliferative tumor, Coats disease and retinal hemangioblastoma.

Cryosurgery is also administered as an adjunct to local excision of conjunctival tumors. After endoresection of choroidal melanoma, cryotherapy is used to treat any entry-site tears and to destroy any seeds at the sclerotomy sites.

In patients with retinoblastoma, cryotherapy can enhance delivery of drugs to the target areas by disrupting the blood barrier.

## PHARMACOTHERAPY

Chemotherapy has become the most important modality in the treatment of retinoblastoma, being administered systemically, intra-arterially, intravitreally and in the sub-Tenon's space. Chemotherapy for retinoblastoma is often combined with local treatments, such as laser therapy, cryosurgery and brachytherapy.

Systemic chemotherapy is also administered for metastases and lymphoma.

Intravitreal chemotherapy and rituximab are effective for retinal lymphoma.

Topical chemotherapy is used extensively for conjunctival melanoma, carcinoma and other tumors.

Intraocular steroids have long been used for inflammation. Although effective for macular edema after radiotherapy, these intraocular steroid injections have largely been superseded by a variety of antiangiogenic agents.

Topical antiseptics, antibiotics, anti-inflammatory agents, meiotic and mydriatics are administered as for other forms of ocular surgery.

## PSYCHOLOGICAL ASPECTS

Besides threatening patients with visual handicap, ocular tumors can also give rise to concerns about disfigurement. Several diseases have implications for the health of the patient well as other family members. These fears give rise to emotional needs, which need to be addressed.

## CONSENT

As with any treatment, it is necessary to obtain informed consent and to ensure that this is well documented.

Informed consent should also be obtained for nontreatment of a potentially-fatal tumor (e.g. "melanocytic tumor of indeterminate malignancy", otherwise known as "suspicious nevus") in case the patient ever develops metastatic disease or other complications attributed to delayed treatment.

Consent should also be obtained routinely for the use of tissues for research and teaching.

Not all centers are able to offer the full range of therapies for a particular condition. Furthermore, many aspects of oncological practice are controversial. For consent to be truly "informed", it is necessary for patients to be told about therapies and opinions that are promoted at other centers.

## COMMUNICATING WITH PATIENTS

Many patients report that their mind "closed" on hearing the word cancer. The author has for many years given patients "live" audio-recordings of their actual consultation and has found this practice to enhance communication, care and the doctor-patient relationship.[10] Some practitioners are concerned about medicolegal implications, but the author is more concerned about what patients forget than what they remember. Printed leaflets are given to patients in case any important points are overlooked in the discussion.

## MULTIDISCIPLINARY CARE

The author's impression is that there is a tendency for some general ophthalmologists to treat ocular malignancies, such as conjunctival melanoma and retinal lymphoma, which do not require special instruments or equipment. However, there is more to treating the patient adequately than just destroying the ocular tumor.

For example, not all general ophthalmologists are aware of the special precautions that are needed to prevent seeding of tumor cells, which can happen all too easily, with fatal consequences. Furthermore, most patients with retinal lymphoma will die of intracranial disease. For these reasons, patients with ocular malignancy are best treated by multidisciplinary teams including oncologists, pathologists, radiotherapists, geneticists and psychologists.

## DEALING WITH UNCERTAINTY

With some tumors, such as uveal melanoma, the impact of ocular treatment on survival is not known. It can therefore be difficult to decide whether to observe, treat or biopsy a tumor of indeterminate malignancy, especially if an intervention is likely to affect vision. Special expertise is required to select the form of management that is optimal for a particular patient, taking into account the individual's needs, wishes and fears.[11] Opinions differ as to whether the "paternalistic" or the "consensual" approach is best. In practice, a combination of the two methods is required. It is necessary to tailor the approach to each individual.

## PEARLS AND PITFALLS

- Ocular treatment is only one aspect of patient care, which must be holistic.
- Informed consent requires the patient to be told about all management options and not only those available at the center attended.
- Failure to document informed consent to nontreatment may have adverse consequences if complications arise.

## REFERENCES

1. Damato B. Does ocular treatment of uveal melanoma influence survival? Br J Cancer. 2010;103(3):285-90.
2. Schalenbourg A, Coupland S, Kacperek A, et al. Iridocyclectomy for neovascular glaucoma caused by proton-beam radiotherapy of pigmented ciliary adenocarcinoma. Graefes Arch Clin Exp Ophthalmol (Albrecht von Graefes Archiv fur klinische und experimentelle Ophthalmologie). 2008;246(10): 1499-501.

3. Damato BE, Groenewald C, Foulds WS. Surgical resection of choroidal melanoma. In: Ryan SJ (Ed). Retina, Vol. 3, 5th edition. Elsevier: London; 2013. pp. 2298-306.
4. Bechrakis NE, Foerster MH. Neoadjuvant proton beam radiotherapy combined with subsequent endoresection of choroidal melanomas. Int Ophthalmol Clin. 2006;46(1):95-107.
5. Damato B, Coupland SE. An audit of conjunctival melanoma treatment in Liverpool. Eye (Lond). 2009;23(4):801-9.
6. Damato B. Adjunctive plaque radiotherapy after local resection of uveal melanoma. Front Radiat Ther Oncol. 1997;30:123-32.
7. Damato B, Groenewald C, McGalliard J, et al. Endoresection of choroidal melanoma. Br J Ophthalmol. 1998;82(3):213-8.
8. Damato B. Vasculopathy after treatment of choroidal melanoma. In: Joussen A, Gardner TW, Kirchhof B, Ryan SJ (Eds). Retinal Vascular Disease. Springer: Berlin; 2007. pp. 582-91.
9. Trichopoulos N, Damato B. Photodynamic therapy for recurrent hyphema after proton beam radiotherapy of iris melanoma. Graefes Arch Clin Exp Ophthalmol (Albrecht von Graefes Archiv fur klinische und experimentelle Ophthalmologie). 2007;245(10):1573-5.
10. Ah-Fat FG, Sharma MC, Damato BE. Taping outpatient consultations: a survey of attitudes and responses of adult patients with ocular malignancy. Eye (Lond). 1998;12(Pt 5):789-91.
11. Damato B, Heimann H. Personalized treatment of uveal melanoma. Eye (Lond). 2013;27(2):172-9.

CHAPTER

# 85

# Biopsy

Bertil Damato, Sarah E Coupland, Heinrich Heimann, Carl Groenewald

## INTRODUCTION

Biopsy of ocular tumors is performed to establish a diagnosis and/or to help determine the prognosis.

## INDICATIONS

- Diagnosis of an intraocular or conjunctival tumor, when clinical examination is inconclusive.
- Differential diagnosis between uveal nevus and melanoma, as an alternative to long-term surveillance.
- Differential diagnosis of conjunctival pigmented lesions, e.g. differentiation between intraepithelial disease (i.e. primary acquired melanosis/conjunctival melanocytic intraepithelial neoplasia) from invasive melanoma.[1,2]
- Differential diagnosis between inflammatory vitreous infiltrate and vitreoretinal lymphoma.[3]
- Confirmation of clinical diagnosis (e.g. uveal metastasis).[4]
- Morphological analysis and genetic typing of an intraocular melanoma, to estimate prognosis (Fig. 85-1).[5]

## CONTRAINDICATIONS

- Possible or definite retinoblastoma, because of risk of tumor dissemination into the orbit and systemically.
- Anticoagulant therapy, if intraocular tumor biopsy is considered, because of the risk of severe intraocular hemorrhage.
- Nodular conjunctival tumor, because of the risk of tumor seeding. Excision biopsy is preferable, if possible.

## PREOPERATIVE CARE

For intraocular tumor biopsy, the pupil is dilated with 1% cyclopentolate and 2.5% phenylephrine.

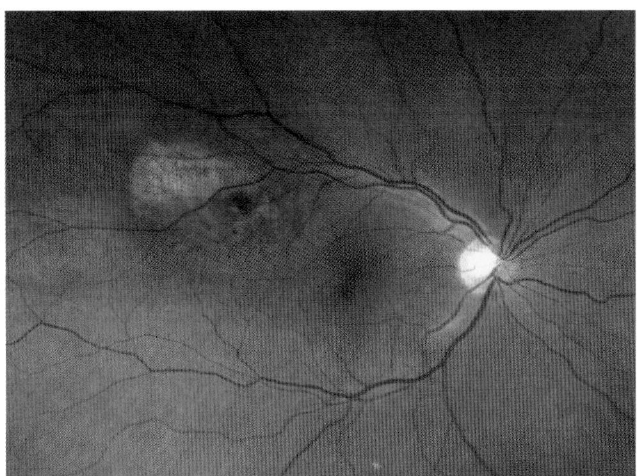

**Figure 85-1** Superotemporal choroidal melanoma in the right eye of a 53-year-old woman after transretinal tumor biopsy performed with a 25-gauge vitreous cutter. The biopsy site is visible as a dark area near the center of the tumor. The tumor had a largest basal diameter of 9.5 mm and a thickness of 2.0 mm, with no epithelioid cells and no chromosome 3 loss. Multivariate analysis using the Liverpool Uveal Melanoma Prognosticator Online (www.ocularmelanomaonline.com) showed the risk of metastatic disease to be minimal.

If intraocular biopsy is performed to diagnose or exclude lymphoma, any steroid therapy must be discontinued at least 5 days prior to biopsy.

## SURGICAL TECHNIQUE

### Aspiration Biopsy

#### *Vitreous Biopsy*

This is best performed with the 25-gauge, 3-port, sutureless, vitrectomy kit. Three ports are inserted, 4 mm from the limbus, for the infusion, light pipe, and vitreous cutter.

The infusion is left closed while the vitreous sample is aspirated into a 10-mL syringe, either allowing the eye to collapse or indenting the eye to maintain a high intraocular pressure. The syringe is attached to the tubing of the vitreous cutter with a T-junction. Once the sample has been obtained, the infusion is turned on.

### *Transretinal Biopsy*

This can be performed with a 25-gauge, 3-port, sutureless vitrectomy kit or with a fine needle (25–30 gauge).

The needle or vitreous cutter is passed through the retina at the tumor apex, avoiding any retinal blood vessels.

When a vitreous cutter is used, the cutting rate is lowered with maximum suction. If hemorrhage occurs on removing the cutter from the tumor, the intraocular pressure is raised until the bleeding stops and then lowered after about a minute. If the hemorrhage recurs, the procedure is repeated. If the tumor is very thin, the retinotomy is placed near the tumor margin and the retina is lifted slightly away from the tumor by moving the vitreous cutter sideways toward the tumor center. The vitreous cutter is rotated so that the port is facing the center of the tumor, before cutting is started.

Vitrectomy, endolaser photocoagulation and internal tamponade are not required.

The surgeon's preferred viewing system is deployed (e.g. noncontact lens system, corneal contact lens or binocular indirect ophthalmoscope).

### *Trans-scleral Biopsy*

A 25–30 gauge needle is passed into the tumor directly through the overlying sclera. The needle is attached to a 10-mL syringe with flexible tubing primed with saline.

The needle is passed obliquely through the sclera to reduce the risk of extraocular tumor seeding. Bipolar cautery or cryotherapy is applied to the needle track to minimize this risk.

Care must be taken not to insert the needle too deeply. If a graduated needle is not available, an ink-mark can be made on the bore of the needle with a felt-pen after scraping the required area of the needle with half-closed artery forceps.

Once the needle is in the desired position, it can be twisted or moved from side-to-side to fragment the tumor, while applying suction, in the hope of increasing the yield. Prolonged aspiration may reduce yield if there is time for clotting to occur in the needle.

The aspirate is back-flushed into a universal container, which is inspected under the operating microscope to ensure that an adequate sample has been obtained. This can be difficult if the specimen is blood-stained. Care must be taken to distinguish tumor fragments from microbubbles.

## Incisional Biopsy

### *Iris Tumor*

Incisional biopsy can be performed with a vitreous cutter or with scissors. When attempting to distinguish nevus from melanoma, it is useful to include the tumor margin with normal tissue. The specimen should be as large as possible, allowing for immunocytochemical and genetic analyses, if required.

### *Choroidal Tumor*

*The first author's technique is as follows*: The tumor margin is defined by transillumination and marked on the sclera with a pen (Figs. 85-2 and 85-3). A lamellar scleral flap is created using a No. 15 Bard-Parker scalpel. A transverse incision is made in the deep sclera, just anterior to the central part of the tumor. Essen biopsy forceps are introduced into the tumor to obtain a tumor pellet, which is flushed into a universal container. This procedure is repeated until the required number of pellets is obtained. Any blood is swabbed without delay to avoid tumor seeding. Any tumor fragments that have scattered into the scleral bed are immediately treated with diathermy. The lamellar scleral flap is glued back in place with tissue adhesive. Two interrupted 6-0 vicryl sutures can be placed to ensure that the flap remains closed but are not usually necessary.

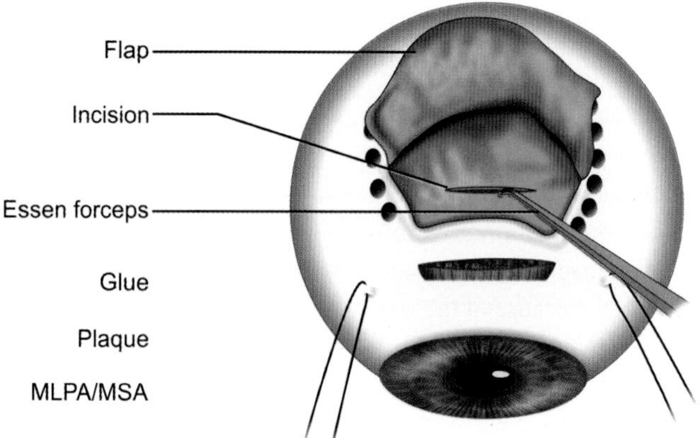


**Figure 85-2** Trans-scleral incisional biopsy of choroidal melanoma with Essen forceps.

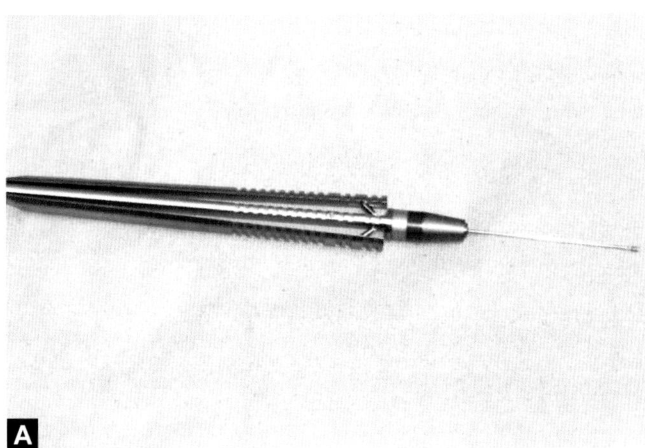


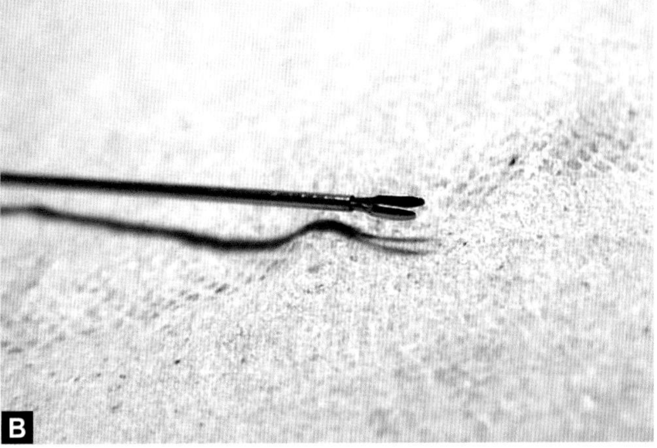


Figures 85-3A and B Essen forceps.

### *Conjunctival Tumor*

Incisional biopsy should not be performed with nodular tumors, which should be removed en bloc using a no-touch technique, to avoid seeding. Microbiopsy is performed for diffuse disease, such as melanosis, C-MIN or carcinoma in situ. The procedure is performed with spring scissors and toothed microforceps. Each biopsy should be triangular or ellipsoid in shape, measuring approximately 4 × 2 mm. The specimen should be placed on a paper mount, taking care not to cause a crush artifact. Multiple specimens should be obtained, starting in areas of normal conjunctiva. Each specimen should be placed in a separate container, which should be labeled to indicate the biopsy site.

## Excisional Biopsy

### *Iris Tumor*

Excision biopsy of a lesion in the mid-zone of the iris or near the pupil margin would require a broad iridectomy, which may require pupilloplasty, an artificial iris or a painted contact lens. If the tumor involves the angle, biopsy requires cycloiridectomy, performed as described elsewhere.

### *Uveal Tumor*

Excision biopsy of a ciliary body and/or choroidal tumor is performed as described in Chapter 90.

### *Conjunctival Tumor*

Excision biopsy of a conjunctival tumor is performed as described in Chapter 93.

# LABORATORY ASPECTS

## Liaison Between Surgeon and Pathologist

Before sending any intraocular sample to the pathology laboratory, the surgeon should check with the pathologist as to what transport medium should be used.[2]

Should it be necessary to send the biopsy fresh, this should be done rapidly with advance notification of the laboratory involved. Special precautions should be taken during weekends.

All specimens must be accompanied by a request form, completed with patient details, the clinical history and the differential diagnoses. Acronyms on the forms should be avoided. A contact number should be provided in case further information is required by the laboratory.

## Transport of Specimen to Laboratory

Aspiration biopsies should be placed in "soft" fixation media, such as Cytolyt, which enables morphological, immunohistochemical and genetic assessment of the samples.

Incisional biopsies can be placed in buffered formalin. Should these be multiple, each specimen should be placed in a separate container.

Excisional biopsies should be placed in buffered formalin. If marking sutures are placed on the sample, these must be explained on the request form, allowing the pathologist to indicate whether tumor cells are extending to a particular surgical margin.

## Laboratory Investigations

Light microscopy is performed on both cytospins and histological sections, following processing of the samples. Whilst conventional morphological stains for cytology include May-Grünwald-Giemsa (MGG), the standard stain for histological sections is hematoxylin and eosin (H&E).

Special stains include:

- Periodic acid Schiff (PAS) is used to highlight particular features in cells, e.g. cytoplasmic granules as well as the presence/absence of microorganisms.
- Grocott stains for the demonstration of microorganisms, particularly fungi.
- Perl's stain for iron.

Immunohistochemistry involves the application of a variety of mono- or polyclonal antibodies onto either cytospins or tissue sections to precisely identify cell types. This involves amplification and visualization steps, which can be applied to both fresh and fixed tissue.

The antibodies used vary according to the differential diagnosis but include:

- Human melanoma black (HMB45), MelanA and S-100P for melanoma.
- Pancytokeratins as well as specialized cytokeratins for carcinomas.
- T-cell markers (CD2, CD3).
- B-cell markers (CD20, CD79a and PAX5) for lymphomas.
- CD68 for macrophages.
- Proliferation markers, which include Ki-67, proliferating cell nuclear antigen (PCNA) and PHH3 (also termed Ser10).

Genetic studies are increasingly being applied for both diagnostic and prognostication purposes.

- *Diagnosis*: For example, the polymerase chain reaction (PCR) is applied for clonality analysis against the B-cell receptor and T-cell receptor in ocular B- and T-cell lymphmas respectively. To perform this analysis, DNA is first extracted from the fresh or fixed sample and assessed for quality and concentration.
- *Prognosis*: In uveal melanoma, chromosomal abnormalities correlate strongly with survival, providing scope for prognostication. Most commonly used techniques include:
  - Fluorescence in situ hybridization (FISH)
  - Microsatellite analysis (MSA)
  - Multiplex ligation dependent probe amplification (MLPA)
  - Comparative genomic hybridization (CGH) array
  - Single-nucleotide polymorphisms arrays
  - Gene expression profiling (GEP).

The tests are performed on tumor cells or on extracted tumor DNA or RNA. They vary with respect to specificity and cost. It is highly recommended that the interpretation of any genetic analysis be made in the context of morphological findings.

## POSTOPERATIVE CARE

Antibiotics as well as any mydriatics and anti-inflammatory agents are prescribed in the usual manner.

## SPECIFIC INSTRUMENTATION

- *Aspiration biopsy*: 25–30G hypodermic needle; 25G vitreous cutter
- *Trans-scleral incisional biopsy*: Essen forceps (DORC, Zuidland, The Netherlands).

## COMPLICATIONS

### Intraoperative Complications

- Inadequate specimens are most likely with aspiration biopsy using a fine needle or vitreous cutter, especially if the tumor is thin (i.e. less than 3-mm thick). Whether the sample size is adequate or not also depends on the amount required for the tests being planned. Other causes of failure are: delay in transporting specimen to laboratory; wrong transport medium; leaking container; and, in the case of lymphomas, prior steroid therapy. With conjunctival biopsies, care must be taken not to cause crush artifact.
- Tumor seeding is most likely to occur with retinoblastoma, with severe consequences. Seeding can also occur after incisional biopsy of melanoma and possibly other nodular malignant tumors, such as carcinoma. Extraocular seeding of uveal melanoma can occur after biopsy (Damato, unpublished data). This complication is especially likely with aggressive tumors showing high-grade malignancy on histology, chromosome 3 loss and/or class 2 gene expression profile.
- Other complications of intraocular biopsy include cataract, hemorrhage, endophthalmitis and rhegmatogenous retinal detachment.

### Postoperative Complications

- Episcleral seeding of uveal melanoma can be treated by excision of any nodules with adjunctive cryotherapy.
- Other complications, such as cataract, hemorrhage, endophthalmitis and rhegmatogenous retinal detachment are treated in the usual fashion.

## SURGICAL OUTCOME: SCIENTIFIC EVIDENCE/METANALYSIS

- Diagnostic biopsy will determine whether a tumor requires treatment, what kind of treatment is required, what

investigations should be undertaken and what long-term surveillance should be planned.
- Prognostic biopsy will guide patient counseling as well as intensity and duration of ocular and systemic monitoring.

## PLACE OF THE TECHNIQUE IN SURGICAL ARMAMENTARIUM

Opinions vary about the scope of ocular tumor biopsy. With suspected intraocular metastases, the author prefers biopsy in the first instance whereas most perform this examination only if extensive systemic investigations are inconclusive (Konstantinides L et al, unpublished data). Immunohistochemical or genetic analyses of intraocular metastases may determine subsequent treatment plans. For example, Her-2 positivity of breast carcinoma metastases and the presence of epidermal growth factor receptor (EGFR) mutations in lung carcinoma metastases would result in particular therapeutic regimens being selected for the patient.

There is also disagreement about whether biopsy should be performed to distinguish intraocular nevus from melanoma, and whether prognostic biopsy should be performed to estimate the survival probability after treatment of uveal melanoma (e.g. following treatment with proton beam or plaque therapy). Our experience demonstrates that reliable genetic information can be obtained postradiotherapy.

## PEARLS AND PITFALLS

- Biopsy requires an experienced surgeon as well as a highly-skilled and well-equipped laboratory team, i.e. experienced ocular pathologist, biomedical scientist preferably dedicated to eye pathology, and molecular technicians.
- Close collaboration and communication between the surgical and pathology teams is essential.
- Clarification of sample media and transport is essential; notification of sample sending to the laboratory prior to its dispatch is desirable, particularly in difficult cases.
- Beware of tumor seeding, especially with conjunctival melanoma.
- Biopsy of retinoblastomas is contraindicated.

## REFERENCES

1. Damato B, Coupland SE. Conjunctival melanoma and melanosis: a reappraisal of terminology, classification and staging. Clin Experiment Ophthalmol. 2008;36(8):786-95.
2. Coupland SE. Analysis of intraocular biopsies. Dev Ophthalmol. 2012;49:96-116.
3. Coupland SE. The pathologist's perspective on vitreous opacities. Eye (Lond). 2008;22(10):1318-29.
4. Sen J, Groenewald C, Hiscott PS, et al. Transretinal choroidal tumor biopsy with a 25-gauge vitrector. Ophthalmology. 2006;113(6):1028-31.
5. Damato B, Eleuteri A, Taktak AF, et al. Estimating prognosis for survival after treatment of choroidal melanoma. Prog Retin Eye Res. 2011;30(5):285-95.

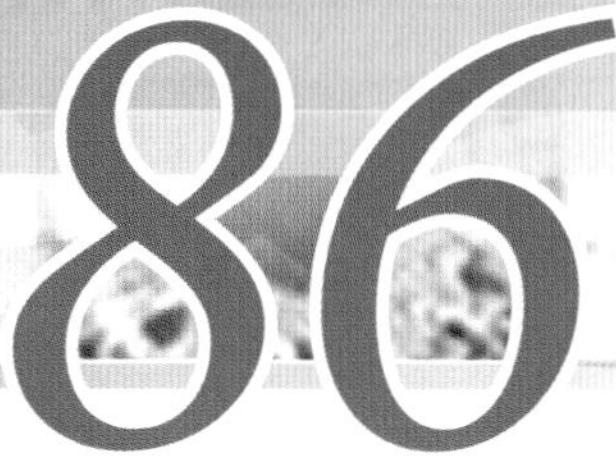

CHAPTER 86

# Phototherapy

Michael I Seider, Paul J Stewart, Bertil Damato

## INTRODUCTION

Phototherapy of ocular tumors includes various forms of photocoagulation, thermotherapy, and photodynamic therapy (PDT).

## INDICATIONS

### Photocoagulation

- Small, retinal hemangioblastomas, not exceeding 4.5 mm in diameter (Figs. 86-1A and B).[1,2]
- Retinoblastoma, as primary treatment if the tumor is small (i.e. diameter and thickness not exceeding 3 and 2 mm, respectively) and posterior. Previously, high-energy photocoagulation was administered around the tumor to deprive it of its blood supply but this method has now been abandoned. (Fig. 86-2).[4] Today, laser is directed at the tumor itself but at a lower energy, to prevent tumor seeding into the vitreous. Intraoperative, adjunctive treatment of choroidal melanoma after endoresection, to destroy any tumor remnants in the scleral bed.[5] Primary photocoagulation of choroidal melanoma has been superseded by other methods.

### Transpupillary Thermotherapy

- As monotherapy for retinoblastoma, if group A and posterior, especially if the retinal pigment epithelium (RPE) is intact as this is where most of the infrared light is absorbed. Thermotherapy is frequently combined with chemotherapy in various ways, usually for small and medium-sized retinoblastomas (Chapters 97 and 98) (Figs. 86-3A and B). Special precautions are taken to avoid seeding of tumor cells into the vitreous.
- Choroidal melanoma, as primary treatment of tumors up to 3 mm in thickness and up to 10 mm in diameter,

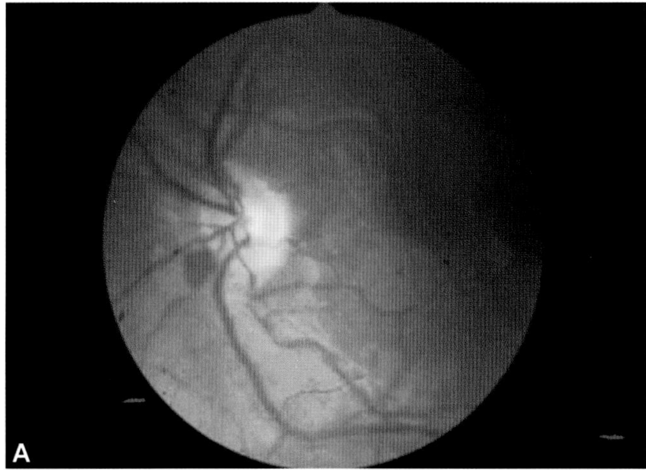

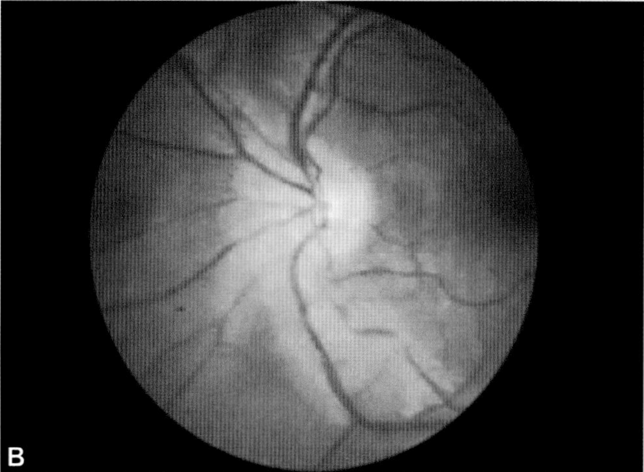

**Figures 86-1A and B** Retinal hemangioblastoma before (A) and after photocoagulation (B). Courtesy of Dr Carol Lane. From Damato.[3]

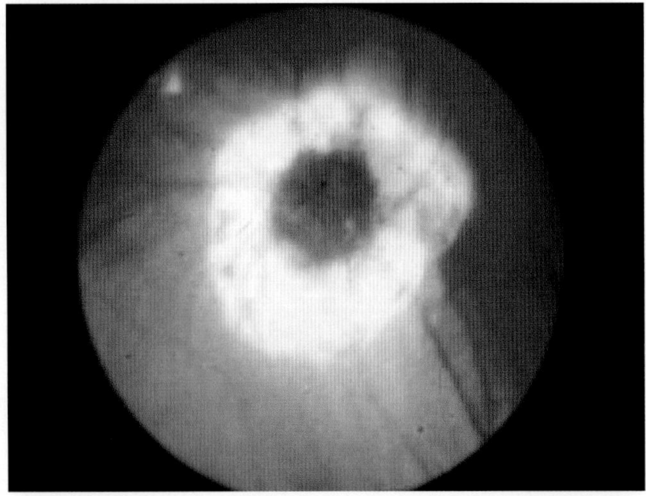

Figure 86-2 Small retinoblastoma after photocoagulation. Courtesy of Dr John Dudgeon.

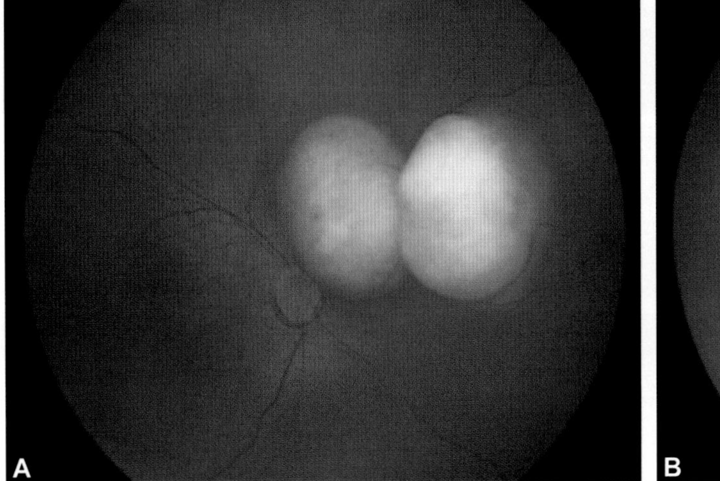

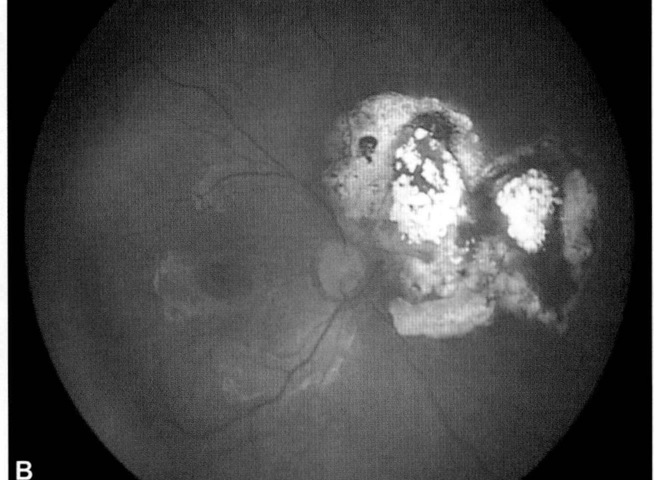

Figures 86-3A and B Retinoblastoma at presentation (A) and after chemotherapy and diode laser phototherapy (B).

if other methods are not appropriate and if the patient accepts an increased risk of local recurrence (Figs. 86-4A and B).[6] Adjunctive transpupillary thermotherapy (TTT) after brachytherapy can avoid local tumor recurrence (Figs. 86-5A and B). Secondary TTT of choroidal melanoma after radiotherapy can reduce exudation, improving vision, temporarily or permanently according to whether collateral damage to optic disk and fovea contributes to any visual loss (Figs. 86-6A and B).[7]

- Choroidal metastasis, if small and posterior and if risk of local recurrence is accepted. Indocyanine green has been used to augment the laser treatment.[8]
- Retinal hemangioblastoma may respond in some cases, but there can be severe exudative reactions if excessive treatment is applied.[2]

## Photodynamic Therapy

- Choroidal haemangioma, as a means of reducing retinal detachment and improving vision (Figs. 86-7A and B).[9] Although most effective with circumscribed tumors, PDT can be useful with some diffuse tumors but may require several treatment sessions.[10]
- Vasoproliferative tumor, as a means of avoiding cryotherapy, which causes vitreous fibrosis and epiretinal membrane formation.[11]
- Retinal hemangioblastoma may respond in some cases.[12]
- Choroidal melanoma, if radiotherapy is unsuitable or unsuccessful. The results of PDT of choroidal melanoma are uncertain so that this is still regarded as an investigational procedure (Figs. 86-8A and B).[13]

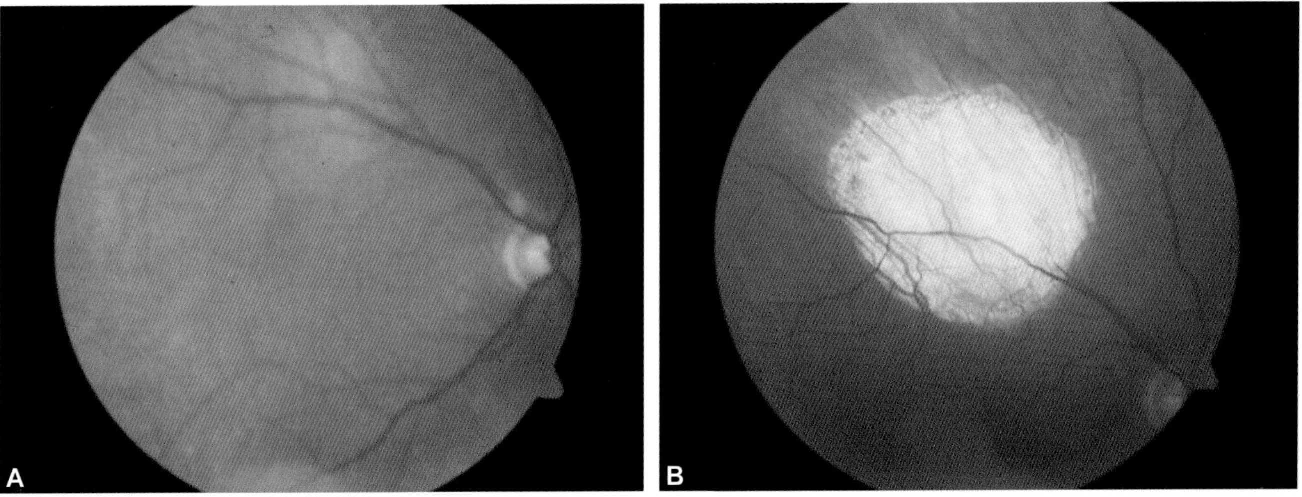

Figures 86-4A and B Choroidal melanoma at presentation (A) and after transpupillary thermotherapy (B). From Damato.[3]

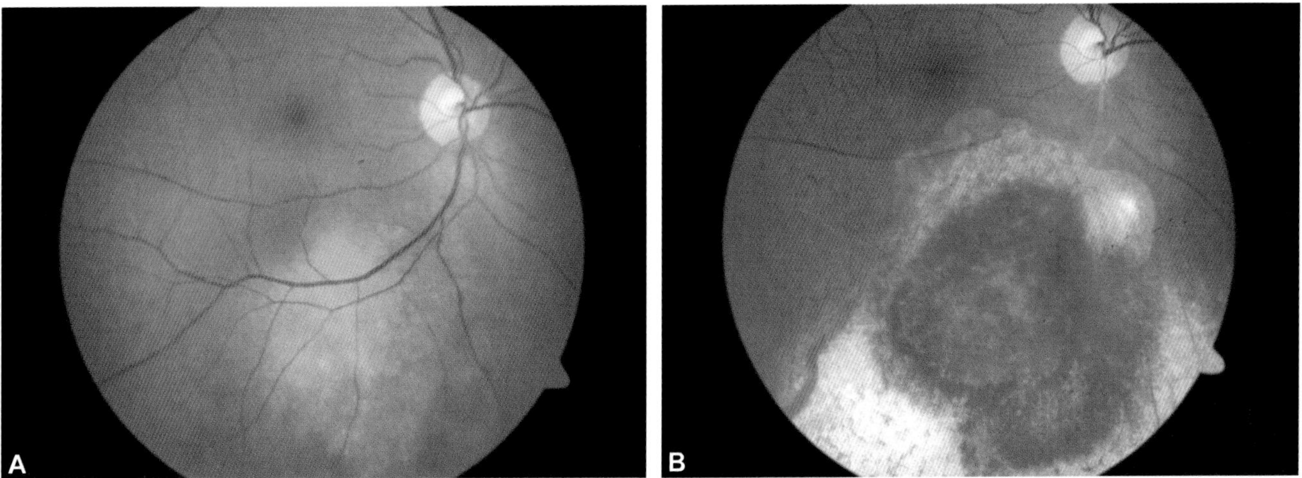

Figures 86-5A and B Choroidal melanoma treated with an eccentrically positioned ruthenium plaque and with adjunctive brachytherapy, before (A) and after treatment (B). More than 10 years later, the visual acuity was 20/20.

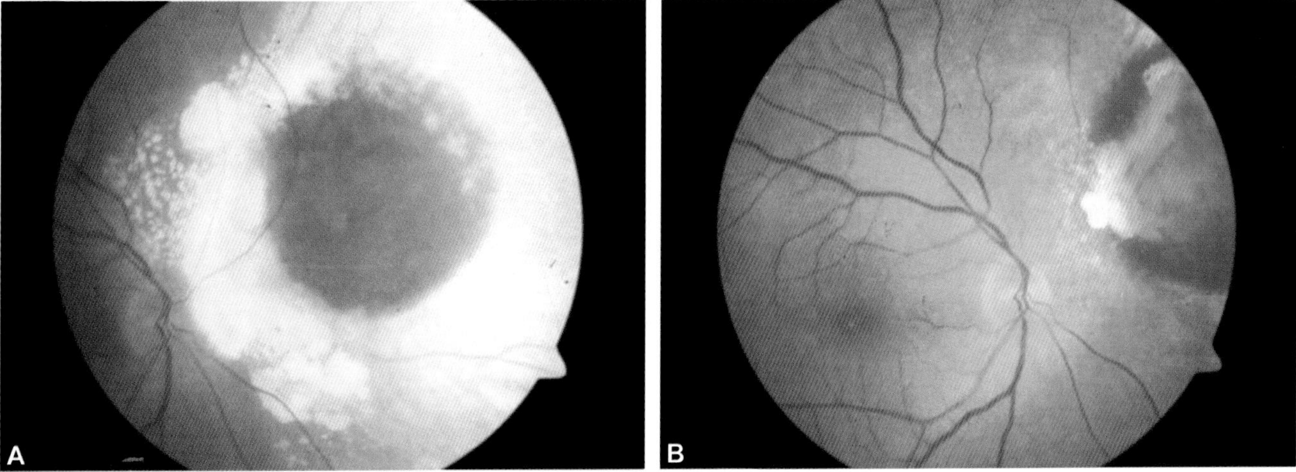

Figures 86-6A and B Choroidal melanoma with exudation after ruthenium plaque radiotherapy (A) showing cessation of exudation after transpupillary thermotherapy (B). From Damato.[7]

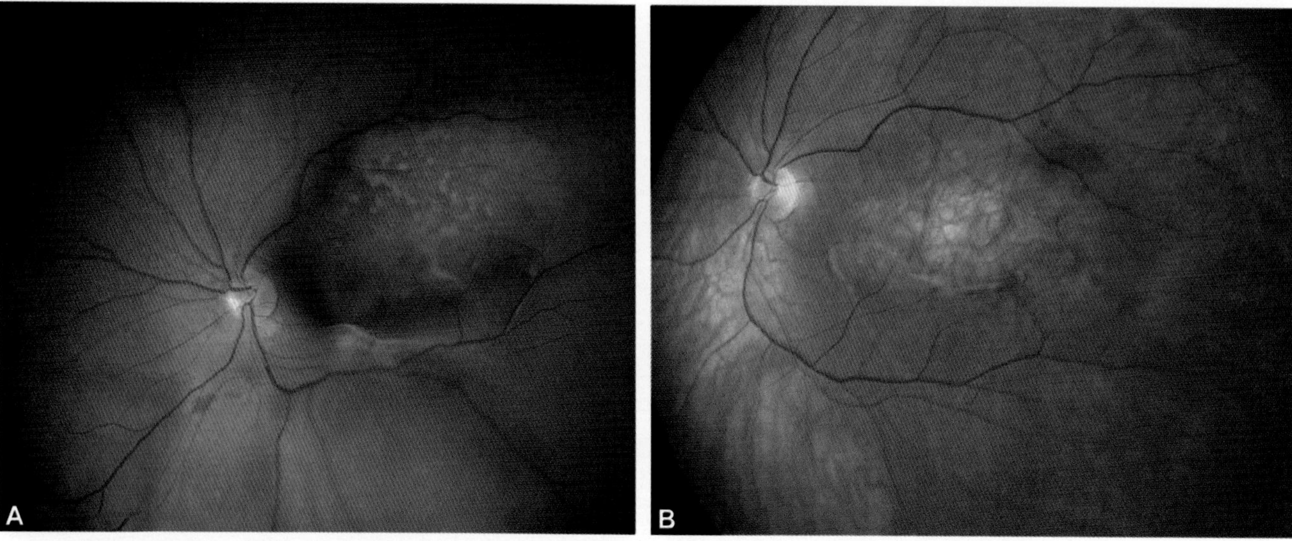

Figures 86-7A and B Circumscribed choroidal hemangioma, before photodynamic therapy (A) and after treatment (B).

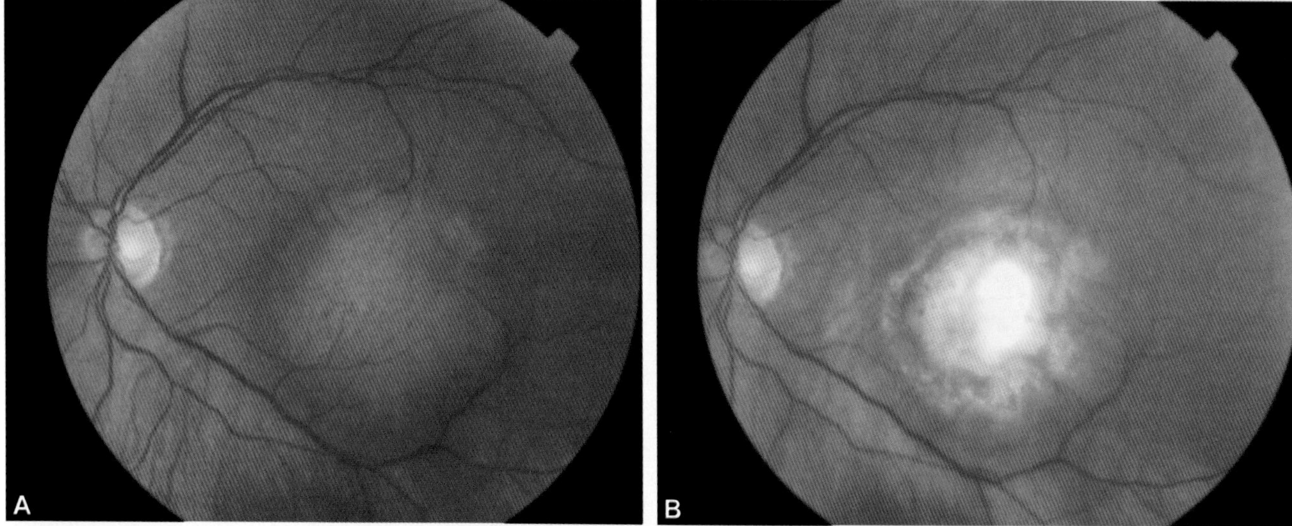

Figures 86-8A and B Amelanotic choroidal melanoma before treatment (A) and after photodynamic therapy (B).

- Exudative choroidal melanoma after radiotherapy.[7]
- Recurrent hyphema from an irradiated iris melanoma.[14]
- Uveal metastasis, as an alternative to radiotherapy.[15]
- Choroidal osteoma, to induce regression of an extrafoveal tumor before vision is lost.[16]

## CONTRAINDICATIONS

- Opaque media.
- Choroidal tumor obscured by excessive overlying retinal detachment.
- Peripheral, posterior-segment tumor.
- Retinoblastoma with vitreous seeding.
- Excessive tumor size.
- Choroidal osteoma involving fovea.

## PREOPERATIVE CARE

Mydriasis, in the usual fashion.

## TECHNIQUE

### Photocoagulation

- *Retinal hemangioblastoma*: The burns are applied to the tumor itself as well as to feeder. With small lesions, it is often possible to achieve tumor control in a single session;

with larger tumors, excessive treatment in a single session can cause a severe reaction.

- *Retinoblastoma*: Argon laser is applied to the entire tumor and adjacent retina (except at the fovea if safe to omit this margin) using an indirect ophthalmoscope or operating microscope to visualize the fundus. The spot size is 200–300 μm with the power initially set at 100 mW and increased in small steps until a visible reaction is achieved, possibly with tiny hemorrhages. Excessive energy is avoided as this may rupture the internal limiting membrane and cause vitreous seeding. Hemorrhages indicate that the maximum power has been reached.

## Transpupillary Thermotherapy

- *Choroidal melanoma*: Infrared, 3 mm, diode laser applications are placed over the entire tumor surface and surrounding choroid with a safety margin of 1.5 mm. Each exposure is 60 seconds long. The power is adjusted so that the retina overlying the tumor begins to blanche at 45 seconds. The power should not be strong enough to close the retinal vessels. The TTT is repeated every 2 months until the tumor is completely atrophic. This may require between two and four sessions. Once the retina has atrophied, after the initial session, it will not blanche so that the power settings should be the same as those used in the first session. If TTT is being administered to arrest exudation from an irradiated tumor, safety margins are not required unless active tumor is suspected
- Choroidal metastasis is treated in a similar fashion to melanoma, except that retinal blanching is less likely to occur if the tumor is amelanotic. The safety margins should be at least 3 mm in diameter because the tumor edges tend to be ill defined
- Retinoblastoma. The diode (810nm) laser treatment is applied just before or after systemic chemotherapy to achieve synergy. About three to four cycles of "chemothermotherapy" (4–6 weeks apart) are required for adequate tumor control (i.e. a flat inactive scar or calcified mass). The laser may be applied via a microscope adaptor with 3-mirror contact lens (spot size adjustable) or using an indirect ophthalmoscope (spot size 1.2 mm).[17] The initial power should be 300 mW for (mean power tends to be 450–500 mW) and should be adjusted according to RPE pigmentation and response to previous treatment. The duration of application should be titrated to treatment endpoints, which include microhemorrhages and slight retinal edema. The required laser duration will vary with the tumor size, from a few seconds for small tumors to > 15 minutes for larger, calcified tumors. Vitreous seeding and extrascleral spread of tumor can occur with excessive energy or many repeat treatments of unresponsive tumor. Indocyanine green can be used to augment the therapeutic effect.[18]

## Photodynamic Therapy

In most patients, PDT is delivered using the standard protocol, although an alternative, high-dose protocol exists.

*The standard protocol is as follows*: Verteporfin is infused at a dose of 6 mg/m$^2$ over 10 minutes. Fifteen minutes after the start of the infusion, each lesion is treated for 83 seconds with a 689 nm laser set at 600 mW/cm$^2$ with total energy density of 50–100 J/cm$^2$.

- *Choroidal hemangioma*: If a circumscribed lesion is small enough, a single spot is used to either cover it entirely. Otherwise, several spots are used in an overlapping fashion to cover the entire lesion.[19] The goal of treatment is to achieve a reduction/elimination in tumor exudation rather than complete involution of the lesion.
- *Choroidal melanoma*: The tumor is treated with a wide safety margin as the microscopic border of the lesion may extend well beyond the visible margins.
- *Choroidal osteoma*: The PDT is delivered following the standard protocol.

# MECHANISM OF ACTION

- Photocoagulation raises the tissue temperature above 60°C to cause coagulation of proteins and immediate cell death.
- TTT causes tumour cell death by raising the temperature to between 45 °C and 60°C for about 60 seconds.
- PDT uses light to activate a photosensitiser, thereby releasing toxic-free radicals, which destroy adjacent tumor cells and cause vaso-occlusion.

# POSTOPERATIVE CARE

Color photography performed immediately after treatment is useful for documenting any visible reaction to the treatment.

# SPECIFIC INSTRUMENTATION

- *Photocoagulation*: Argon green laser (532 nm), indirect ophthalmoscope/condensing lens (usually 20 diopter), or attachment on slit-lamp or operating microscope.
- *TTT*: Diode laser (810 nm), indirect ophthalmoscope/condensing lens (usually 20 diopter), or slit-lamp/operating microscope attachment.

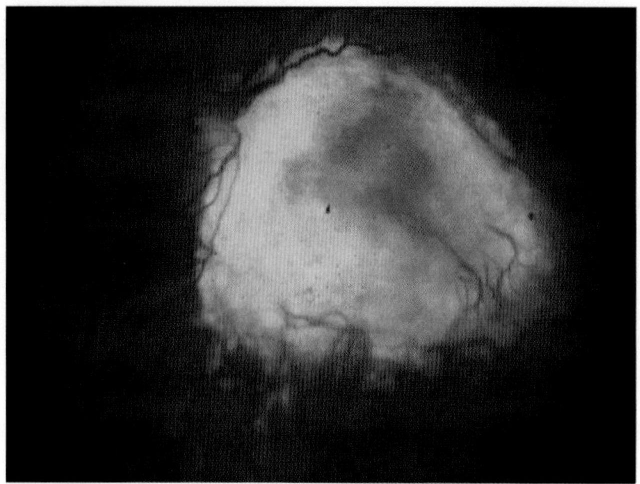

Figure 86-9 Vascular occlusion, choroidal neovascularization, and subretinal hemorrhage after low-energy, long-duration phototherapy of a choroidal melanoma.

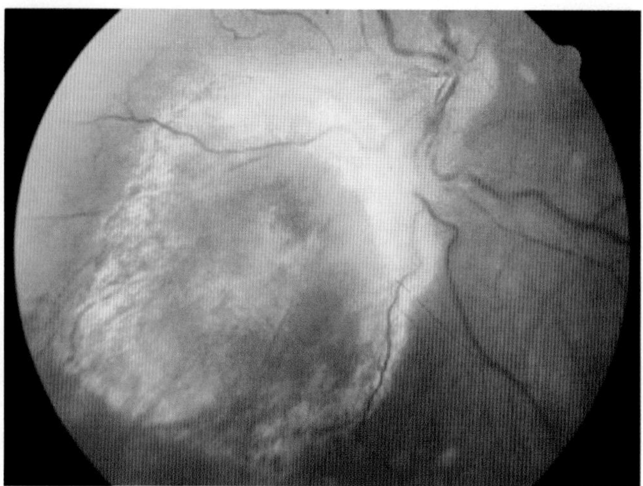

Figure 86-10 Retinal traction after low-energy, long-duration phototherapy of a choroidal melanoma.

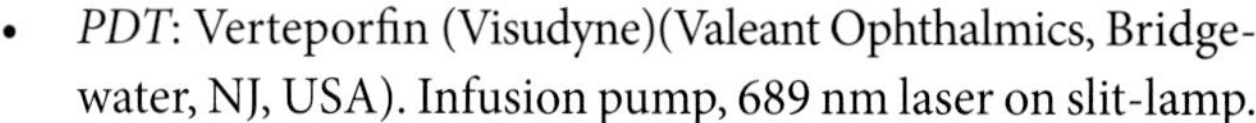

- *PDT*: Verteporfin (Visudyne)(Valeant Ophthalmics, Bridgewater, NJ, USA). Infusion pump, 689 nm laser on slit-lamp.

## COMPLICATIONS

- Recurrent or persistent tumor can occur if treatment is insufficient or if the tumor extent is underestimated.
- Seeding of retinoblastoma cells can occur if excessive light energy is used.
- Thermal complications include:
  - Retinal vascular occlusion, possibly with neovascularization (Fig. 86-9).
  - Retinal traction if excessive energy is used (Fig. 86-10).
  - Iris burns, causing posterior synechiae and cataract.
  - Choroidal atrophy and visual loss if PDT is administered to the fovea.[20]
- Complications from photodynamic agents can occur.[21] These include:
  - Edema/pain/hemorrhage at the injection site.
  - Photosensitivity reaction (sunburn).
  - Infusion-related back pain.

## SURGICAL OUTCOME: SCIENTIFIC EVIDENCE/META-ANALYSIS

### Photocoagulation

- Selected retinoblastomas usually respond to photocoagulation, either administered alone or in combination with chemotherapy.[22]
- Small choroidal melanomas may respond to photocoagulation but with high rate of local tumor recurrence, neovascularization, retinal traction, and other complications.[23,24]
- Small retinal hemangioblastomas usually undergo fibrosis with photocoagulation but treatment may need to be repeated several times.[2]

### Transpupillary Thermotherapy

- Retinoblastoma is widely treated with TTT, usually but not always administered in association with chemotherapy.[25-27]
- Choroidal melanoma usually responds to TTT, if small, but there is a significant recurrence rate.[6]

### Photodynamic Therapy

- Choroidal hemangioma is widely treated with PDT, having become the first-line treatment in most centers.[28] This treatment can also be effective with some diffuse choroidal hemangiomas.[10]
- Amelanotic choroidal melanoma has been treated successfully with PDT but experience is limited.[13]
- Choroidal osteoma can regress after PDT, which has been used to prevent foveal involvement.[16] PDT may also be effective for choroidal neovascular membranes arising from osteoma.

## PLACE OF THE TECHNIQUE IN SURGICAL ARMAMENTARIUM

- *Primary treatment*: The various forms of phototherapy are useful for selected, small tumors in the hope of avoiding the need for more harmful modalities such as radiotherapy and local resection.

- *Secondary treatment*: The different forms of phototherapy can be useful for treating radiation-induced complications, such as macular edema and recurrent hyphema, as an alternative to intravitreal injections of antiangiogenic agents.

## PEARLS AND PITFALLS

- Wide safety margins are required for malignant tumors, unless previous radiotherapy has been administered.
- Assuming proper case selection, complications arise because of excessive energy or an insufficient number of treatment sessions.

## REFERENCES


1. Palmer JD, Gragoudas ES. Advances in treatment of retinal angiomas. Int Ophthalmol Clin. 1997;37(4):159-70.
2. Singh AD, Shields CL, Shields JA. von Hippel-Lindau disease. Surv Ophthalmol. 2001;46(2):117-42.
3. Damato B. Ocular Tumours: Diagnosis and Treatment. Oxford: Butterworth-Heinemann; 2000.
4. Shields JA, Shields CL, De Potter P. Photocoagulation of retinoblastoma. Int Ophthalmol Clin. 1993;33(3):95-9.
5. Damato B, Groenewald C, McGalliard J, et al. Endoresection of choroidal melanoma. Br J Ophthalmol 1998; 82(3):213-8.
6. Shields CL, Shields JA, Perez N, et al. Primary transpupillary thermotherapy for small choroidal melanoma in 256 consecutive cases: outcomes and limitations. Ophthalmology. 2002; 109(2):225-34.
7. Damato B. Vasculopathy After Treatment of Choroidal Melanoma. In: Joussen A, Gardner TW, Kirchhof B, Ryan SJ. (eds). Retinal Vascular Disease. Berlin: Springer; 2007. pp. 582-91.
8. Puri P, Gupta M, Rundle PA, et al. Indocyanine green augmented transpupillary thermotherapy in the management of choroidal metastasis from breast carcinoma. Eye (Lond). 2001;15 (Pt 4):515-8.
9. Blasi MA, Tiberti AC, Scupola A, et al. Photodynamic therapy with verteporfin for symptomatic circumscribed choroidal hemangioma: five-year outcomes. Ophthalmology. 2010; 117(8):1630-37.
10. Ang M, Lee SY. Multifocal photodynamic therapy for diffuse choroidal hemangioma. Clin Ophthalmol. 2012;6:1467-9.
11. Blasi MA, Scupola A, Tiberti AC, et al. Photodynamic therapy for vasoproliferative retinal tumors. Retina. 2006;26(4):404-9.
12. Papastefanou VP, Pilli S, Stinghe A, et al. Photodynamic therapy for retinal capillary hemangioma. Eye (Lond). 2013;27(3):438-42.
13. Tuncer S, Kir N, Shields CL. Dramatic regression of amelanotic choroidal melanoma with PDT following poor response to brachytherapy. Ophthalmic Surg Lasers Imaging: The Official journal of the International Society for Imaging in the Eye. 2012;43(3):e38-40.
14. Trichopoulos N, Damato B. Photodynamic therapy for recurrent hyphema after proton beam radiotherapy of iris melanoma. Graefe's Arch Clin Exp Ophthalmol = Albrecht von Graefes Archiv fur klinische und experimentelle Ophthalmologie. 2007;245(10):1573-5.
15. Isola V, Pece A, Pierro L. Photodynamic therapy with verteporfin of choroidal malignancy from breast cancer. Am J Ophthalmol. 2006;142(5):885-7.
16. Shields CL, Materin MA, Mehta S, et al. Regression of extrafoveal choroidal osteoma following photodynamic therapy. Arch Ophthalmol. 2008;126(1):135-7.
17. Shields CL, Shields JA. Retinoblastoma management: advances in enucleation, intravenous chemoreduction, and intra-arterial chemotherapy. Curr Opin Ophthalmol. 2010;21(3):203-12.
18. Francis JH1, Abramson DH, Brodie SE, et al. Indocyanine green enhanced transpupillary thermotherapy in combination with ophthalmic artery chemosurgery for retinoblastoma. Br J Ophthalmol. 2013 Feb;97(2):164-8.
19. Tsipursky MS, Golchet PR, Jampol LM. Photodynamic therapy of choroidal hemangioma in Sturge-Weber syndrome, with a review of treatments for diffuse and circumscribed choroidal hemangiomas. Surv Ophthalmol. 2011;56(1):68-85.
20. Figurska M, Wierzbowska J, Robaszkiewicz J. Severe decrease in visual acuity with choroidal hypoperfusion after photodynamic therapy. Med Sci Monit: International Medical Journal of Experimental and Clinical Research. 2011;17(6): CS75-79.
21. Verteporfin Roundtable P. Guidelines for using verteporfin (Visudyne) in photodynamic therapy for choroidal neovascularization due to age-related macular degeneration and other causes: update. Retina. 2005;25(2):119-34.
22. Shields JA, Shields CL, Parsons H, et al. The role of photocoagulation in the management of retinoblastoma. Arch Ophthalmol. 1990;108(2):205-8.
23. Shields JA, Glazer LC, Mieler WF, et al. Comparison of xenon arc and argon laser photocoagulation in the treatment of choroidal melanomas. Am J Ophthalmol. 1990;109(6):647-55.
24. Foulds WS, Damato BE. Low-energy long-exposure laser therapy in the management of choroidal melanoma. Graefe's Arch Clin Exp Ophthalmol. = Albrecht von Graefes Archiv fur klinische und experimentelle Ophthalmologie 1986;224(1):26-31.
25. Shields CL, Palamar M, Sharma P, et al. Retinoblastoma regression patterns following chemoreduction and adjuvant therapy in 557 tumors. Arch Ophthalmol. 2009;127(3):282-90.
26. Lumbroso L, Doz F, Levy C, et al. [Diode laser thermotherapy and chemothermotherapy in the treatment of retinoblastoma]. J Francais d'Ophtalmologie 2003;26(2):154-9.
27. Abramson DH, Schefler AC. Transpupillary thermotherapy as initial treatment for small intraocular retinoblastoma: technique and predictors of success. Ophthalmology. 2004;111(5):984-91.
28. Elizalde J, Vasquez L, Iyo F, Abengoechea S. Photodynamic therapy in the management of circumscribed choroidal hemangioma. Can J Ophthalmol. Journal Canadien d'ophtalmologie. 2012;47(1):16-20.

CHAPTER

87

# Brachytherapy

Sonia Callejo, Bertil Damato

## INTRODUCTION

Brachytherapy is defined as radiotherapy in which the source of radiation is placed close to the target. Most ocular brachytherapy is delivered with a plaque-shaped applicator, which is placed adjacent to the tumor. The objective is to administer high doses of radiation to the tumor while sparing adjacent healthy tissues.

A variety of radioactive isotopes are used, which include strontium-90, ruthenium-106, iodine-125 and palladium-103.[1-6]

Much of the success of brachytherapy depends on the skills of the surgeon and the techniques used to position the plaque accurately in relation to the tumor.

## INDICATIONS

- *Uveal melanomas*: Primary therapy for small-sized uveal melanoma with documented growth and medium-sized choroidal and ciliary body melanomas; in some centers, iris melanomas deemed unsuitable for resection;[7] adjunctive treatment after transpupillary thermotherapy (i.e. "sandwich technique") or local resection.[8,9]
- *Invasive conjunctival melanomas and carcinomas*: Adjunctive therapy after excision.[10]
- *Retinoblastoma*: Primary or secondary treatment of tumor greater than 4 mm in thickness with or without localized vitreous seeding.[11,12]
- *Retinal hemangioblastomas*: Large tumors unlikely to respond to phototherapy.[13]
- *Vasoproliferative tumors*: Salvage therapy if photodynamic therapy fails.[14]
- *Choroidal metastases*: Brachytherapy has the advantage of being completed in a few days, avoiding the need for a prolonged course of external beam radiotherapy.[15]

## CONTRAINDICATIONS

- *Choroidal melanoma*: Extensive diffuse tumor; bulky extraocular spread, unless this tumor is resectable;[16] optic disk involvement, unless adjunctive transpupillary thermotherapy is administered or a notched plaque used;[17] extensive, diffuse iris melanoma.
- *Retinoblastoma*: Tumor exceeding 18 mm in diameter and/or thickness greater than 8 mm; proximity to optic disk and/or fovea; widespread vitreous seeding.[12,18]
- *Conjunctival tumors*: Noninvasive tumors; tumors involving fornix unless an unshielded iodine plaque is used; caruncular and tarsal conjunctival tumors, which are treated more easily by some form of teletherapy.

## PREOPERATIVE CARE

Accurate measurements of longitudinal basal diameter and tumor thickness by standardized A-scan and/or B-scan ultrasonography are essential. It is also useful to measure the distance between the tumor and the optic disk.

### Plaque Selection

Ruthenium plaques are used for tumors not exceeding 5 mm in thickness. Iodine plaques enable treatment of tumors up to 10 mm in thickness.

The size of a plaque is generally 4 mm larger than the largest tumor dimension to include tapering tumor edges and allow for imprecision in plaque placement and plaque movement.[19] We select a 15 mm ruthenium CCA plaque for tumors up to 11 mm in basal diameter, a 20 mm CCB plaque for tumors having a basal diameter of 10–16 mm, and a 25 mm CCC plaque for tumors up to 21 mm in diameter (BEBIG GmbH, Berlin, Germany) (Fig. 87-1).

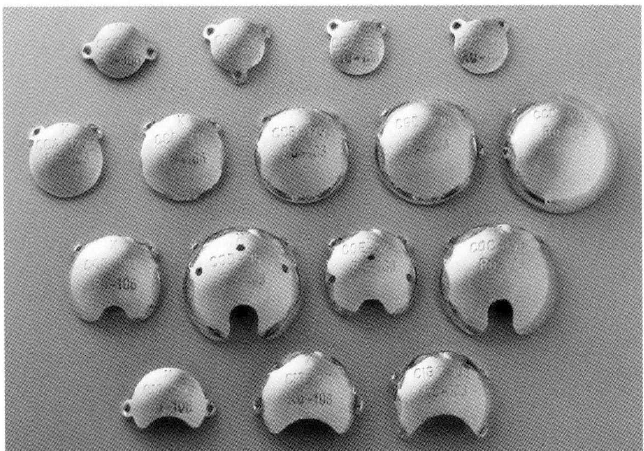

**Figure 87-1** Ruthenium-106 plaques, with diameters ranging from 11.6 mm to 25.4 mm. Some plaques have a crescent for the ciliary body or a notch for the optic nerve. The total thickness of the ruthenium plaque is 1 mm.

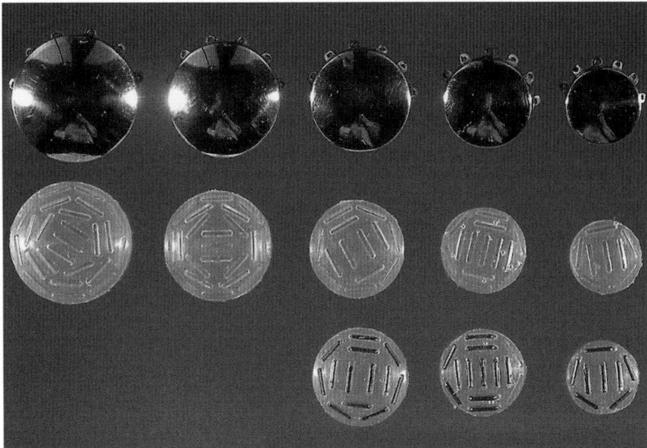

**Figure 87-2** Iodine-125 COMS plaques: are available in diameters of 12, 14, 16, 18 and 20 mm. (Upper row) they are composed of a circular outer bowl-shape surface lined with gold to prevent radiating tissues outside the eye. The lugs at the anterior border of the plaque are used to suture the plaque to the sclera. (Middle row) corresponding circular siliastic carrier with linear striations. (Bottom row) three siliastic carriers loaded with I-125 seeds on inside surface.
*Source* Photo courtesy of Dr Christine Corriveau, Montreal, Canada.

Iodine-125 Collaborative Ocular Melanoma Study (COMS) plaques are circular and are available in diameters of 12, 14, 16, 18 and 20 mm (Fig. 87-2). Notched iodine or ruthenium plaques can be used for the treatment of peripapillary tumors. Crescent-shaped plaques are also available for the management of ciliary body lesions.

## Dosimetry

Historically, 100 Gy to the apex of the tumor (or to a 5-mm depth for a tumor less than 5 mm in height) was prescribed until 1995, when the dose was reduced to 85 Gy to the apex.

The dosimetry for ruthenium treatment is performed using software such as the Astrahan program.[20] We prescribe a minimum of 350 Gy to the scleral surface and a minimum of 85 Gy to the tumor apex. This scleral dose ensures that visible choroidal atrophy develops after a few months.

Iodine-125 was the only isotope used in the COMS. An updated version of the original COMS calculations system still remains as the most commonly-used planning tool for iodine treatment. The COMS dose is 85 Gy to the tumor apex allowing for a dose rate between 0.60 and 1.05 Gy/h to the prescription point. The total dose is delivered in 3–7 consecutive days. The COMS dosimetry included point source approximation, no anisotropy and no effects from the gold shield or the silastic insert. Planning systems such as Plaque Simulator (227 BEBIG GmbH, Berlin, Germany) are now commonly used and take into account all variables that were excluded from the original COMS calculations.

If the brachytherapy is administered as an adjunct to excision of a uveal or conjunctival melanoma, we administer a dose of 100 Gy to a depth of 1 mm.

## Preplanning

Ruthenium has a half-life of 368 days. Plaques can be reused during this period and are, therefore, readily available.

Iodine has a half-life of 59.4 days and plaques are custom-made for individual treatments. During the pretreatment planning, the number and strength of the seeds, tumor coverage and duration of the treatment are estimated. By varying the number and/or strength of each seed, the duration of the treatment can be manipulated to take into account, for instance, of operating room availability. The plaques can be loaded symmetrically with single activity seeds or asymmetrically with seed activity ranging from 0.5 to 7 millicurie. The seed arrangement and strength can be adjusted to minimize radiation to critical structures or to ensure adequate radiation dose along the posterior plaque edge. I-125 seeds are placed in a silastic insert and cemented into a gold shield using methyl methacrylate. The plaque undergoes gas or steam sterilization prior to insertion. The preplanning process may take between 2 and 4 weeks depending on seed availability.

# SURGICAL TECHNIQUE

## Ruthenium Plaque

The pupil is dilated with 1% cyclopentolate and 2.5% phenylephrine.

*Anesthesia:* Plaque insertion can be done under general anesthesia to facilitate correct positioning. Local anesthesia is preferred by some surgeons. Local radiation safety regulations will dictate whether brachytherapy can be performed as an outpatient or inpatient procedure.

*Exposure:* A 180° conjunctival peritomy is made. Two traction sutures are placed in the sclera, 4 mm from limbus.

Any rectus or inferior oblique muscles impeding accurate plaque placement are retracted or disinserted after measuring the distance between the muscle knot and the limbus. The superior oblique muscle is thin and can usually be compressed against the globe using a mattress suture over the plaque.

*Tumor delineation:* The tumor limits are defined by trans-pupillary and trans-scleral transillumination, using a 20-gauge, vitrectomy transilluminator with the tip pre-bent 90°. Care is taken to avoid oblique transillumination, which exaggerates the apparent tumor extent.

*Template placement:* Templates have the same shape and size as the radioactive plaque and allow for surgical manipulations without exposing the surgical team to unnecessary radiation. With tumors extending far posteriorly, we prefer to position the plaque eccentrically, with its posterior edge aligned with the posterior tumor margin.[3,21] This allows a higher dose of radiation to be given while reducing the risk of collateral damage to optic disk and fovea. Eccentric plaque placement is safe only if the applicator can be positioned precisely in relation to the tumor. This section describes our technique for achieving such precision.

The intended location of the anterior plaque edge is marked on the sclera with a pen. This is determined by subtracting the longitudinal basal tumor diameter from the plaque diameter and then adjusting for the desired physical overlap of the tumor by the plaque posteriorly. For example, if the longitudinal tumor diameter is 9 mm and the plaque diameter is 15 mm, then the mark on the sclera should be placed 6 mm anterior to the anterior tumor margin if no posterior safety margin is intended. If a 2-mm posterior safety margin is desired, this mark should be placed 4 mm anterior to the anterior tumor margin.

A plaque template is sutured to the sclera so that its anterior edge is aligned with the scleral ink-mark. The position of the template in relation to the tumor is checked by transillumination. This is performed by placing the tip of a right-angled, 20-gauge fiberoptic light through a hole near the posterior margin of the template and performing binocular indirect ophthalmoscopy (Figs. 87-3A to C). If no safety margin is intended, the fiberoptic light is visible at the posterior tumor margin ("sunset sign"). If a 2-mm safety margin is intended, this transilluminated spot of light is visible 2 mm posterior to the posterior tumor margin.

*Trans-scleral biopsy:* Any trans-scleral tumor biopsy is performed at this stage.

*Radioactive plaque insertion:* The radioactive plaque is tethered to the sclera using the same sutures as used to fix the template. First, the plaque is fixed in place with the mattress suture, so that its anterior edge is aligned with the scleral ink-mark. Next, the lug sutures are tightened and adjusted to ensure that the plaque is fixed in its desired position (Fig. 87-4A).

The usual purpose of the mattress suture is to ensure that the entire plaque is tightly apposed to the globe. This happens if the mattress suture is located at the plaque equator or more posteriorly. If the mattress suture is anterior to the plaque equator, it can flatten that part of the globe so that the posterior part of the plaque is "levered" away from the ocular surface. This plaque "tilting" effect can be exploited so as to reduce the dose to the fovea if the posterior tumor margin is tapering and thin.

*Muscle repositioning:* Any disinserted muscles are sutured to their original insertions so that the distances from the intramuscular knots to the limbus are the same as before disinsertion.

*Transretinal biopsy:* If transretinal biopsy is preferred, it can be performed at this stage, when any vitreous hemorrhage would not interfere with the plaque placement.

*Conjunctival closure:* The conjunctiva is closed in the usual fashion.

*Plaque removal:* The conjunctival sutures are removed. If necessary, the muscle sutures are divided so as to enhance access to the plaque. Fresh muscle sutures are placed around the old suture knots. The old sutures are left in the muscle to prevent the muscle from fraying.

One lug of the plaque is grasped with St Martin's forceps and the eye is rotated while retracting the conjunctiva. The mattress suture and then the two lug sutures are cut and removed. The plaque is removed. Any disinserted muscles are reinserted, respecting the original knot-to-limbus distances. The inferior oblique muscle is not reinserted. The conjunctiva is closed, ensuring that no sclera is left exposed.

## Iodine Plaque

*Dilation, anesthesia, exposure and tumor delineation*: These are achieved as described for ruthenium plaques.

*Template placement:* The template is placed on the sclera with its anterior edge overhanging the anterior edge of the tumor by 2 mm. Two or three out of six small lugs that cover the anterior half of the plaque are used to secure the plaque to the sclera using releasable knots.

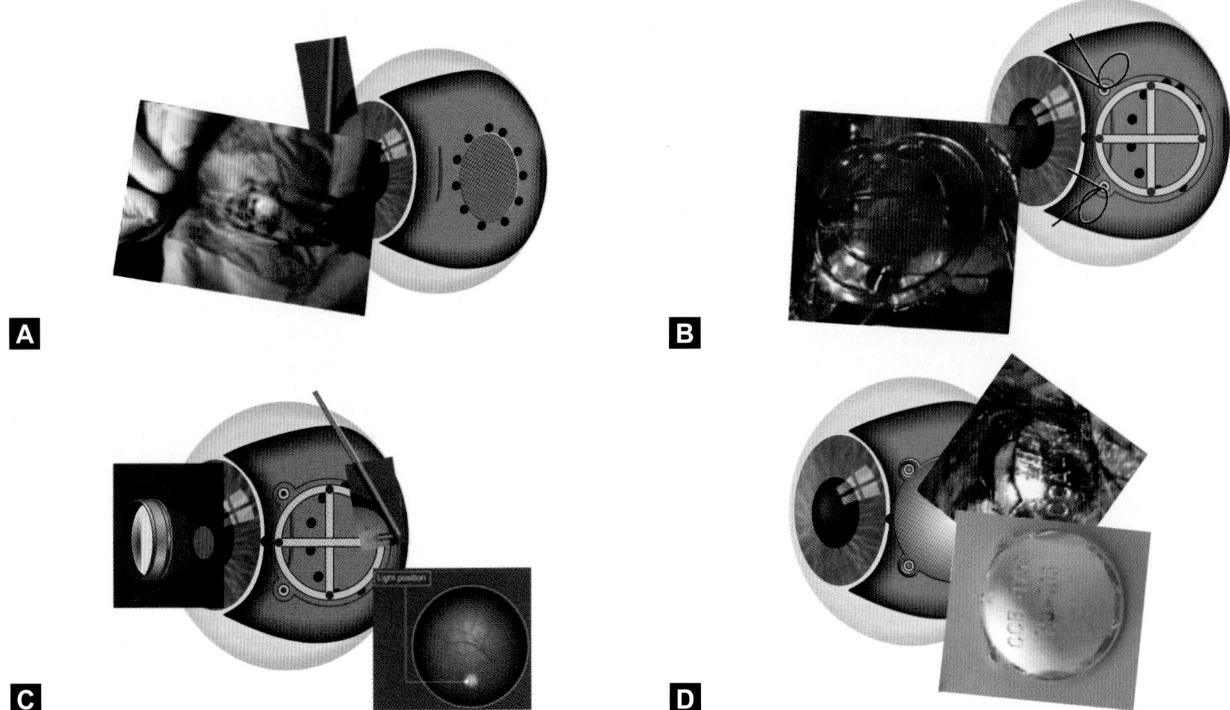


**Figures 87-3A to D** Ruthenium plaque template with perforations and grooves for positioning a right-angled 20-gauge transilluminator. (A) The tumor is localized by shining a light through the pupil with a right-angled transilluminator; (B) A transparent dummy plaque is placed over the tumor and sutured to the eye with a bow; (C) The right-angled transilluminator is shone through each hole in the dummy plaque and binocular indirect ophthalmoscopy is performed so that a light is visible at the back of the eye near the tumor edge; (D) The dummy plaque is replaced with the radioactive plaque (The color photographs are only to show the real thing. Please shift to look beneath).

The position of the template in relation to the tumor is assessed by intraoperative ultrasound with the probe in direct contact with the globe under sterile conditions. The plaque produces a well-demarcated orbital shadow with distinct borders. The relationship between this orbital shadowing and the tumor margins can be assessed in both transverse and longitudinal views.

*Trans-scleral biopsy:* can be performed at this stage as previously described.

*Radioactive plaque insertion:* When the position of the template is satisfactory, the template can be replaced by the radioactive plaque using the preplaced releasable sutures (Fig. 87-4B). At this stage, intraoperative ultrasound can be repeated.

*Muscle repositioning and conjunctival closure:* These are achieved as described for ruthenium plaques. The eye may be covered with a lead shield.

*Plaque removal:* The surgical procedure is as described for ruthenium plaques. Immediately following removal of the plaque, the level of radioactivity is verified to ensure complete removal of all radioactive material. The iodine plaque is also examined to ensure that all seeds have remained attached to the silastic insert.

## MECHANISM OF ACTION

Brachytherapy delivers continuous radiation at a low dose and with a conformal dose distribution, which minimizes collateral damage to the surrounding normal tissue. Ruthenium is mostly a beta-ray emitter as opposed to I-125 sources, which emit gamma irradiation with deeper penetration.

The effects of the plaque depend on the distance from the internal plaque surface. Near the tumor apex, the ionizing radiation mostly affects the tumor DNA, preventing tumor cell proliferation and inducing senescence and apoptosis. Closer to the plaque, where the tumor doses are higher, there is more membrane disruption, inducing immediate cell death. With very high basal doses, particularly with ruthenium plaque radiotherapy, there is also vascular obliteration, resulting in tumor infarction. Lower doses of radiation cause delayed vascular incompetence, with ischemia and exudation, resulting in exudation, macular edema, hard exudates, retinal detachment, and possibly neovascular glaucoma (i.e. "toxic tumor syndrome").

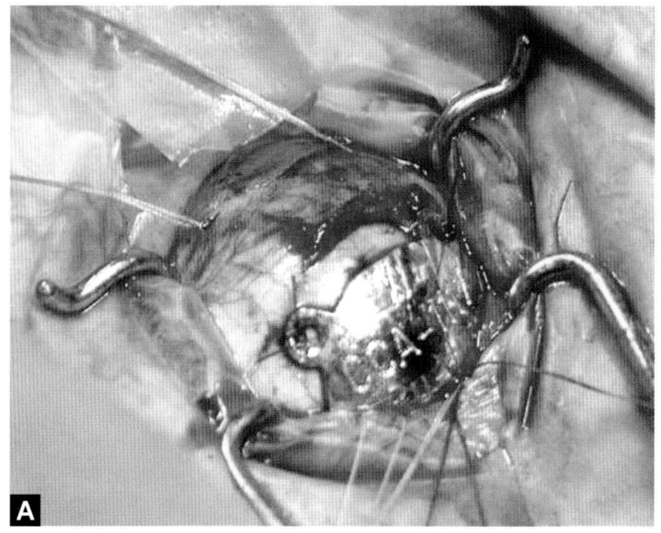
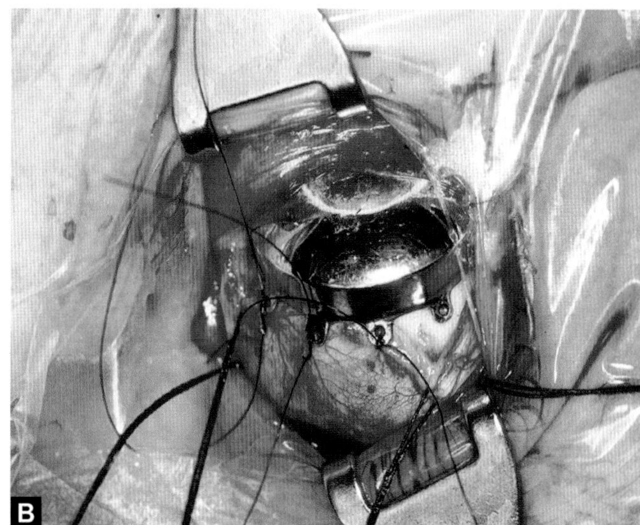

Figures 87-4A and B Intraoperative photographs showing a ruthenium-106 plaque (A) and an iodine-125 plaque in position.
*Source* Photo courtesy of Dr Christine Corriveau, Montreal, Canada (B).

## POSTOPERATIVE CARE

At the end of the surgical procedure, antibiotic and mydriatic drops are instilled. A long-acting local anesthetic is injected under the conjunctival flap to reduce postoperative pain.

Follow-up examinations are scheduled 4 weeks postoperatively and every 3 months during the first year, every 6 months for 5 years and yearly thereafter. Tumor regression may not be apparent in the first 3–6 months following treatment.

Long-term surveillance for tumor recurrence and radiation-induced complications is performed as usual. The tumor margins and thickness are monitored by sequential color photography and ultrasonography respectively.

Psychological support and systemic screening for metastatic disease are undertaken in the usual manner.

## SPECIFIC INSTRUMENTATION

### Radioactive Applicators

- *Ruthenium plaque*: This plaque has an outer silver shell (0.9-mm thick) and a layer of ruthenium-106 painted on the inner surface of the shell, sealed with a 0.1-mm coating of silver.
- *Iodine plaque*: This has a gold or steel shell housing an average of 13 radioactive seeds. The seeds are kept in place by resin or a silastic insert. A lip at the shell margin collimates the radiation to reduce side scatter.
- *Other isotopes*: These include strontium, palladium and iridium.

Templates are widely used to reduce exposure of staff to radiation.

## COMPLICATIONS

### Intraoperative Complications

- Inaccurate localization of tumor, because of poor ultrasonography or transillumination technique.
- Scleral perforation and retinal tear if any scleral sutures are placed too deeply. Cryotherapy or binocular indirect laser retinopexy is then performed to prevent retinal detachment.
- *Damage to a ruthenium plaque*: Special care must be taken to avoid scratching the inner ruthenium plaque surface.

### Postoperative Complications

- *Local tumor recurrence*: This can be central, if the tumor apex has received an inadequate dose of radiation, or marginal if the plaque was inadequately positioned in relation to the tumor ("geographic miss").[22,23] This complication is treated by repeating the brachytherapy or by administering proton beam radiotherapy. Enucleation may be necessary if the recurrence is too extensive or if it involves the optic disk. Tumor recurrence is defined as a total regrowth of at least 30% of tumor thickness or at least 500 microns of tumor base recorded within two successive post-treatment visits. By these criteria, transient postirradiation tumor swelling secondary to radiation vasculopathy-induced hemorrhage are excluded.

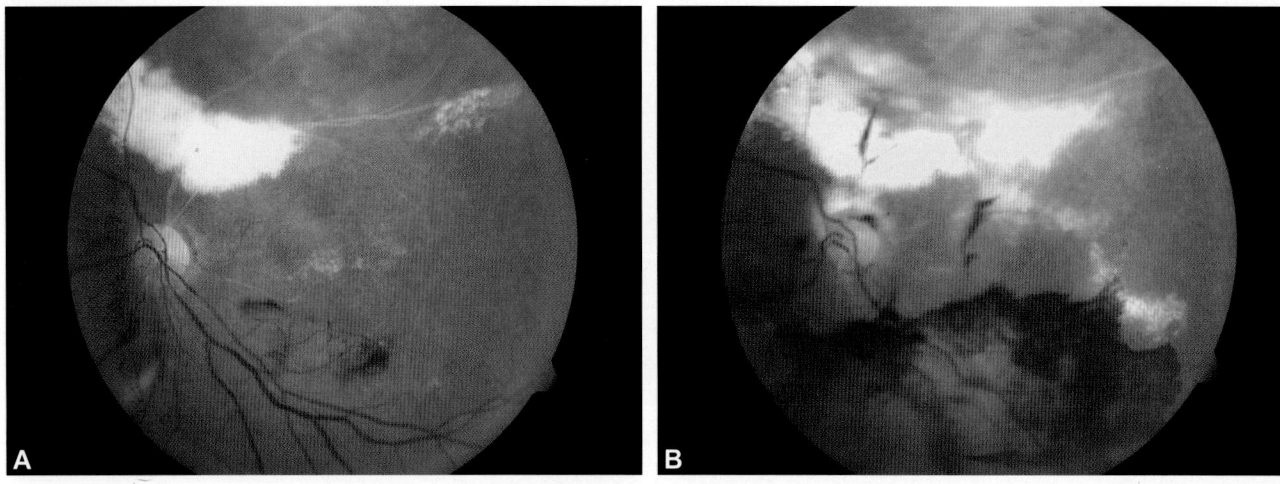


Figures 87-5A and B Fundus photograph of the left eye showing radiation retinopathy 3 years after iodine plaque radiotherapy of a superior choroidal melanoma (A). There is marked vascular attenuation along the superior arcade, neovascularization along the inferior arcade as well as retinal hemorrhages and cotton wool spots inferonasal to the disk. Subretinal exudates are also present around the tumor. The patient presented shortly after with areas of preretinal hemorrhages arising from areas of neovascularization (B).

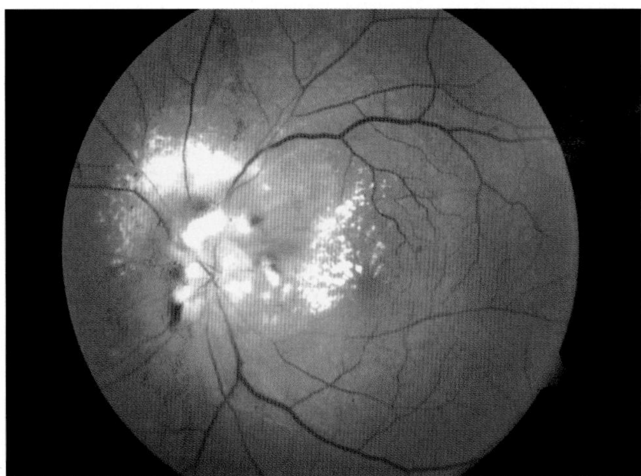

Figure 87-6 Radiation-induced optic neuropathy following treatment of a juxtapapillary choroidal melanoma located beneath the superotemporal arcade. Note the presence of cotton wool spots and hemorrhages surrounding the optic nerve, as well as associated areas of subretinal exudates. The tumor responded well to treatment.

- *Secondary enucleation*: The main causes of enucleation are local tumor recurrence and painful neovascular glaucoma.
- Radiation-induced retinopathy and maculopathy can be detected as early as 4 months after treatment, with a peak incidence between 12 and 18 months.[24] The causes of maculopathy include: (1) macular involvement by tumor; (2) collateral damage by high doses of radiation and (3) foveal damage caused by edema or exudates (Fig. 87-5). Macular edema/exudation can be treated by laser photocoagulation, photodynamic therapy, and intravitreal antiangiogenic agents. Intravitreal steroids can also be effective, but can cause cataract and/or glaucoma.
- *Radiation-induced optic neuropathy*: This is manifested by optic disk swelling, peripapillary hemorrhage, cotton wool spots, exudates and/or disk pallor (Fig. 87-6).[25] The visual outcome is usually disappointing.
- *Iris neovascularization and neovascular glaucoma*: Following I-125 brachytherapy, neovascularization of the iris correlates with larger tumor size.[24,26,27] The optimal treatment is not yet known, but panretinal photocoagulation and intraocular injections of antiangiogenic agents have been advocated.[28]
- *Toxic tumor syndrome*: It is hypothesized that the radiation vasculopathy within the residual tumor results in ischemia, exudation and production of vascular endothelial growth factor, which causes maculopathy, retinal detachment, rubeosis iridis, and neovascular glaucoma.[24] It is more commonly associated with large tumor size.
- *Radiation-induced cataract*: The incidence is highest in patients with larger tumors and tumor located anterior to the equator.
- Persistent diplopia can be managed with prisms, botulin toxic injection or surgery.
- Scleral thinning and perforation can occur if high doses of radiation are delivered to anterior sclera or if irradiated sclera is exposed because the conjunctiva is not closed properly.

## SURGICAL OUTCOMES: SCIENTIFIC EVIDENCE/METANALYSIS

Conservation of visual acuity is most likely if the tumor is small and located far from the optic disk and fovea (Fig. 87-7).[3,5] The impact of radiation on visual acuity and

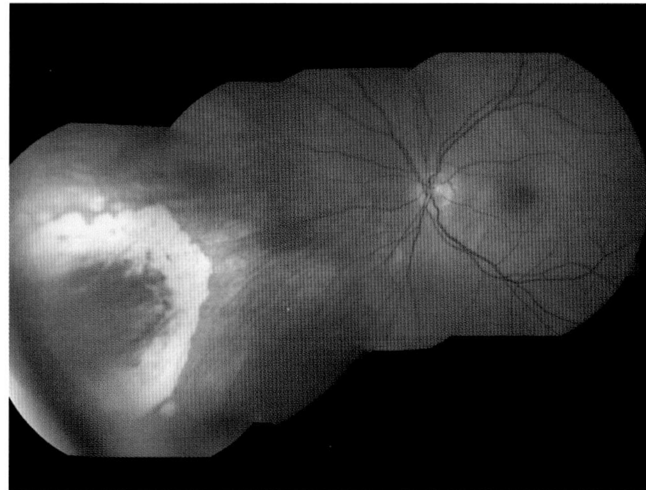

Figure 87-7 Medium-sized choroidal melanoma treated with iodine brachytherapy: Amelanotic, dome-shaped melanoma in the inferotemporal quadrant of the right eye. The tumor measured 4.3 mm in thickness and was treated with iodine plaque. One year later, the tumor exhibited signs of tumor regression evident in B-scan ultrasonography. Two years following treatment, the lesion was minimally elevated clinically and by ultrasonography.
*Source* Photos courtesy of Dr Christine Corriveau, Montreal, Canada.

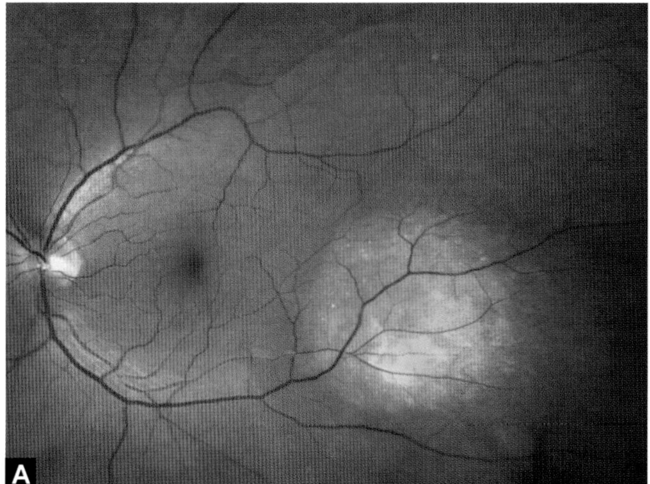


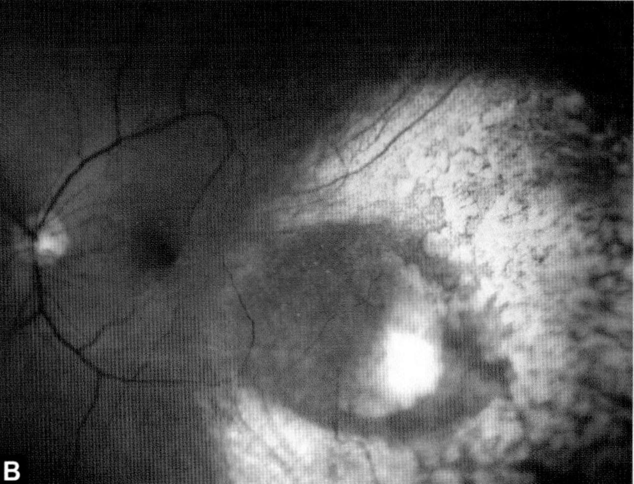


Figures 87-8A and B Choroidal melanoma in the left eye of a 65-year-old man. The tumor had a basal diameter of 11.6 mm and a thickness of 2.7 mm (A) Biopsy confirmed that the tumor was a melanoma with epithelioid cells. The patient was treated with a 20-mm ruthenium plaque, positioned eccentrically. (B) More than 2 years postoperatively, there was good local tumor control and the visual acuity was 20/30.

vision-related functioning remains a concern with I-125 treatment, with substantial visual loss of six or more lines of visual acuity from baseline in a large group of COMS-treated patients. Ru-106 brachytherapy achieves good conservation of vision if the tumor does not extend close to the optic nerve or fovea, unless eccentric plaque positioning is possible (Figs. 87-8A and B). The main risk factors associated with visual acuity loss following Ru-106 treatment are reduced initial visual acuity, posterior tumor extension, temporal tumor location, increased tumor height, and older age at treatment.

The COMS reported a 5-year local recurrence rate of 10.3% with I-125 brachytherapy. Risk factors for tumor recurrence included greater tumor thickness and proximity of the tumor to the foveal avascular zone. Tumor recurrence following Ru-106 is more common with large tumors and with tumors extending close to optic disk. A careful selection of patients will decrease the risk of tumor recurrences.

Local tumor recurrence is associated with increased mortality but it is not known whether the recurrence is the cause of the metastatic disease or merely an indicator of increased tumor malignancy.[29] Rapid tumor regression after brachytherapy is also associated with increased mortality, probably because more malignant tumors are more radiosensitive.[30,31]

The COMS demonstrated no significant difference in mortality between I-125 brachytherapy and enucleation;[4] however, the number of patients and of patients with recurrence were too small for the study to have sufficient statistical power to identify a difference.[32]

## PLACE OF THE TECHNIQUE IN SURGICAL ARMAMENTARIUM

Ruthenium plaque radiotherapy is more widely used in Europe than in other parts of the world, where iodine applicators are preferred.

Brachytherapy is our first choice of treatment for choroidal melanomas. If the risk of local tumor recurrence is considered to be greater than 5%, because of the tumor size or location, then proton beam radiotherapy or another form of treatment is selected.

When comparing plaque brachytherapy with proton beam radiotherapy, the latter has the advantage of a more homogenous dose and more sparing of normal tissue close to the tumor. Proton beam radiotherapy can cause significant damage to eyelids and canaliculus, resulting in troublesome keratitis and epiphora.

## PEARLS AND PITFALLS

- Brachytherapy of juxtapapillary tumors is difficult so that the risks of visual loss and local tumor recurrence are greater.
- With juxtafoveal tumors, eccentric placement of a ruthenium plaque can result in a better visual outcome.
- Local tumor recurrence is a more severe complication than diplopia. Any extraocular muscle interfering with accurate plaque placement should therefore be disinserted. The risk of diplopia is reduced by measuring the muscle "knot-to-limbus" distances when disinserting and reinserting muscles.
- Different methods of assessing the accuracy of plaque placement have been described. These include various forms of transillumination and ultrasonography.
- Brachytherapy implies a readiness to deal with any radiation-induced morbidity.
- Inadequate conjunctival closure may result in exposed sclera, which if irradiated can undergo necrosis and perforation.
- Safety guidelines suggest that a single surgeon can perform around 100 Ru-106 plaques and 50 Iodine I-125 plaque procedures per year.

## REFERENCES


1. Missotten L, Dirven W, Van der Schueren A, et al. Results of treatment of choroidal malignant melanoma with high-dose-rate strontium-90 brachytherapy. A retrospective study of 46 patients treated between 1983 and 1995. Graefes Arch Clin Exp Ophthalmol (Albrecht von Graefes Archiv fur klinische und experimentelle Ophthalmologie). 1998;236(3):164-73.
2. Lommatzsch PK, Werschnik C, Schuster E. Long-term follow-up of Ru-106/Rh-106 brachytherapy for posterior uveal melanoma. Graefes Arch Clin Exp Ophthalmol (Albrecht von Graefes Archiv fur klinische und experimentelle Ophthalmologie). 2000;238(2):129-37.
3. Damato B, Patel I, Campbell IR, et al. Visual acuity after Ruthenium (106) brachytherapy of choroidal melanomas. Int J Radiat Oncol Biol Phys. 2005;63(2):392-400.
4. Collaborative Ocular Melanoma Study Group. The COMS randomized trial of iodine 125 brachytherapy for choroidal melanoma: V. Twelve-year mortality rates and prognostic factors: COMS report No. 28. Arch Ophthalmol. 2006;124(12):1684-93.
5. Shields CL, Shields JA, Cater J, et al. Plaque radiotherapy for uveal melanoma: long-term visual outcome in 1106 consecutive patients. Arch Ophthalmol. 2000;118(9):1219-28.
6. Finger PT, Chin KJ, Duvall G, et al. Palladium-103 ophthalmic plaque radiation therapy for choroidal melanoma: 400 treated patients. Ophthalmol. 2009;116(4):790-6, 796 e791.
7. Shields CL, Shields JA, De Potter P, et al. Treatment of non-resectable malignant iris tumours with custom designed plaque radiotherapy. Br J Ophthalmol. 1995;79(4):306-12.
8. Bartlema YM, Oosterhuis JA, Journee-De Korver JG, et al. Combined plaque radiotherapy and transpupillary thermotherapy in choroidal melanoma: 5 years' experience. Br J Ophthalmol. 2003;87(11):1370-3.
9. Damato B. Adjunctive plaque radiotherapy after local resection of uveal melanoma. Front Radiat Ther Oncol. 1997;30:123-32.
10. Damato B, Coupland SE. An audit of conjunctival melanoma treatment in Liverpool. Eye (Lond). 2009;23(4):801-9.
11. Abouzeid H, Moeckli R, Gaillard MC, et al. (106)Ruthenium brachytherapy for retinoblastoma. Int J Radiat Oncol Biol Phys. 2008;71(3):821-8.
12. Shields CL, Mashayekhi A, Sun H, et al. Iodine 125 plaque radiotherapy as salvage treatment for retinoblastoma recurrence after chemoreduction in 84 tumors. Ophthalmology. 2006;113(11):2087-92.
13. Bastos-Carvalho A, Damato B. Images in clinical medicine. Retinal hemangioblastoma in von Hippel-Lindau disease. N Engl J Med. 2010;363(7):663.
14. Anastassiou G, Bornfeld N, Schueler AO, et al. Ruthenium-106 plaque brachytherapy for symptomatic vasoproliferative tumours of the retina. Br J Ophthalmol. 2006;90(4):447-50.
15. Shields CL, Shields JA, De Potter P, et al. Plaque radiotherapy for the management of uveal metastasis. Arch Ophthalmol. 1997;115(2):203-9.
16. Muen WJ, Damato BE. Uveal malignant melanoma with extrascleral extension, treated with plaque radiotherapy. Eye (Lond). 2007;21(2):307-8.
17. Sagoo MS, Shields CL, Mashayekhi A, et al. Plaque radiotherapy for juxtapapillary choroidal melanoma: tumor control in 650 co nsecutive cases. Ophthalmology. 2011;118(2):402-7.
18. Shields CL, Shields JA, De Potter P, et al. Plaque radiotherapy in the management of retinoblastoma. Use as a primary and secondary treatment. Ophthalmology. 1993;100(2):216-24.
19. Nag S, Quivey JM, Earle JD, et al. The American Brachytherapy Society recommendations for brachytherapy of uveal melanomas. Int J Radiat Oncol Biol Phys. 2003;56(2):544-55.

20. Astrahan MA, Luxton G, Jozsef G, et al. An interactive treatment planning system for ophthalmic plaque radiotherapy. Int J Radiat Oncol Biol Phys. 1990;18(3):679-87.
21. Russo A, Laguardia M, Damato B. Eccentric ruthenium plaque radiotherapy of posterior choroidal melanoma. Graefes Arch Clin Exp Ophthalmol (Albrecht von Graefes Archiv fur klinische und experimentelle Ophthalmologie). 2012;250(10):1533-40.
22. Jampol LM, Moy CS, Murray TG, et al. The COMS randomized trial of iodine 125 brachytherapy for choroidal melanoma: IV. Local treatment failure and enucleation in the first 5 years after brachytherapy. COMS report no. 19. Ophthalmology. 2002;109(12):2197-206.
23. Damato B, Patel I, Campbell IR, et al. Local tumor control after 106Ru brachytherapy of choroidal melanoma. Int J Radiat Oncol Biol Phys. 2005;63(2):385-91.
24. Groenewald C, Konstantinidis L, Damato B. Effects of radiotherapy on uveal melanomas and adjacent tissues. Eye (Lond). 2013;27(2):163-71.
25. Kellner U, Bornfeld N, Foerster MH. Radiation-induced optic neuropathy following brachytherapy of uveal melanomas. Graefes Arch Clin Exp Ophthalmol (Albrecht von Graefes Archiv fur klinische und experimentelle Ophthalmologie). 1993;231(5):267-70.
26. Summanen P, Immonen I, Kivela T, et al. Radiation related complications after ruthenium plaque radiotherapy of uveal melanoma. Br J Ophthalmol. 1996;80(8):732-9.
27. Detorakis ET, Engstrom RE Jr, Wallace R, et al. Iris and anterior chamber angle neovascularization after iodine 125 brachytherapy for uveal melanoma. Ophthalmology. 2005;112(3):505-10.
28. Bianciotto C, Shields CL, Kang B, et al. Treatment of iris melanoma and secondary neovascular glaucoma using bevacizumab and plaque radiotherapy. Arch Ophthalmol. 2008;126(4):578-9.
29. Vrabec TR, Augsburger JJ, Gamel JW, et al. Impact of local tumor relapse on patient survival after cobalt 60 plaque radiotherapy. Ophthalmology. 1991;98(6):984-8.
30. Augsburger JJ, Gamel JW, Shields JA, et al. Post-irradiation regression of choroidal melanomas as a risk factor for death from metastatic disease. Ophthalmology. 1987;94(9):1173-7.
31. Chappell MC, Char DH, Cole TB, et al. Uveal melanoma: molecular pattern, clinical features, and radiation response. Am J Ophthalmol. 2012;154(2):227-32.e2.
32. Damato B. Legacy of the collaborative ocular melanoma study. Arch Ophthalmol. 2007;125(7):966-8.

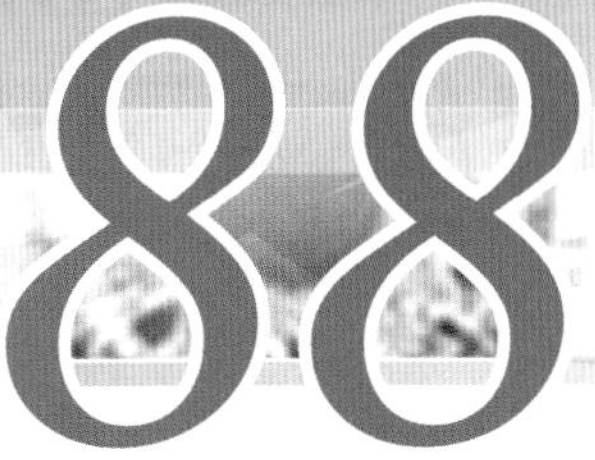


# Proton Beam Radiotherapy

Andrea Russo, Bertil Damato

## INTRODUCTION

Proton beams are highly collimated, minimizing collateral damage to adjacent healthy tissues. Furthermore, protons cause most tissue damage only at the point where they stop moving, with relative sparing of deeper and more superficial tissues from ionizing damage (i.e. Bragg Peak). Proton beam radiotherapy is becoming available in a growing number of centers around the world.

## INDICATIONS

- *Choroidal melanoma*: Some centers deploy proton beam radiotherapy for all tumors whereas others reserve this modality for tumors that cannot readily be treated with plaque radiotherapy (Figs. 88-1A and B).[1,2]
- *Iris melanoma*: Proton beam radiotherapy causes less morbidity than iridectomy and provides better dosimetry than brachytherapy.[3] For diffuse iris melanomas, some centers administer proton beam radiotherapy to the entire anterior segment of the eye, as far posterior as the ora serrata.[4]
- *Choroidal hemangioma*: Proton beam radiotherapy is effective for these tumors.[5] In many centers, however, this modality has been superseded by photodynamic therapy.
- Conjunctival melanoma, as an adjunct to excision and as an alternative to brachytherapy.[6]
- Juxtapapillary hemangioblastoma, albeit with a small chance of conserving vision.

## CONTRAINDICATIONS

- As mentioned before, some would consider proton beam radiotherapy to be contraindicated if brachytherapy is likely to provide a good result.
- Extensive uveal melanomas, if the chances of recurrent tumor and the toxic tumor syndrome are considered unacceptable.
- Juxtapapillary melanomas, if the high risk of visual loss is not accepted by the patient.

## PREOPERATIVE CARE

With choroidal melanomas, accurate measurements of basal tumor dimensions and the tumor-to-disk distance are required. Wide-angle photographs are also helpful.

Pupillary dilatation is required to enable ophthalmoscopic localization of the markers in relation to choroidal tumor margins.

## TECHNIQUE

### Marker Insertion

The tumor is localized by transillumination and/or indentation. Damato has designed a disposable transilluminator that shines light through the perforations of the tantalum markers, facilitating localization by binocular indirect ophthalmoscopy (Fig. 88-2) (Altomed, Tyne and Wear, UK). Between 3 and 5 tantalum markers are sutured to the sclera at known distances from the tumor margin, from each other, and from the limbus (Figs. 88-3A to E).

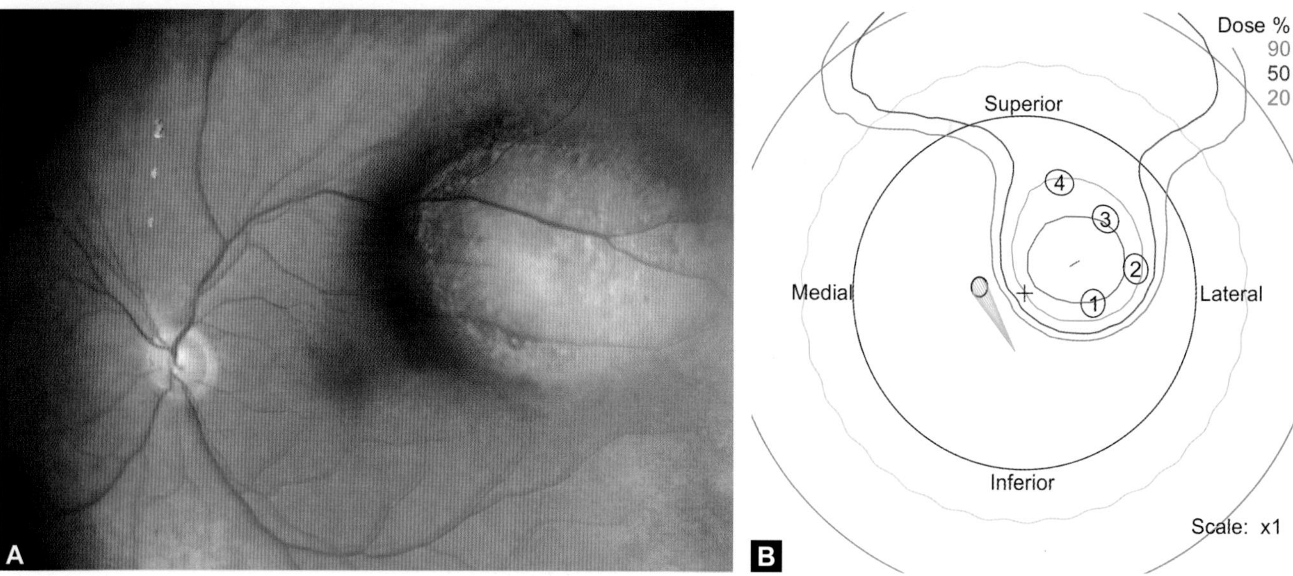


**Figures 88-1A and B** Left fundus of a 67-year-old man with a superotemporal choroidal melanoma with a basal diameter of 9.1 mm and a thickness of 2.8 mm (A). The patient received proton beam radiotherapy, which was delivered through the closed upper eyelid so as not to irradiate the lid margin, thereby preventing keratinization of the superior tarsal conjunctiva, which is painful on blinking (B). Biopsy was performed on completion of the radiotherapy and showed the tumor to be of mixed cell type. Genetic studies showed chromosome 6p gain with no chromosome 3 loss and no chromosome 8q gain, hence indicating an excellent prognosis for survival. More than 3.5 years after radiotherapy, the visual acuity was 20/20 and the tumor was inactive.
*Source* Treatment plans courtesy of The National Centre for Eye Proton Therapy at The Clatterbridge Cancer Centre, UK.

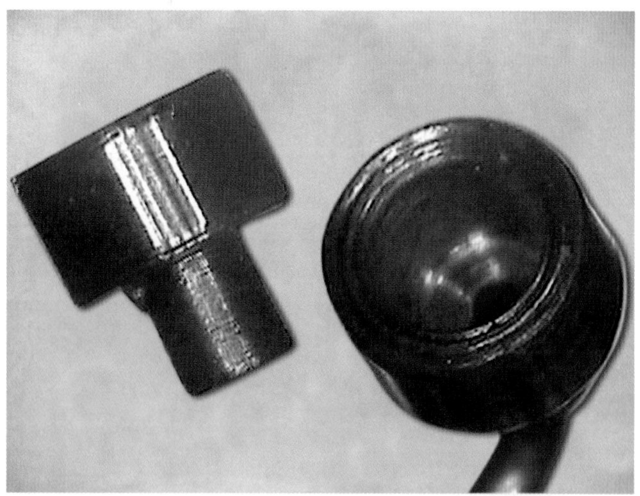

**Figure 88-2** Disposable, right-angled fiberoptic transilluminator (developed by Damato), which is designed to fit over the tantalum marker, so that the marker can be localized intraoperatively by binocular indirect ophthalmoscopy.

### Simulation

A 3-D computer model of the eye is created, complete with tumor, markers and proton beam. The modeling is based on echographic measurements of tumor and ocular dimensions as well as radiographic and intraoperative localization of tantalum markers (Figs. 88-4A to D). With iris melanomas, the tumor localization is based on color photographs without using tantalum markers (Figs. 88-5A to D).

### Treatment

The protocol varies between centers. In Liverpool, the proton beam radiotherapy is delivered in four fractions, administered on consecutive days, to a total dose of 53–70 Gy. During each treatment, the patient is asked to gaze at a fixation target, with the treated eye or the fellow eye. The ocular position is monitored with a closed-circuit TV camera. The tumor is treated together with a 2.5-mm surround of healthy tissue.

## MECHANISM OF ACTION

As with other forms of radiotherapy, protons kill target cells by ionizing molecules of DNA and cell membranes.

## POSTOPERATIVE CARE

In some centers, prognostic biopsy is performed as described in Chapter 85. This is done on the last day of the proton beam radiotherapy, or within a week afterwards to avoid any risk of tumor seeding and to prevent any hemorrhage from disrupting the radiotherapy.

Patients are followed up as for other forms of treatment.

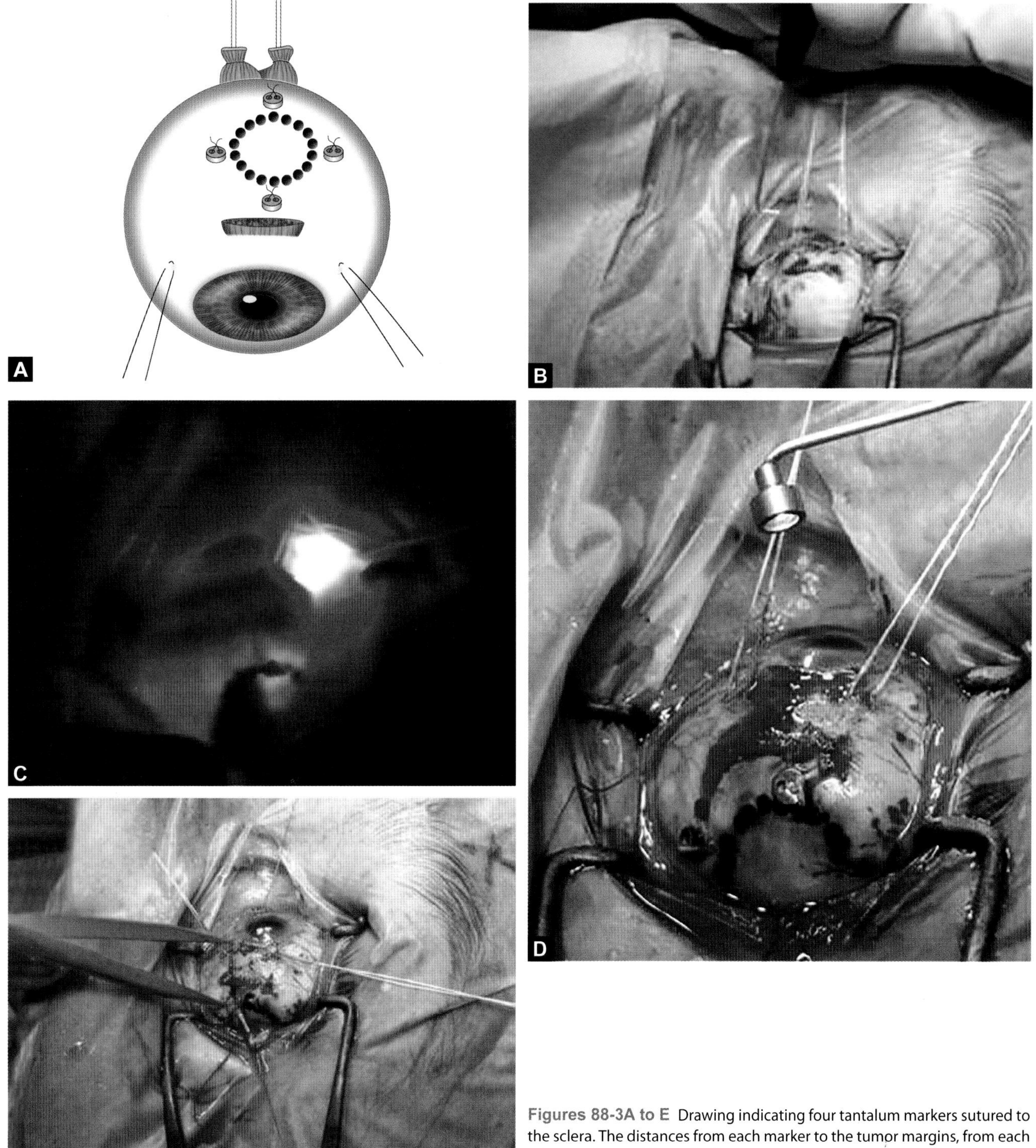


Figures 88-3A to E Drawing indicating four tantalum markers sutured to the sclera. The distances from each marker to the tumor margins, from each other marker and from the limbus are measured to enable a 3-D computer model of the eye to be generated.

## SPECIFIC INSTRUMENTATION

- Tantalum markers
- Transilluminators
- Callipers.

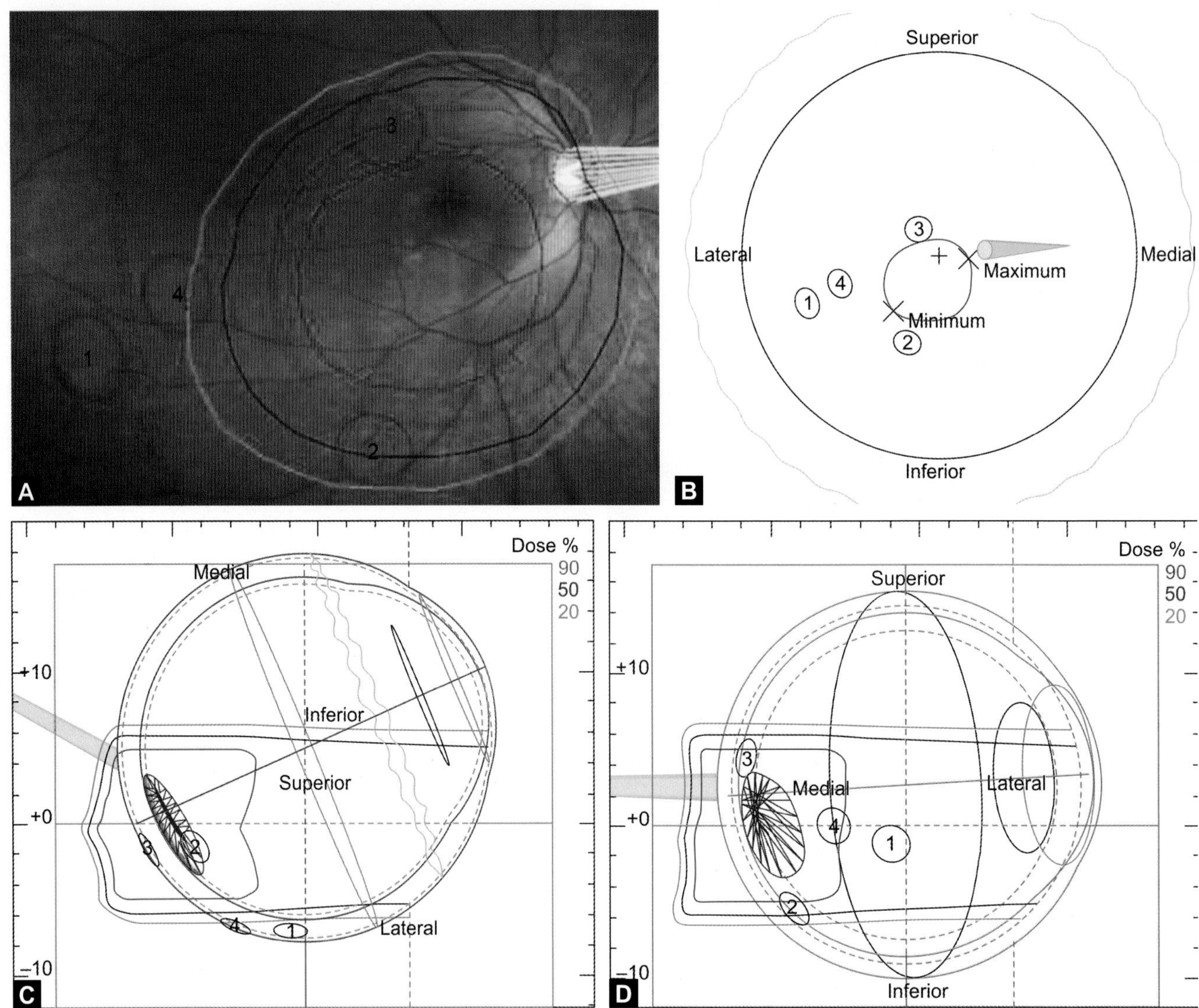


**Figures 88-4A to D** Treatment plans for a macular melanoma in the right eye.
*Source* Treatment plans courtesy of The National Centre for Eye Proton Therapy at The Clatterbridge Cancer Centre, UK.

## COMPLICATIONS

- Optic neuropathy is most likely to occur if the tumor extends to within one disk diameter of the optic disk margin (Fig. 88-6).[7]
- Maculopathy can be caused by direct collateral damage to the fovea or by exudation from the irradiated tumor.[1]
- Cataract is likely if the proton beam involves the lens.
- Serous retinal detachment, which is most likely to develop after radiotherapy of a bulky tumor. This can be treated by excising the irradiated tumor.
- Neovascular glaucoma can occur as a result of optic neuropathy or extensive exudative retinal detachment.[8] The neovascularization tends to regress after intraocular injection of antiangiogenic agents, such as bevacizumab.[9]
- Keratopathy can be secondary to limbal stem cell failure or superior tarsal conjunctival metaplasia with keratinization.
- Local tumor recurrence can develop because of undetected lateral tumor extension or because of inaccurate tumor localization. Marginal tumor recurrence is most likely to occur with diffuse iris melanomas (which is why whole anterior segment radiotherapy is advocated in such cases) and with ciliary body melanomas.[4,10]
- Eyelid damage can occur if the lid margin cannot be completely retracted out of the proton beam. This results in madarosis, poliosis, and squamous metaplasia of the tarsal conjunctiva, with keratinization, which causes painful

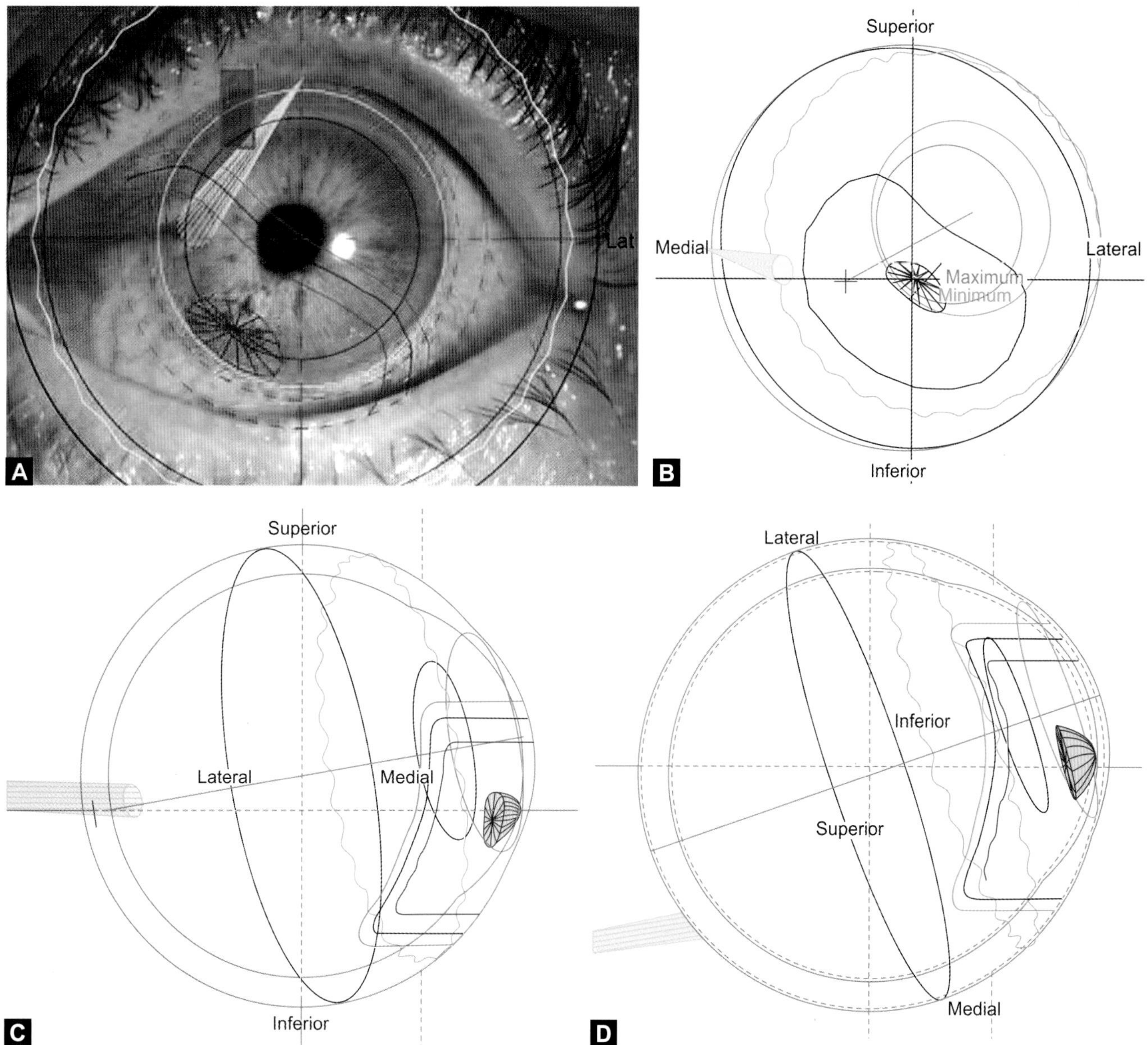


**Figures 88-5A to D** Treatment plans for an inferonasal iris melanoma in the left eye.
*Source* Treatment plans courtesy of The National Centre for Eye Proton Therapy at The Clatterbridge Cancer Centre, UK.

corneal abrasion with every blink. These problems can be avoided by treating the intraocular tumor through closed lids, ensuring that the upper eyelid margin is out of the beam.

## SURGICAL OUTCOMES: SCIENTIFIC EVIDENCE/METANALYSIS

Compared to brachytherapy, proton beam radiotherapy has relatively high rates of local tumor control. This is because computer modeling can adjust for minor errors in marker placement so that there is less reliance on surgical expertise.

Despite the Bragg peak, high doses of radiation are received by intervening tissues, such as the eyelids, conjunctiva, cornea and lens, so that side-effects affecting these structures commonly occur.

With tumors extending close to optic disk and fovea, visual loss tends to be caused by direct collateral damage to these structures. When these receive minimal or no radiation, any visual loss is likely to be caused by fluid leaking from the residual, irradiated tumor.

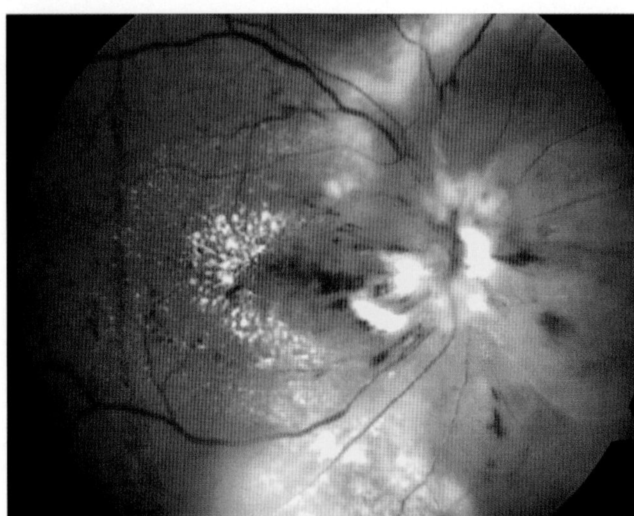

Figure 88-6 Radiation-induced optic neuropathy and maculopathy after proton beam radiotherapy of a medial, juxtapapillary choroidal melanoma in the right eye.

Neovascular glaucoma is often induced by vasproliferative factors produced by bulky, residual tumor and extensive, detached retina, both of which are ischemic. Such neovascular glaucoma can resolve if the irradiated tumor is removed and if the retinal detachment resolves.[11,12]

## PLACE OF THE TECHNIQUE IN SURGICAL ARMAMENTARIUM

In some centers, proton beam radiotherapy is advocated as the best eye-conserving therapy for all uveal melanomas. In other centers, plaque radiotherapy is the first choice of treatment, resorting to proton beam treatment only if such brachytherapy is considered unlikely to succeed, that is, (1) large melanomas, (2) small, posterior melanomas extending close to optic disk, and (3) iris melanomas.

With large tumors, some surgeons skilled in local resection prefer this form of treatment as a means of avoiding the toxic tumor syndrome. Others prefer to consider proton beam radiotherapy as neoadjuvant therapy, performing endoresection as planned therapy at an early stage, before toxic tumor complications develop.[13]

To the author's knowledge, there have been no direct comparisons between proton beam radiotherapy and stereotactic radiotherapy. The latter form of treatment tends to be deployed in centers where proton beam radiotherapy is not available.

## PEARLS AND PITFALLS

- Proton beam radiotherapy targets tumors precisely, providing high rates of local tumor control while limiting collateral damage to healthy tissues.
- Most recurrences develop because the tumor extent is underestimated.

## REFERENCES


1. Gragoudas ES. Proton beam irradiation of uveal melanomas: the first 30 years. The Weisenfeld Lecture. Invest Ophthalmol Vis Sci. 2006;47(11):4666-73.
2. Damato B, Kacperek A, Chopra M, et al. Proton beam radiotherapy of choroidal melanoma: the Liverpool-Clatterbridge experience. Int J Radiat Oncol Biol Phys. 2005;62(5):1405-11.
3. Damato B, Kacperek A, Chopra M, et al. Proton beam radiotherapy of iris melanoma. Int J Radiat Oncol Biol Phys. 2005; 63(1):109-15.
4. Konstantinidis L, Roberts D, Errington RD, et al. Whole anterior segment proton beam radiotherapy for diffuse iris melanoma. Br J Ophthalmol. 2013;97(4):471-4.
5. Zografos L, Egger E, Bercher L, et al. Proton beam irradiation of choroidal hemangiomas. Am J Ophthalmol. 1998;126(2):261-8.
6. Zografos L, Uffer S, Bercher L, et al. Combined surgery, cryocoagulation and radiotherapy for treatment of melanoma of the conjunctiva. Klinische Monatsblatter fur Augenheilkunde. 1994;204(5):385-90.
7. Kim IK, Lane AM, Egan KM, et al. Natural history of radiation papillopathy after proton beam irradiation of parapapillary melanoma. Ophthalmology. 2010;117(8):1617-22.
8. Boyd SR, Gittos A, Richter M, et al. Proton beam therapy and iris neovascularisation in uveal melanoma. Eye (Lond). 2006; 20(7):832-6.
9. Groenewald C, Konstantinidis L, Damato B. Effects of radiotherapy on uveal melanomas and adjacent tissues. Eye (Lond). 2013;27(2):163-71.
10. Gragoudas ES, Lane AM, Munzenrider J, et al. Long-term risk of local failure after proton therapy for choroidal/ciliary body melanoma. Trans Am Ophthalmol Soc. 2002;100:43-8; discussion 48-9.
11. Damato BE, Groenewald C, Foulds WS. Surgical resection of choroidal melanoma. In: Ryan SJ (Ed). Retina, Vol. 3, 5th edition. Elsevier: London; 2013. pp. 2298-306.
12. Konstantinidis L, Groenewald C, Coupland SE, et al. Transscleral local resection of toxic choroidal melanoma after proton beam radiotherapy. Br J Ophthalmol. 2014 Feb 25. doi: 10.1136/bjophthalmol-2013-304501. [Epub ahead of print].
13. Bechrakis NE, Foerster MH. Neoadjuvant proton beam radiotherapy combined with subsequent endoresection of choroidal melanomas. Int Ophthalmol Clin. 2006;46(1):95-107.

CHAPTER

89

# Stereotactic Photon Beam Radiation

Bertil Damato, Martin Zehetmayer

## INTRODUCTION

With stereotactic external beam irradiation, ionizing radiation is directed at the tumor from many different directions. It is termed stereotactic radiosurgery (SRS) if delivered in a single fraction and stereotactic radiotherapy (SRT) if fractionated over several days.

## INDICATIONS

Uveal melanomas considered unsuitable for ruthenium plaque radiotherapy because of tumor size or location.

## CONTRAINDICATIONS

Extra-large tumors (> 12–14 mm thickness), pre-existing uncontrolled neovascular glaucoma better treated with enucleation.

## PREOPERATIVE CARE

Tumor size and extent are determined by computerized tomography and magnetic resonance imaging to create a 3D computerized model of the eye and tumor.

## TECHNIQUE

### Stereotactic Radiotherapy

- The patient's face is immobilized by means of a mask, made from thermoplastic material (Fig. 89-1).
- The eye position is monitored with a closed circuit television (CCTV) system, with the patient gazing at a fixation target during CT/MRI delineation and radiotherapy.

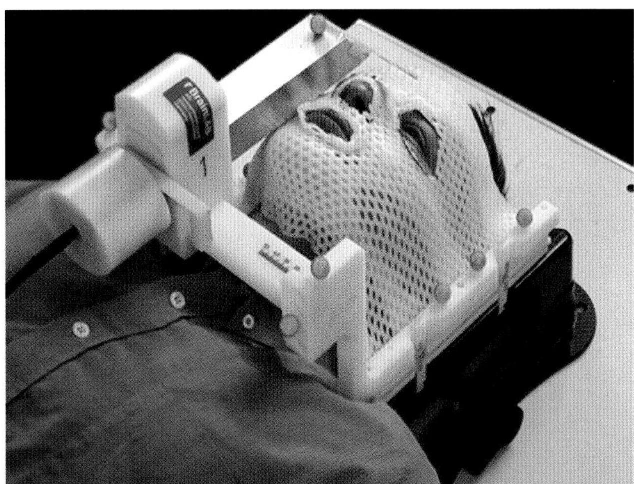

Figure 89-1 Patient's set-up prior to CT/MRI delineation and radiotherapy. The patient's head is immobilized with a thermoplastic head mask system, consisting of an anterior and a posterior half. On the left mask margin three grey spheres are visible, used for 3D localization and alignment. In front of the tumor-containing eye, an eye fixation system is mounted; it contains infrared illumination diodes, a flashing red light diode and a TV camera. The patient will look into a 45° mirror. All parts and wiring are MRI-compatible.

- The radiotherapy is administered with a linear accelerator (LINAC). This aims a single beam of radiation at the tumor from multiple directions sequentially (Fig. 89-2).
- Micro-multileaf collimators or round circular collimators (arc rotation) are used to adjust the beam shape (static field).
- A total dose of 50–70 Gy is delivered in multiple, usually five, fractions administered over 5–10 days.
- A safety margin of 2.0–2.5 mm is added to the clinical tumor margins.

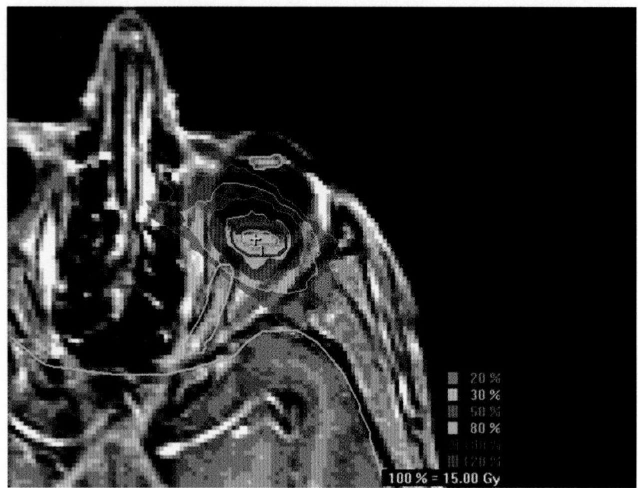


Figure 89-2 Linear accelerator treatment plan for a macular melanoma. Tumor margins will be included within the 12 Gy isodose line. Five fractions within 7–10 days will be administered (= total dose 60 Gy).

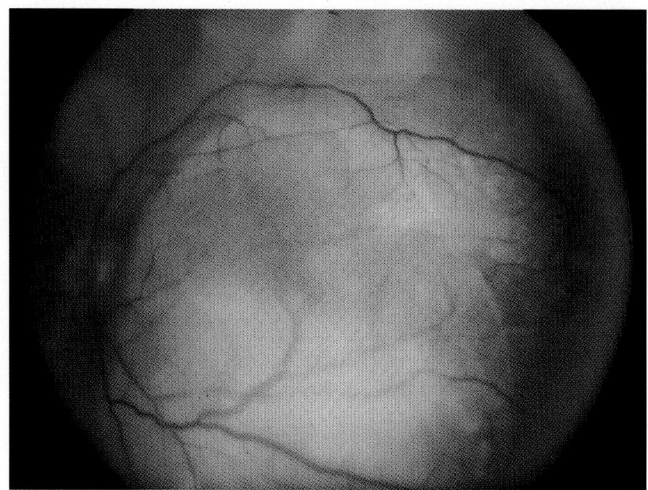

Figure 89-3 Macular melanoma, prior to stereotactic radiotherapy.

### Stereotactic Radiosurgery

- The patient's head is positioned in a rigid Leksell head frame.
- The eye is immobilized with a retrobulbar injection of anesthetic, often combined with rectus muscle sutures or a suction-assisted contact lens.
- This is usually delivered with a Leksell gamma knife, which comprises 201 cobalt sources placed in a metal hemispheric device positioned around the patient's head so that the highly collimated beams of radiation converge in the tumor volume.
- A total dose of 25–40 Gy is delivered with a safety margin of 1–2 mm.

## MECHANISM OF ACTION

The objective is to focus a high dose of radiation at the tumor with limited irradiation of surrounding tissues.

## POSTOPERATIVE CARE

Postoperative care is performed as for other forms of conservative therapy. During the first 3 months, local cycloplegic and anti-inflammatory medications are advisable.

## SPECIFIC INSTRUMENTATION

- *Stereotactic radiotherapy*: Linear accelerator; usually fractionated treatment.
- *Stereotactic radiosurgery*: Leksell gamma knife; contact lens suction device for ocular immobilization; usually single fraction treatment.

## COMPLICATIONS

- Acute effects are minimal.
- Rates of local tumor recurrence are low (i.e. approximately 5% at 5 years).
- *Long-term side effects include*: Optic neuropathy, maculopathy, cataract, exudative retinal detachment and neovascular glaucoma. Long-term overall eye retention rate is about 70–75% (Figs. 89-3 and 89-4).

## SURGICAL OUTCOMES: SCIENTIFIC EVIDENCE/METANALYSIS

Stereotactic photon beam irradiation has been under clinical investigation for the treatment of uveal melanoma for over 15 years. The therapeutic single dose for Single-fraction stereotactic radiosurgery (SRS) has been reduced to as low as 35 Gy over the past few years without reduction in tumor control. Studies have shown that doses of 40 Gy delivered at the 50% isodose result in good local tumor control and acceptable toxicity.

Fractionated stereotactic radiotherapy (SRT) has gained additional interest lately. Fractionation allows for increased tumor control and reduced toxicity. Linear accelerators (LINAC) have the advantage of a feasible fractionation. Most

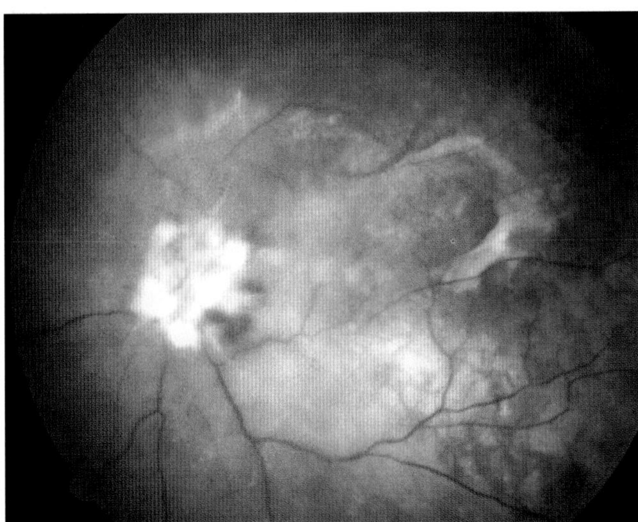

Figure 89-4 Same patient as Figure 89-3, 30 months after radiotherapy. Good local tumor control, but optic neuropathy with exudation and neovascularization on disk margins is visible (radiogenic optic neuropathy)

LINAC studies employ a hypofractionated scheme of 4-5 fractions and total doses between 50 and 70 Gy.

The efficacy of SRT for uveal melanoma has been proven in different studies with local tumor control rates reported over 90%, 5 and 10 years after treatment. Side effects after SRT are similarly to other forms of radiotherapy such as cataract, radiation retinopathy, optic neuropathy and neovascular glaucoma. Overall, SRS and SRT are considered effective treatment modalities for uveal melanoma, with promising late tumor control and toxicity rates.[1-8]

## PLACE OF THE TECHNIQUE IN SURGICAL ARMAMENTARIUM

Fractionated LINAC SRT is increasingly being used as an alternative to proton beam radiotherapy when brachytherapy is not considered appropriate.

For bulky tumors, some authors advocate stereotactic photon irradiation as neoadjuvant therapy before endoresection so as to avoid the toxic tumor syndrome while minimizing any risk of tumor seeding around the eye and systemically.

## PEARLS AND PITFALLS

- As with other forms of therapy, it is essential for the patient to understand the likely outcomes in terms of visual acuity, local tumor control and comfort.
- Patients should be aware and agree in consent that this treatment, similar to other forms of radiotherapy, is an attempt to conservatively sterilize the malignant intraocular tumor.
- Regular follow-up should be arranged.
- Most eyes will experience reduction of vision acuity.
- Additional treatment may be necessary. Long-term overall eye retention rate is about 70–75%. Some eyes may be lost after some years due to intractable complications (especially due to neovascular glaucoma).

## REFERENCES

1. Zehetmayer M, Kitz K, Menapace R, et al. Local tumor control and morbidity after one to three fractions of stereotactic external beam irradiation for uvela melanoma. Radiother Oncol. 2000;55:135-44.
2. Mueller AJ, Talies S, Schaller UC, et al. Stereotactic radiosurgery of large uveal melanomas with the gamma-knife. Ophthalmol. 2000;107:1381-7.
3. Modorati G, Miserocchi E, Galli L, et al. Gamma knife radiosurgery for uveal melanoma: 12 years of experience. Br J Ophthalmol. 2009;93:40-4.
4. Krema H, Somani S, Sahgal A, et al. Stereotactic radiotherapy for treatment of juxtapapillary choroidal melanoma: 3-year follow-up. Br J Ophthalmol. 2009;93:1172-6.
5. Dunavoelgyi R, Dieckmann K, Gleiss A, et al. Local tumor control, visual acuity, and survival after hypofractionated stereotactic photon radiotherapy of choroidal melanoma in 212 patients treated between 1997 and 2007. Int J Radiat Oncol Biol Phys. 2011;81:199-205.
6. Dunavoelgyi R, Dieckmann K, Gleiss A, et al. Radiogenic side effects after hypofractionated stereotactic photon radiotherapy of choroidal melanoma in 212 patients treated between 1997 and 2007. Int J Radiat Oncol Biol Phys. 2012;83:121-8.
7. Muller K, Naus N, Nowak PJ, et al. Fractionated stereotactic radiotherapy for uveal melanoma, late clinical results. Radiother Oncol. 2012;102:219-24.
8. Suesskind D, Scheiderbauer J, Buchgeister M, et al. Retrospective evaluation of patients with uveal melanoma treated by stereotactic radiosurgery with and without tumor resection. JAMA Ophthalmol. 2013;14:1-8.

# Exoresection of Choroidal Melanoma

Bertil Damato

## INTRODUCTION

Exoresection of choroidal melanoma is also known as "partial choroidectomy", "trans-scleral resection", "eye-wall resection", and "sclerouvectomy". There are many variations in technique.[1-5] The aim of this operation is to remove the tumor en bloc, if possible without damaging the adjacent retina. Exoresection can be performed as a primary procedure or as a secondary, salvage procedure after radiotherapy, as a treatment of local tumor recurrence or the toxic tumor syndrome. This chapter focuses on the author's methods, most of which he has developed himself, having been trained by Wallace S Foulds.

## INDICATIONS

- Choroidal or ciliochoroidal melanoma considered unsuitable for any form of radiotherapy because of tumor bulk and/or extensive exudative retinal detachment (Figs. 90-1A and B).
- Patient highly motivated to retain the eye, for occupational reasons or because of poor vision in the fellow eye.
- Bulky residual tumor after radiotherapy, with severe exudative retinal detachment, iris neovascularization, and neovascular glaucoma (i.e. "toxic tumor syndrome").[2]

## CONTRAINDICATIONS

- Tumor involving optic disk and/or more than 2 clock hours of pars plicata.
- Diffuse melanoma.
- Bulky extraocular spread, unless this can be resected en bloc.[6]
- Retinal perforation by tumor, if subsequent retinopexy and internal tamponade are not possible.
- Systemic disease precluding hypotensive anesthesia (e.g. cerebrovascular disease).
- Inexperience with surgical and anesthetic techniques.

## PREOPERATIVE CARE

Antibiotics are administered and the pupil is dilated in the usual manner.

## SURGICAL TECHNIQUE

### Exposure

The lashes are trimmed and the lids are retracted both with traction sutures and a wire speculum. A 180° conjunctival peritomy is made. Any rectus and/or oblique muscle overlying the tumor is disinserted. Before dividing any rectus muscle, the distance between the suture knots and the limbus is measured and recorded. Two traction sutures are placed in the sclera, 4 mm from limbus.

### Tumor Delineation

The tumor limits are defined by transpupillary and transscleral transillumination, using a 20-gauge vitrectomy transilluminator with the tip pre-bent 90°. Care is taken to avoid oblique transillumination, which exaggerates the apparent tumor extent. The tumor margins are marked on the sclera with a pen.

### Superficial Lamellar Scleral Flap

A lamellar scleral flap is prepared, which is hinged posteriorly. This has a polygonal shape anteriorly, to facilitate apposition during closure, and is wider posteriorly so that the radial

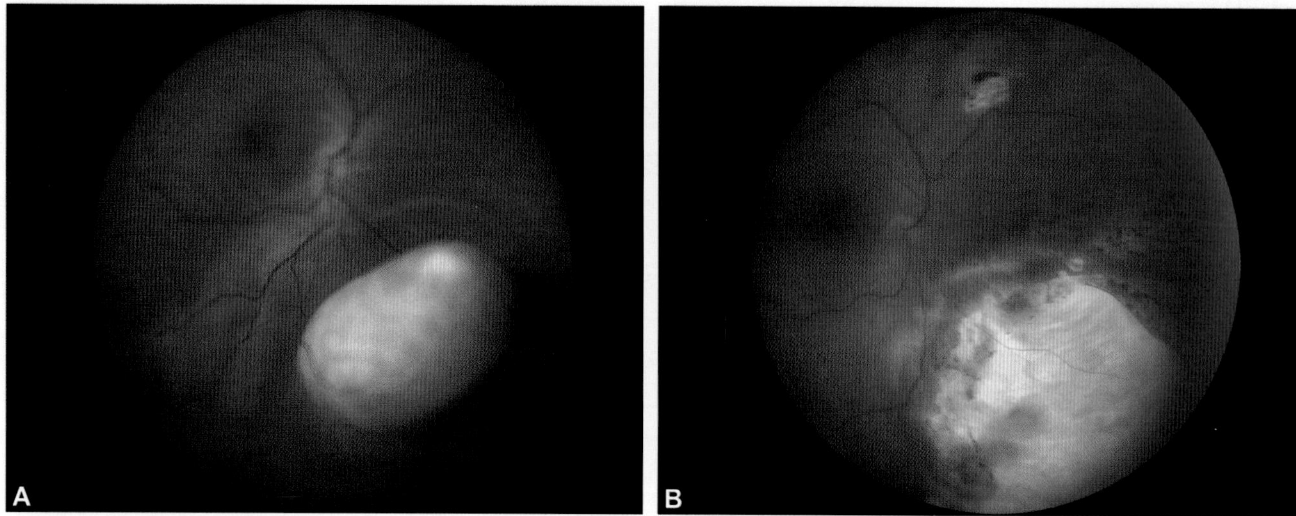


**Figures 90-1A and B** Right eye of a 44-year-old man with an inferonasal choroidal melanoma measuring 11.9 mm basally with a thickness of 7.6 mm (A). Postoperative appearance showing a surgical coloboma, a flat retina, and a healthy macula (B). Almost 3 years postoperatively, the visual acuity was 20/30. The survival prognosis was good because laboratory studies showed the tumor to have no chromosome 3 loss.

incisions can be shortened. The flap is as thick as possible, to provide strength. The superficial scleral incisions clear the tumor margins by about 4 mm.

Any vortex veins and long posterior ciliary arteries are closed by applying bipolar diathermy, both to the extraocular and intrascleral portions of the blood vessels. This diathermy is applied before dividing the blood vessels.

If the superficial scleral lamella is inadvertently perforated (i.e. "buttonholed"), this defect is immediately closed with a purse-string suture, using 8-0 nylon. If the deep sclera is inadvertently sutured, so that tumor or uveal tissue begins to prolapse through the defect, then the opening is closed with sutures or covered with a plastic square that has been cut from the drape.

If cyclectomy is planned, the anterior scleral incision is placed along the limbus. After completing the superficial scleral flap, a partial thickness incision is made in the deep sclera, which is split into a further two layers by lamellar dissection that extends anteriorly into peripheral cornea. This makes it possible to excise deep sclera and peripheral cornea with the tumor while leaving a scleral "skirt" along the anterior wound edge, preventing leakage.

## Ocular Decompression

The eye is decompressed to prevent retinal prolapse through the scleral window as the tumor is excised. Ocular decompression also facilitates access to postequatorial regions of the globe. It can be performed before or after dissection of the superficial scleral flap is completed. The decompression is achieved by performing a limited core vitrectomy through a single sclerotomy placed 4 mm from the limbus, using a corneal contact lens and illumination from the operating microscope. Instead of infusion, the eye is indented at a point diametrically opposite to the tumor.

## Closure of Short Posterior Ciliary Arteries

Gentle bipolar diathermy is applied to the short posterior ciliary arteries adjacent to the optic nerve in the quadrant of the tumor. The blood vessels are pulled away from the nerve before applying the diathermy to prevent collateral damage to the nerve itself. After diathermy, the closed blood vessels are divided with blunt-tipped, spring scissors to expose any residual patent blood vessels in that quadrant.

## Deep Scleral Incisions

A deep sclerotomy is made on each side of the tumor. This is done by pinching the sclera with colibri forceps and shaving the sclera with a feather blade, with the blade angled away from the choroid so as not to damage the adjacent uveal tissue. These incisions are extended with blunt-tipped spring scissors, first along the lateral tumor margins, then posteriorly and finally anteriorly. These incisions should overlie the tumor margins. As the scleral incision is extended, gentle bipolar cautery can be applied to the choroid to reduce hemorrhage, albeit at the risk of inducing retinal burns.

## Tumor Excision

This is performed under hypotensive anesthesia, lowering the systolic blood pressure to approximately 50–60 mm Hg, as described elsewhere.[7]

A uveal opening is made, posterior to the ora serrata so as to preserve the integrity of the ciliary epithelium over the pars plana. This is done by gently grasping the uvea with two pairs of notched, colibri microforceps and stretching the intervening uveal tissue until it rips. The tumor is lifted out of the eye with the left hand, using the deep scleral lamella as a handle. As the choroid separates from the retina, it is divided with the spring scissors.

If the tumor excision extends anterior to the ora serrata, it is important to conserve the ciliary epithelium so as to prevent retinal dialysis and detachment. This is achieved by first perforating the uvea posterior to the ora serrata, as mentioned before, then separating the ciliary epithelium from the uvea by blunt dissection before dividing the uvea with blunt-tipped spring scissors.

Any blood collecting in the operative field is mopped away before it clots, taking care not to touch the retina. If the bleeding is excessive, the blood is sucked away with an aspiration device, again taking care not to damage the retina.

If the tumor is adherent to retina, adhesions are divided using a No.15 Bard Parker scalpel. These adhesions are usually invisible and located approximately 2 mm away from the apparent point of contact between retina and tumor.

If the tumor has invaded retina, the apex of the tumor is "top-sliced" with the scalpel and left in situ, to be treated with brachytherapy. If there is bulky transretinal growth of the tumor, then the entire tumor is excised, leaving a large defect in the retina, which is treated at the end of the resection procedure.

## Closure

As soon as the tumor is removed, the scleral flap is closed, using fresh instruments. Two wicks are wedged posterior to the excision area to prevent any potential space, in which subretinal hematoma might form, and to compress the uveal blood vessels, preventing further hemorrhage. The superficial scleral flap is sutured in place with interrupted, 8-0 nylon sutures, first anteriorly and then laterally.

## Ocular Reformation

As soon as suturing of the scleral flap has been completed, balanced salt solution is injected intraocularly through the sclerotomy (which was used for the ocular decompression). The wicks are removed. Care is taken not to induce dehiscence of the wound by overinflating the eye. The sclerotomy is sutured in the usual manner.

## Adjunctive Brachytherapy

A plaque is inserted as soon as the globe is reformed, unless cyclochoroidectomy has been performed, in which case the brachytherapy is delayed by 1 month to avoid hypotony. The author's preference is to use a 25 mm CCC ruthenium plaque. First, a transparent template ("dummy plaque") is inserted and sutured to the sclera in the appropriate position. This is done by placing a posterior ink-mark on the outer surface of the template at a distance from the posterior edge corresponding to the intended posterior safety margin, then placing a second ink-mark anteriorly at a point corresponding to the previous location of the anterior margin (i.e. separated from the first ink-mark by a distance corresponding to the longitudinal basal tumor diameter). Next, the template is placed on the eye so that the anterior ink-mark overlies the previous location of the anterior tumor margin (marked on the sclera before the scleral flap dissection). Then, the template is sutured in place with two releasable bows. If necessary, the position of the template can be checked ophthalmoscopically, as described in Chapter 87. Finally, the template is replaced by the radioactive plaque, using the same sutures. The plaque is removed about a day later, once a dose of 100 Gy has been delivered to a depth of 1 mm.

## Muscle Repositioning

The oblique muscles are left loose without re-insertion. Any disinserted rectus muscles are sutured to their original insertions or attached to the anterior sclera by slings so that the distances from the intra-muscular knots to the limbus are the same as before disinsertion.

## Conjunctival Closure

The conjunctiva is closed in the standard manner. If performed by an experienced surgeon, exoresection is completed in approximately 2 hours (Figs. 90-2A to L).

# MECHANISM OF ACTION

Less than 5% of patients with a class 1/disomy 3 melanoma develop metastatic disease after exoresection. It is not known how many tumors would have transformed to class 2/monosomy 3 and metastasized, without successful ocular treatment.[8,9]

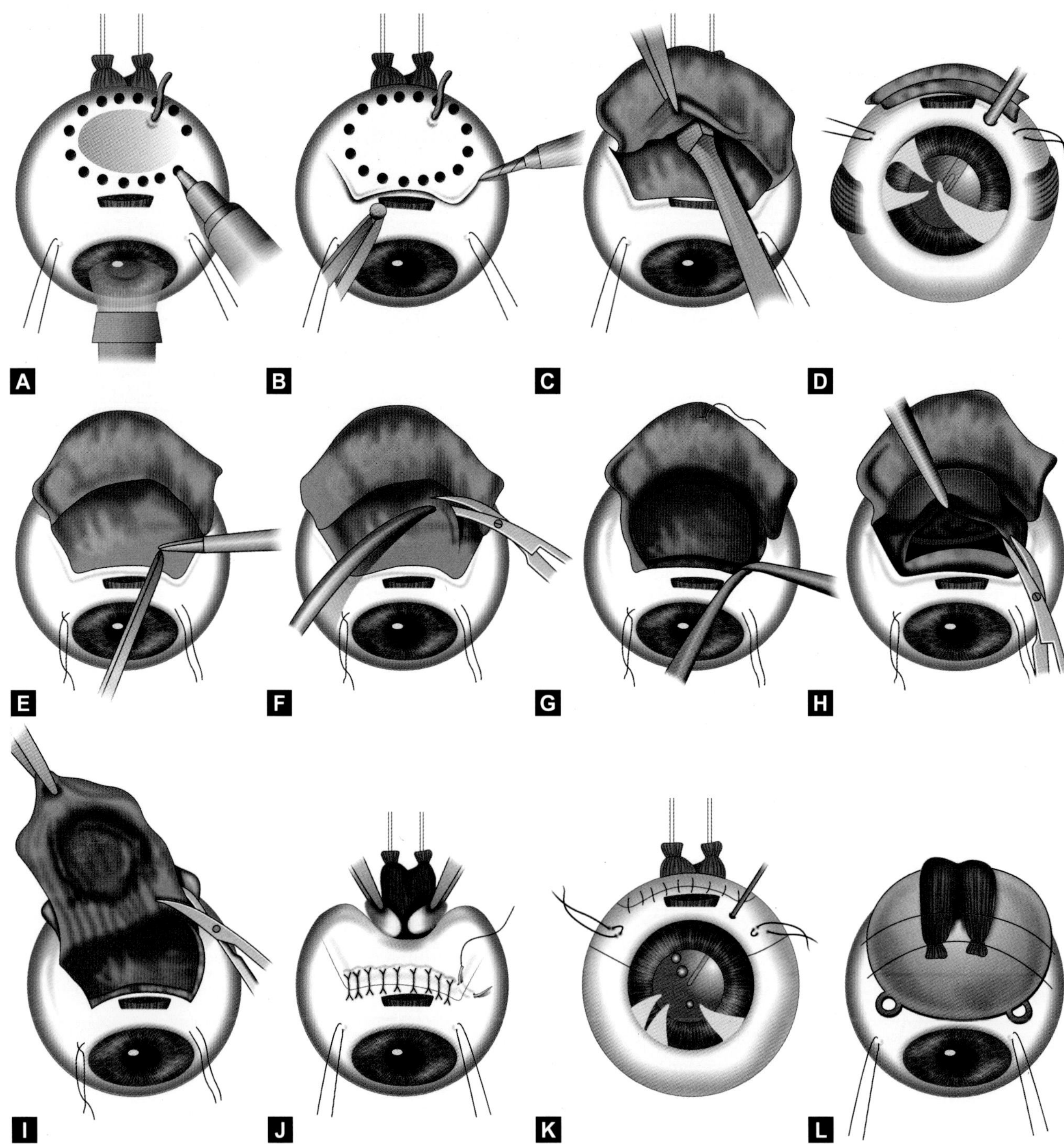


**Figures 90-2A to L** Technique for exoresection of choroidal melanoma (A to L).

Almost all patients with a class 2/monosomy 3 melanoma develop metastatic disease despite successful excision of the ocular tumor, so that the main benefit is conservation of a useful eye.[8,9] What is deemed to be a useful eye varies from one patient to another. Some patients are satisfied if they merely retain a comfortable and cosmetically satisfactory eye whereas others also need conservation of useful vision for the procedure to be considered worthwhile.

In eyes with the toxic tumor syndrome, excision removes the ischemic and exudative tumor tissue, resulting in immediate retinal reattachment, regression of the iris neovascularization and, possibly, improved aqueous outflow so that in some patients the intraocular pressure returns to normal, even without antiglaucoma therapy.[2]

### Postoperative Care

At the end of the surgical procedure, subconjunctival antibiotic and steroid injections are administered together with atropine 1% drops. Systemic antibiotics are given, either as an intravenous bolus or orally for 1 week. Oral steroids are also given, tapering the dose after 1 week.

The patient is postured for 24 hours so that any blood arising from the margins of the surgical coloboma gravitates away from the fovea. The patient is nursed in a general ophthalmic ward and is discharged from hospital 1 day after the operation to remove the tumor or the plaque.

Approximately 4 weeks postoperatively, the patient is reviewed at the oncology center, to assess the operated eye. The patient is informed of the survival probability, which is based on the clinical stage of the ocular tumor, the histologic grade of malignancy, and the genetic tumor type. An online tool has been developed for multivariate analysis of all major predictors, also taking the patient's age and sex into account.

If adjunctive brachytherapy was not administered at the time of the primary exoresection and if the tumor shows high-grade malignancy or extends to the resection margins, then plaque radiotherapy can be administered at this time. Long-term surveillance is performed as for other forms of treatment for uveal melanoma. Psychological support and systemic screening for metastatic disease are undertaken in the usual manner.

## SPECIFIC INSTRUMENTATION

Forceps:
- Artery forceps for eyelid sutures
- Forceps for conjunctiva
- Toothed forceps for sclera
- Toothed colibri (×2), for closure of scleral flap
- Notched colibri (×2), for tearing uvea

Scissors:
- Spring scissors, for conjunctiva
- Pointed scissors, for muscles
- Blunt-tipped spring scissors, for uvea

Blades:
- Feather ("supersharp") blade
- Number 15 Bard-Parker knife
- Desmarres scarifier.

Sutures:
- 6-0 vicryl sutures, for muscles and conjunctiva
- 8-0 nylon sutures, for scleral flap
- 7-0 vicryl sutures, for sclerotomy

Retractors:
- Fison's
- Malleable.

Miscellaneous:
- Barraquer wire speculum
- Barraquer needle holder
- Castroviejo needle holder
- Two strabismus hooks
- Nettleship dilator
- 90° 20-gauge transilluminator, to localize tumor margins
- Scleral pen, to mark tumor extent
- Calipers, to measure knot-to-limbus distances when disinserting and reinserting rectus muscles
- Bipolar cautery
- 20-gauge vitreous cutter
- O'Malley contact lens
- Tissue glue, in case tumor separates from deep scleral lamella during excision
- 20 mL syringe with 25-gauge needle and filter, for injecting balanced salt solution intraocularly
- 25 mm ruthenium plaque, unless another form of adjunctive radiotherapy is preferred.

## COMPLICATIONS

### Intraoperative Complications

- Malposition of flap.
- Superficial scleral buttonhole. This requires a purse-string suture. Adjunctive brachytherapy should be delayed by a minimum of 4 weeks to allow healing.
- Inadvertent deep scleral perforation. This results in prolapsed of tumor or uvea when dissecting the posterior sclera. This perforation should be sutured or covered with a plastic patch cut from the eye drape.
- Lens and/or retinal damage during vitrectomy.
- Optic nerve damage while cauterizing short posterior ciliary arteries. The power should be turned down and the cautery applied while pulling the blood vessels away from the nerve.
- Uveal and retinal perforation during deep sclerotomy. This is avoided by shaving the sclera with the sharp edge of the blade pointing away from the uvea.
- Uncontrolled hemorrhage, if a vortex vein is divided without adequate bipolar cautery.

- Retinal damage when excising tumor. This requires immediate vitreoretinal surgery before proliferative vitreoretinopathy develops. The procedure requires total vitrectomy, removal of subretinal blood, retinopexy, and silicone oil tamponade.
- Choroidal tear, from excessive traction when lifting the tumor out of the eye.
- Expulsive hemorrhage, which is rare unless exoresection is attempted without hypotensive anesthesia.
- Incomplete tumor excision, which is treatable by adjunctive brachytherapy.
- Scleral wound dehiscence or leakage. This is avoided by using interrupted nonabsorbable sutures and preparing a stepped wound edge.
- Incorrect placement of plaque.
- Inaccurate reinsertion of muscles.
- Inadequate conjunctival wound closure, with scleral exposure. If irradiated sclera is left exposed, it may undergo necrosis and perforation.

### Postoperative Complications

- Subretinal hematoma, which can cause visual loss if the macula is involved.
- Vitreous hemorrhage, which usually indicates a retinal break and which is therefore an indication for immediate vitreoretinal surgery.
- Rhegmatogenous retinal detachment, which occurs if a retinal break is not detected and treated at the time of the exoresection.[10]
- Local tumor recurrence, which has become much less common since the introduction of routine adjunctive brachytherapy using an adequately sized applicators (i.e. 25 mm for large tumors). Recurrences tend to occur in nonirradiated areas: within the coloboma, at the margins of the coloboma and, rarely, in distant parts of the uvea.[11,12]
- Orbital tumor recurrence is exceedingly rare unless exoresection is performed without adjunctive brachytherapy. This complication usually occurs if an intraocular recurrence is not immediately detected and treated.
- Disciform macular degeneration from neovascularization arising from the margins of the coloboma or from a choroidal tear.
- Cataract, which is rare unless the lens has been irradiated or damaged by surgical instruments or silicone oil.
- Lens subluxation, if extensive cyclectomy is performed.
- Ocular hypotony, if adjunctive brachytherapy is administered at the time of primary cyclectomy.
- Phthisis is rare if ocular hypotony and retinal detachment are prevented.
- Diplopia, if the rectus muscles are not reinserted accurately.

## SURGICAL OUTCOMES: SCIENTIFIC EVIDENCE

If performed by an experienced surgeon in well-selected cases, intraoperative complications are rare. The visual outcome depends on the distance of the tumor from the fovea and on the avoidance of complications such as subretinal hematoma, retinal detachment, and local tumor recurrence.[13]

Ocular conservation is achieved in approximately 90% of patients. The survival probability is approximately the same as other forms of conservative therapy, after taking all predictors into account.[14,15] Recurrent tumor can show a higher grade of malignancy than the initial tumor.[16] Although no data are available, this suggests that local tumor recurrence may increase the risk of metastasis.

## PLACE OF THE TECHNIQUE IN SURGICAL ARMAMENTARIUM

Because of its technical complexity, exoresection of choroidal melanoma is performed only when the tumor is considered unsuitable for radiotherapy and when the patient is very reluctant to avoid enucleation.

## PEARLS AND PITFALLS

- Use a sharp blade to separate tumor from retina. This is safer than blunt dissection.
- Avoid wide safety margins, which cause increased morbidity, especially when cyclectomy is performed. Residual tumor should respond to adjunctive brachytherapy.
- Measure the knot-to-limbus distances before disinserting any rectus muscles; this will prevent postoperative diplopia.
- Postoperative vitreous hemorrhage indicates a retinal tear and a high risk of rhegmatogenous retinal detachment.
- Exoresection is more difficult in young patients, in whom hypotensive anesthesia is less effective at preventing hemorrhage. Conversely, older individuals do not require such profound hypotension to control bleeding.
- Scleral invasion is helpful because it allows the deep scleral lamella to be used as a handle when lifting the tumor out of the eye.
- Serous retinal detachment facilitates the tumor resection because it reduces the risk of retinal damage.

## REFERENCES


1. Peyman GA, Gremillion CM. Eye wall resection in the management of uveal neoplasms. Jpn J Ophthalmol. 1989;33(4):458-71.
2. Damato BE, Groenewald C, Foulds WS. Surgical resection of choroidal melanoma. In: Ryan SJ (ed.), Retina. Vol. 3, 5th edn. London: Elsevier; 2013. pp 2298-2306.
3. Shields JA, Shields CL, Shah P, et al. Partial lamellar sclerouvectomy for ciliary body and choroidal tumors. Ophthalmology. 1991;98(6):971-83.
4. Char DH, Miller T, Crawford JB. Uveal tumour resection. Br J Ophthalmol. 2001;85(10):1213-9.
5. Bechrakis NE, Petousis V, Willerding G, et al. Ten-year results of transscleral resection of large uveal melanomas: local tumour control and metastatic rate. Br J Ophthalmol. 2010;94(4):460-66.
6. Muen WJ, Damato BE. Uveal malignant melanoma with extrascleral extension, treated with plaque radiotherapy. Eye (Lond). 2007;21(2):307-8.
7. Damato B, Jones AG. Uveal melanoma: resection techniques. Ophthalmol Clin North Am. 2005;18(1):119-128, ix.
8. Damato B, Dopierala JA, Coupland SE. Genotypic profiling of 452 choroidal melanomas with multiplex ligation-dependent probe amplification. Clin Cancer Res: An Official Journal of the American Association for Cancer Research. 2010;16(24):6083-92.
9. Onken MD, Worley LA, Char DH, et al. Collaborative ocular oncology group report number 1: prospective validation of a multi-gene prognostic assay in uveal melanoma. Ophthalmology. 2012;119(8):1596-603.
10. Damato B, Groenewald CP, McGalliard JN, et al. Rhegmatogenous retinal detachment after transscleral local resection of choroidal melanoma. Ophthalmology. 2002;109(11):2137-43.
11. Damato BE, Paul J, Foulds WS. Risk factors for residual and recurrent uveal melanoma after trans-scleral local resection. Br J Ophthalmol. 1996;80(2):102-8.
12. Kim JW, Damato BE, Hiscott P. Noncontiguous tumor recurrence of posterior uveal melanoma after transscleral local resection. Arch Ophthalmol. 2002;120(12):1659-64.
13. Damato BE, Paul J, Foulds WS. Predictive factors of visual outcome after local resection of choroidal melanoma. Br J Ophthalmol. 1993;77(10):616-23.
14. Foulds WS, Damato BE, Burton RL. Local resection versus enucleation in the management of choroidal melanoma. Eye (Lond). 1987;1(Pt 6):676-9.
15. Damato BE, Paul J, Foulds WS. Risk factors for metastatic uveal melanoma after trans-scleral local resection. Br J Ophthalmol. 1996;80(2):109-16.
16. Bechrakis NE, Sehu KW, Lee WR, et al. Transformation of cell type in uveal melanomas: a quantitative histologic analysis. Arch Ophthalmol. 2000;118(10):1406-12.

CHAPTER

91

# Iridocyclectomy

Iwona Rospond-Kubiak, Bertil Damato

## INTRODUCTION

Iridocyclectomy has been performed for many years.[1-3] The technique is not particularly demanding and does not require hypotensive anesthesia. Besides removing the offending lesion, this procedure also provides the entire tumor specimen for diagnosis and prognostication. The standard technique is to dilate the pupil preoperatively and to perform iridocyclectomy in an anteroposterior direction.[4] The authors have found that results are better if the procedure is performed "back-to-front", first constricting the pupil and then excising the tumor in a posteroanterior or circumferential direction.[5]

## INDICATIONS

- Primary treatment of melanoma involving the peripheral iris, angle and/or ciliary body.
- Excision biopsy of an undiagnosed tumor involving peripheral iris and/or ciliary body.
- Treatment of persistent uveitis after treatment of a peripheral and/or ciliary body tumor (i.e. "toxic tumor syndrome").

## CONTRAINDICATIONS

- Involvement of more than 2 clock hours of iris, angle or ciliary body.
- Diffuse spread or seeding.
- Anticoagulation.

## PREOPERATIVE CARE

The pupil is constricted with 1% pilocarpine drops.

## SURGICAL TECHNIQUE

### Exposure

A 180° conjunctival peritomy is made. Two traction sutures are placed in the sclera, 4 mm from limbus.

### Tumor Delineation

The tumor limits are defined by transpupillary and trans-scleral transillumination, using a 20-gauge, vitrectomy transilluminator with the tip pre-bent 90°. Care is taken to avoid oblique transillumination, which exaggerates the apparent tumor extent. The tumor margins and the ora serrata are marked on the sclera with a pen.

### Superficial Lamellar Scleral Flap

A lamellar scleral flap is prepared, which is hinged anteriorly. This has a polygonal shape posteriorly (Fig. 91-1A), to facilitate apposition during closure. The flap is as thick as possible, to provide strength (Figs. 91-1B and C). The superficial scleral incisions clear the tumor margins by about 4 mm.

If necessary, the superficial flap is extended into cornea until the anterior tumor margin is visible through the deep cornea.

### Ocular Decompression

Ocular decompression is not required unless there is excessive bulging of vitreous, during or after tumor excision and if conservation of an intact vitreous is considered desirable. A limited core vitrectomy can be performed through a sclerotomy placed 2–3 mm away from the large scleral opening.

An O'Malley contact lens is used. Infusion and endoillumination are not required.

## Deep Scleral Incisions

A deep sclerotomy is made on each side of the tumor, using a feather blade (Fig. 91-1D). These incisions are extended with spring scissors, first along the lateral tumor margins, then posteriorly and finally anteriorly, within cornea.

## Tumor Excision

This is performed under mild hypotensive anesthesia, lowering the systolic blood pressure to approximately 70–80 mm Hg.[6]

If the tumor involves both iris and ciliary body, the uveal opening is made in the peripheral iris. If the tumor is located entirely in the ciliary body, this opening is made over pars plana. This is done by grasping the uvea with toothed colibri forceps and dividing the tissue with spring scissors. It is not usually possible to conserve the ciliary epithelium, but this is of no consequence if the excision does not extend posterior to ora serrata. The uveal incision is extended first posterior to the tumor, with blunt-tipped spring scissors, then along the anterior tumor margin with fine, pointed, spring scissors (e.g. Ong's scissors) (Fig. 91-1E). A safety margin of approximately 1 mm is adequate. Some ciliary body tumors peel away from the posterior surface of the iris, which can be left intact.

Care is taken to avoid touching the lens with any instruments. The procedure is facilitated by lifting the tumor out of the eye as it is excised, so that the scissors do not need to be introduced into the eye.

If there is vitreous loss, a limited but adequate open-sky vitrectomy is performed until the wound edges are clear of vitreous (Fig. 91-1F).

## Closure

As soon as the tumor is removed, the scleral flap is closed, using fresh instruments. If an intact vitreous face is prolapsing through the scleral window, it can gently be pushed back into the eye by suturing the scleral flap in a zip-like fashion (i.e. commencing the suturing at the limbus and placing each successive suture adjacent to the previous suture until the limbus is reached again and the flap is closed) (Fig. 91-1G). Interrupted 8-0 nylon sutures are used. Care is taken not to induce astigmatism when tightening the scleral sutures near the limbus.

## Ocular Reformation

If there has been vitreous loss, the volume of the eye is reconstituted by injecting balanced salt solution into the eye with a 25-gauge needle placed 4 mm from the limbus, about 2 mm lateral to the scleral flap.

## Adjunctive Brachytherapy

The brachytherapy is delayed by 1 month to avoid hypotony. If the tumor diameter is less than 10 mm, the author's preference is to use a 15-mm CCC ruthenium plaque; otherwise, a larger applicator is needed. The plaque is removed about a day later, once a dose of 100 Gy has been delivered to a depth of 1 mm.

## Muscle Repositioning

It is not usually necessary to disinsert any rectus muscles. However, any disinserted rectus muscles are sutured to their original insertions so that the distances from the intramuscular knots to the limbus are the same as before disinsertion.

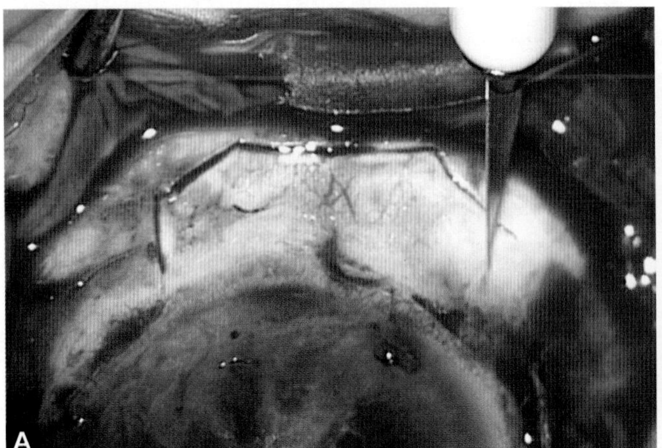


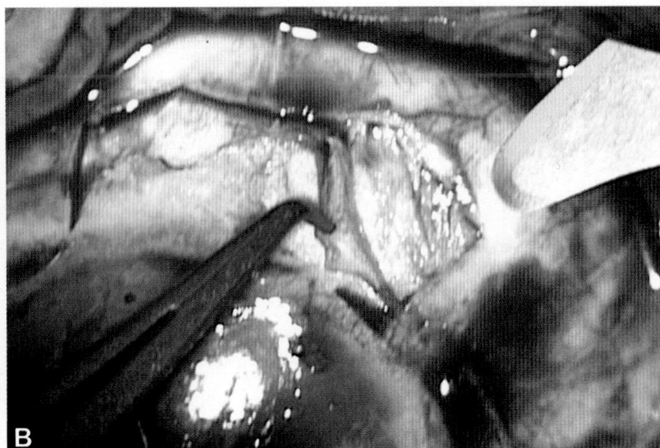


**Figures 91-1A and B** Iridocyclectomy of an inferior, iridociliary tumor in a 76-year-old man. The tumor proved to be a melanoma with epithelioid cells and chromosome 3 loss. Six weeks postoperatively, the visual acuity was 6/19. The operation involves the following steps: (A) A scleral incision is made to prepare a polyhedral superficial scleral flap, hinged anteriorly; (B) The flap is dissected with a Desmarres scarifier.

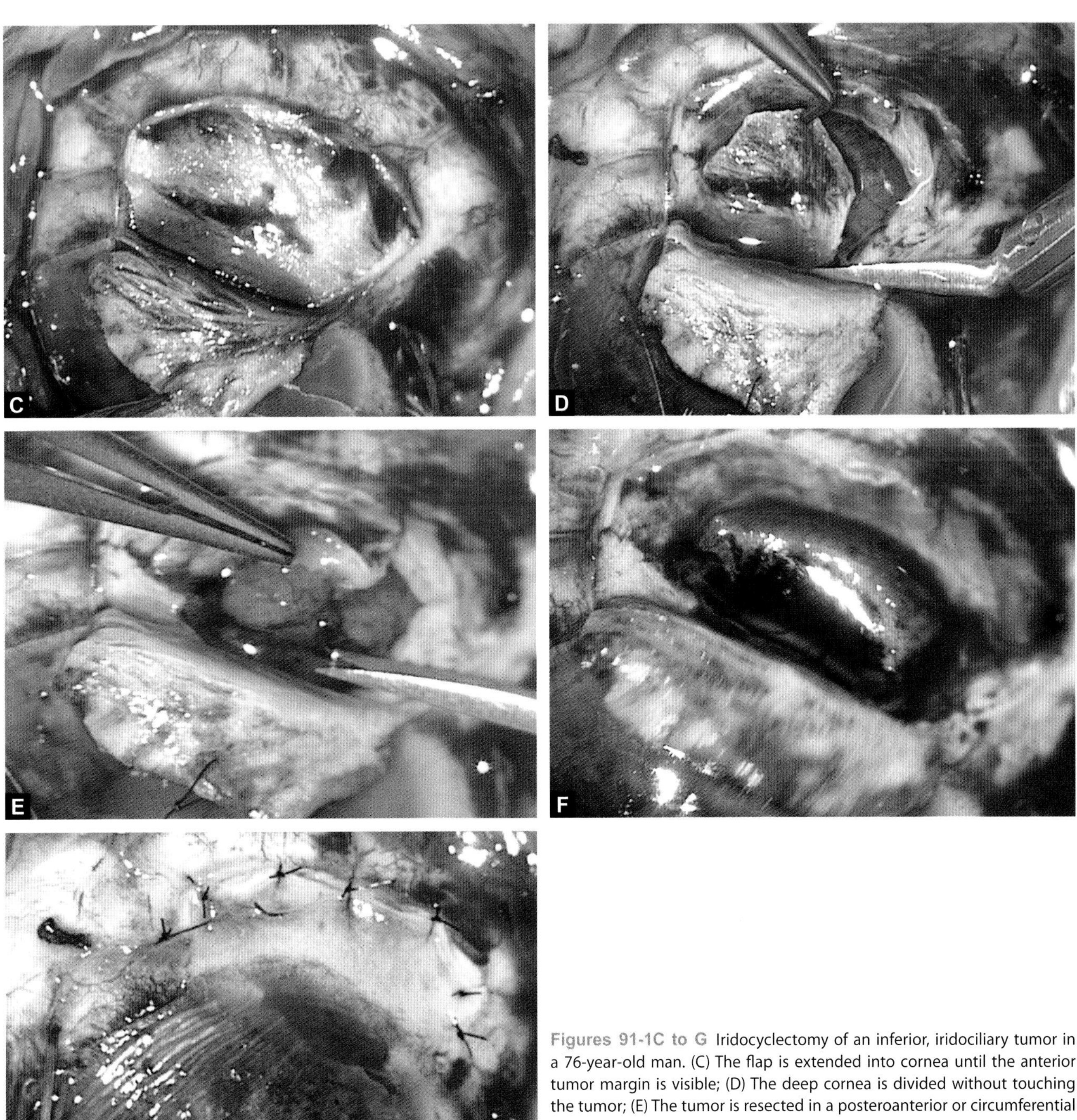


Figures 91-1C to G Iridocyclectomy of an inferior, iridociliary tumor in a 76-year-old man. (C) The flap is extended into cornea until the anterior tumor margin is visible; (D) The deep cornea is divided without touching the tumor; (E) The tumor is resected in a posteroanterior or circumferential direction, using the deep sclera as a handle; (F) Any prolapsed vitreous is either pushed back into the eye or removed by open-sky vitrectomy, according to whether or not its face is intact; (G) The sclera is closed with nonabsorbable nylon sutures, in case adjunctive brachytherapy is required within the next few weeks.

### Conjunctival Closure

The conjunctiva is closed in the standard manner.

If performed by an experienced surgeon, iridocyclectomy is completed in less than 1 hour.

## MECHANISM OF ACTION

If the diagnosis is uncertain, iridocyclectomy provides ample tissue for histological examination and immunohistochemistry.

If the diagnosis of melanoma is beyond doubt, iridocyclectomy also provides tissue for genetic studies, which greatly enhance prognostication.[7]

Whether excision of a melanoma actually prolongs life depends on whether or not metastatic spread has already occurred by the time the patient undergoes this surgery. It is not known how many disomy 3/class 1 melanomas transform to monosomy 3/class 2 tumors if left untreated.

After radiotherapy, uveal melanomas and even adenocarcinomas can give rise to the "toxic tumor syndrome", which should respond to excision of the offending tumor.[8]

## POSTOPERATIVE CARE

At the end of the surgical procedure, subconjunctival antiobiotic and steroid injections are administered together with atropine 1% drops.

Approximately 4 weeks postoperatively, the patient is reviewed at the oncology center, to assess the operated eye. The patient is informed of the survival probability, which is based on the clinical stage of the ocular tumor, the histologic grade of malignancy and the genetic tumor type. An online tool has been developed for multivariate analysis of all major predictors, also taking the patient's age and sex into account.[9]

If adjunctive brachytherapy was not administered at the time of the primary exoresection and if the tumor shows high-grade malignancy or extends to the resection margins, plaque radiotherapy can be administered at this time.

Long-term surveillance is performed as for other forms of treatment for uveal melanoma.

Psychological support and systemic screening for metastatic disease are undertaken in the usual manner.

## SPECIFIC INSTRUMENTATION

### Forceps

- Moorfields forceps for conjunctiva
- Toothed colibri forceps for sclera (with fresh forceps for closure)

### Scissors

- Spring scissors for conjunctiva
- Blunt-tipped spring scissors for uvea
- Ong's scissors for iris

### Blades

- Feather blade for incising sclera
- Number 15 Bard-Parker knife for clearing scleral surface
- Desmarres scarifier for preparation of scleral flap.

### Sutures

- 6-0 vicryl sutures for muscles and conjunctiva
- 8-0 nylon sutures for scleral flap
- 7-0 vicryl sutures for sclerotomy

### Retractors

- Fison's retractor

### Miscellaneous

- Needle holder
- 90° 20-gauge transilluminator, to localize tumor margins
- Scleral pen, to mark tumor extent
- Calipers, to measure knot-to-limbus distances if disinserting and reinserting rectus muscles
- Bipolar cautery
- 20-gauge vitreous cutter
- 20-mL syringe with 25-gauge needle and filter, for injecting balanced salt solution intraocularly, should vitreous loss occur.

## COMPLICATIONS

### Intraoperative Complications

- Malposition of flap
- Superficial scleral buttonhole
- Inadvertent deep scleral perforation, which is most likely to occur at limbus
- Vitreous loss does not seem to have any adverse outcomes if managed adequately, and may even reduce the (small) risk of malignant glaucoma
- Lens damage, if the tumor is excised without being lifted out of the eye during dissection
- Incomplete tumor excision, which is treatable by adjunctive brachytherapy
- Scleral wound dehiscence or leakage, particularly if brachytherapy is administered
- Incorrect placement of plaque
- Inaccurate reinsertion of muscles
- Inadequate conjunctival wound closure, with scleral exposure. If irradiated sclera is left exposed, it may undergo necrosis and perforation.

### Postoperative Complications

- Vitreous hemorrhage, which is usually mild, resolving spontaneously.
- Rhegmatogenous retinal detachment, which might occur only if the excision extends posterior to ora serrata.

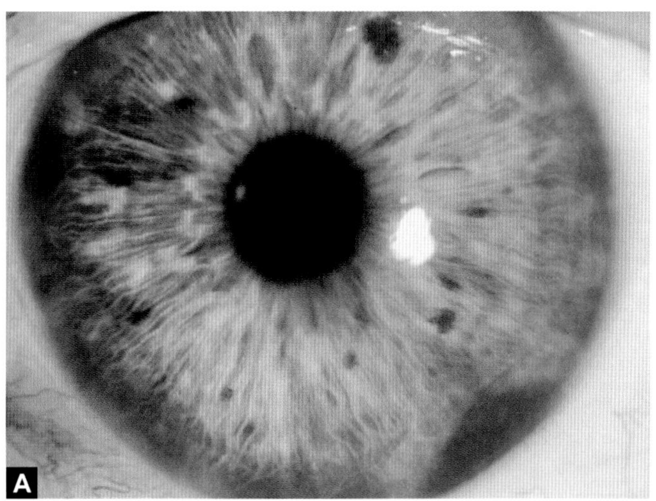


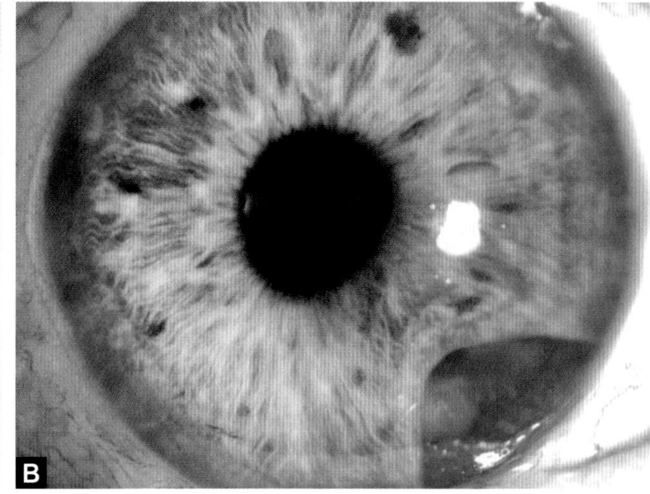


**Figures 91-2A and B** Iris and ciliary body melanoma in the left eye of a 78-year-old woman, photographed preoperatively (A) and 6 weeks after local resection, when the visual acuity was 20/30 (B). The tumor was a spindle-cell, disomy 3 melanoma.

- Local tumor recurrence, which is rare if adjunctive radiotherapy is administered for aggressive histology or tumor extension to surgical margins.
- Orbital tumor recurrence is exceedingly rare.
- Cataract, which is rare unless the lens has been irradiated or damaged by surgical instruments or silicone oil.
- Lens subluxation, if extensive cyclectomy is performed. This can occur even if the zonule is conserved.
- Ocular hypotony, if adjunctive brachytherapy is administered at the time of primary cyclectomy.
- Phthisis is rare if ocular hypotony and retinal detachment are prevented.
- Diplopia, if the rectus muscles are not reinserted accurately.

## SURGICAL OUTCOMES: SCIENTIFIC EVIDENCE/METANALYSIS

- If performed by an experienced surgeon in well-selected cases, intraoperative complications are rare (Figs. 91-2A and B).[10]
- The most common problem is ocular hypotony, which usually resolves with a pressure bandage if the patient has not received immediate adjunctive brachytherapy.
- Secondary enucleation is rare.

## PLACE OF THE TECHNIQUE IN SURGICAL ARMAMENTARIUM

Iridocyclectomy provides the best results if the iris sphincter is preserved and if not more than 2 clock hours of ciliary body requires excision. When the tumor involves sphincter or if the tumor is diffuse or shows extensive involvement of the ciliary body or angle then radiotherapy seems superior, although randomized, prospective studies have yet to be performed.[5,11]

## PEARLS AND PITFALLS

- Pupil constriction preoperatively makes it easier to conserve the iris sphincter.
- Conservation of ocular function is more likely to be achieved if the tumor is excised in a posteroanterior or circumferential direction.
- Inadvertent perforation of the deep sclera can happen all too easily at the sclerocorneal junction, directly over the tumor.
- A wide scleral step facilitates scleral suturing during closure.
- Delay brachytherapy for 1 month to prevent hypotony. Such radiotherapy may not be required if the tumor is not a melanoma or if a melanoma is of low-grade malignancy with no extension to surgical margins.

## REFERENCES


1. Memmen JE, McLean IW. The long term outcome of patients undergoing iridocyclectomy. Ophthalmology. 1990;97:429-32.
2. Damato BE, Foulds WS. Cilary body tumours and their management. Trans Ophthalmol Soc UK. 1986;105:257-64.
3. Daubner D, Prokosch V, Busse H, et al. Long-term results of iridocyclectomy for iris tumours. Klin Monbl Augenheilkd. 2008;225(12):1045-50.
4. Zografos L. Excision chirurgicale des tumeurs intraoculaires. Tumeurs intraoculaires. Société Française d'Ophthalmologie et Masson: Paris; 2002. pp. 59-63.

5. Damato BE. Local resection of uveal melanoma. Dev Ophthalmol. 2012;49:66-80.
6. Damato B, Jones AG. Uveal melanoma: resection techniques. Ophthalmol Clin North Am. 2005;18(1):119-28.
7. Damato EM, Damato B, Sibbring JS, et al. Ciliary body melanoma with partial deletion of chromosome 3 detected with multiplex ligation-dependent probe amplification. Graefes Arch Clin Exp Ophthalmol. 2008;246(11):1637-40.
8. Schalenbourg A, Coupland S, Kacperek A, et al. Iridocyclectomy for neovascular glaucoma caused by proton-beam radiotherapy of pigmented ciliary adenocarcinoma. Graefes Arch Clin Exp Ophthalmol. 2008;246(10):1499-501.
9. Damato B, Eleuteri A, Taktak AF, et al. Estimating prognosis for survival after treatment of choroidal melanoma. Prog Retin Eye Res. 2011;30(5):285-95.
10. Rospond-Kubiak I, Damato B. The surgical approach to the management of anterior uveal melanomas. Eye (Lond). 2014 Jun;28(6):741-7.
11. Damato BE. Treatment Selection for uveal melanoma. Dev Ophthalmol. 2012;49:16-26.

CHAPTER

# 92

# Endoresection of Choroidal Melanoma

Carl Groenewald, Bertil Damato

## INTRODUCTION

Endoresection of choroidal melanoma involves piecemeal tumor removal with a vitreous cutter. This can be performed as a primary procedure or after radiotherapy.

## INDICATIONS

- Primary endoresection is performed for juxtapapillary melanomas when other methods are unlikely to conserve vision (Figs. 92-1A and B).
- Secondary endoresection is performed as a treatment for sight-threatening retinal detachment or exudation from an irradiated choroidal melanoma ("toxic tumor syndrome") or for local tumor recurrence.

## CONTRAINDICATIONS

### Primary Endoresection

- Tumor involving more than 6 clock hours of optic disk margin
- Basal tumor diameter exceeding 10 mm
- Extraocular tumor spread
- Diffuse melanoma
- Ciliary body involvement
- Tumor treatable with less controversial methods.

## PREOPERATIVE CARE

- Ultrasonography and biometry are performed to exclude extraocular tumor growth and in anticipation of cataract surgery after silicone oil removal.

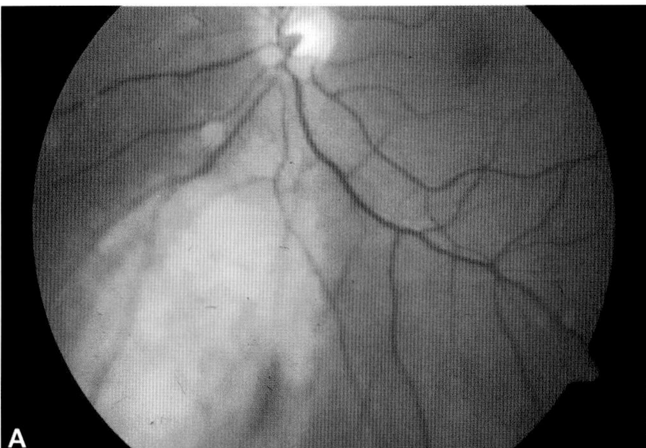


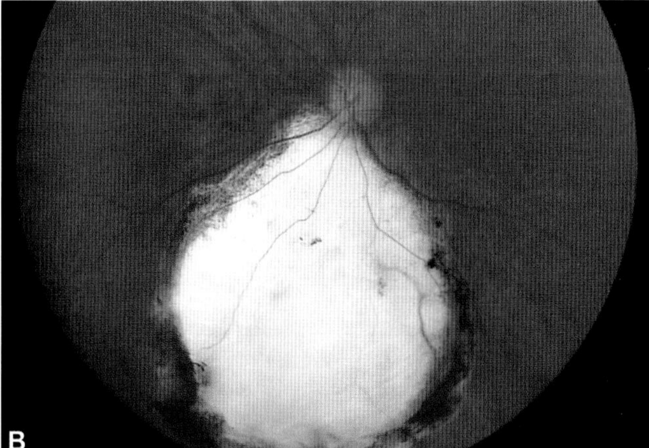


**Figures 92-1A and B** Left fundus of a 38-year-old woman with an inferonasal choroidal melanoma having a basal diameter of 9.9 mm and a thickness of 2.5 mm (A). Postoperative photograph showing the surgical coloboma with a small retinal defect at its center and a healthy macula. The visual acuity more than 10 years after surgery was 20/30. The tumor was of mixed, spindle-epithelioid type. There was no evidence of local tumor recurrence or seeding despite not administering neoadjuvant or adjunctive radiotherapy.

- Antibiotics and mydriatics are administered in the conventional manner.

## SURGICAL TECHNIQUE

*Vitrectomy*: Total 3-port vitrectomy is performed in the usual manner.

*Tumor endoresection*: The tumor is removed with a 20-gauge vitreous cutter, which is passed through the retina at the tumor apex. The entire tumor is removed together with a 1-mm surround of apparently-healthy choroid (Fig. 92-2A).

*Endolaser photocoagulation*: The surgical coloboma is treated with endophotocoagulation to destroy any tumor remnants.

*Retinopexy*: Fluid-heavy liquid (perfluorocarbon liquid) exchange is performed (Fig. 92-2B). When the retina is flat, endolaser burns are applied around the coloboma to achieve retinopexy (Fig. 92-2C).

*Perfluorocarbon liquid-silicone exchange*: The eye is filled with silicone, which prevents retinal detachment and vitreous hemorrhage (Fig. 92-2D).

*Treatment of entry-site tears*: The eye is indented with a cryoprobe to identify any entry-site tears, which are treated with cryotherapy.

*Closure of sclerotomies*: The sclerotomies are sutured and treated with cryotherapy in case tumor seeding has occurred.

*Adjunctive radiotherapy*: Adjunctive brachytherapy or proton beam radiotherapy can be administered if histological and genetic studies indicate that the tumor is highly malignant.

*Conjunctival closure*: The conjunctiva is closed in the usual manner.

## MECHANISM OF ACTION

- Primary endoresection of the tumor is performed to conserve the eye and vision while preventing metastatic spread.
- Secondary endoresection of a toxic melanoma after radiotherapy is aimed at eliminating the source of exudation.

## POSTOPERATIVE CARE

- The patient is postured so that any hemorrhage gravitates away from the fovea.
- The silicone oil is removed after 12 weeks, when phacoemulsification is performed.

## SPECIFIC INSTRUMENTATION

Standard vitrectomy equipment.

## COMPLICATIONS

### Intraoperative Complications

*Vitrectomy*: These include complications common to any vitrectomy procedure, such as lens touch, entry-site tears.

*Endoresection*: The main complication is residual tumor, particularly if not visible because of its location beneath healthy retinal pigment epithelium or within sclera. Tumor dissemination is probably inevitable but only rarely seems to result in tumor recurrence. Hemorrhage is controlled by raising the intraocular pressure and lowering the systemic blood pressure. There have been reports of fatal air embolism so that the use of air has been abandoned in favor of heavy liquid.

### Postoperative Complications

- *Local tumor recurrence*: Rates of recurrence are similar to those achieved with other modalities.[1,2] Seeding of tumor around the eye is rare but can arise from residual uveal tumor if this is not detected and treated in a timely manner.[3] Residual intrascleral tumor can spread extraocularly.[4] Some authors have advocated neoadjuvant radiotherapy as a means of preventing tumor seeding.[5,6] However, in view of the rarity of local tumor recurrence, such radiotherapy and any associated iatrogenic complications are unnecessary in most patients.
- *Rhegmatogenous retinal detachment*: This can arise as a result of entry-site tears or because the retinopexy around the surgical coloboma is inadequate. Proliferative vitreoretinopathy is rare in the absence of rhegmatogenous retinal detachment.
- *Ocular hypotony*: This can occur if the endoresection is extensive, unless it is possible to preserve most of the retina over the coloboma. This is because the retina is relatively waterproof.
- *Maculopathy*: This is likely to occur if the coloboma extends close to the fovea and arises as a result of retinal distortion, macular excision or the formation of a neovascular membrane.
- *Vitrectomy complications*: These are the same as for other vitrectomy procedures and include cataract, glaucoma and endophthalmitis.

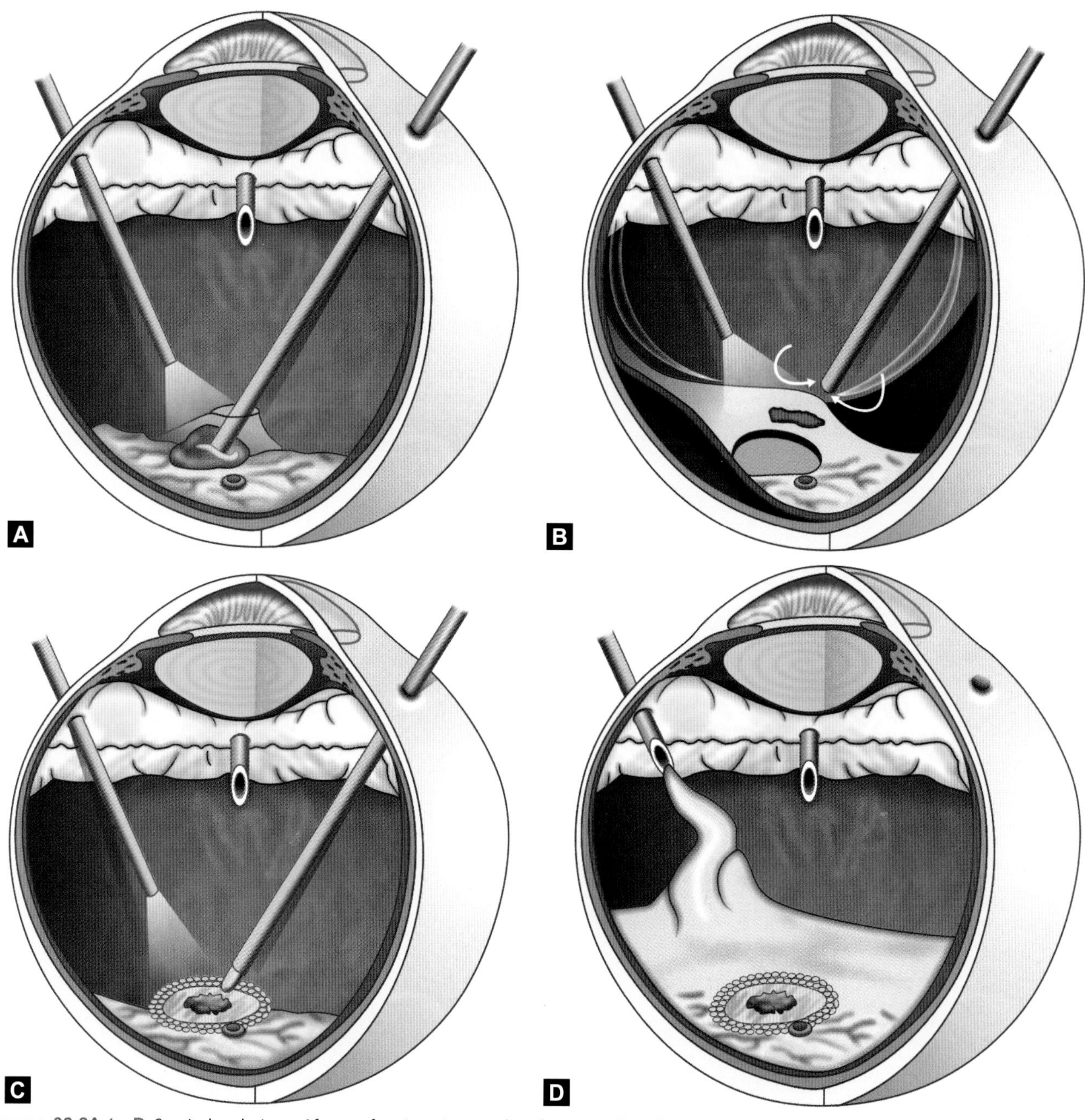


Figures 92-2A to D Surgical technique. After performing vitreous detachment and total vitrectomy, the tumor is removed through a retinal hole over the tumor apex (A); The retina is reattached by performing a fluid-heavy liquid exchange (B); Endolaser photocoagulation is administered to destroy any tumor remnants and to achieve retinopexy (C); Heavy liquid-silicone exchange is performed for postoperative tamponade, which prevents retinal detachment and hemorrhage (D).

## SURGICAL OUTCOMES: SCIENTIFIC EVIDENCE/METANALYSIS

Several authors have reported outcomes after endoresection.[1,2,7] There are fears that piecemeal removal of melanoma can disseminate tumor around the eye and systemically; however, such concerns are mostly based on intuition and not on outcomes analysis.[8] Of concern are recent reports of fatal intra-operative air embolism, which have resulted in air being replaced with heavy liquid.[9]

## PLACE OF THE TECHNIQUE IN SURGICAL ARMAMENTARIUM

Endoresection is useful when radiotherapy is expected to cause optic neuropathy. It is also useful as a treatment for the toxic tumor syndrome after radiotherapy.

## PEARLS AND PITFALLS

- Endoresection can conserve vision when radiotherapy is likely to cause optic neuropathy.
- Seeding of tumor is rare unless residual uveal tumor is not detected and treated without delay. This is because of the defect in the retina, which acts as a barrier to transvitreal tumor spread.

## REFERENCES

1. Damato B, Groenewald C, McGalliard J, et al. Endoresection of choroidal melanoma. Br J Ophthalmol. 1998;82(3):213-8.
2. Garcia-Arumi J, Zapata MA, Balaguer O, et al. Endoresection in high posterior choroidal melanomas: long-term outcome. Br J Ophthalmol. 2008;92(8):1040-5.
3. Hadden PW, Hiscott PS, Damato BE. Histopathology of eyes enucleated after endoresection of choroidal melanoma. Ophthalmology. 2004;111(1):154-60.
4. Damato B, Wong D, Green FD, et al. Intrascleral recurrence of uveal melanoma after transretinal "endoresection". Br J Ophthalmol. 2001;85(1):114-5.
5. Bechrakis NE, Foerster MH. Neoadjuvant proton beam radiotherapy combined with subsequent endoresection of choroidal melanomas. Int Ophthalmol Clin. 2006;46(1):95-107.
6. Schilling H, Bornfeld N, Talies S, et al. Endoresection of large uveal melanomas after pretreatment by single-dose stereotactic convergence irradiation with the leksell gamma knife—first experience on 46 cases. Klinische Monatsblatter fur Augenheilkunde. 2006;223(6):513-20.
7. Kertes PJ, Johnson JC, Peyman GA. Internal resection of posterior uveal melanomas. Br J Ophthalmol. 1998;82(10):1147-53.
8. Damato B. Choroidal melanoma endoresection, dandelions and allegory-based medicine. Br J Ophthalmol. 2008;92(8):1013-4.
9. Rice JC, Liebenberg L, Scholtz RP, et al. Fatal air embolism during endoresection of choroidal melanoma. Retinal Cases & Brief Reports. 2014; 8: 127-9.

# CHAPTER 93

# Conjunctival Tumor Excision

Nihal Kenawy, Sarah E Coupland, Bertil Damato

## INTRODUCTION

Excision is the primary form of treatment for nodular conjunctival tumors and some diffuse tumors. It is often performed together with adjunctive cryotherapy, radiotherapy and/or topical chemotherapy.

## INDICATIONS

- *Benign tumors*: Excision is indicated for a wide variety of benign tumors, the most common being melanocytic nevi and papillomas.
- *Malignant tumors*: The most common nodular tumors are melanoma, squamous cell carcinoma, sebaceous gland carcinoma and lymphoma. The diffuse, intraepithelial counterparts of these neoplasms include conjunctival melanocytic intraepithelial neoplasia, in situ carcinoma and pagetoid spread of sebaceous gland carcinoma are usually too extensive for surgical excision and tend to be treated by topical chemotherapy and/or radiotherapy.

## CONTRAINDICATIONS

- Lymphangiomas and racemose hemangiomas are not treated surgically.
- Extensive intraepithelial melanocytic neoplasia is not resectable.

## PREOPERATIVE CARE

- Full conjunctival examination must be performed with color photographs and drawings. It is important to examine the superior tarsal conjunctiva and fornix. These can be assessed with a binocular indirect ophthalmoscope and a 20D lens for magnification, gently pulling the eyelid away from the eye. Tumor location and extent are documented on a conjunctival mapping chart (Fig. 93-1).[1]
- The regional lymph nodes are palpated.
- High-frequency B-scan ultrasonography is performed if any primary or secondary intraocular tumor is suspected.
- The tumor is staged according to the 7th edition of the tumor node metastasis (TNM) system by the American Joint Committee on Cancer.

## TECHNIQUE

Local anesthesia is adequate for small tumors. General anesthesia is required for uncooperative patients, children and advanced tumors requiring extensive excision.

### Bulbar Conjunctival Tumor

- The conjunctival excision site is marked with bipolar diathermy with minimal safety margins. A subconjunctival injection of lidocaine 2% with epinephrine 1:200,000 can be administered to facilitate surgery and reduce hemorrhage. Corneal epithelial debridement is performed with a Bard-Parker knife after devitalizing the epithelium with alcohol so as to excise any corneal extension of the tumor. Tumor nodules are excised, using blunt-tipped spring scissors and applying the no-touch technique to avoid dissemination of tumor cells. This is done without lamellar scleral excision; instead, bipolar diathermy is applied to any suspicious areas. Meticulous hemostasis is maintained. The specimen is mounted on paper, taking care to avoid crush artifact (Fig. 93-2).[1-3]

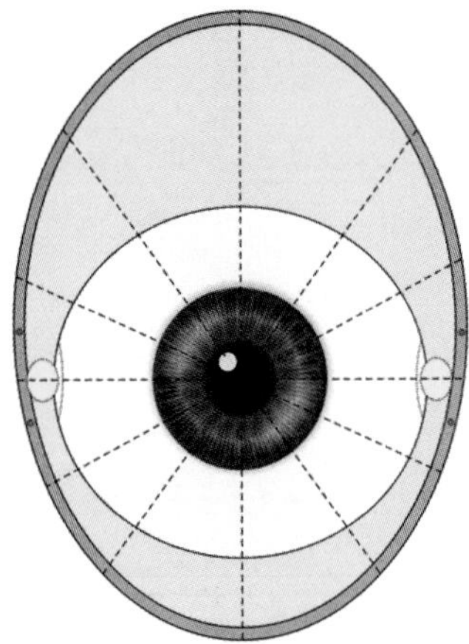

Figure 93-1 Conjunctival mapping. Conjunctival diagram for tumor mapping displaying the conjunctiva as a flat surface. The conjunctiva is divided into quadrants. The center of the conjunctiva is the center of the cornea. The limbus, bulbar conjunctiva, fornix, tarsal conjunctiva, eyelid margin and skin are progressively more peripheral.

- Irrigating the resection area with balanced salt solution is best avoided to minimize seeding of tumor cells with the irrigating solution.[3]
- Care should be taken to avoid reusing microsurgical swabs in the operative field to prevent carriage of cells to nontumor area.
- Wound closure is performed using a fresh set of instruments undermining the conjunctiva and using 7/0 absorbable sutures. Buried sutures are recommended to avoid discomfort from sutures ends.
- In cases where wide resection has been performed, an amniotic membrane or mucous membrane graft can be used to close the defect using absorbable sutures.[4,5] A graft can be harvested from the contralateral superotemporal fornix.[6]
- If incisional biopsy is to be performed, marking of the tumor with diathermy is not required. Snip biopsies do not require suturing unless more than 3–4 mm long. Fresh instruments are used for closure as mentioned previously.
- The transport medium or fixative should be agreed with the pathologist before the biopsy or excision is performed. Genetic analysis may be undertaken to identify mutations that might influence systemic treatment for metastasis (e.g. BRAF inhibitors). The orientation of some specimens may require marking.

## Forniceal Tumor

- To adequately expose the area of interest, it is necessary to apply traction sutures on the sclera, away from the excision area so that the eye is rotated away from the tumor site.

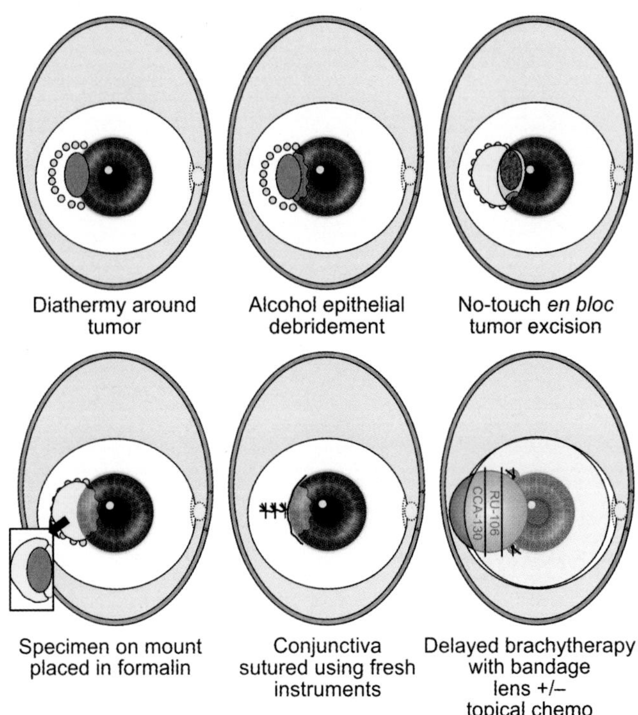


Figure 93-2 Excision of a bulbar conjunctival tumor.

- Excision is performed as previously described. Healing is usually good (Figs. 93-3A and B).
- Some authors recommend wide excision with application of alcohol to the scleral bed and cryotherapy to the excision edges.[6]

## Caruncular Tumor

Excision of caruncular tumors is performed as described above, with few differences:

- The safety margin may need to be reduced.
- A superficial plane of conjunctival dissection is maintained and excessive traction is avoided to prevent prolapse of retro-orbital fat, which can result in enophthalmos, ptosis and diplopia.
- Closure of large defects may necessitate grafting to avoid adhesions, which can cause diplopia.

## Conjunctival Tumor with Orbital Spread

- Orbital exenteration is the treatment of choice for primary, malignant, conjunctival tumors invading the orbit. If the eyelids are not involved by the tumor, lid sparing produces better cosmetic results and faster rehabilitation. When exenteration is not possible, proton beam radiotherapy or external beam radiotherapy should be employed.[2,3,7]

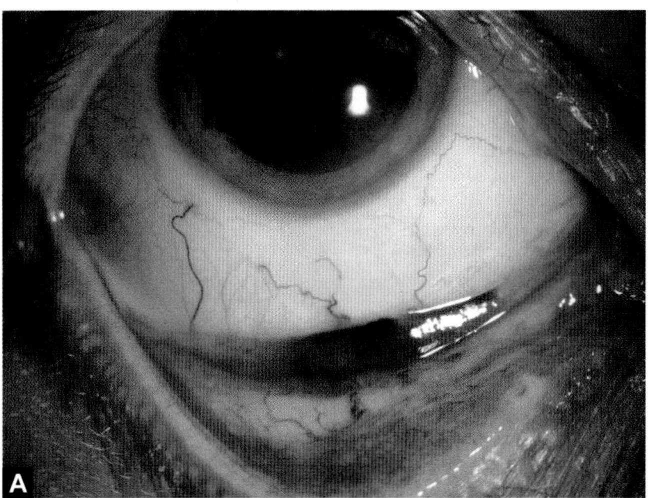


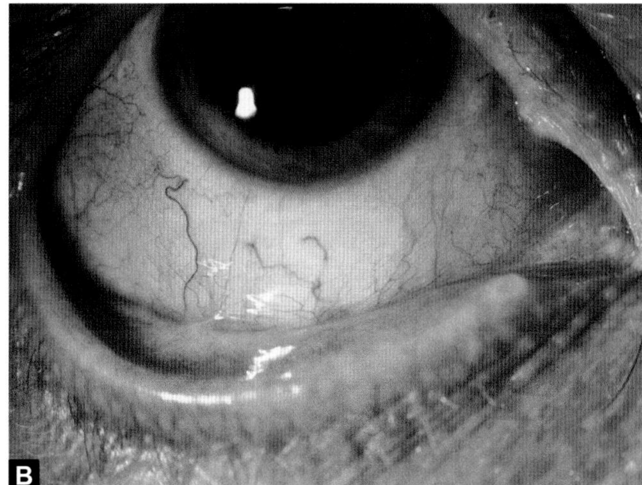


**Figures 93-3A and B** Microinvasive conjunctival melanoma of the lower fornix of the right eye (A). Appearance several months after treatment with excision and topical mitomycin C (B).

## MECHANISM OF ACTION

- As with malignancies elsewhere, excision of conjunctival tumors is aimed at alleviating or avoiding local morbidity as well as preventing invasion of adjacent tissues and metastasis. It also enables histopathological assessment of the entire lesion.
- Removal of the nodular part of the tumor enhances tumor control with topical chemotherapy, which is effective only for intraepithelial disease.

## POSTOPERATIVE CARE

- Topical antibiotic drops are prescribed for 1–2 weeks. Topical ointment is preferred if the excision site is adjacent to the medial limbus, to prevent formation of corneal dellen.
- A bandage contact lens or symblepharon rings may be required in grafted conjunctiva with topical antibiotics for longer periods.
- Adjunctive therapy in the form of chemotherapeutic drops is prescribed in cases of residual melanocytic or squamous intraepithelial disease. Cryotherapy is advocated if chemotherapy fails.
- Local radiotherapy is administered if deep invasion or incomplete clearance is histologically evident or in selected cases of lymphoma.
- Proton beam therapy may be the adjunctive treatment of choice for caruncular and forniceal invasive tumors when brachytherapy is not possible.
- After treatment of a malignant tumor, patients are reviewed every 4–6 months for 4 or 5 years then yearly to ensure early detection of any recurrence.

## SPECIFIC INSTRUMENTATION

- *For conjunctival biopsy*: Clark's speculum (for exposure), nontoothed forceps (e.g. Moorefields forceps), and spring scissors.
- *For corneal debridement*: Alcohol swabs folded and mounted on a blunt forceps, Bard Parker No. 15 blade.
- *For the transport of the specimen to the laboratory*: sterile tissue paper, cassettes for specimen laid flat on tissue paper (e.g. Cellsafe biopsy insert) placed into histopathology container.
- Fresh set of instruments for wound closure and 7/0 absorbable sutures.

## COMPLICATIONS

Postoperative complications are uncommon especially when proper surgical techniques are followed. Possible complications include:

- Infection
- Bleeding
- Wound dehiscence
- Tenon's cyst
- Pyogenic granuloma
- Excessive scarring
- Adhesions and symblepharon leading to restrictive strabismus

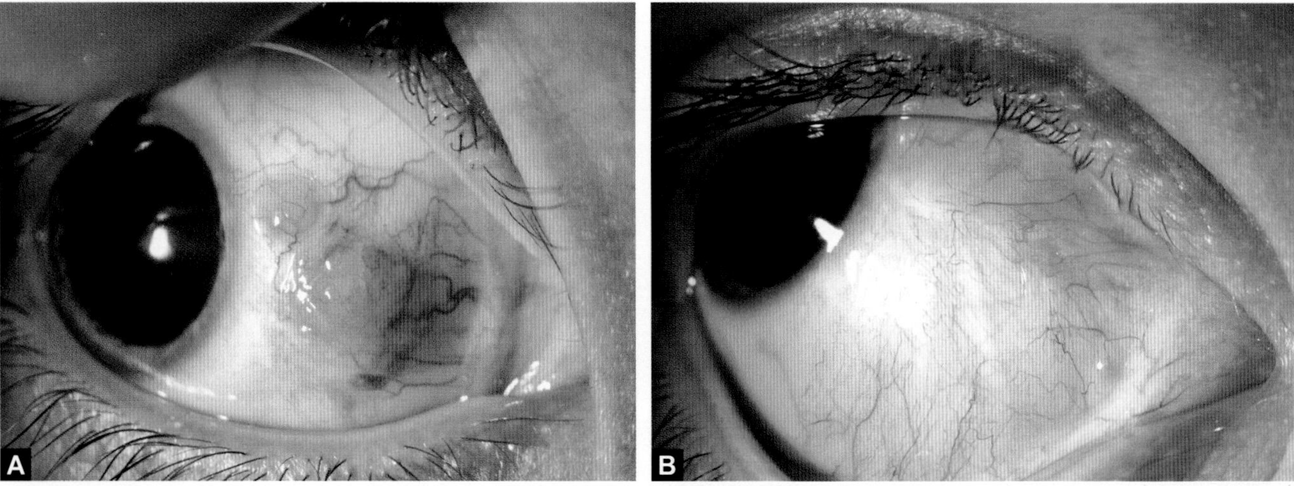

Figures 93-4A and B Invasive conjunctival melanoma in the right eye (A). Appearance several months after treatment by excision, ruthenium brachytherapy and topical mitomycin C (B).

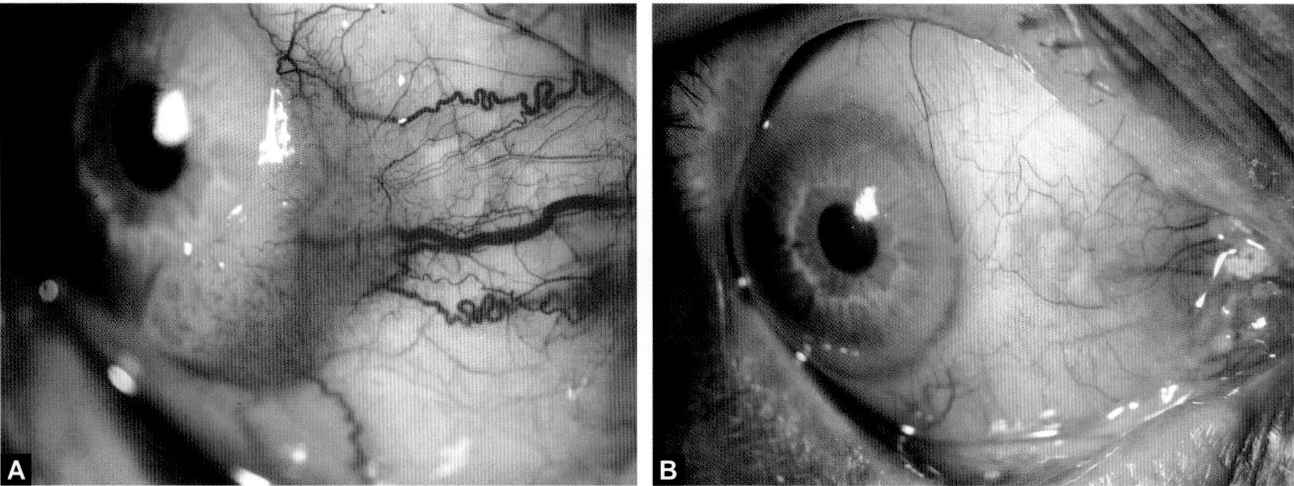

Figures 93-5A and B Squamous cell carcinoma in the right eye (A). Appearance after treatment by local excision, ruthenium brachytherapy and topical 5-fluorouracil chemotherapy (B)

- Tumor seeding, which can be caused by incisional biopsy or failure to use a fresh set of instruments for wound closure.

## SURGICAL OUTCOMES: SCIENTIFIC EVIDENCE/METANALYSIS

- En bloc excision is the technique of choice in localized tumors (Figs. 93-4 and 93-5). Local tumor control is achieved when following the abovementioned principles.[2,6-9] The authors have shown 100% success rate of controlling melanocytic disease when proper surgical techniques are applied accompanied by adjuvant therapy, such as brachytherapy irrespective of deep histological clearance.[2,7,10] Recurrences in distant parts of the conjunctiva have occurred as a result of seeding because of incomplete excision or biopsy before referral to our center. Incisional biopsy is best avoided in localized lesions and should be reserved for widespread disease.[7,8]
- Proton beam radiotherapy has been described in the successful management of extensive, unresectable tumors in place of exenteration. This applies to forniceal and caruncular tumors where extensive surgery is not feasible and complete excision is unlikely.[2,7,11] Other forms of radiotherapy are also possible.
- Simple local excision is performed in symptomatic dermoids and osseous choristomas, but may necessitate corneal grafts or superficial scleral dissection if adherent to the deep tissues.[3]

## Metastasis

- Without adjunctive therapy, surgical excision is associated with an increased risk of recurrence. Hence, brachytherapy and/or topical chemotherapy are recommended.[8,12]
- Systemic screening is required in cases suspected of metastasis or in high-risk invasive melanoma (nasal and caruncular tumors ≥2 mm in thickness). This generally involves full medical examination, chest radiography, liver function tests and liver imaging. The tests are performed every 6 months for 10 years and are undertaken routinely in some centers.[13]
- The role of whole-body positron emission tomography (PET)/CT is still controversial albeit being reported as superior to other imaging. The use of PET scans is limited by their high cost, nonspecificity and false negative results.[14,15]
- The value of sentinel lymph node biopsy (SLNB) in detecting micrometastasis to the regional lymph nodes has yet to be established. The technique requires special expertise and currently the evidence is unclear as to the patient selection criteria and the stage at which SLNB should be undertaken.[14,16-18]

## PLACE OF THE TECHNIQUE IN SURGICAL ARMAMENTARIUM

- Surgical margins as wide as 5 mm have been reported.[6,19,20] We do not exceed 3 mm to reduce the risk of compromised ocular function from shortened conjunctiva.[2,7]
- Cryotherapy applied intraoperatively to the margins of resection is a routine practice in many centers; however, evidence does not support its role as an adjuvant modality.[6,8,12,21-23] We have substituted cryotherapy for ruthenium brachytherapy and topical chemotherapy, which give high rates of local tumor control.[2,7]
- Brachytherapy has proven beneficial as adjunctive treatment in invasive conjunctival melanoma and squamous cell carcinoma. Conventional radiotherapy has been shown to be inferior in such cases and should be only employed when local resection is contra-indicated.[7,24-26]

## PEARLS AND PITFALLS

- En bloc excision is the treatment of choice in most localized tumors. This minimizes the risk of recurrence and iatrogenic dissemination of cells in cases of malignancy.
- The specimen should not be crushed and should be laid with the epithelial side facing upwards to facilitate histopathologic assessment.
- Discussion with the pathologist prior to surgery is advised for best processing of the sample.
- We do not advocate superficial dissection of the scleral tissue unless there is visible invasion by the tumor.
- We do not administer cryotherapy at the time of primary excision but this can be used as a secondary treatment following complete conjunctival healing and when other methods fail or are not possible.
- Topical antibiotic ointment is best after excisions around the medial limbal area to prevent formation of corneal dellen.
- Symblepharon rings are recommended with conjunctival grafts involving the fornices to avoid retraction and adhesions.
- Adjuvant brachytherapy and/or topical chemotherapy are effective with most malignant lesions but should be employed only after complete conjunctival healing.

## REFERENCES


1. Damato B, Coupland SE. Clinical mapping of conjunctival melanomas. Br J Ophthalmol. 2008;92:1545-9.
2. Damato B, Coupland SE. An audit of conjunctival melanoma treatment in Liverpool. Eye (Lond). 2009;23:801-9.
3. Shields CL, Shields JA. Tumors of the conjunctiva and cornea. Surv Ophthalmol. 2004;49:3-24.
4. Dalla Pozza G, Ghirlando A, Busato F, et al. Reconstruction of conjunctiva with amniotic membrane after excision of large conjunctival melanoma: a long-term study. Eur J Ophthalmol. 2005;15:446-50.
5. Paridaens D, Beekhuis H, van Den Bosch W, et al. Amniotic membrane transplantation in the management of conjunctival malignant melanoma and primary acquired melanosis with atypia. Br J Ophthalmol. 2001;85:658-61.
6. Shields JA, Shields CL, De Potter P. Surgical management of circumscribed conjunctival melanomas. Ophthal Plast Reconstr Surg. 1998;14:208-15.
7. Damato B, Coupland SE. Management of conjunctival melanoma. Expert Rev Anticancer Ther. 2009;9:1227-39.
8. Shields CL, Shields JA, Gunduz K, et al. Conjunctival melanoma: risk factors for recurrence, exenteration, metastasis, and death in 150 consecutive patients. Arch Ophthalmol. 2000;118:1497-507.
9. Shields CL, Shields JA, Armstrong T. Management of conjunctival and corneal melanoma with surgical excision, amniotic membrane allograft, and topical chemotherapy. Am J Ophthalmol. 2001;132:576-8.
10. Fraunfelder FT, Wingfield D. Management of intraepithelial conjunctival tumors and squamous cell carcinomas. Am J Ophthalmol. 1983;95:359-63.
11. Wuestemeyer H, Sauerwein W, Meller D, et al. Proton radiotherapy as an alternative to exenteration in the management of extended conjunctival melanoma. Graefes Arch Clin Exp Ophthalmol. 2006;244:438-46.

12. De Potter P, Shields CL, Shields JA, et al. Clinical predictive factors for development of recurrence and metastasis in conjunctival melanoma: a review of 68 cases. Br J Ophthalmol. 1993; 77:624-30.
13. Kenawy N, Lake SL, Coupland SE, et al. Conjunctival melanoma and melanocytic intraepithelial neoplasia. Eye (Lond). 2013; 27(2):142-52.
14. Esmaeli B. Regional lymph node assessment for conjunctival melanoma: sentinel lymph node biopsy and positron emission tomography. Br J Ophthalmol. 2008;92:443-5.
15. Patel P, Finger PT. Whole-body 18F FDG positron emission tomography/computed tomography evaluation of patients with uveal metastasis. Am J Ophthalmol. 2012;153:661-8.
16. Tuomaala S, Kivela T. Sentinel lymph node biopsy guidelines for conjunctival melanoma. Melanoma Res. 2008;18:235.
17. Savar A, Ross MI, Prieto VG, et al. Sentinel lymph node biopsy for ocular adnexal melanoma: experience in 30 patients. Ophthalmology. 2009;116:2217-23.
18. Tuomaala S, Kivela T. Metastatic pattern and survival in disseminated conjunctival melanoma—Implications for sentinel lymph node biopsy. Ophthalmology. 2004;111:816-21.
19. Paridaens AD, McCartney AC, Minassian DC, et al. Orbital exenteration in 95 cases of primary conjunctival malignant melanoma. Br J Ophthalmol. 1994;78:520-8.
20. Shields JA, Shields CL, De Potter P. Surgical management of conjunctival tumors. The 1994 Lynn B. McMahan Lecture. Arch Ophthalmol. 1997;115:808-15.
21. Jakobiec FA, Brownstein S, Wilkinson RD, et al. Adjuvant cryotherapy for focal nodular melanoma of the conjunctiva. Arch Ophthalmol. 1982;100:115-8.
22. Brownstein S, Jakobiec FA, Wilkinson RD, et al. Cryotherapy for precancerous melanosis (atypical melanocytic hyperplasia) of the conjunctiva. Arch Ophthalmol. 1981;99:1224-31.
23. Finger PT. "Finger-tip" cryotherapy probes: treatment of squamous and melanocytic conjunctival neoplasia. Br J Ophthalmol. 2005;89:942-5.
24. Layton C, Glasson W. Clinical aspects of conjunctival melanoma. Clin Experiment Ophthalmol. 2002;30:72-9.
25. Stannard CE, Sealy GR, Hering ER, et al. Malignant melanoma of the eyelid and palpebral conjunctiva treated with iodine-125 brachytherapy. Ophthalmology. 2000;107:951-8.
26. Lommatzsch PK, Lommatzsch RE, Kirsch I, et al. Therapeutic outcome of patients suffering from malignant melanomas of the conjunctiva. Br J Ophthalmol. 1990;74:615-9.

CHAPTER

94

# Cryosurgery

Bertil Damato

## INTRODUCTION

Cryosurgery (also known as cryotherapy) is widely used to treat tumors. It kills tumor cells by creating ice crystals, which physically disrupt cell membranes.

## INDICATIONS

### Retinoblastoma

- Pre-equatorial tumors up to 2–3 mm in diameter and 1–2 mm thick (Figs. 94-1A and B).[1]
- Localized subretinal seeding.
- Selected cases of systemic chemotherapy, as a means of enhancing drug penetration into the vitreous.

### Vasoproliferative Tumor

Cryosurgery is the first choice of treatment in some centers but there are concerns that it can aggravate epiretinal membrane formation.[2] Photodynamic therapy can avoid this problem and in some centers has replaced cryotherapy.[3]

### Retinal Hemangioblastoma

As with vasoproliferative tumors, cryosurgery is effective.[4] In some centers, cryosurgery has been replaced by methods that are considered less likely to cause fibrosis.[5]

### Coats Disease

Cryosurgery is indicated for telangiectasia causing retinal detachment and/or exudation if laser photocoagulation has failed.[6]

### Conjunctival Tumors

- After excision of nodular conjunctival tumors, such as melanoma, adjunctive cryotherapy is administered by some authors as a means of preventing local tumor recurrence.[7]

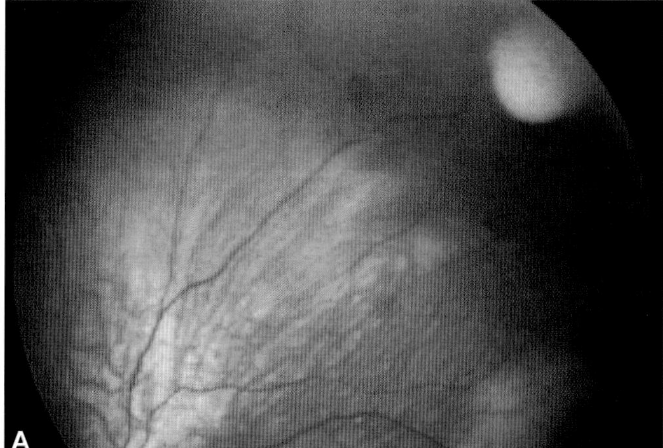


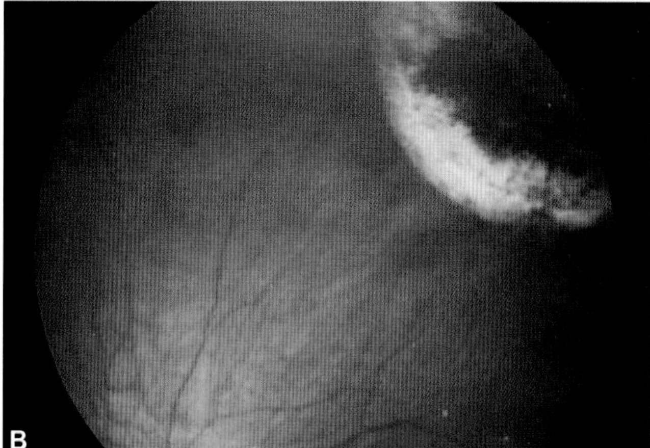


**Figures 94-1A and B** Peripheral retinoblastoma before treatment (A) and after cryosurgery (B)
*Source* Courtesy of T Hadjistilianou, Siena, Italy

The author has abandoned this procedure in favor of adjunctive radiotherapy and topical chemotherapy.[8]

- Conjunctival melanocytic intraepithelial neoplasia with atypia (otherwise known as primary acquired melanosis with atypia) has widely been treated with cryosurgery.[7] The author prefers topical chemotherapy, which seems more effective with less morbidity, except perhaps with tarsal conjunctival disease when cryosurgery is useful for neoplasia that is resistant to topical chemotherapy.[8,9]

## CONTRAINDICATIONS

- *Retinoblastoma*: Cryosurgery is unlikely to succeed with large tumors, vitreous seeding, and extensive subretinal seeding.[1] Cryosurgery with concurrent subtenon carboplatin injections increases the risk of ocular toxicity. Treatment of postequatorial tumors with this modality risks optic nerve and macular damage.
- *Retinal hemangioblastoma and vasoproliferative tumor*: Some authors consider cryosurgery to be contraindicated if other methods are possible, because of the risk of fibrosis.
- Coats disease does not require cryosurgery if the retina is flat or if laser photocoagulation is successful.
- *Conjunctival neoplasia*: There is no consensus as to whether cryosurgery is superior to other methods.

## PREOPERATIVE CARE

Preoperative care is the same as that recommended for other modalities.

## SURGICAL TECHNIQUE

### Intraocular Cryotherapy

The target tissue is frozen and thawed two or three times. The freeze is continued until the entire target is enveloped by the iceball. The thawing is allowed to occur spontaneously, without accelerating the process with warm water. Care must be taken not to move the probe until complete thawing has occurred.

With intraocular cryosurgery, the formation of the iceball is observed by binocular indirect ophthalmoscopy.

The cryotherapy may need to be repeated in several sessions. Indeed, overenthusiastic cryotherapy can cause severe complications. This is particularly the case with retinal hemangioblastomas, because severe exudation and edema may occur.[4] With Coats disease, not more than two quadrants of the retina should be treated at the same time if possible (unless glaucoma is imminent because of advanced disease) and care should be taken to avoid damage to ciliary body.

In selected patients with retinoblastoma, laser retinopexy may be performed to avoid rhegmatogenous retinal detachment. With Coats disease, drainage of subretinal fluid may be necessary if the retinal detachment is severe.

### Conjunctival Cryotherapy

With extraocular cryosurgery, naked-eye inspection is adequate. Some authors have recommended the use of a subconjunctival thermocouple but with experience, the author found this to be unnecessary, having learnt to recognize the appearances when the required temperature is reached (i.e. confluent and solid whitening of the conjunctiva).

To treat the tarsal conjunctiva and fornices, the author first everts the lid with a chalazion clamp, and then grasps the forniceal conjunctiva with forceps, pulling this down toward the limbus where it is more easily treated.

To avoid damaging the intraocular tissues when administering cryotherapy to the bulbar conjunctiva, some authors have recommended injecting air subconjunctivally to insulate the globe from the cryoprobe. This is not usually possible when the cryotherapy is repeated, because of adhesions.

If the entire conjunctiva is being treated with cryotherapy, for example, in a patient with conjunctival melanocytic intraepithelial neoplasia with atypia, or melanoma in situ, the conventional practice is to treat not more than 50–60% of the conjunctiva in the same session.

## MECHANISM OF ACTION

Expanding gases cool, to induce the formation of ice crystals, which destroy frozen tissues. Cryosurgery can be performed with closed probes or by delivering spray to the target tissue.

## POSTOPERATIVE CARE

Intraocular cryosurgery is followed by surveillance to ensure that an adequate response has been achieved and that any recurrence is detected and treated promptly.

Conjunctival cryotherapy is followed by topical antibiotics and steroids. Biopsy is usually performed after several months to ensure that the tumor has indeed been eradicated.

## SPECIFIC INSTRUMENTATION

Intraocular cryosurgery uses carbon dioxide whereas for conjunctival disease, some authors have advised liquid nitrogen, which produces lower temperatures.

With extraocular tumors, the freezing can be achieved with a closed probe or with spray. A thermocouple has been recommended for conjunctival cryosurgery to ensure that a temperature of –20°C is achieved.

When administering conjunctival cryotherapy, the author uses a wooden spatula to protect the cornea. A syringe of tepid water is available in case the iceball inadvertently involves the cornea so that rapid thawing is required.

## COMPLICATIONS

Intraocular cryosurgery can be complicated by:

- Persistent or recurrent tumor
- Macular edema
- Epiretinal membrane formation
- Retinal tear formation with rhegmatogenous retinal detachment, especially with calcified retinoblastomas[10]
- Proliferative vitreoretinopathy
- Exudative retinal detachment
- Vitreous hemorrhage
- Uveal effusion
- Cataract
- Scleral atrophy
- Eyelid swelling

Conjunctival cryosurgery complications include:

- Persistent or recurrent tumor
- Uveitis and macular edema, in the case of bulbar tumors
- Eyelid damage with loss of lashes, after treatment of tarsal conjunctival lesions

## SURGICAL OUTCOMES: SCIENTIFIC EVIDENCE/METANALYSIS

The current literature on the efficacy of cryosurgery is scanty, and to the author's knowledge, there have not been randomized studies comparing this modality with rival therapies.

## PLACE OF THE TECHNIQUE IN SURGICAL ARMAMENTARIUM

With retinoblastoma, cryosurgery is useful for small, pre-equatorial tumors after chemotherapy. It is also useful to enhance penetration of chemotherapeutic agents into the retina and vitreous.

With vasoproliferative tumors and retinal hemangioblastomas, cryosurgery may be useful as adjunctive therapy to other methods but must be delivered "gently" to avoid inducing harmful reactions.

Cryosurgery has in some centers been replaced by other methods, such as photodynamic therapy for vasoproliferative tumors and retinal angiomas, and topical chemotherapy or radiotherapy for conjunctival neoplastic disease.

With conjunctival tumors, cryosurgery can control superficial disease when topical chemotherapy fails.

Cryosurgery of choroidal melanoma has been performed but has not gained widespread acceptance.[11]

## PEARLS AND PITFALLS

- Consider cryotherapy for small, pre-equatorial retinoblastomas as an adjunct to systemic chemotherapy.
- Beware of administering cryotherapy postequatorially, because of the risk of damage to optic nerve and fovea.
- Overzealous cryotherapy of intraocular tumors can cause severe ocular morbidity.
- Bulbar conjunctival cryotherapy can cause uveitis, hypotony and macular edema.
- Tarsal conjunctival cryosurgery may help control superficial disease that is resistant to chemotherapy.

## REFERENCES


1. Shields JA, Shields CL. Treatment of retinoblastoma with cryotherapy. Trans Pa Acad Ophthalmol Otolaryngol. 1990;42:977-80.
2. Heimann H, Bornfeld N, Vij O, et al. Vasoproliferative tumours of the retina. Br J Ophthalmol. 2000;84(10):1162-9.
3. Barbezetto IA, Smith RT. Vasoproliferative tumor of the retina treated with PDT. Retina. 2003;23(4):565-7.
4. Chew EY, Schachat AP. Capillary hemangioblastoma of the retina and von Hippel-Lindau disease. In: Ryan SJ (Ed). Retina, Vol. 3. Elsevier Saunders: New York; 2013. pp. 2156-63.
5. Papastefanou VP, Pilli S, Stinghe A, et al. Photodynamic therapy for retinal capillary hemangioma. Eye (Lond). 2013;27(3):438-42.
6. Shields JA, Shields CL, Honavar SG, et al. Classification and management of Coats disease: the 2000 Proctor Lecture. Am J Ophthalmol. 2001;131(5):572-83.
7. Jakobiec FA, Rini FJ, Fraunfelder FT, et al. Cryotherapy for conjunctival primary acquired melanosis and malignant melanoma. Experience with 62 cases. Ophthalmology. 1988;95(8):1058-70.
8. Damato B, Coupland SE. An audit of conjunctival melanoma treatment in Liverpool. Eye (Lond). 2009;23(4):801-9.
9. Kurli M, Finger PT. Topical mitomycin chemotherapy for conjunctival malignant melanoma and primary acquired melanosis with atypia: 12 years' experience. Graefes Arch Clin Exp Ophthalmol (Albrecht von Graefes Archiv fur klinische und experimentelle Ophthalmologie). 2005;243(11):1108-14.
10. Mullaney PB, Abboud EB, Al-Mesfer SA. Retinal detachment associated with type III retinoblastoma regression after cryotherapy and external-beam radiotherapy. Am J Ophthalmol. 1997;123(1):140-2.
11. Wilson DJ, Klein ML. Cryotherapy as a primary treatment for choroidal melanoma. Arch Ophthalmol. 2002;120(3):400-3.

CHAPTER

# 95

# Enucleation for Intraocular Tumors

Sachin Salvi, Naz Raoof, Bertil Damato

## INTRODUCTION

Many patients with uveal melanoma, retinoblastoma and other tumors require enucleation, either as a primary procedure or because of complications. In enucleation surgery, the complete eyeball is removed (as opposed to the contents of the eyeball removed in evisceration), thus avoiding any disturbance of the intraocular tumor. In the event that there is any extraocular spread, special measures must be taken to ensure total tumor excision. In some centers, a tumor sample is also harvested for laboratory investigations after the eye is enucleated. In this chapter, we discuss oncological aspects of enucleation and describe the first author's preferred technique.

## INDICATIONS

### Uveal Melanoma

- *Primary enucleation* is indicated when conservative therapy is unlikely to succeed or preserve a useful eye because of large tumor size and/or extensive involvement of optic disk, ciliary body, iris, angle or extraocular tissues.[1] Primary enucleation is also performed when the patient is not motivated to undergo conservative therapy.
- *Secondary enucleation* is required for local tumor recurrence unamenable to conservative management, as well as for complications of treatment such as retinal detachment and neovascular glaucoma.[1]

### Retinoblastoma

- Primary enucleation is performed when the tumor is not treatable conservatively because of size, extent or location (e.g. anterior segment involvement). Some authors consider primary enucleation to be the first choice of treatment for patients with extensive unilateral retinoblastoma [International Retinoblastoma Classification (IRC) groups D and E when the fellow eye is healthy]. Features indicating enucleation include: rubeosis iridis; anterior chamber involvement by tumor; tumor seeding into pars plana; tumor involvement of optic nerve or orbit; persistent retinal detachment and poor visual prognosis.
- Secondary enucleation is undertaken for persistent disease or painful complications. This happens in approximately 50% of eyes with IC Group D retinoblastoma and up to 10% of eyes with less extensive disease.

### Other Tumors

- A variety of benign and malignant tumors can cause extensive ocular disorganization, preventing conservative therapy (e.g. uveal metastases, retinal hemangioblastoma, choroidal hemangioma).
- Patients with longstanding poor vision who develop a painful blind eye should be considered for enucleation (rather than evisceration) in case they harbor an intraocular malignancy.

## CONTRAINDICATIONS

There are many contraindications to enucleation, which vary between tumors and from one center to another. Only a few general principles will therefore be mentioned.

- *Uncertain diagnosis*: Enucleation may cause patient dissatisfaction unless the patient accepts such uncertainty beforehand this being documented clearly in the charts. If the clinical diagnosis is in doubt, it is prudent to perform a biopsy.

- *Alternative treatment options*: Enucleation should be avoided in cases where the tumor can be treated completely with other conservative treatment options, thus increasing the likelihood of maintaining some useful vision.
- *Intuitive impressions about impact of treatment on survival*: Many patients with uveal melanoma imagine that enucleation is safer than conservative therapy. Several studies suggest that survival after enucleation is no worse than after other forms of treatment.[2] Whether local tumor control is achieved by conservative therapy or enucleation in similar sized uveal melanomas, it is likely that survival is similar. However, local treatment failure is associated with increased mortality.[3,4] Whether the recurrent tumor is the cause of metastatic disease or whether it is merely an indicator of increased tumor malignancy is uncertain. The authors believe that the clinician should attempt to communicate this information to patients when deciding between enucleation and less aggressive treatment.
- *Lack of regular experience with enucleation*: As with other operations, severe complications can arise if the procedure is not performed correctly.
- *Inadequate multidisciplinary support*: Ocular treatment is only one aspect of patient care, which involves prognostication, psychological support and systemic investigation requiring the involvement of different specialists.

## PREOPERATIVE CARE

Preoperative care is the same as for other forms of treatment. It is imperative to ensure that the correct eye is removed. In addition to standard procedures, the authors perform binocular indirect ophthalmoscopy for choroidal melanoma, ensuring that this is done after taping the fellow eye and draping the patient.

In patients with retinoblastoma and buphthalmos, some authors have recommended systemic chemotherapy to induce tumor regression and to soften the eye, thereby reducing the risk of globe perforation during enucleation.[5]

With uveal melanoma, opinions vary as to the indications for systemic screening, with some centers screening all patients prior to enucleation surgery and others investigating only high-risk patients after enucleation.[6]

It is essential to identify any extraocular tumor spread, with the aid of investigations such as B-scan ultrasonography and MRI, in case the surgical technique needs to be modified (Figs. 95-1A to C).

## SURGICAL TECHNIQUE

One drop of 5% povidone iodine is instilled to prevent infection.

### Conventional Procedure

The enucleation can be performed in the usual manner. Briefly, a 360° conjunctival peritomy is performed followed by blunt dissection of the conjunctiva and Tenon's capsule from the globe in all quadrants (Fig. 95-2). The extraocular muscles are disinserted (Fig. 95-3). The medial rectus stump is held with artery forceps to rotate the globe and the optic nerve is divided with scissors or a snare (Fig. 95-4). Sizing balls are used to decide the correct size of the implant (Fig. 95-5). The surgeon's preferred implant is inserted into the orbit, possibly using a slide or wrapped in a finger of sterile glove to prevent Tenon's capsule from being dragged posteriorly and to prevent the implant from touching eyelashes and other contaminants (Figs. 95-6A to C). The rectus muscles are sutured either to the implant or to each other in front of the implant (conventional muscle imbrication technique). In some centers, the inferior oblique muscle (or both oblique muscles) is sutured to the implant posterior to the equator. Tenon's capsule is closed with 4-0 absorbable sutures. The conjunctiva is sutured with a 7-0 absorbable suture. A conformer is placed into the socket with antibiotic ointment. A pressure bandage is applied for 24–48 hours.

### Myoconjunctival Technique Modification

This modification, in which the four recti muscles are sutured to the conjunctiva close to the corresponding fornices (instead of imbricating them to each other or suturing onto the implant), is preferred by the first author as a means of improving the motility of the artificial eye, as demonstrated in some studies.[7] With this technique, the enucleation is performed initially according to the conventional methods. After the preferred orbital implant is inserted deep into the orbit, the posterior Tenon's is closed with interrupted 5.0 vicryl to prevent anterior migration of the implant (Fig. 95-7). The sutures on the four recti muscles are then passed out through the conjunctiva onto the conjunctival surface close to the corresponding fornices (superior rectus close to superior fornix, inferior rectus close to inferior fornix, medial rectus and lateral rectus close to the inner and outer canthus respectively and outside the peritomy wound edge) (Fig. 95-8). The anterior Tenon's capsule then closed with 6.0 vicryl to allow the conjunctival edges to rest against each other (Fig. 95-9).

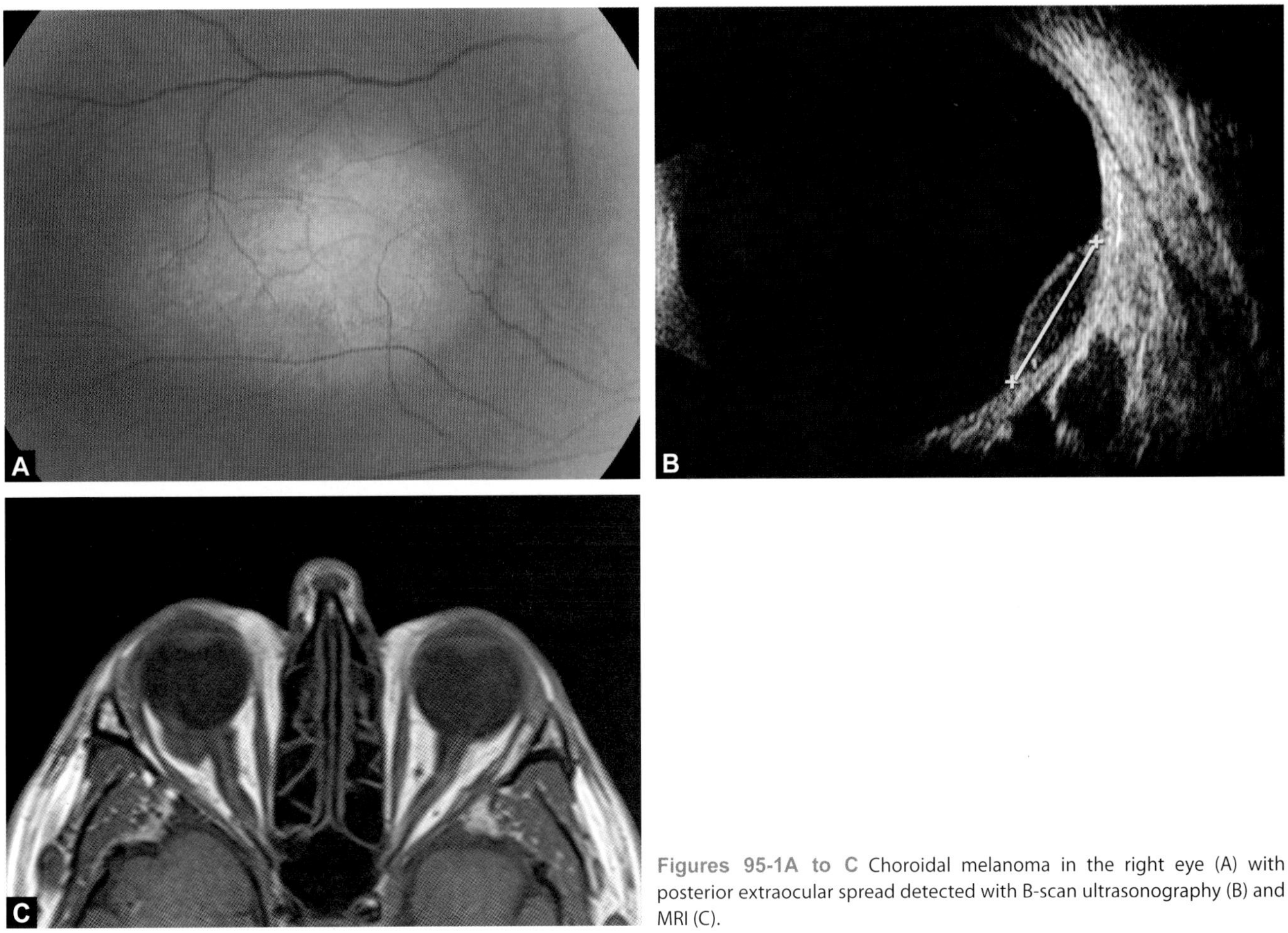

**Figures 95-1A to C** Choroidal melanoma in the right eye (A) with posterior extraocular spread detected with B-scan ultrasonography (B) and MRI (C).

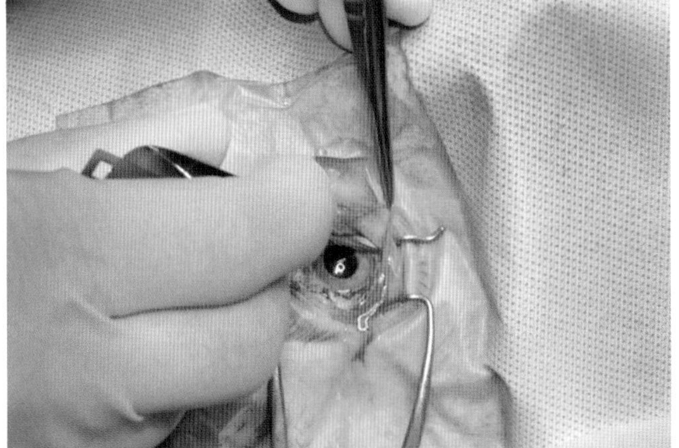

**Figure 95-2** Dissection of conjunctiva and Tenon's from the globe after 360° peritomy.

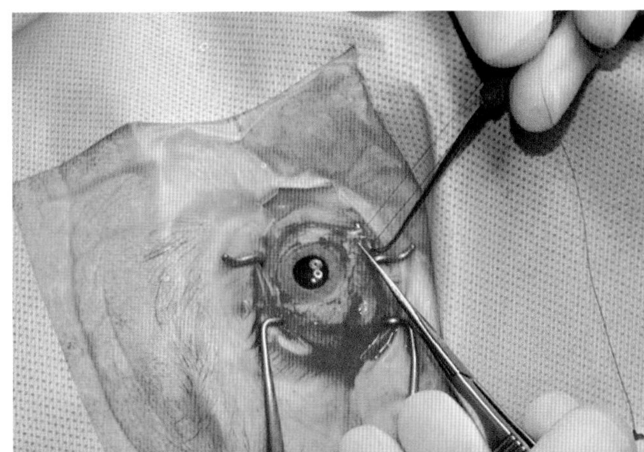

**Figure 95-3** Disinsertion of inferior rectus muscle.

The conjunctiva is then closed with a continuous 7.0 vicryl suture (Fig. 95-10). The sutures on the four recti are tied over the conjunctiva (Fig. 95-11). A conformer is then inserted. A 3–5 mL volume of 0.5% bupivacaine with epinephrine is injected via the skin approach into the lower lid to exert pressure onto the surgical site.

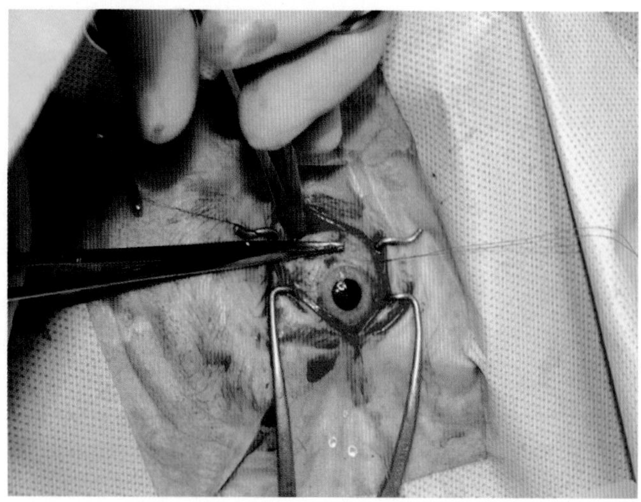

Figure 95-4 The optic nerve is cut from medial aspect while rotating the globe laterally by exerting traction on medial rectus muscle stump. Note that the medial orbital approach is taken to cut the nerve as extraocular spread is lateral to the optic nerve in the posterior orbit in this patient.

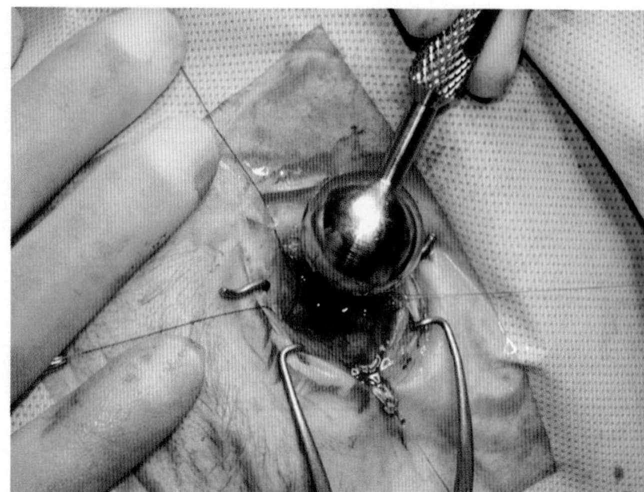

Figure 95-5 A sizing ball is used to select an orbital implant of the appropriate size.

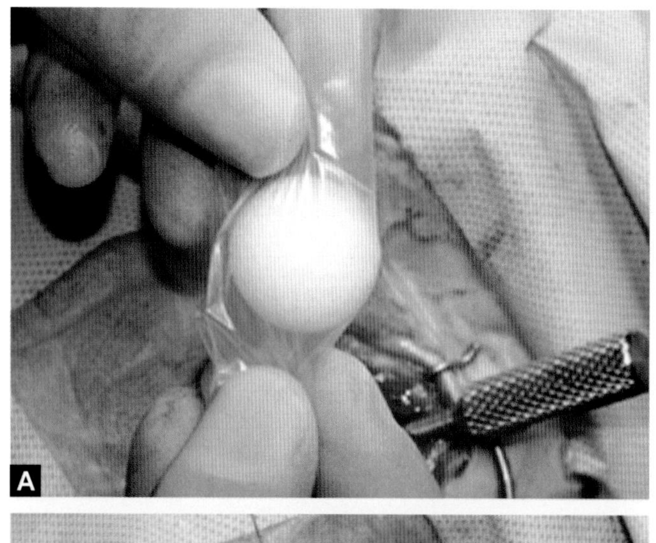

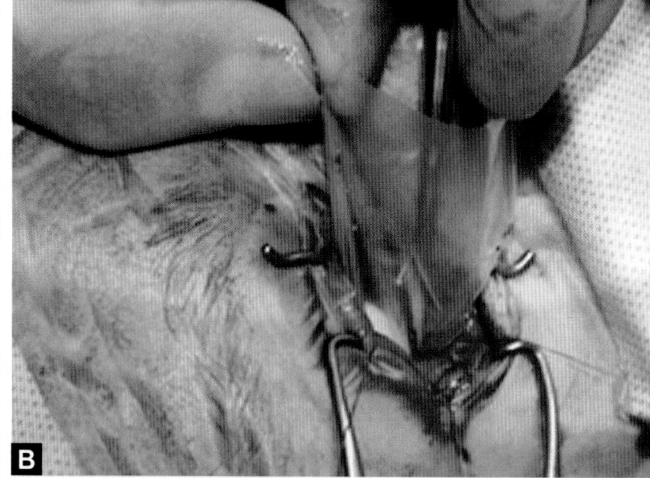

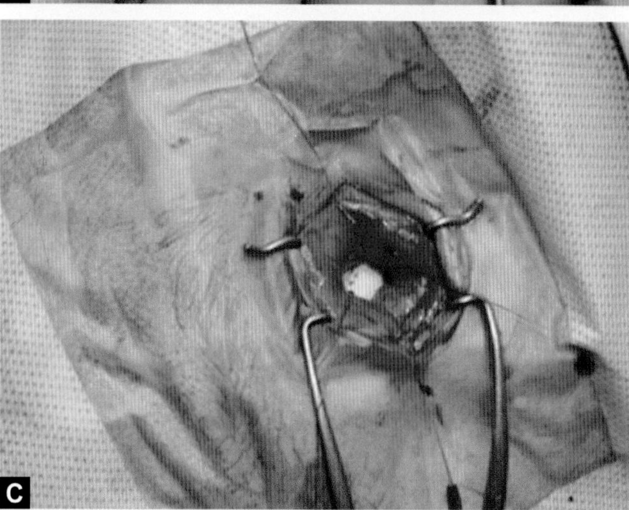

Figures 95-6A to C A 22-mm Medpore orbital implant is wrapped in the finger of a sterile glove to be inserted deep into the orbit without dragging the Tenon's capsule posteriorly and to avoid the implant from touching any lashes.

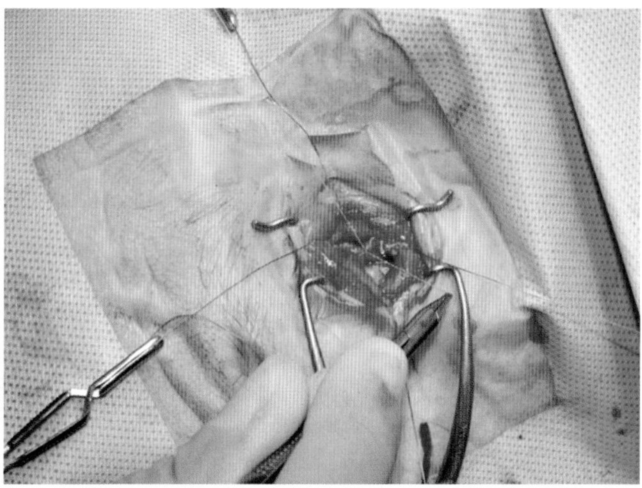

Figure 95-7 The posterior Tenon's is sutured over the orbital implant with interrupted 5.0 vicryl sutures to ensure complete implant coverage.

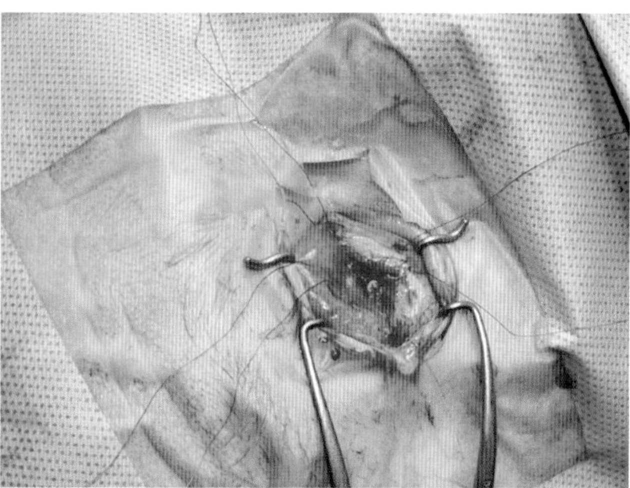

Figure 95-8 The sutures on the four recti muscles are passed through the conjunctiva close to their respective fornices.

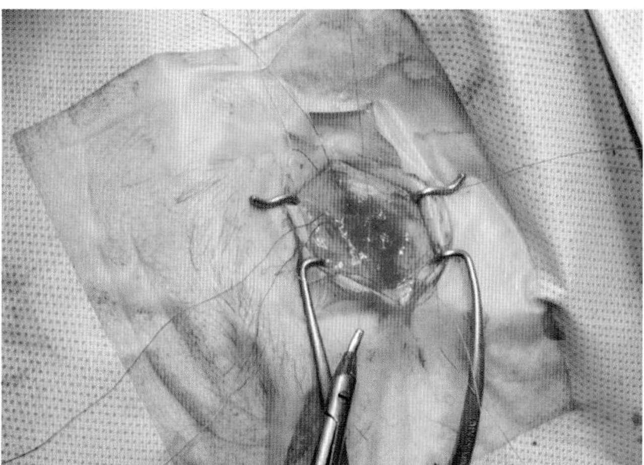

Figure 95-9 The anterior Tenon's is closed with interrupted 6.0 vicryl suture.

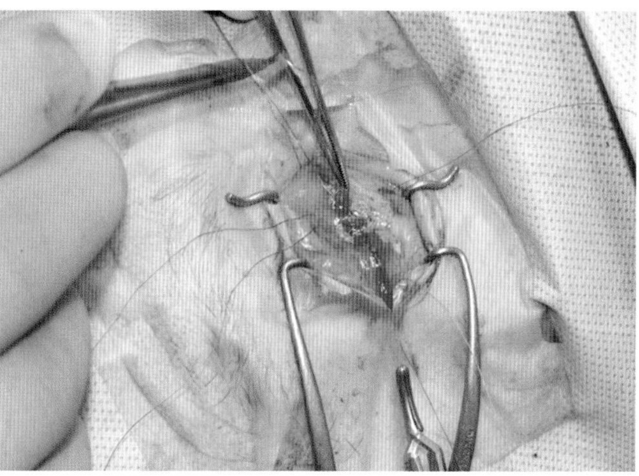

Figure 95-10 The conjunctiva is closed with a continuous 7.0 vicryl suture.

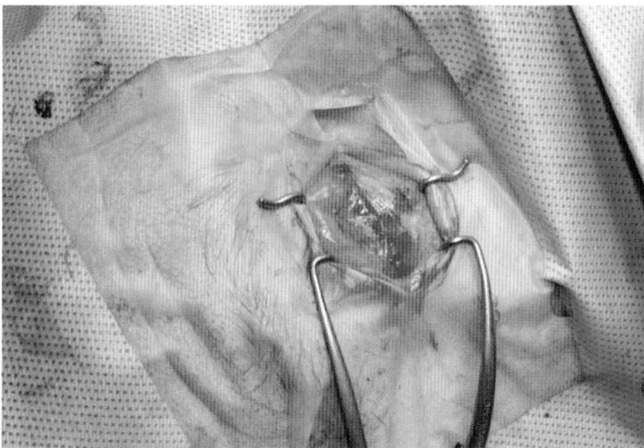

Figure 95-11 In the myoconjunctival technique of muscle insertion, the four rectus muscles are sutured onto the conjunctival surface, thus allowing the muscles to move the conjunctiva and fornices, thereby helping to increase motility of the artificial eye.

As the muscles are directly inserted onto the conjunctiva, the muscle action is translated directly into the movement of the conjunctiva and fornix, thus allowing improved movement of the artificial eye.

## Modification in Patients with Extraocular Extension

The extraocular extension size and site should be clearly confirmed prior to surgery. During surgery, this area should be avoided. If the extension is anterior, as in cases with ciliary body melanoma, the overlying conjunctiva with a 2-mm margin should be incorporated into the peritomy. With posterior extraocular extensions, care should be taken not to disrupt the pseudocapsule around the tumor. Dissection of the Tenon's from the globe in the quadrant of extension should be gentle. Cutting of the optic nerve should be performed in

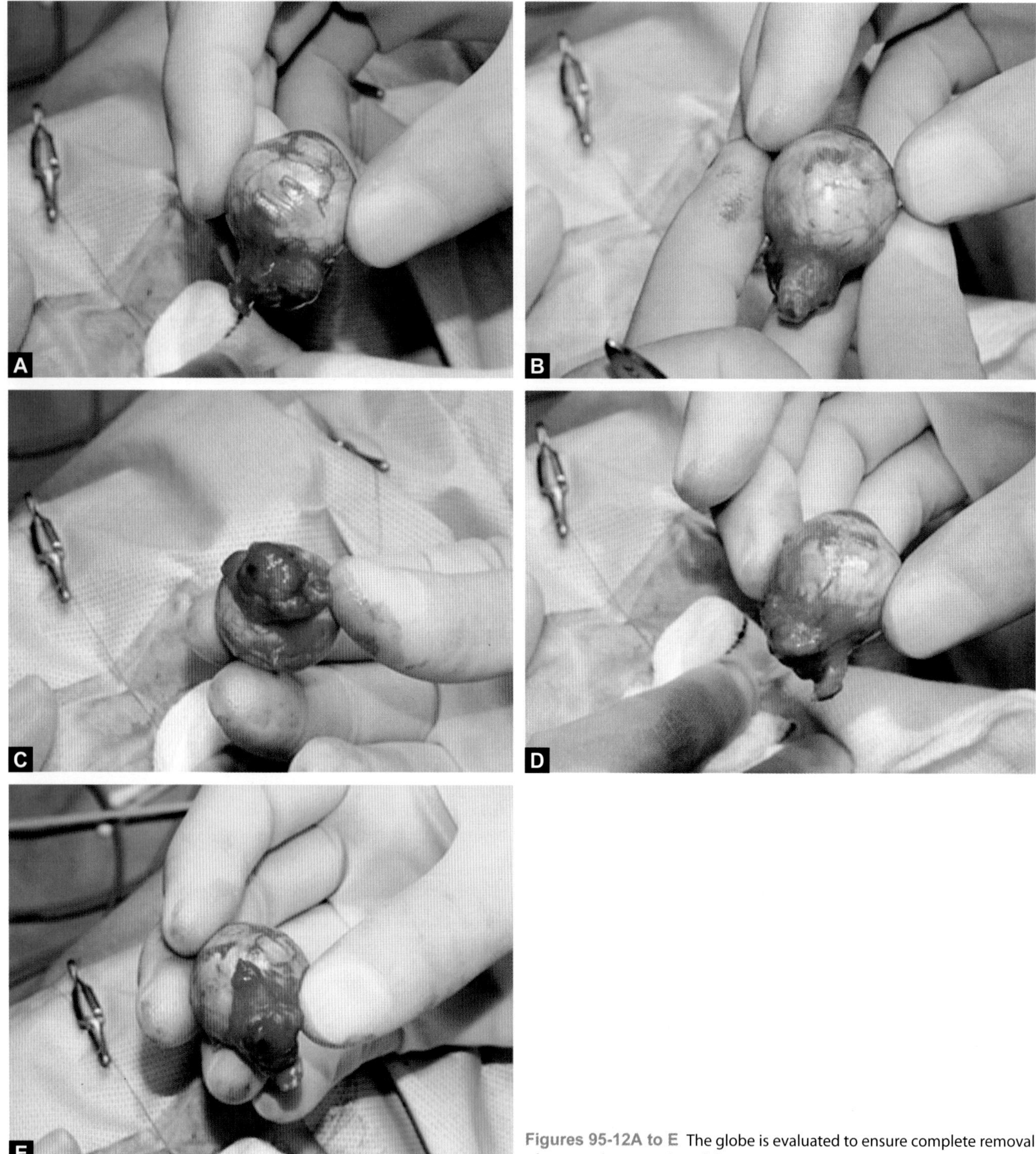


Figures 95-12A to E The globe is evaluated to ensure complete removal of extraocular extension of the tumor.

a quadrant away from the site of extension. After the eye is removed, the globe should be examined to confirm that the pseudocapsule around the extraocular extension is intact (Figs. 95-12A to E). The orbit should be examined to confirm that there is no residual tumor. If any tumor remnants are suspected, biopsies from the orbital tissue should be taken.

To reduce postoperative pain, an injection of bupivacaine 0.5% is given either at the beginning or at the end of the operation. With melanoma, pre-enucleation injection prevents the oculocardiac reflex and, if combined with 1:80,000 adrenaline, the intraoperative hemorrhage is reduced. With retinoblastoma, postenucleation injection is preferred, so as to avoid any risk of perforating the globe. In babies, excessive doses of bupivacaine can cause cardiotoxicity.

With retinoblastoma, it is especially important remove the eye with at least 12 mm of optic nerve, and to avoid rupturing the globe. This is achieved with scissors or a snare. It has been shown that any crush artifact caused by the snare does not compromise histological examination for retinoblastoma extension into the nerve.

Precautions should be taken to avoid wound dehiscence if healing may be compromised by chemotherapy or radiotherapy.

Tumor tissue can be harvested after the eye is enucleated but before immersion into formalin, for cytogenetic analysis and research, in cooperation with the pathologist. With retinoblastoma, such harvesting should be performed after excising the optic nerve and placing this in a formalin container with the distal or proximal end marked with ink or a suture.

## MECHANISM OF ACTION

One of the main objectives of enucleation is to prevent metastatic spread. With some tumors, such as retinoblastoma, this is highly effective. With uveal melanoma, many patients go on to develop metastatic disease because the tumor has disseminated at an early stage, years before detection and treatment of the ocular tumor.[8] It has previously been suggested that enucleation accelerates metastatic death.[9] This hypothesis has, however, gone out of favor, mostly because pre-enucleation radiotherapy was reported by the Collaborative Ocular Melanoma Study (COMS) not to improve survival.[10] Although influential, the COMS results were inconclusive because of insufficient data.[11]

## POSTOPERATIVE CARE

Postoperative management is similar to other forms of treatment. Postoperative compression over 24–48 hours followed by ice packs reduces the postoperative swelling. Nonsteroidal anti-inflammatory medications should be avoided in the early postoperative period.

## SPECIFIC INSTRUMENTATION

Some centers deploy single use instruments for enucleation surgery, because of concerns about prion disease.

## COMPLICATIONS

These include:

- Globe rupture with tumor dissemination into the orbit.
- Incomplete tumor excision because an inadequate length of optic nerve has been removed. When extensive optic nerve invasion is known to be present, pre-enucleation chemotherapy may reduce the risk of this complication.
- Rarely, retinoblastoma patients with orbital recurrence may present with signs suggestive of orbital cellulitis months after enucleation surgery. A high index of suspicion should be maintained especially with tumor extension to the cut end of the optic nerve or extraocular spread at enucleation surgery. An urgent MRI scan should be performed.
- Other complications are the same as enucleation performed for other reasons. These include postenucleation socket syndrome, implant exposure, granuloma formation, shortening of the inferior fornix, implant problems, lower lid laxity and phantom eye syndrome.

## SURGICAL OUTCOMES: SCIENTIFIC EVIDENCE/METANALYSIS

Understandably, most patients are reluctant to undergo enucleation. The large majority, however, are pleasantly surprised once a few weeks have elapsed since the operation. This is especially the case with older individuals once they receive their permanent artificial eye.

The author's impression is that the patient's well-being is greatly influenced by the counseling received. Cultural influences are also important, with loss of the eye having a greater stigma in some countries than in others.

## PLACE OF THE TECHNIQUE IN SURGICAL ARMAMENTARIUM

Enucleation has an important place in the management of ocular tumors, both as primary treatment and to relieve or prevent painful ocular complications after conservative therapy.

## PEARLS AND PITFALLS

- Enucleation is an efficacious method of eliminating the primary tumor and in selected patients is preferable to conservative forms of treatment.
- Even with skin marking, the correct eye for enucleation should be confirmed by indirect ophthalmoscopy before proceeding with surgery.

- The myoconjunctival technique of muscle insertion at enucleation surgery may help improve artificial eye motility.
- Extraocular spread should be identified preoperatively and appropriate measures should be taken at enucleation.
- Gentle handling of tissues with the instruments is the key to a successful outcome.

## REFERENCES

1. Damato B, Lecuona K. Conservation of eyes with choroidal melanoma by a multimodality approach to treatment: an audit of 1632 patients. Ophthalmology. 2004;111(5):977-83.
2. Collaborative Ocular Melanoma Study Group. The COMS randomized trial of iodine 125 brachytherapy for choroidal melanoma: V. Twelve-year mortality rates and prognostic factors: COMS report No. 28. Arch Ophthalmol. 2006;124(12):1684-93.
3. Vrabec TR, Augsburger JJ, Gamel JW, et al. Impact of local tumor relapse on patient survival after cobalt 60 plaque radiotherapy. Ophthalmology. 1991;98(6):984-8.
4. Gragoudas ES, Lane AM, Munzenrider J, et al. Long-term risk of local failure after proton therapy for choroidal/ciliary body melanoma. Trans Am Ophthalmol Soc. 2002;100:43-8; discussion 48-9.
5. Aerts I, Sastre-Garau X, Savignoni A, et al. Results of a multicenter prospective study on the postoperative treatment of unilateral retinoblastoma following primary enucleation. J Clin Oncol. 2013;31(11):1458-63.
6. Marshall E, Romaniuk C, Ghaneh P, et al. MRI in the detection of hepatic metastases from high-risk uveal melanoma: a prospective study in 188 patients. Br J Ophthalmol. 2013;97(2):159-63.
7. Shome D, Honavar SG, Raizada K, et al. Implant and prosthesis movement after enucleation: a randomized controlled trial. Ophthalmology. 2010;117(8):1638-44.
8. Kujala E, Makitie T, Kivela T. Very long-term prognosis of patients with malignant uveal melanoma. Invest Ophthalmol Vis Sci. 2003;44(11):4651-9.
9. Zimmerman LE, McLean IW, Foster WD. Does enucleation of the eye containing a malignant melanoma prevent or accelerate the dissemination of tumour cells. Br J Ophthalmol. 1978;62(6):420-5.
10. Hawkins BS, Collaborative Ocular Melanoma Study Group. The Collaborative Ocular Melanoma Study (COMS) randomized trial of pre-enucleation radiation of large choroidal melanoma: IV. Ten-year mortality findings and prognostic factors. COMS report number 24. Am J Ophthalmol. 2004;138(6):936-51.
11. Damato B. Legacy of the collaborative ocular melanoma study. Arch Ophthalmol. 2007;125(7):966-8.

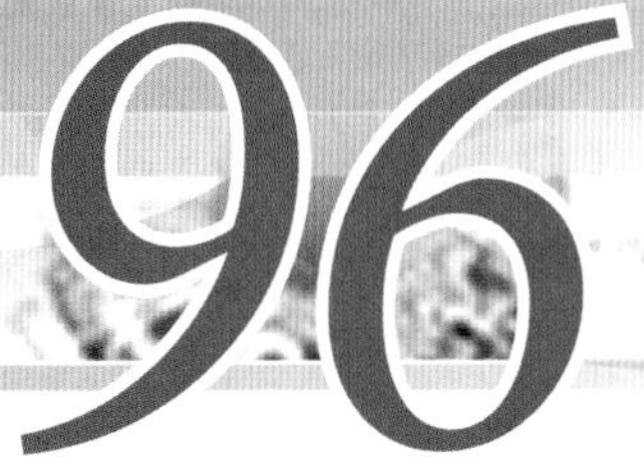


# Topical Therapy for Conjunctival Tumors

Nihal Kenawy, Bertil Damato

## INTRODUCTION

Topical chemotherapy has gained wide acceptance in the treatment of malignant and premalignant tumors of the conjunctiva, delivering a high concentration of the therapeutic agent to the ocular surface without systemic adverse effects.

## INDICATIONS

### Melanocytic Tumors

- Conjunctival intraepithelial neoplasia (C-MIN), synonym PAM, is the main indication.
- Invasive melanomas (CoM) have also been rarely treated with topical chemotherapeutics.

### Squamous Neoplasia

- Conjunctival squamous intraepithelial neoplasia (C-SIN), including carcinoma in situ.
- Less commonly invasive squamous cell carcinoma (SCC).

### Sebaceous Carcinoma

- Pagetoid spread of sebaceous gland carcinoma and residual tumor following excision.

## MECHANISM OF ACTION

### Mitomycin C

- Mitomycin C (MMC) is an alkylating agent that causes cross-linking of DNA and inhibition of DNA synthesis.
- At high concentrations, MMC also suppresses cellular RNA and protein synthesis.[1]

### 5-Fluorouracil

- 5-Fluorouracil (5-FU) is an antimetabolite. It is a pyrimidine analog that inhibits thymidylate synthetase, an enzyme required in the synthesis of thymidine, preventing DNA replication.[2]

### Interferon Alpha 2-β

- Interferon alpha 2β (Intron) is a cytokine that directly inhibits the proliferation of normal and tumor cells. Intron downregulates oncogene expression and induces tumor suppressor genes, which can contribute to the antiproliferative activity and the increase of MHC class I expression, enhancing immune recognition.[3]

### All Transretinoic Acid

- Retinoids bind to the retinoic acid receptors and downregulate matrix metalloproteinases.[4]
- The combination of interferon and retinoic acid has been shown to have antiproliferative function.[5]

## TECHNIQUE OF APPLICATION

- The drops should be instilled using disposable gloves, which must be discarded after use.
- Cheek skin is protected prior to instillation of the drops by applying a light covering of petroleum jelly (such as Vaseline).
- One drop is instilled in the lower fornix by pulling down the lower lid to form a pocket.
- Any spillage of drops onto the skin is wiped immediately and the affected area washed with warm water and soap.

- Should other drops be used, at least 5 minutes separation time between the drops is needed to prevent dilution.
- The used gloves and all other waste (i.e. any tissues used to wipe the eye after instilling the drops) should also be disposed of in a special container.
- On completion of the treatment, the container should be sealed and disposed of using appropriate methods.
- The drops are stored in the fridge.
- Handling of drops is not recommended during pregnancy. Care should be taken if there is any risk of pregnancy or if the patient is breastfeeding.
- Both men and women should use birth control methods during the treatment with topical chemotherapy and for 3 months afterward.

## COMPLICATIONS

### Mitomycin C

- Transient side effects include delayed wound healing, conjunctival injection, chemosis, and/or keratitis.
- Permanent side effects are rare and are secondary to limbal stem cell failure. They include recurrent corneal epithelial defects, pannus, and epiphora.[6-9]
- Cataract may rarely occur, possibly as a result of intraocular absorption.[8]

### 5-Fluorouracil

- Rarely, keratoconjunctivitis develops after prolonged application.[10]

### Interferon

- Superficial punctate keratopathy, conjunctival injection, and folliculitis may occur through the preparation vehicle.[11]
- Temporary myalgia and fever have been reported with subconjunctival application.[12]

### Retinoic Acid

- Transient blepharoconjunctivitis or irritation with topical application.[13]

## SURGICAL OUTCOMES: SCIENTIFIC EVIDENCE/META-ANALYSIS

### Melanocytic Tumors

- MMC has shown efficacy mainly in the treatment of C-MIN (PAM), while the evidence of success in CoM is not convincing.
- The widely used concentration is 0.02–0.04%. Topical chemotherapy is administered in 2 to 4 cycles with the treatment phase with the treatment phase lasting 1–2 weeks and the rest period lasting between 2 and 3 weeks.[6,8,14-21]
- Interferon alpha 2ß has been used for prolonged periods to treat invasive CoM. The dose is 1 million IU/mL drops and applied four times daily until complete regression.[22,23]

### Squamous Neoplasia

- 5-FU 1%, interferon alpha 2ß, and retinoic acid have been used in treating both C-SIN and SCC, with minimal side effects to the ocular surface as compared with MMC.[7,10-13,24-48]
- MMC 0.02–0.04% has been used as adjunctive therapy after excision and cryotherapy, with the treatment duration ranging from 2–14 weeks.[24,37,40,42]
- In few instances, MMC was applied preoperatively for chemoreduction. The concentration used was 0.04%. The drops were administered four times daily for 7–14-day cycles until tumor regression or no further regression was achieved or until ocular toxicity occurred.[26,33]
- MMC 0.4 mg/mL has been applied for 3 minutes intraoperatively to prevent tumor recurrence after excision.[33]
- The efficacy of topical 5-FU 1% has been demonstrated in the treatment of limited cases of C-SIN with variable treatment protocols.[27,38,39]
- 5-FU1% was rarely used as a primary treatment of invasive SCC; however, a high rate of failure has been reported so that this approach is not recommended.[10,38]
- Interferon alpha 2ß has been administered as the sole treatment of primary C-SIN or in recurrent cases following excision for extended periods of time. The treatment is given in the form of 1 million IU/mL drops four times daily.[11,12,35,41,44]
- Interferon alpha 2ß has also been used as subconjunctival perilesional injection (3 million international units (IU) in 0.5 mL) in combination with the topical form as an alternative to surgical excision.[12]
- Retinoic acid 0.01% has also been described as effectively treating C-SIN when used once every second day in combination with interferon alpha 2ß on surgery-naive eyes until complete resolution occurred.[13]
- Subconjunctival Ranibizumab has also been advocated a successful treatment option in refractory SCC but the evidence is insufficient for validating its potential advantage.[49]

### Sebaceous Carcinoma

- Topical MMC has been shown to be the efficacious adjunctive topical therapy in residual intraepithelial disease

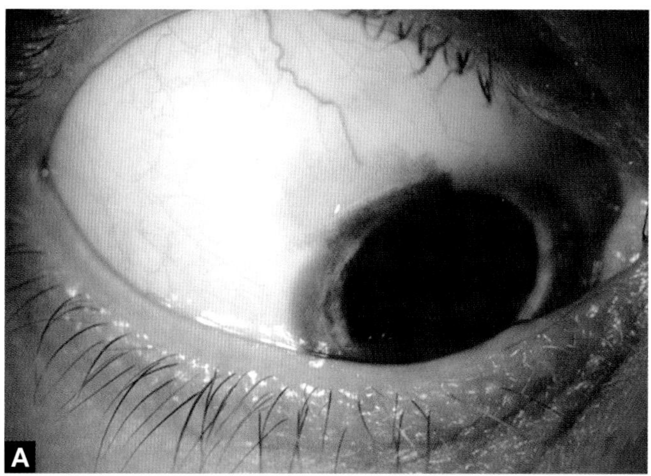


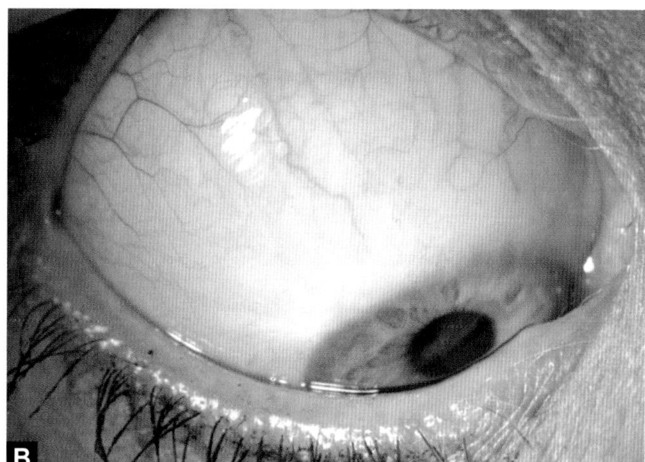


Figures 96-1A and B Conjunctival melanocytic intraepithelial neoplasia score 4 of the right eye of a 49-year-old woman (A). Appearance 8 months after excision and topical mitomycin C 0.04% (B).

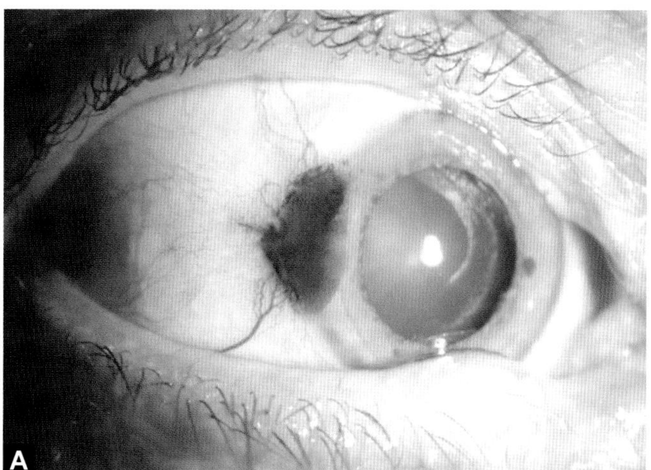


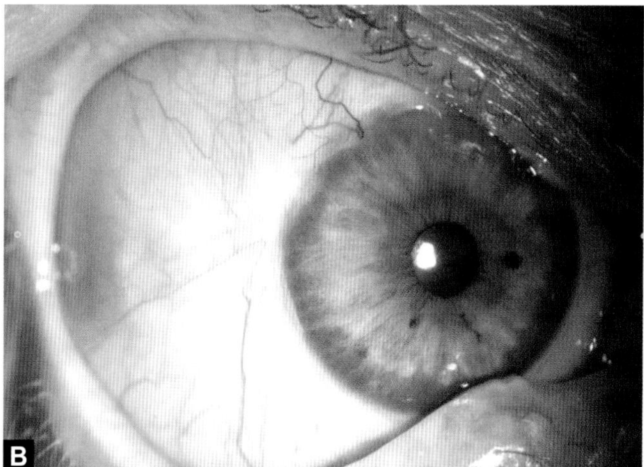


Figures 96-2A and B Invasive conjunctival melanoma of the conjunctiva of the right eye of a 72-year-old woman (A). Appearance 6 months after excision, ruthenium brachytherapy, and topical mitomycin C 0.04% (B).

following the excision of the invasive tumor.[33,50,51] MMC 0.02–0.04% has been prescribed in 7-day cycles until biopsy-proven clearance of the disease was achieved.

- As a chemoreduction agent, topical MMC 0.04% four times for 4 weeks has also been applied prior to surgical excision together with intraoperative application of 0.4 mg/mL for 3 minutes in a single case.[33]

## PLACE OF THE TECHNIQUE IN SURGICAL ARMAMENTARIUM

### Melanoma

- MMC has shown efficacy mainly in the treatment of C-MIN, while the evidence of success in CoM is not convincing.
- At the authors' institution, MMC is reserved for the treatment of C-MIN proven by biopsy or as adjuvant therapy for residual intraepithelial disease following the excision of invasive melanomas with high success rate[52] (Figs. 96-1 and 96-2).

### Squamous Carcinoma

- MMC is the most widely used chemotherapeutic in squamous neoplasia; however, 5-FU 1%, interferon alpha 2ß, and retinoic acid have been used less commonly with success. The long-term outcome is still not known.[7,10-13,24-48]
- 5-FU 1% was rarely used as a primary treatment of invasive SCC with high rate of failure and, therefore, based on the available evidence, the use of 5-FU 1% in SCC is not recommended.[10,38]

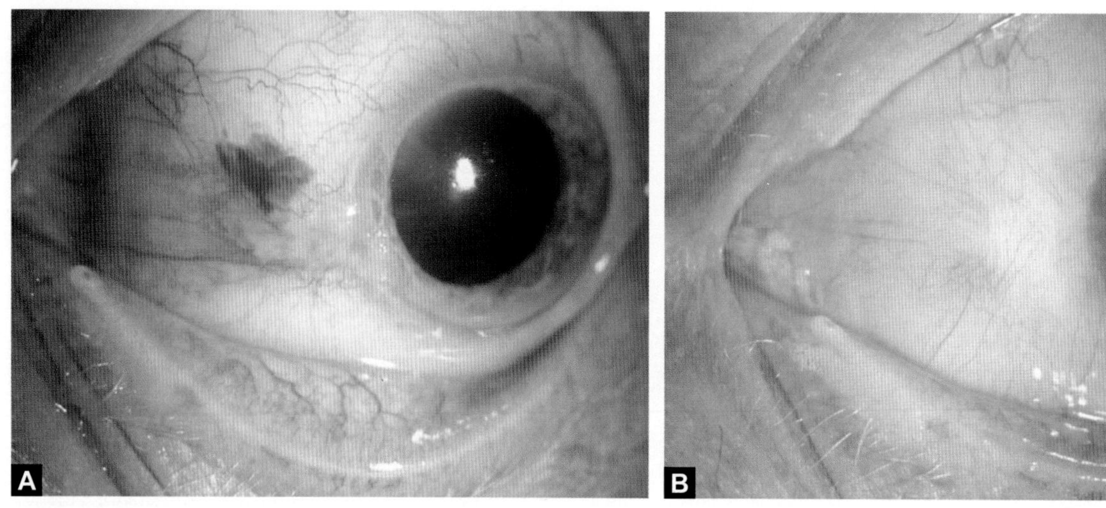


Figures 96-3A and B Squamous cell carcinoma of the left eye of a 46-year-old woman (A). Appearance 4 months following excision, Ruthenium brachytherapy and topical 5-fluoruracil 1% (B).

- The authors employ 5-FU 1%; four times for 4-day cycles separated by 3 weeks interval and for a total of 4 cycles, in managing C-SIN or residual intraepithelial disease following SCC excision (Figs. 96-3A and B).

## Sebaceous Carcinoma

- The treatment of choice in sebaceous gland carcinoma is wide surgical excision.
- Pagetoid extension into the conjunctiva is a recognized part of the disease process and determining its extent can be quite challenging despite mapping biopsies and requires topical adjuvant therapy.
- Topical MMC has been shown to be the efficacious adjunctive topical therapy in residual intra-epithelial disease following the excision of the invasive tumor.[33,50,51]
- It is advisable to administer MMC in treating selected cases of residual intraepithelial disease of sebaceous carcinoma and after complete healing of the surgical site using the lower concentration of MMC to avoid significant ocular surface complications. Caution should be warranted in cases that undergo extensive lids surgery as surface abnormalities frequently occur with lids malfunction.[53]
- It has also been suggested that excision and preservation of part of the limbal stem cells, prior to commencing any treatment, to be reimbedded following the end of the treatment may beneficial in reducing stem cell deficiency especially with higher concentrations of MMC.
- Adjunctive topical steroids such as fluorometholone 0.1% can be applied four times daily to minimize the side effects of chemotherapeutic agents.

## PEARLS AND PITFALLS

- Topical chemotherapeutic agents are best applied after the conjunctiva has completely healed following surgical excision of the tumor.
- Due to lack of robust evidence of success in invasive disease, chemotherapy is best employed in treating intraepithelial disease only.
- Lower concentration of MMC of 0.02% may be used in cases intolerant of the higher concentrations but with increase risk of recurrence.
- To reduce the risk of punctual stenosis and damage to the nasopharyngeal epithelium, punctual plugs can be placed temporarily. Manual punctual occlusion has also been advised.

## REFERENCES

1. McKelvie PA, Daniell M. Impression cytology following mitomycin C therapy for ocular surface squamous neoplasia. Br J Ophthalmol. 2001;85:1115-9.
2. Longley DB, Harkin DP, Johnston PG. 5-fluorouracil: mechanisms of action and clinical strategies. Nat Rev Cancer. 2003; 3:330-8.
3. Ferrantini M, Capone I, Belardelli F. Interferon-alpha and cancer: mechanisms of action and new perspectives of clinical use. Biochimie. 2007;89:884-93.
4. Uchida G, Yoshimura K, Kitano Y, et al. Tretinoin reverses upregulation of matrix metalloproteinase-13 in human keloid-derived fibroblasts. Exp Dermatol. 2003;12 Suppl 2:35-42.

5. Marth C, Daxenbichler G, Dapunt O. Synergistic antiproliferative effect of human recombinant interferons and retinoic acid in cultured breast cancer cells. J Natl Cancer Inst. 1986;77: 1197-202.
6. Demirci H, McCormick SA, Finger PT. Topical mitomycin chemotherapy for conjunctival malignant melanoma and primary acquired melanosis with atypia: clinical experience with histopathologic observations. Arch Ophthalmol. 2000; 118:885-91.
7. Frucht-Pery J, Rozenman Y, Pe'er J. Topical mitomycin-C for partially excised conjunctival squamous cell carcinoma. Ophthalmology. 2002;109:548-52.
8. Kurli M, Finger PT. Topical mitomycin chemotherapy for conjunctival malignant melanoma and primary acquired melanosis with atypia: 12 years' experience. Graefes Arch Clin Exp Ophthalmol. 2005;243:1108-14.
9. Khong JJ, Muecke J. Complications of mitomycin C therapy in 100 eyes with ocular surface neoplasia. Br J Ophthalmol. 2006; 90:819-22.
10. Midena E, Angeli CD, Valenti M, et al. Treatment of conjunctival squamous cell carcinoma with topical 5-fluorouracil. Br J Ophthalmol. 2000;84:268-72.
11. Schechter BA, Koreishi AF, Karp CL, et al. Long-term follow-up of conjunctival and corneal intraepithelial neoplasia treated with topical interferon alfa-2b. Ophthalmology. 2008;115:1291-6,6 e1.
12. Vann RR, Karp CL. Perilesional and topical interferon alfa-2b for conjunctival and corneal neoplasia. Ophthalmology. 1999; 106:91-7.
13. Krilis M, Tsang H, Coroneo M. Treatment of conjunctival and corneal epithelial neoplasia with retinoic acid and topical interferon alfa-2b: long-term follow-up. Ophthalmology. 2012;119: 1969-73.
14. Finger PT, Milner MS, McCormick SA. Topical chemotherapy for conjunctival melanoma. Br J Ophthalmol. 1993;77:751-3.
15. Shields CL, Shields JA, Armstrong T. Management of conjunctival and corneal melanoma with surgical excision, amniotic membrane allograft, and topical chemotherapy. Am J Ophthalmol. 2001;132:576-8.
16. Rodriguez-Ares T, Tourino R, De Rojas V, et al. Topical mitomycin C in the treatment of pigmented conjunctival lesions. Cornea. 2003;22:114-7.
17. Yuen VH, Jordan DR, Brownstein S, et al. Topical mitomycin treatment for primary acquired melanosis of the conjunctiva. Ophthal Plast Reconstr Surg. 2003;19:149-51.
18. Ditta LC, Shildkrot Y, Wilson MW. Outcomes in 15 patients with conjunctival melanoma treated with adjuvant topical mitomycin C: complications and recurrences. Ophthalmology. 2011;118:1754-9.
19. Pe'er J, Frucht-Pery J. The treatment of primary acquired melanosis (PAM) with atypia by topical Mitomycin C. Am J Ophthalmol. 2005;139:229-34.
20. Damato B, Coupland SE. Management of conjunctival melanoma. Expert Rev Anticancer Ther. 2009;9:1227-39.
21. Frucht-Pery J, Pe'er J: Use of mitomycin C in the treatment of conjunctival primary acquired melanosis with atypia. Arch Ophthalmol. 1996;114:1261-4.
22. Herold TR, Hintschich C. Interferon alpha for the treatment of melanocytic conjunctival lesions. Graefes Arch Clin Exp Ophthalmol. 2010;248:111-5.
23. Finger PT, Sedeek RW, Chin KJ. Topical interferon alfa in the treatment of conjunctival melanoma and primary acquired melanosis complex. Am J Ophthalmol. 2008;145:124-9.
24. Frucht-Pery J, Sugar J, Baum J, et al. Mitomycin C treatment for conjunctival-corneal intraepithelial neoplasia: a multicenter experience. Ophthalmology. 1997;104:2085-93.
25. Al-Barrag A, Al-Shaer M, Al-Matary N, et al. 5-Fluorouracil for the treatment of intraepithelial neoplasia and squamous cell carcinoma of the conjunctiva, and cornea. Clin Ophthalmol. 2010;4:801-8.
26. Shields CL, Demirci H, Marr BP, et al. Chemoreduction with topical mitomycin C prior to resection of extensive squamous cell carcinoma of the conjunctiva. Arch Ophthalmol. 2005; 123:109-13.
27. Yeatts RP, Engelbrecht NE, Curry CD, et al. 5-Fluorouracil for the treatment of intraepithelial neoplasia of the conjunctiva and cornea. Ophthalmology. 2000;107:2190-5.
28. Karpova AY, Ronco LV, Howley PM. Functional characterization of interferon regulatory factor 3a (IRF-3a), an alternative splice isoform of IRF-3. Mol Cell Biol. 2001;21:4169-76.
29. Chen C, Louis D, Dodd T, Muecke J. Mitomycin C as an adjunct in the treatment of localised ocular surface squamous neoplasia. Br J Ophthalmol. 2004;88:17-8.
30. Stone DU, Butt AL, Chodosh J. Ocular surface squamous neoplasia: a standard of care survey. Cornea. 2005;24:297-300.
31. Grossniklaus HE, Aaberg TM, Sr. Mitomycin C treatment of conjunctival intraepithelial neoplasia. Am J Ophthalmol. 1997; 124:381-3.
32. Akpek EK, Ertoy D, Kalayci D, et al. Postoperative topical mitomycin C in conjunctival squamous cell neoplasia. Cornea. 1999; 18:59-62.
33. Kemp EG, Harnett AN, Chatterjee S. Preoperative topical and intraoperative local mitomycin C adjuvant therapy in the management of ocular surface neoplasias. Br J Ophthalmol. 2002; 86:31-4.
34. Hirst LW. Randomized controlled trial of topical mitomycin C for ocular surface squamous neoplasia: early resolution. Ophthalmology. 2007;114:976-82.
35. Maskin SL. Regression of limbal epithelial dysplasia with topical interferon. Arch Ophthalmol. 1994;112:1145-6.
36. Tseng SH, Tsai YY, Chen FK. Successful treatment of recurrent corneal intraepithelial neoplasia with topical mitomycin C. Cornea. 1997;16:595-7.
37. Prabhasawat P, Tarinvorakup P, Tesavibul N, et al.: Topical 0.002% mitomycin C for the treatment of conjunctival-corneal intraepithelial neoplasia and squamous cell carcinoma. Cornea. 2005;24:443-8.
38. Yeatts RP, Ford JG, Stanton CA, et al. Topical 5-fluorouracil in treating epithelial neoplasia of the conjunctiva and cornea. Ophthalmology. 1995;102:1338-44.
39. de Keizer RJ, de Wolff-Rouendaal D, van Delft JL. Topical application of 5-fluorouracil in premalignant lesions of cornea, conjunctiva and eyelid. Doc Ophthalmol. Advances in Ophthalmology. 1986;64:31-42.

40. Wilson MW, Hungerford JL, George SM, et al. Topical mitomycin C for the treatment of conjunctival and corneal epithelial dysplasia and neoplasia. Am J Ophthalmol. 1997;124:303-11.
41. Karp CL, Moore JK, Rosa RH, Jr. Treatment of conjunctival and corneal intraepithelial neoplasia with topical interferon alpha-2b. Ophthalmology. 2001;108:1093-8.
42. Rozenman Y, Frucht-Pery J. Treatment of conjunctival intraepithelial neoplasia with topical drops of mitomycin C. Cornea. 2000;19:1-6.
43. Gupta A, Muecke J. Treatment of ocular surface squamous neoplasia with Mitomycin C. Br J Ophthalmol. 2010;94:555-8.
44. Boehm MD, Huang AJ. Treatment of recurrent corneal and conjunctival intraepithelial neoplasia with topical interferon alfa 2b. Ophthalmology. 2004;111:1755-61.
45. Holcombe DJ, Lee GA. Topical interferon alfa-2b for the treatment of recalcitrant ocular surface squamous neoplasia. Am J Ophthalmol. 2006;142:568-71.
46. Sturges A, Butt AL, Lai JE, et al. Topical interferon or surgical excision for the management of primary ocular surface squamous neoplasia. Ophthalmology. 2008;115:1297-302, 302 e1.
47. Karp CL, Galor A, Chhabra S, et al. Subconjunctival/perilesional recombinant interferon alpha2b for ocular surface squamous neoplasia: a 10-year review. Ophthalmology. 2010;117:2241-6.
48. Kim HJ, Shields CL, Shah SU, et al. Giant ocular surface squamous neoplasia managed with interferon alpha-2b as immunotherapy or immunoreduction. Ophthalmology. 2012;119:938-44.
49. Finger PT, Chin KJ. Refractory squamous cell carcinoma of the conjunctiva treated with subconjunctival ranibizumab (Lucentis): a two-year study. Ophthal Plast Reconstr Surg. 2012;28:85-9.
50. Putterman AM. Conjunctival map biopsy to determine pagetoid spread. Am J Ophthalmol. 1986;102:87-90.
51. Shields CL, Naseripour M, Shields JA, et al. Topical mitomycin-C for pagetoid invasion of the conjunctiva by eyelid sebaceous gland carcinoma. Ophthalmology. 2002;109:2129-33.
52. Damato B, Coupland SE. Management of conjunctival melanoma. Expert Rev Anticancer Ther. 2009;9:1227-39.
53. Tumuluri K, Kourt G, Martin P. Mitomycin C in sebaceous gland carcinoma with pagetoid spread. Br J Ophthalmol. 2004; 88:718-9.

CHAPTER

97

# Systemic Therapy for Retinoblastoma

Laurence Desjardins, Christine Levy-Gabriel, Livia Lumbroso Le-Rouic, Nathalie Cassoux, Isabelle Aerts

## INTRODUCTION

This chapter will focus on systemic chemotherapy of retinoblastoma. Systemic therapy may be administered before, during or after local treatment of the ocular tumor or it may be the only treatment although with very limited indications.

Patients with the *Rb* gene mutation have a high risk of second cancer. In such patients, chemotherapy avoids the need for external beam radiation but is itself mutagenic so that the lowest possible doses are used.

Systemic therapy is likely to play an ever-increasing role in ocular oncology as more effective agents are developed.

## INDICATIONS

### Intraocular Tumors

- Macular tumor, as a means of avoiding or reducing local therapy.[1]
- Chemoreduction in combination with local therapy (Fig. 97-1).[2,3]
- In case of buphthalmos, chemotherapy is used first to induce tumor shrinkage and softening of the eye thereby reducing the risk of scleral perforation during enucleation. The chemotherapy is continued after enucleation for at least four cycles even if no histological risk factor is found after the first two cycles.[4]
- After primary enucleation, in case of identification of histopathological risk factors in order to prevent local relapse and metastasis.[5,6]
- In bilateral Retinoblastoma to reduce risk of primitive neuroectodermal tumor (which is controversial).[7]

### Extraocular Disease

- Extraocular spread to orbit
- Optic nerve involvement, demonstrated radiologically[6]
- Systemic metastasis[8]

## CONTRAINDICATIONS

- As a general principle, systemic chemotherapy is contraindicated if the malignancy is localized to the eye(s) and if local therapy is likely to achieve adequate tumor control without excessive morbidity.
- Some would consider systemic chemotherapy to be contraindicated in patients with extensive unilateral retinoblastoma (where enucleation is the treatment of choice) nevertheless in case of buphthalmos we prefer to administer chemotherapy before the enucleation.
- There may also be systemic problems with a need to reduce or adapt the doses.

## INVESTIGATIONS

Investigations have the following objectives:

- To stage the malignancy and hence to assess the response to systemic therapy with greater sensitivity.
- To detect disorders that might be aggravated by systemic chemotherapy, such as deafness, which can be aggravated by carboplatin.

## TECHNIQUE

After being found to be effective in the treatment of extraocular retinoblastoma, the combination of carboplatin, vincristine and etoposide was subsequently used for intraocular tumors.

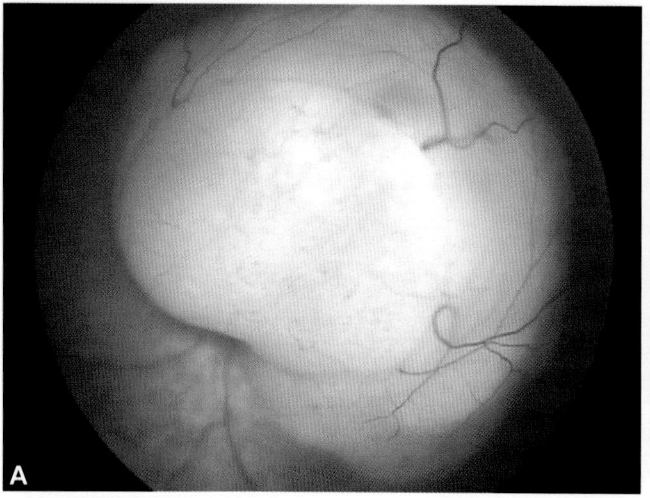


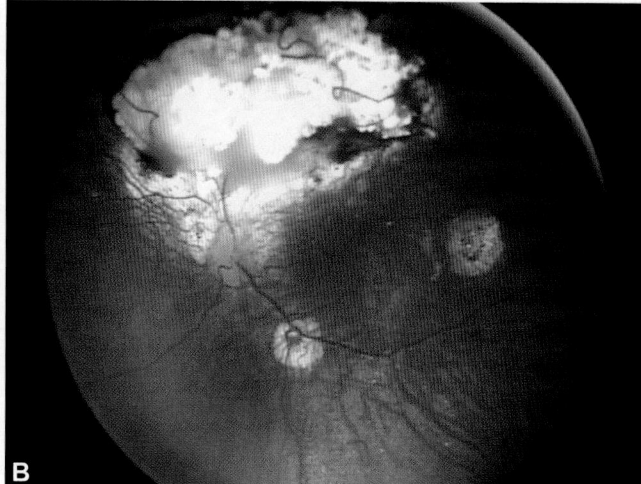


**Figures 97-1A and B** (A) Large retinoblastoma before treatment and (B) after two courses of carboplatin and etoposide followed by chemothermotherapy plus local forms of therapy.

Lynn Murphree was the first to treat selected intraocular retinoblastoma with a combination of intravenous carboplatin and heat, which was delivered to the tumor with a diode laser (chemothermotherapy).[9] Since 1995, we have been using chemothermotherapy for the treatment of intraocular retinoblastoma, with good results.[3,10]

- *Chemothermotherapy*: An intravenous infusion of carboplatin alone is followed by diode laser treatment, which is administered 2 or 3 hours later. This is often preceded by two cycles of carboplatin and etoposide to reduce tumor volume and avoid dissemination of viable tumor cells during laser treatment.
- *Chemotherapy alone*: This can be curative with some large, macular tumors but has a significant failure rate.[1] Small tumors are more chemoresistant, probably because they are less vascular. We treat such macular tumors with six cycles of carboplatin, etoposide and vincristine in the hope of avoiding destructive laser treatment, especially if there is bilateral macular involvement.
- *Chemoreduction*: Protocols vary between centers. At the Curie Institute, for Group B and C eyes, we prescribe two courses of carboplatin and etoposide followed by three cycles of chemothermotherapy (i.e. carboplatin alone with transpupillary thermotherapy) (Figs. 97-2A to D). Some centers administer two agents (i.e. carboplatin with etoposide or vincristine) for Group B eyes and all three agents for Groups C and D eyes, prescribing six cycles and administering local therapy as early as the third cycle (Figs. 97-3A and B) (most, centers use six courses of 3 drugs + local treatments for bilateral group D). Such local therapy can consist of thermotherapy, cryotherapy, plaque brachytherapy and/or intravitreal melphalan injection.
- Chemoprophylaxis in patients with histological risk factors for metastasis (i.e. optic nerve invasion and massive choroidal invasion). Some authors have recommended the same protocol as for chemoreduction.[11,12]
- *Metastatic disease*: High-dose chemotherapy with high dose of alkylating agent (thiotepa), etoposide and carboplatin followed by stem cell rescue.[8]

## PATIENT MONITORING

The objectives of patient monitoring are to:

- Identify any side-effects or complications caused by the systemic treatment (e.g. hearing loss).
- Assess the tumor response to the systemic treatment.
- Detect tumor recurrence.
- Detect second tumor

## COMPLICATIONS

Chemotherapy can cause a wide variety of complications.[13] These include:

- Alopecia
- Bone marrow suppression
- Mucositis
- Hepatotoxicity
- Diarrhea
- Constipation, caused by vincristine
- Tissue pain caused by leakage of vincristine
- Neuropathic pain

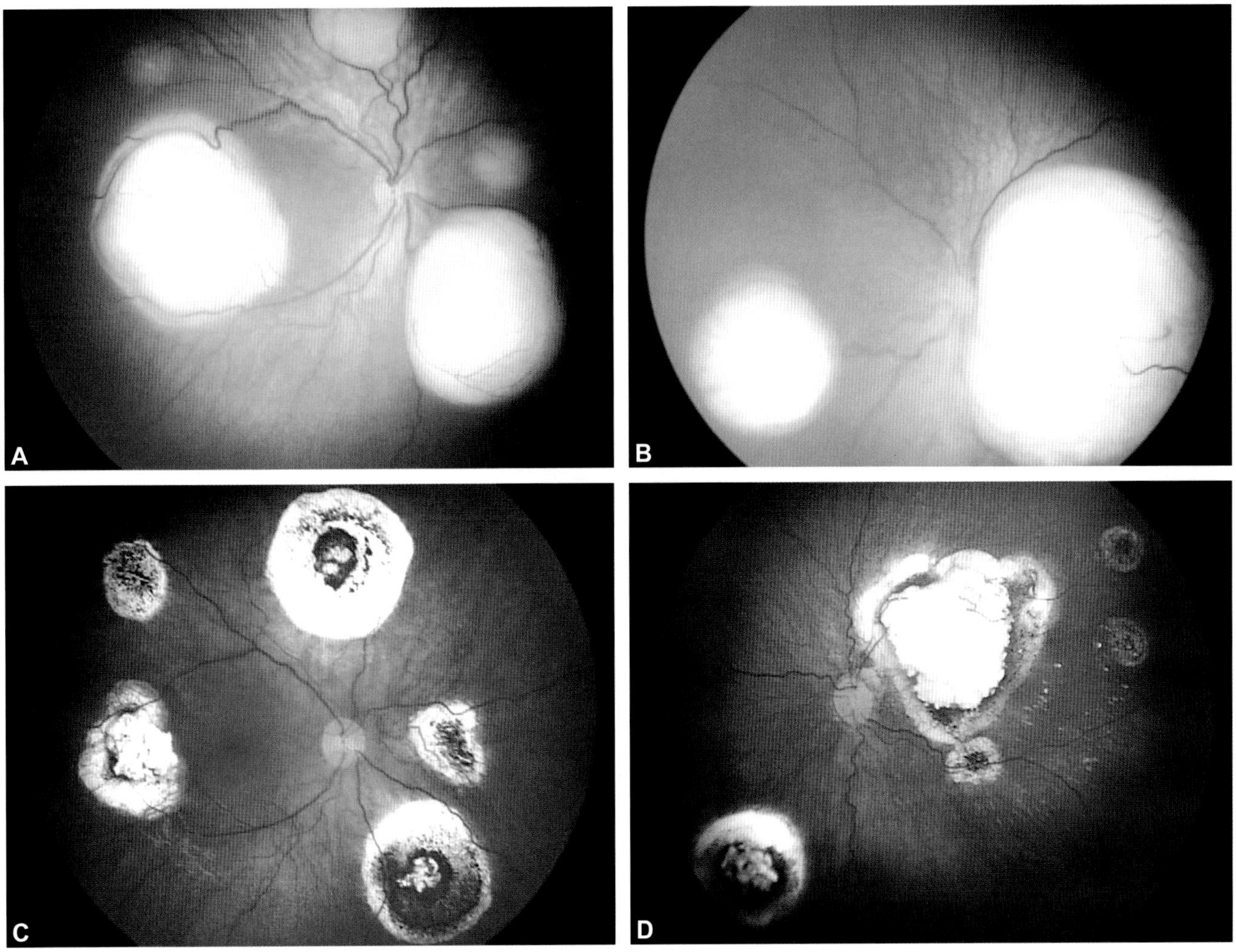

**Figures 97-2A to D** (A and B) Macular tumors in the right and left eyes before treatment and (C and D) after six cycles of triple-agent chemotherapy and local therapy.

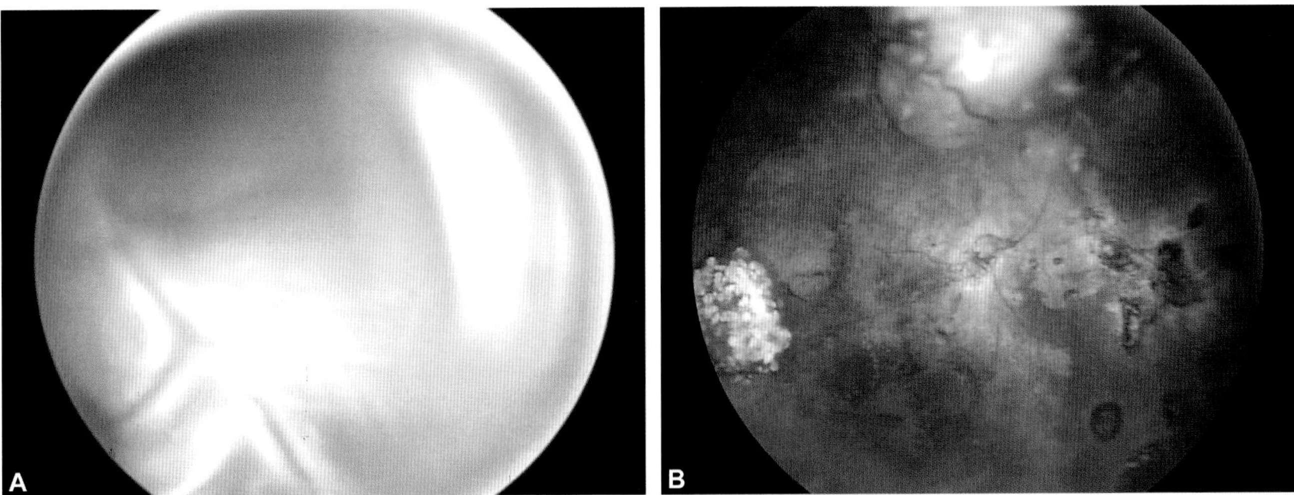


**Figures 97-3A and B** (A) Group D eye with retinoblastoma causing total retinal detachment before treatment and (B) after six cycles of triple-agent chemotherapy and local therapy.

- Acute myeloid leukemia, very rarely, after etoposide treatment[14]
- Second primary tumors
- Hearing loss, rarely, after carboplatin treatment[15]
- Infertility is extremely rare
- Allergic reactions to etoposide vehicle or carboplatin

## SURGICAL OUTCOMES: SCIENTIFIC EVIDENCE/META-ANALYSIS

- *Macular tumor*: Success rates of 84% have been reported with chemotherapy alone.[1]
- *Chemoreduction*: Eye salvage rates are 100%, 93%, 90% and 47% for Groups A to D.[16] Group E eyes may be salvaged if low-dose external beam radiotherapy is also administered.[17]
- The use of chemothermotherapy gives good visual results if the tumor is away from the macula.[18]
- *Orbital involvement*: Neoadjuvant chemotherapy with postoperative chemotherapy and radiotherapy may make it possible to perform enucleation instead of exenteration.[12]
- *Metastatic disease*: Encouraging survival rates have been reported.[19] Central nervous system (CNS) involvement has a poor prognosis although survival may be improved by intrathecal agents such as cytarabine and topotecan.[20]
- Prophylaxis in high-risk patients. Adjuvant chemotherapy in patients with Rb at cut end of optic nerve has reduced the rate of metastatic disease from around 75–25%.[21]
- Prevention of primitive neuroectodermal tumor.[7] The efficacy of treatment in preventing disease is uncertain.

## PEARLS AND PITFALLS

- Systemic chemotherapy for retinoblastoma, and indeed other malignancies, requires multidisciplinary collaboration.
- Any center administering systemic therapy must be fully equipped to detect and treat any iatrogenic morbidity.
- Systemic therapy can reduce iatrogenic morbidity by avoiding the need for external beam radiation and allowing less aggressive local therapy.
- Chemotherapy can delay wound healing, increasing the risk of wound dehiscence after enucleation.

## REFERENCES


1. Gombos DS, Kelly A, Coen PG, et al. Retinoblastoma treated with primary chemotherapy alone: the significance of tumor size, location, and age. Br J Ophthalmol. 2002;86(1):80-3.
2. Shields CL, Mashayekhi A, Cater J, et al. Chemoreduction for retinoblastoma: analysis of tumor control and risks for recurrence in 457 tumors. Trans Am Ophthalmol Soc. 2004;102: 35-44.
3. Lumbroso-Le Rouic L, Aerts I, Lévy-Gabriel C, et al. Conservative treatments of intraocular retinoblastoma. Ophthalmology. 2008;115(8):1405-10.
4. Bellaton E, Bertozzi AI, Behar C, et al. Neoadjuvant chemotherapy for extensive unilateral retinoblastoma. Br J Ophthalmol. 2003;87(3):327-9.
5. Honavar SG, Singh AD, Shields CL, et al. Postenucleation adjuvant therapy in high-risk retinoblastoma. Arch Ophthalmol. 2002;120(7):923-31.
6. Aerts I, Sastre-Garau X, Savignoni A, et al. Results of a multicenter prospective study on the postoperative treatment of unilateral retinoblastoma after primary enucleation. J Clin Oncol. 2013;31(11):1458-63.
7. Shields CL, Meadows AT, Shields JA, et al. Chemoreduction for retinoblastoma may prevent intracranial neuroblastic malignancy (trilateral retinoblastoma). Arch Ophthalmol. 2001; 119(9): 1269-72.
8. Rodriguez-Galindo C, Wilson MW, Haik BG, et al. Treatment of metastatic retinoblastoma. Ophthalmology. 2003;110(6): 1237-40.
9. Murphree AL, Villablanca JG, Deegan WF, et al. Chemotherapy plus local treatment in the management of intraocular retinoblastoma. Arch Ophthalmol. 1996;114(11):1348-56.
10. Levy C, Doz F, Quintana E, et al. Role of chemotherapy alone or in combination with hyperthermia in the primary treatment of intraocular retinoblastoma: preliminary results. Br J Ophthalmol. 1998;82(10):1154-8.
11. Kaliki S, Shields CL, Shah SU, et al. Postenucleation adjuvant chemotherapy with vincristine, etoposide, and carboplatin for the treatment of high-risk retinoblastoma. Arch Ophthalmol. 2011;129(11):1422-7.
12. Chantada G, Fandiño A, Casak S, et al. Treatment of overt extraocular retinoblastoma. Med Pediatr Oncol. 2003;40(3): 158-61.
13. Leahey A. Systemic chemotherapy: a pediatric oncology perspective. In: Ramasubramanian A, Shields CL (Eds). Retinoblastoma. New Delhi, India: Jaypee Brothers Medical Publishers (P) Ltd; 2012. pp. 81-5.
14. Gombos DS, Hungerford J, Abramson DH, et al. Secondary acute myelogenous leukemia in patients with retinoblastoma: is chemotherapy a factor? Ophthalmology. 2007;114(7):1378-83.
15. Jehanne M, Lumbroso-Le Rouic L, Savignoni A, et al. Analysis of ototoxicity in young children receiving carboplatin in the context of conservative management of unilateral or bilateral retinoblastoma. Pediatr Blood Cancer. 2009;52(5):637-43.
16. Shields CL, Mashayekhi A, Au AK, et al. The international classification of retinoblastoma predicts chemoreduction success. Ophthalmology. 2006;113(12):2276-80.
17. Shields CL, Ramasubramanian A, Thangappan A, et al. Chemoreduction for group E retinoblastoma: comparison of chemoreduction alone versus chemoreduction plus low-dose external radiotherapy in 76 eyes. Ophthalmology. 2009;116(3):544-51.e1.

18. Desjardins L, Chefchaouni MC, Lumbroso L, et al. Functional results after treatment of retinoblastoma. J AAPOS. 2002;6(2):108-11.

19. Kremens B, Wieland R, Reinhard H, et al. High-dose chemotherapy with autologous stem cell rescue in children with retinoblastoma. Bone Marrow Transplant. 2003;31(4):281-4.

20. Dimaras H, Héon E, Budning A, et al. Retinoblastoma CSF metastasis cured by multimodality chemotherapy without radiation. Ophthalmic Genet. 2009;30(3):121-6.

21. Uusitalo MS, Van Quill KR, Scott IU, et al. Evaluation of chemoprophylaxis in patients with unilateral retinoblastoma with high-risk features on histopathologic examination. Arch Ophthalmol. 2001;119(1):41-8.

CHAPTER

# 98

# Intra-arterial Chemotherapy for Retinoblastoma

Doris Hadjistilianou

## INTRODUCTION

At present, intra-arterial (IA) chemotherapy (also known as superselective IA chemotherapy or chemosurgery) is restricted to retinoblastoma. IA chemotherapy for the treatment of intraocular retinoblastoma was first performed by Algernon B. Reese with direct internal carotid artery injection of the alkylating agent triethylene melamine (TEM) in 1954.[1] The idea of local delivery for retinoblastoma was later revisited by Yamane and Kaneko[2]; they described the technique of "selective ophthalmic artery infusion" (SOAI) using a microballoon catheter positioned distal to the ostium of the ophthalmic artery and injecting chemotherapy with flow directed into the ophthalmic artery. The SOAI Japanese technique was further developed into "direct intra-arterial ophthalmic artery infusion" by Abramson and Gobin.[3]

IA chemotherapy is a promising, primary, and salvage treatment for moderate and advanced retinoblastoma, particularly in eyes that would otherwise require enucleation. The technique furthers the trend toward localized drug delivery to an ocular target and has forged new partnerships between ocular oncologists and interventional neuroradiologists.[4-6]

## INDICATIONS

- Primary treatment of unilateral advanced retinoblastoma that cannot be treated by thermoablation or cryotherapy alone, that is, Reese-Ellsworth Stage II, III, IV, Va and Vb (ABC Stage B, C, and D).
- Adjunctive treatment after systemic chemotherapy, with or without focal therapy.
- Incomplete response to conservative therapy.
- Local tumor recurrence after conservative therapy.[6-9]

## CONTRAINDICATIONS

- Anterior chamber invasion
- Secondary glaucoma
- Vitreous hemorrhage
- Iris heterochromia
- Suspected invasion of postlaminar optic nerve and sclera (MRI)
- Extraocular disease.

## PREOPERATIVE CARE

### Ophthalmological Examination to Assess Stage of Retinoblastoma

- Examination under anesthesia
- Fundus photography (Ret-Cam)
- Ocular ultrasonography (A and B scan)
- UBM (Ultrasound biomicroscopy)
- ERG (Electroretinogram).

### MRI

This imaging is required to exclude extraocular disease (Fig. 98-1). Some centers also perform MRA (magnetic resonance angiography) to assess the vasculature before treatment).

### Pediatric Evaluation of Systemic Disease

Special measures include complete history, general medical examination, assessment of neuromotor development, and detection of dysmorphisms. Examination of lymph nodes, liver, and spleen is mandatory. Lumbar puncture and bone marrow biopsy are performed when necessary.

Complete clinical examination and blood tests are needed before each procedure. After each procedure, support therapy,

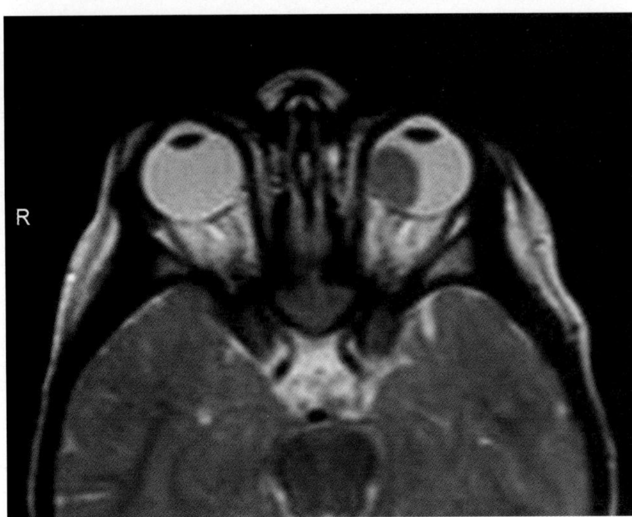


Figure 98-1 MRI scan of a nasal retinoblastoma in the left eye.

antiemetic therapy, and rehydration may be required. At the end of each IA chemotherapy cycle, the patient should be assessed for short- and long-term systemic side effects.

## SURGICAL TECHNIQUE

Interventional neuroendovascular procedures represent an important and evolving part of the management of pediatric patients.[10,11] Appropriately trained physicians can safely perform pediatric cerebral angiography.

A proper procedure for IA chemotherapy requires the cooperation of skilled specialists including ocular oncologist, neurointerventional radiologist, pediatric anesthesiologist, pediatric oncologist, neuroradiologist, pharmacist, and specialized nurses.

### General Anesthesia

This is administered in the conventional fashion.

### Chemotherapy Infusion

This involves the following steps:

- The femoral artery (at each session, alternating between right and left side) is punctured (Figs. 97-2A and B).
- Intravenous heparin is administered to prevent thrombosis, initially as a bolus followed by a continuous infusion to maintain an activated partial thromboplastin time of at least twice the normal value throughout the procedure.
- Nonionic contrast medium (Iopamidol) is used in all patients.
- The internal carotid artery ipsilateral to the eye to be treated is then catheterized by a four-F (1.3 mm diameter) guide catheter and a 0.035-inch hydrophilic polymer-coated guide wire through a display of the vessels by "roadmapping".
- Using fluoroscopy and roadmapping, the ophthalmic artery arising from the internal carotid artery is then superselectively catheterized using a flow-directed microcatheter whose outer diameter at the distal tip is 1.5 F.
- A 30-min superselective infusion is then performed, by a pulsatile injection to avoid streaming and inhomogenous drug delivery. If more than one drug is injected, the different agents are delivered sequentially and not simultaneously.
- A lateral arteriogram is then performed, to exclude procedure-related complications such as vasospasm, embolism, or arterial dissection.
- The catheter system is then withdrawn.
- Haemostasis of the femoral artery is achieved by manual compression.[12]

When the ophthalmic artery cannot be catheterized, there are other routes of treatment. While the ophthalmic artery usually branches off the internal carotid artery, it may also branch off the middle meningeal artery; in such cases, catheterizing the external carotid artery and passing the catheter tip into the middle meningeal artery from the internal maxillary artery is safe and successful.[13]

IA chemotherapy sessions are repeated every 3–4 weeks. Decisions regarding the number of sessions are not standardized but depend on the findings of the examinations under anesthesia and responses to previous treatments.

### Bridge Chemotherapy

Bridge IV-IA chemotherapy is a promising strategy to treat retinoblastoma in neonates and young infants. Initial single-agent intravenous chemotherapy acts to bridge the time from diagnosis to when threshold criteria are met for IA chemotherapy. Patients < 3 months old are treated with intravenous carboplatin every 3–4 weeks. This strategy allows immediate treatment while postponing IA chemotherapy, further avoiding potential toxicity of multiagent chemotherapy in very young patients.[14]

### Tandem Therapy

Patients with bilateral disease can have both eyes treated in a single session. Different agents are used for each eye to prevent systemic complications that might occur if a patient receives a double dose of a single agent.[15]

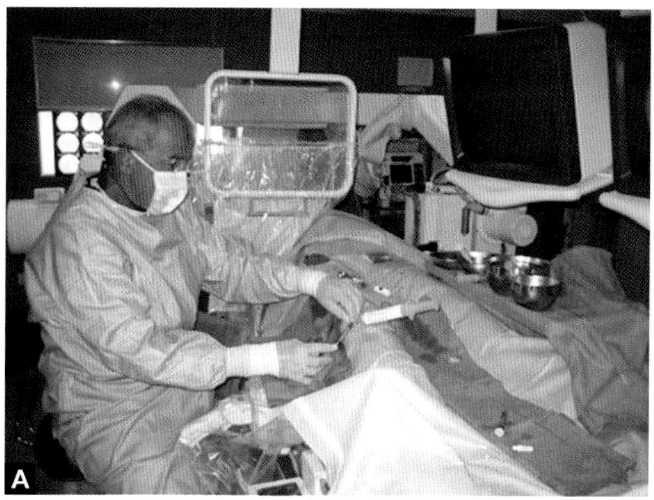
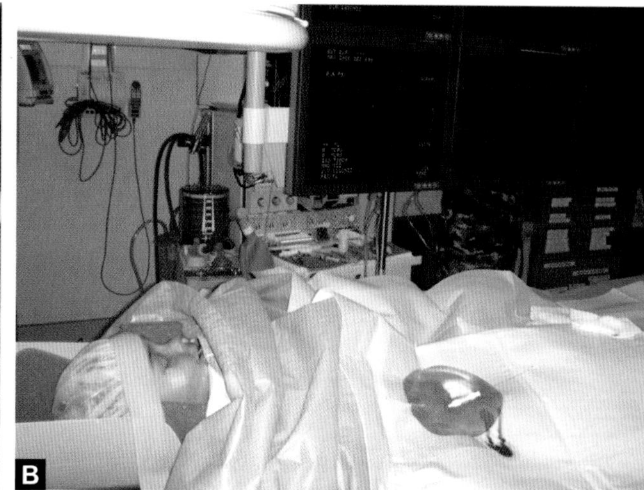

Figures 98-2A and B Neurointerventional radiology theatre (A). Puncture of the femoral artery and catheterization (B).

## MECHANISM OF ACTION

The objective of IA chemotherapy is to deliver a high dose of melphalan and/or topotecan to the tumor while avoiding the side effects and risks of systemic chemotherapy. IA chemotherapy also avoids the risks of external beam radiotherapy, which include midfacial contracture, cataract, radiation retinopathy and, in patients with germinal mutations, the development of second malignant neoplasms.[16,17]

Interestingly, the tumor response to IA chemotherapy, in most cases, is dramatic, with an immediate tumor shrinkage after the first infusion. Additional treatment, usually consisting of laser therapy and/or cryotherapy, may usefully increase the permeability of the blood–retina barrier prior to IA chemotherapy if no retinal detachment is present.

## POSTOPERATIVE CARE

- Pediatric evaluation includes:
  - Complete blood count with platelets is recommended 8–10 days after the procedure to monitor for myelosuppression (particularly neutropenia).
  - Interval history, weight and height measurements.
  - Head and orbit gadolinium-enhanced MRI, when clinically indicated by the multidisciplinary group.
  - Complete ophthalmic examination every 3–4 weeks, RetCam digital photography, B-Scan ultrasonography, and ERG to monitor retinal toxicity.[18,19]

The efficacy of treatment is evaluated by examination under anesthesia performed 3–4 weeks after each treatment. Efficacy is assessed according to tumor shrinkage and regression, disappearance, or calcifications of vitreous seeds and subretinal seeds, and absence of new tumor growth. Retinal toxicity is estimated from ERG results.

## SPECIFIC DRUGS AND INSTRUMENTATION

- Heparin
- Melphalan
- Topotecan
- Carboplatin
- Cerebral angiography equipment
- 4-F guide catheter
- 1.2 or 1.5 microcatheters
- 0.08-inch hydrophilic guide wire.

The three principal chemotherapeutic agents used in IA chemotherapy are as follows:

- *Melphalan*: Melphalan, an alkylating agent, has been the agent most extensively used in IA chemotherapy for the treatment of retinoblastoma. The rationale of the use of this drug is based on in vitro studies with human cultured retinoblastoma cells, using clonogenic assays, which showed that in comparison with other commonly used drugs melphalan had the greatest effect on retinoblastoma cells. The dose of melphalan is chosen according to the territory infused, i.e. the size of the eye at ultrasound and not the body surface area or body weight.[3,17,20]
- *Topotecan*: This topoisomerase inhibitor has increasingly been used in IA chemotherapy for aggressive tumors that are unresponsive to melphalan alone. Superselective ophthalmic artery infusion of topotecan results in a significantly higher vitreous concentration.

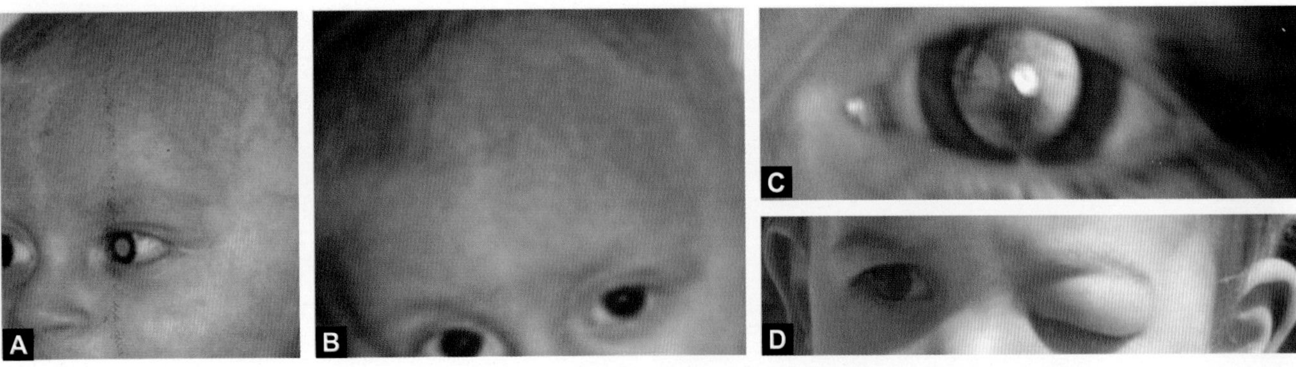

Figures 98-3A to D Ipsilateral eyelid and frontal rash (A), alopecia (B) lash loss (C), and eyelid edema (D), which are transient.

- *Carboplatin*: This alkylating agent has been used with tumors that do not respond to melphalan and/or topotecan. It has usually been administered as part of a simultaneous triple therapy in eyes that have failed single- or double-agent IA chemotherapy or systemic intravenous chemotherapy.

Gobin et al. reported the dose regimen of the three chemotherapeutics.[20]

When IA chemosurgery is repeated, the chemotherapy dose is adjusted according to:

- Size of the eye on ultrasonography
- Response to previous IA chemotherapy
- Persistent seeds
- Presence of large extraocular branches of the ophthalmic artery.

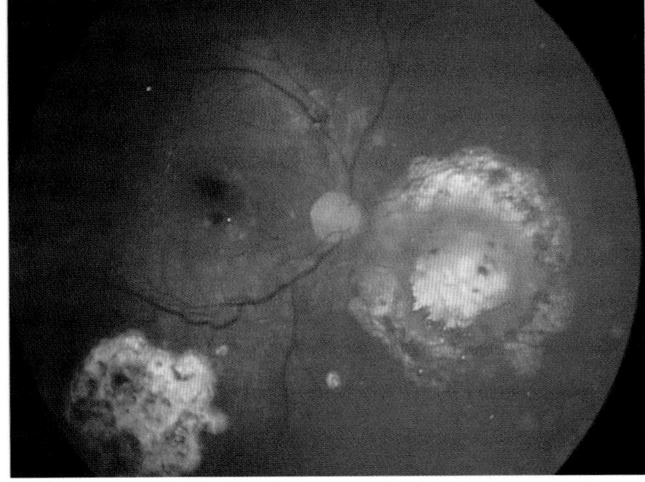

Figure 98-4 Roth spot after first session of intra-arterial chemotherapy for recurrent retinoblastoma. The tumor had shown dramatic regression.

## COMPLICATIONS

In literature there have been no reports of death. Stroke and other neurological complications have been rare.[21,22]

## TRANSIENT

### Ocular[23]

- Periocular erythema in the distribution of the supraorbital or supratrochlear artery (Fig. 98-3A).
- Frontal alopecia (Fig. 98-3B).
- Temporary lash loss (madarosis), especially in medial third of the upper eyelid (Fig. 98-3C).
- Upper eyelid edema and redness (Fig. 98-3D).
- Rectus muscle inflammation.
- Ophthalmic artery stenosis.
- Roth spots (Fig. 98-4).
- Macular hemorrhage (Figs. 98-5A and B).
- Vitreous hemorrhage.
- Retinal arteriolar embolization.
- Purtscher-like retinopathy with peripapillary cotton wool spots and scattered intraretinal hemorrhages (most likely due to an embolic event).[22]

Most side effects are transient. They are more evident at the first infusion and less pronounced in the following cycles. The etiology of thrombotic events is still controversial and includes possible crystallization of chemotherapeutic agents and foreign bodies introduced during the catheterization procedure, as documented by Eagle et al.[24]

### Systemic

- Anesthetic complications, such as bronchospasm and bradycardia, as a result of the vagal reflex.
- Nonperfusion brain defects.
- Hematoma at the femoral puncture site.
- Neutropenia and/or anemia, especially with higher doses of chemotherapy.

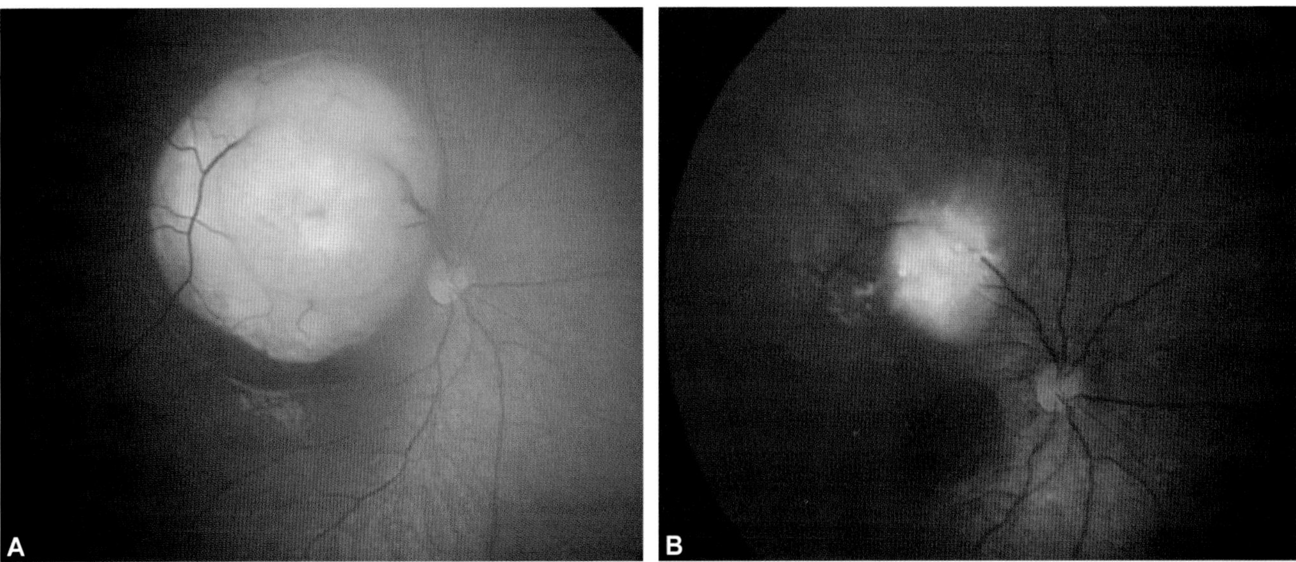


Figures 98-5A and B Pretreatment photograph of the right fundus showing stage B retinoblastoma (A). Dramatic shrinkage and calcification after the first infusion, with a macular hemorrhage, which resolved within 1 week (B).

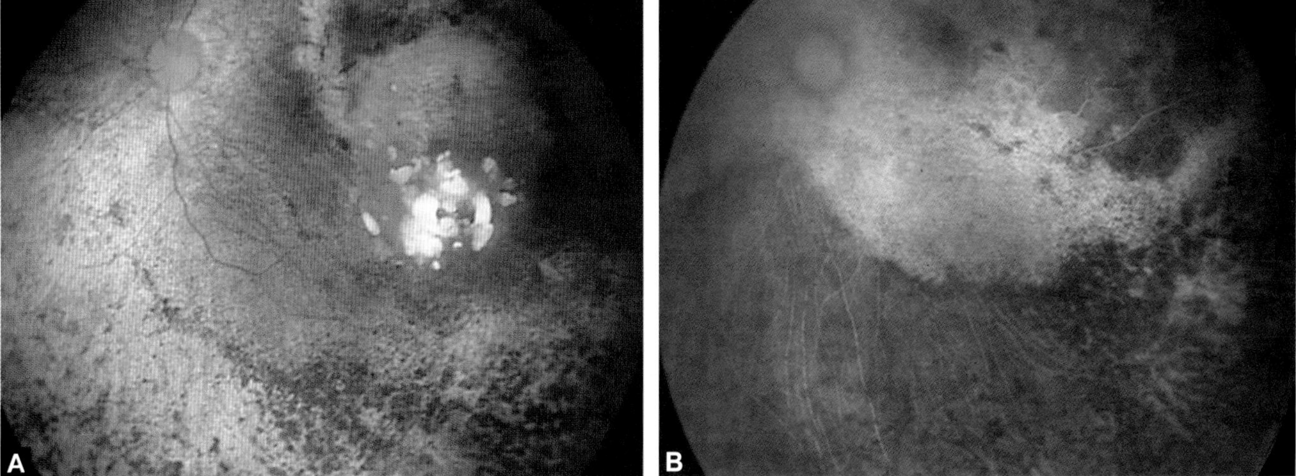


Figures 98.6A and B Chorioretinal atrophy after intra-arterial chemotherapy demonstrated by color photography (A) and fluorescein angiography (B).

## Permanent

### *Ocular*[12,21,25,26]

- Retinal pigment epithelium changes (mottling).
- Choroidal occlusive vasculopathy (Fig. 98-6A). This atrophy can be due to toxic effects on the endothelium, catheter-related damage to the vessel walls, chemotherapy precipitation, or foreign body embolization. Munier et al. reported fluoroangiography findings in a series of 13 eyes after IA, in which choroidal occlusive vasculopathy developed in 2 (15%) and retinal arterial emboli developed in 1 (8%) after a total of 29 catheterizations. In two cases, progression of choroidal occlusion to choroidal atrophy is described. Gobin et al. reported ischemic retinopathy in 9% of catheterizations.
- Using high-resolution fluorescein angiography, Bianciotto et al. documented choroidal sectors of diffuse nonperfusion (Fig. 98-6B).[21,26,27]
- Ptosis (Fig. 98-7A).
- Strabismus (Fig. 98-7B).

## Systemic

Another concern with IA chemotherapy is the cumulative toxic effect from repeated exposure to ionizing radiations.

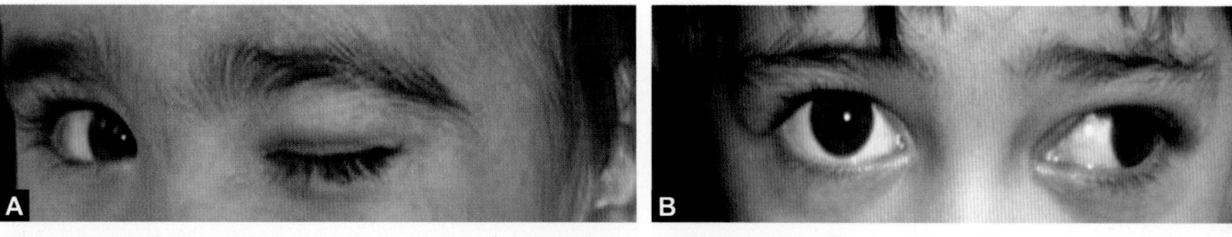

Figures 98-7A and B Permanent complications of intra-arterial chemotherapy include ptosis (A) and strabismus (B).

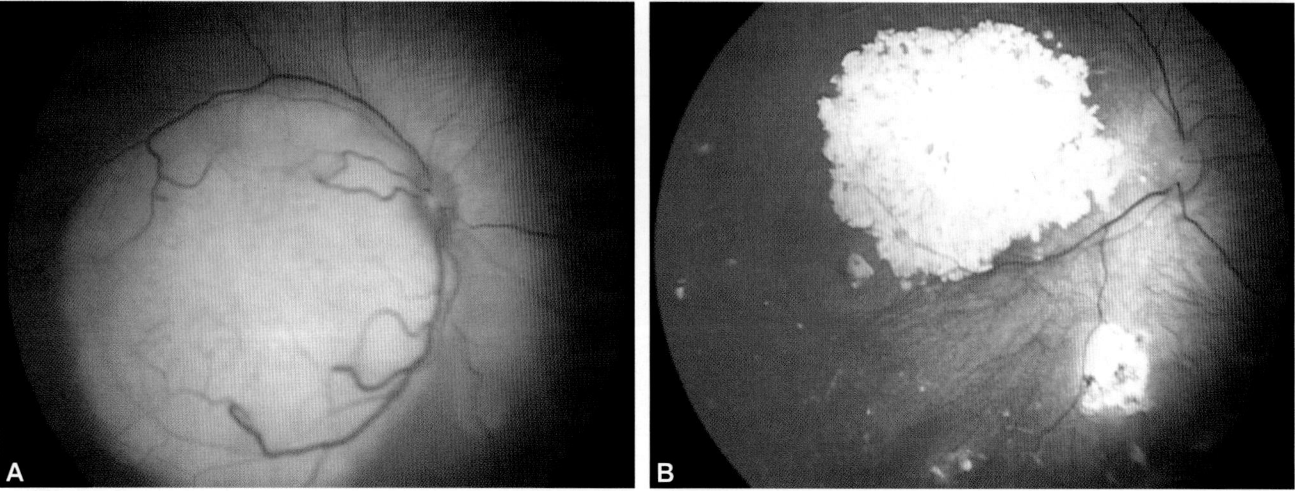

Figures 98-8A and B Large macular tumor in the right eye before treatment (A) and after a single dose of intra-arterial chemotherapy (B).

It has been reported that radiation doses remained far below toxic levels for gonads, thyroid and bone marrow but were possibly cataractogenic.[28] The effects of even low-dose radiation in retinoblastoma children with germ line mutations could be more serious. Thus, a careful use of fluoroscopy during IA chemotherapy with limited irradiation exposure is required.

## SURGICAL OUTCOMES: SCIENTIFIC EVIDENCE

- Tumor control in 100% eyes if stage C or D and 80% if stage E disease (Figs. 98-8A and B)
- Disease control in approximately 50% of eyes with subretinal seeds and approximately 67% of eyes with vitreous seeds.
- Tumor control with chemotherapy alone (i.e. without adjunctive treatment) in approximately 30% of eyes.
- Flat retina in 100% eyes if partial retinal detachment and 50% eyes if total retinal detachment (Figs. 98-9A and B).
- Ocular conservation in approximately 70% of eyes receiving IA chemosurgery as primary treatment and 50% of eyes receiving such treatment after failed radiotherapy and systemic chemotherapy.
- Successful local control of relapsed tumors (Figs. 98-10A and B).

## PLACE OF THE TECHNIQUE IN SURGICAL ARMAMENTARIUM

IA chemosurgery conserves many eyes with retinoblastoma that would otherwise require enucleation, at the same time avoiding the risks of radiotherapy and systemic chemotherapy.

## PEARLS AND PITFALLS

### Pearls

Intra-arterial chemosurgery delivering chemotherapeutic drugs selectively into the ophthalmic artery:

- Minimizes systemic absorption and drug-related toxicity, such as neutropenia, infection, and secondary neoplasms.
- Decreases the need for hospitalization.
- Reduces the risk of resistance to IA melphalan in recurrent retinoblastoma, since this drug is not used in protocols of intravenous chemotherapy.
- Administers significantly higher doses of chemotherapy directly to the tumor and to any seeds, thereby increasing

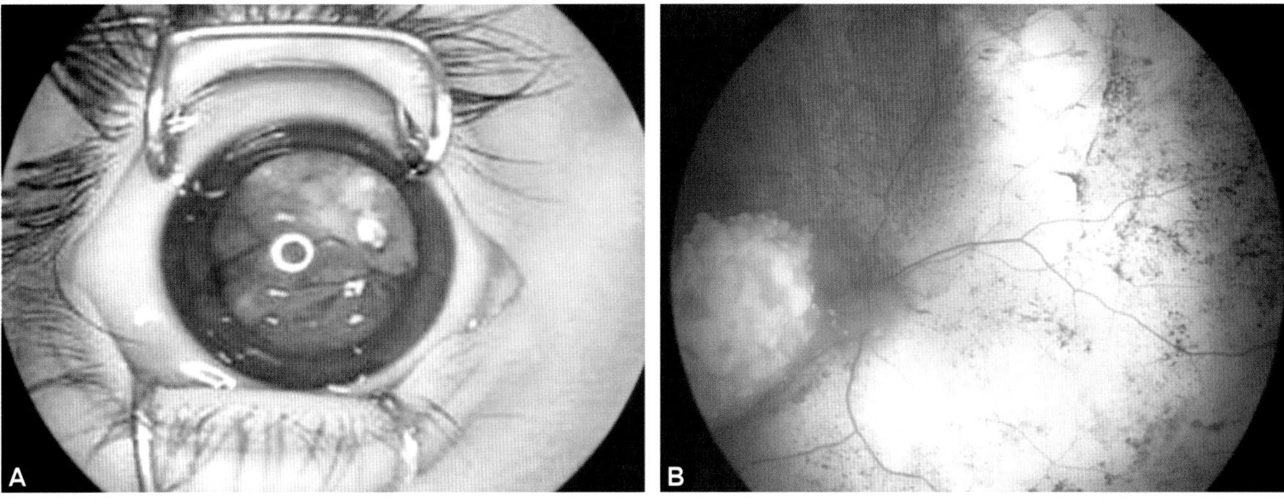


Figures 98-9A and B Advanced retinoblastoma (Group V) with total retinal detachment before treatment (A). After three courses of intra-arterial chemotherapy, there was type I tumor regression with a flat retina and a sectorial area of choroidal atrophy (B).

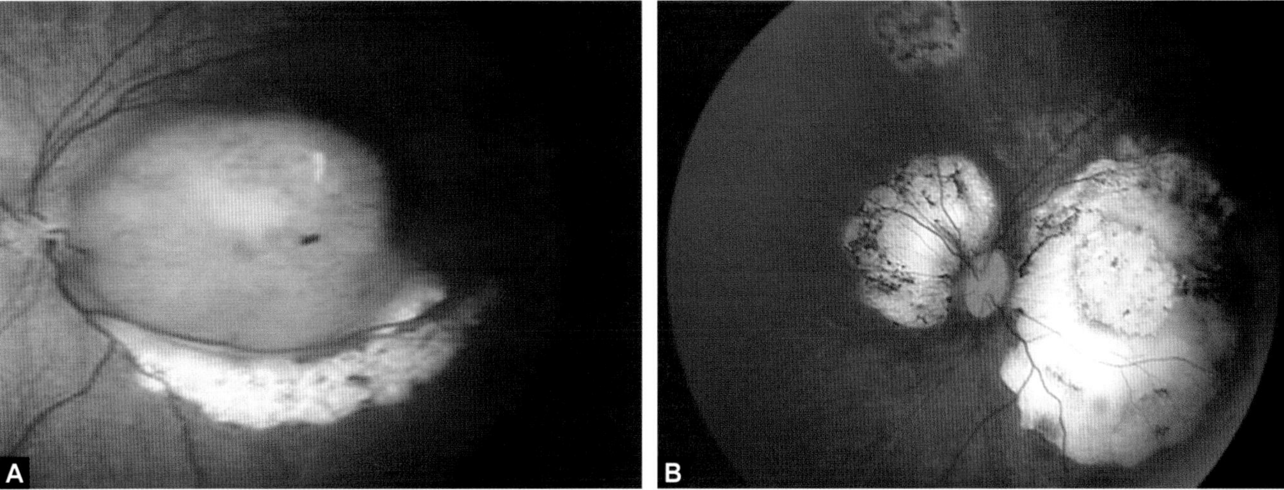


Figures 98-10A and B Recurrent retinoblastoma after systemic chemotherapy and focal therapy (A). Complete regression of the recurrent tumor with three cycles of intra-arterial chemotherapy (B).

the biological effect, enhancing tumor control, and reducing the rate of recurrence.[5,29,30]

- All the above contribute to a dramatic reduction in en cleation in advanced and treatment-resistant retinoblastoma.[6]

## Pitfalls

- Vitreous seeds are the most common indications for enucleation in eyes treated with IA chemotherapy.
- Lack of effect on subclinical systemic disease.
- Most adverse side effects are transient, but choroidal vasculopathy is permanent and in some cases progressive.[12,31,32]

## REFERENCES

1. Reese AB, Hyman G, Tapley N, et al. The treatment of retinoblastoma by X-Ray and triethylene melamine. AMA Arch Ophthalmol. 1958;60:897-906.
2. Yamane T, Kaneko A, Mohri M. The technique of ophthalmic arterial infusion therapy for patients with intraocular retinoblastoma. Int J Clin Oncol. 2004;9(2):69-73.
3. Abramson DH, Dunkel IJ, Brodie SE, et al. A phase I/II study of direct intraarterial (ophthalmic artery) chemotherapy with melphalan for intraocular retinoblastoma initial results. Ophthalmology. 2008;115(8):1398-404.
4. Shields CL, Ramasubramanian A, Rosenwasser R, et al. Superselective catheterization of the ophthalmic artery for intraarterial chemotherapy for retinoblastoma. Retina. 2009;29(8):1207-9.

5. Shields CL, Shields JA. Intra-arterial chemotherapy for retinoblastoma: the beginning of a long journey. Clin Experiment Ophthalmol. 2010;38(6):638-43.
6. Peterson EC, Elhammady MS, Quintero-Wolfe S, et al. Selective ophthalmic artery infusion of chemotherapy for advanced intraocular retinoblastoma: initial experience with 17 tumors. J Neurosurg. 2011;114(6):1603-8. Epub 2011 Feb 4.
7. Aziz HA, Boutrid H, Murray TG, et al. Supraselective injection of intraarterial melphalan as the primary treatment for late presentation unilateral multifocal stage Vb retinoblastoma. Retina. 2010;30(4 Suppl):S63-5.
8. Shields CL, Shields JA. Retinoblastoma management: advances in enucleation, intravenous chemoreduction, and intra-arterial chemotherapy. Curr Opin Ophthalmol. 2010;21(3):203-12.
9. Abramson DH, Dunkel IJ, Brodie SE, et al. Superselective ophthalmic artery chemotherapy as primary treatment for retinoblastoma (chemosurgery). Ophthalmology. 2010;117(8):1623-9.
10. Berenstein A, Ortiz R, Niimi Y, et al. Endovascular management of arteriovenous malformations and other intracranial arteriovenous shunts in neonates, infants, and children. Childs Nerv Syst. 2010;26:1345-58.
11. Stiefel MF, Heuer GG, Basil AK, et al. Endovascular and surgical treatment of ruptured cerebral aneurysms in pediatric patients. Neurosurgery. 2008;63:859-5; discussion 865-6.
12. Venturi C, Bracco S, Cerase A, et al. Superselective ophthalmic artery infusion of melphalan for intraocular retinoblastoma: preliminary results from 140 treatments. Acta Ophthalmol. 2013;91(4):335-42.
13. Klufas MA, Gobin YP, Marr B, et al. Intra-arterial chemotherapy as a treatment for intraocular retinoblastoma: alternatives to direct ophthalmic artery catheterization. Am J Neuroradiol. 2012;33:1608-14.
14. Gobin YP, Dunkel IJ, Marr BP, et al. Combined, sequential intravenous and intra-arterial chemotherapy (bridge chemotherapy) for young infants with retinoblastoma. PLOS ONE. 2012;7(9):e44322.doi:10.1371/journal.pone.0044322.Epub2012 Sep 18.
15. Abramson DH, Dunkel IJ, Brodie SE, et al. Bilateral superselective ophthalmic artery chemotherapy for bilateral retinoblastoma: tandem therapy. Arch Ophthalmol. 2010;128(3):370-2.
16. Abramson DH. Super selective ophthalmic artery delivery of chemotherapy for intraocular retinoblastoma: 'chemosurgery' the first Stallard lecture. Br J Ophthalmol. 2010;94(4):396-9.
17. Abramson DH. Chemosurgery for retinoblastoma: what we know after 5 years. Arch Ophthalmol. 2011;129(11):1492-4.
18. Brodie SE, Gobin YP, Dunkel IJ, et al. Persistence of retinal function after selective ophthalmic artery chemotherapy infusion for retinoblastoma. Doc Ophthalmol. 2009;119(1):13-22.
19. Brodie S, Paulus Y, Patel M, et al. ERG monitoring of retinal function during systemic chemotherapy for retinoblastoma. Br J Ophthalmol. 2012;96:877-80.
20. Gobin YP, Dunkel IJ, Marr BP, et al. Intra-arterial chemotherapy for the management of retinoblastoma four-year experience. Arch Opthalmol. 2011;129(6):732-7.
21. Shields CL, Bianciotto CG, Jabbour P, et al. Intra-arterial chemotherapy for retinoblastoma: report No. 2, treatment complications. Arch Ophthalmol. 2011;129(11):1407-15. Epub 2011 Jun 13.
22. Vajzovic LM, Murray TG, Aziz-Sultan MA, et al. Supraselective intra-arterial chemotherapy: evaluation of treatment-related complications in advanced retinoblastoma. Clin Ophthalmol. 2010;5:171-6.
23. Marr B, Gobin PY, Dunkel IJ, et al. Spontaneously resolving periocular erythema and ciliary Madarosis following intra-arterial chemotherapy for retinoblastoma. Middle East Afr J Ophthalmol. 2010;17(3):207-9.
24. Eagle RC Jr, Shields CL, Bianciotto C, et al. Histopathologic observations after intra-arterial chemotherapy for retinoblastoma. Arch Ophthalmol. 2011;129(11):1416-21. Epub 2011 Jul 11.
25. Munier FL, Beck-Popovic M, Balmer A. Occurrence of sectoral choroidal occlusive vasculopathy and retinal arteriolar embolization after superselective ophthalmic artery chemotherapy for advanced intraocular retinoblastoma. Retina. 2011;31(3): 566-73.
26. Muen WJ, Kingston JE, Robertson F, et al. Efficacy and complications of super-selective intra-ophthalmic artery melphalan for the treatment of refractory retinoblastoma. Ophthalmology. 2011;118(10):2081-7
27. Bianciotto C, Shields CL, Iturralde JC, et al. Fluorescein angiographic findings after intra-arterial chemotherapy for retinoblastoma. Ophthalmology. 2012;119(4):843-9.
28. Vijayakrishnan R, Shields CL, Ramasubramanian A, et al. Irradiation toxic effects during intra-arterial chemotherapy for retinoblastoma: should we be concerned? Arch Ophthalmol. 2010;128(11):1427-31.
29. Jabbour P, Chalouhi N, Tjoumakaris S, et al. Pearls and pitfalls of intraarterial chemotherapy for retinoblastoma. J Neurosurg Pediatr. 2012;10(3):175-81.
30. Suzuki S, Yamane T, Mohri M, et al. Selective ophthalmic arterial injection therapy for intraocular retinoblastoma: the long-term prognosis. Ophthalmology. 2011;118:2081-7
31. Hadjistilianou T, De Francesco S, De Luca M, et al. Superselective intraarterial chemotherapy complications in advanced retinoblastoma. Acta Ophthalmol. Article first published online: 11 AUG 2011, doi: 10.1111/j.1755-3768.2011.4163.x.
32. Hadjistilianou T, De Francesco S, Venturi C, et al. Direct intra-arterial (ophthalmic artery) chemotherapy with melphalan for advanced intraocular retinoblastoma: the Italian experience. Acta ophthalmologica. Article first published online : 23 SEP 2010, doi: 10.1111/j.1755-3768.2010.4364.x.

CHAPTER

# 99

# Intravitreal Injections in Oncology

Lazaros Konstantinidis, Francis Munier, Bertil Damato

## INTRODUCTION

Intravitreal injections are increasingly being administered as treatment for retinal lymphoma, retinoblastoma, radiation-induced complications and other conditions.[1-5]

## INDICATIONS

### Retinoblastoma

- Recurrent or resistant vitreous seeds after treatment of retinoblastoma (Figs. 99-1A and B)
- Iatrogenic vitreous seeding after phototherapy or plaque radiotherapy
- Group C and D eyes as adjunctive treatment after conservative therapy
- Group B eyes with ruptured internal limiting membrane, because of the high risk of vitreous seeding if other forms of conservative therapy are administered alone.

### Lymphoma

Retinal lymphoma, either as primary treatment or after failed external beam radiotherapy.

### Radiation-induced Complications

- Macular edema
- Exudative retinal detachment
- Optic neuropathy
- Neovascular glaucoma.

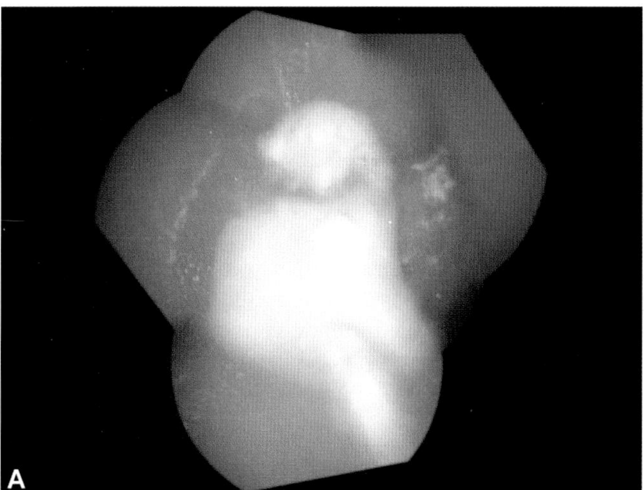

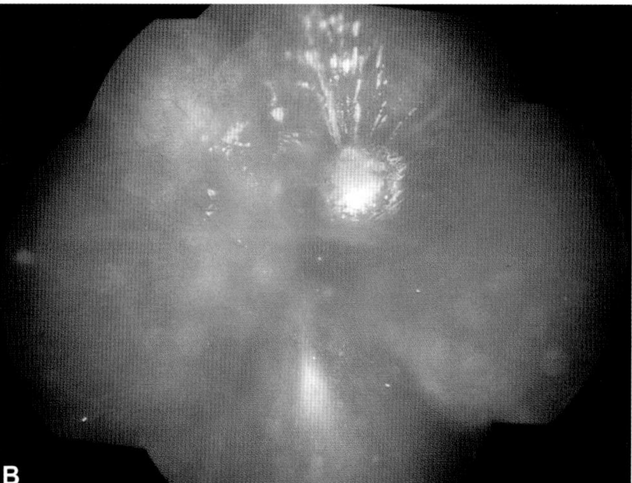

**Figures 99-1A and B** Retinoblastoma with vitreous seeds before (A) and after (B) intravitreal injections of Melphalan

## CONTRAINDICATIONS

### Retinoblastoma

- Vitreous seeding, retinal detachment or anterior hyaloid detachment at injection site
- Anterior chamber involvement by tumor
- Intra-retinal or uveal tumor at injection site.

### Retinal Lymphoma

- Ocular or periocular infections
- Caution should be exercised in case of keratoconjunctivitis sicca due to the high incidence of corneal epitheliopathy.

### Radiation-induced Complications

- Ocular or periocular infections, hypersensitivity to the injected agent.
- Caution should be exercised in case of history of stroke, cardiac arrest, uncontrolled hypertension as there is a potential risk of arterial thromboembolic events following intravitreal use of vascular endothelial growth factor (VEGF) inhibitors.
- Caution should be exercised in case of pregnancy as VEGF inhibitors may pose a risk to fetal development.
- Corticosteroids are contraindicated in patients with systemic fungal infections, active ocular herpes simplex and hypersensitivity to corticosteroids. Caution should be exercised in case of glaucoma as well as in pregnancy due to potential hazard to the fetus.

## PREOPERATIVE CARE

### Retinoblastoma

- High-frequency ultrasonography is performed to ensure that the injection site is free of active retinoblastoma, retinal detachment and undetached vitreous.

### Retinal Lymphoma

- Cytologic evidence of malignant lymphocytes on vitreous biopsy is generally required before ocular treatment.

### Radiation-induced Complications

Fluorescein angiogram (FA) can be useful in highlighting retinal microvascular changes and assessing the extent and degree of capillary malformation, incompetence and closure. Indocyanine green angiography can reveal precapillary arteriolar occlusion and areas of choroidal hypoperfusion. Optical coherence tomography (OCT) can be helpful in evaluating macular edema.

## SURGICAL TECHNIQUE

### Retinoblastoma

- *Anterior chamber paracentesis*: Aqueous is drained from the anterior chamber to reduce the intraocular pressure (IOP) and, hence, the risk of vitreous leakage through the scleral injection site. This is performed by aspirating 0.1–0.15 mL of aqueous fluid (i.e. the same amount as the injection volume). This sample is sent to the cytopathology laboratory for analysis, to exclude the presence of tumor cells.
- *Intravitreal injection*: A dose of 20–30 µg of melphalan is injected into the vitreous with a 32-gauge needle inserted 3.0–3.5 mm from the limbus.
- *Cryotherapy*: As soon as the needle is withdrawn, the cryoprobe is placed over the injection site and triple freeze-thaw cryotherapy is applied.
- *Drug dispersion*: The conjunctiva at the limbus is grasped with forceps and the eye is shaken for 10–20 seconds to disperse the drug throughout the vitreous cavity.

### Retinal Lymphoma

- A dose of 400 µg/0.1 mL of methotrexate (MTX) is injected intravitreally at the level of the pars plana using a 30-gauge needle, under topical anesthesia. Methotrexate is injected twice weekly as an induction phase for 4 weeks, then weekly for 1 month or 2 months as consolidation therapy, followed by once monthly injection for 1 year as maintenance therapy.
- A dose of 1 mg/0.1 mL rituximab is injected intravitreally at the level of the pars plana.[6]

### Radiation-induced Complications

- The intravitreal injection procedure should be carried out under controlled aseptic conditions. Adequate local anesthesia and broad-spectrum microbicide should be given prior to the injection.
- The pharmacologic agent is injected 3.5–4 mm from the limbus with a 30-gauge needle for anti-VEGF agents and 27-gauge needle for steroids.

- Confirm hand motion vision and consider measuring IOP using tonometry 30 minutes following the intravitreal injection. Monitoring may also consist of a check for perfusion of the optic nerve head immediately after the injection.

## MECHANISM OF ACTION

### Retinoblastoma

- Intravitreal administration of chemotherapy for vitreous disease offers the opportunity of delivering the desired tumoricidal drug concentration within the vitreous cavity.
- Melphalan, a mechlorethamine derivative, is an alkylating antineoplastic agent. It forms carbonium ions, resulting in deoxyribonucleic acid (DNA) and ribonucleic acid (RNA) synthesis inhibition. It cross-links DNA strands and acts on both resting and rapidly dividing tumor cells.

### Retinal Lymphoma

- Methotrexate is a folate analog that inhibits dihydrofolate reductase, thereby blocking de novo purine synthesis.
- Methotrexate acts specifically during DNA and RNA synthesis and, thus, it is cytotoxic during the S-phase of the cell cycle. It, therefore, has a greater toxic effect on rapidly dividing cells, which replicate their DNA more frequently.
- How rituximab can lead to depletion of B cells is not completely known.

### Radiation-induced Complications

#### *Anti-VEGF*

- Ranibizumab binds to the receptor binding site of active forms of VEGF-A, including the biologically active, cleaved form of this molecule, VEGF110.
- VEGF-A has been shown to cause neovascularization and leakage and is thought to contribute to pathophysiology of macular edema following radiation. The binding of ranibizumab, bevacizumab to VEGF-A prevents the interaction of VEGF-A with its receptors on the surface of endothelial cells, reducing endothelial cell proliferation, vascular leakage and new blood vessel formation.

#### *Steroids*

Although these glucocorticoids mediate their effects through modulation of inflammatory cytokines and their anti-VEGF effect to achieve a clinical outcome, they also affect both common and unique gene expression pathways involving oxidative stress and neuroprotection. It has been proposed that triamcinolone acetonide (TA), a synthetic glucocorticoid, decreases macular edema by means of its antiangiogenic, anti-inflammatory, and blood-retinal barrier (BRB)-stabilizing effects increasing the levels of tight-junction proteins and, thus, diminishing vessel leakage.

## POSTOPERATIVE CARE

### Retinoblastoma

- The eye is protected by a transparent plastic shield and treated with topical antibiotics and steroids three times a day for 1 week.
- The ocular status at each follow-up is objectively monitored under anesthesia with fundus photography and, in select cases, B-scan ultrasonography. At each visit, the residual vitreous tumor burden is reassessed and intravitreal chemotherapy (IViC) is administered every 7–10 days up to eight injections, if a response could be documented, until complete seed fragmentation is observed or complete response is achieved.

### Retinal Lymphoma

- Monitor IOP after the injection
- Immediately after the injection, all patients are examined by dilated funduscopy and, eventually slit-lamp biomicroscopy
- At each visit, patient examinations include measurement of visual acuity (VA) and IOP, slit-lamp biomicroscopy to view individual cells within the vitreous cavity, and dilated funduscopy to see malignant cellular infiltrates involving the retina and/or optic nerve head. A gonioscopic examination may be performed in order to identify iris and anterior chamber angle neovascularization.

### Radiation-induced Complications

Prescribe topical antibiotics for at-home patient use. Patients should also be monitored for and instructed to report any symptoms suggestive of endophthalmitis without delay following the injection. Patients are reviewed every 4–6 weeks. At each visit, patient examinations include measurement of VA and IOP, slit-lamp biomicroscopy, OCT and occasionally FA.

## SPECIFIC INSTRUMENTATION

- Instrumentation could include lid speculum, conjunctival forceps, calipers
- Furthermore, various intravitreal injection-guiding instruments have been developed and used in some centers in order to facilitate intravitreal injection procedure, stabilizing the eye and needle, whilst accurately positioning the needle.

## COMPLICATIONS

Serious adverse reactions related to the injection procedure of intravitreal injections, include rhegmatogenous retinal detachment and iatrogenic traumatic cataract.

### *Drug-specific Complications*

*Methotrexate*: The most commonly reported ocular side-effects associated with intravitreal injection of methotrexate include cataract, conjunctival hyperemia and transient keratopathy ranging from mild punctuate epithelial erosions to severe epitheliopathy.

*Rituximab*: Early evidence suggests that intravitreal rituximab may have fewer side-effects than methotrexate. The major ocular complications of intravitreal rituximab include elevated IOP with severe anterior segment inflammation and mutton-fat keratic precipitates.

*Steroids*: The most commonly reported adverse events following administration of intraocular steroids is elevated IOP and cataract progression. These events have been reported to occur in 20–60% of patients. Less common reactions include, hypopyon, injection site reactions, vitreous floaters and detachment of the retinal pigment epithelium, retinal vasculopathy, eye inflammation, conjunctival hemorrhage, and reduced visual acuity.

*Anti-VEGF*: There is a theoretical risk of arterial thromboembolic events following intravitreal use of inhibitors of VEGF. A potential relationship between fatal events and intravitreal use of VEGF inhibitors could not be excluded in patients with diabetic macular edema.

## OUTCOME SCIENTIFIC EVIDENCE

### Retinoblastoma

The use of intravitreal melphalan for vitreous seeding was first introduced in the 1990s by Kaneko and Suzuki, who treated 41 eyes with 8 mg melphalan and simultaneous hyperthermia using a Lagendijk applicator. At 50 months of follow-up, the eye preservation rate was 51.3%.[7]

Since their initial pioneering report, Kaneko and Suzuki have performed 896 IViCs in 237 eyes of 227 patients.[8] They reported the occurrence of extraocular subconjunctival extension in one eye (0.4%), which had anterior chamber involvement and dense vitreous seeds. The patient received adjuvant chemotherapy after enucleation was in complete remission at the study close. Among the 10 patients (4.4%) who developed metastases, IViC was potentially related to 1 (0.4%).

Munier et al. reported a retrospective study of 23 consecutive heavily pretreated retinoblastoma patients (23 eyes) with active vitreous seeding.[3] They received a total of 122 intravitreal injections of melphalan (20–30 mg) given every 7–10 days. All patients were alive without evidence of extraocular spread (95% CI, 82.19–100%). Concomitant treatments, including other chemotherapeutic modalities, were used until complete sterilization of the retinal seeding source and subretinal seeds. Globe retention was achieved in 87% (20/23) of cases. All retained eyes were in complete remission after a median follow-up period of 22 months (range 9–31 months). The Kaplan Meier estimate of ocular survival rates at 2 years was 84% (95% CI, 62–95%). A localized peripheral salt-and-pepper retinopathy was noted in 10 eyes (43%) at the site of injection.

### Retinal Lymphoma

Randomized-controlled clinical trials have not been performed for primary vitreoretinal lymphoma (PVRL) and are unlikely. Published recommendations from the International Primary Central Nervous System Lymphoma Collaborative Group (IPCG) symposium on PVRL[4] and from the British Neuro-Oncology Society differ in recommendations for the management of PVRL without concomitant brain lymphoma. The IPCG symposium on PVRL specifies local treatment for uniocular disease and local treatment with or without systemic chemotherapy for bilateral ocular disease, whereas the British guidelines specify systemic chemotherapy incorporating high-dose methotrexate with whole-globe irradiation for ocular only disease.[2]

Intravitreal methotrexate was shown to be efficacious in small nonrandomized trials [23, 69–73]. Frenkel et al.[9] reported on the largest series of 44 eyes of 26 patients with PVRL. They demonstrated clinical remission after a mean of 6.4 ± 3.4 (range, 2–16) injections of methotrexate.

Intravitreal rituximab was shown to penetrate the entire retina. Small, nonrandomized reports have demonstrated the efficacy of intravitreal rituximab monotherapy for PVRL.[5]

In a series by Ohguro et al., two patients received four, weekly injections of rituximab (1 mg/0.1 mL) and have remained tumor free for a limited follow-up time of 2 months. Itty and Pulido presented a patient who received 11 intraocular injections of rituximab (1 mg/0.1 mL) and maintained 20/20 vision and no evidence of retinal toxicity on examination after 8 months of follow-up.[5]

## Radiation-induced Complications

### *Corticosteroids*

Intravitreal steroids are effective in reducing radiation-induced macular edema. Their efficacy was first reported by Sutter in 2003.[10] Shields et al. treated 31 patients with symptomatic radiation-induced maculopathy with a single intravitreal TA injection (4 mg/0.1 mL). The visual acuity was stable or improved in 91% of patients by 1 month and in 45% by 6 months. Mean foveal thickness by OCT was 417 μm at injection, 207 μm at 1 month and 292 μm 6 months after injection.[11] Complications included transient elevation in IOP (16%), persistent glaucoma requiring topical medications (10%) and cataract (10%). In a randomized clinical trial, Horgan et al. administered periocular triamcinolone injections to 108 patients, who had received iodine-125 plaque radiotherapy for uveal melanoma. Injections given at the time of the plaque application, and 4 and 8 months later reduced macular edema for up to 18 months, improving vision without significant rates of glaucoma and cataract.[12] More recently, Russo et al. reported functional and anatomic improvement 4 weeks after a single intravitreal injection of dexamethasone 0.7 mg (Ozurdex) in a case of radiation-induced macular edema following ruthenium-106 plaque brachytherapy for a choroidal melanoma.[13]

### *Anti-vascular Endothelial Growth Factor Agents (anti-VEGF)*

Several studies have reported promising results with the use of anti-VEGF agents in the treatment of radiation-induced macular edema. Mason et al., in a retrospective case series of ten consecutive patients, evaluated the effect of a single intravitreal injection of bevacizumab after the development of radiation-induced macular edema. The mean visual acuity improved from 20/100 to 20/86 at 6 weeks and to 20/95 at 4 months. The mean foveal thickness measured by OCT was 482 μm before injection, 284 μm 6 weeks after injection, and 449 μm 4 months after injection.[14] Finger et al. reported the results of intravitreal injections of bevacizumab (1.25 mg in 0.05 mL) repeated every 6–12 weeks in 21 patients with radiation retinopathy. They noted reduction in retinal hemorrhage and exudation while visual acuity was maintained in 86% of patients, with 14% regaining two or more lines of visual acuity.[15] Gupta et al. reported five patients who developed radiation-induced macular edema after Ru-106 plaque radiotherapy for choroidal melanoma, suggesting that younger patients with shorter duration of macular edema may benefit the most after intravitreal injections of bevacizumab.[16] A phase 1, open-label, Genentech-sponsored study of five consecutive patients with macular edema after Pd-103 plaque radiotherapy for uveal melanoma showed visual acuity improvement in four patients and decreased foveal thickness in all cases after monthly intravitreal ranibizumab (0.5 mg) injections for at least four cycles.[17] In summary, most published studies suggest that anti-VEGF agents reduce radiation-induced macular edema and retinal neovascularization, although not all studies demonstrate improvement in visual acuity.[18] The optimal treatment regime has yet to be defined.

Shields reported the results of intravitreal TA (4 mg/0.1 mL) in 9 patients with radiation optic neuropathy (RON) after plaque radiotherapy for choroidal melanoma. They observed rapid resolution of optic disk hyperemia and edema with modest improvement of visual acuity.[19]

Encouraging results have been reported with antiangiogenic agents. Finger et al. evaluated intravitreal administration of bevacizumab in 14 patients with RON related to plaque radiotherapy for choroidal melanoma. They observed reduction in optic disk hemorrhage and edema in all patients while visual acuity was stable or improved in 9 of the 14 patients.[20]

The literature on the effect of anti-VEGF on exudative retinal detachment is inconsistent. Newman et al. reported complete resolution of the exudative retinal detachment secondary to choroidal melanoma in 2 patients after systemic treatment with bevacizumab (10 mg/kg intravenous bevacizumab every 2 weeks for 3 or 4 cycles) after plaque radiotherapy.[21] Parrozzani et al. evaluated the efficacy and safety of prompt intravitreal TA injection (4 mg/0.1 mL) vs intravitreal bevacizumab injection (1.25 mg/0.05 mL) vs observation in the management of extensive exudative retinal detachment secondary to posterior uveal melanoma. After a follow-up of approximately 37 months, marked exudative retinal detachment regression was documented in 22 (69%) of eyes treated with intravitreal triamcinolone vs 11 (34%) treated with intravitreal bevacizumab and 9 (28%) untreated eyes. No statistical significance was found between intravitreal bevacizumab group and the observation group ($P = .45$).[22] Vásquez et al.

reported resolution of exudative retinal detachment after intracameral bevacizumab in a case of neovascular glaucoma after brachytherapy for choroidal melanoma.[23] Similarly, Dunavoelgyi et al. described a case of successful management of exudative retinal detachment and neovascular glaucoma of a radiation-induced exudative retinal detachment and neovascular glaucoma with intravitreal ranibizumab.[24]

## PLACE OF THE TECHNIQUE IN SURGICAL ARMAMENTARIUM

### Retinoblastoma

Intravitreal chemotherapy for retinoblastoma with vitreous seeding can avoid radiotherapy or enucleation; however, a good surgical technique is required to avoid iatrogenic dissemination of tumor extraocularly.

### Retinal Lymphoma

Vitreoretinal involvement of lymphoma can be controlled effectively and without serious adverse reactions by intravitreal MTX injections.[25]

### Radiation-induced Complications

Several studies have reported promising results with the use of anti-VEGF and steroid agents in the treatment of radiation-induced macular edema and neovascular glaucoma. The role of these agents on exudative retinal detachment and optic neuropathy is less conclusive.

## PEARLS AND PITFALLS

- Injection of anti-VEGF and steroid agents through an oblique, tunneled fashion incision through the sclera instead of rectangular radial incision may reduce vitreous or drug reflux under the conjunctiva.
- A "z"-shaped puncture track by penetrating the conjunctiva first and then moving the needle slightly before penetrating the sclera might be of advantage regarding endophthalmitis.
- Early recognition of endophthalmitis is critical, therefore, it is very important that patients know the signs and symptoms and are able to self-report issues.
- In case of retinal lymphoma, continued observation and co-management with the oncologist or neuro-oncologist is advised because of the high likelihood of eventual CNS disease.[2]

## REFERENCES


1. Groenewald C, Konstantinidis L, Damato B. Effects of radiotherapy on uveal melanomas and adjacent tissues. Eye (Lond). 2013;27(2):163-71.
2. Davis JL. Intraocular lymphoma: a clinical perspective. Eye (Lond). 2013;27(2):153-62.
3. Munier FL, Gaillard MC, Balmer A, et al. Intravitreal chemotherapy for vitreous disease in retinoblastoma revisited: from prohibition to conditional indications. Br J Ophthalmol. 2012;96(8):1078-83.
4. Chan CC, Rubenstein JL, Coupland SE, et al. Primary vitreoretinal lymphoma: a report from an International Primary Central Nervous System Lymphoma Collaborative Group symposium. Oncologist. 2011;16(11):1589-99.
5. Itty S, Pulido JS. Rituximab for intraocular lymphoma. Retina. 2009;29(2):129-32.
6. Ohguro N, Hashida N, Tano Y. Effect of intravitreous rituximab injections in patients with recurrent ocular lesions associated with central nervous system lymphoma. Arch Ophthalmol. 2008;126(7):1002-3.
7. Kaneko A, Suzuki S. Eye-preservation treatment of retinoblastoma with vitreous seeding. Jpn J Clin Oncol. 2003;33(12): 601-7.
8. Suzuki S KA. Vitreous injection therapy of melphalan for retinoblastoma. In: XVth Biannual meeting of the International Society of Ocular Oncology (ISOO), 14-17 November 2011; Buenos Aires.
9. Frenkel S, Hendler K, Siegal T, et al. Intravitreal methotrexate for treating vitreoretinal lymphoma: 10 years of experience. Br J Ophthalmol. 2008;92(3):383-8.
10. Sutter FK, Gillies MC. Intravitreal triamcinolone for radiation-induced macular edema. Arch Ophthalmol. 2003;121(10): 1491-3.
11. Shields CL, Demirci H, Dai V, et al. Intravitreal triamcinolone acetonide for radiation maculopathy after plaque radiotherapy for choroidal melanoma. Retina. 2005;25(7):868-74.
12. Horgan N, Shields CL, Mashayekhi A, et al. Periocular triamcinolone for prevention of macular edema after plaque radiotherapy of uveal melanoma: a randomized controlled trial. Ophthalmology. 2009;116(7):1383-90.
13. Russo A, Avitabile T, Uva M, et al. Radiation Macular Edema after Ru-106 Plaque Brachytherapy for Choroidal Melanoma Resolved by an Intravitreal Dexamethasone 0.7-mg Implant. Case Rep Ophthalmol. 2012;3(1):71-6.
14. Mason JO, Albert MA, Persaud TO, et al. Intravitreal bevacizumab treatment for radiation macular edema after plaque radiotherapy for choroidal melanoma. Retina. 2007;27(7):903-7.
15. Finger PT. Radiation retinopathy is treatable with anti-vascular endothelial growth factor bevacizumab (Avastin). Int J Radiat Oncol Biol Phys. 2008;70(4):974-7.
16. Gupta A, Muecke JS. Treatment of radiation maculopathy with intravitreal injection of bevacizumab (Avastin). Retina. 2008;28(7):964-8.
17. Finger PT, Chin KJ. Intravitreous ranibizumab (lucentis) for radiation maculopathy. Arch Ophthalmol. 2010;128(2):249-52.

18. Giuliari GP, Sadaka A, Hinkle DM, et al. Current treatments for radiation retinopathy. Acta Oncol. 2011;50(1):6-13.
19. Shields CL, Demirci H, Marr BP, et al. Intravitreal triamcinolone acetonide for acute radiation papillopathy. Retina. 2006;26(5):537-44.
20. Finger PT, Chin KJ. Antivascular endothelial growth factor bevacizumab for radiation optic neuropathy: secondary to plaque radiotherapy. Int J Radiat Oncol Biol Phys. 2012;82(2):789-98.
21. Newman H, Finger PT, Chin KJ, et al. Systemic bevacizumab (Avastin) for exudative retinal detachment secondary to choroidal melanoma. Eur J Ophthalmol. 2011;21(6):796-801.
22. Parrozzani R, Pilotto E, Dario A, et al. Intravitreal triamcinolone versus intravitreal bevacizumab in the treatment of exudative retinal detachment secondary to posterior uveal melanoma. Am J Ophthalmol. 2013;155(1):127-33.
23. Vásquez LM, Somani S, Altomare F, et al. Intracameral bevacizumab in the treatment of neovascular glaucoma and exudative retinal detachment after brachytherapy in choroidal melanoma. Can J Ophthalmol. 2009;44(1):106-7.
24. Dunavoelgyi R, Zehetmayer M, Simader C, et al. Rapid improvement of radiation-induced neovascular glaucoma and exudative retinal detachment after a single intravitreal ranibizumab injection. Clin Experiment Ophthalmol. 2007;35(9):878-80.
25. Chan CC, Sen HN. Current concepts in diagnosing and managing primary vitreoretinal (intraocular) lymphoma. Discov Med. 2013;15(81):93-100.

# *Section* 8

# Extraocular Muscle Surgery

*Section Editors* Aparna Ramasubramanian, Deborah K Vanderveen

CHAPTER

# 100

# Principles of Strabismus Surgery

Aparna Ramasubramanian, Deborah K Vanderveen

## INTRODUCTION

This chapter discusses the general principles of strabismus surgery. The surgical anatomy is discussed in chapter 101 and the details of specific muscle surgery are discussed in later chapters.

## PREOPERATIVE EVALUATION

Preoperative planning should encompass an ophthalmologic evaluation including visual acuity, cycloplegic retinoscopy, anterior segment and fundus examination. Detailed strabismus evaluation is pivotal to surgical outcome but is beyond the scope of this book.

### Fusion and Stereopsis

Testing fixation behavior is the first step in evaluating binocular function. Fusion is graded as first degree—retinal correspondence; second degree—motor fusion; and third degree—stereopsis. Stereopsis is most commonly tested with the Titmus test but other tests include Lang test and Frisbie test. In patients with negative stereoacuity, Worth 4 dot test can be used to assess fusion and also to evaluate diplopia.

### Ductions and Versions

Duction refers to movement of each eye alone. Testing of ductions alone can be misleading to assess overactions and underactions and hence, comparison with the contralateral yoke is important which can be done with versions.

### Angle of Strabismus

It is very important to assess the angle of strabismus accurately and in most cases, at least two sets of measurements should be obtained prior to surgery. The methods to assess the angle of strabismus include cover-uncover test, alternate cover test, simultaneous cover test and Krimsky test. The measurements should be obtained at distance and near and also in the nine cardinal gazes. Hirschberg test is a crude way to test the amount of strabismus by looking at the light reflex but is useful to evaluate Angle Kappa. In cases of intermittent exotropia, a patch test can be performed to assess the total amount of deviation.

## ANESTHESIA FOR STRABISMUS SURGERY

### General Anesthesia

In children, general anesthesia is always the preferred choice. The risk of postoperative nausea and vomiting is high after strabismus surgery and hence, routine use of antiemetics is advised and it is preferable to avoid narcotics which increase nausea and vomiting.

### Local Anesthesia

Retrobulbar anesthesia or sub-Tenon anesthesia can be used for older cooperative patients. Retrobulbar anesthesia can successfully anesthetize the anterior orbit and the extraocular muscles but the area of ligament of Zinn is not completely anesthetized. Hence, with local anesthesia during a resection

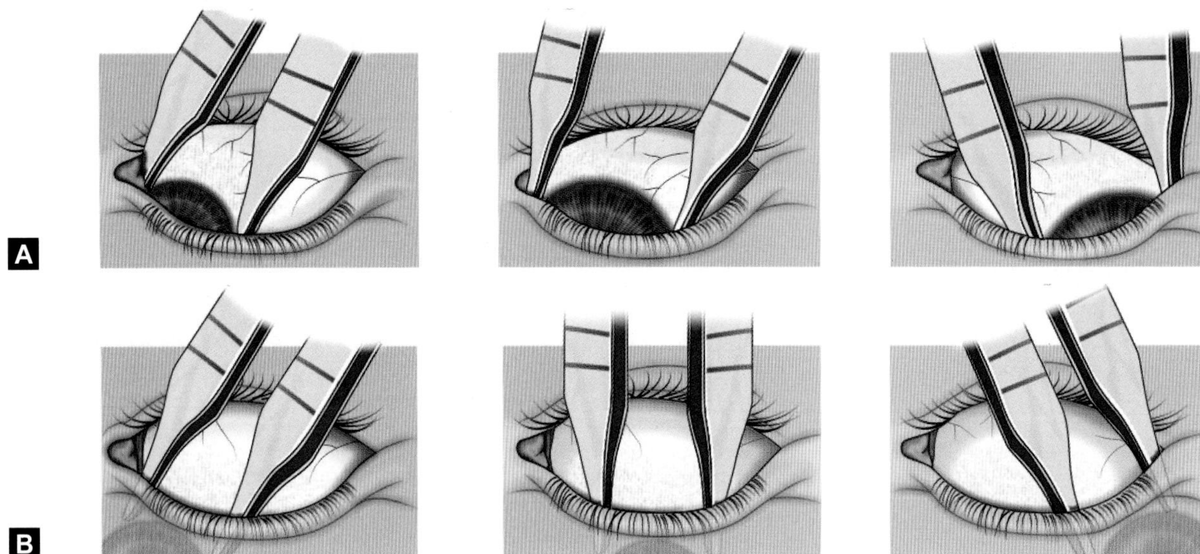


**Figures 100-1A and B** Superior oblique forced duction test (surgeon's view). (A) Superior oblique traction test in a normal eye showing the popping of the eye as it passes over the superior oblique tendon; (B) Traction test in a patient with a lax superior oblique tendon showing the eye sliding to the orbit.

procedure, the patient may still feel pain. For adjustable sutures, a sufficient amount of time needs to be given when local anesthesia is used for the muscles to regain their action. Adjustment after surgery should be performed after clinical assessment of full ductions.

### Topical Anesthesia

Topical anesthesia is rarely used for strabismus surgery but can be considered for a very cooperative patient. It allows for suture adjustment on the table.

## FORCED DUCTION TEST

Forced duction testing should be performed in all patients ideally after anesthesia, before surgery is started. It is especially important in restrictive strabismus.

### Rectus Muscle

The conjunctiva-episclera is grasped with a toothed forceps close to the limbus and the eye is proptosed. Alternately, two toothed forceps can be used to move the muscles medially, laterally, superiorly and inferiorly to rule out muscle restriction.

### Superior Oblique

Using toothed forceps, the eye is grabbed at 4 and 10 o'clock position for the right eye and 2 and 8 o'clock for the left eye. The eye is pushed down to the orbit and is adducted. The eye is then rotated temporally passing over the superior oblique tendon. In a normal eye, the eye pops up as it passes over the tendon, and this can be felt and seen and can be graded by surgeon experience. In the case of a lax tendon, the pop would not be felt and the eye will further slide back to the orbit (Figs. 100-1A and B).[1]

### Inferior Oblique

This test is useful to assess the completeness of inferior oblique weakening. Similar to the superior oblique test, the eye is grasped at the limbus, retropulsed and rotated nasally. The eye is then rotated temporally passing over the inferior oblique tendon and a pop is felt. If no pop is felt, the inferior oblique is sufficiently weakened (Figs. 100-2A and B).[1]

## INSTRUMENTS FOR STRABISMUS SURGERY

The surgeon should use his or her preferred instruments for strabismus surgery. A suggested typical set includes some combination of the following (Fig. 100-3):

- Surgeon's choice of lid speculum
- Steven's muscle hook
- Jameson/Green/Graefe muscle hook
- Desmarres retractor
- Bishop-Harmon dressing forceps—serrated
- Two Castroviejo fixation forceps

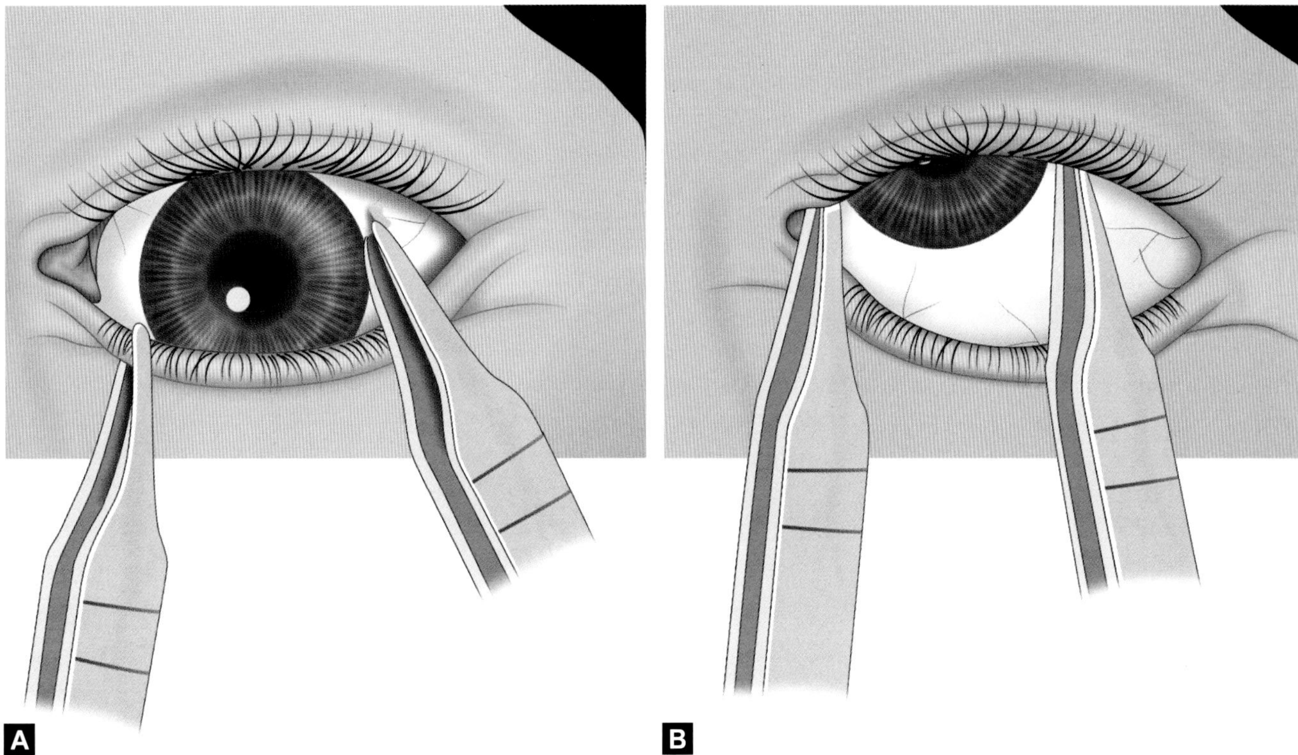


**Figures 100-2A and B** Inferior oblique forced duction test (surgeon's view). (A) The eye is grasped at the limbus; (B) The pop is felt as the eye passes over the inferior oblique tendon.

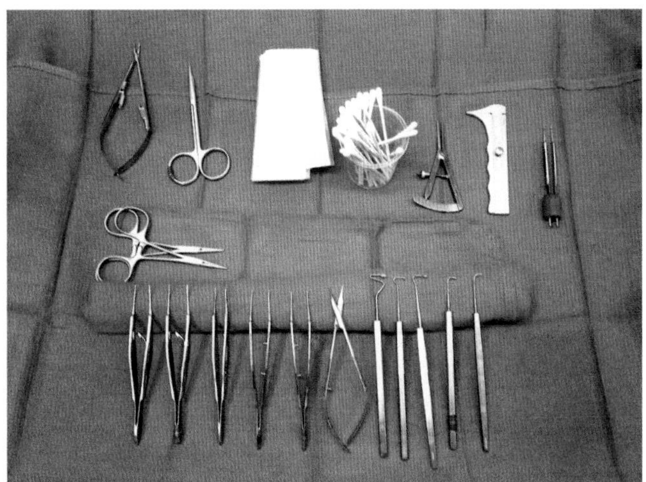

**Figure 100-3** Instruments commonly used for strabismus surgery.

- Castroviejo caliper—20 mm scale straight
- Stevens tenotomy scissors—standard blunt and straight
- Westcott tenotomy scissors—blunt, right
- Flexible stainless steel rule
- Castroviejo needle holders
- Serrefine—straight, large or small
- Halstead mosquito forceps.

Different kinds of muscle hooks are available to modify the surgical technique. Guyton devised an "S"-shaped hook that can be used with the fornix incision to keep the incision small.[2] In cases of restrictive strabismus where the risk of scleral perforation is high, a grooved muscle hook can be used.[3]

For the measurement of the amount of surgery, either regular calipers can be used or curved rulers can be used in which case the measurement can be taken from the limbus. Curved rulers are especially of benefit in large recessions or for Fadenoperation.[4]

*Magnification*: Operating microscope is rarely used for strabismus surgery, and most commonly surgical loupes are used. Most commonly used loupes have a magnification of 2.5 as higher magnification decreases the operative field of vision and depth perception.

## SUTURES AND NEEDLES FOR STRABISMUS SURGERY

### Suture

Synthetic absorbable suture is most commonly used for muscle anchoring. The most commonly used suture is

Vicryl™ (polyglactin 910). The braided suture is 50% absorbed by 3 weeks and completely absorbed in 56–70 days. The suture provides good tensile support till the muscle adheres to the sclera and incites minimal tissue reaction. For muscle suturing, usually 6-0 vicryl is used and for conjunctival closure, 8-0 vicryl is utilized. The main drawback of this suture is that because it is braided tissue, especially the Tenon's tissue can get engaged in the suture material.

Nonabsorbable suture such as 5-0 or 6-0 dacron or mersilene are used for superior oblique tuck, Fadenoperation and transposition surgeries. Mersilene™ polyester fiber suture is a nonabsorbable, braided suture composed of poly(ethylene terephthalate), and dacron is a polymer of ethylene glycol and terephthalic acid.

Black silk suture either 5-0 or 6-0 is used for traction during the surgical procedure.

### Needles

The kind of needle used is based on surgeon preference, the characteristics of the eye and the availability of the needle on the required suture material. For scleral passes, either a spatulated or side-cutting needle is preferred. A vertically cutting needle will either cause deep pass (if cutting down) or will cheese wire (if cutting up). A study was conducted to determine the ultrasound biomicroscopy profile of scleral tunnels created with needles commonly used during strabismus surgery, namely S14, S24, S28 and TG100.[5] Needle design had a definite impact on the characteristics of scleral tunnels, but the differences were not such as to predicate for or against the general use of any of these four needles for strabismus surgery.[5]

## INCISION

Conjunctival incisions should provide adequate exposure of extraocular muscles but at the same time produce minimal scarring. All incisions have to go through conjunctiva and Tenon's capsule to get to bare sclera. Mikhail et al. surveyed American Association for Pediatric Ophthalmology and Strabismus (AAPOS) members regarding preference for strabismus incisions and reported that limbal incisions were preferred for greater intraoperative exposure and better teaching of junior surgeons.[6] Fornix incisions on the other hand caused less postoperative pain and inflammation and led to more rapid soft tissue healing.[6]

### Limbal Incisions

Limbal incision provides good exposure of all the rectus muscles and is easy to perform for beginners. The disadvantage is that it requires careful closure, since the conjunctiva is disrupted near the limbus and can cause visible scarring. The risks of corneal dellen are also more common with the limbal incision. Some surgeons prefer to use the limbal incision for reoperations.

### Fornix Incisions

It was devised by Marshall Parks and is the most commonly performed incision for primary strabismus surgery. The advantage is that the incision is hidden causing minimal visible scarring. It is also postulated that forniceal incisions have a lower occurrence of anterior segment ischemia. The incision need not be sutured and the overall patient comfort is better with the fornix incision.

## SECURING MUSCLE

Appropriate muscle suturing is critical to the success of strabismus surgery and to avoid slipped and lost muscles. The authors' technique is described below though there can be many modifications to the technique (all surgeons employ the locking bites on the edge). With gentle traction on the muscle insertion with the Jameson hook, a double-armed synthetic absorbable suture (6-0 vicryl) on a fine spatulated needle is woven through the tendon 1 mm from its insertion to make a central full-thickness bite including the central one-third of the muscle. This is followed by weaving of the suture through partial thickness of the muscle from the center exiting at the edge of the muscle. The locking bite is then made by passing the suture full thickness backwards from the edge of the muscle (Fig. 100-4A). It is important to engage the deeper muscle tissues also to make a full-thickness locking bite (Fig. 100-4B). It is advised to take only approximately 2 mm of the edge of the muscle in the locking bite. Making a larger pass during the locking bite would cause the tendon width to narrow. Some surgeons use a double-locking bite but in most cases that is not required.

## SCLERAL PASS

Scleral passes can be made directly at the point of recession or muscle can be allowed to hang-back by attaching the muscle to the original insertion. Scleral pass should be at least 1.5 mm or longer and at least 0.2 mm in depth to be stable and effective. The distance between the two points of scleral entrance should optimally be at least 10 mm to ensure adequate spacing of the muscle, and both points of entrance must be parallel to the limbus. Some surgeons prefer to use a cross-swords technique. The needles should be advanced in the direction of the

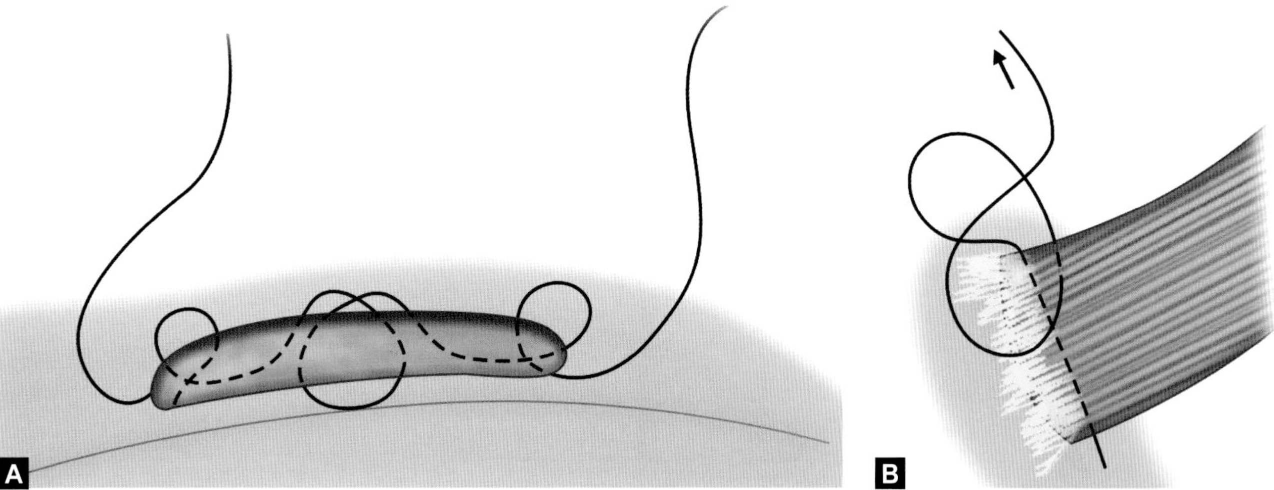


**Figures 100-4A and B** Diagram representing securing of the rectus muscle (A). Locking bite for securing the muscle (B).

movement and should not be forced through the tissues. It is important to view the needle as it passes intrasclerally as this ensures that the pass is not deep. Bigger needles such as the S14 needle lead to deeper passes as the needle can be easily visualized even when it is deep in the sclera. The author's preference is to use S28, S29 or RD-1 needles. The suture is then tied with a surgeon's knot with at least three throws.

## MECHANISM OF ACTION OF STRABISMUS SURGERY

The mechanism of action of extraocular muscles and the effect of surgery on these muscles is not well understood. It has been thought that the mechanism of action of strabismus surgery follows the Starling's law. Recession of a muscle shifts the muscle length to point where the elastic and contractile forces are reduced. Similarly, resection of a muscle increases both the elastic and contractile force.[7] This simplistic explanation of mechanism of surgery is questionable as with the correction of strabismus, the rotation of the eye changes and this in turn modifies the force-length relationship. This phenomenon is known as induced advancement.[8] A newer concept evaluated the role of pulleys in muscle recession. This newer theory postulates that as the rectus muscles are anchored to orbital pulleys, recession changes the force vector.[8]

The amount of surgery and the surgical result are variable dependent on multiple of partially understood factors. Some of the surgical factors include amount of stretching of the muscle during surgery; intraoperative bleeding; muscle suturing; muscle adhesion to sclera; separation of check ligaments etc. The healing process also influences the final outcome including amount of scarring, adhesions and conjunctival elasticity. Hence, the surgical normograms are only a guideline and need to be modified based on patient characteristics and surgeon's technique.

## REFERENCES

1. Guyton DL. Exaggerated traction test for the oblique muscles. Ophthalmology. 1981;88(10):1035-40.
2. Guyton DL. A small-incision muscle hook for the Parks cul-de-sac approach for strabismus surgery. Binocul Vis Strabismus Q. 2005;20(3):147-50.
3. Wright KW. Color Atlas of Strabismus Surgery: Strategies and Techniques. New York: Springer; 2007. p. 110.
4. Scott WE, Martin-Casal A, Braverman DE. Curved ruler for measurement along the surface of the globe. Arch Ophthalmol. 1978;96(6):1084.
5. Hussein MA, Coats DK, Harris LD, et al. Ultrasound biomicroscopy (UBM) characteristics of scleral tunnels created with suture needles commonly used during strabismus surgery. Binocul Vis Strabismus Q. 2007;22(2):102-8.
6. Mikhail M, Verran R, Farrokhyar F, et al. Choice of conjunctival incisions for horizontal rectus muscle surgery-a survey of American Association for Pediatric Ophthalmology and Strabismus members. J AAPOS. 2013;17(2):184-7.
7. Porter JD, Baker RS, Ragusa RJ, et al. Extraocular muscles: basic and clinical aspects of structure and function. Surv Ophthalmol. 1995;39(6):451-84.
8. Kushner BJ. Perspective on strabismus, 2006. Arch Ophthalmol. 2006;124(9):1321-6.

CHAPTER

# 101

# Anatomical Considerations

Steven J Ryder, Richard L Levy

## INTRODUCTION

Successful strabismus surgery requires a keen understanding of orbital anatomy. Within the tight, closed space of the orbit, the extraocular muscles are surrounded by a network of connective tissues, nerves, vasculature, and fat. The surgeon should always have these relationships in mind when isolating and moving the extraocular muscles.

The position of the eyes is determined by the orbital walls, the distribution and tension of the six oculorotary muscles, the musculofibroelastic suspensory network, and the surrounding fat. The orbits are oriented at a 45° angle, such that without any muscle tension, the eyes would lie in an abducted position. Under normal waking conditions the medial recti tonically pull the eyes into primary position so that the visual axis is parallel with the sagittal plane and 23° away from the orbital axis (Fig. 101-1). Under general anesthesia, when the tonic convergence force of the medial recti is suspended, the eyes will often drift back into a mild abduction.

Even before the first incision, the surgeon examines the position of the eyes and the tone of the extraocular muscles. Abnormal eye position under anesthesia may demonstrate chronic changes in extraocular muscle length or tone that correlate to clinical findings and help guide choice of procedure.

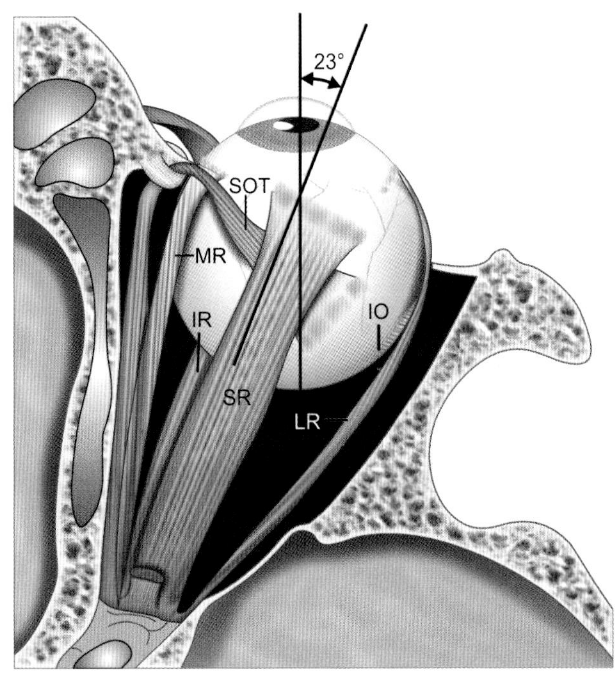


**Figure 101-1** The axis of the muscle cone is rotated 23 outward from the optical axis.
(MR: Medial rectus; SR: Superior rectus; LR: Lateral rectus; IR: Inferior rectus; SO: Superior oblique muscle; SOT: Superior oblique tendon; IO: Inferior oblique).

## SURGICAL ANATOMY

### Conjunctiva

The conjunctiva is the elastic, clear mucous membrane lining the anterior surface of the globe and reflecting onto the eyelids. In adults, conjunctiva, Tenon's capsule, and sclera form a fused structure extending 2 mm posterior to the limbus. This number is slightly smaller in children. Under normal conditions, there are no other connections between conjunctiva and the underlying structures of the globe, until more posteriorly where it fuses to forniceal and eyelid structures. It is for this reason that strabismus surgery may be carried out through small, buttonhole incisions in the conjunctiva that may be stretched and manipulated to provide exposure. In older patients, the conjunctiva is more friable and may easily

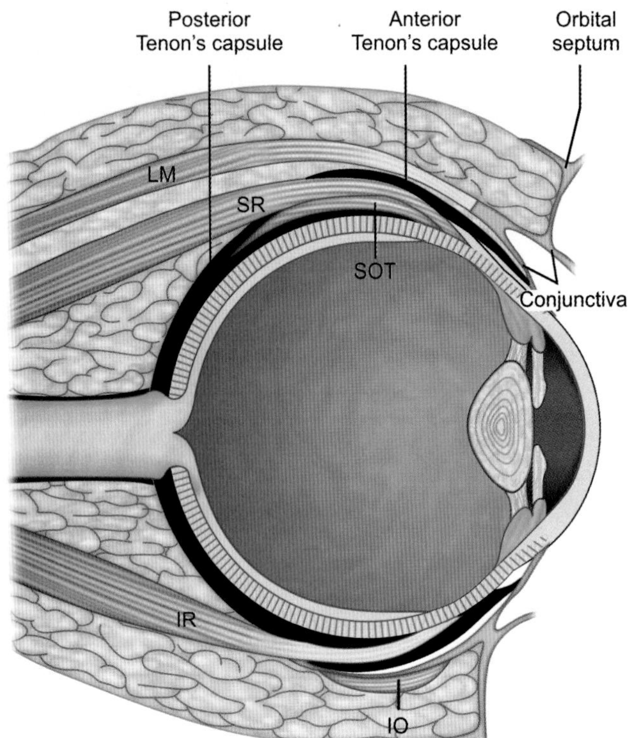


**Figure 101-2** The extraocular muscles divide anterior and posterior Tenon's capsule.
(SR: Superior rectus; IR: Inferior rectus; SOT: Superior oblique tendon; IO: Inferior oblique; LM: Levator muscle).

tear under the forces required for smaller incision strabismus surgery. Similarly, where there is scarring from prior surgery, attention must be paid to dissect conjunctiva into freely mobile flaps, thereby gaining exposure and avoiding propagating incisions.

## Tenon's Capsule and Intermuscular Septum

Tenon's capsule, or fascia bulba, is a dense, white, connective tissue membrane that envelops the eye, extending from the limbus and fusing posteriorly to the optic nerve. It becomes thinner and more translucent as we age. The extraocular muscles penetrate Tenon's capsule just anterior to the equator of the eye, dividing it into anterior and posterior segments (Fig. 101-2). Tenon's capsule is readily distinguished from conjunctiva due to its location and appearance. If there is doubt, it readily hydrates when irrigated into a fluffy, white protrusion through the incision (Figs. 101-3A to C).

Posterior Tenon's capsule separates the globe and extraocular muscles from adipose tissue within the orbit. Fat adherence syndrome, a feared complication of extraocular muscle surgery, is a progressive restrictive strabismus due to intrusion of extraconal fat after damage to posterior Tenon's capsule, with adherence to the sclera. Once created, fat adherence syndrome carries a grim prognosis for re-establishing normal ocular motility. It is therefore important, when operating posterior to the muscle insertions, to dissect close to the globe and muscles to avoid encountering fat.

The intermuscular septum, a thin fascial plane, connects the rectus muscles from the point at which they pierce Tenon's capsule and fuses with Tenon's capsule anteriorly (Figs. 101-4A and B).

## Sclera

The thickness of the sclera varies according to location (Fig. 101-5). At the limbus, the sclera is 0.8-mm thick. Anterior to the rectus muscle insertions, it is 0.6-mm thick. Posterior to the rectus muscle insertions, it is 0.3-mm thick. At the equator, it is 0.5- to 0.8-mm thick. At the posterior pole, it is > 1-mm thick. The area of greatest surgical activity for the extraocular muscle surgeon coincides with the thinnest area of the sclera.

## Rectus Muscles

The four rectus muscles originate at the orbital apex at the annulus of Zinn and course anteriorly to insert on the anterior aspect of the globe. The rectus muscle insertions form an imaginary structure termed the spiral of Tillaux around the limbus. The medial rectus insertion is the nearest to the limbus, and the insertions then spiral posteriorly in the direction of incyclotorsion (Fig. 101-6).

The medial rectus is the primary adductor of the eye, forming a 6- to 7-mm arc of contact with the globe. Its tendon is the shortest of the recti at 4.5 mm. The lateral rectus is the primary abductor, inserting onto the globe with a 10- to 12-mm arc of contact. In contrast with the medial rectus, the tendon of the lateral rectus is the longest of the recti at 7–8 mm. In primary gaze, these muscles each provide only a single, horizontal action. However, when the eye is in elevation or depression, the tendon of the muscle rotates superiorly or inferiorly, thereby creating a secondary, vertical force. Surgery that offsets the horizontal recti takes advantage of this principle to correct small vertical deviations.

The inferior rectus functions primarily as a depressor, but also as an excyclotorter and adductor. When the eye is rotated 23° into abduction, the tendon is aligned with the axis of the muscle cone and the muscle becomes a pure depressor. The inferior rectus and oblique muscles are intimately connected with inferior forniceal and eyelid structures. Attachments between the inferior rectus muscle and the lower eyelid retractors can be identified as white bands on the orbital surface of the muscle about 5 mm posterior to its insertion (Fig. 101-7). These bands are continuous with the

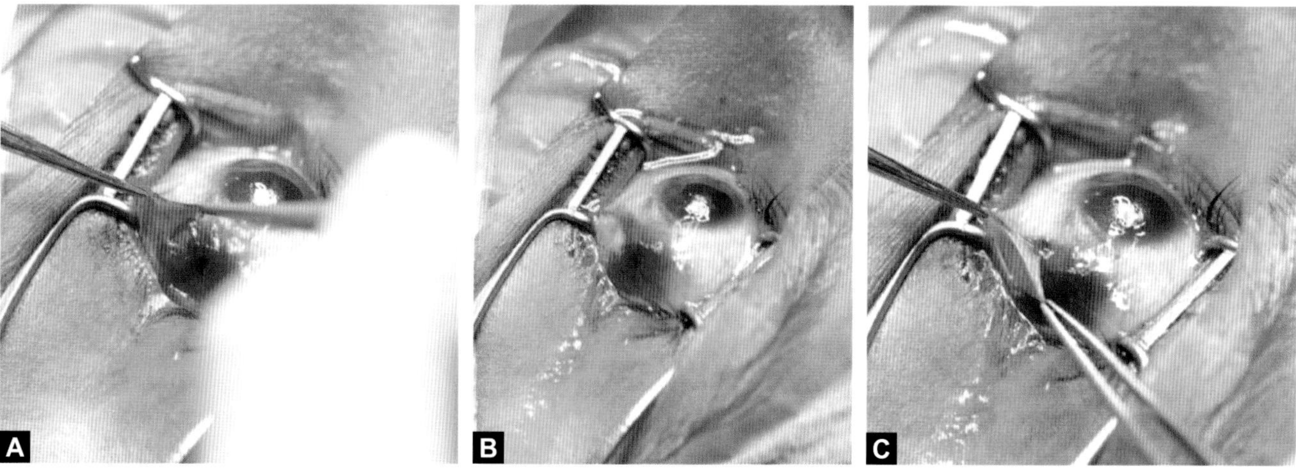

**Figures 101-3A to C** (A) Tenon's pulled from under a conjunctival flap. The two layers appear similar. (B) When hydrated, Tenon's becomes fluffy and white, easily differentiating it from the surrounding conjunctival incision. (C) The same hydrated Tenon's flap again pulled from underneath the conjunctiva.

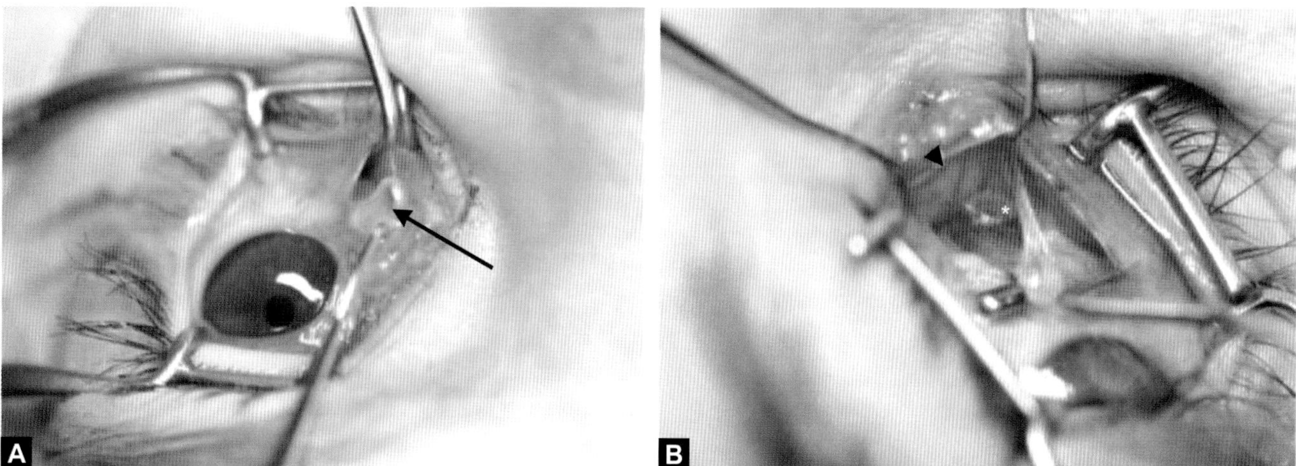

**Figures 101-4A and B** (A) A thin intermuscular septum, shown here tented up on a Guyton muscle hook. (B) After isolating the right medial rectus, a check ligament (asterisk) appears. Posterior Tenon's (arrowhead) is visible on nasal exposure.

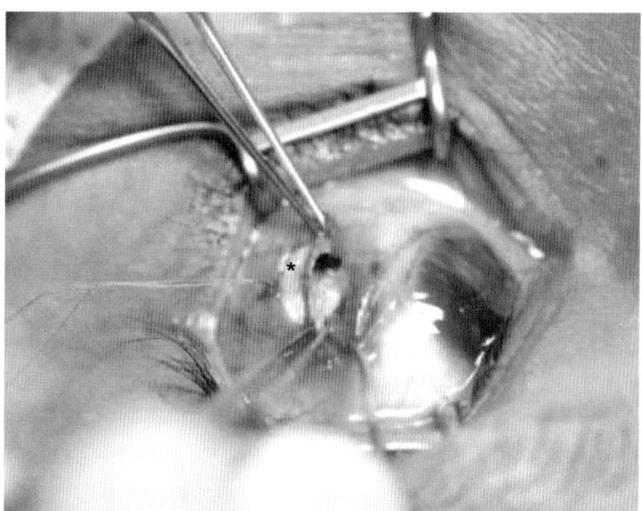

**Figure 101-5** The sclera varies in thickness according to location. Shown here a rectus muscle has been secured on a suture and disinserted from the sclera. The muscle is retracted into the orbit, with the sutures protruding from the conjunctival incision. The midpoint of the muscle insertion has been marked with a marking pen. Forceps are used to grasp the insertion, demonstrating a shelf created in the sclera in the prior position of the muscle, with very thin sclera posterior to the insertion (asterisk).

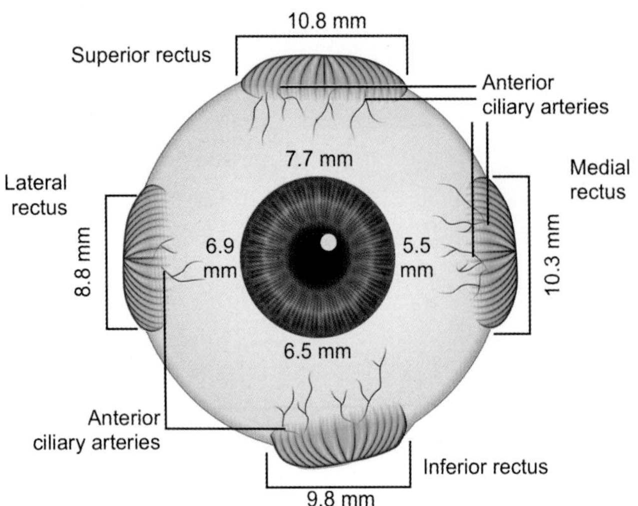


**Figure 101-6** The spiral of Tillaux and the width of the rectus muscle insertions.

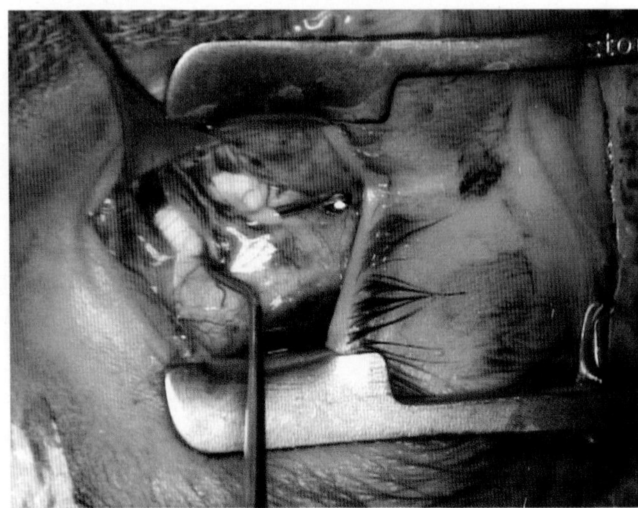

**Figure 101-7** Surgeon's view. Connections to the eyelid retractors are seen on the orbital surface of the inferior rectus muscle, deep within the conjunctival incision.
*Courtesy*: Dr Ankoor Shah.

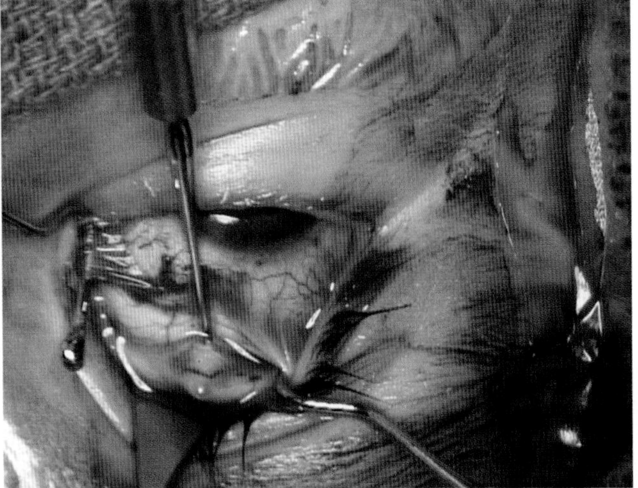

**Figure 101-8** Surgeon's view. When isolated between the medial and superior recti, the superior oblique tendon appears as a white cord within its sheath.
*Courtesy*: Dr Ankoor Shah.

capsulopalpebral fascia, which envelops the inferior oblique muscle and then coalesces anteriorly to form Lockwood's ligament. Via the inferior tarsal muscle, these structures contribute to lower eyelid positioning. When operating on the inferior rectus, it is therefore important to lyse connections to the eyelid retractors. In some settings, such as in thyroid eye disease, lower eyelid repositioning can still occur even after the most thorough dissection.

The superior rectus is primarily an elevator, but it also performs incyclotorsion and adduction. Similar to the inferior rectus, the superior rectus is a pure elevator when the eye is abducted 23°. Also similar to the inferior rectus, fascial attachments connect the superior rectus and the levator aponeurosis and superior tarsus, and it is important to dissect these connections carefully with large recessions and resections of the muscle to avoid upper eyelid repositioning.

## Superior Oblique Muscle

The superior oblique muscle arises from the orbital apex above the annulus of Zinn and passes anteriorly and upward along the superomedial wall of the orbit. The muscle itself is not encountered during traditional strabismus surgery. The muscle becomes tendinous before journeying through the trochlea, then redirects inferiorly, posteriorly, and laterally. The trochlea acts as its functional origin. The tendon of the superior oblique penetrates Tenon's capsule 2 mm nasally and 5 mm posteriorly to the nasal insertion of the superior rectus muscle. It passes under the superior rectus muscle to insert in the posterosuperior quadrant of the globe. When isolated from a superonasal approach, the superior oblique muscle is a cord that may be seen or palpated as a "bump" as it dives under the superior rectus (Fig. 101-8). As it passes underneath the superior rectus, the superior oblique tendon fans out into a 7- to 18-mm array of translucent white fibers that can be difficult to distinguish from the globe and surrounding connective tissue (Fig. 101-9).

The anterior fibers of the tendon provide the primary action of incyclotorsion, whereas the posterior fibers serve the secondary and tertiary actions of depression and abduction. Procedures such as the Harada–Ito procedure are performed on only part of the tendon to take advantage of this specialization.

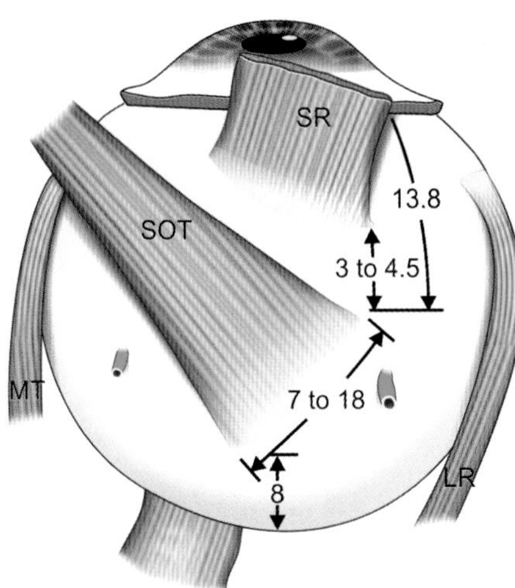


Figure 101-9 Relationships of the superior oblique tendon. Measurements are in millimeters. The superior rectus muscle (SR) is cut and reflected. The vortex veins lie on either side of the tendon insertion.
(SOT: Superior oblique tendon; MR: Medial rectus; LR: Lateral rectus).

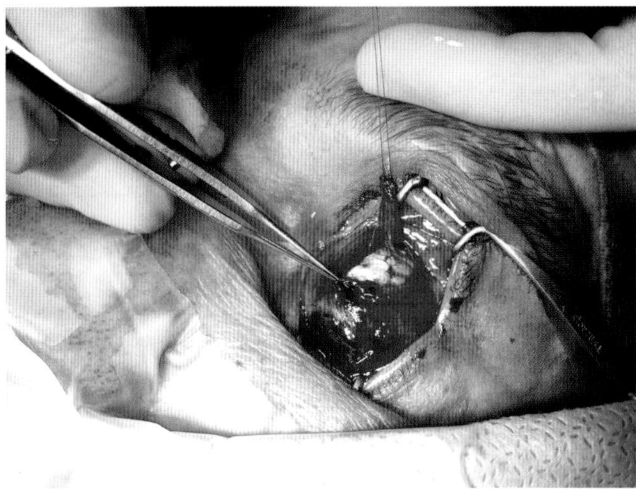

Figure 101-10 The superior rectus muscle is detached and reflected to reveal the frenulum connecting it to the superior oblique tendon sheath. The superior oblique tendon is discernable as white fibers running parallel to the limbus.

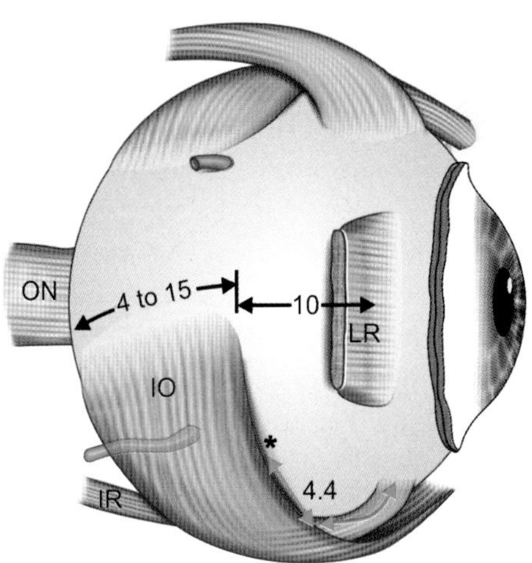


Figure 101-11 Course of the inferior oblique muscle. The lateral rectus muscle has been cut. Fink's point is shown with an asterisk.

The superior oblique tendon is connected to the superior rectus muscle via a fibrous band sometimes called the frenulum (Fig. 101-10). With small superior rectus recessions, the superior oblique fibers will bow posteriorly via the frenulum, without affecting the action of either muscle. For large recessions, however, it may be necessary to lyse the frenulum to avoid tethering the superior rectus anterior to its desired location. In general, when operating on the superior rectus muscle, the surgeon should be cognizant of the location of the superior oblique and keep instruments relatively anterior and away from it, to avoid accidental lysing its fibers or incarceration them into a suture.

## Inferior Oblique Muscle

The inferior oblique originates from the periosteum of the maxillary bone, just posterior to the orbital rim and lateral to the orifice of the lacrimal fossa. It passes laterally, superiorly, and posteriorly, going inferior to the inferior rectus muscle and inserting under the lateral rectus muscle in the posterolateral portion of the globe. There is virtually no tendinous component – some argue <1 mm – only muscle. The width of the insertion is about 9 mm, but it may range from 4 mm to 15 mm, and the posterior aspect overlies the macula (Fig. 101-11).

A shared fibroneurovascular bundle between inferior rectus and inferior oblique enters the oblique as it passes beneath the nasal border of the inferior rectus. This bundle is important for several reasons. First, it innervates the pupillary sphincter and ciliary body, and large resections of the oblique may create a permanent mydriasis. This complication can be avoided by observing the pupil after clamping the muscle, and repositioning as needed. Second, if the inferior oblique is anteriorized, the fibrovascular bundle becomes the effective origin of the muscle. A large anteriorization will therefore create a "J-deformity", greatly changing the action of the muscle and even restricting elevation. Third, this shared connective tissue limits the amount of recession of the inferior oblique via a temporal approach; when the muscle is transected during a myectomy, the proximal end will likely reattach to the globe near the lateral border of the inferior rectus, creating effectively a 13-mm recession. Eliminating all action of the inferior oblique muscle therefore requires extirpating it via a nasal approach.

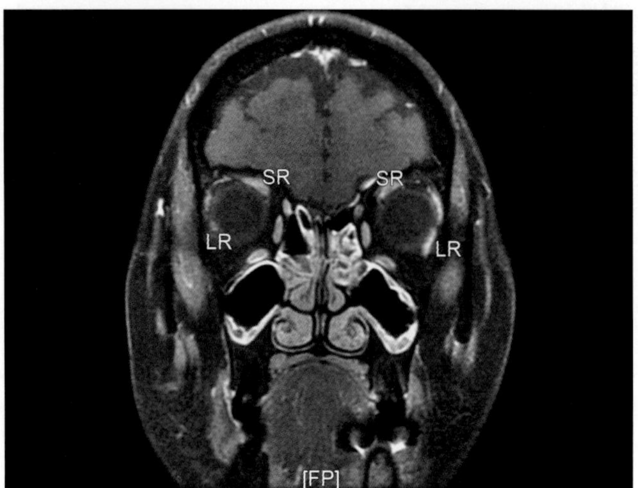


Figure 101-12 Coronal magnetic resonance image of the orbits, in a patient with esotropia and high myopia. The lateral rectus (LR) and superior rectus (SR) muscle bellies are displaced inferiorly and nasally.

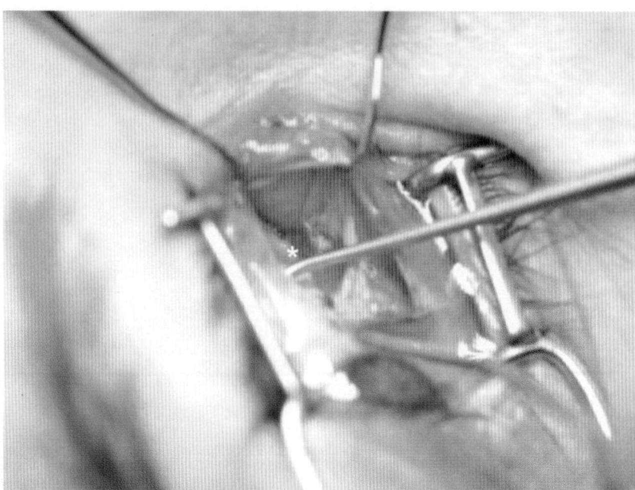


Figure 101-13 The fibromuscular sleeve (or "pulley") associated with the medial rectus muscle. The eye is rotated medially using a hook underneath the medial rectus muscle, and conjunctiva and Tenon's capsule are retracted with hooks to reveal the muscle and check ligaments. At the superior border of the muscle belly, the pulley is seen as a thick white band of connective tissue (asterisk).

In general, the lateral border of inferior rectus serves as a reference for repositioning the inferior oblique. Cadaver studies demonstrate that the inferior oblique passes under the inferior rectus about 4 mm posterior its insertion. The point 4.0 mm posterior and 4.4 mm lateral to the lateral border of the inferior rectus insertion is called Fink's point, which estimates an 8.0-mm recession of the muscle along its normal course (Fig. 101-11). Other desired amounts of recession can be obtained by using these landmarks as a guide; placement of the inferior oblique closer to the inferior rectus insertion, therefore, creates an anteriorization.

It is also important to realize that the inferior oblique insertion is 2 mm superior to the inferior border of the lateral rectus. Aggressive posterior manipulations during lateral rectus surgery may, therefore, inadvertently involve the inferior oblique.

## PULLEY SYSTEM

The globe is suspended in a thick and complex musculofibroelastic network that serves to maintain the position of the extraocular muscles relative to the orbit and stabilize the muscle paths. Specific structures within this network, now referred to as pulleys, consist of a continuous sleeve that surrounds the horizontal recti about 6 mm posterior to their insertions. Our understanding of these pulleys is evolving. Pulleys are theorized to serve as functional origins of the muscle tendons, and adjustments of the position and tension of the pulleys may play a significant role in extraocular function.

Defects in the pulleys may be the etiology of some forms of strabismus. For example, heterotopy of the rectus muscle pulleys may cause incomitant strabismus and mimic oblique muscle dysfunction. Changes with age and pathology such as axial elongation of the globes also affect the pulley system. In axial high myopia, the connective tissue between the superior and lateral recti may become lax, allowing the posterior globe to prolapse out of the muscle cone and create a strabismus fixus. The abnormal course of the rectus muscles can be seen on magnetic resonance imaging (Fig. 101-12).

During surgery, pulleys may be visualized as thick bands associated with posterior Tenon's capsule extending to either side of the rectus muscles (Fig. 101-13).

Surgery just on the pulleys themselves, rather than on the muscles directly, is being investigated.

## EXTRAOCULAR MUSCLE MICROANATOMY

Histologically, extraocular muscles are voluntary, striated muscle and should thus be categorized as skeletal muscle. However, they are innervated at a ratio of nerve fiber to muscle fiber up to 10 times that of skeletal muscle, allowing for finely controlled, highly accurate eye movements.

Oculorotatory muscles consist of two distinct layers, the inner, or deeper, global layer and the outer, or more superficial, orbital layer. The tendon of the global layer inserts on the sclera to move the globe. The orbital layer acts on the

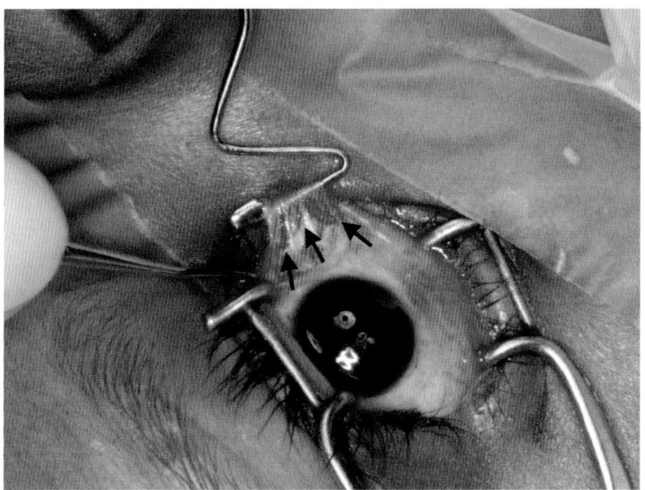

Figure 101-14 Prominent ciliary vessels (arrows) on the surface of the medial rectus muscle.

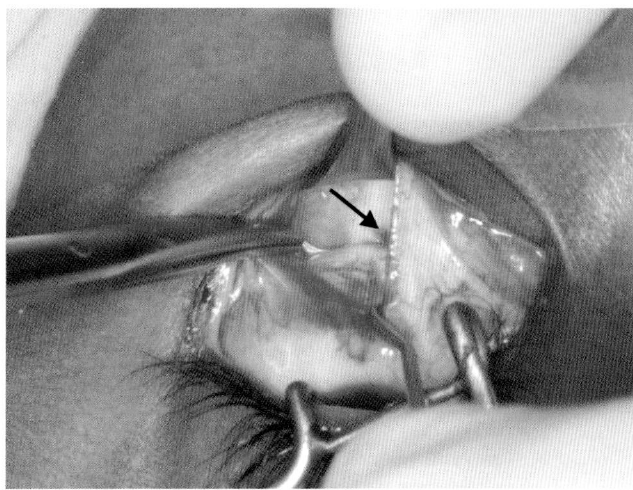

Figure 101-15 In the surgeon's view, an inferior vertex vein (arrow) is visualized in the relatively avascular white septum between the inferior oblique muscle to the left and the inferior rectus. The inferior rectus is retracted by a muscle hook and hidden underneath the conjunctival flap to the right.

aforementioned connective tissue pulleys to maintain ocular position and relative tension within the orbit.

The extraocular muscle fibers are divided based on pattern of innervation and mitochondrial content. The orbital layer is generally considered to have a large majority (80%) of singly innervated fibers (SIFs) and a smaller set of multiply innervated fibers (MIFs). The orbital SIFs are considered the major contributor to sustained extraocular muscle force. The other 20% are composed of MIFs, which demonstrate slower contraction. The larger percentages (90%) of muscle fibers comprising the global layer are SIFs. Over one third of fibers in the global layer are termed red SIFs due to high mitochondrial content. These fibers are considered fast twitch and fatigue resistant. Intermediate SIFs comprise one quarter of fibers in the global layer. Lastly, pale, or white, SIFs constitute about another one quarter of the global layer and exhibit low fatigue resistance. The remaining 10% is composed of global MIFs, exhibiting a slow-graded, nonpropagated response following activation. Clinically speaking, SIFs are most affected by denervation to motor nerves and motor end plates, as is the case with injection of botulinum toxin.

## VASCULAR SUPPLY TO THE EXTRAOCULAR MUSCLES

The muscular branches of the ophthalmic artery provide the most important blood supply for the extraocular muscles. The lateral muscular branch supplies the lateral rectus, superior rectus, superior oblique, and levator palpebrae superioris muscles. The lateral rectus is partially supplied by the lacrimal artery. The medial muscular branch, the larger of the two, supplies the inferior rectus, medial rectus, and inferior oblique muscles. The inferior oblique and inferior rectus muscles are partially supplied by the infraorbital artery. The muscular branches give rise to the anterior ciliary arteries accompanying the rectus muscles; each rectus muscle has 1–3 anterior ciliary arteries (Fig. 101-14). Operating on three or more extraocular muscles may, therefore, lead to anterior segment ischemia.

Generally, four vortex veins are located posterior to the equator (Fig. 101-15). They are usually found near the nasal and temporal margins of the superior rectus and inferior rectus muscles.

## GROWTH CONSIDERATIONS

The rectus muscles in infants are slightly smaller than those of adults but grow rapidly before reaching adult dimensions at 20 months of age. On average, the rectus muscle insertions in neonates are approximately 2.5–3.0 mm narrower than those in adults. At birth, the insertion–limbal distance of the rectus muscles is roughly 2 mm less than that in adults (Table 101-1). That disparity is cut in half by 9 months. At 20 months of age, the adult dimensions may be used as estimates.

The positioning of the oblique insertions in neonates is considerably different than in older children and adults. For one, the insertions are closer together, starting near the horizontal meridian and the posterior pole. The posterior

**TABLE 101-1** Comparative measurements of the medial and lateral rectus muscles in adults and newborns. Measurements are in millimeters

| | MR (adult) | MR (newborn) | LR (adult) | LR (newborn) |
|---|---|---|---|---|
| Length | 37.7 | 28 | 36.3 | 31.6 |
| Width | 10.4 | 7.9 | 9.6 | 6.9 |
| Distance from limbus (middle of insertion) | 5.7 | 3.9 | 7.5 | 4.8 |

edge of the insertion of the inferior oblique begins within 1 mm of the optic nerve and migrates temporally toward the macula, its adult residence.

## SUGGESTED READING

1. Apt L, Call NB. An anatomical reevaluation of rectus muscle insertions. Ophthalmic Surg. 1982;13(2):108-12.
2. Apt L, Call NB. Inferior oblique muscle recession. Am J Ophthalmol. 1978;85:95-100.
3. Christensen LE, Wright KW. Surgical anatomy. In: Wright KW (ed.), Color atlas of ophthalmic surgery. Philadelphia, PA: Lippincott, 1991.
4. Clark RA, Ariyasu R, Demer JL. Medial rectus pulley posterior fixation is as effective as scleral posterior fixation for acquired esotropia with a high AC/A ratio. Am J Ophthalmol. 2004;137(6):1026-33.
5. Demer JL, Clark RA, Miller JM. Heterotopy of extraocular muscle pulleys causes incomitant strabismus. In: Lennerstrand G (ed.), Advances in strabismology. Buren (Netherlands): Aeolus Press, 1999:91-4.
6. Fink WH. Surgery of the vertical muscles of the eyes, 2nd edn. Springfield, IL: Charles C Thomas, 1962.
7. Guyton DL. Exaggerated traction test for the oblique muscles. Ophthalmology. 1981;88(10):1035-40.
8. Helveston, EM. Surgical management of strabismus: a practical and updated approach, 5th edn. Wayenborgh Publishing, Oostende, Belgium 2005; Ch2: Lecture 1-22.
9. Last RJ. Wolff's anatomy of the eye and orbit, 6 edn. Philadelphia, PA: HK Lewis & Co, 1968.
10. Mims J, Wood RC. Bilateral anterior transposition of the inferior obliques. Arch Ophthalmol. 1989;107:41-4.
11. Swan KC, Wilkins JH. Extraocular muscle surgery in early infancy–anatomical factors. J Pediatr Ophthalmol Strabismus. 1984;21:44-9.
12. Taylor D, Hoyt C. Peditaric ophthalmology and strabismus. 3rd edn. Edinburgh, UK: Elsevier Saunders, 2005:200-12.
13. von Noorden GK. Campos EC. Binocular vision and ocular motility: theory and management of strabismus, 6th edn. St Louis, MO: Mosby–Year Book, 2002:38-49.
14. Wright KW, Strube YNJ. Pediatric ophthalmology and strabismus. 3rd edn. New York: Oxford University Press, 2012:86-98.
15. Yanoff M, Duker JS. Ophthalmology. 3rd edn. St Louis, MO: Mosby. 2009.

CHAPTER

102

# Rectus Muscle Recession

Marielle P Young

## INTRODUCTION

Rectus muscle recession involves weakening the muscle by disinserting it from the globe and replacing it more posteriorly. Rectus muscle recession is often preferred over resection because it is a reversible procedure that is better tolerated in the immediate postoperative period. Access to the muscle can be attained through a fornix or limbal conjunctival incision.

## INCISION

### Fornix Incision

The fornix incision has the advantage of being partially or completely hidden behind the eyelids. It is initiated in the bulbar conjunctiva 2–3 mm posterior to the limbus midway between rectus muscles and extended posteriorly 5–6 mm (Fig. 102-1). The conjunctival incision can alternatively be made 1 or 2 mm to the bulbar side of the cul-de-sac and extended in an arc on a course parallel to the cul-de-sac.[1] The medial and lateral rectus muscles are usually accessed from an inferior approach. After incising the conjunctiva, an additional cut through Tenon's capsule is necessary to expose bare sclera. Spreading Westcott scissors posteriorly in the same quadrant opens the pocket to allow for visualization and dissection. The muscle is engaged using a series of muscle hooks (i.e. starting with a small Stevens and progressing to a Jameson, Guyton or Green hook) that hug the sclera as they sweep posteriorly around the muscle (Fig. 102-2). The conjunctiva is stretched over the end of the hook that has traveled across the length of the muscle insertion. The intermuscular septum on the superior edge of the muscle is incised just under the tip of the hook and the hook visualized.

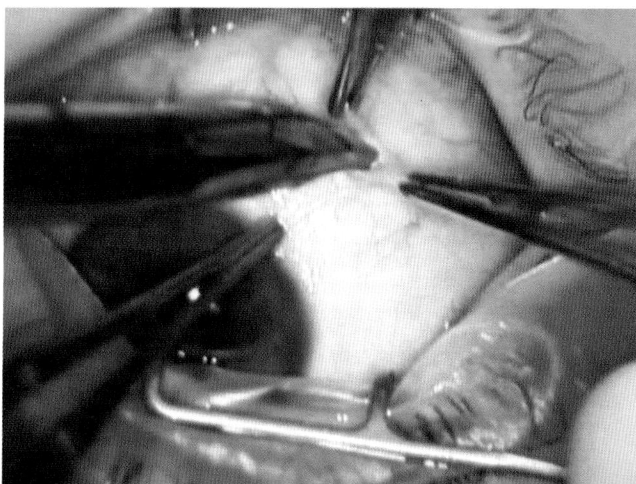

**Figure 102-1** Inferotemporal fornix incision for lateral rectus recession.

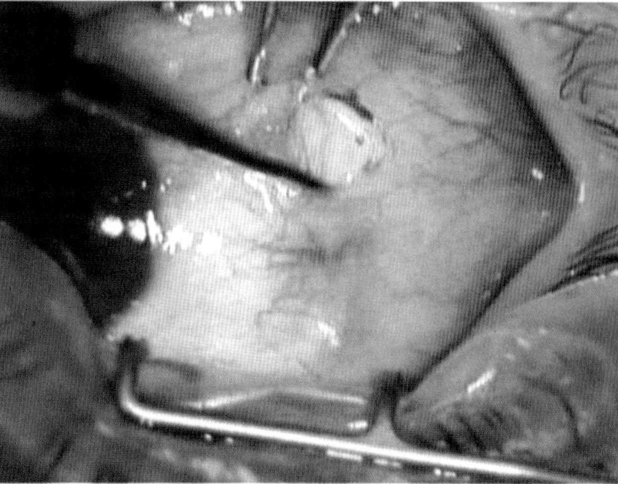

**Figure 102-2** Isolating the lateral rectus muscle using a Stevens hook.

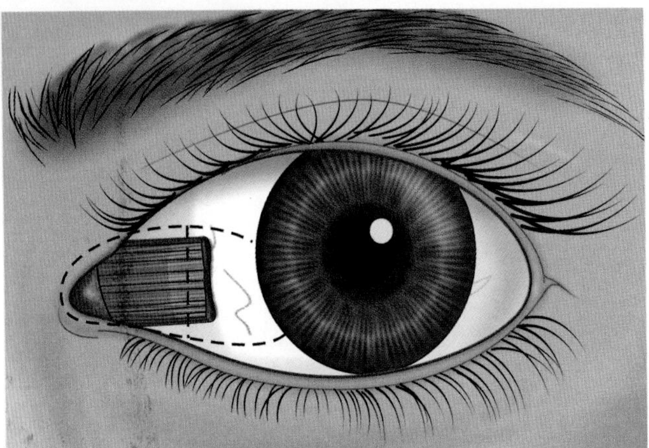

**Figure 102-3** Limbal incision for medial rectus recession.

## Limbal Incision

The limbal incision for strabismus surgery is initiated in the perilimbal tissue where conjunctiva and Tenon's are fused.[2] A limbal peritomy is made extending approximately 3 clock hours around the muscle to be recessed. Relaxing incisions oriented perpendicular to the limbus are extended posteriorly 3–4 mm in the quadrants between rectus muscles (Fig. 102-3). Incisions may need to be enlarged for large recessions. The flap of fused conjunctiva and Tenon's is reflected posteriorly to allow exposure of the rectus muscle. A Graefe and then Jameson hook can be used to isolate the muscle.

## MUSCLE RECESSION

The muscle is cleaned of adherent connective tissue and Tenon's capsule using Westcott scissors. If a large recession is to be performed, it is important to dissect posteriorly to free the muscle from the intermuscular septum and check ligaments. The removal of Tenon's capsule allows for easier exposure, but the removal of too much Tenon's can also lead to unsightly postoperative scarring.

The rectus muscle is secured using an absorbable suture on a spatulated, double-armed needle while the muscle is held on a muscle hook. This suture is placed using a full-thickness bite through the central third of the muscle and tied using a square knot (Fig. 102-4A). The remaining suture ends are woven through the muscle and secured with locking bites at each end (Figs. 102-4B and C). Some surgeons prefer to make a central loop instead of the central knot.

The muscle is then disinserted from the eye using Westcott scissors. Making a cut flush with the sclera allows for a better cosmetic result as well as for easier suture placement in the case of hang-back recession. Bipolar or low-temperature cautery is used to obtain hemostasis. The muscle is then allowed to retract posteriorly. A caliper is used to measure the desired amount of recession from the posterior edge of the muscle insertion. The suture ends are then passed through the sclera using partial-thickness scleral bites (Fig. 102-5). These passes can be oriented in either a crossed-swords fashion to allow the sutures to exit at the same location or perpendicular to the muscle insertion to avoid the area of scleral thinning just posterior to the insertion. If the second technique is used, an instrument may be necessary to hold the first tie of the square knot to assure that it does not slip prior to being firmly secured. A third option is to pass the suture ends through the original insertion and allow the muscle to hang back the desired amount of recession. This approach is somewhat safer as the needles are being passed more anteriorly, thus minimizing the risk of damage to the choroid or retina. If the scleral passes are too close together there may some central sag of the rectus muscle. This can increase the recession effect and should be accounted for in determining the final position of the muscle.

The amount of recession performed depends on the surgeon and the technique used. See Table 102-1 for a standard table of bilateral recessions for esotropia or exotropia from David G Hunter's book, Learning Strabismus Surgery: A Case-Based Approach. For vertical deviations, 1 mm of recession corrects about 3 prism diopters of deviation.

Instead of securing the muscle down with a square knot, a temporary or sliding knot can be placed that allow the position of the muscle to be adjusted postoperatively. This can be achieved using either a bow tie or sliding noose technique.[3] Adjustable sutures may be particularly useful in fine-tuning the amount of recession in patients with restrictive strabismus, previous trauma, slipped or lost muscles, incomitant deviations or those with longstanding, complex strabismus.

## MYOTOMY

Another technique used to weaken a rectus muscle is marginal or Z-myotomy.[4] After application of a mosquito hemostat, the muscle is cut 70% of the way across from above and below using Westcott scissors or thermocautery (Fig. 102-6A). It is important to perform the distal myectomy first. After completion of the myectomies, the muscle has been lengthened or weakened (Fig. 102-6B). Reoperation following a marginal or Z-myotomy can be challenging.

**TABLE 102-1** Amount of rectus recession for esotropia and exotropia

| Esotropia<br>Bilateral medial rectus recession | | Exotropia<br>Bilateral lateral rectus recession | |
|---|---|---|---|
| 15Δ | 3 mm | 15Δ | 4 mm |
| 20Δ | 3.5 mm | 20Δ | 5 mm |
| 25Δ | 4 mm | 25Δ | 6 mm |
| 30Δ | 4.5 mm | 30Δ | 7 mm |
| 35Δ | 5 mm | 35Δ | 7.5 mm |
| 40Δ | 5.5 mm | 40Δ | 8 mm |
| 50Δ | 6 mm | 50Δ | Perform R/R |
| 60Δ | 6.5 mm | 60Δ | Perform R/R |

*Source* Reprinted with permission from Cestari DM, Hunter DG (Eds). Learning Strabismus Surgery: A Case-Based Approach. Philadelphia, PA: Lippincott Williams and Wilkins; 2013. Appendix 1.

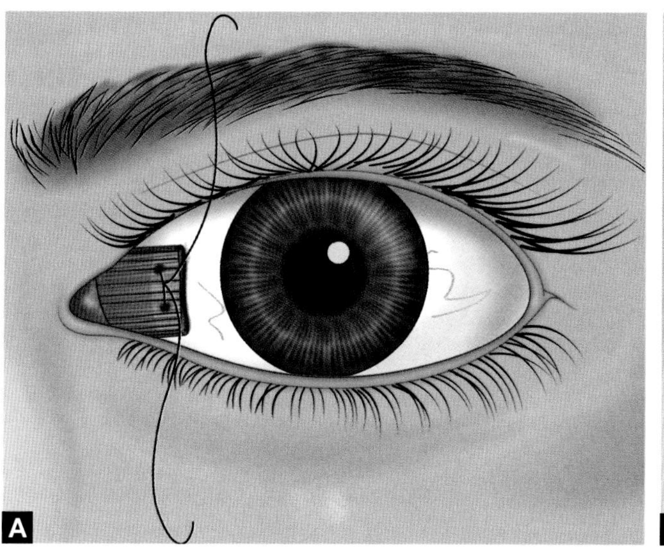


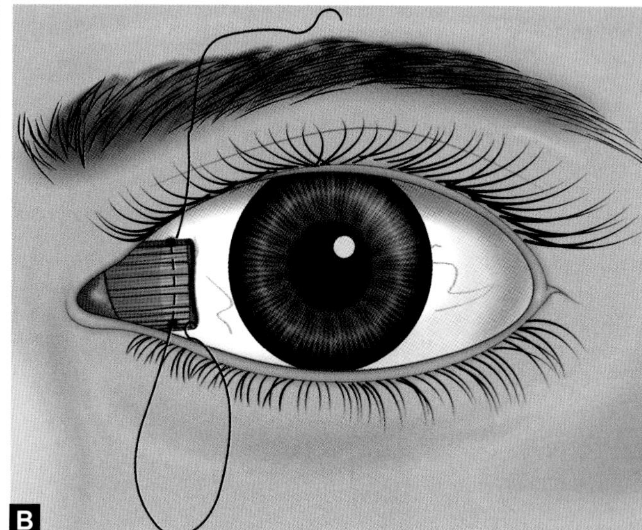


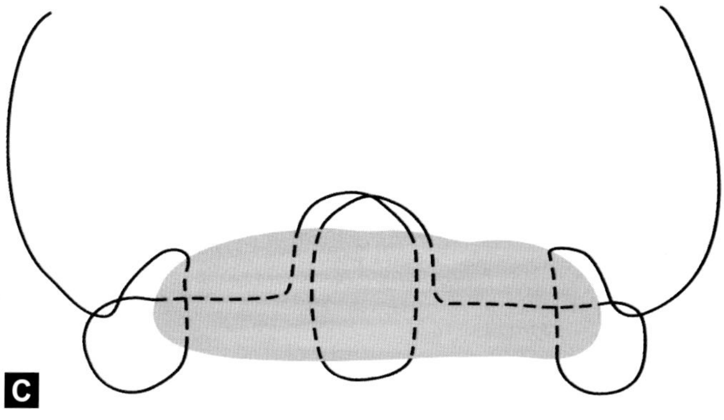


**Figures 102-4A to C** Securing a rectus muscle. (A) Central locking bite; (B) Locking loops at each end; (C) Muscle appearance after securing the muscle.

## CONJUNCTIVAL CLOSURE

The final step in strabismus surgery is to close the conjunctiva. In cases where a fornix incision is used, it may not be necessary to suture the incision if the rectus muscle sutures are covered and no Tenon's is exposed. This can be particularly helpful in cases using adjustable sutures. If the incision does require closure, 8-0 absorbable suture (i.e. Vicryl$^{TM}$) is used to

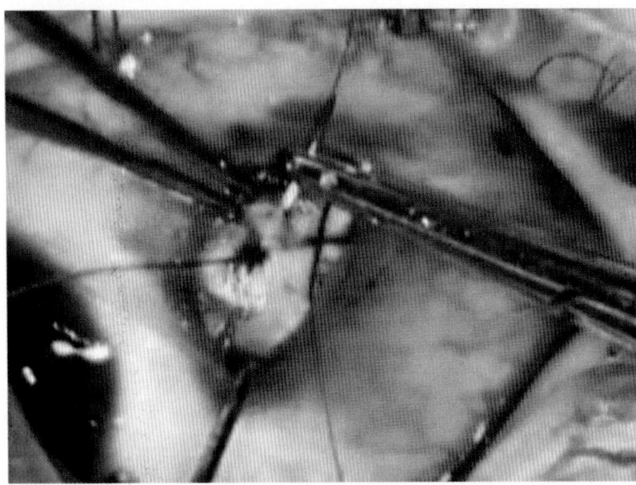

**Figure 102-5** Reattaching the muscle to the original insertion in a crossed-swords fashion. The purple mark is the center of the original insertion and the desired exit point of the needles.

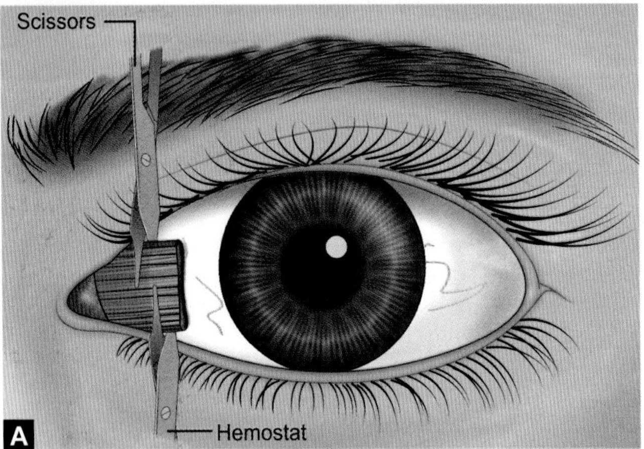


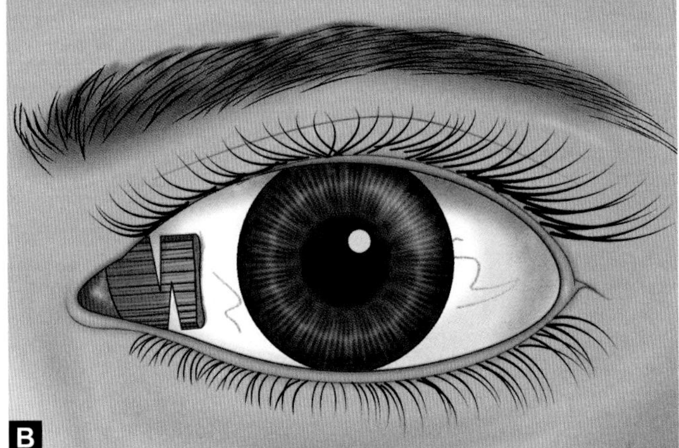


**Figures 102-6A and B** A marginal myotomy of 70% is performed using Westcott scissors to make two parallel incisions (one superiorly and one inferiorly) (A) through 70% of the muscle belly (B) to lengthen (or weaken) the muscle.

reapproximate the conjunctival edges. If a limbal incision is used, the wound is closed with two interrupted stitches that secure the flap corners to the perilimbal episclera.

## SPECIAL CONSIDERATIONS

To avoid inducing incomitance or a deviation that varies in different positions of gaze, recessions are either balanced with a bilateral recession or a recess/resect procedure on one eye. Depending on which muscle is recessed, there are several other factors to keep in mind.

### Medial Rectus

The medial rectus is usually found 5.5 mm behind the limbus. Although its proximity to the limbus makes it relatively easy to identify, it can also make postoperative scarring more apparent. When closing the conjunctiva after a medial rectus recession, it is important to avoid incorporating the plica or pulling the tissues too tight and inducing restriction. After hooking the muscle, careful inspection of the superior and inferior poles of the insertion is necessary to make sure that the whole muscle is isolated prior to recession. In cases of a "lost" muscle, the superior, inferior and lateral rectus muscles have attachments to oblique muscles or lid retractors that can make recovery easier. Finding a "lost" medial rectus muscle can prove more difficult. In one study, Plager and Parks reported that 67% of lost superior, inferior and lateral rectus muscles were retrievable, while this was possible in only 10% of cases involving the medial rectus muscle.[5]

### Superior Rectus

When hooking the superior rectus muscle, it is important to isolate only the rectus muscle and to avoid also catching some or all of the superior oblique muscle fibers or tendon.

**TABLE 102-2** Amount of surgery for nystagmus.

| Right face turn | | | | Left face turn | | | |
|---|---|---|---|---|---|---|---|
| Degrees of face turn | 20° | 20–45° | 45° | Degrees of face turn | 20° | 20–45° | 45° |
| Recess right medial rectus (mm) | 6 | 6.5 | 7 | Resect right medial rectus (mm) | 7.5 | 7.75 | 8.5 |
| Resect right lateral rectus (mm) | 9.5 | 10.5 | 11.25 | Recess right lateral rectus (mm) | 8.5 | 9 | 9.75 |
| Resect left medial rectus (mm) | 7.25 | 7.75 | 8.5 | Recess left medial rectus (mm) | 6 | 6.5 | 7 |
| Recess left lateral rectus (mm) | 8.5 | 9 | 9.75 | Resect left lateral rectus (mm) | 9.5 | 10.5 | 11.25 |

*Source* Reprinted with permission from Cestari DM, Hunter DG (Eds). Learning Strabismus Surgery: A Case-Based Approach. Philadelphia, PA: Lippincott Williams and Wilkins; 2013. Appendix 3.

Inadvertently incorporating the superior oblique can lead to restrictive postoperative hypertropia and incyclotorsion.[6] After the rectus muscle has been removed from its insertion, it should be reflected superiorly and the frenulum connecting the rectus and oblique muscle severed. In cases of large recessions for dissociated vertical deviation, posterior dissection must be completed to release attachments to the levator and prevent postoperative lid retraction.

### Lateral Rectus

Similar to the superior rectus, care must be taken when hooking the lateral rectus muscle to avoid also catching the inferior oblique. This risk can be minimized by not sweeping the hook too far posteriorly as well as by passing a few different hooks in succession. Again, posterior dissection is important, particularly in cases requiring a large recession.

### Inferior Rectus

Failure to adequately release the lower lid retractors from the inferior rectus can lead to postoperative lower lid retraction. Although the exact mechanism is not fully understood, the inferior rectus muscle is prone to late overcorrection after recession surgery.[7,8] The use of nonabsorbable sutures (e.g. Mersilene™) or the use of "semiadjustable" techniques for recession may help minimize this risk.[9,10]

### A- and V-Pattern Strabismus

In cases of small A- or V-patterns without significant oblique dysfunction, the lateral and medial rectus muscles can be offset to treat the incomitance between upgaze and downgaze. The medial recti muscles are shifted toward the apex of the pattern (i.e. inferiorly in cases of V-pattern) and the lateral rectus muscles are shifted away from the apex of the pattern (i.e. superiorly in cases of A-pattern). The amount of offset can be up to one-tendon-width and depends on the size of the pattern. Care must be taken, however, because such shifts can worsen torsion.

## KESTENBAUM-ANDERSON PROCEDURE

Patients with congenital nystagmus will often adopt a face turn to put their eyes in a position where they shake less (null point) to attain better acuity. Strabismus surgery combining recessions (Anderson's contribution) and resections (Kestenbaum's contribution) can be performed to shift the eyes toward the direction of the face turn so that the null position is as close to primary as possible. When strabismus is also present, the numbers can be combined in an effort to treat both problems (Table 102-2).

## PEARLS AND PITFALLS

- When performing strabismus surgery in a child, it is important to treat associated amblyopia first to ensure the best outcome. In patients where amblyopia therapy is challenging, timing of surgery should be carefully balanced with ongoing therapy in an effort to regain binocular vision as early as possible.
- Findings from the Congenital Esotropia Observational Study indicate that esotropia in early infancy frequently resolves, particularly in infants examined prior to 20 weeks of age and with angles of deviation less than 40 prism diopters, and suggest that these patients should be examined over a period of time prior to undergoing surgery.[11]
- Surgical tables are recommendations; surgeons may need to modify these numbers based on their technique and outcomes.

## REFERENCES

1. Parks MM. Fornix incision for horizontal rectus muscle surgery. Am J Ophthalmol. 1968;65:907-15.

2. Von Noorden GK. The limbal approach to surgery of the rectus muscles. Arch Ophthalmol. 1968;80:94-7.
3. Nihalani BR, Hunter DG. Adjustable suture strabismus surgery. Eye (Lond). 2011;25(10):1262-76.
4. Von Noorden GK, Campos EC (Eds). Binocular Vision and Ocular Motility: Theory and Management of Strabismus, 6th edition. St. Louis, MO: Mosby; 2002. pp. 597-8.
5. Plager DA, Parks MM. Recognition and repair of the "lost" rectus muscle. A report of 25 cases. Ophthalmology. 1990;97:131-7.
6. Kushner BJ. Superior oblique tendon incarceration syndrome. Arch Ophthalmol. 2007;125(8):1070-6.
7. Sprunger DT, Helveston EM. Progressive overcorrection after inferior rectus recession. J Pediatr Ophthalmol Strabismus. 1993;30:145-8.
8. Wright KW. Late overcorrection after inferior rectus recession. Ophthalmology. 1996;103:1503-7.
9. Kerr NC. The role of thyroid eye disease and other factors in the overcorrection of hypotropia following unilateral adjustable suture recession of the inferior rectus (an American Ophthalmological Society thesis). Trans Am Ophthalmol Soc. 2011;109:168-200.
10. Spielmann A. Association of fixed suspensions of the capsulopalpebral head of the inferior rectus muscle to minimize complications. In: Kaufmann H (Ed). Transactions of the 21st Meeting of the European Strabismological Association. Giessen: GahmigDruck; 1993. pp. 175-80.
11. Pediatric Eye Disease Investigator Group. Spontaneous resolution of early-onset esotropia: experience of the Congenital Esotropia Observational Study. Am J Ophthalmol. 2002;133(1):109-18.

CHAPTER

103

# Rectus Muscle Resection

Sudha Nallasamy

## INTRODUCTION

Resection (shortening) of a rectus muscle is the most common method employed to "strengthen" the muscle. Rather than truly "strengthening" the muscle, resection and other tightening procedures are thought to alter the length-tension curve and result in a tethering effect, without causing a clinically significant change in the movement of the eye.

Rectus muscle resection is typically performed following a weakening procedure of the antagonist muscle (performed in a previous surgery or in the same surgery). This is because resections may be less effective and technically more difficult if performed alone. Patients are typically more uncomfortable after a resection compared to a recession, and have more swelling and conjunctival injection in the area. Also, muscle that is sutured to the original insertion site after the resection has taken place is usually thicker than the tendon and may appear bulkier.

With rectus muscle resection, it is especially important to assure firm suture bites into muscle and sclera, since the increased tension required to reattach the shortened muscle at the insertion increases the risk of suture breakage and inadvertent muscle loss.

## HORIZONTAL RECTUS MUSCLE RESECTION

With any rectus muscle resection procedure, it is important to do a thorough job of releasing attachments above the muscle to prevent unsightly dragging of tissues forward.

With a lateral rectus resection, it is important to also ensure that the inferior oblique muscle was not inadvertently incorporated with the lateral rectus muscle. It may be prudent to slide a large hook along the ocular surface of the muscle as far back as possible to release any potential attachments to the inferior oblique muscle. This can help avoid inadvertently dragging the inferior oblique muscle anteriorly and altering its action in any way.

## VERTICAL RECTUS MUSCLE RESECTION

When planning a vertical rectus muscle resection, it is important to take into account the potential effects on torsional and horizontal alignment that may result. This is important not only in determining the optimal surgical approach, but also in preoperatively preparing the patient for potential inadvertent alignment outcomes. Large superior rectus resections may result in incyclotorsion as well as esotropia in upgaze (A-pattern). Large inferior rectus resections may result in excyclotorsion and esotropia in downgaze (V-pattern).

In addition, it is important to carefully dissect away attachments to the eyelid as far back as possible when performing a resection on a vertical rectus muscle. If this is not properly performed, a large superior rectus resection can result in ptosis and a large inferior rectus resection can result in lower eyelid elevation.

When performing a superior rectus resection, it is important to dissect away attachments to the superior oblique tendon, as there is the possibility of dragging it forward and altering its action.

When performing an inferior rectus resection, one should avoid rupturing a vortex vein. A vortex vein pierces the sclera adjacent to the inferior rectus border on both the medial and temporal sides, 8–12 mm posterior to the muscle insertion. Rupture of a vortex vein can cause pronounced bleeding, but can be controlled with pressure.

## SURGICAL TECHNIQUE

Rectus muscle resection through a fornix incision using a double-armed 6-0 coated Vicryl™ suture with S-29 needles is shown in Figures 103-1 to 103-6.

The author prefers fornix incisions for patients of all ages. Compared to limbal incisions, fornix incisions create less postoperative discomfort, less scarring, and better cosmetic results. Limbal incisions may be employed in cases with extensive scarring or presence of external hardware (glaucoma implant or scleral buckle) for improved exposure.

A standard 2-plane fornix incision is made in the inferotemporal fornix for lateral rectus resection (this typically does not require suture closure at the end of the case). The assistant grasps the conjunctiva and Tenon's capsule adjacent to the inferotemporal limbus with a toothed forceps and elevates and adducts the eye. The conjunctiva is examined to identify the location of the lateral and inferior rectus muscles based on their anterior ciliary vessels. The open blades of a blunt Westcott scissors are placed firmly down on the relatively avascular conjunctiva against the globe between the two muscles parallel to the lower lid margin and squeezed closed. This creates an incision through the conjunctiva only. The incision may be enlarged as necessary. Next, two toothed forceps (one held by the surgeon and one by the assistant) are used to grasp and lift the Tenon's capsule visible beneath the conjunctival incision. The surgeon then uses blunt Westcott scissors pressed firmly against the globe to cut through Tenon's down to bare sclera perpendicular to the conjunctival incision. Blunt dissection can be performed in the inferotemporal quadrant to ensure that bare sclera has been exposed.

Next, the rectus muscle is isolated on a small hook (e.g. Stevens), followed by a large hook (e.g. Jameson, Green, Guyton, etc.). The large hook is rotated toward the limbus to ensure that all muscle fibers have been hooked. Next, Tenon's capsule is dissected away from the insertion and adjacent sclera using Westcott scissors. Posterior dissection along the orbital surface of the muscle is then performed to remove intermuscular septum and check ligaments (Fig. 103-1). This is an important step in rectus muscle strengthening procedures to prevent dragging of these tissues forward with the muscle and producing a cosmetically unsatisfactory result. The intermuscular septum is lifted off the sclera and stretched out by the assistant using two small hooks, and it is dissected posteriorly by cutting as close to the muscle as possible to avoid penetrating fat (which could result in a restrictive strabismus due to fat adherence syndrome). Once the surface of the rectus muscle has been cleaned, a second large hook is placed beneath the muscle belly in the opposite direction to expose the segment of muscle to be resected. Using a caliper that has been inked with a sterile marking pen on the measuring side, the desired length of resection is measured from just behind the large hook at the muscle insertion and the muscle is marked (Fig. 103-2). By measuring from behind the large hook, this places the resection point (in front of the suture line) at the correct distance from the insertion.

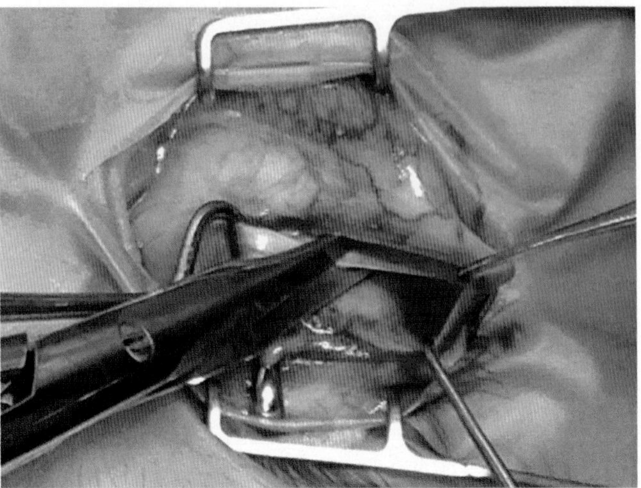

**Figure 103-1** Dissection of intermuscular septum and check ligaments.

A small full-thickness bite is taken at the center of the mark made on the muscle using a 6-0 double-armed absorbable suture (e.g. polyglactin 910/coated Vicryl™) with spatula needles (e.g. S-29, S-14, RD-1, etc.). The suture is pulled halfway through and a square knot is placed for a central locking bite. One of the needles is imbricated half thickness through the muscle belly from just above the central knot to one edge of the muscle at the mark. Next, a full-thickness locking bite is placed at the pole of the muscle proximal to the half-thickness bite to incorporate approximately 2 mm of peripheral muscle tissue. The identical procedure is then performed with the other arm of the suture to secure the remaining pole of the muscle (Fig. 103-3). The sutures are held up along with the large hook and the muscle is then clamped anterior to the suture (carefully avoiding the suture track), and left in place for 30–60 seconds to provide hemostasis (Fig. 103-4). The clamp is then removed and the muscle is then cut in this crushed area of tissue, carefully avoiding the suture. The remaining muscle stump is then cut from its original scleral insertion using Westcott scissors, taking care to not leave residual stump for best cosmesis and ease of reattaching the muscle (Fig. 103-5).

The original scleral insertion is secured by placing a locking forceps (e.g. 0.5 mm locking Castroviejo or Moody forceps) at each end of the original insertion. The muscle is

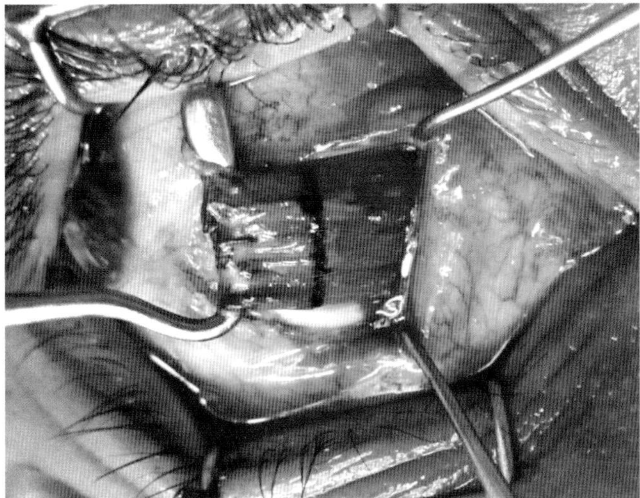

**Figure 103-2** Muscle marked at suture line for resection.

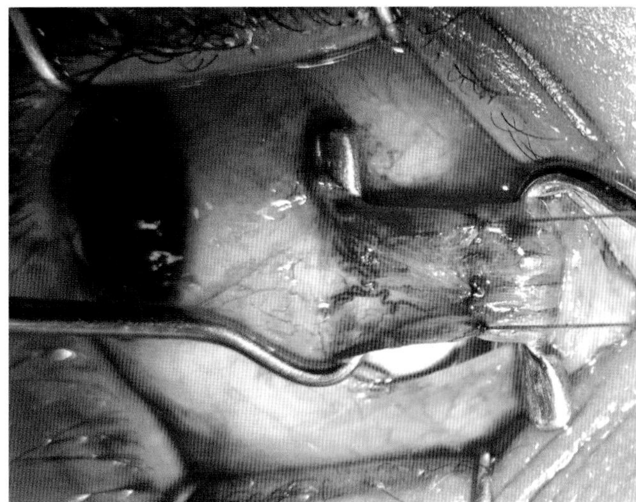

**Figure 103-3** 6-0 double-armed coated Vicryl™ suture placed at marked line.

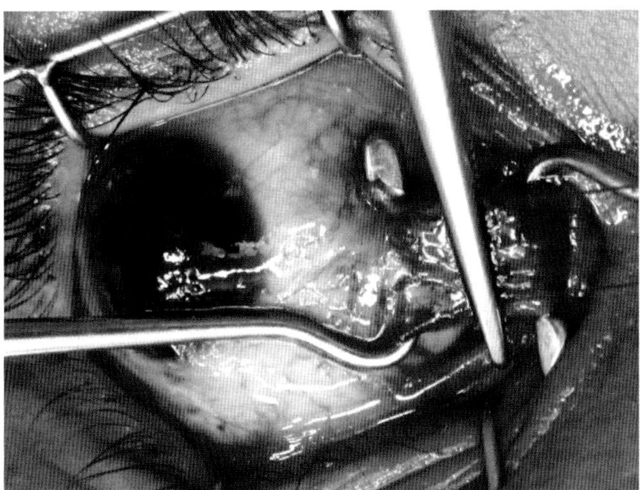

**Figure 103-4** Straight clamp placed anterior to the suture line.

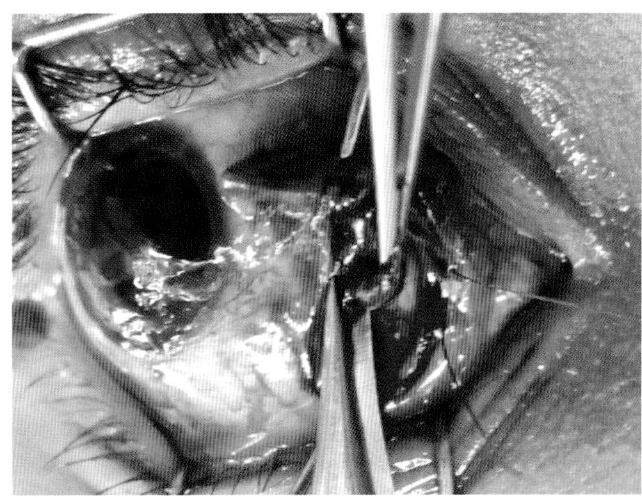

**Figure 103-5** Removal of residual muscle stump.

then secured to the original insertion in a crossed-swords fashion with partial-thickness scleral bites. Each pole suture needle should enter immediately posterior to the ridge of the insertion as far laterally (close to the locking forceps) as possible and exit the sclera centrally and 1–2 mm anterior to the ridge of the insertion. It is best if the two sutures exit the sclera at nearly the same point, making it easier to hold the muscle tight against the original insertion. It is important to attach each pole of the muscle at the insertion as far laterally as possible in order to prevent central sag, which is commonly encountered after rectus muscle resection. If central sag does occur, despite one's best efforts, it can be alleviated by passing the needle under the central edge of the muscle to pull the muscle up toward the insertion and then tied down in place.

In order to advance the muscle to the original insertion, the assistant holds the two locking forceps to rotate the globe toward the muscle while the surgeon uses slow, firm traction on each pole suture to advance the muscle forward. The sutures should be pulled in the direction of the scleral bites to avoid tearing through sclera.

The two arms of the suture are then tied together with a triple throw. If there appears to be any slippage of either pole of the muscle, the globe should be rotated toward the muscle again and the sutures gently pulled upward prior to tightening the triple throw. Next, two single throws are placed, squared on each previous throw. The sutures are then trimmed. Figure 103-6 shows the final result prior to massaging the conjunctiva back in place.

**TABLE 103-1** Suggested surgical guidelines for bilateral lateral rectus resection for esotropia (typically performed for residual esotropia after maximal bilateral medial rectus recession).

| Esotropic deviation (prism diopters) | Bilateral lateral rectus resection (mm) |
|---|---|
| 15 | 3.5 |
| 20 | 4.5 |
| 25 | 5.5 |
| 30 | 6.0 |
| 35 | 6.5 |
| 40 | 7.0 |
| 50 | 8.0 |

**TABLE 103-2** Suggested surgical guidelines for bilateral medial rectus resection for exotropia (typically performed for residual exotropia after maximal bilateral lateral rectus recession).

| Exotropic deviation (prism diopters) | Bilateral medial rectus resection (mm) |
|---|---|
| 15 | 3.0 |
| 20 | 4.0 |
| 25 | 5.0 |
| 30 | 5.5 |
| 35 | 6.0 |
| 40 | 6.5 |

**TABLE 103-3** Suggested surgical guidelines for unilateral recess-resect to treat esotropia.

| Esotropic deviation (prism diopters) | Medial rectus recession (mm) | Lateral rectus resection (mm) |
|---|---|---|
| 15 | 3.0 | 3.5 |
| 20 | 3.5 | 4.0 |
| 25 | 4.0 | 5.0 |
| 30 | 4.5 | 6.0 |
| 35 | 5.0 | 7.0 |
| 40 | 5.5 | 7.5 |
| 50 | 6.0 | 8.0 |
| 60 | 6.5 | 8.5 |

**TABLE 103-4** Suggested surgical guidelines for unilateral recess-resect to treat exotropia.

| Exotropic deviation (prism diopters) | Lateral rectus recession (mm) | Medial rectus resection (mm) |
|---|---|---|
| 15 | 4.0 | 3.0 |
| 20 | 5.0 | 4.0 |
| 25 | 6.0 | 4.5 |
| 30 | 7.0 | 5.0 |
| 35 | 7.5 | 5.5 |
| 40 | 8.0 | 6.0 |
| 50 | 9.0 | 6.5 |

Surgical dosing guidelines for bilateral resections in the treatment of esotropia and exotropia are presented in Tables 103-1 and 103-2. Surgical dosing guidelines for unilateral recess-resect procedures in the treatment of esotropia and exotropia are presented in Tables 103-3 and 103-4. These are sample tables based on the author's experience and should be modified based on one's technique and experience.

For vertical rectus muscle resection, each millimeter corrects approximately 3 prism diopters of deviation.

For A- or V-pattern strabismus (differences from upgaze to downgaze of 10 or more prism diopters) without significant inferior oblique overaction, vertical offsets of the horizontal muscles have been shown to collapse the pattern. Usually, this is done in the context of a bilateral medial or lateral rectus recession, but has also been shown to be effective in unilateral horizontal recess-resect procedures.[1] For an A-pattern, the medial rectus is transposed superiorly and the lateral rectus is transposed inferiorly, regardless of which muscle is recessed or resected. Similarly, for a V-pattern, the medial rectus is transposed inferiorly and the lateral rectus is transposed superiorly, regardless of which muscle is recessed or resected. Typically, half-tendon transpositions are effective for patterns less than 20 prism diopters, and full-tendon width deviations are effective for larger patterns. A greater pattern collapse is seen with greater initial deviations.[1]

When performing a unilateral horizontal rectus muscle recess-resect procedure on a patient who also has a small vertical deviation, both the medial and lateral rectus muscles can be vertically shifted to treat the vertical deviation. For a hyperdeviation, the muscles should be transposed inferiorly, and for a hypodeviation, the muscles should be transposed superiorly. Vertical transposition of both the medial and lateral rectus muscles by 1 mm for each prism diopter of vertical deviation has a high success rate.[2]

## ALTERNATIVE "STRENGTHENING" PROCEDURES

### Rectus Muscle Advancement

Advancement of a rectus muscle toward the limbus can be performed when a muscle has been previously recessed in order to strengthen the muscle. Often, advancement of a

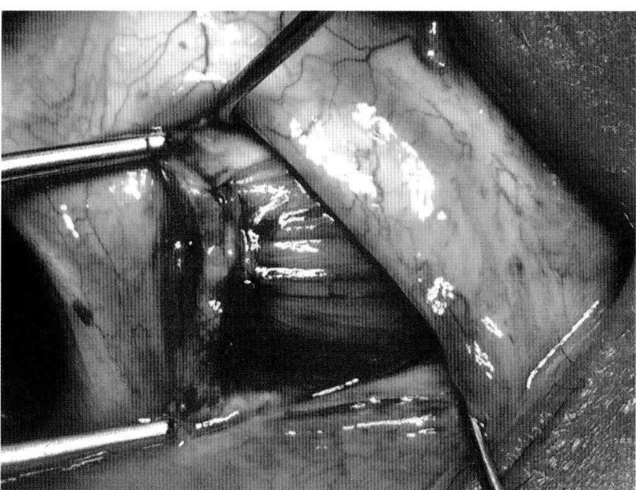

**Figure 103-6** Final result after resection, prior to massaging conjunctiva back in place.

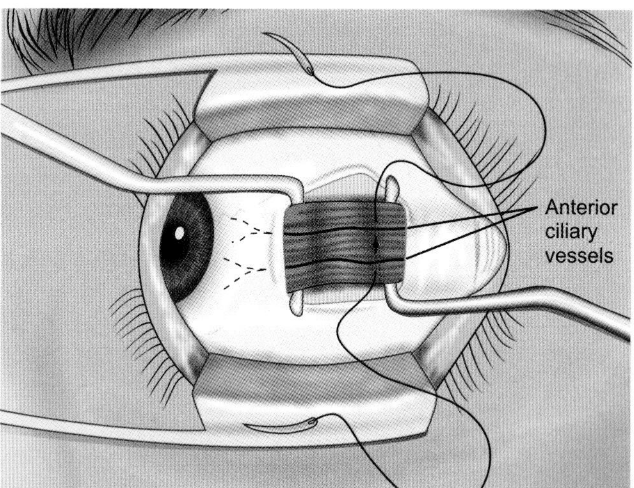


**Figure 103-7** In rectus muscle plication, suture tracks should avoid the anterior ciliary arteries in order to preserve circulation.

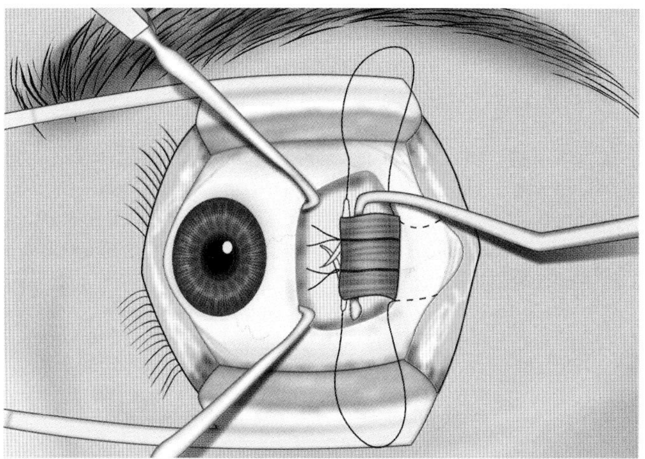

**Figure 103-8** Needles are placed partial thickness through sclera in a crossed-swords fashion, avoiding branching ciliary vessels.

rectus muscle is combined with a small resection. The sum of the millimeters of resection and millimeters of advancement is roughly equivalent to the total number of millimeters needed if resection was to be performed alone. The surgical technique for advancement of a rectus muscle is identical to resection except that the sutures are placed at the site of the intended new insertion rather than at the current insertion site.

## Rectus Muscle Plication (Tuck)

Plication is an alternative procedure used to strengthen a rectus muscle. This procedure may be useful in a complicated case as it can easily be completely reversed in the early postoperative period (within first few days) by cutting the suture and allowing the muscle to return to its original location. Rectus muscle plication is especially valuable in eyes which have already had operations on two or more rectus muscles, as it is possible to leave the anterior ciliary arteries intact, reducing the risk of anterior segment ischemia.[3,4] Another advantage of plication is its relative safety, as there is virtually no chance of losing the muscle.

In rectus muscle plication, the distal portion of the rectus muscle to be plicated is isolated, cleaned, exposed and secured with a double-armed 5-0 or 6-0 nonabsorbable suture (e.g. Mersilene™ or Ethibond™ polyester) as previously described for rectus muscle resection. The same number of millimeters is used as would be required for rectus muscle resection. A nonabsorbable suture is used since there will be no cut surface for the muscle to heal to. It is important to identify the anterior ciliary arteries prior to suturing and carefully avoid them by passing the half-thickness bites beneath them and taking care to avoid including them within the locking bites (Fig. 103-7). If necessary, a blunt-tipped instrument can be used to retract each ciliary artery while placing the locking bites.

Once the suture is secured to the muscle at the desired location, the needles are placed through the anterior sclera in a crossed-swords fashion, each suture needle entering just adjacent or slightly anterior to the pole of the muscle insertion and exiting centrally, 1–2 mm anterior to the insertion (Fig. 103-8). In order to preserve as much anterior segment circulation as possible, try to avoid any finer branching ciliary vessels during suture placement. Exiting with both suture needles at nearly the same point reduces the risk of damage to the anterior ciliary vessels. Next, while the sclera is grasped with locking forceps adjacent to each pole of the muscle insertion, the globe is rotated toward the muscle being

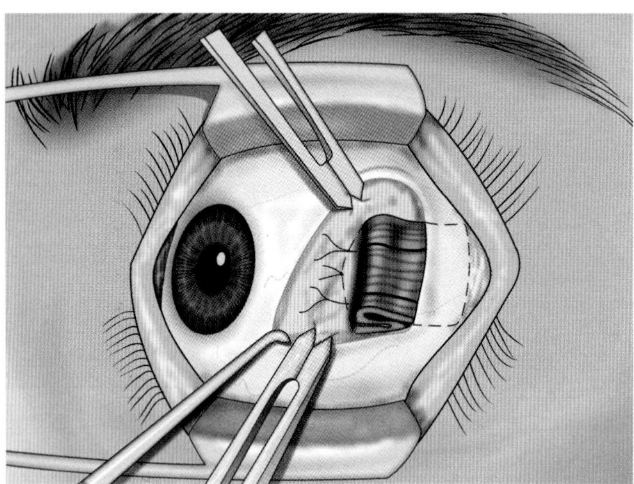

**Figure 103-9** Final result after rectus muscle plication, with tucked muscle directed beneath advancing muscle.

plicated, and the posterior muscle is advanced and tucked by firm traction on the two pole sutures (Fig. 103-9). Muscle to muscle union is not recommended as it is not as reliable and tends to loosen over time. (However, tendon to tendon union, as in a superior oblique tuck, works very well.)

Cosmesis is improved if the tucked portion of muscle is directed beneath rather than above the advancing muscle. This is not always easy to do, as the tucked portion may be short. Regardless, the small bulge of tissue will flatten out over a period of 6–8 weeks. A triple throw is placed, followed by two single throws, squared on each previous throw to permanently secure the plicated muscle in place.

## PEARLS AND PITFALLS

- With rectus muscle resection, it is especially important to assure firm suture bites into muscle and sclera, since the increased tension required to reattach the shortened muscle at the insertion increases the risk of suture breakage and inadvertent muscle loss.
- Large vertical rectus resections can result in change in eyelid position if dissection of lid attachments is not properly performed.
- Large vertical rectus resections may induce torsional diplopia and result in pattern horizontal deviations if not properly planned.
- Rectus muscle plication is a nice alternative to resection that can be employed to preserve anterior ciliary circulation.

## REFERENCES

1. Scott WE, Drummond GT, Keech RV. Vertical offsets of horizontal recti muscles in the management of A and V pattern strabismus. Aust N Z J Ophthalmol. 1989;17:281-8.
2. Metz HS. The use of vertical offsets with horizontal strabismus surgery. Ophthalmology. 1988;95:1094-7.
3. Park C, Min BM, Wright KW. Effect of a modified rectus tuck on anterior ciliary artery perfusion. Korean J Ophthalmol. 1991;5:15-25.
4. Wright KW, Lanier AB. Effect of a modified rectus tuck on anterior segment circulation in monkeys. J Pediatr Ophthalmol Strabismus. 1991;28:77-81.

CHAPTER 104

# Faden Operation

Melanie Kazlas

## BACKGROUND

Cüppers introduced a unique procedure into the surgical armamentarium of strabismus surgeons he called Faden Operation.[1] Ideally suited to treat incomitant strabismus, the Faden operation diminishes the ability of an operated rectus muscle to function in its field of action with little or no effect on the operated muscle's function in primary position or in other fields of gaze. The meaning of the German word "Faden" is thread. Since most strabismus surgery is performed with suture, a type of thread, Von Noorden applied the term posterior fixation procedure to emphasize the posterior placement of the suture. Another term for this procedure is retroequatorial myopexy, which highlights the muscle to globe adhesion created posterior to the equator. This adhesion functions as a new insertion for the operated muscle. The mechanical advantage of the rectus muscle acting on the globe is reduced, similar to creating an artificial paresis.

## MECHANISM OF ACTION

Cüppers classically described the mechanical effect of Faden operation using a lever system model. Placement of the suture posterior to the equator decreases the arc of contact between the muscle and globe (Figs. 104-1A to C). This decreased arc of contact produces a reduction in the amount of torque exerted by that muscle in its field of action. Torque is a measure of the extent a force produces rotation about an axis. Torque is equal to the product of a radius vector, which is measured from the center of rotation of the eye to the point of application of the force and the force vector. Applying a posterior fixation suture to adhere a portion of the muscle to the globe creates a new functional insertion of the rectus muscle. The radius vector, also known as the moment arm, is shortened, with a corresponding reduction in torque if the force vector remains the same. Therefore, additional innervation is required to rotate the globe, i.e. the force vector must

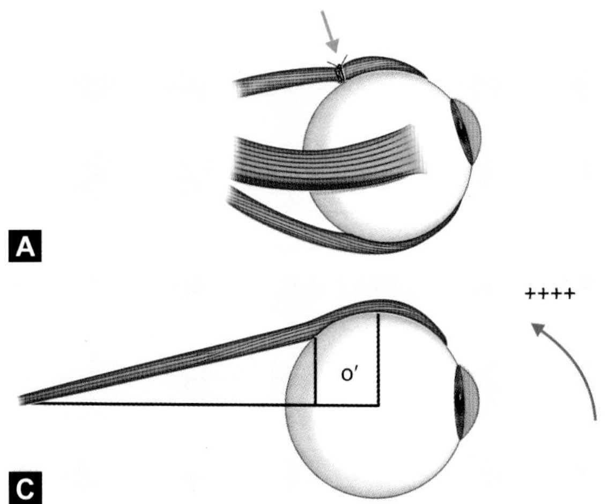


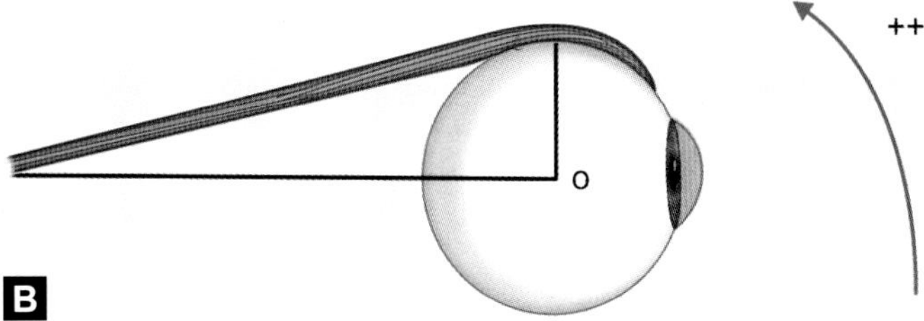


**Figures 104-1A to C** Schematic diagram of Faden Operation and geometric model of mechanism of action. (A) Muscle secured to the sclera behind the equator; (B) The new effective insertion for the muscle decreases the lever arm; (C) The decrease in the lever arm causes increased innervation to produce the muscle action.

increase. This increased innervational stimulus is transmitted to the contralateral yoke muscle, in accordance with Hering's law of reciprocal innervation and can be useful in creating comitance.

Clark and coworkers, in 1999, called into question the lever system model. They demonstrated with magnetic resonance imaging (MRI) of the orbits that no significant reduction in torque occurred in patients who had a Faden operation. Much less angular displacement occurs than predicted by a geometric model.

## INDICATIONS FOR FADEN OPERATION (BOX 104-1)

### Nystagmus

As with many strabismus surgeons who develop a surgical innovation, Cüppers needed a better approach for his patients who exhibited a constellation of findings he described as nystagmus blockage syndrome. Thus, the initial indication for Faden Operation was nystagmus blockage syndrome. Cüppers and Adelstein in 1966 described the hallmarks of this condition as early onset esotropia, pseudoabducens paralysis, head turn toward the side of the fixating eye, absence of nystagmus when the fixating eye is in adduction and increased amplitude of nystagmus in abduction. The theory is that convergence dampens the nystagmus and the persistent convergence tonus induces esotropia. Von Noorden studied the syndrome and described the surgical management, which usually includes large bimedial rectus recessions with or without the addition of Faden Operation. Reinecke studied three patients with organic causes of poor vision in one eye whom he suspected had nystagmus blockage as the reason for their variable esotropia and mild head turn to keep the fixating eye in adduction. Reinecke recommended a small (3.0 mm) bimedial rectus recession with Faden Operation and a resection of the lateral rectus to improve the head posture as well as the variable esotropia.[2]

The head posture in congenital motor nystagmus usually is ameliorated with a Kestenbaum procedure, grading the amount of surgery per eye according to the degree of head posture. However, larger amounts of surgery performed with the "40%" and "60%" modifications can result in limited motility. Isenberg addressed this problem in a study with nine patients with infantile nystagmus, 20–35° of head turn and no strabismus. He performed a "classic plus one" Kestenbaum procedure and added a Faden Operation to the recessed muscles, 11 mm posterior to the insertion for the recessed medial and 13 mm posterior to the insertion for the recessed lateral. Seventy eight percent achieved improvement of head posture to less than 10° with a mean follow-up of 29 months and no induced strabismus. Mild limitation of gaze into the field of action of the recessed muscle with Faden Operation was seen in 33%.[3]

**BOX 104-1** Indications for Faden Operation.

Strabismus:

- Nonparalytic
  - Congenital esotropia
  - Partially accommodative esotropia
    - With high AC/A ratio
    - Convergence excess
  - Intermittent exotropia
    - With high AC/A ratio
  - Dissociated vertical deviation
  - Dissociated horizontal deviation
- Duane's retraction syndrome
- Paralytic
  - Sixth nerve palsy
  - Fourth nerve palsy
  - Third nerve palsy
- Restrictive
  - Thyroid eye disease
  - Orbital fractures
  - Post scleral buckle
  - Post glaucoma implant
  - Post cataract surgery
  - Post strabismus surgery

Nystagmus:

- Nystagmus blockage syndrome
- Manifest latent nystagmus with head turn
- Idiopathic infantile nystagmus with anomalous head posture

[Accommodative convergence/accommodation (AC/A) ratio].

### Incomitant Strabismus

Faden Operation is particularly useful in treating incomitant strabismus. Primary position deviation may be minimal, but a significant incomitance can result in double vision in a functional field of gaze, such as downgaze. By trying to match a duction deficit by creating one in the unaffected eye, the field of binocular single vision can be expanded without compromising primary position.

### Incomitant Vertical Strabismus

#### *Inferior Rectus Weakness*

Orbital blowout fractures or surgical trauma can produce troublesome diplopia in downgaze with little or no vertical deviation in primary position. The inferior rectus behaves as a weakened muscle, similar to a paresis. Use of a Faden

Operation to the normal inferior rectus of the contralateral eye can create limitation of depression in the sound eye to match the impaired infraduction of the affected eye, thereby increasing the field of single binocular vision.

### *Thyroid Eye Disease*

The mechanical strabismus seen in thyroid eye disease often requires recession of a tight inferior rectus muscle. Late overcorrection after recession of an inferior rectus has been described. In a paper published by Buckley and Meekins, seven patients with Graves' disease who experienced late overcorrection after recession of the inferior rectus were helped with a Faden Operation to the more normally functioning inferior rectus.[4]

### *Monocular Elevation Deficiency*

Comitance can be promoted in monocular elevation deficiency by Faden Operation on the contralateral superior rectus with or without a small recession. Similarly, for monocular depression deficiency, a rare form of strabismus, a Faden Operation could be performed on the inferior rectus of the unaffected eye with or without a small recession.

### *Antielevation Syndrome*

Anteriorization of the inferior oblique may be performed for dissociated vertical deviation (DVD) associated with inferior oblique overaction. Some surgeons will anteriorize the ipsilateral inferior oblique for a superior oblique palsy. Occasionally, an antielevation syndrome will be induced in which the patient will see double in up and in adduction ipsilateral to the operated inferior oblique. To treat this troublesome postoperative result, a Faden Operation to the contralateral superior rectus could improve diplopia.

### *Duane's Retraction Syndrome*

Faden Operation can treat upshoots or downshoots seen with a tight lateral rectus in Duane's retraction syndrome by applying a posterior fixation suture to the lateral rectus.

### *Dissociated Vertical Deviation*

Dissociated vertical deviation is an occasional epiphenomenon of congenital strabismus, which may require surgery to improve binocularity or improve eye contact with others. Surgical results of asymmetrical superior rectus recession, inferior oblique anteriorization, or inferior rectus resection, have been variable. Faden Operation of the superior rectus alone was found to be effective for small unilateral DVD of less than 14 prism diopters (PD) in a study by Lorenz.[5] For larger measured DVD, a Faden in conjunction with small superior rectus recession was found to result in a satisfactory outcome of 9 PD or less of vertical deviation. However, limitations of their study included its retrospective nature and short follow-up period of 2 months.

## Incomitant Horizontal Strabismus

### *High Accommodative Convergence/Accommodation Ratio*

The Faden Operation has been successfully applied in the treatment of patients with a high accommodative convergence/accommodation (AC/A) ratio. If weaning the bifocal is unsuccessful in the older child, Faden Operation could be considered. Peterseim and Buckley studied 16 consecutive children who underwent a Faden Operation for accommodative esotropia with high AC/A ratio.[6] The preoperative mean distance esotropia was 8.8 PD and the near mean esotropia was 33 PD, with an average AC/A ratio of 7.4, using the gradient method. Postoperatively the mean distance deviation was 3.2 PD of esotropia and the mean near deviation was 10.3 PD of esotropia, with an average AC/A ratio of 2.9. Stereopsis was present in 70% of patients postoperatively compared with 44% preoperatively.

Usually intermittent exotropia will exhibit a low or normal AC/A ratio. For those patients who demonstrate a high AC/A ratio, the potential for a postoperative esotropia at near is significant, especially if the surgeon aims to correct the distance exotropia fully. A Faden Operation to the medial rectus muscles simultaneously with recessing the lateral rectus muscles is an approach Brodsky reviewed in six patients.[7] They found a reduction in the distance near disparity, but not the AC/A ratio. Five out of six patients did not require bifocals.

### *Sixth Nerve Palsies*

A Faden Operation could be performed on the contralateral medial rectus. According to Hering's law, increased innervation required to adduct the eye with the medial rectus Faden would be transmitted to the paretic lateral rectus, to maximize its function and decrease incomitance.

### *Duane's Retraction Syndrome*

Incomitant horizontal strabismus is a hallmark of Duane's retraction syndrome, in which a branch of the third nerve aberrantly innervates the lateral rectus. For type I Duane's, a Faden Operation on the contralateral medial rectus could be useful to expand the field of binocular vision.

### *Third Nerve Palsies*

There are numerous clinical presentations of third nerve paresis depending on the extent and specific muscles involved. In theory, a Faden Operation to the contralateral lateral rectus could expand the binocular field of vision horizontally. However, the arc of contact of the lateral rectus to the globe is quite posterior, and to shorten the arc of contact, a Faden Operation would need to be performed far posterior with placement of a scleral suture over the macula, with its attendant risks. However, Holmes and Leske performed adjustable suture recessions with Faden Operation to the lateral rectus of three patients with contralateral adduction deficit with good results.

## SURGICAL TECHNIQUE

To perform a Faden Operation, one must have excellent exposure. Faden Operation has been performed both with limbal peritomy and fornix peritomy. Dissection of check ligaments and intermuscular septa must proceed several millimeters beyond anticipated placement of sutures. Consider using an operating microscope or surgical headlight (Box 104-2). Keep the globe retracted maximally to increase surgical exposure with traction sutures or locking forceps. Choosing and using the appropriate retractor will keep Tenon's capsule and orbital fat out of the surgical field and facilitate exposure and safe needle passage. Most Faden Operations are performed with a nonabsorbable suture on a spatula needle. To complete a partial thickness scleral pass, use the safest approach. Make sure that you are able to forward pass, reverse pass or use your nondominant hand based on the unique characteristics of the operated muscle. One can complete the scleral pass prior or after muscle capture. Capture one-third of the muscle as far posterior as possible by passing suture through muscle. To measure far posterior to the rectus insertion, consider using a curved caliper, which follows the curvature of the globe. Another option to capture a portion of the rectus is to create a slit in the muscle with small Stevens hook at the desired location and exteriorize the hook with the aid of a smooth Bishop-Harmon forceps. Feed the suture through the opening in the captured muscle with a fenestrated Gass muscle hook. Secure the captured muscle to the scleral site by tying the ends of the suture with a surgeon's knot. Repeat this procedure of scleral pass and muscle capture on the opposite pole of the muscle. A variation of the Faden Operation includes disinserting the rectus muscle, placing the scleral pass at the desired location posterior to the insertion under the muscle, incorporating the central one-third of muscle with the suture and then tying the suture down over the captured middle one-third of muscle.

**BOX 104-2** Surgical instrumentation and supplies for Faden Operation.

- Consider surgical headlight or operating microscope
- Retractors
  - Small Desmarres
  - Conway
  - Helveston "Barbie"
  - Fison
  - Ribbon
- Calipers
  - Curved
  - Flexible plastic ruler
- Needle holder
  - Non-locking Castroviejo to make scleral pass
- Sutures (5-0 or 6-0)
  - Non-absorbable (preferable)
    - Mersilen
    - Dacron
    - Supramid Extra
  - Absorbable
    - Vicryl

Suture material chosen for Faden Operation must incite enough of a reaction to create a firm adhesion between the globe and captured portion of muscle. One study in a rabbit model of Faden Operation demonstrated a strong adhesion between muscle and globe with an application of talc or doxycycline allowing for a sutureless type of Faden Operation. Mersilene (braided polyester on an S-24 needle which is 8.0 mm, ¼ circle) is the most common type of suture used for Faden Operation, although some have used Dacron, Supramid Extra, nylon or even absorbable Vicryl.

Mojon described a novel technique he called minimally invasive strabismus surgery (MISS) for rectus muscle posterior fixation in 19 patients.[8] The posterior fixation sutures were placed on medial rectus 13 mm posterior to the insertion, inferior rectus 14 mm posterior to the insertion and on lateral rectus 15–18 mm posterior to the insertion. He used an operating microscope and created a small keyhole conjunctival incision at the location of where he wanted to place the muscular scleral suture at each pole of the muscle. He touted the reduced discomfort and reduced visible redness of this approach and found similar success rates for his variation on the Faden Operation.

Faden Operation can be combined with a fixed recession of the rectus muscle. However, one criticism of Faden Operation has been that it is difficult to combine with simultaneous adjustable recession of the operated muscle. Recent studies address this criticism. Combined adjustable suture and Faden Operation of a vertical rectus muscle to treat incomitant vertical strabismus was described in seven patients operated by Hoover.[9] Diagnoses included superior oblique palsy, inferior oblique palsy and inferior rectus palsy. All patients had constant diplopia in primary position and in the field of the palsied muscle. Bowtie adjustable suture was placed on the Mersilene posterior fixation suture as well as on the Vicryl suture securing the recessed muscle. Scleral sutures were placed prior to recession of the muscle. The average placement of the Faden suture was 13 mm posterior to the insertion. Although resolution of diplopia was successful, Hoover noted increased patient discomfort with this technique. He adjusted six of the seven patients in this study. To minimize discomfort, he placed a Faden suture only on one pole of the muscle, or if the vortex vein was quite anterior, he placed the Faden suture under the disinserted rectus and came up through the middle one-third of the muscle and secured the suture with a bowtie that was tied permanently at the time of adjustment.

## SELECTED COMPLICATIONS OF FADEN OPERATION

A greater incidence of certain complications has been reported with the Faden Operation. Due to the technical difficulty of placing the suture far posteriorly in a tight space, the risk of scleral penetration or perforation is theoretically increased. Alio and coworkers confirmed an increased prevalence of scleral penetration in a study of 187 eyes which underwent uneventful Faden Operation.[10] Binocular indirect ophthalmoscopy was performed prior and just after surgery, as well as at 2 weeks, 4 weeks and 3 months postoperatively. Twenty-nine eyes or 15.5% of the eyes examined, revealed chorioretinal scars in the area of the muscle to globe suture. One eye displayed a triangular area of choroidal ischemia. No retinal tears were found. This incidence is in contrast with a recent study of extraocular muscle recessions, resections and Faden Operations by Isenberg. Their study of consecutive eyes operated on revealed an incidence per muscle operated of 4.3% for scleral penetration and 1.9% for scleral perforation.

The incidence of postoperative nausea and emesis is 37–80% across all strabismus procedures. A prospective double-blind study was conducted to determine the effect of surgical technique on the incidence of postoperative emesis.[11] One hundred twenty children age 2–12 years old who underwent strabismus surgery by one surgeon with total intravenous anesthesia were studied. Perioperative oculocardiac reflex, procedure performed, total surgical time and incidence of emesis during 48 hours postoperatively were recorded. The incidence of vomiting in the Faden group was 53% compared with 12% ($p < 0.05$) in the non-Faden group. The incidence of perioperative oculocardiac reflex was similar as well as the dose of intravenous anesthetics and the postoperative requirements for analgesics. The patients in the Faden group had a longer operative time and were younger and weighed less than the non-Faden group ($p < 0.05$).

## FADEN OPERATION ANALOGS

### Scott Procedure

Given the technical difficulties of Faden Operation, Alan Scott developed a procedure with Faden-like effect.[12] Scott described a resect/recess procedure in which a portion of the rectus is rendered ineffective, thereby changing the functional insertion of the muscle similar to traditional Faden Operation (Figs. 104-2A to C). Scott meant not to replace the Faden Operation, but to give the surgeon the option of performing his procedure on the lateral rectus or in situations where a combined Faden and recession is indicated for incomitant strabismus with clinically significant primary position strabismus. The change in ocular alignment is more sensitive to small changes in recession in contrast to the amount of resection performed. Clinical pearls include: lateral rectus' final position on the globe be at least 13 mm posterior to the original insertion and the medial at least 9–10 mm posterior to the original insertion. Freedman and coworkers examined the results of the Scott procedure on 12 patients with incomitant strabismus, including incomitant vertical and horizontal strabismus, dissociated horizontal deviation and distance/near disparity, in which one muscle was recessed more than it was resected.[13] Five patients had adjustable recessions and seven patients had fixed amounts of recession. The change in incomitance in PD was calculated and was reduced in both groups. Eight out of 12 patients had this procedure on the lateral rectus muscle. Too few other rectus muscles were operated to comment on the efficacy of the Scott procedure compared with traditional Faden Operation. Freedman and coworkers performed smaller amounts of resection than advocated by Scott in his original paper because of a fear of an unknown effect on the long-term functioning of the muscle and fear of overcorrection.

Lee and coworkers studied 22 patients who underwent the Scott procedure for primary position deviation and incomitance with symptomatic diplopia.[14] Their study confirmed reduction in incomitance and expanded field of single vision in over half their patients. The ease of the procedure compared with the Faden Operation on the lateral rectus indicated for incomitant exotropia associated with contralateral adduction weakness is emphasized.

## Pulley Surgery

Contributions to the understanding of extraocular muscle biomechanics with MRI continue to be made by Demer, Clark and colleagues. The traditional explanation for Faden Operation's effect has been revised based on their demonstration that a scleral posterior fixation suture creates a mechanical restriction, preventing the muscle from telescoping normally through its pulley. Building on this new model, a surgical technique was proposed to create a Faden effect without the risk of passing scleral sutures. The usual location of rectus muscle pulleys is near the equator of the globe. Geometric modeling, cadaveric studies, high resolution MRI and intraoperative forced duction testing, suggest that scleral posterior fixation suture impedes the telescoping of the extraocular muscle through its pulley sleeve, creating a mechanical restriction, which impairs the contraction of the muscle in its field of action. Based on this revised mechanical explanation for Faden Operation, they developed a new surgical technique called "pulley posterior fixation".[15] Kowal and Mitchell reviewed 26 patients with accommodative and partially accommodative esotropia with convergence excess.[16] Traditional bimedial rectus recession was performed aiming for correction of the mean of the corrected distance and near deviation. A pulley posterior fixation procedure was done on both medial rectus muscles at the same surgery (Figs. 104-3A to D). With a mean follow-up of 12.7 months, all had a statistically significant decrease in near/distance disparity with only two overcorrections and two undercorrections at last follow-up.

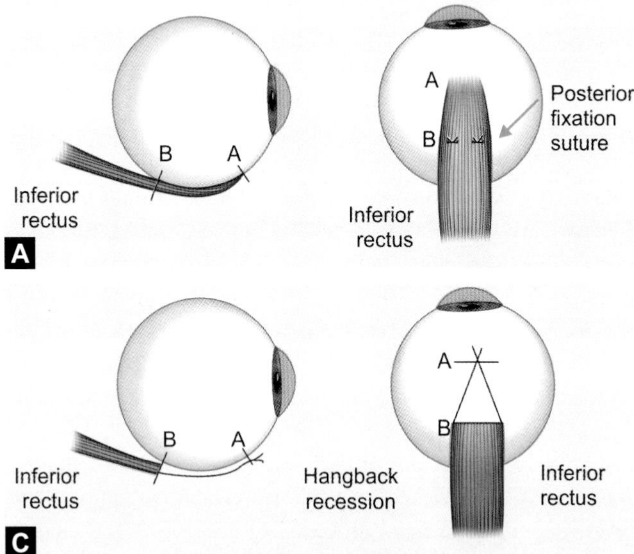


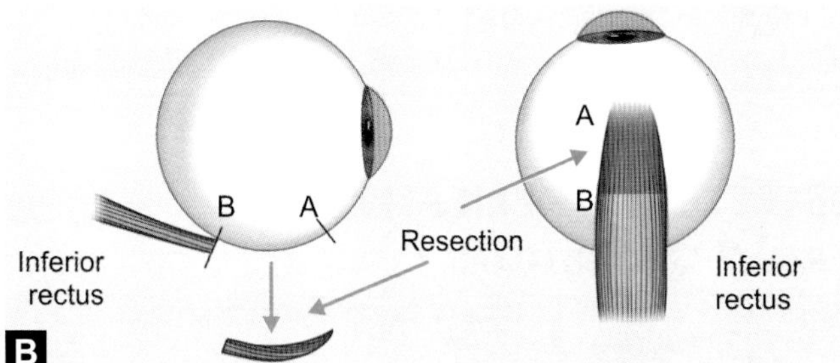


**Figures 104-2A to C** Schematic diagram of Scott procedure. (A) Diagram representing the Faden Operation. Point A shows the original insertion and point B is the site of the Faden which behaves as the effective new insertion; (B) Representation of the Scott procedure (recess-resect procedure)—the muscle in between points A and B is excised and the muscle is recessed to point B; (C) Representation of the Scott procedure (recess-resect procedure)—after resection of the muscle it is allowed to hang back to obtain the desired recession.

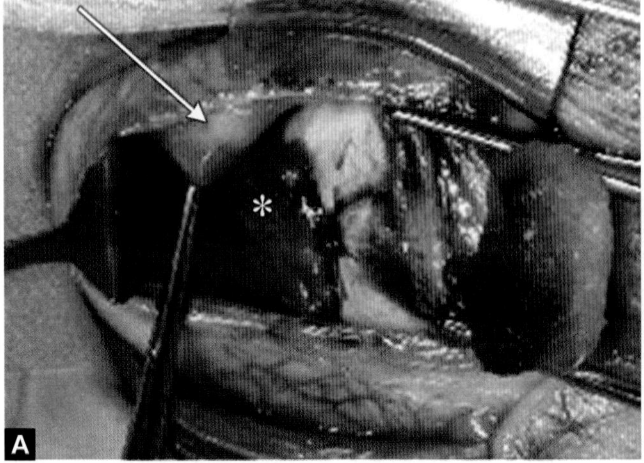


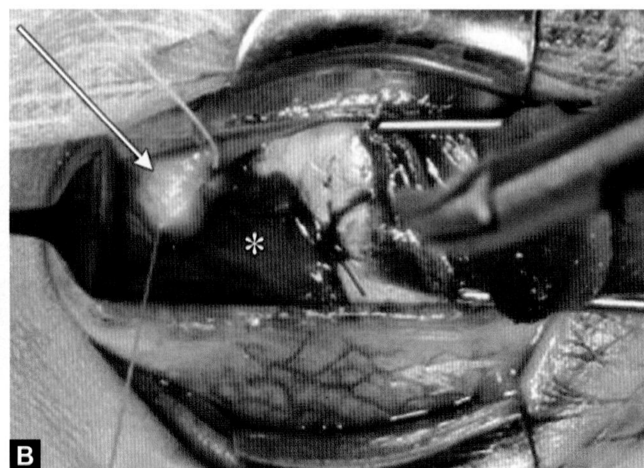


**Figures 104-3A and B** Pulley posterior fixation suture surgery on the medial rectus muscle with recession. (A) Medial rectus pulley (arrow) hooked with a muscle hook; (B) Medial rectus pulley secured with polyester suture.

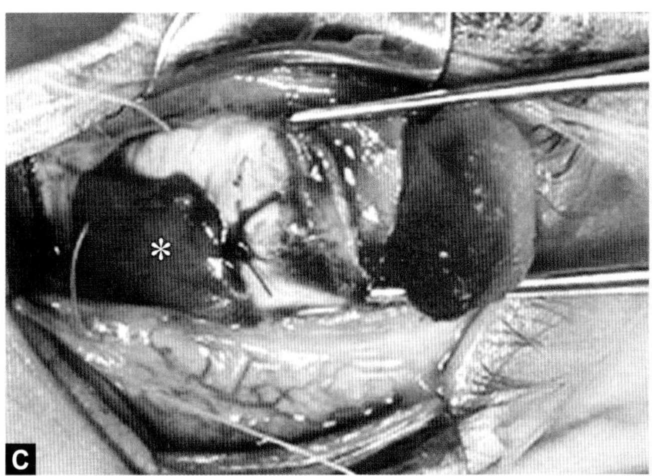


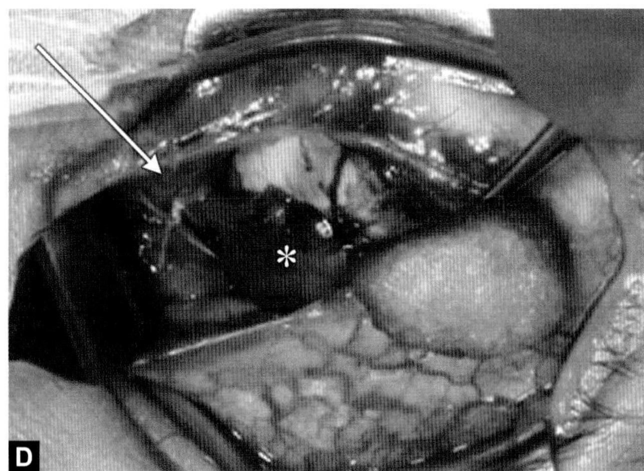


**Figures 104-3C and D** Pulley posterior fixation suture surgery on the medial rectus muscle with recession. (C) Suture passed through the medial rectus muscle belly as posteriorly as possible; (D) Suture tied to fix the pulley to the muscle belly.
*Source* Reproduced with permission from Mitchell L, Kowal L. Medial rectus muscle pulley posterior fixation sutures in accommodative and partially accommodative esotropia with convergence excess. J AAPOS. 2012;16(2):125-30.

## PEARLS AND PITFALLS

- Faden Operation and Faden-like operations are useful procedures which can effectively treat incomitant strabismus associated with childhood strabismus, as well as paralytic and mechanical strabismus in adults.
- It ameliorates anomalous head posture, and expands the field of single binocular vision in properly selected patients.
- The surgical procedure is challenging in view of the placement of the posterior sclera bites but with a careful technique the complications rates are low.

## REFERENCES


1. Cüppers C. The so-called "Faden Operation" (surgical corrections by well-defined changes in the arc of contact). The Second Congress of the International Strabismological Association. 1976;395-400.
2. Reinecke RD. Nystagmus blockage syndrome in the unilaterally blind patient. Doc Ophthalmol. 1984;58:125-30.
3. Kang NY, Isenberg SJ. Kestenbaum procedure with posterior fixation suture for anomalous head posture in infantile nystagmus. Graefes Arch Clin Exp Ophthalmol. 2009;24:981-7.
4. Buckley EG, Meekins BB. Faden Operation for the management of complicated incomitant vertical strabismus. Am J Ophthalmol. 1988;105:304-12.
5. Lorenz B, Raab I, Boergen KP. Dissociated vertical deviation: what is the most effective surgical approach? J Pediatr Ophthalmol Strabismus. 1992;29:21-9.
6. Millicent M, Peterseim W, Buckley EG. Medial rectus Faden Operation for esotropia only at near fixation. J AAPOS. 1997;1:129-33.
7. Brodsky MC, Fray KJ. Surgical management of intermittent exotropia with high AC/A ratio. J AAPOS. 1998;2:330-2.
8. Mojon DS. Minimally invasive strabismus surgery for rectus muscle posterior fixation. Ophthalmologica. 2009;223:111-5.
9. Hoover DL. Results of a combined adjustable recession and posterior fixation suture of the same vertical rectus muscle for incomitant vertical strabismus. J AAPOS. 1998;2:336-9.
10. Alio JL, Faci A. Fundus changes following Faden operation. Arch Ophthalmol. 1984;102:211-3.
11. Saiah M, Borgeat A, Ruetsch YA, et al. Myopexy (Faden) results in more postoperative vomiting after strabismus surgery in children. Acta Anaesthesiol Scand. 2001;45:59-64.
12. Scott A. Posterior fixation: adjustable and without posterior sutures. In: Lennerstrand G (Ed). Proceedings VIIth Congress International Strabismological Association. Boca Raton, FL: CRC Press; 1995.
13. Bock CJ, Buckley EG, Freedman SF. Combined resection and recession of a single rectus muscle for the treatment of incomitant strabismus. J AAPOS. 1999;3:263-8.
14. Dawson E, Boyle N, Taherian K, et al. Use of the combined recession and resection of a rectus muscle procedure in the management of incomitant strabismus. J AAPOS. 2007;11:131-4.
15. Clark RA, Ariyasu R, Demer JL. Medial rectus pulley posterior fixation: a novel technique to augment recession. J AAPOS. 2004;8:451-6.
16. Mitchell L, Kowal L. Medial rectus muscle pulley posterior fixation sutures in accommodative and partially accommodative esotropia with convergence excess. J AAPOS. 2012;16(2):125-30.


## SUGGESTED READING


1. de Decker W. The Faden operation. When and how to do it. Trans Ophthalmol Soc U K. 1981;101:264-70.
2. Guyton DL. The posterior fixation procedure: mechanism and indications. Int Ophthalmol Clin. 1985;25:79-88.
3. Von Noorden G, Campos EC (Eds). Binocular Vision and Ocular Motility: Theory and Management of Strabismus, 6th edition. St. Louis: Mosby; 2001. pp. 574-7.

CHAPTER

# 105

# Inferior Oblique Muscle Surgery

Ankoor S Shah, Aristomenis Thanos

## INTRODUCTION

The inferior oblique (IO) muscle elevates the eye in adduction and provides the globe with extorsional forces, which are important in the ocular counter roll mechanism with head tilt. IO muscle surgery typically weakens an overaction of this muscle. There are strengthening procedures for "weakness" of this muscle, but this is beyond the scope of this chapter and basic strabismus surgery techniques.

## INDICATIONS

- IO muscle overaction associated with horizontal and/or vertical ocular misalignments with or without V-patterns.
- Superior oblique (SO) muscle palsy, acquired or congenital
- Dissociated vertical deviation (DVD).

## CONTRAINDICATIONS

SO muscle overaction is a contraindication to IO surgery as weakening the IO muscle will simply worsen the situation.

## SURGICAL TECHNIQUE

Several types of IO muscle weakening surgeries have been described including myectomy at the origin (orbital floor),[1,2] tenotomy,[3-6] myectomy at the insertion (sclera),[1,7-13] recession,[3,14-20] anterior transposition,[21-23] anterior and nasal transposition,[24-26] and denervation and extirpation.[27] The indication for each varies based on the type of strabismus and the preference of the surgeon. This chapter will focus on the basic IO surgeries of tenotomy (or myotomy as referenced by some),[28] myectomy at its insertion on the globe, recession, and anterior transposition. These are the most common IO muscle surgeries performed today. The approach to isolating the IO muscle is similar in each surgery, but the post-isolation technique varies slightly.

### Isolating the IO Muscle

The IO muscle insertion is isolated for surgery from the inferior temporal quadrant of the eye. After creating a sterile field, an exaggerated traction test should be performed to grade the tightness of the IO muscle.[29] The eye is then grasped at the inferior temporal limbus with a 0.5 forcep and rotated superonasally. A 7 mm incision perpendicular to and 4 mm posterior to the limbus is made through conjunctiva and Tenon's capsule half way between the inferior border of the lateral rectus (LR) muscle and the temporal border of the inferior rectus (IR) muscle (Fig. 105-1A). Westcott scissors are utilized to dissect connective tissue within the quadrant bluntly. A small muscle hook is passed through the incision, juxtaposed to the sclera, and directed superiorly to hook the LR muscle. This hook is exchanged for a Gass muscle hook, and the end of the Gass hook is lifted off the scleral surface after it has cleared the superior aspect of the LR muscle in the superior temporal quadrant. A 4-0 silk suture on a taper-point needle is passed through the conjunctiva and through the hole in the Gass muscle hook in a fashion that the needle is always pointed away from the globe (Fig. 105-1B). The needle is cut off the silk suture, and the Gass hook is retracted through the inferior nasal incision pulling the former needle-end of the silk suture with it. This end of the suture is recovered from the conjunctival incision, and an overhand knot is placed on the two ends of the suture. This creates a sling around the LR muscle that allows the surgeon to rotate the globe superonasally, and the sling can be affixed to the sterile drapes on the contralateral forehead with a hemostat.

Identifying the IO muscle in the inferior temporal quadrant is the next step of surgery. A Conway retractor is used to open the conjunctival incision inferior temporally. A small muscle hook pointed nasally is then used to gently depress the sclera in the inferior temporal quadrant. The Conway retractor is advanced posteriorly as well. Once the equator is reached, the IO muscle, a band of pink tissue traversing the conjunctival side of the incision from the nasal to temporal side, will be visible. Gentle pressure on the Conway retractor inferior and temporally will retract the IO muscle off the globe, and the vortex vein should be visualized temporally, the intermuscular septum posteriorly, and the IO muscle anteriorly within a triangular configuration (Fig. 105-1C). Next, the small muscle hook is rotated such that the tip captures the posterior aspect of the IO muscle and lifts it out of the incision. Care must be taken throughout this step to avoid lacerating the vortex vein, violating the orbital fat, or splitting the IO muscle. Once the muscle is isolated, the traction suture around the LR muscle can be released to allow the eye to return to primary position.

Isolating the IO muscle from the intermuscular septum and orbital fat is next. The region posterior to the IO muscle band is inspected to ensure that the entire muscle is isolated. If there are red fibers coursing in the same direction as the band, a second small muscle hook is used to lift these onto the original small muscle hook. If there is a "white triangle" of connective tissue, the entire IO muscle has been isolated (*see* Fig. 105-1C). Once all of the visible fibers are hooked, the Tenon's capsule and underlying orbital fat is lifted off the tip of muscle hook with serrated tissue forceps (Fig. 105-1D). The small muscle hook tip is exposed with a small incision into intermuscular septum, and a Jameson muscle hook can then be placed laterally to ensure that the IO does not slip. The small muscle hook and Jameson hook can be separated laterally to further isolate the IO muscle from the intermuscular septum and Tenon's capsule. Care must be taken not to pull to greatly on the IO muscle as the nerve to this muscle carries the pupillary fibers for constriction and accommodation. Excessive pulling may lead to damage to the ciliary ganglion.[30]

The next step is determined based on the type of IO procedure being performed, but it is often helpful to use the silk sling to adduct and elevate the eye. This also displaces the LR muscle slightly superior to expose the IO insertion.

## Performing a Tenotomy/Myotomy

A tenotomy has been described by numerous authors for any amount of IO muscle overaction.[3-6] It is roughly equivalent to myotomy or myomectomy, terms used by Dunlap based on arguments that IO muscle did not have a tendon.[28] However, later light microscopy of the IO muscle insertion did show a 1 mm tendon at its insertion to the sclera.[7]

The tenotomy of the IO muscle proceeds from the IO muscle isolation described above. The IO muscle is traced to its scleral insertion, which is located approximately 10–12 mm posterior to the insertion of the LR muscle along the inferior border. The Jameson hook capturing the IO muscle is gently advanced to this location by moving it temporally and bluntly lysing the intermuscular septum. A curved mosquito clamp is applied near the insertion of the IO muscle with the curve away from the sclera. Westcott scissors are utilized to disinsert the tendon from the globe with small snips. Care must be taken to avoid cutting the sclera, LR muscle, and orbital fat. Since the tendon is incised, there should be minimal bleeding, but gentle cautery to the distal IO muscle in the clamp is advised. The tendon and muscle are allowed to retract into the IO muscle sheath.

Once the muscle has been released, an exaggerated traction test is performed to ensure that the entire IO muscle has been tenotomized. Any tightness or "bump" in this test indicates that residual fibers are still inserted on the sclera, and this will result in an undercorrection. If this happens, the steps to the isolate the IO muscle must be repeated to find the residual fibers.

## Performing a Myectomy (At the Insertion)

A myectomy has been described to correct IO muscle overaction associated with horizontal strabismus with and without a V-pattern, unilateral hypertropia, or SO palsy.[1,7,12,13,16]

A myectomy is performed by isolating the muscle as described above. The intermuscular septum attachments are cleaned toward the insertion near the posterior LR muscle by separating the two muscle hooks capturing the IO band. The muscle sheath is then lifted off the muscle and, and it is stripped with blunt Westcott scissors towards the scleral insertion of the muscle. Approximately 8–10 mm of the IO muscle must be exposed. A curved mosquito clamp is placed on the IO muscle near its scleral insertion and a straight mosquito clamp is placed at least 5 mm toward the IO muscle origin. The tissue between the two clamps is excised, and cautery is applied to the cut ends prior to releasing the clamps. The two cuts ends are released and allowed to retract.

An exaggerated traction test is performed to ensure that the entire IO muscle is myectomized. Any residual fibers will promote undercorrection.

## Performing a Recession

A recession of the IO muscle can be performed for the same indications as the tenotomy and myectomy.[14-18] The early

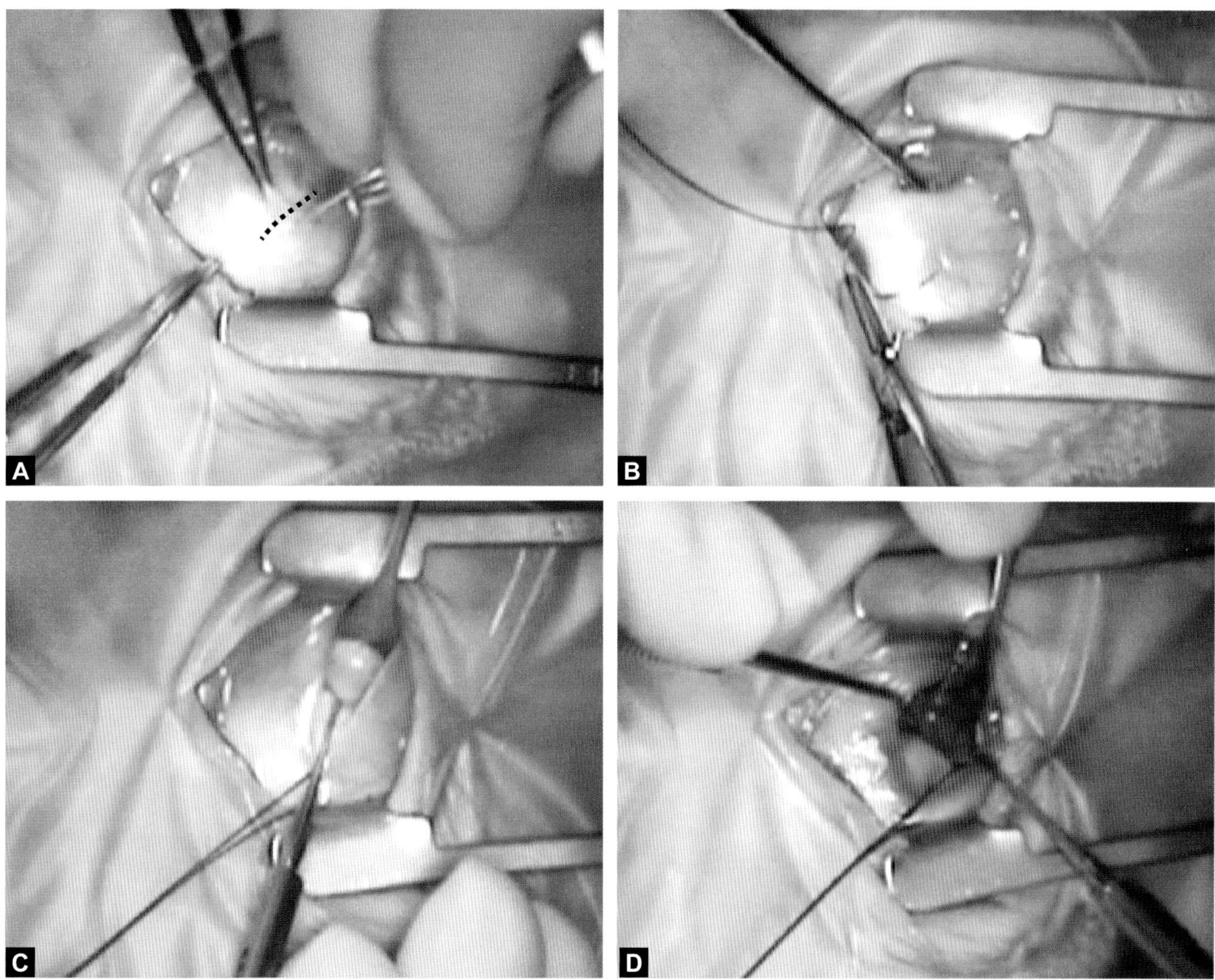


**Figures 105-1A to D** Isolating the inferior oblique muscle of the right eye (surgeon's view). (A) A speculum retracts the eyelids, and the eye is rotated superior nasally with a forcep. A radial 7 mm conjunctival fornix incision is made between the inferior rectus (IR) and lateral rectus (LR) muscles. (B). A Gass muscle hook engages the LR muscle, and a silk suture is passed through the conjunctiva and the hole in the muscle hook. The needle of the silk suture is always pointed away from the globe. Not shown: Once the needle is placed through the hook, it is cut off, and the Gass hook is retracted through the conjunctival incision with the silk suture creating a sling around the LR muscle. (C). A Conway retractor is inserted into the conjunctival incision while the globe is rotated superior nasally using the silk sling around the LR muscle. The sclera is gently depressed using a small hook placed flush against its surface. A pink band of tissue, the inferior oblique (IO) muscle, should be seen coursing nasal to temporal with the intermuscular septum posterior and the vortex vein temporal to it. The small muscle tip is then rotated off the scleral surface to hook this band of tissue. (D) The IO muscle is lifted out of the incision, and the adherent Tenon's capsule is gently lifted off the muscle band with serrated forceps. Care is taken to avoid exposing the underlying fat, which can lead to postoperative fat adherence and restricted motility.

descriptions of IO muscle recession come from White,[18] comments from Dunnington and Berrens in White's 1942 paper,[18] and Berens et al.[14] In these studies, the exact amount of recession is not clearly delineated, but Berens expounds that 3–7 mm of recession is possible. Parks later describes the procedure in detail initially prescribing 8 mm recessions[16,17] and then suggesting graded recessions of 10, 12, and 14 mm.[19,31] There is still considerable debate on graded recession with some surgeons varying their recession based on the amount of IO overaction.[20] For purposes of this chapter and for the ease of execution for novice IO muscle surgeons, this section will focus on a standard 12 mm recession.

A recession of the IO muscle is performed by isolating the IO muscle as described previously and then cleaning the attachments to the intermuscular septum and Tenon's capsule toward the scleral insertion. Separating the two hooks

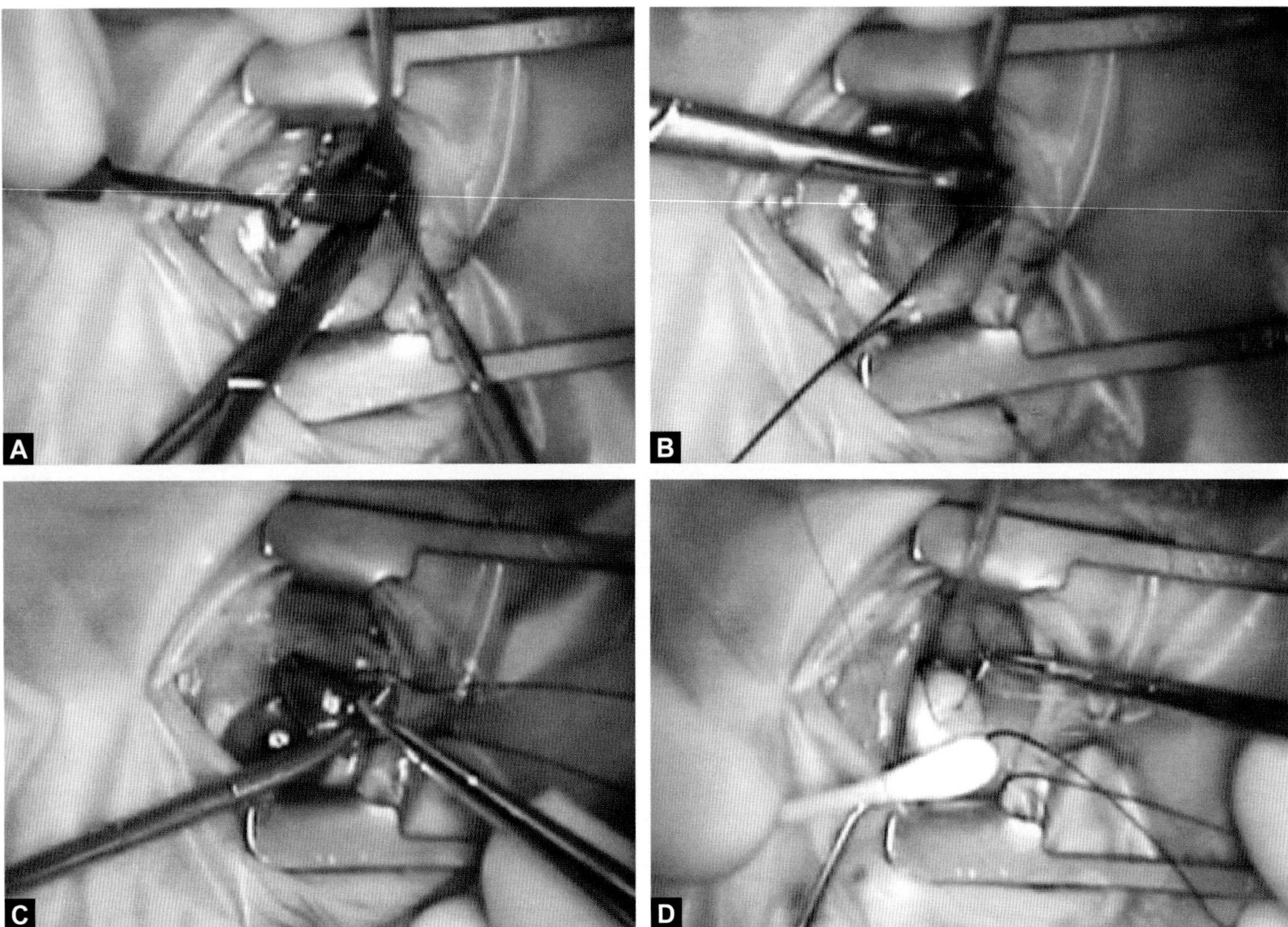


**Figures 105-2A to D** Recession of the inferior oblique (IO) muscle from the surgeon's view of the right eye. (A and B). The IO muscle is clamped near its insertion on the sclera and disinserted. Cautery is applied to cut end (not shown), and a 6-0 polyglactin 910 suture secures the muscle proximal to the clamp. (C). The muscle is secured to the sclera with the anterior nasal pole suture affixed to the sclera 2 mm lateral and 6 mm posterior to the lateral insertion of the inferior rectus muscle. The posterior temporal pole suture is affixed to the sclera posteriorly and temporally such that the IO muscle insertion is splayed across the sclera in its natural orientation (D).

around the IO muscle bluntly dissects the attachments to the muscle sheath and intermuscular septum. A serrated forcep is then used to lift the muscle sheath approximately 5 mm from the insertion, and a small snip of the Westcott scissors is used to expose the muscle. The muscle sheath is then striped with the Westcott scissors to the insertion. Once the entire muscle is exposed distally, a curved mosquito clamp is placed on the IO muscle near its insertion. The muscle is disinserted from the sclera, and the proximal end is cauterized. Care must be taken to avoid cutting the LR muscle and the unexposed orbital fat posteriorly. An exaggerated traction test is performed to confirm that all fibers have been disinserted.

The IO muscle is now sutured back to the sclera with a recessed insertion. A double-armed, 6-0 polyglactin 910 suture on spatulated needles is imbricated across the anterior and posterior two-thirds of the muscle and locked on each end (Fig. 105-2A). The silk traction suture is released allowing the eye to return to primary position, and the IR muscle is hooked. The globe is rotated superiorly without inducing torsion, adduction, or abduction; otherwise, the landmark for grading the recession, which is the lateral border of the IR muscle, will be distorted (Fig. 105-2B). The sclera is marked 6 mm posterior to and 2 mm temporal to the temporal insertion of the IR muscle (Fig. 105-2C). The anterior nasal pole suture of the IO muscle is passed through the sclera at this location, and the pass should follow the natural course of the muscle. The posterior lateral pole suture of the IO muscle is then passed through the sclera at a location posterior temporal to this such that the muscle is splayed appropriately across the globe. The sutures ends are tied, and the pole sutures are cut leaving a 2 mm tail on the muscle (Fig. 105-2D). An exaggerated traction test is repeated to confirm that the IO muscle is reattached to the globe.

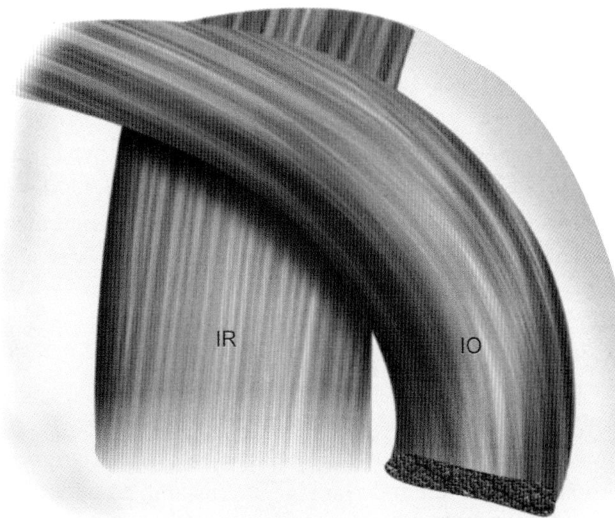


**Figure 105-3** Anterior transposition of the inferior oblique (IO) muscle from the surgeon's view of the right eye. The inferior rectus (IR) muscle is hooked, and the eye is placed in supraduction. The IO muscle is sutured to the sclera at the temporal insertion of the IR muscle. The anterior IO muscle should be kept compact on the sclera.

### Performing an Anterior Transposition

An anterior transposition of the IO muscle is performed for an antielevation effect, and it is most useful in cases of DVD or marked IO muscle overaction from horizontal strabismus or SOP palsy.[21-23] Since this procedure causes marked limitation of elevation in adduction, one should use the procedure unilaterally only if there is a marked asymmetry in IO overaction or DVD.

The approach to the anterior transposition is very similar to the IO mucle recession noted above, but the new insertion of the IO muscle is adjacent to the temporal insertion of the IR muscle (Fig. 105-3). The IO muscle insertion should not be splayed in this location as it will have a more profound antielevation effect. Instead, the pole sutures should be kept close to each other to keep the new insertion of the IO muscle tight. The effect can be enhanced with an IO myectomy as necessary if the overaction or DVD is excessive.[32]

### Closing the Conjunctival Incision

Once the IO muscle surgery is complete, the silk suture sling around the LR muscle is cut on one side and removed. The inferior temporal conjunctival incision is closed with 8-0 polyglactin 910 suture. Care should be taken to remove or reposit any prolapsed Tenon's capsule. Also, if there is any fat exposed, one should close the defect in the Tenon's capsule overlying this fat to decrease the likelihood of fat adherence.

## MECHANISM OF ACTION

The IO muscle weakening procedures work by changing the point of contact to the sclera. The tenotomy and myectomy release the muscle from its scleral insertion, and they permit a freelance recession. These two surgeries are thought to "self-adjust" allowing the muscle or its fascial connections to the IR muscle to guide its residual activity. Recession of the IO muscle performs a similar function. In each of these three surgeries, the recessed point of contact to the globe decreases the extortion and elevation forces of the muscle. This is similar to recessing a rectus muscle; the larger the recession, the weaker the effective force. The anterior transposition of the IO muscle, on the other hand, not only weakens the extortion and elevation forces but also tethers the globe in elevation and adduction preventing full excursion. This tethering occurs because the neurovascular bundle, which joins the IO muscle as it is crossing the IR muscle, is stretched and limits the muscle action in adduction and elevation.[24,33]

## COMPLICATIONS

Intraoperative
- Scleral perforation
- LR or IR muscle damage
  - Hemorrhage
  - Laceration
  - Contusion.
- Orbital fat exposure
- Retrobulbar hemorrhage (from the vortex vein or the muscle itself).

Postoperative (or typically noted postoperatively):
- Submacular hemorrhage
- Pupillary dilation
- Paresis of the ciliary muscle with loss of accommodation
- Orbital cellulitis/infection
- Fat adhesion causing restricted motility.

## SURGICAL OUTCOMES: SCIENTIFIC EVIDENCE

### Tenotomy/Myotomy

Tenotomies are relatively easy and quick surgeries that may be used for any amount of IO overaction.[4-6] Dyer et al. reported its use in 45 eyes (43 patients). All patients had hyperdeviations in primary gaze and an increase in this deviation in adduction of the ipsilateral eye. The hypertropias varied from < 5–40 prism diopters (Δ), and the surgical effect was related directly to the pre-operative overaction of the IO muscle with greater overaction predicting greater effect. Forty-one of the 45 eyes (91%) had a resultant postoperative hypertropia of $<10^{\Delta}$, and he had neither overcorrections nor any reoperations (though the time of follow-up is not reported). Posey[6] and Dunnington[5] also reported good results with this method.

In contrast, a controlled, comparative study by Parks evaluating disinsertion of the IO muscle (loosely similar to Dyer's tenotomy) to other IO weakening procedures showed approximately 53% recurrence of IO muscle overaction and only 43% resolution of the IO overaction.[16] Moreover, Dunlap argued that tenotomy is unpredictable, though he did not provide any data to back his claim.[28]

## Myectomy

Myectomy is another relatively quick surgery to weaken the IO muscle.[7] Davis et al. reported their experience with 130 surgeries in 81 patients. They included patients with IO muscle overaction in horizontal strabismus with or without a V-pattern, unilateral hypertropia of $<10^{\Delta}$, and unilateral fourth nerve palsy. All IO overaction was graded as 3+ or greater (0 is normal and 4+ is $25^{\Delta}$ or more). The surgeries resulted in resolution of the IO overaction in 119 of 130 (91%), residual overaction in 6 (5%), and underaction (overcorrection) in 4 (3%). There were no cases of induced vertical deviations in primary position.

In contrast to the high success rate reported by Davis et al., both Harcourt and Parks had less success. Harcourt et al. noted good efficacy of the procedure in 68%, residual overaction in 12.2%, and underaction (or overcorrection) in 19.9%.[12] Parks' comparative study examined myectomy versus recession, and he took all comers with IO overaction (slight, moderate, and marked). He found that the myectomy resulted in resolution of IO overaction in 49%, residual overaction in 37%, underaction in 8%, and primary position hypotropia in 6%.[16] Parks, however, used an 8 mm myectomy, in comparison to the 5 mm done by Harcourt and Freedman and Davis et al.; thus, it may not be fair to compare the results.

## Recession

Recession of the IO muscle adds complexity but the results have been studied systematically.[16] Parks performed the surgery on 444 cases of "slight, moderate, and marked" IO overaction, and he showed that 81% of surgeries resulted in resolution of the overaction, 15% resulted in residual overaction, and 4% resulted in underaction. The merits of IO recession have also been touted to correct the lateral incomitance of hyperdeviations in unilateral SO palsy,[34] a finding not so unexpected given Parks' findings. Others have shown that IO recession is "self-adjusting" in SO palsy patients,[35,36] as has been claimed with myectomy. However, at least one study shows that a primary position hypertropia of $<15^{\Delta}$ is more consistently corrected with myectomy as opposed to recession even though all other measurements such as diplopia and overaction in adduction were equivalent between the two subsets.[37]

## Anterior Transposition

Anterior transposition moves the contact point of the IO muscle anteriorly to provide an antielevation effect. Originally proposed by Elliott and Nankin,[21] Mims and Wood showed its efficacy in children with infantile esotropia, who are prone to developing DVD.[33] They placed the insertion of the IO muscle 2 mm anterior to the lateral border of the IR muscle insertion instead of at the insertion itself, as is described above and advocated by Parks[16] and Elliott and Nankin.[21] With this slight modification, Mims and Wood showed that only 1 child developed DVD requiring further surgery out of 61 children undergoing infantile esotropia surgery and IO overaction surgery treated with concurrent IO anterior transposition. This was in contrast to a group of 60 children with a similar condition but no anterior transposition of the IO muscle; of these, 9 children developed DVD later requiring further surgery. Thus, there seemed to be a prophylactic effect against development of DVD in the children treated with IO anterior transposition. Second, they identified significant reduction in DVD in 9 patients who had DVD ranging from $8^{\Delta}$ to $25^{\Delta}$ with the anterior transposition. They followed all of these patients slightly over 2 years.

# PLACE OF THE TECHNIQUE IN SURGICAL ARMAMENTARIUM

There are many methods to weaken the IO muscle, and the most common techniques are described above. Unfortunately, even master strabismus surgeons differ vastly in their choice of surgery in each case. Thus, for the beginning strabismus surgeon, the following guidelines may be useful.

The tenotomy procedure is quick, easy, and bloodless, but it has fallen out of favor because of its unpredictable nature despite Dyer's results.[4] It is better to avoid this procedure.

The myectomy is a fast, effective weakening procedure that can have a large effect. The concern is that profound weakening or paralysis of IO muscle function may occur without ability to reoperate on the IO muscle and reverse the effect. Thus, this technique may be best utilized in instances where there is $\geq 10^{\Delta}$ of hyperphoria or -tropia in primary position, $\geq$ 3+ IO overaction (defined as 0 being normal and 4+ being severe overaction with $25^{\Delta}$ of hypertropia), or 3- to 4- SO underaction (again defined as 0 being normal and 4- being severe underaction). If the patient has a congenital strabismus, it may be wise to avoid this procedure since the IO muscle will not be amenable to anteriorization in future to correct DVD.

The recession is a slightly more complicated procedure that has a lower rate of overcorrection. The advantage of this technique is that the muscle may be found at the surgeon's prescribed location in the future for additional weakening procedures or anteriorization should DVD result. The recession can be used for hyperphorias and -tropias of $<10^{\Delta}$ in primary position, 2-3+ IO overactions, or 1- to 2- SO underactions.

The anteriorization procedure is most effective in limiting elevation of the eye in adduction. It has a profound effect and should be used unilaterally with pause. Thus, it is best reserved for cases of bilateral DVD or IO overaction.

## PEARLS AND PITFALLS

- Careful dissection in the inferior temporal quadrant is necessary to isolate the IO muscle easily and visualize it quickly.
- Damaging the vortex vein, LR, IR, or IO muscles can cause significant bleeding making isolation of the IO muscle difficult.
- Creating an inadvertent hole in the Tenon's capsule posteriorly will allow orbital fat prolapse, which leads to restricted motility in the future from adhesions. This should be corrected when it occurs.
- An exaggerated traction test is useful before and during IO muscle surgery to ensure that the entire muscle has been isolated. Once the IO muscle is disinserted, this test should confirm no IO muscle attachment.

## REFERENCES


1. Rubinstein K, Dixon J. Myectomy of the inferior oblique; report on 100 cases. Br J Ophthalmol. 1959;43(1):21-8.
2. White JW. Paralysis of the superior rectus muscle. Trans Am Ophthalmol Soc. 1933;31:551-84.
3. Brown HW. Surgery of the oblique muscles. In Allen JH (ed.), Strabismus ophthalmic symposium (I). St. Louis: The C. V. Mosby Company; 1950. pp. 401-22.
4. Dyer JA. Tenotomy of the inferior oblique muscle at its scleral insertion. An easy and effective procedure. Arch Ophthalmol. 1962;68:176-81.
5. Dunnington JH. Tenotomy of the inferior oblique. Trans Am Ophthalmol Soc. 1929;27:277-96.
6. Posey WC. Tenotomy of the inferior oblique muscle. Trans Am Ophthalmol Soc. 1915;14(Pt 1):65-88.
7. Davis G, McNeer KW, Spencer RF. Myectomy of the inferior oblique muscle. Arch Ophthalmol. 1986;104(6):855-8.
8. McNeer KW, Scott AB, Jampolsky A. A technique for surgically weakening the inferior oblique muscle. Arch Ophthalmol. 1965;73:87-8.
9. Loutfallah M. The surgery of the inferior oblique muscle. Part III. Presentation of cases, comment, conclusions. Eye Ear Nose Throat Mon. 1950;29(12):678-86.
10. Loutfallah M. The surgery of the inferior oblique muscle. II Surgical anatomy and operative techniques. Eye Ear Nose Throat Mon. 1950;29(11):613-21.
11. Loutfallah M. The surgery of the inferior oblique muscle; clinical physiology and operative indications. Eye Ear Nose Throat Mon. 1950;29(10):543-50.
12. Harcourt BAS, Freedman H. The efficacy of inferior oblique myectomy. Orthoptics, Research and Practice: Transactions of the Fourth International Congress. London: Henry Kimpton Publishers; 1981.
13. Schlossman A. Surgery of the inferior oblique. Eye Ear Nose Throat Mon. 1955;34(5):328-9.
14. Berens C, Cole HG, Chamichian S, et al. Retroplacement of the inferior oblique at its scleral insertion. Am J Ophthalmol. 1952; 35(2):217-27.
15. Benedict WL (ed.). Recession of the Inferior Oblique Muscle. In: Society Transactions, New York Academy of Medicine, Section of Ophthalmology. Arch Ophthalmol. 1943;1033-38.
16. Parks MM. A study of the weakening surgical procedures for eliminating overaction of the inferior oblique. Trans Am Ophthalmol Soc. 1971;69:163-87.
17. Parks MM. The weakening surgical procedures for eliminating overaction of the inferior oblique muscle. Am J Ophthalmol. 1972;73(1):107-22.
18. White JW. Surgery of the inferior oblique at or near the insertion. Trans Am Ophthalmol Soc. 1942;40:118-26.
19. Parks MM. Atlas of Strabismus Surgery. Philadelphia: Harper & Row; 1983.
20. Plager DA. Inferior oblique overaction. In: Plager DA (ed.), Strabismus Surgery: Basic and Advanced Strategies. New York: Oxford University Press, Inc.; 2004. pp. 40-5.
21. Elliott RL, Nankin SJ. Anterior transposition of the inferior oblique. J Pediatr Ophthalmol Strabismus. 1981;18(3):35-8.
22. Farvardin M, Nazarpoor S. Anterior transposition of the inferior oblique muscle for treatment of superior oblique palsy. J Pediatr Ophthalmol Strabismus. 2002;39(2):100-4.
23. Jiffer AJ, Isenberg SJ, Elliott RL, et al. The effect of anterior transposition of the inferior oblique muscle. Am J Ophthalmol. 1993;116(2):224-7.
24. Stager DR. Costenbader lecture. Anatomy and surgery of the inferior oblique muscle: recent findings. J AAPOS. 2001;5(4): 203-8.

25. Stager DR, Sr., Beauchamp GR, Stager, Jr. DR. Anterior and nasal transposition of the inferior oblique muscle: a preliminary case report on a new procedure. Binocul Vis Strabismus Q. 2001;16(1):43-4.
26. Stager DR, Beauchamp GR, Wright WW, et al. Anterior and nasal transposition of the inferior oblique muscles. J Am Assoc Pediatr Ophthalmol Strabismus. 2003;7(3):167-73.
27. Del Monte MA, Parks MM. Denervation and extirpation of the inferior oblique. An improved weakening procedure for marked overaction. Ophthalmology. 1983;90(10):1178-85.
28. Dunlap EA. Selection of operative procedures in vertical muscle deviations. Arch Ophthalmol. 1960;64:167-74.
29. Guyton DL. Exaggerated traction test for the oblique muscles. Ophthalmology. 1981;88(10):1035-40.
30. Bajart AM, Robb RM. Internal ophthalmoplegia following inferior oblique myectomy: a report of three cases. Ophthalmology. 1979;86(8):1401-6.
31. McKeown CA, Cavuoto K, Morris R. Inferior Oblique Surgery. In: CS Hoyt, D Taylor (eds), Chapter 85: Strabismus Surgery, Pediatric Ophthalmology and Strabismus.
32. Snir M, Axer-Siegel R, Cotlear D, et al. Combined resection and anterior transposition of the inferior oblique muscle for asymmetric double dissociated vertical deviation. Ophthalmology. 1999;106(12):2372-6.
33. Mims JL 3rd, Wood RC. Bilateral anterior transposition of the inferior obliques. Arch Ophthalmol. 1989;107(1):41-4.
34. Hendler K, Pineles SL, Demer JL, et al. Does inferior oblique recession cause overcorrections in laterally incomitant small hypertropias due to superior oblique palsy? Br J Ophthalmol. 2013;97(1):88-91.
35. Shipman T, Burke J. Unilateral inferior oblique muscle myectomy and recession in the treatment of inferior oblique muscle overaction: a longitudinal study. Eye (Lond). 2003;17(9):1013-8.
36. Yoo JH, Kim SH, Seo JW, et al. Self-grading effect of inferior oblique recession. J Pediatr Ophthalmol Strabismus. 2013; 50(2):102-5.
37. Bahl RS, Marcotty A, Rychwalski PJ, et al. Comparison of inferior oblique myectomy to recession for the treatment of superior oblique palsy. Br J Ophthalmol. 2013;97(2):184-8.

CHAPTER

# 106

# Superior Oblique Surgery

Christopher M Fecarotta, Jonathan H Salvin

## INTRODUCTION

Marshall Parks once referred to dysfunction of the oblique muscles as "the last bastion of motility disorders to be conquered".[1] The superior oblique muscle was the "chief offender" and had famously been labeled in the 19th century by von Graefe as a *noli me tangere* (never to be touched).[2] In 1946, Berke described a procedure where a muscle hook was blindly used in the sub-Tenon's space to engage the superior oblique and pull it into view.[3] This procedure was frequently complicated by hemorrhage after disruption of the vortex vein, adherence syndrome after rupturing Tenon's capsule and permanent ptosis. In 1970, Parks described his technique of directly visualizing the superior oblique insertion temporal to the superior rectus and reflecting the conjunctiva nasally to access the tendon.[4] Widespread acceptance of direct visualization has made superior oblique surgery much safer and both weakening and strengthening procedures are performed regularly today.

## INDICATIONS

### Weakening Procedures

- Superior oblique tenotomy, posterior tenectomy, suture elongation (chicken suture) and expander placement are effective treatments for patients with superior oblique overaction associated with Brown syndrome, A-pattern strabismus and inferior oblique palsy.[5]
- Superior oblique myokymia has also been treated effectively with weakening procedures.[6]
- Other less commonly used procedures to weaken an overacting superior oblique include superior oblique recession, split tendon lengthening and Z-tenotomy.

### Strengthening Procedures

- Superior oblique tucks work well for patients that exhibit superior oblique underaction without inferior oblique overaction.
- Superior oblique tucks are also effective for congenital superior oblique palsies with a lax tendon on forced duction testing.[7]
- The Harada-Ito is the procedure of choice in patients with only symptomatic excyclotorsional diplopia but no significant vertical deviation.[8]

## CONTRAINDICATIONS

### Weakening Procedures

Bifoveal fixation is a relative contraindication, as intractable torsional diplopia from induced excyclotorsion can result.[9] Posterior tenectomy can be carefully performed in bifoveal fixators, as the anterior fibers, which control torsion, are left undisturbed in this procedure.

### Strengthening Procedures

Previous surgery on the superior oblique muscle can make strengthening procedures very difficult to perform due to scarring.

## SURGICAL TECHNIQUE FOR WEAKENING PROCEDURES

Superior oblique weakening procedures usually are performed nasal to the superior rectus muscle through a conjunctival incision approximately 8 mm posterior to the limbus at the nasal border of the superior rectus muscle.[4] Forced duction testing of the superior oblique tendon should be performed

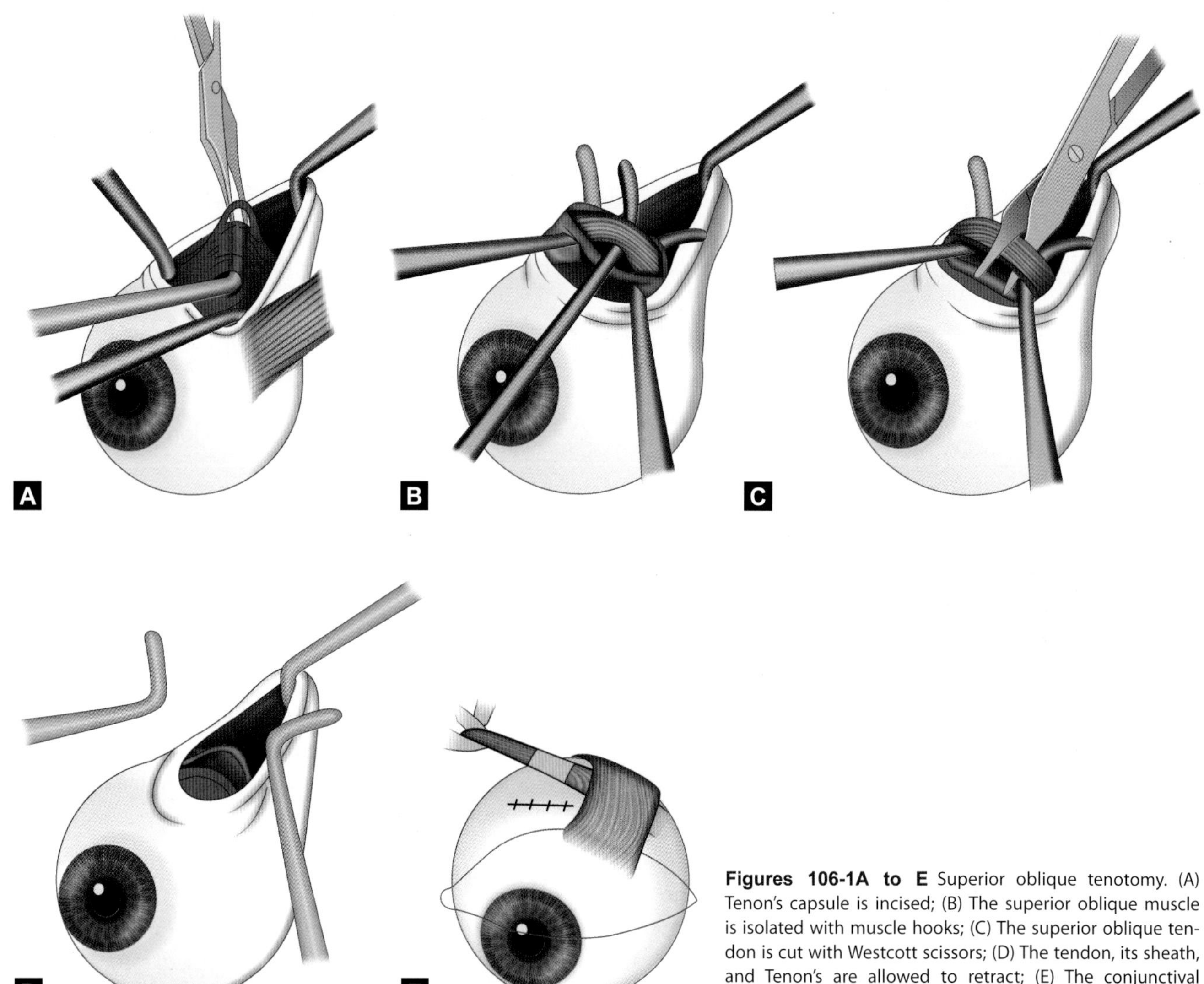

**Figures 106-1A to E** Superior oblique tenotomy. (A) Tenon's capsule is incised; (B) The superior oblique muscle is isolated with muscle hooks; (C) The superior oblique tendon is cut with Westcott scissors; (D) The tendon, its sheath, and Tenon's are allowed to retract; (E) The conjunctival wound is closed.

before beginning the procedure.[10] Tenon's capsule is incised after the conjunctival incision and the superior rectus muscle is isolated with a muscle hook. Tenon's and conjunctiva are then reflected temporally across the superior rectus insertion, leaving the intermuscular septum intact. A Desmarres retractor is then placed along the nasal border of the superior rectus and the superior oblique tendon with its fascial sheath can be directly visualized. A small incision is then made over the fascial sheath and the superior oblique muscle is hooked with two small Stevens hooks. The surgeon can then proceed with the preferred weakening procedure. Once the weakening procedure has been performed, forced duction testing should be repeated prior to completion of the procedure to confirm the desired anatomic effect.[10] The conjunctiva should then be closed with the surgeon's preferred suture.

*Tenotomy*: The superior oblique tendon is cut in between the two Stevens hooks and allowed to retract. It is important to sever the entire tendon, as incomplete tenotomy is a common cause of residual superior oblique overaction[11] (Figs. 106-1A to E).

*Tenectomy*: The superior oblique tendon is followed nasally, beneath the superior rectus. Two hemostats are placed across the tendon and the portion between the hemostats is removed.[5]

*Suture elongation (chicken suture)*: This procedure involves using a suture to connect the two ends of a tenotomized superior oblique, in case future surgery is necessary. After isolation of the superior oblique tendon, a nonabsorbable suture is placed through the proximal end. A loop is created and a similar pass is made 2–3 mm distal to the first suture. The tendon is then cut in between the two sutures, and both

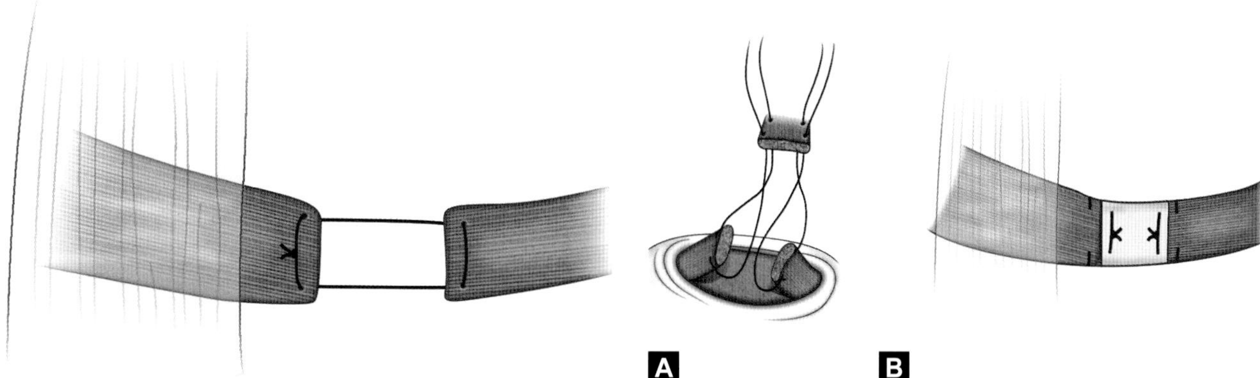


**Figure 106-2** The appearance of the weakened superior oblique tendon after the suture elongation ("chicken suture") procedure.

**Figures 106-3A and B** Wright procedure. (A) Appearance of the superior oblique before tying down the silicon band; (B) Final appearance of the weakened superior oblique tendon after performing an expander placement procedure.

suture and superior oblique are allowed to retract. Sutures can be tied on a temporary basis and adjusted if necessary to match the desired forced ductions[5] (Fig. 106-2).

*Expander placement (Wright procedure)*: This procedure allows a controlled lengthening of the superior oblique tendon, so the amount of weakening can be titrated based on the amount needed. A nonabsorbable double-armed suture is placed in the superior oblique tendon 3 mm nasal to the superior rectus muscle with locking bites on both anterior and posterior ends. Another nonabsorbable double-armed suture is placed in the superior oblique tendon 2 mm nasal to the first suture. The tendon is then cut in between the two sutures. A 240 or 40 retinal band, presoaked in antibiotic, is then measured to the desired length, generally between 4 mm and 7 mm depending on the clinical overaction of the superior oblique seen and forced duction testing. The double-armed sutures in the superior oblique tendon are sutured to the ends of the band. The sutures are trimmed and both tendon capsule and conjunctiva are closed with the surgeon's preferred suture[11] (Figs. 106-3A and B).

## SURGICAL TECHNIQUE FOR STRENGTHENING PROCEDURES

The technique to access the superior oblique tendon is similar to that described above for weakening procedures; however, most strengthening procedures are performed temporal to the superior rectus. Forced duction testing of the superior oblique tendon should be performed before beginning the procedure. A conjunctival incision is made approximately 10 mm behind the limbus temporal to the border of the superior rectus. Tenon's capsule is incised and the superior rectus muscle is isolated with a muscle hook. Tenon's and conjunctiva are then reflected nasally across the superior rectus insertion, leaving the intermuscular septum intact. A Desmarres retractor is then placed along the temporal border of the superior rectus and the superior oblique tendon with its fascial sheath can be directly visualized. A small incision is then made over the fascial sheath and the superior oblique muscle is hooked with two small Stevens hooks. Some surgeons prefer to pass a 5-0 nylon or silk suture under the tendon, the needle is removed, and the suture is then passed under the superior oblique tendon to the temporal side of the superior rectus. This maneuver ensures that the entire superior oblique tendon insertion is included in the chosen procedure. The surgeon can then proceed with the preferred strengthening procedure. The conjunctiva should then be closed with the surgeon's preferred suture.

*Superior oblique tuck*: Using either a muscle hook or a tendon tucker, the superior oblique tendon is lifted temporal to the superior rectus and the desired amount of tuck is measured with a caliper. The total amount of tuck depends on the amount of slack felt on forced duction testing. The tendon is folded on itself, so only half the amount of the desired tuck length should be used when measuring. Mattress sutures are then placed to suture the folded tendon to itself. These sutures are tied with releasable slipped knots. Once the tuck has been performed, forced duction testing should be repeated to confirm the desired anatomic effect. Once the desired affect is achieved, the slip knots are tied permanently. The surgeon should take care to avoid excessive tightening, as an induced Brown syndrome can result[11] (Figs. 106-4A to F).

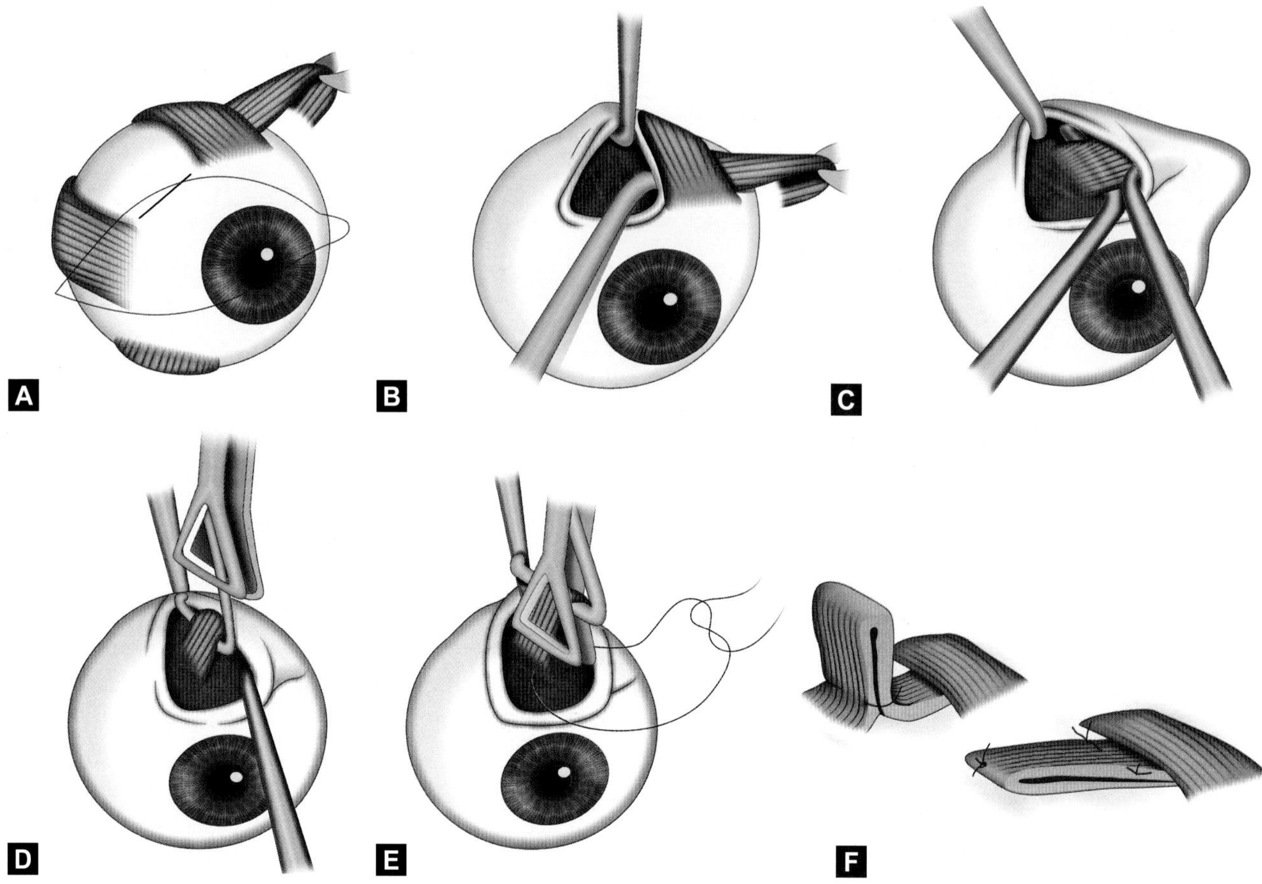


**Figures 106-4A to F** Superior oblique tuck. (A) The superior oblique passing through the trochlea and underneath the superior rectus; (B) Reflection of conjunctiva and Tenon's capsule and isolation of the superior rectus; (C) Isolation of the superior oblique tendon; (D) Engagement of the superior oblique with the tendon tucker; (E) Mattress sutures placed in the folded tendon; (F) Final appearance of the tucked superior oblique tendon.

*Harada-Ito*: The incision is extended temporally in a circumferential direction. The superior oblique tendon sheath is incised and attachments to the superior rectus muscle are severed. Westcott scissors are used to split the tendon lengthwise approximately 5 mm from the anterior edge. This split is extended to the midportion of the superior rectus. A double-armed 6-0 suture is then placed with locking bites on both ends of the anterior portion of the tendon. The anterior fibers are then disinserted from the globe. Muscle hooks are used to isolate the lateral rectus muscle and the superior border is directly visualized. The anterior fibers of the superior oblique tendon are then transposed approximately 8 mm posterior to the lateral rectus and directly superior to its border[5] (Figs. 106-5A to D).

## POSTOPERATIVE CARE

After the procedure, the surgeon should place combination antibiotic/steroid drops or ointment in the conjunctival fornix of the operated eye. Some surgeons also place povidone-iodine and topical anesthetic for immediate postoperative comfort. There is no need to place a patch over the operative eye. Postoperative nausea and vomiting are common after strabismus surgery and should be managed with the help of an anesthesiologist. Oral intake should be advanced slowly.

Some surgeons choose to put patients on topical antibiotic/steroid drops or ointment after surgery, while others do not. Most surgeons advise their patients to avoid swimming or head submersion for at least 1 week after strabismus surgery, but shower and gentle cleaning around the eye are allowed. Eye rubbing should be discouraged as much as possible. The first postoperative visit should be within 1 week after surgery and the patient and/or parents should know the signs and symptoms of infection. Foreign body sensation, injection, subconjunctival hemorrhage, blood-tinged tears, eyelid crusting, mild discomfort and blurry vision are all normal in the first few days after strabismus surgery.

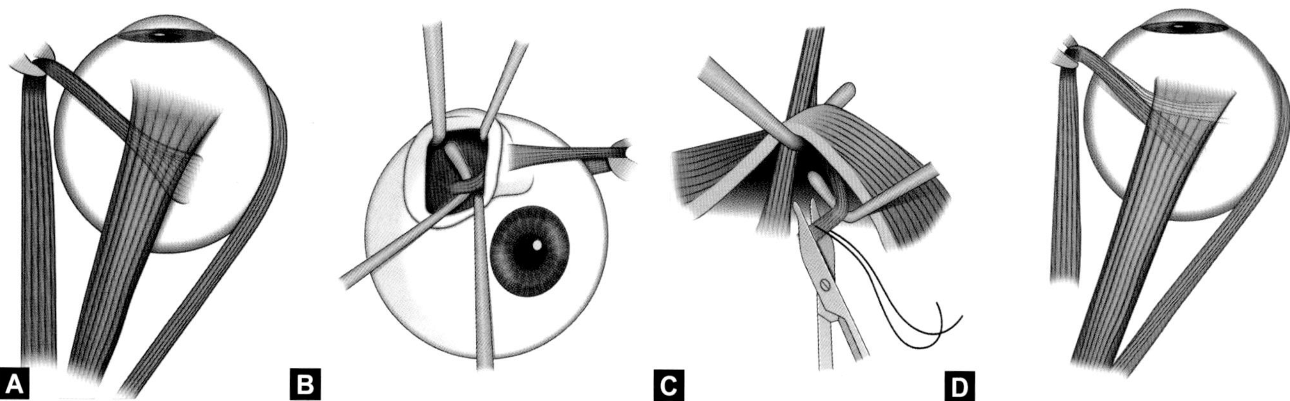


**Figures 106-5A to D** The Harada-Ito procedure. (A) Appearance of the superior oblique tendon as it courses through the trochlea and underneath the superior rectus muscle; (B) Isolation of the superior rectus and superior oblique tendon; (C) Suture placement in the anterior fibers and removal from the globe with Westcott scissors (D) Final appearance of the transposed anterior fibers of the superior oblique tendon after the Harada-Ito procedure.

## COMPLICATIONS

All strabismus surgeries carry a risk of over- or undercorrection, orbital cellulitis, a lost or slipped muscle and endophthalmitis. Any strabismus surgery that involves scleral sutures carries a risk of retinal tear or detachment if the globe is inadvertently punctured. Superior oblique surgeries carry an added risk of excessive bleeding from rupture of a vortex vein. Excessive fibrosis, restriction, lid edema and ptosis can occur if the surgeon excessively dissects in the superior fornix and fat adherence syndrome results from inadvertent posterior violation of Tenon's capsule. Each superior oblique weakening and strengthening procedure has the potential for other unique complications.

### Weakening Procedures

The most common complication of superior oblique weakening procedures is residual superior oblique overaction (undercorrection) from failure to completely identify the entire tendon.[9,12] This complication can be avoided by performing traction testing on the superior oblique at the end of surgery prior to waking the patient from anesthesia and adjusting the procedure as necessary. Symptomatic superior oblique palsy (overcorrection) is another common complication after a weakening procedure.[13,14] Intractable excyclotorsional diplopia is the presenting symptom and can occur up to 2 years after the procedure. Some surgeons choose to simultaneously weaken the inferior oblique muscles, but this option does not eliminate the possibility of superior oblique palsy. Placement of an expander allows the surgeon to return for an adjustment if an over- or undercorrection occurs. If the underside of the superior oblique capsule is violated, the expander can scar directly to the sclera and cause a downgaze restriction. Other complications of expander placement include discomfort in the superior fornix and a small chance of extrusion.

### Strengthening Procedures

An excessively tight tuck can cause an iatrogenic Brown syndrome and an inability to elevate in adduction.[15,16] This complication can be avoided by carefully performing a traction test of the superior oblique after the tuck and adjusting to match the forced ductions if necessary. The tendon should be mildly tight at the end of the procedure, but the surgeon should relieve excessive tightness if present. If a significant Brown syndrome occurs postoperatively, the surgeon should bring the patient back to the operating room in the immediate postoperative period to revise the tuck. Undercorrection and residual superior oblique underaction can also occur if the tuck is not large enough. Rarely, a Harada-Ito procedure can also cause an iatrogenic Brown syndrome.[17,18]

## PLACE IN SURGICAL ARMAMENTARIUM

Superior oblique procedures are an important part of any strabismologist's armamentarium. Many forms of ocular misalignment will not resolve without addressing under- or overaction of the superior oblique. Such forms of strabismus include A-pattern with superior oblique overaction, Brown syndrome and large symptomatic excyclotorsion from bilateral superior oblique palsies. Advances in surgical technique and careful planning have minimized the risk of disastrous complications that previously plagued attempts to alter the superior oblique and as Marshall Parks said, the superior oblique is "no longer a *noli me tangere*".

## PEARLS AND PITFALLS

- The actions of the superior oblique include incyclotorsion, depression and abduction. Superior oblique surgeries either weaken or strengthen the action of the muscle and choice of procedure depends on whether the muscle is overacting or underacting.
- Procedures on the superior oblique should be performed cautiously, as proper identification of the surgical anatomy may be difficult for a surgeon without superior oblique experience.
- The most common complications from superior oblique procedures include residual under- or overaction. Other significant complications include bleeding from a ruptured vortex vein, fibrosis from excessive dissection and fat adherence from inadvertent posterior violation of Tenon's capsule.
- Superior oblique weakening procedures include tenotomy, posterior tenectomy, suture elongation and spacer placement. Weakening procedures should be cautiously performed in patients with high-grade stereopsis, as debilitating excyclotorsional diplopia may result.
- Strengthening procedures include the tuck and Harada-Ito. Overcorrection with a strengthening procedure can lead to iatrogenic Brown syndrome, which should be corrected in the immediate postoperative period if present.
- The surgeon should perform intraoperative superior oblique traction testing, as described by Guyton,[19] at the beginning and end of any procedure on the superior oblique. This technique will minimize the risk of incomplete identification of the entire superior oblique tendon during a weakening procedure or an excessively tight tendon after a strengthening procedure.

## REFERENCES

1. Plager DA (Ed). Strabismus Surgery: Basic and Advanced Strategies—the American Academy of Ophthalmology Monographs 17. New York: Oxford University Press; 2004. p. 51.
2. McGuire WP. Present concepts of surgery of the superior oblique muscle. Am J Ophthalmol. 1953;36:1237-41.
3. Berke RN. Tenotomy of the superior oblique muscle for hypertropia. Arch Ophthal. 1947;38:605-44.
4. Parks MM, Helveston EM. Direct visualization of the superior oblique tendon. Arch Ophthalmol. 1970;84:491-4.
5. Lozano MJ, Rosenbaum AL, Santiago AP. Superior oblique procedures. In: Rosenbaum AL, Santiago AP (Eds). Clinical Strabismus Management: Principles and Surgical Techniques. Philadelphia: WB Saunders Company; 1999. pp. 459-75.
6. Brazis PW, Miller NR, Henderer JD, et al. The natural history and results of treatment of superior oblique myokymia. Arch Ophthalmol. 1994;112:1063-7.
7. Plager DA. Tendon laxity in superior oblique palsy. Ophthalmology. 1992;99:1032-8.
8. Finkelman SG, Mazow ML. Surgical management of excyclotorsion. Am Orthopt J. 1991;41:81.
9. Parks MM. Management of overacting superior oblique muscles. Trans New Orleans Acad Ophthalmol. 1986;34:409-18.
10. Plager DA. Traction testing in superior oblique palsy. J Pediatr Ophthalmol Strabismus. 1990;27:136-40.
11. Wright KW. Color Atlas of Strabismus Surgery: Strategies and Techniques, 2nd edition. Torrance, CA: Wright Publishing; 2000. pp. 205-14.
12. Frey T. Isolated paresis of the inferior oblique. Ophthalmic Surg. 1982;13:936-8.
13. Crawford JS, Orton RB, Labow-Daily L. Late results of superior oblique muscle tenotomy in true Brown's syndrome. Am J Ophthalmol. 1980;89:824-9.
14. Eustis HS, O'Reilly C, Crawford JS. Management of superior oblique palsy after surgery for true Brown's syndrome. J Pediatr Ophthalmol Strabismus. 1987;24:10-6.
15. Morris RJ, Scott WE, Keech RV. Superior oblique tuck surgery in the management of superior oblique palsies. J Pediatr Ophthalmol Strabismus. 1992;29:337-46.
16. Saunders RA. Treatment of superior oblique palsy with superior oblique tendon tuck and inferior oblique muscle myectomy. Ophthalmology. 1986;93:1023-7.
17. Elsas FJ. Vertical effect of the adjustable Harada-Ito procedure. J Pediatr Ophthalmol Strabismus. 1988;25:164-6.
18. Ohtsuki H, Hasebe S, Hanabusa K, et al. Intraoperative adjustable suture surgery for bilateral superior oblique palsy. Ophthalmology. 1994;101:188-93.
19. Guyton DL. Exaggerated traction test for the superior oblique muscles. Ophthalmology. 1981;88(10):1035-40.

CHAPTER

# 107

# Adjustable Sutures

Bharti Nihalani-Gangwani

## INTRODUCTION

Strabismus is an enigma, an ocular misalignment caused by loss of central control of binocular alignment. There is no way to reprogram the brain to align the eyes, instead we treat this neurological problem with eye muscle surgery. This may be one of the major reasons for unpredictable outcomes after strabismus surgery. In the quest to improve the outcomes of strabismus surgery, an approach that allowed adjustment in the early postoperative period was developed. The concept of having a "second chance" to change the position of the eye after initial surgery is very appealing to many surgeons. Most published studies have shown better short-term success rates when using adjustable sutures versus conventional sutures in strabismus surgery. Newer modifications of adjustable sutures allow delayed adjustment and provide an option of "no adjustment" in children and adults with satisfactory alignment in the postoperative recovery period. Improved outcomes combined with increased options in surgical technique make adjustable sutures, an attractive option, even in children.

Adjustable suture strabismus surgery was first described by Bielschowsky in the German literature in 1907.[1] The first modern account of adjustable sutures was presented by Jampolsky in 1975.[2] The basic principle of the adjustable suture technique is to secure the extraocular muscle to the sclera using a temporary or a sliding knot. After the patient has recovered from anesthesia, the alignment of the eyes is checked. The length of the suture between the attachment site and muscle may be shortened or lengthened to fine tune the alignment in an awake cooperative patient or under brief sedation patient.

This chapter discusses various aspects of adjustable suture strabismus surgery.

## INDICATIONS

- Restrictive strabismus (thyroid ophthalmopathy, scleral buckle)
- Previous surgery or trauma
- Slipped, lost or disinserted muscles
- Incomitant deviations (Duane syndrome, Moebius syndrome, myasthenia gravis or paralytic strabismus)
- Any long-standing complex strabismus
- Combined horizontal, vertical and torsional deviations.

The ideal candidates for adjustable sutures are patients in whom standard strabismus surgical dosages do not apply. They are particularly useful in patients with risk of postoperative diplopia. Tripathi et al.[3] suggested that adjustable sutures can be used in virtually all types of patients who can cooperate.

"Q-tip" test can be used to identify patients who will cooperate for the adjustment procedure. The test consists of touching a Q-tip or a twirled tissue end to the medial and/or lateral aspect of the unanesthetized bulbar conjunctiva. If the patient is able to tolerate this manipulation, then he or she should be able to tolerate the adjustment procedure.

## ANESTHESIA AND ANALGESIA

Adjustable suture surgery can be performed under general or local anesthesia depending on the surgeon's preference.

### General Anesthesia

General anesthesia is preferred as it allows for assessment of the position of the eyes under anesthesia,[4] forced duction testing without any concern of discomfort and earlier suture adjustment on the day of surgery. Induction with intravenous propofol and maintenance with short-acting intravenous

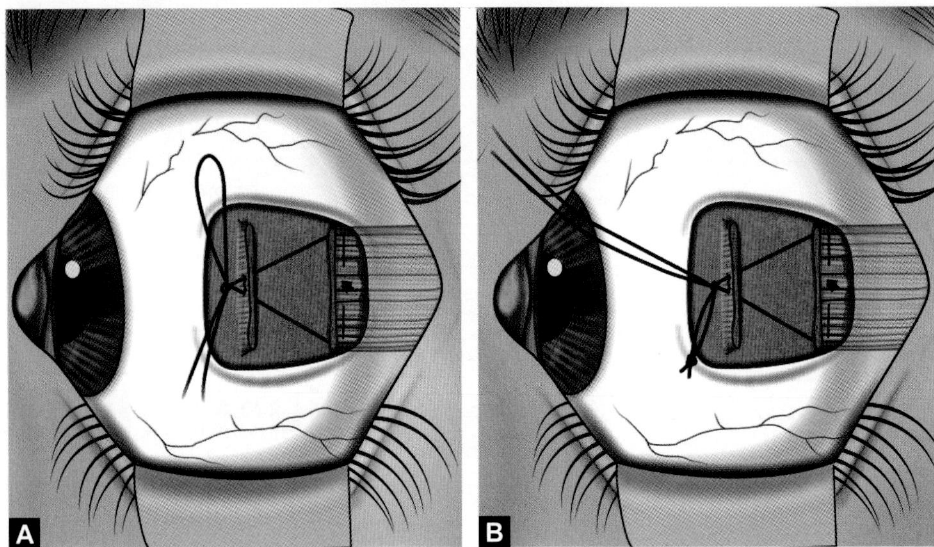


**Figures 107-1A and B** (A) Bow tie technique: the sutures are tied together in a bow tie like a shoelace; (B) Sliding noose technique: a noose is created by tying a separate piece of suture around the pole sutures.

agents, such as propofol or dexmedetomidine, is recommended.[5] Premedication with anticholinergics, anxiolytics and antiemetics is preferred. Long-acting muscle relaxants should be avoided as they may interfere with postoperative adjustment. It is important to avoid older inhalational anesthestics, such as isoflurane and halothane, as they cause postoperative nausea, vomiting and more sedation, which make accurate postoperative examination nearly impossible. Narcotics, such as morphine and opoid analgesics, should be avoided owing to the risk of postoperative nausea and vomiting.[6]

### Local Anesthesia

Local anesthesia may be used in patients in whom general anesthesia is contraindicated or in ambulatory settings that do not allow for general anesthesia. When local anesthesia is used, long-acting local anesthetics, such as bupivacaine, should be avoided. Even with short-acting local anesthetics, such as lidocaine, a minimum of 5 hours are required for the motility to recover. When local anesthesia is required, I prefer sub-tenon administration under brief propofol sedation, using 4% lidocaine to reduce the volume of anesthetic in the retrobulbar space.

## SURGICAL TECHNIQUES

### Limbal versus Fornix Approach

The limbal approach provides broad exposure during surgery and suture adjustment; however, it requires preplaced conjunctival sutures, as it is difficult to cover the suture knot with conjunctiva after the adjustment. Compared to the limbal approach, the exposure is limited with fornix approach, which may increase the technical difficulty of surgery and suture adjustment. The advantages of fornix approach include a hidden incision under the eyelid, improved patient comfort and excellent cosmetic results in most cases making it my preferred approach.

### Muscle Reattachment Technique

There are two methods for muscle reattachment (Figs. 107-1A and B).

#### *Bow-Tie Technique*

After scleral passes, the sutures are tied together in a single loop bow tie, as with a shoe lace. During adjustment, the bow is untied, the muscle position is adjusted and the bow is retied. Once the desired alignment is achieved, the bow is cut and converted to a square knot.

#### *Cinch or Sliding-Noose Technique*

The pole sutures are positioned to emerge from the scleral tunnels less than 1 mm apart. A noose is created by tying a separate piece of suture around the pole sutures with a square knot. The ends of the noose suture are tied together to provide a bucket handle for manipulation of the noose during adjustment. Once the desired alignment is achieved, most surgeons secure the pole sutures to each other with a permanent square knot and trim the noose.

### Timing of Adjustment

The adjustment can be performed intraoperatively or postoperatively from 1 hour to 2 weeks after surgery. Intraoperative adjustment allows for immediate correction of a major postoperative misalignment but is less likely to allow for more refined adjustment, which requires an alert patient. Adjustment is generally performed as per surgeon's preference however most surgeons typically perform the adjustment within 24 hours.

## DO ADJUSTABLE SUTURES INCREASE THE SUCCESS RATES?

A number of studies on outcomes of adjustable sutures have been published over the years. It is beyond the scope of this chapter to discuss all those studies; however, Nihalani and Hunter have published an extensive review on outcomes of adjustable sutures.[7] Most of the studies have compared the results of adjustable sutures with historic controls.[3,8-14] Some of the newer studies have compared patients with adjustable sutures versus non-adjustable sutures operated in the same institution and among the same surgeon or group of surgeons.[15-17] Most published studies show an advantage of adjustable sutures in primary surgery as well as complicated strabismus. Despite continued and widespread skepticism about the effect of adjustable suture surgery, there are no "gold standard" prospective, randomized, controlled trials addressing this topic.[18]

## OPTIONAL AND DELAYED SUTURE ADJUSTMENT

In conventional adjustable suture surgery, a second stage is required to tie and trim the suture ends whether or not patients require adjustment. This is of particular concern in children as they require second stage of anesthesia for suture adjustment. The techniques with optional suture adjustment seem logical not only in children but also in adults. Hence adjustable suture techniques continue to be modified to meet these criteria. Saunders and O'Neill[19] described a technique in which adjustable suture was left untied. There was no incidence of muscle slippage in their study. With these encouraging results, various modifications of conventional adjustable sutures have been described.[20-28]

The postoperative healing process causes adhesions and inhibits delayed adjustment in patients with late postoperative drift. Most of the current techniques allow delayed adjustment up to 1–2 weeks after surgery, especially in elderly patients. The younger the patient, the sooner the muscle becomes firmly adherent to the globe. It is usually not possible to adjust children more than 2 days after surgery without sedation in the operating room. After 2 weeks, it is not recommended to even attempt an adjustment out of concern that the now dissolving polyglactin 910 suture will break before the muscle has readhered to the globe. Various materials and drugs[29-31] are being evaluated in animal models to facilitate delayed adjustment up to 5 weeks postoperatively which appear intriguing; however, trials to evaluate safety and efficacy in humans are still awaited.

## MY PREFERRED SURGICAL TECHNIQUE

I perform the sliding noose adjustable suture technique (and short tag noose technique for optional suture adjustment) described by Hunter et al.[32]

The adjustable suture surgery is performed under general anesthesia in all patients, unless it is contraindicated. The muscle is secured with a double-armed 6-0 polyglactin 910 (Vicryl, Ethicon Inc., Johnson & Johnson) suture and disinserted from the sclera as in traditional strabismus surgery. The muscle insertion is identified and grasped with 0.5 Castroviejo forceps. Spatulated needles from the sutures are passed one after the other, through the original insertion, at half-thickness depth. The needles are passed in a "V" configuration. For recessions, the scleral passes are separated by 1–2 mm where they enter sclera, but are nearly touching where they exit. For resections, this "V" separation is exaggerated to 3–5 mm at the entry site, but the sutures are still nearly touching at the exit site.

For an adjustable recession, the standard hang-back approach and surgical dosages are used. For an adjustable resection, an extra 1–3 mm of muscle is resected. The muscle is then allowed to hang back by the same amount. This allows for either advancement or recession of the resected muscle at adjustment. This also avoids the sometimes unsightly appearing muscle stump at the insertion site.

It is important to pull the muscle up to the original insertion. The pole sutures are then secured to each other using an overhand knot, with care being taken not to allow either pole of the muscle to fall back asymmetrically. The extra suture is cut just above the overhand knot. A 5 cm fragment of polyglactin 910 suture (Vicryl, Ethicon, Johnson & Johnson, NJ) is used for the adjustable noose (Figs. 107-2A to C). This piece of suture is placed underneath the pole sutures and wrapped around a second time. A square knot is then tied to ensure a tight noose, which prevents inadvertent slippage. It is critical that the noose should be as tight as possible. The ends

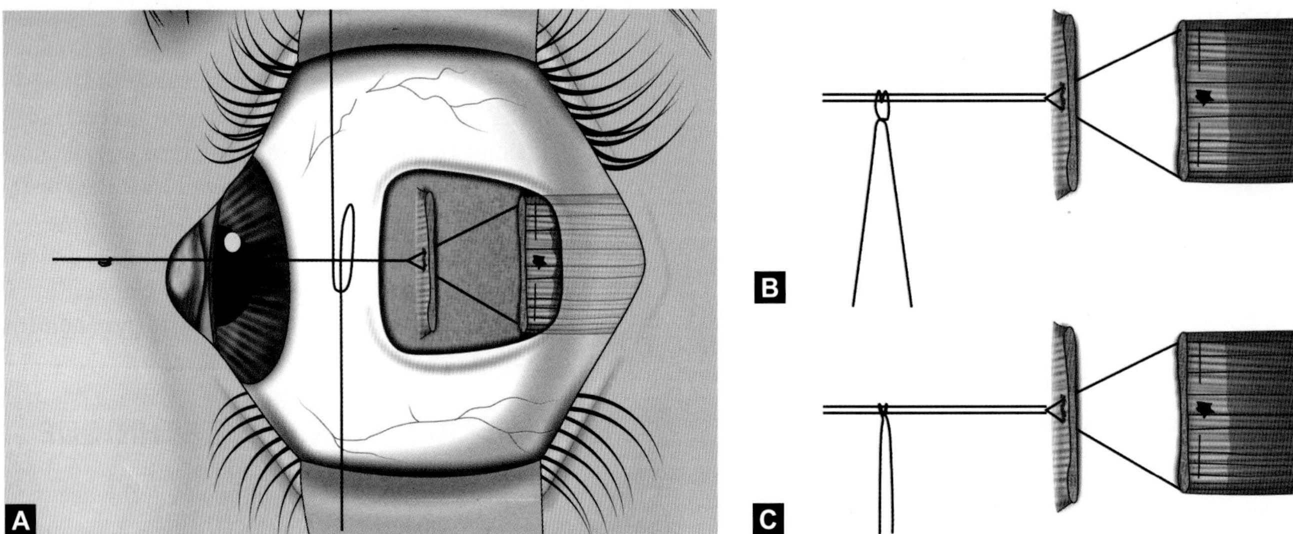


**Figures 107-2A to C** Technique of applying the noose. (A) A piece of suture is placed underneath the pole sutures, wrapped around a second time. (B) It is tied using a square knot. (C) The ends of the noose are tied together in an overhand knot.

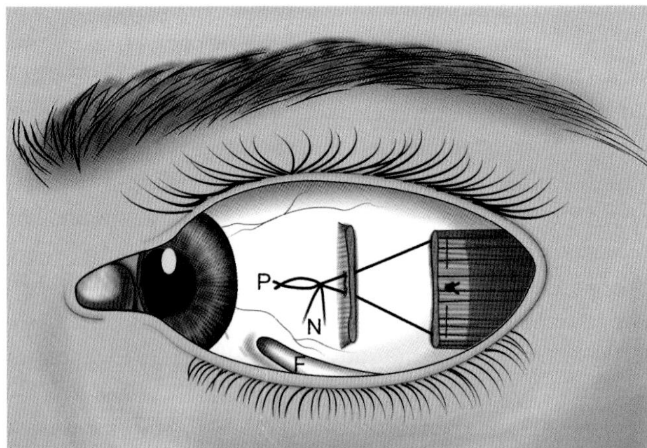


**Figure 107-3** Short tag noose technique showing the fornix incision (F), trimmed pole sutures (P) and trimmed noose (N) buried under the conjunctiva.

of this noose are tied together in an overhand knot to obtain a noose length of 5 cm. The extra suture above the overhand knot is trimmed. The noose is slid forward or backward to the desired location. If the pole sutures are nearly touching where they exit, the noose is placed at the exact desired recession (e.g. 5 mm from the exit site for a 5 mm recession). If the pole sutures are separated where they exit, an additional "fudge factor" is added (e.g. 5.5 mm for a 5 mm recession if the pole sutures exit 1 mm apart). The new muscle position is confirmed by measuring its distance from the scleral insertion. A 5-0 polyester (Mersilene, Ethicon Inc., Johnson & Johnson) traction suture helps in manipulating the globe and retracting conjunctiva during suture adjustment.

The excess Tenon's tissue is excised to prevent the formation of conjunctival cyst or pyogenic granuloma. The incision is irrigated with saline and the protruding tissue is grasped and excised. The conjunctiva is not routinely sutured as the small incision self-seals under the eyelid. If the conjunctival incision has enlarged inadvertently during surgery, it is partly closed with a 6-0 fast absorbing gut or 8-0 polyglactin 910 suture. (Vicryl, Ethicon, Johnson & Johnson, NJ) The incision must be left large enough to allow for suture adjustment even if it is partially closed with sutures. An eye patch is not necessary unless there is an epithelial defect. Antibiotic or steroid drops are preferred over ointment to avoid blurring the vision during the adjustment. The long suture ends are folded and taped over the medial surface of the noose or just lateral to the lateral canthus with a 1/2" steri-strip.

For pediatric patients I perform short tag noose adjustable suture technique[26] where the pole sutures and noose are cut to "short tags" and tucked under the conjunctiva (Fig. 107-3). No polyester traction suture is placed. An overhand knot is placed 5 mm away from the suture exit site on pole sutures, allowing for an additional 5 mm recession. An overhand knot is also placed on the noose suture at 5 mm, but it is trimmed with longer whiskers to distinguish it from the pole sutures at the time of adjustment.

## ADJUSTMENT

The adjustment is performed 1–2 hours after surgery in the recovery room when the surgery is performed under general

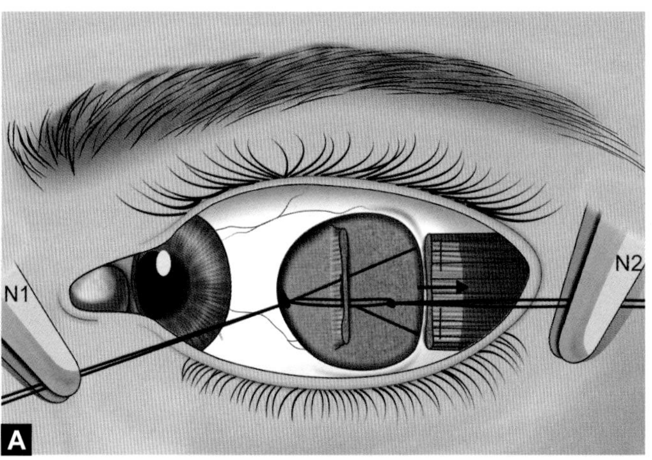


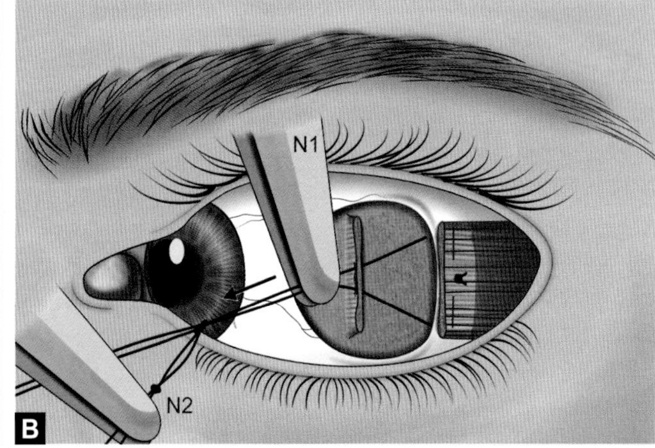


**Figures 107-4A and B** Adjustment Technique. (A) To tighten or decrease the recession, the pole sutures are stabilized with a needle holder (N1) clamped in front of the noose and the noose is slid posteriorly to the sclera (arrow) with another needle holder (N2). (B) To loosen or increase the recession, the pole sutures are stabilized by clamping behind the noose with N1. The noose is grasped and moved away from the muscle (arrow) with N2.

anesthesia. Topical proparacaine drops are instilled at least thrice at 2–3 minute intervals. To assure that the patient is sufficiently alert, I ask the patient to sit without back support on the edge of the bed with legs dangling. The alignment is assessed with corrective glasses in place, if indicated. If the patient had required prisms preoperatively, care should be taken to assure that the glasses used during adjustment do not have a prism! For patients with high refractive error who wear contact lenses, the alignment can be assessed by applying topical anesthesia and inserting the contact lenses for the adjustment session.

First, the ductions and versions are carefully assessed. Then cover testing is performed at distance and near. The goal of adjustment in cases of esotropia and hypertropia is to achieve orthotropia. The only exception is to undercorrect the superior oblique (SO) palsy patient who has had an inferior oblique weakening procedure in combination with a vertical rectus muscle recession. The goal of adjustment for exotropia cases is to overcorrect so that the patient is diplopic at distance (ET 10-15 PD) with no shift at 1/3rd meter.

In very young, less cooperative children I maintain nil per os (NPO) status in the recovery room with the intravenous line left in place. I advise the anesthesiologist in advance about the possible need for sedation in the recovery room. Sedation with propofol supplemented with topical proparacaine is recommended for suture adjustment in children.

To access the noose for an adjustment, the pole sutures are always grasped first to avoid inadvertent sliding of the noose. To tighten or decrease the recession, the pole sutures are pulled up to draw the muscle anteriorly while the patient is asked to look toward the muscle (or, if the patient is sedated, the globe is rotated toward the muscle using a traction suture). This pulls the noose suture up and away from the sclera. The pole sutures are stabilized with a needle holder clamped in front of the noose and the noose is slid posteriorly to the sclera with another needle holder. To loosen or increase the recession, the pole sutures are again pulled forward with a needle holder, this time stabilizing the pole sutures by clamping behind the noose. With the second needle holder, the noose is grasped and moved away from the muscle. Once the noose is adjusted, the sutures are released and the patient is asked to look toward the recessed muscle while the eye is stabilized or pulled away from the muscle. This will retract the muscle posteriorly and force the noose firmly against the sclera (Figs. 107-4A and B).

To permanently secure the suture after completing the adjustment, the distal overhand knot is cut to separate the pole sutures. The sutures are then firmly tied to each other. Care is taken not to pull up on the pole sutures while tying the sutures, as this may change the position of the muscle. Both the pole and noose sutures are trimmed and the polyester traction suture is removed. The sutures are tucked under the conjunctiva which generally covers the suture ends without the need for closure.

A different completion step is used on the day of surgery to allow for readjustment up to 7 days later. A second overhand knot is tied on the pole suture to reduce its length to 5 mm. The noose sutures are then trimmed to a 5 mm length (short tag noose) with longer whiskers on overhand knot. The polyester suture is removed and the suture ends tucked under conjunctiva. If the sliding noose is tied securely with a good square knot, it does not usually move during the healing period.

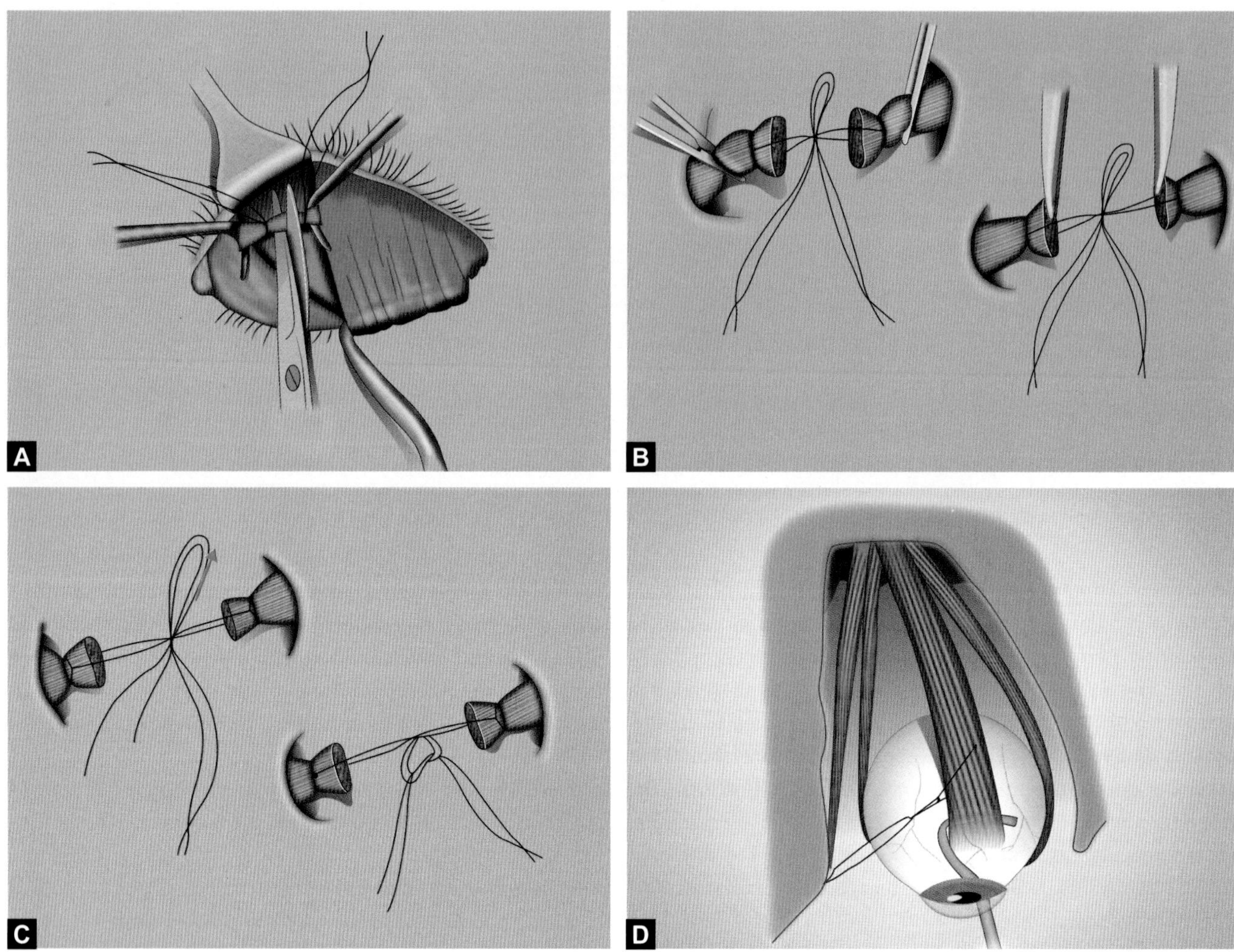


**Figures 107-5A to D** Surgical technique of adjustable SO suture spacer. (A) Exposure of the SO tendon and placement of sutures. (B) Sutures tied, leaving a gap of 2–8 mm. (C) The slipknot is converted into a square knot by cutting one of the pairs of sutures and passing this pair through the knot. The sutures are then secured with a permanent square knot. (D) Final position of SO tendon, with suture spacer in place.

It is crucial that the surgeon should not ignore the original numbers and should know when to stop adjusting. Adjustments greater than 2 mm should be avoided except in unusual cases such as severe restrictive strabismus. If there is no change in alignment after an adjustment, it may be due to other factors such as orbital restriction and there is no point in trying to adjust further.

## SPECIAL CIRCUMSTANCES

### Adjustable Superior Oblique Surgery

The adjustable SO suture spacer[33] is a modification of Knapp's "chicken suture"[34] and Wright's superior oblique "tendon expander"[35] techniques. The procedure allows for partial, reversible and intraoperatively adjustable SO weakening using a nonabsorbable suture to separate the cut ends of the SO tendon. The suture allows the separation to be adjusted intraoperatively after performing the exaggerated traction test and fundus torsion assessment. A sliding noose adjustable SO weakening and Harada-Ito procedure[36-38] that allow postoperative adjustment have shown good results in a small number of patients (Figs. 107-5A to D).

### Semi-adjustable Sutures

The incidence of inferior rectus muscle slippage is between 7% and 41%,[39] both in adjustable and nonadjustable cases. Kushner[40] described a "semi-adjustable" technique that secures the muscle more firmly to the globe, thus reducing

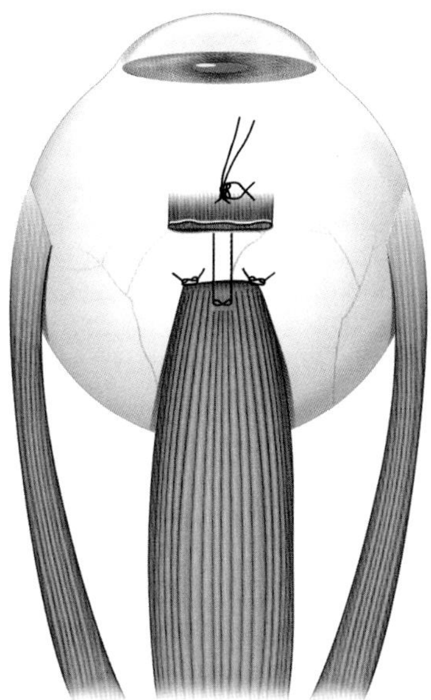

Figure 107-6 Semi-adjustable sutures showing that the corners of inferior rectus muscle are sutured firmly to the sclera and the center of the muscle is placed on an adjustable suture.

the incidence of muscle slippage (Fig. 107-6). The technique involves suturing the corners of the muscle firmly to the sclera and placing the center of the muscle on an adjustable suture. The disadvantage of this procedure is that it limits the capability to increase the amount of recession at the time of adjustment; which can be overcome by targeting an initial overcorrection.

### Adjustable Suture for Transposed Muscles

Guyton and co-authors[41] has developed an innovative technique for transposition of the vertical muscles in sixth nerve palsy that reduces the need for the ipsilateral medial rectus to be recessed and also eliminates a foster suture. The transposed muscles are placed on an adjustable suture with a noose. The superior rectus can be adjusted with the noose located inferior to the lateral rectus, and the inferior rectus can be adjusted with the noose located superior to the lateral rectus. This technique allows for further tightening of the vertical muscles by allowing them to cross underneath the lateral rectus muscle, thus, increasing abduction.

## ADVANTAGES AND DISADVANTAGES

### Advantages

- Reduce the rate of reoperations by providing a "second chance" to refine alignment.

### Disadvantages

- Complex surgery requiring greater operating time
- Increased patient anxiety
- More suture material left in the eye
- Postoperative drift.

## POSTOPERATIVE DRIFT

The extent of postoperative drift that occurs after suture adjustment is unpredictable. Eino and Kraft[12] found that both esotropia and exotropia groups had equal tendency to drift toward either undercorrection or overcorrection. Isenberg et al.[42] found that most exotropia patients developed a general drift toward undercorrection. In our short tag noose study,[26] the postoperative drift was toward undercorrection in patients with esotropia, exotropia and vertical deviation. Mean vertical drift toward undercorrection was less than mean horizontal drift.

## COMPLICATIONS

Any complication that can occur in strabismus surgery can also occur with adjustable suture surgery. Complications unique to the adjustable suture technique include:

- Vagal reactions during suture adjustment
- Increased postoperative inflammation due to excessive suture material
- Exposed sutures
- Slipped adjustable suture knot.

## CONCLUSION

The concept of adjustable sutures makes intellectual sense; however, it has not gained universal acceptance, particularly in children, due to difficulties in examining and judging the postoperative drift. Most published studies suggest improved outcomes with adjustable sutures in adults and children. Newer techniques allow the option of "no adjustment" in patients who do not require adjustment in the postoperative recovery period and allow greater time to elapse between completion of primary surgery and suture adjustment. With the additional time to evaluate the results of primary surgery and perform modifications, it seems logical that the accuracy of surgery should further improve. These developments should lead more surgeons to use adjustable sutures at least in patients with complex strabismus where the surgical outcomes are unpredictable.[43]

## PEARLS AND PITFALLS

- Adjustable sutures provide a "second chance" to improve the outcome of first strabismus surgery.
- Ideal candidates are patients in whom the standard strabismus dosages do not apply.
- The noose should be tied as tight as possible to prevent inadvertent slippage.
- Assure that the patient is sufficiently alert for adjustment.
- Do not ignore the original numbers. Know when to stop adjustment.
- Short tag noose technique is useful for children as it avoids the need for sedation in those with satisfactory postoperative alignment.
- Adjustable sutures may reduce the need for reoperations but add to the time and complexity of surgery.

## REFERENCES


1. Bielschowsky A. Die neueren Anschauungen uber sen und Behandlung des Schielens. Med Klin. 1907;3:335-6.
2. Jampolsky A. Strabismus reoperation techniques. Trans Sect Ophthalmol Am Acad Ophthalmol Otolaryngol. 1975;79:704-17.
3. Tripathi A, Haslett R, Marsh IB. Strabismus surgery: adjustable sutures-good for all? Eye (Lond). 2003;17:739-42.
4. Castelbuono AC, White JE, Guyton DL. The use of (a)symmetry of the rest position of the eyes under general anesthesia or sedation-hypnosis in the design of strabismus surgery: a favorable pilot study in 51 exotropia cases. Binocul Vis Strabismus Q. 1999;14:285-90.
5. Cogen MS, Guthrie ME, Vinik HR. The immediate postoperative adjustment of sutures in strabismus surgery with comaintenance of anesthesia using propofol and midazolam. J AAPOS. 2002;6:241-5.
6. Haynes GR, Bailey MK. Postoperative nausea and vomiting: review and clinical approaches. South Med J. 1996;89:940-9.
7. Nihalani BR, Hunter DG. Adjustable suture strabismus surgery. Eye (Lond). 2011;25:1262-76.
8. Rosenbaum AL, Metz HS, Carlson M, et al. Adjustable rectus muscle recession surgery: a follow-up study. Arch Ophthalmol. 1977;95:817-20.
9. Keech RV, Scott WE, Christensen LE. Adjustable suture strabismus surgery. J Pediatr Ophthalmol Strabismus. 1987;24:97-102.
10. Wisnicki HJ, Repka MX, Guyton DL. Reoperation rate in adjustable strabismus surgery. J Pediatr Ophthalmol Strabismus. 1988;25:112-4.
11. Leuder GT, Scott WE, Kutschke PJ, et al. Long term results of adjustable suture surgery for strabismus secondary to thyroid ophthalmopathy. Ophthalmology. 1992;99:993-7.
12. Eino D, Kraft SP. Postoperative drifts after adjustable suture strabismus surgery. Can J Ophthalmol. 1997;32:163-9.
13. Ogut MS, Onal S, Demirtas S. Adjustable suture surgery for correction of various types of strabismus. Ophthalmic Surg Lasers Imaging. 2007;38:196-202.
14. Kraus DJ, Bullock JD. Treatment of thyroid ocular myopathy with adjustable and non-adjustable suture strabismus surgery. Trans Am Ophthalmol Soc. 1993;91:67-79.
15. Awadein A, Sharma M, Bazemore MG, et al. Adjustable suture strabismus surgery in infants and children. J AAPOS. 2008;12:585-90.
16. Zhang MS, Hutchinson AK, Drack AV, et al. Improved ocular alignment with adjustable sutures in adults undergoing strabismus surgery. Ophthalmology 2012;119:396-402.
17. Mireskandari K, Cotesta M, Scho eld J, et al. Utility of adjustable sutures in primary strabismus surgery and reoperation. Ophthalmology. 2012;119:629-33.
18. Haridas A, Sundaram V. Adjustable versus non-adjustable sutures for strabismus. Cochrane Database Syst Rev. 2005;(1): CD004240.
19. Saunders RA, O'Neill JW. Tying the knot: is it always necessary? Arch Ophthalmol. 1992;110:1318-21.
20. Eustis HS, Elmer TR Jr., Ellis G Jr. Postoperative results of absorbable, subconjunctival adjustable sutures. J AAPOS. 2004; 8:240-2.
21. Kipioti A, George ND, Taylor RH. Tied and tidy: closing the conjunctiva over adjustable sutures. J Pediatr Ophthalmol Strabismus. 2004;41:226-9.
22. Engel JM, Rousta ST. Adjustable sutures in children using a modified technique. J AAPOS. 2004;8:2438.
23. Nguyen DQ, Hale J, Von Lany H, et al. Releasable conjunctival suture for adjustable suture surgery. J Pediatr Ophthalmol Strabismus. 2007;44:35-8.
24. Hakim OM, El-Hag YG, Haikal MA. Releasable adjustable suture technique for children. J AAPOS. 2005;9:386-90.
25. Coats DK. Ripcord adjustable suture technique for use in strabismus surgery. Arch Ophthalmol. 2001;119:1364-7.
26. Nihalani BR, Whitman MC, Salgado CM, et al. Short tag noose technique for optional and late suture adjustment in strabismus surgery. Arch Ophthalmol. 2009;127:1584-90.
27. Robbins SL, Granet DB, Burns C, et al. Delayed adjustable sutures: a multicentred clinical review. Br J Ophthalmol. 2010; 94:1169-73.
28. Budning AS, Day C, Nguyen A. The short adjustable suture. Can J Ophthalmol. 2010;45:359-62.
29. Choi MY, Auh SJ, Choi DG, et al. Effect of ADCON-L on adjustable strabismus surgery in rabbits. Br J Ophthalmol. 2001;85:80-4.
30. Choung HK, Jin SE, Lee MJ, et al. Slow-releasing paclitaxel in polytetrafluoroethylene/polylactide-co-glycolide laminate delays adjustment after strabismus surgery in rabbit model. Invest Ophthalmol Vis Sci. 2008;49:5340-5.
31. Lee MJ, Jin SE, Kim CK, et al. Effect of slow-releasing all-trans-retinoic-acid in bioabsorbable polymer on delayed adjustable strabismus surgery in a rabbit model. Am J Ophthalmol. 2009;148:566-72.

32. Hunter DG, Dingeman RS, Nihalani BR. Adjustable sutures in strabismus surgery. In: Wilson ME, Saunders RA, Trivedi RH (Eds). Pediatric Ophthalmology: Current Thought and a Practical Guide. Germany: Springer-Heidelberg; 2008. pp. 213-26.
33. Suh DW, Guyton DL, Hunter DG. An adjustable superior oblique tendon spacer with the use of nonabsorbable suture. J AAPOS. 2001;5:164-71.
34. Jampolsky A. The Philip Knapp Lectureship. J AAPOS. 1998;2:131-2.
35. Wright KW. Superior oblique silicone expander for Brown syndrome and superior oblique overaction. J Pediatr Ophthalmol Strabismus. 1991;28:101-7.
36. Goldenberg-Cohen N, Tarczy-Hornock K, Klink DF, et al. Postoperative adjustable surgery of the superior oblique tendon. Strabismus. 2005;13:5-10.
37. Metz HS, Lerner H. The adjustable Harada-Ito procedure. Arch Ophthalmol. 1981;99:624-6.
38. Nishimura JK, Rosenbaum AL. The long-term torsion effect of the adjustable Harada-Ito procedure. J AAPOS. 2002;6:141-4.
39. Sprunger DT, Helveston EM. Progressive overcorrection after inferior rectus recession. J Pediatr Ophthalmol Strabismus. 1993;30:145-8.
40. Kushner BJ. An evaluation of the semiadjustable suture strabismus surgical procedure. J AAPOS. 2004;8:481-7.
41. Phamonvaechavan P, Anwar D, Guyton DL. Adjustable suture technique for enhanced transposition surgery for extraocular muscles. J AAPOS. 2010;14:399-405.
42. Isenberg SJ, Abdarbashi P. Drift of ocular alignment following strabismus surgery. Part 2: using adjustable sutures. Br J Ophthalmol. 2009;93:443-7.
43. Engel JM. Adjustable sutures: an update. Curr Opin Ophthalmol. 2012;23:373-6.

CHAPTER

108

# Transposition Surgery

Manoj V Parulekar

## INTRODUCTION

The term transpose comes from transposen (Middle English) that means to transform, and from transposer (Old French) that means alteration. Transposition strabismus surgery refers to procedures that involve alteration of the position as well as direction of action of the extraocular muscles. This includes:

- Moving the insertion of the horizontal recti up or down the spiral of Tillaux toward the insertion of the vertical recti.
- Moving the insertion of the vertical recti along the spiral of Tillaux laterally or medially toward the insertion of the horizontal recti.
- Transposition of the oblique muscles includes transposition of the superior oblique tendon to the medial rectus insertion, or anterior transposition of the inferior oblique muscle.

The discussion in this chapter will be restricted to full transposition surgery. Partial transposition of the horizontal or vertical muscles to deal with alphabetic pattern (A, V, X, or Y) strabismus or small horizontal or vertical deviations will be dealt with in Chapters 3 and 4, and oblique muscle surgery in Chapters 6 and 7.

## ANATOMICAL CONSIDERATIONS AND PRINCIPLE BEHIND TRANSPOSITIONS

All four rectus muscles arise from the annulus of Zinn at the apex of the orbit, and insert along the spiral of Tillaux. The muscles are connected by a complex system of intermuscular septa and pulleys.

Movement of the insertion of a rectus muscle in a given direction will alter the net vector of pull in that direction due to the viscous drag of the muscles and surrounding tissues, and the complex pulley system. This effect is insignificant with movement less than half the tendon width, and increases incrementally thereafter.

This has two effects:

1. Static change—the resting position of the eye is altered, in the direction of transposition.
2. Dynamic change—the range of movement in the direction of transposition increases.

It follows that vertical transposition of the horizontal recti will alter the vertical alignment as well as expand the range of vertical movement in the direction of transposition, and horizontal transposition of the vertical recti will affect the horizontal alignment and range of horizontal movement.

The aim of transposition surgery therefore is to:

1. Improve the range of movement.
2. Expand the field of binocular vision, and move it to a more usable position, e.g. downgaze.

## HISTORY

Hummelsheim described the first partial tendon transposition procedure on the vertical recti for lateral rectus palsy in 1907. Several variations were subsequently reported by O'Connor, Wener, and Berens and Girard.[1] Carlson and Jampolsky described an adjustable technique for partial tendon transposition.[2] Jensen described a rectus muscle unionoperation where the muscle was split rather than disinserted to minimize the risk of anterior segment ischemia.[3] However, the risk remained due to constriction of ciliary vessels from the sutures.

The first full tendon transposition was described by O'Connor[1] and was associated with significant induced

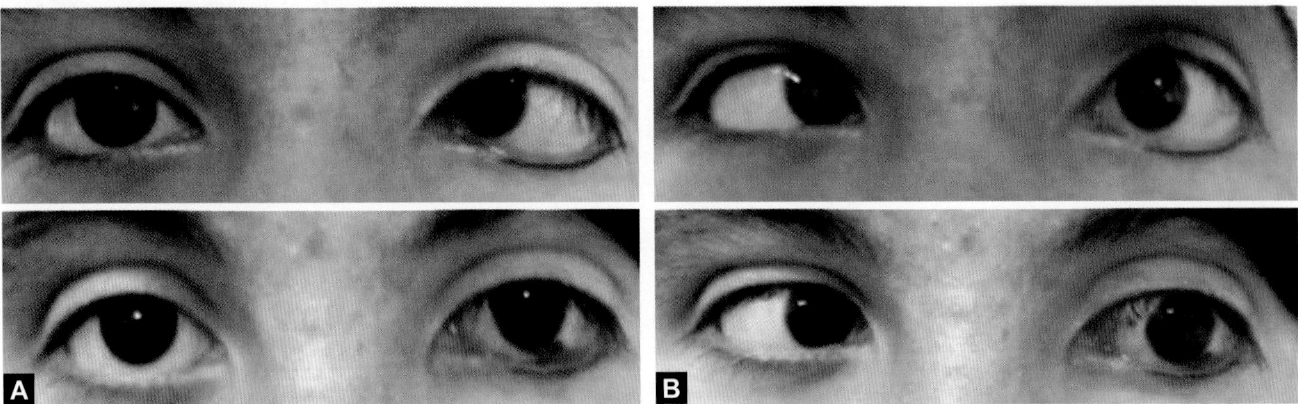

**Figures 108-1A and B** Left sixth nerve palsy preoperative appearance in (A) – primary gaze, (B) – left gaze. Following – Left medial rectus recession and temporal transposition of the superior rectus (A) – primary gaze, (B) – left gaze showing improvement in esotropia and left eye abduction.

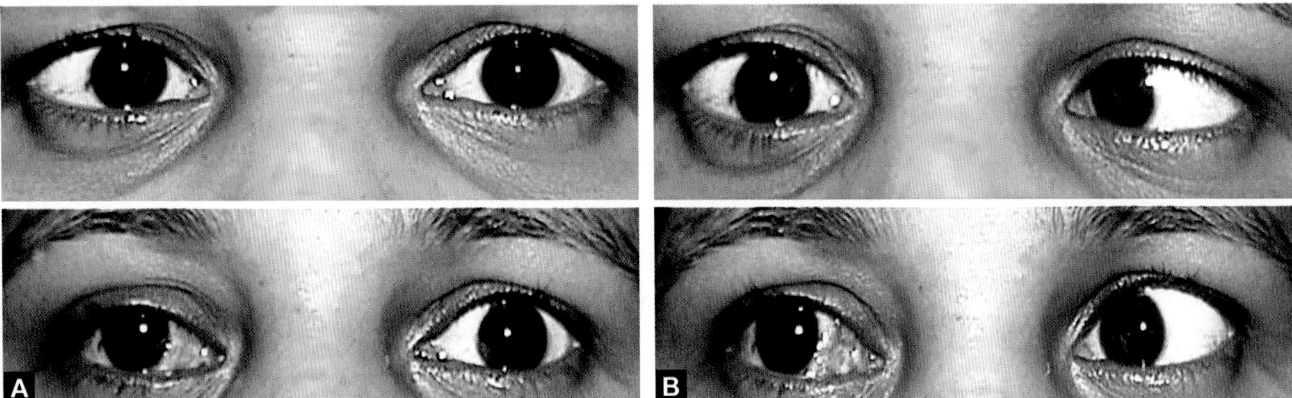

**Figures 108-2A and B** Right sixth nerve palsy preoperative appearance in (A) – primary gaze, (B) – right gaze. Following temporal transposition of the left superior and inferior rectus, with open sky injection of botulinum toxin into the left medial rectus (A) – primary gaze, (B) – right gaze showing improvement in esotropia and right eye abduction.

vertical deviations. Rosenbaum described an adjustable technique to minimize the risk, placing the superior rectus insertion parallel to the long axis of the lateral rectus.[4] McManaway et al. suggested moving the muscle along the spiral of Tillaux. The addition of botulinum toxin weakening of the medial rectus was described later,[5] and Foster described the technique of lateral fixation suture to attach the transposed muscle to sclera to augment the effect of the transposition procedure.[6]

## INDICATIONS (FIGS. 108-1 AND 108-2)

Transposition surgery is indicated when there is significant limitation of the range of movement of the eye in one direction of gaze, with minimal or no muscle function resulting in an incomitant strabismus. The aim of surgery is to improve the alignment in primary position or to improve the range of movement in the intended direction, thereby reducing the incomitance, or both. It must be emphasized that such operations can improve but not restore the full range of movement of the weak muscle.

Common indications include:

- Paralytic strabismus
  - Lateral rectus palsy—one or both vertical recti are transposed laterally toward the insertion of the lateral rectus to improve the convergent strabismus and the range of abduction of the affected eye.
  - Superior division of 3rd nerve palsy—both horizontal recti are transposed up toward the superior rectus insertion to improve the vertical alignment and range of elevation (Knapp procedure).
  - Inferior rectus paralysis—typically following blowout fracture of the orbit. Both horizontal recti are transposed toward the inferior rectus to improve the vertical alignment, and augment the range of depression (inverse Knapp procedure).
- Dysinnervation (Duane syndrome or Möbius syndrome)—If there is virtually no action in the lateral rectus muscle,

lateral transposition of the vertical recti can increase the range of abduction to or beyond the vertical midline and improve the esotropia.
- Congenital hypoinnervation (Monocular elevation deficiency)—In this condition, there is limitation of elevation of the affected eye, with or without hypotropia in the primary position, and accompanying mild upper lid ptosis.
- Muscle trauma (blowout fracture), lost muscle (surgical complication), or congenital absence of muscle—typically affects the medial or inferior rectus. Transposition muscle surgery can restore some of the lost function in such cases.

## ASSESSMENT OF SUITABILITY OF TRANSPOSITION PROCEDURES

The decision to consider transposition strabismus surgery is based on the degree of residual function in the affected muscle. This can be determined by assessing the range of saccadic versions. If the affected eye can move past the midline in the direction of action of the weak muscle, standard recess-resect procedures should be sufficient, and transposition is not necessary. If, however, the rotations stop short of the midline, the force-generation test can be used in cooperative adults to assess how much force the affected muscle can generate. If minimal or no force is generated, transposition surgery should be considered.

It is important to determine that the muscles to be transposed have sufficient function as conditions like 3rd cranial nerve palsy can affect horizontal as well as vertical rectus muscles, and transposition of a palsied muscle will give an inadequate result.

## SURGICAL TECHNIQUE

The technique for temporal transposition of the vertical recti to correct lateral rectus underaction is described below. A similar technique can be used for superior transposition of the horizontal recti (Knapp procedure) or inferior transposition (inverse Knapp procedure). It is important to perform the forced duction test at the beginning to look for contracture of the antagonist muscle. If there is limitation in the direction of the paretic muscle, botulinum toxin injection to the antagonist muscle should be considered to maximize the effect of surgery.

Although adequate exposure can be obtained with the Moody Locking forceps, the author prefers the use of 5/0 or 6/0 silk traction sutures placed in oblique quadrants between the superior rectus and the lateral rectus, and between the inferior and the lateral rectus to maximize exposure. Conjunctival incisions are made in the superotemporal and inferotemporal quadrants, 7 mm posterior to and parallel to the limbus to facilitate access to both superior and lateral rectus, and inferior and lateral rectus, respectively. The superior rectus is isolated and double-armed locked 6/0 polyglactin sutures are passed through the tendon posterior to and close to the insertion before detaching it from the sclera. The intermuscular septa attaching it to the underlying superior oblique muscle are carefully separated. The superior rectus is then moved laterally along the spiral of Tillaux and sutured to the sclera 7 mm behind the limbus, adjacent to the insertion of the lateral rectus.

The inferior rectus is isolated through the inferotemporal quadrant, and a similar procedure is repeated, moving the inferior rectus superiorly and sutured to the spiral of Tillaux adjacent to the lateral rectus insertion.

### Augmented Transposition Surgery

If Foster augmentation sutures[6] are required, 5/0 or 6/0 nonabsorbable suture such as Dacron is passed through the lateral one-fourth of the transposed vertical rectus muscle to unite the border adjoining the lateral rectus with the sclera 5–6 mm posterior to the spiral of Tillaux (*see* Chapter 1).

### Adjustable Transposition Surgery

If there are concerns about inducing vertical deviation, the superior and inferior rectus can be sutured with the new insertion parallel to and 1 mm from the superior and inferior border of the lateral rectus, respectively.[4] The sutures are tied on a slipknot as with other adjustable strabismus surgery (*see* Chapter 8), and the conjunctiva left unsutured, allowing for adjustment the following day.

If there is a vertical deviation postoperatively, the appropriate vertical rectus can be recessed to correct the deviation. If there is a horizontal overcorrection, both the vertical recti can be recessed the same amount. If the medial rectus is tight on forced duction testing, it can be weakened at the same time as transposition surgery with botulinum toxin injection, or a few months later with a medial rectus recession.

### Knapp Procedure

The Knapp procedure[7] involves transposition of the medial and lateral rectus tendons superiorly adjacent to the underacting superior rectus insertion to improve the range of elevation and/or correct any hypotropia. The usual indication would be monocular elevation deficiency, but other indications include absent superior rectus in craniofacial syndromes, palsy of the superior division of the 3rd nerve, and traumatic injury to the superior rectus. It is quite an effective procedure on its own, but may be combined with the Foster augmentation sutures to enhance the effect and correct large vertical deviations.

### Inverse Knapp Procedure

The inverse Knapp procedure[8] involves transposition of the medial and lateral rectus tendons inferiorly adjacent to the underacting inferior rectus insertion to improve the range of depression and/or correct any hypotropia. The usual indication would be traumatic injury to the inferior rectus following blowout fractures, monocular depression deficiency (double depressor palsy), absent superior rectus in craniofacial syndromes, and palsy of the inferior division of the 3rd nerve.

It is quite an effective procedure on its own, but may be combined with the Foster augmentation sutures to enhance the effect and correct large vertical deviations. The use of augmentation sutures does carry a significant risk of overcorrection, and must be used with caution.

### Single Rectus Transposition Surgery

This is a very useful modification[9,10] described for lateral rectus underaction where the medial rectus has developed contracture, and needs to be recessed. The technique involves temporal transposition of the superior rectus alone, combined with an adjustable recession of the ipsilateral medial rectus. The edges of the superior and lateral rectus muscle bellies are united with a loop suture 8–12 mm posterior to the muscle insertion. As only 1 vertical rectus is transposed, the medial rectus can be safely recessed without fear of inducing anterior segment ischemia. Undercorrections can be dealt with by subsequent temporal transposition of the inferior rectus.

## COMPLICATIONS AND THEIR MANAGEMENT

### Overcorrections

Early postoperative overcorrections following temporal transposition for lateral rectus palsy may be due to botulinum toxin-induced paralysis of the medial rectus. If botulinum toxin denervation of the medial rectus has not been used, the adjustable technique described above can be used to correct early postoperative overcorrections by recessing both the vertical recti by the same amount. Late overcorrections may be due to return of lateral rectus function, and can be avoided by waiting at least 6 months before considering such surgery.

### Undercorrections

Undercorrections are common with transposition of the vertical recti to the medial rectus in cases with isolated medial rectus weakness. This is usually due to unopposed action or contracture of the lateral rectus, and can be minimized by maximal recession of the lateral rectus beyond the functional equator, i.e. >17 mm from the limbus. The effect of transposition can be augmented by resecting both the vertical recti. Undercorrections are rare with transposition of vertical recti to the lateral rectus as the process of temporal transposition puts the vertical recti on stretch and the resultant increased tone enhances the effect.

### Induced Vertical Deviations

Vertical deviations can occur in up to a third of patients undergoing temporal transposition of the vertical recti, commonly hyperdeviations.[11] This can be minimized by recessing the superior rectus by 2 mm. The adjustable technique described above can be used to correct any induced vertical deviations.

### Ptosis

Temporal transposition of the vertical recti can result in narrowing of the palpebral fissure and ptosis. This is because temporal transfer causes tightening of the vertical recti, and the attachments between the superior rectus and the levator muscle, and inferior rectus and capsule-palpebral fascia cause lowering of the upper lid and raise the lower lid.

### Anterior Segment Ischemia

There is a small but recognized risk of anterior segment ischemia if more than two recti muscles are detached from the globe at the same time. If 2-muscle transposition is performed, weakening of the ipsilateral antagonist, i.e. medial rectus in case of lateral rectus weakness is best performed by chemodenervation (botulinum) or performed at least 3, preferably 6 months later.[12]

### Restriction of Ocular Movements

Transposition surgery can result in limitation of range of eye movements in the opposite direction; e.g. temporal transposition will result in limited adduction of the operated eye. This may be desirable in some cases to ensure long-term stability of the surgical result, but may be progressive due to scarring and contracture resulting in late overcorrections.

## PEARLS AND PITFALLS

- Transposition strabismus surgery can be very effective in improving the range of movement of the eye as well as improving ocular alignment in cases where one or more muscles are underacting.
- Careful case selection is key to a successful outcome.
- Anterior segment ischemia can occur after transposition surgery, preoperative planning is required and chemodenervation can be considered.

## ACKNOWLEDGMENTS

I am grateful to Dr Eduardo Villaseca, Staff at the Hospital CalvoMackenna (children hospital) and Chief Adult Strabismus Department Hospital Salvador Santiago, Chile, for contributing clinical photos for this chapter.

## REFERENCES

1. O'Connor R. Transplantation of ocular muscles. Am J Ophthalmol. 1921;4:838.
2. Carlson MR, Jampolsky A. An adjustable transposition procedure for abduction deficiencies. Am J Ophthalmol. 1979;87(3): 382-7.
3. Jensen CDF. Rectus muscle union: a new operation for paralysis of the rectus muscles. Trans Pac Coast Ophthalmol Soc. 1964;45:359
4. Laby DM, Rosenbaum AL. Adjustable vertical rectus muscle transposition surgery. J Pediatr Ophthalmol Strabismus. 1994; 31(2):75-8.
5. McManaway JW 3rd, Buckley EG, Brodsky MC. Vertical rectus muscle transposition with intraoperative botulinum injection for treatment of chronic sixth nerve palsy. Graefes Arch Clin Exp Ophthalmol. 1990;228(5):401-6.
6. Foster RS. Vertical muscle transposition augmented with lateral fixation. J AAPOS. 1997;1(1):20-30.
7. Knapp P. The surgical treatment of double-elevator paralysis. Trans Am Ophthalmol Soc. 1969;67:304-23.
8. Burke JP, Keech RV. Effectiveness of inferior transposition of the horizontal rectus muscles for acquired inferior rectus paresis. J Pediatr Ophthalmol Strabismus. 1995;32(3):172-7.
9. Mehendale RA, Dagi LR, Wu C, et al. Superior rectus transposition and medial rectus recession for Duane syndrome and sixth nerve palsy. Arch Ophthalmol. 2012;130(2):195-201.
10. Johnston SC, Crouch ER Jr, Crouch ER. An innovative approach to transposition surgery is effective in treatment of Duane's syndrome with esotropia [ARVOabstract]. Invest Ophthalmol Vis Sci. 2006;47:e-abstract 2475.
11. Ruth AL, Velez FG, Rosenbaum AL. Management of vertical deviations after vertical rectus transposition surgery. J AAPOS. 2009;13(1):16-9.
12. Keech RV, Morris RJ, Ruben JB, et al. Anterior segment ischemia following vertical muscle transposition and botulinum toxin injection. Arch Ophthalmol. 1990;108(2):176.

CHAPTER

109

# Complications of Strabismus Surgery

Aparna Ramasubramanian, Ashwin Mallipatna

## INTRODUCTION

Complications during and after surgery are inevitable but fortunately serious complications are rare after strabismus surgery. Bradbury and Taylor analyzed severe complications after strabismus surgery in 24,000 surgeries and reported an overall incidence of 1 in 400 operations with poor clinical outcome recorded as 1 operation per 2,400. The most common reported complication was perforation of the globe (0.08%), followed by a suspected slipped muscle (0.07%), severe infection (0.06%), scleritis (0.02%), and lost muscle (0.02%).[1]

The complications after strabismus surgery can vary based on the type of surgery and the patient characteristics. It is important to discuss the potential complications with the patient and their family in detail prior to the procedure. In this chapter, we will discuss the complications that can occur with strabismus surgery, the ways to avoid them, and the management of the complications.

## NONOCULAR COMPLICATIONS

### Oculocardiac Reflex

It is defined as a 20% decrease in heart rate with or without dysrhythmia and sinoatrial arrest associated with ocular muscle traction.[2] The afferent limb of this reflex is the ophthalmic division of the trigeminal nerve that goes to the Gasserian ganglion and then to the main sensory nucleus of the trigeminal nerve. The efferent fibers travel through the vagus nerve.[3] The incidence varies from 14% to 90% based on the study population, the type of anesthetic use, and the definition of oculocardiac reflex.[4] The oculorespiratory reflex is a similar reflex with its effects being reduction in tidal volume and respiratory rate.

#### *Predisposing Factors*

Children are at higher risk of developing oculocardiac reflex in view of the high vagal tone. Other predisposing factors are depth of anesthesia, type of anesthetic, hypoxia, hypercarbia, and acidosis. It is postulated that traction on the medial rectus induces the reflex more commonly than the other extraocular muscles.[5] The oculocardiac reflex can also be stimulated postoperatively in the adjustable suture technique.

#### *Prevention*

Gentle handling of the muscle is advised. Sevoflurane with its vagolytic effect decreases the incidence of oculocardiac reflex. Some studies have demonstrated that topical lidocaine decreases the reflex. Pretreatment with atropine or glycopyrrolate decreases the incidence, though its routine clinical use is controversial.[4]

#### *Treatment*

The initial response is to stop surgical manipulation immediately. It is important for the surgeon to pay attention to the heart rate while handling extraocular muscles by keeping the monitor on sound alert. It is also imperative to assess the depth of anesthesia and to rule out hypercarbia or hypoxia. The heart rate usually normalizes after the surgical stimulation is suspended. The vagal reflex has a fatigue component, and hence after repeated stimulation the degree of bradycardia is usually less. In cases of recurrent bradycardia or severe dysrhythmia, atropine or glycopyrrolate can be administered.

### Malignant Hyperthermia

Historically strabismus was considered a risk factor for malignant hyperthermia but a review by Hopkins negated this association.[6] It is an autosomal dominant condition, and hence a obtaining a detailed family history is very important. In patients with a positive family history testing for mutation in the ryanodine receptor may be useful. The earliest sign of malignant hyperthermia is masseter muscle spasm along with increase in end-tidal carbon dioxide. Other signs include tachycardia, muscle rigidity, and increase in body temperature (late sign). Treatment includes discontinuation of all anesthetic agents, ventilatory support, body cooling, and dantrolene.

### Postoperative Nausea and Vomiting

Postoperative nausea and vomiting is a major limitation after strabismus surgery leading to discomfort, dehydration, prolonged hospital stay, and increased hospital costs. The incidence of nausea and vomiting after strabismus surgery varies from 37% to 80%.[7] The factors influencing nausea and vomiting are age, type of surgery, duration of surgery, type of anesthetic used, and personal history of nausea and vomiting. The most commonly used antiemetics are dexamethasone and ondansetron and the combination is more effective than singular agent.[4]

## INTRAOPERATIVE OCULAR COMPLICATIONS

### Surgery to the Wrong Muscle/Wrong Procedure

In spite of the Joint Commission on Accreditation of Healthcare Organizations (JCAHO) established universal protocol to minimize surgical errors, wrong muscle surgery can still happen in strabismus as multiple muscles can be operated on the same marked eye and the terminology recession/resection can often be confused. Shen et al. surveyed 517 strabismus surgeons and 33% of surgeons self-reported having operated on the wrong eye or muscle or performed the wrong procedure at least once.[8] The mean error rate was 1 in 2506 operations and the inferior rectus was the most common "wrong muscle". In this survey, the most common contributing factors were confusion between the type of deviation and/or surgical procedure (30%), globe torsion or anatomical difficulties (17%), and inattention and/or distraction (17%).

#### *Prevention*

Suggested methods to avoid operating on the wrong muscle or performing wrong procedure:

- Clearly written notes with the deviation and full surgical plan visible to the surgeon and other staff in the operating room.
- Time out with the surgical assistant modified to strabismus including the preoperative deviation, the specific eye muscles, and whether strengthening or weakening would be performed.[8]
- Site marking including whether recession or resection would be performed.
- The symmetry of the globe and rotation should be verified prior to surgery to avoid inadvertent hooking of the wrong muscle.
- Normal position of the four recti can be confirmed prior to the conjunctival incision by gently rotating the globe under anesthesia with fixation forceps. During the torsion movement, we get a clue about the true position of the recti by observing for the anterior ciliary vessels coming from the recti that will rotate along with the globe, while the conjunctival vessels will not rotate as much.
- Special attention should be applied intraoperatively when identifying the extraocular muscles in patients with facial dysmorphism, as muscle displacement from the normal clock hour axis or an axially displaced insertion may occur. In situations where changes are expected in the anatomy of the extraocular muscles, imaging might help preoperatively to identify the position of the extraocular muscles.[9]

#### *Management*

As soon as an error is recognized, corrective surgery must be performed. If a recession is performed instead of a resection, it can be reversed but in the opposite scenario the muscle is permanently shortened and the force–length relationship is altered. In all scenarios, full disclosure to the patient and family is mandatory.

## INTRAOPERATIVE MUSCLE COMPLICATIONS

### Slipped/lost Muscle

A slipped muscle occurs when the muscle retracts back into the capsule that remains attached to the globe. In a lost muscle, the capsule also loses its attachment to the globe. The causes include inadvertent transection during surgery, suture breakage, slippage from muscle clamp, or direct trauma. It is more commonly encountered in patients with previous eye muscle surgery, history of retinal detachment surgery, and in older individuals.[10] The medial rectus has no attachments to other muscles and hence is the most common muscle to be lost. The superior and lateral recti have attachments to the oblique muscles and hence are less likely to retract. The inferior rectus is slightly easier to find than the medial rectus due to possible connections to the inferior oblique.

### *Prevention*

Maneuvers to avoid muscle loss include:

- Careful handling of the muscle, especially in eyes with history of trauma or history of previous surgery.
  - Ensure that adequate muscle tissue is incorporated in the full-thickness suture bites.
  - Careful passage of needles, to avoid cutting previously passed sutures.
- Careful secure tying of the suture with square knots.
- Cautious use of cautery to avoid damage to the sutures.
- Adequate depth of the scleral pass.
- Preservation of posterior Tenon's capsule to avoid posterior retraction of lost muscle.[10]

### *Management*

When the muscle is lost during surgery, careful examination of the surgical site with adequate illumination and good exposure is needed. An illuminated headlamp or an operating microscope can be used and malleable retractors are very useful to provide the much needed exposure. The lost muscle is usually adherent to the Tenon's capsule, and hence hand over hand grasping of Tenon's capsule enables visualization of the muscle. Irrigation of the wound also helps differentiate the pink muscle from the white-ballooned Tenon's capsule. When visualized a suture should be passed through the muscle.

### Pulled in Two Syndrome (PITS)

PITS describes an intraoperative tear of the rectus muscle usually at the muscle–tendon junction. It can be caused by excessive tension on the muscle during surgery, inherent weakness of the muscle, or combination of both. The medial rectus is most commonly involved followed by the inferior rectus.[10] The risk factors for PITS include advanced age, extraocular muscle (EOM) pathology (like metastasis, thyroid disease, radiation), and previous EOM surgery.[11] The treatment of PITS involves immediate isolation of the muscle stump, securing it with full-thickness bites and reattaching to sclera.

## GLOBE PERFORATION

The incidence of scleral perforation varies in reported literature from 1% to 3%.[12-13] Most of these go unrecognized and are detected only when routine indirect ophthalmoscopy is performed. Anatomically the sclera is thinnest behind the insertion of the rectus muscles measuring approximately 0.3 mm. Globe perforations most commonly occur during muscle reattachment but they have been noted to occur at any step of the procedure including muscle disinsertion, muscle suturing, or tissue dissection. They are also noted to occur more commonly with recessions than resections.[12] Risk factors include myopia, prior strabmismus surgery, thyroid ophthalmopathy, posterior scleral passes, and surgical inexperience. Perforations mostly have no long-term sequelae but can cause retinal detachment in 2%, endophthalmitis in 0.5%, and rare complications like vitreous hemorrhage, choroidal detachment, hyphema, lens dislocation, and phthisis.[14]

### Prevention

- Use of adequate magnification and illumination during strabismus surgery with loupes or microscope.
- Extra caution in patients with thin sclera and in reoperations and patients with restrictive strabismus In scenarios where posterior sclera pass is difficult, hang-back recession is safer.
- Scleral passes should be made at a depth of 1/3 to 1/2 using a fine spatulated needle. The spatulated cutting needle (S-24 needle, Ethicon) that is pointed at the top has a high incidence of perforations,[12] and hence the authors preference is to use a conventional spatulated cutting needle (S-29 needle, Ethicon) that is pointed at the bottom.
- The most preferred suture material is 6-0 vicryl in view of its high tensile strength and minimal tissue reaction.[13]

### Management

Indirect ophthalmoscopy should be performed intraoperatively in all patients suspected to have a deep sclera pass. If a perforation is detected, management is controversial. Traditionally either cryotherapy or laser photocoagulation was recommended. Clinical and experimental studies have demonstrated the safety of observation.[15] In all patient topical antibiotics should be administered and some authors suggest the use of subconjunctival antibiotic or systemic antibiotic in view of the risk of endophthalmitis. These patients should be monitored closely in the postoperative period to look for signs of infection and retinal detachment.

## SCLERAL WOUND

Scleral wounds are rarely seen after strabismus surgery but can occur during muscle disinsertion especially in patients with restrictive strabismus and thin sclera. It can be prevented by applying only gentle traction on the muscle hook and ensuring good visualization during muscle disinsertion. In all patients, indirect ophthalmoscopy should be performed. For small wounds direct suturing can be attempted, but for large defects a scleral patch graft is often required.[16]

## HEMORRHAGE

Hemorrhage is usually mild in strabismus surgery but can interfere with visualization and suture placement. Hemorrhage is encountered more frequently in reoperations. In the United States and United Kingdom, routinely topical phenylephrine and topical diluted epinephrine are used respectively prior to strabismus surgery. More recently topical brimonidine and apraclonidine have been noted to be as efficacious to limit bleeding.[17] During surgery light diathermy can be used to control the bleeding. Surgery to the inferior oblique muscle is more prone for bleeding either from the cut muscle or from damage to the vortex vein.

## POSTOPERATIVE COMPLICATIONS

### Eyelid Changes

Vertical rectus muscle surgery can cause significant altering of the lid configuration and contour. It has been reported that 91% of the patients develop upper lid retraction with superior rectus recession, 94% of patients develop lower lid retraction with inferior rectus recession, and patients with inferior rectus resection develop lower lid advancement with accompanying flattening.[18] Kushner reported that anterior transposition of the inferior oblique muscle causes a narrowing of the palpebral fissure and a deformity of the lower eyelid on upgaze especially when combined with superior rectus recession for dissociated vertical deviation.[19] The lower eyelid retraction with inferior rectus recession is noticeable when the recession exceeds 4 mm and is especially of concern in patients with thyroid eye disease. Multiple techniques have been described to minimize this complications including lysis of surrounding check ligaments and fascial attachments, advancement of the capsulopalpebral head, and complete detachment of the fascia of the capsulopalpebral head.[20]

## DELLEN

### Scleral Dellen

It can occur after strabismus surgery if the sclera is left exposed. This occurs when the conjunctiva is resected, or when adjustable suture is done with the limbal approach and a conjunctival retraction suture is placed for exposure.[21] Excessive use of cautery also contributes to this complication. Ensuring that conjunctival closure is complete avoids this complication. Treatment consists of intense lubrication and in refractory cases surgical conjunctival procedures can be considered.

### Corneal Dellen

It is described as a sausage-shaped excavation of the peripheral cornea secondary to local dehydration. It is reported to occur with high frequency in reoperations and in transposition surgeries utilizing the limbal incision.[22] It can be avoided by ensuring good conjunctival closure and burying of the sutures at the limbus. The disease is self-limited and responds to lubrication and bandage contact lenses.

## WOUND COMPLICATIONS

### Conjunctival Cyst

The incidence of conjunctival cysts after strabismus surgery has been reported to be 0.25%.[23] Most cysts are small but large conjunctival and orbital cysts can occur that can lead to restrictive strabismus.[24] The risk factor to the formation of cyst is young patients in whom the Tenon's tissue is exuberant. It also occurs more commonly with recession because of the dragging of Tenon's during surgery.[23] It can be avoided by closure of the conjunctiva using the edge and not allowing the conjunctiva to roll under the wound. In cases of orbital cyst, orbital imaging is important to localize the extent of the cyst prior to treatment. Treatment can include thermal cauterization or injection of sclerosing agent but in most cases surgical excision is preferred.

### Suture Granuloma

They occur rarely with the advent of modern absorbable sutures like polyglycolic acid (vicryl). It can still occur in procedures like posterior fixation suture or superior oblique tuck where nonabsorbable suture is used. Theoretically with the adjustable suture technique, there is more suture material in the eye to incite inflammation but in clinical practice this is not encountered.

### Prolapsed Tenon's Capsule

Prolapsed Tenon's capsule leads to an unsightly scar and makes the eye prone to infection. It can be avoided by careful conjunctival closure and removal of the Tenon's tissue at the wound prior to closure. Postoperatively if noticed can be treated by excision of the redundant tissue in the office in adults and in the operating room in children.

### Advancement of Plica Semilunaris

This leads to an unsightly red scar medially. Care should be taken to differentiate the plica from the conjunctiva during closure after medial rectus surgery especially after resections.

## REFRACTIVE CHANGES

There has been a wide variation in the reports of refractive changes after strabismus surgery. Most studies have noted a shift toward "with the rule" astigmatism in patients undergoing horizontal muscle surgery. Vertical muscle surgery has a lower tendency to cause refractive shift. Though myopic changes have been reported more consistently than other changes in spherical equivalent, a consistent shift has not been reported. The mechanism of the refractive change is also debatable, but it is thought to be secondary to the tension of the extraocular muscles exerted on the sclera that is transmitted to the cornea.[25] Most of these changes are transient but as some of the refractive changes are more permanent a cycloplegic retinoscopy 3 months after strabismus surgery is recommended.

## INFECTIONS

Infections after strabismus surgery are not very common and are mostly limited to the superficial tissues. Studies have documented that the postoperative use of antibiotic does not alter the frequency of infections, and hence in most cases use of povidone iodine at the end of surgery alone is sufficient for prophylaxis.[26] The risk of infection in higher in reoperations and extensive surgeries and in those patients an antibiotic may be beneficial postoperatively.

### Conjunctivitis

It is usually mild and self-limiting. It is difficult to differentiate infective conjunctivitis from allergic reaction to suture material. Conjunctivitis responds well to topical antibiotics and has no long-term sequelae.

### Periocular Infection

Periocular infections are rare after strabismus surgery but can be severe. Kivlin and Wilson surveyed 419 pediatric ophthalmologists in 1995 and reported 25 patients with documented orbital cellulitis.[27] In their report *Staphylococcus aureus* was the most common organism and all patients responded to treatment with no long-term sequelae. Orbital cellulitis is more common in children with undetected sinus disease and usually presents with pain, lid swelling, and pyrexia. Most of the patients do not respond to oral antibiotics and need hospitalization for intravenous antibiotics. Orbital imaging is critical in the management of these patients to rule out an abscess collection and to delineate the extent of the infection. On computed tomography of the orbits, an abscess would show a tubular rim-enhancing lesion at the site of muscle insertion, usually associated with a thickened rectus muscle and subtle scleral thickening.[28] Prompt recognition and treatment usually lead to good response with no effect on the outcome of the strabismus surgery.

### Endophthalmitis

Poststrabismus surgery endophthalmitis is exceedingly rare, with an estimated incidence of 1:185,000 strabismus surgeries.[29] The anatomical outcome and visual prognosis following endophthalmitis has been noted to be very poor in post strabismus cases and very few eyes obtain visual acuity of 20/200 or better. As the incidence is very low routine prophylaxis with antibiotics is not required. Pre and post procedure instillation of povidone iodine in the cul-de-sac could be of benefit.[26] The risk is higher if the sclera is perforated during the procedure and in these patients subconjunctival antibiotics or systemic antibiotics are advised.

## NECROTISING SCLERITIS

Necrotising scleritis can occur following any ocular surgery and has been rarely reported after strabismus surgery. It occurs in higher frequency in adults with autoimmune disease or thyroid eye disease but has been reported in children also.[30] Infective etiology needs to be ruled out prior to treating these eyes as surgically induced necrotizing scleritis with systemic steroids or immunosuppression.

## ANTERIOR SEGMENT ISCHEMIA

The blood supply to the anterior segment of the eye including the iris and ciliary body is from the anterior ciliary arteries (~70%) and posterior ciliary arteries (~30%). The anterior ciliary arteries traverse through the extraocular muscles with two vessels each in the medial, superior, and inferior rectus and one vessel in the lateral rectus muscle. The superior and inferior oblique muscles do not carry any blood vessel, and hence surgery to these muscles does not pose a risk for ischemia. Anterior segment ischemia (ASI) is rare after strabismus surgery in view of the extensive collateral circulation. The incidence is estimated to be 1 case in 13,000 strabismus surgeries.[31]

### Risk Factors

It is postulated that though clinical ASI is rare, subclinical cases occur with much greater frequency. In an experimental human study using fluorescein angiography, it was found that surgery on horizontal recti did not have any circulatory change in the iris.[32] But surgery on the vertical recti induced a localized circulatory delay in the temporal quadrant. Hence, surgery on the two vertical recti and the lateral rectus poses a higher risk for ASI.[33] The most important risk factor for ASI is advancing age with very few reported cases in children. The other risk factors include atherosclerotic disease, thyroid eye disease, blood dyscrasia, and carotid disease.[31] Most of the circulatory disturbances after rectus muscle surgery are transient and collaterals develop mainly via the long posterior ciliary artery. Though the safe time period between multiple surgeries is not clearly determined, most surgeons advise to wait for 6 months to operate on the vertical recti after horizontal muscle surgery.

### Clinical Features

The clinical features can vary from mild anterior chamber flare to severe ischemia with eventual phthisis. The most consistent features are corneal epithelial edema, cellular aqueous reaction, keratic precipitates, hypotony, iris atrophy, and pupillary abnormalities. Late complications include rubeosis iridis, cataract, and glaucoma.[32]

### Treatment

ASI is treated with topical and systemic corticosteroids. Most mild cases resolve over few weeks. Hyperbaric oxygen has been noted to improve circulation in severe cases.[33]

### Prevention

Strategies to avoid the occurrence of ASI include:

- Staged surgery with an interval of 3–6 months. Most reports of ASI have occurred after three or four recti muscle are operated simultneously. Some patients have been reported to develop ASI even after two rectus muscle surgery but those eyes usually are at high risk and in those eyes caution is advised.
- If more than three muscles need to be operated on for the correction of the strabismus, botulinum toxin can be considered as a temporizing measure.
- Forniceal incision has been noted to have a lower incidence of ASI as it preserves the perilimbal circulation.[34]
- Microsurgical preservation of the anterior ciliary vessels during surgery can avoid interruption of the circulation.[35]

## STRABISMUS OUTCOME

### Overcorrection

Undercorrection and overcorrection are the most common complications of strabismus surgery. Though the definition is variable based on the preoperative goal of surgery, most surgeons define surgical success as within 10 prism diopters of motor alignment. In some situations like intermittent exotropia, surgical overcorrection is the goal as over time orthophoria is reached. The reported occurrence of overcorrection is variable ranging from 3% to 38%.[14] Some causes of overcorrection are inaccurate preoperative measurement, slipped muscle in a recession, and resection of a tight muscle. Overcorrections can be avoided by careful preoperative evaluation with at least two sets of measurements obtained on different days. Adjustable suture technique gives room for postoperative adjustment and should be considered in at-risk patients.

### Undercorrection

Undercorrection is more common than overcorrection especially for congenital esotropia in which it is reported to occur in 14% of surgeries.[14] Schutte et al. reported that approximately half of the reoperations in strabismus surgery are caused by inaccuracy in the measurement of the angle of strabismus, variability in surgical strategy and imprecise surgery.[36] Hence, careful preoperative assessment and surgical planning are of utmost importance and adjustable sutures can also be considered.

Esotropia surgery in children with developmental disorders needs a careful approach. In one study, bimedial recess procedures were found to have a greater effect per millimeter of recession, while recess-resect surgeries did not demonstrate the same effect.[37] Habot-Wilner Z et al. reported a 38% success rate in correction of esotropia in children with developmental delay after a single surgery, and two-thirds of the failures were undercorrections.[38] Proper patient (or parent) counseling

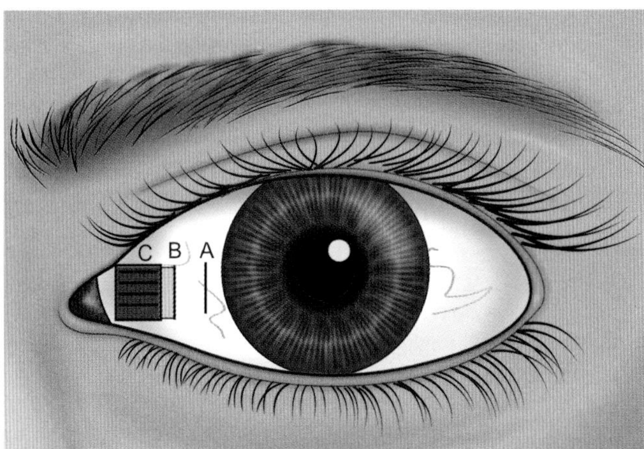


**Figure 109-1** Diagrammatic representation of a slipped medial rectus causing increase in intended recession. (A) Original insertion. (B) Intended new insertion with only muscle capsule sutured to that point. (C) Position of muscle fibers that are retracted in the capsule.

should precede surgery in those who are known to be at risk of a second surgical procedure.

## Slipped Muscle

A slipped muscle causes an increase in the effect of a recession. It occurs more commonly when the muscle suture does not include muscle fibers and only the muscle capsule is sutured to the insertion. With movement of the eye, the muscle fibers contract backward to the capsule (Fig. 109-1). Rarely one of the scleral bites tears through causing increased slipping of the muscle. When both the scleral bites are torn, the muscle is lost. Clinically the patient would have a weakness of duction and a deviation away from the affected muscle. This complication can be avoided by careful placement of muscle suture and ensuring that the scleral bites are of adequate depth. Treatment of a slipped muscle involves anchoring the muscle including substance of the muscle and then advancing it to a point anterior to the originally intended insertion.

## Fat Adherence

Fat adherence occurs when the Tenon's tissue is violated and orbital fat pads are exposed during surgery leading to restrictive strabismus. It is most commonly seen with inferior oblique surgery, causing hypotropia in primary position and limitation of elevation on adduction. It can be avoided by careful hooking of the muscle under direct visualization. If fat is encountered during surgery, the defect should be very carefully closed with Tenon's tissue with absorbable suture. If large defects are encountered, amniotic membrane grafts can be used.

## Diplopia

The occurrence of diplopia depends on the preoperative diagnosis and it would be useful to do prism adaptation test prior to surgery to detect the patients at risk for postoperative diplopia. Mostly postoperative diplopia is transient and resolves by 6–8 weeks. In spite of motor alignment, 0.8% of patients will have persistent diplopia.[39] Treatment involves prisms, surgery, or botulinum toxin.

## PEARLS AND PITFALLS

- Complications of strabismus surgery occur in 1 in 400 surgeries.
- Undercorrection and overcorrection are the most common complication and can be avoided by careful preoperative measurement and surgical planning.
- Muscle complications are more common in restrictive strabismus and in thyroid eye disease and in these patients extra caution is advised.
- Anterior segment ischemia is a serious complication that can be avoided by identifying the risk factors and by performing staged surgery.

## REFERENCES

1. Bradbury JA, Taylor RH. Severe complications of strabismus surgery. J AAPOS. 2013;17:59-63.
2. Allison CE, De Lange JJ, Koole FD, et al. A comparison of the incidence of the oculocardiac and oculorespiratory reflexes during sevoflurane or halothane anesthesia for strabismus surgery in children. Anesth Analg. 2000;90:306-10.
3. Dewar KMS. The oculocardiac reflex. Proc Roy Soc Med. 1976; 6:13-14.
4. Rodgers A, Cox RG. Anesthetic management for pediatric strabismus surgery: continuing professional development. Can J Anaesth. 2010;57(6):602-17.
5. Ohashi T, Kase M, Yokoi M. Quantitative analysis of the oculocardiac reflex by traction on human extraocular muscle. Invest Ophthalmol Vis Sci. 1986;27:1160-4.
6. Hopkins PM. Malignant hyperthermia: advances in clinical management and diagnosis. Br J Anaesth. 2000;85:118-28.
7. Kuhn I, Scheifler G, Wissing H. Incidence of nausea and vomiting in children after strabismus surgery following desflurane anaesthesia. Paediatr Anaesth. 1999;9:521-6.
8. Shen E, Porco T, Rutar T. Errors in strabismus surgery. JAMA Ophthalmol. 2013;131:75-9.
9. Somani S, Mackeen LD, Morad Y, et al. Assessment of extraocular muscles position and anatomy by 3-dimensional ultrasonography: a trial in craniosynostosis patients. J AAPOS. 2003;7(1):54-9.
10. Cherfan CG, Traboulsi EI. Slipped, severed, torn and lost extraocular muscles. Can J Ophthalmol. 2011;46:501-9.

11. Wallace DK, Steven RV, Mukherji SK. Strabismus surgery complicated by "pulled-in-two syndrome" in a case of breast carcinoma metastatic to the medial rectus muscle. J AAPOS. 2000;4:117-9.
12. Dang Y, Racu C, Isenberg SJ. Scleral penetrations and perforations in strabismus surgery and associated risk factors. J AAPOS. 2004;8:325-31.
13. Morris RJ, Rosen PH, Fells P. Incidence of inadvertent globe perforation during strabismus surgery. Br J Ophthalmol. 1990;74:490-3.
14. Larson SA, Petersen DB, Scott WE. Strabismus surgery complications: prevention and management. Comp Ophthalmol Update. 2003;4:255-63.
15. Bagheri A, Erfanian-Salim R, Ahmadieh H, et al. Globe perforation during strabismus surgery in an animal model: treatment versus observation. J AAPOS. 2011;15:144-7.
16. Awad AH, Mullaney PB, Al-Hazmi A, et al. Recognized globe perforation during strabismus surgery: incidence, risk factors, and sequelae. J AAPOS. 2000;4:150-3.
17. Dahlmann-Noor AH, Cosgrave E, Lowe S, et al. Brimonidine and apraclonidine as vasoconstrictors in adjustable strabismus surgery. J AAPOS. 2009;13:123-6.
18. Pacheco EM, Guyton DL, Repka MX. Changes in eyelid position accompanying vertical rectus muscle surgery and prevention of lower lid retraction with adjustable surgery. J Pediatr Ophthalmol Strabismus. 1992;29:265-72.
19. Kushner BJ. The effect of anterior transposition of the inferior oblique muscle on the palpebral fissure. Arch Ophthalmol. 2000;118:1542-6.
20. Liao SL, Shih MJ, Lin LL. A procedure to minimize lower lid retraction during large inferior rectus recession in graves ophthalmopathy. Am J Ophthalmol. 2006;141(2):340-45.
21. Perez I. The "scleral dellen," a complication of adjustable strabismus surgery. J AAPOS. 2002;6(5):332-3.
22. Fresina M, Campos EC. Corneal "dellen" as a complication of strabismus surgery. Eye (Lond). 2009;23:161-3.
23. Guadilla AM, de Liaño PG, Merino P, et al. Conjunctival cysts as a complication after strabismus surgery. J Pediatr Ophthalmol Strabismus. 2011;48(5):298-300.
24. Song JJ, Finger PT, Kurli M, et al. Giant secondary conjunctival inclusion cysts: a late complication of strabismus surgery. Ophthalmology. 2006;113:1049.e1-2.
25. Bagheri A, Farahi A, Guyton DL. Astigmatism induced by simultaneous recession of both horizontal rectus muscles. J AAPOS. 2003;7:42-6.
26. Koederitz NM, Neely DE, Plager DA, et al. Postoperative povidone-iodine prophylaxis in strabismus surgery. J AAPOS. 2008;12(4):396-400.
27. Kivlin JD, Wilson ME Jr. Periocular infection after strabismus surgery. The Periocular Infection Study Group. J Pediatr Ophthalmol Strabismus. 1995;32(1):42-9.
28. Brenner C, Ashwin M, Smith D, et al. Sub-Tenon's space abscess after strabismus surgery. J AAPOS. 2009;13(2):198-9.
29. Simon JW, Lininger LL, Scheraga JL. Recognized scleral perforation during eye muscle surgery: incidence and sequelae. J Pediatr Ophthalmol Strabismus. 1992;29(5):273-5.
30. Kearney FM, Blaikie AJ, Gole GA. Anterior necrotizing scleritis after strabismus surgery in a child. J AAPOS. 2007;11(2):197-8.
31. Saunders RA, Bluestein EC, Wilson ME, et al. Anterior segment ischemia after strabismus surgery. Surv Ophthalmol. 1994; 38(5):456-66.
32. Hayreh SS, Scott WE. Fluorescein iris angiography. II. Disturbances in iris circulation following strabismus operation on the various recti. Arch Ophthalmol. 1978;96:1390-400.
33. Oguz H, Sobaci G. The use of hyperbaric oxygen therapy in ophthalmology. Surv Ophthalmol. 2008;53(2):112-20.
34. Fishman PH, Repka MX, Green WR, et al. A primate model of anterior segment ischemia after strabismus surgery. The role of the conjunctival circulation. Ophthalmology. 1990;97(4): 456-61.
35. McKeown CA, Lambert HM, Shore JW. Preservation of the anterior ciliary vessels during extraocular muscle surgery. Ophthalmology. 1989;96(4):498-506.
36. Schutte S, Polling JR, van der Helm FC, et al. Human error in strabismus surgery: quantification with a sensitivity analysis. Graefes Arch Clin Exp Ophthalmol. 2009;247(3):399-409.
37. van Rijn LJ, Langenhorst AE, Krijnen JS, et al. Predictability of strabismus surgery in children with developmental disorders and/or psychomotor retardation. Strabismus. 2009;17(3): 117-27.
38. Habot-Wilner Z, Spierer A, Barequet IS, et al. Long-term results of esotropia surgery in children with developmental delay. J AAPOS. 2012;16(1):32-5.
39. Kushner BJ. Intractable diplopia after strabismus surgery in adults. Arch Ophthalmol. 2002;120(11):1498-504.

CHAPTER

110

# Chemodenervation for Strabismus

Mohammad Ali A Sadiq

## BOTULINUM TOXIN

## INTRODUCTION

Type A botulinum toxin produced by *Clostridium botulinum* causes temporary muscle paralysis in humans, and injection with toxin in extraocular muscles as an alternative to strabismus surgery was first described by Alan Scott in 1973.[1] The indications for use of this technique were not very clear initially; however, with increasing use and further study, botulinum has been shown to be a viable alternative to incisional surgery for particular types of strabismus or particular types of patients.

## OCULAR INDICATIONS

### Diagnostic

- To evaluate postoperative diplopia prior to strabismus surgery.[2,3]
- To assess the likelihood of reducing the abnormal head posture and reducing the diplopia by increasing the field of binocular single vision in Duane's retraction syndrome as a precursor to surgery.[4]
- To evaluate binocular potential.

### Therapeutic

#### *Strabismic indications*

- Small and moderate angle, comitant strabismus with potential for binocular vision.[5,6]
- Adjuvant procedure after overcorrection or undercorrection following incisional strabismus surgery.[7]
- In paralytic strabismus, to relieve diplopia and to prevent contraction of the antagonist muscle, e.g. 6th nerve palsy[8,9] superior oblique palsy[10] and traumatic 3rd nerve palsy.[11,12]
- Restrictive strabismus, e.g. thyroid eye disease.[13,14]
- Congenital and acquired nystagmus and oscillopsia with retrobulbar injection of botulinum toxin.[15]
- Internuclear ophthalmoplegia (INO).[16]
- Convergence spasm.[17]

#### *Nonstrabismic indications*

- Muscular spasm, e.g. blepharospasm and hemifacial spasm, and Meige syndrome.[18,19]
- Lid retraction in thyroid eye disease.[20-22]
- Compressive optic neuropathy in Graves disease following failed orbital decompression.[23]
- Chemical tarsorrhaphy by injecting botulinum toxin in the levator muscle to prevent exposure keratopathy.[24,25]
- Entropion correction.[26,27]
- Severe dry eyes.[28]
- Apraxia of eyelid opening (blepharospastic apraxia).[29,30]
- Elevated intraocular pressure (IOP) from restrictive myopathy.[31]
- Eyelid myokymia.[32,33]
- Lacrimal gland hypersecretion.[34,35]

## CONTRAINDICATIONS

- Hypersensitivity to any botulinum toxin preparation.
- Conjunctivitis.

## SURGICAL TECHNIQUE

In adult patients, the injection can be given in the clinic with topical proparacaine drops. Most children require sedation. Ketamine is used as the preferred anesthetic as muscle tone is not lost with this agent, thus allowing use of an electromyography (EMG) for directed injection.

### Preparation of Botulinum Toxin for Injection

The efficacy and safety of botulinum toxin depends on the proper storage, selection of the right dose, and proper reconstitution. Botulinum toxin comes in the form of onabotulinumtoxinA (Botox; Allergan, Inc. Irvine, CA), rimabotulinumtoxinB (Myobloc; Solstice Neurosciences, CA), abobotulinumtoxinA (Dysport Ipsen, France), and incobotulinumtoxinA (Xeomin Merz Pharmaceuticals, GmbH, Germany).[36] The proprietary unit of each is noninterchangeable as they have been made of different strains of bacteria.

Botox is used in a single use 100 units or 200 units per vial. However, it retains effectiveness for at least 3 months if frozen and for at least 2 weeks if refrigerated. It may be inactivated with shaking and rapid injection. Each vacuum dried vial is reconstituted with sterile, nonpreserved 0.9% sodium chloride injection. The proper amount of diluent is drawn up in a 5 cc syringe and slowly injected into the vial. Botox is mixed with the saline by gently rotating the vial. An amount slightly more than the intended dose of reconstituted toxin is drawn into a 1cc syringe and is then attached to a 27-gauge needle of the EMG recorder and then air bubbles from the syringe barrel are expelled.

Some practitioners prefer to inject without EMG guidance. This requires a higher level of experience and skill on the part of the physician, in addition to knowledge of the anatomy of the eye and the extraocular muscle location, and good cooperation from the patient.[37-39]

### Dosages Used

For the treatment of strabismus, the concentration of Botox ranges from 2.5 to 7.5 International units/0.1 mL of solution depending on the degree of strabismus (Table 110-1). Strabismus <20PD is usually injected with 2.5 International units while those between 20 PD and 50PD with 5 International units, and deviations >50PD with 7.5 International units. Injection can be used in one or both eyes.

### Specific Instrumentation (Electromyogram)

Electromyography (EMG) amplifies the extracellular potential of the muscles when a Teflon-plated electrode needle is inserted into the muscle. The electric signals are detected by the tip of the Teflon-plated electrode needle.[40,41] The amplifier magnifies the electrical impulses and makes them audible through the speaker or earphone of the unit. The amplifier signal is designed in such a way that it filters all background noise. The Teflon-plated needle is connected to the amplifier through a cable, while the ground cable is attached to the skin of the patient, usually the forehead.

**TABLE 110-1** Recommended dosage of Botox per injection

| Deviation | Units injected |
|---|---|
| <20 PD | 2.5 I.U in one or two muscles |
| 20–50 PD | 5.0 I.U in one or two muscles |
| >50 PD | 7.5 I.U in one or two muscles |

### Method of Injecting a Rectus Muscle

The eye is anesthetized by using topical proparacaine drops. Topical phenylephrine drops 2.5% may be used to reduce vascularity of the tissues. A cotton tip applicator is then soaked in topical proparacaine and applied on the site of the muscle for 5–10 seconds. A monopolar, Teflon-coated 27-gauge needle attached to the EMG unit[40,41] is passed through the conjunctiva just posterior to the muscle insertion (2.5 mm). The needle should enter with the bevel away from the sclera, and is advanced along the orbital side of the muscle with the patient looking in the direction opposite to the muscle being injected or looking straight ahead (depending on surgeon preference) while listening for the high-level EMG signal for the evidence of the needle entry into the muscle belly. The patient is then asked to slowly look in the field of action of the muscle. Botulinum is then injected into the muscle belly. The electromyographic recorder signal reduces as the injected fluid buffers contact between the muscle fibers and the needle. The needle is then withdrawn from the eye (Fig. 110-1). A toothed forcep is used to stabilize and move the eye in the desired position when injecting children under anesthesia.

### Method of Injecting the Inferior Oblique Muscle

After anesthetizing the eye and instilling 2.5% phenylephrine drops, the patient is asked to look superiorly in adduction (superonasally). The needle, bevel away from the sclera, is introduced into the conjunctiva 10 mm from the limbus inferotemporally, and advanced 10mm to reach the site of the belly of inferior oblique while listening for the EMG signal (Fig. 110-2). Once the inferior oblique muscle belly is entered, the botulinum toxin is injected. The needle is then withdrawn from the eye.[10]

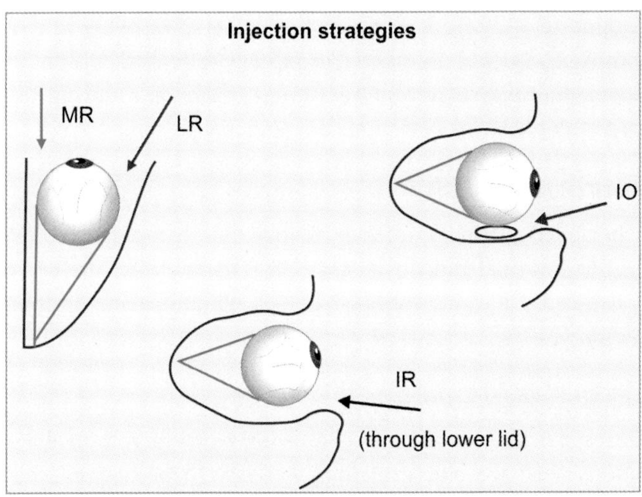


**Figure 110-1** Direction of the needle during botulinum injection to the extraocular muscles. (MR: Medial rectus muscle; LR: Lateral rectus muscle; IR: Inferior rectus muscle; IO: Inferior oblique).

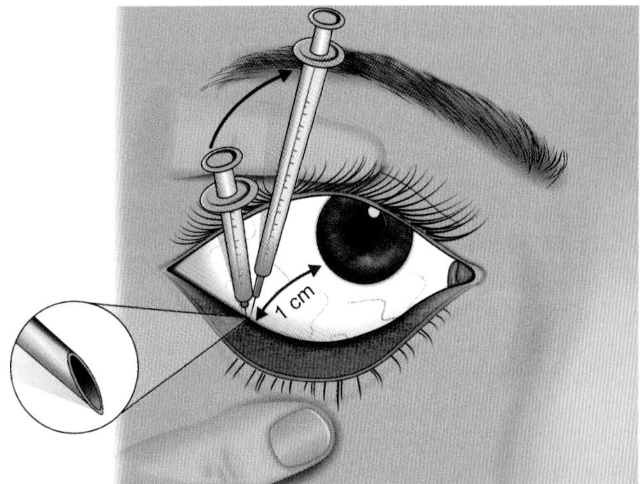


**Figure 110-2** Anterior view of botulinum toxin injection in the inferior oblique muscle. Magnified view: the direction of the bevel of the needle.

**TABLE 110-2** Proposed follow-up schedule after injection of botulinum toxin

| Time | 1st week | 12 weeks | 24 weeks |
|---|---|---|---|
| Deviation | Maximum change in deviation (possible overcorrection) | Decrease in change in deviation | Final alignment (maximum reduction in change in deviation) |
| Motility | Weakness in direction of muscle injected | Recovery of motility | Full motility |
| Complication | Possible ptosis | Recovery of ptosis | No ptosis |

Injections under anesthesia must be done without EMG guidance unless ketamine is used, since other anesthetic agents will suppress muscle firing responses detected by the EMG.

### Postoperative Care

After the injection, topical antibiotics/steroid drops are instilled in the eye, and continued three to four times daily for 5–7 days.

### Proposed Follow-Up Time After Injection

Based on the effect of the injection, we propose a follow-up after 1 week of injection followed by after 3 months and then 6 months (Table 110-2).

## MECHANISM OF ACTION

Botulinum toxin interferes with the release of acetylcholine at the neuromuscular junction of striated muscle. Toxin seems to act upon individual motor nerve terminals but does not block the propagation of the nerve impulse. It has been suggested that the toxin antagonizes calcium ion transport by serotonin. After calcium ion depletion, there is no release of acetylcholine from the endplate and the muscle fiber fails to contract. Eventually there is denervation. Eventually axons resprout after 3 months. Treatment of developing extraocular muscle with botulinum toxin causes acute reduction in muscle strength and mitochondrial densities, but minimal changes in muscle fiber diameter and neuromuscular junction structures. The permanent therapeutic effects most likely do not cause permanent changes at the level of the peripheral effector organ, but rather involve central (CNS) adaptive responses.[42]

## EFFECT ON ALIGNMENT

After injection of botulinum toxin, there is a delay in onset of alignment change and paralysis that is observed. The onset of paralysis begins after 2–3 days with the peak effect being seen after 5–6 days (1 week), which often causes the eyes to deviate in the opposite direction. Thus, the maximum effect is attained around the first week and gradually lessens thereafter. The paralytic effect of the toxin remains for 3–4 months. Injections can be repeated if needed. The maximum number of reported injections to one individual has been 68 without any side effect with the time interval between injection increasing and the angle of deviation decreasing with repeated injections.[43]

## COMPLICATIONS

- Ptosis
- Vertical deviation
- Diplopia
- Subconjunctival hemorrhage
- Infection
- Pupillary dilation (tonic pupil)[44]
- Scleral perforation
- Acute angle closure glaucoma, thought to result from mydriasis from parasympathetic effect at the ciliary ganglion[45]
- Accommodative insufficiency due to deep posterior orbital effects on the ciliary ganglion[46]
- Retinal detachment[47]

## OUTCOMES AFTER BOTULINUM INJECTION

### *Small and Moderate Angle Comitant Strabismus*

It has been demonstrated that early intervention using simultaneous bimedial rectus injection can reestablish motor and sensory fusion with good long term results comparable with those reported with surgical corrections[15,48-50] Carruther showed that the effect of botulinum toxin was not comparable to surgery in patients with no potential for binocularity,[51] but increased success rates were seen with repeated injections in children with acquired esotropia, many of whom achieved at least peripheral fusion. Larger doses are required for large angle deviations, which are then associated with higher incidence of complications such as ptosis.

### *Adjuvant to Surgery*

Botulinum toxin is also equally effective to surgery as a retreatment modality. Tejedor in a prospective comparative study showed that in children requiring retreatment for infantile esotropia, 67.8% of children who underwent reoperation and 59.2% of those treated with botulinum injection attained orthotropia at the 3-year visit ($p = 0.72$) thus depicting a similar success rate.[7]

### *Sixth Nerve Palsy*

Improved rates of recovery of normal alignment after use of Botox range from 38% to 70%, especially if treated within 6 months of onset, compared to the expected spontaneous recovery rate of 12–54%.[52] Thus, Botox has been used to weaken the antagonistic medial rectus muscle in patients with traumatic, ischemic, inflammatory, and tumor-related 6th nerve palsy. However, prospective studies carried out by Holmes et al.[53] and Lee et al.[54] showed equal recovery rate in Botox treated and nontreated groups. Despite this, botulinum toxin may play a role in alleviation of diplopia during the recovery phase for deviations due to nerve palsies.

### *Fourth Nerve Palsy*

Chemodenervation of inferior oblique muscle rapidly restores a more normal binocular status in patients with 4th nerve palsy causing a substantial relief of symptoms in the long term.[10]

### *Restrictive Myopathy*

For restrictive myopathies, Botox may play a role in deviations that are still evolving, and it is hypothesized that it may be helpful in halting the muscle fibrosis of thyroid ophthalmopathy if injected in the acute phase of the disease.

Botox has also been used to treat increased IOP caused by restrictive myopathies.[31] The increased IOP, mostly evident with up gaze, is difficult to treat with topical medication, and occasionally requires orbital decompression to relieve the coexisting vascular congestion. The IOP lowering effect lasts for 2–4 months, and requires repeat injections in the hypertrophied muscle/s.

### *Congenital and Acquired Nystagmus*

Botulinum toxin in multiple rectus muscles has been used to treat nystagmus.[55-58] A decrease in amplitude of congenital nystagmus in 42.9% of patients with nystagmus and esotropia, 50% with exotropia and nystagmus, and 28.6% with horizontal and vertical nystagmus has been reported.[59] Improved visual acuity in up to 66% of patients with nystagmus was seen after retrobulbar injection of the toxin.[60-62] However, symptomatic diplopia and ptosis was more frequent with the retrobulbar injections.[63,64]

### *Internuclear Ophthalmoplegia*

Internuclear ophthalmoplegia (INO) is caused by lesions of the medial longitudinal fasciculus (MLF) causing limitation of adduction. The most disconcerting symptom of this condition is diplopia that can be horizontal, vertical, or oblique. In most patients, the symptoms reduce or resolve completely either due to recovery of function of MLF axons or because of central adaptive mechanism. Injection of botulinum toxin in one or both the lateral rectus muscles has been used to treat symptomatic INO of >6 months in duration. The effect of the injection is transient and so maintenance injections may be required to relieve symptoms. It is hypothesized that repeated injections may have a longer effect and the disease-free interval may increase, necessitating fewer injections.[16]

# BUPIVACAINE

## INTRODUCTION

Bupivacaine used for local anesthesia in cataract surgery results in strabismus if the anesthetic enters the muscle. Injection into the fast muscle fibers of laboratory animals resulted in immediate and massive degeneration of muscle fibers within minutes, probably by allowing excess calcium ions to enter the cytoplasm from the sarcoplasmic reticulum resulting in dissolution of myofibrils at the Z-band,[65] while other structures including the basal lamina and satellite cells and nearby nerves and vasculature remain unchanged.[66-68] After 2 days of injection, the satellite cells are activated and regeneration begins with the muscle reaching preinjection size and strength around day 21.[65,69] The satellite cells continue to elaborate new fibers, with the resulting hypertrophy continuing for many days and the muscle remaining enlarged for up to 500 days.[70] In extraocular muscles, proliferation continues on to build a muscle having greater contractile strength, intrinsic elastic stiffness, and size than before, with consequent effects on eye alignment.[71] Alan Scott was able to successfully harness the muscle response to improve eye alignment and correct strabismus.[70] Magnetic resonance imaging (MRI) of eye muscles showed an average muscle size increase ranging from 5.8% to 6.2%.[72] The same increase in muscle thickness was also seen with ultrasonography.[73]

## STRABISMIC INDICATIONS

- Small and moderate angle comitant strabismus.
- To treat strabismus due to paralytic muscles.
- As an adjunct to surgery when there is under or overcorrection.
- As an adjunct to botulinum toxin injection. The effect attained with both is double the effect with either injection bupivacaine or injection botulinum toxin alone.[71]

## CONTRAINDICATIONS

Restrictive myopathy, e.g. thyroid ophthalmopathy for fear of causing compressive optic neuropathy and increased IOP.

## SURGICAL TECHNIQUE

Magnetic resonance imaging (MRI) studies have shown that bupivacaine diffuses poorly along the muscle,[74] so Scott et al. advocate using EMG guidance to fill the whole muscle by injecting most of the bupivacaine in the posterior third and the remainder in the middle of the muscle, allowing some bupivacaine to move anteriorly along the needle track. Scott et al. showed that the best effects on comitant strabismus treatment are achieved with bupivacaine in concentrations of 3.0%, 2.0%, and 1.5% and a volume of between 2 and 4 mL injected into the target muscle.[71] After the injection, topical antibiotics/steroid drops are instilled in the eye.

## EFFECT ON ALIGNMENT

Immediately after the injection, there is an increase in deviation and motility weakness due to underaction of the injected muscle for 7 days according to one report. This was followed by recovery of motility and then reduction in deviation reaching a maximum reduction in deviation at 33 days. The deviation remained constant till the final follow-up exam at 54 days after injection.[70]

## COMPLICATIONS

- Mild proptosis[70]
- Subconjuctival hemorrhage[70]
- Motility deficit[70]
- Transient vertical deviation[70,71,73]
- Significant swelling and discomfort[71]
- Retrobulbar hemorrhage[73]
- Orbital inflammation[71]

## PEARLS AND PITFALLS

- Good anatomical knowledge of anatomy of extraocular muscle is necessary.
- Superior rectus muscle should not be injected due to the risk of causing ptosis in all patients.
- Superior oblique muscle is not injected due to its difficult approach.

## REFERENCES


1. Scott AB, Rosenbaum A, Collins CC. Pharmacologic weakening of extraocular muscles. Invest Ophthalmol. 1973;12(12):924-7.
2. Rayner SA, Hollick EJ, Lee JP. Botulinum toxin in childhood strabismus. Strabismus. 1999;7(2):103-11.
3. Khan J, Kumar I, Marsh IB. Botulinum toxin injection for postoperative diplopia testing in adult strabismus. J Aapos. 2008;12(1):46-8.

4. Dawson EL, Maino A, Lee JP. Diagnostic use of botulinum toxin in patients with Duane syndrome. Strabismus. 2010;18(1):21-3.
5. de Alba Campomanes AG, Binenbaum G, Campomanes Eguiarte G. Comparison of botulinum toxin with surgery as primary treatment for infantile esotropia. J Aapos. 2010;14(2):111-6.
6. Tejedor J, Rodriguez JM. Long-term outcome and predictor variables in the treatment of acquired esotropia with botulinum toxin. Invest Ophthalmol Vis Sci. 2001;42(11):2542-6.
7. Tejedor J, Rodriguez JM. Early retreatment of infantile esotropia: comparison of reoperation and botulinum toxin. Br J Ophthalmol. 1999;83(7):783-7.
8. Owens PL, Strominger MB, Rubin PA, Veronneau-Troutman S. Large-angle exotropia corrected by intraoperative botulinum toxin A and monocular recession resection surgery. J Aapos. 1998;2(3):144-6.
9. Metz HS, Mazow M. Botulinum toxin treatment of acute sixth and third nerve palsy. Graefe's archive for clinical and experimental ophthalmology = Albrecht von Graefes Archiv fur klinische und experimentelle Ophthalmologie. 1988;226(2):141-4.
10. Bagheri A, Eshaghi M. Botulinum toxin injection of the inferior oblique muscle for the treatment of superior oblique muscle palsy. J Aapos. 2006;10(5):385-8.
11. Talebnejad MR, Sharifi M, Nowroozzadeh MH. The role of Botulinum toxin in management of acute traumatic third-nerve palsy. J Aapos. 2008;12(5):510-3.
12. Elston JS. Traumatic third nerve palsy. Br J Ophthalmol. 1984; 68(8):538-43.
13. Dunn WJ, Arnold AC, O'Connor PS. Botulinum toxin for the treatment of dysthyroid ocular myopathy. Ophthalmology. 1986;93(4):470-5.
14. Lyons CJ, Vickers SF, Lee JP. Botulinum toxin therapy in dysthyroid strabismus. Eye (London, England). 1990;4 (Pt 4):538-42.
15. Lennerstrand G, Nordbo OA, Tian S, et al. Treatment of strabismus and nystagmus with botulinum toxin type A. An evaluation of effects and complications. Acta ophthalmologica Scandinavica. 1998;76(1):27-7.
16. Murthy R, Dawson E, Khan S, et al. Botulinum toxin in the management of internuclear ophthalmoplegia. J Aapos. 2007; 11(5):456-9.
17. Kaczmarek BB, Dawson E, Lee JP. Convergence spasm treated with botulinum toxin. Strabismus. 2009;17(1):49-51.
18. Arand M. [Ameliorating strabismus, preventing blepharospasm: botulinum toxin can do more than smooth wrinkles]. MMW Fortschritte der Medizin. 2008;150(47):16.
19. Cohen DA, Savino PJ, Stern MB, et al. Botulinum injection therapy for blepharospasm: a review and report of 75 patients. Clin Neuropharmacol. 1986;9(5):415-29.
20. Uddin JM, Davies PD. Treatment of upper eyelid retraction associated with thyroid eye disease with subconjunctival botulinum toxin injection. Ophthalmology. 2002;109(6):1183-7.
21. Salour H, Bagheri B, Aletaha M, et al. Transcutaneous dysport injection for treatment of upper eyelid retraction associated with thyroid eye disease. Orbit (Amsterdam, Netherlands). 2010;29(2):114-8.
22. Shih MJ, Liao SL, Lu HY. A single transcutaneous injection with Botox for dysthyroid lid retraction. Eye (London, England). 2004;18(5):466-9.
23. Simonsz HJ, Vingerling JR. Botulinum toxin as adjunct for refractory compressive optic neuropathy in Graves' disease. Orbit (Amsterdam, Netherlands). 1998;17(3):173-8.
24. Ellis MF, Daniell M. An evaluation of the safety and efficacy of botulinum toxin type A (BOTOX) when used to produce a protective ptosis. Clin Experiment Ophthalmol. 2001;29(6):394-9.
25. Mackie IA. Successful management of three consecutive cases of recurrent corneal erosion with botulinum toxin injections. Eye (London, England). 2004;18(7):734-7.
26. Deka A, Saikia SP. Botulinum toxin for lower lid entropion correction. Orbit (Amsterdam, Netherlands). 2011;30(1):40-2.
27. Christiansen G, Mohney BG, Baratz KH, et al. Botulinum toxin for the treatment of congenital entropion. Am J Ophthalmol. 2004;138(1):153-5.
28. Sahlin S, Chen E, Kaugesaar T, et al. Effect of eyelid botulinum toxin injection on lacrimal drainage. Am J Ophthalmol. 2000;129(4):481-6.
29. Boghen D, Tozlovanu V, Iancu A, et al. Botulinum toxin therapy for apraxia of lid opening. Ann NY AcadSci. 2002;956: 482-3.
30. Piccione F, Mancini E, Tonin P, et al. Botulinum toxin treatment of apraxia of eyelid opening in progressive supranuclear palsy: report of two cases. Arch Phys Med Rehabil. 1997;78(5):525-9.
31. Kikkawa DO, Cruz RC, Jr., Christian WK, et al. Botulinum A toxin injection for restrictive myopathy of thyroid-related orbitopathy: effects on intraocular pressure. Am J Ophthalmol. 2003;135(4):427-31.
32. Jordan DR, Anderson RL, Thiese SM. Intractable orbicularis myokymia: treatment alternatives. Ophthalmic Surg. 1989;20(4):280-3.
33. Sedano MJ, Trejo JM, Macarron JL, et al. Continuous facial myokymia in multiple sclerosis: treatment with botulinum toxin. Eur Neurol. 2000;43(3):137-40.
34. Hofmann RJ. Treatment of Frey's syndrome (gustatory sweating) and 'crocodile tears' (gustatory epiphora) with purified botulinum toxin. Ophthal Plast Reconstr Surg. 2000;16(4): 289-91.
35. Keegan DJ, Geerling G, Lee JP, et al. Botulinum toxin treatment for hyperlacrimation secondary to aberrant regenerated seventh nerve palsy or salivary gland transplantation. Br J Ophthalmol. 2002;86(1):43-6.
36. Albanese A. Terminology for preparations of botulinum neurotoxins: what a difference a name makes. Jama. 2011;305(1): 89-90.
37. Jankovic J. Needle EMG guidance for injection of botulinum toxin. Needle EMG guidance is rarely required. Muscle Nerve. 2001;24(11):1568-70.
38. Sanjari MS, Falavarjani KG, Kashkouli MB, et al. Botulinum toxin injection with and without electromyographic assistance for treatment of abducens nerve palsy: a pilot study. J Aapos. 2008;12(3):259-62.
39. Benabent EC, Garcia Hermosa P, Arrazola MT, et al. Botulinum toxin injection without electromyographic assistance. J Pediatr Ophthalmol Strabismus. 2002;39(4):231-4.
40. Barbano RL. Needle EMG guidance for injection of botulinum toxin. Needle EMG guidance is useful. Muscle Nerve. 2001;24(11):1567-8.

41. Shaari CM, Sanders I. Quantifying how location and dose of botulinum toxin injections affect muscle paralysis. Muscle Nerve. 1993;16(9):964-9.
42. Croes SA, Baryshnikova LM, Kaluskar SS, et al. Acute and long-term effects of botulinum neurotoxin on the function and structure of developing extraocular muscles. Neurobiol Dis. 2007;25(3):649-64.
43. Gardner R, Dawson EL, Adams GG, et al. Long-term management of strabismus with multiple repeated injections of botulinum toxin. J Aapos. 2008;12(6):569-75.
44. Speeg-Schatz C. Persistent mydriasis after botulinum toxin injection for congenital esotropia. J Aapos. 2008;12(3):307-8.
45. Corridan P, Nightingale S, Mashoudi N, et al. Acute angle-closure glaucoma following botulinum toxin injection for blepharospasm. Br J Ophthalmol. 1990;74(5):309-10.
46. Levy Y, Kremer I, Shavit S, Korczyn AD. The pupillary effects of retrobulbar injection of botulinum toxin A (oculinum) in albino rats. Invest Ophthalmol Vis Sci. 1991;32(1):122-5.
47. Liu M, Lee HC, Hertle RW, et al. Retinal detachment from inadvertent intraocular injection of botulinum toxin A. Am J Ophthalmol. 2004;137(1):201-2.
48. McNeer KW, Tucker MG, Guerry CH, et al. Incidence of stereopsis after treatment of infantile esotropia with botulinum toxin A. J Pediatr Ophthalmol Strabismus. 2003;40(5):288-92.
49. Tengtrisorn S, Treyapun N, Tantisarasart T. Botulinum A toxin therapy on esotropia in children. J Med Assoc Thai = Chotmaihet thangphaet. 2002;85(11):1189-97.
50. Ruiz MF, Moreno M, Sanchez-Garrido CM, et al. Botulinum treatment of infantile esotropia with abduction nystagmus. J Pediatr Ophthalmol Strabismus. 2000;37(4):196-205.
51. Carruthers JD, Kennedy RA, Bagaric D. Botulinum vs adjustable suture surgery in the treatment of horizontal misalignment in adult patients lacking fusion. Arch Ophthalmol. 1990; 108(10):1432-5.
52. Chuenkongkaew W, Dulayajinda D, Deetae R. Botulinum toxin treatment of the sixth nerve palsy: an experience of 5-year duration in Thailand. J Med Assoc Thai= Chotmaihet thangphaet. 2001;84(2):171-6.
53. Holmes JM, Droste PJ, Beck RW. The natural history of acute traumatic sixth nerve palsy or paresis. J Aapos. 1998;2(5): 265-8.
54. Lee J, Harris S, Cohen J, et al. Results of a prospective randomized trial of botulinum toxin therapy in acute unilateral sixth nerve palsy. J Pediatr Ophthalmol Strabismus. 1994;31(5): 283-6.
55. Carruthers J. The treatment of congenital nystagmus with Botox. J Pediatr Ophthalmol Strabismus. 1995;32(5):306-8.
56. Crone RA, de Jong PT, Notermans G. [Treatment of nystagmus using injections of botulinum toxins into the eye muscles]. Klinische Monatsblatter fur Augenheilkunde. 1984;184(3): 216-7.
57. Leigh RJ, Tomsak RL, Grant MP, et al. Effectiveness of botulinum toxin administered to abolish acquired nystagmus. Ann Neurol. 1992;32(5):633-42.
58. Repka MX, Savino PJ, Reinecke RD. Treatment of acquired nystagmus with botulinum neurotoxin A. Arch Ophthalmol. 1994;112(10):1320-4.
59. Oleszczynska-Prost E. [Botulinum toxin A in the treatment of congenital nystagmus in children]. Klinika oczna. 2004;106 (4-5):625-8.
60. Helveston EM, Pogrebniak AE. Treatment of acquired nystagmus with botulinum A toxin. Am J Ophthalmol. 1988; 106(5):584-6.
61. Ruben S, Dunlop IS, Elston J. Retrobulbar botulinum toxin for treatment of oscillopsia. Aust N Z J Ophthalmol. 1994;22(1): 65-7.
62. Ruben ST, Lee JP, O'Neil D, et al. The use of botulinum toxin for treatment of acquired nystagmus and oscillopsia. Ophthalmology. 1994;101(4):783-7.
63. Thesleff S, Molgo J, Tagerud S. Trophic interrelations at the neuromuscular junction as revealed by the use of botulinal neurotoxins. Journal de physiologie. 1990;84(2):167-73.
64. Tomsak RL, Remler BF, Averbuch-Heller L, et al Leigh RJ. Unsatisfactory treatment of acquired nystagmus with retrobulbar injection of botulinum toxin. Am J Ophthalmol. 1995; 119(4):489-96.
65. Hall-Craggs EC. Early ultrastructural changes in skeletal muscle exposed to the local anaesthetic bupivacaine (Marcaine). Br J Experiment Pathol. 1980;61(2):139-49.
66. Hall-Craggs EC. Survival of satellite cells following exposure to the local anesthetic bupivacaine (Marcaine). Cell Tissue Res. 1980;209(1):131-5.
67. Nonaka I, Takagi A, Ishiura S, et al. Pathophysiology of muscle fiber necrosis induced by bupivacaine hydrochloride (Marcaine). Acta Neuropathol. 1983;60(3-4):167-74.
68. Komorowski TE, Shepard B, Okland S, et al. An electron microscopic study of local anesthetic-induced skeletal muscle fiber degeneration and regeneration in the monkey. J Orthop Res. 1990;8(4):495-503.
69. Park CY, Park SE, Oh SY. Acute effect of bupivacaine and ricin mAb 35 on extraocular muscle in the rabbit. Curr Eye Res. 2004;29(4-5):293-301.
70. Scott AB, Alexander DE, Miller JM. Bupivacaine injection of eye muscles to treat strabismus. Br J Ophthalmol. 2007;91(2): 146-8.
71. Scott AB, Miller JM, Shieh KR. Treating strabismus by injecting the agonist muscle with bupivacaine and the antagonist with botulinum toxin. Trans Am Ophthalmol Soc. 2009 ;107:104-9.
72. Scott AB, Miller JM, Shieh KR. Bupivacaine injection of the lateral rectus muscle to treat esotropia. J Aapos. 2009;13(2): 119-22.
73. Hopker LM, Zaupa PF, Lima Filho AA, et al. Bupivacaine and botulinum toxin to treat comitant strabismus. Arq Bras Oftalmol. 2012;75(2):111-5.
74. Capo H, Roth E, Johnson T, et al. Vertical strabismus after cataract surgery. Ophthalmology. 1996;103(6):918-21.

# Section 9

# Open Globe Injuries

*Section Editor* Rupesh Agrawal

CHAPTER

111

# Open Globe Injuries: Evaluation and Management

Rupesh Agrawal, Sumita Phatak

## INTRODUCTION

Ocular trauma is a major cause of monocular visual impairment and blindness worldwide, either as a direct result of the trauma itself, or due to the devastating sequelae, most of them avoidable by timely and proper management. The importance of initial management comes into the forefront when we see higher prevalence of ocular trauma, especially open globe injuries, among people in the most productive age group, compounded by the fact that the more underprivileged and illiterate population with lesser access to eye care services bears its major burden.

Over the past few decades, ophthalmology has truncated into subspecialties with major paradigm shifts in ophthalmic practice patterns and training world over. However, ocular trauma, as an exclusive specialty have found place in only a few tertiary care centers especially in developing nations. The biggest concern with open globe injuries is the loss of anatomical landmarks, and repair of such an eye is no mean task, as it involves restoring the eye to best possible anatomical perfection, a delicate and precise task in itself. This surgical intervention needs skill, patience and knowledge. Most importantly, it needs an understanding of the priority that these eyes need.

Factors affecting the outcome of an injured eye can be the nature of trauma, immediate effects on ocular tissues, presence of intraocular foreign body and/or infection. An immediate anatomical restoration of the ocular coats and prevention (and/or treatment) of post-traumatic endophthalmitis remain the emergency goals along the continuum of management of ocular trauma. Management of sequelae requires a multidisciplinary approach with prioritization in the treatment plan.

## EVALUATION OF A PATIENT WITH OPEN GLOBE INJURY

Unless emergency ocular intervention is indicated as in fire cracker injury or chemical injury, the patient's systemic condition should be evaluated along the ophthalmic assessment of trauma. The primary goal of the evaluation process is to obtain essential information about the patient in order to triage the patient into systemic emergency requiring primary multispecialty trauma intervention or primary ophthalmic intervention. Evaluation should be sufficiently comprehensive so that appropriate management decisions can be based on it, yet it must be limited to relevant information to avoid possible delay in primary intervention. Following the systemic check, a detailed evaluation of the injured eye is essential to prioritize and strategically plan treatment, either as a single sitting or a multistage procedure.

The immediate goal of ophthalmic evaluation is to assess the extent of injury and categorize it into the Ocular Trauma Score (OTS).

*A word of caution*: The written record and the test results are important evidence in any patient with history of trauma as these are potential medicolegal cases. This step therefore holds equal importance for the ophthalmologist and the patient. One should try and achieve meticulous listing of every minor tissue lesion, as it may have a bearing on eventual prognosis. For example, an innocuous iris knuckle may trigger sympathetic ophthalmia.

## The Ophthalmic Workup of a Patient with Open Globe Injury

### History

Details about the incidence leading to injury should be elucidated as it can prepare the surgeon about nature or extent of injury and the treatment can be planned before reaching the operating theatre. The most important history to be taken is the duration since injury, as the extent of inflammation, chances of secondary infection and development of sympathetic ophthalmia depend on the time elapsed since injury. A good history is particularly useful in cases of retained intraocular foreign bodies where it can help detail the type and size of foreign body and whether it is single or multiple. History of trauma with vegetative matter pushes the focus toward possible devastating infections.

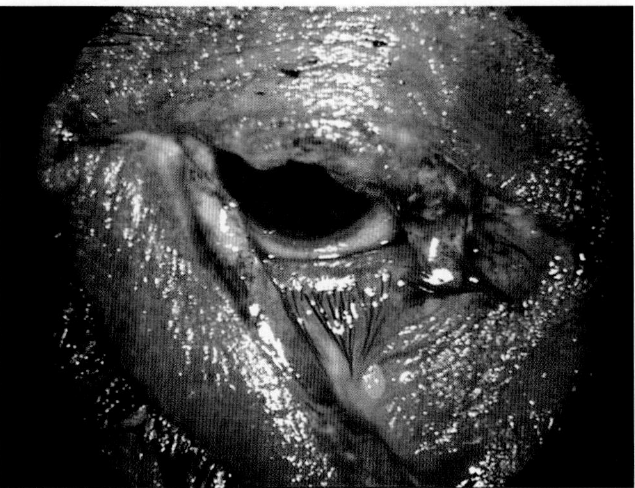

**Figure 111-1** External photograph of the upper lid showing presence of full thickness lid laceration involving lid margin.

### Visual Acuity

It is essential to determine the visual acuity in both the injured and the fellow eye. If for some reason, ophthalmologist or emergency physician is not able to assess visual acuity, the reason should be documented. It is imperative to know if the pre-injury visual acuity was normal or whether the patient had amblyopia or reduced visual acuity prior to injury. Importantly, even if the injured eye does not perceive bright light, one should try and reconstruct the eye anatomically, with special focus on uveal tissue. No perception of light by itself is not an indication for primary enucleation or evisceration of the eye, as in some occasions, dense vitreous hemorrhage and optic nerve contusion may cause the patient to not be able to perceive light.

### Pupil

Testing the pupils for direct and consensual light reflex and checking for relative afferent pupillary defect is one of the essential steps in evaluation of traumatized eyes. In cases with badly traumatized eye where the pupil may be distorted and invisible, the consensual reflex in the fellow eye can be used to check the integrity of optic nerve in the injured eye. Similarly, presence of relative afferent pupillary defect in cases of blunt ocular trauma is the only clinical indicator of traumatic optic neuropathy besides subnormal visual acuity.

### Extraocular Motility

Extraocular motility should never be checked in open globe injury as it can further extend the trauma by shear injury to the tissues. The only indication of motility testing is a suspected orbital or cranial nerve injury, and that too should be deferred in case of associated open globe. Direct muscle or cranial nerve trauma is rare, and if the ophthalmoplegia cannot be explained by adnexal or orbital injury, a neurosurgeon should be consulted to rule out a central origin. In certain situations like severe lid edema, orbital hemorrhage or lack of patient cooperation, motility test may be impossible to conduct.

### Eyeball

Detailed systematic examination of the lids and adnexa, cornea and sclera should be carried out with torch light and on slit lamp followed by fundus examination with indirect ophthalmoscope. Photographic documentation or diagrammatic representation of type and extent of injury should be done in all cases.

### Sequential Examination of the Traumatized Globe with Illustrative Clinical Photographs:

*Lids:*

- Edema, Ecchymosis, Raccoon or panda eyes
- *Laceration*: Extent of involvement, full or partial thickness, involvement of canaliculi and/or lid margin (Fig. 111-1).

*Orbit:*

- Proptosis or Enopthalmos, rule out orbital fracture
- *Bony orbital margin*: Crepitus on palpation, tenderness.

*Conjunctiva*:

- Bogginess, presence of air or subconjunctival pigmentation
- *Subconjunctival hemorrhage*: Always look for posterior extent
- Episcleral tissue.

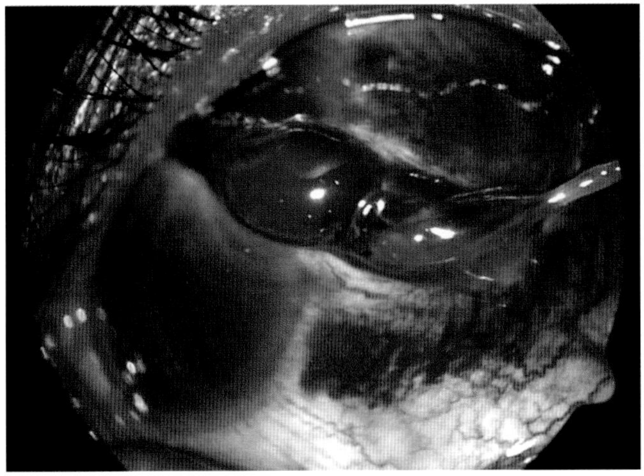

**Figure 111-2** Slit lamp photograph of corneoscleral laceration with vitreous knuckle.

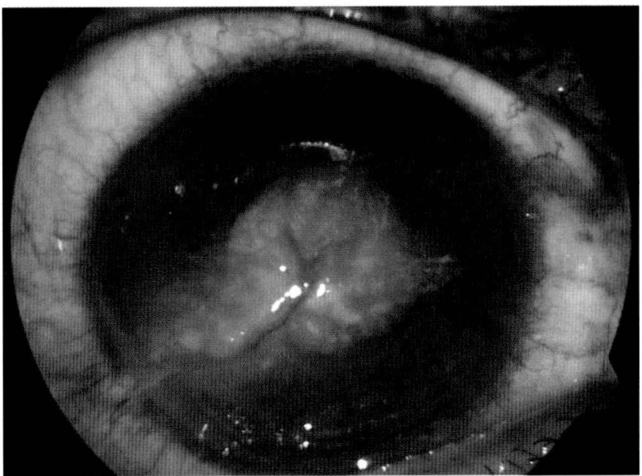

**Figure 111-3** Stellate corneal laceration with traumatic cataract.

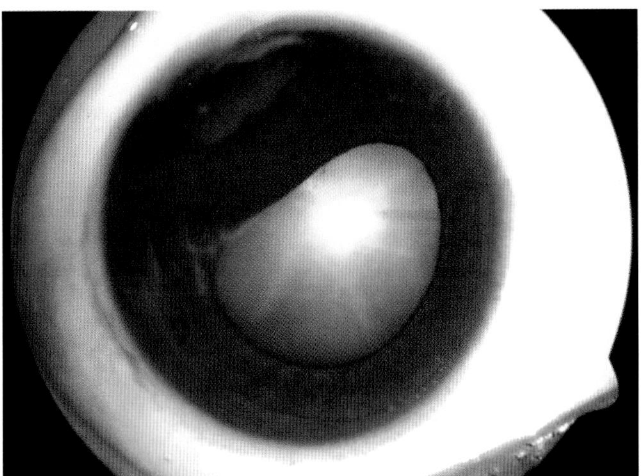

**Figure 111-4** Slit lamp photograph of superior iridodialysis with traumatic cataract.

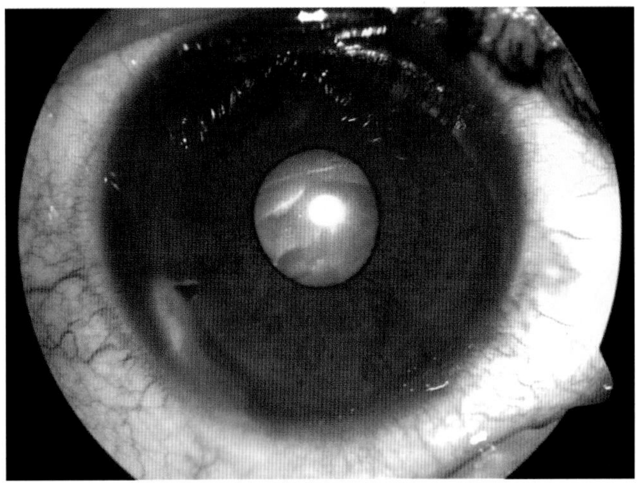

**Figure 111-5** Slit lamp photograph showing presence of iris hole, one of the imminent sign of retained intraocular foreign body.

*Sclera:*

- Full thickness scleral laceration with or without uveal tissue prolapse (Fig. 111-2).
- Vitreous prolapse/retinal tissue prolapse
- *Occult scleral dehiscence*: Subconjunctival hemorrhage, dispersed pigment.

*Cornea:*

- *Extent of injury*: Full or partial thickness wound. In case of doubt, performing Siedel's test using sterile 2% fluorescein may help in detecting full thickness corneal wounds.
- Siedel's test need not be performed if there is uveal tissue plugging the wound or vitreous or lens matter plugging the wound as it will be falsely negative, any intraocular tissue incarcerated into corneal wound require surgical intervention.
- *Type of wound*: Stellate, perpendicular, irregular or clean edges.
- *Associated tissue prolapse*: Tissue viability needs to be checked. If prolapsed iris looks discolored, lusterless with feathery surface, it indicates non-viability and it is best to be abscissed.
- *Iris*: Iridodialysis extent in clock hours (Fig. 111-4) sphincter tears with associated papillary irregularity, viability of prolapsed iris, iris holes (Fig. 111-5).

*Anterior chamber depth and its contents:*

- *Shallow anterior chamber*: Open globe injury, traumatic intumescent cataractous lens or even occult scleral dehiscence.
- *Deep or irregular depth anterior chamber*: Angle recession or posterior occult scleral dehiscence.

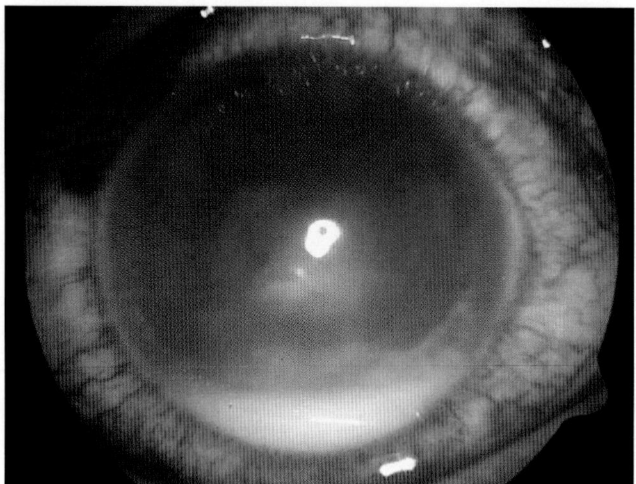

**Figure 111-6** Slit lamp photograph of patient with ocular trauma showing hypopyon in the anterior chamber.

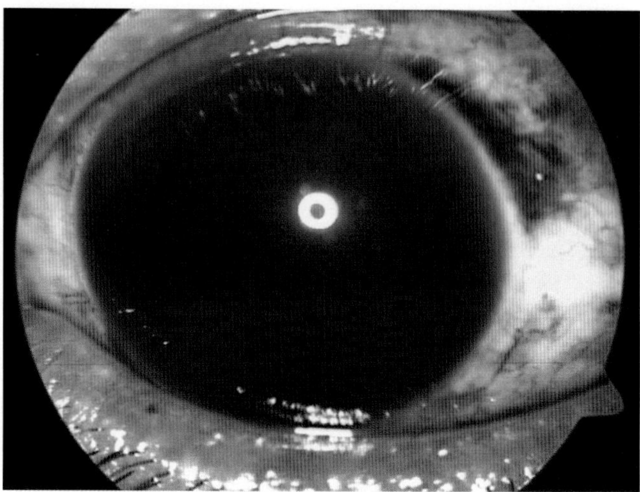

**Figure 111-7** Slit lamp photograph of patient with ocular trauma showing hyphema.

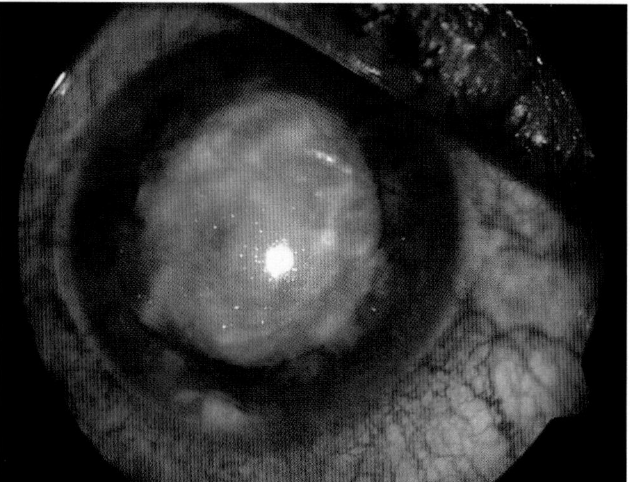

**Figure 111-8** Slit lamp photograph of patient with ocular trauma showing ruptured lens matter with foreign body in the anterior chamber.

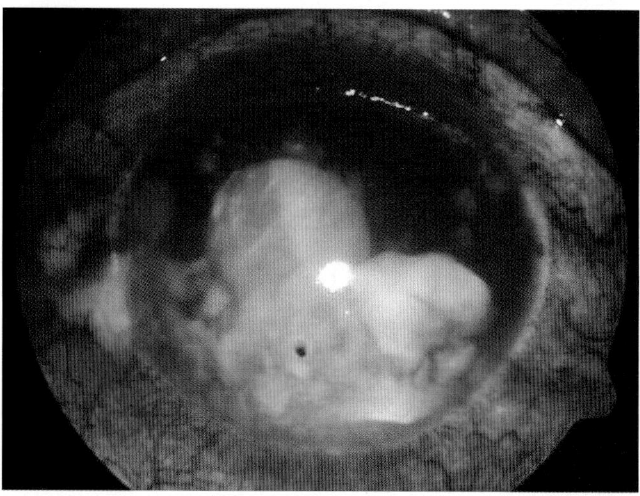

**Figure 111-9** Slit lamp photograph showing lens vitreous admixture following trauma.

- Anterior chamber can show presence of hypopyon (Fig. 111-6), hyphema (Fig. 111-7), traumatic fibrinous uveitis, intraocular foreign body, loose lens matter or vitreous strands secondary to zonular disruption or ruptured lens capsule.

*Lens:*

- Traumatic cataract with intact or torn anterior or posterior capsule (Fig. 111-8).
- Lens matter can be compact or can be loose or flocculent and can be admixed with vitreous in cases with posterior capsular rupture (Fig. 111-9).
- *Lens position*: Subluxated or dislocated. In such situations, it is imperative to look for the location of the dislocated lens (Fig. 111-10).
- Posterior capsular status: attempt to assess for on slit lamp. Look for lens matter in vitreous cavity or posterior bowing of lens matter in vitreous or lens vitreous admixture indicates presence of posterior capsular rupture (Fig. 111-11).
- In cases with long standing traumatic cataract there can be calcification and fibrosis of the membrane (Fig. 111-12).

*Fundus examination*: The earliest possible opportunity should be taken to examine the fundus for any posterior segment manifestation of trauma in the form of Berlin's edema (Fig. 111-13) vitreous hemorrhage, subhyaloid hemorrhage (Fig. 111-14) retinal tears and detachment, choroidal rupture (Fig. 111-15), macular hole (Fig. 111-16), optic nerve avulsion, etc. Direct visualization of the fundus can locate and identify IOFBs in cases with minimal vitreous hemorrhage

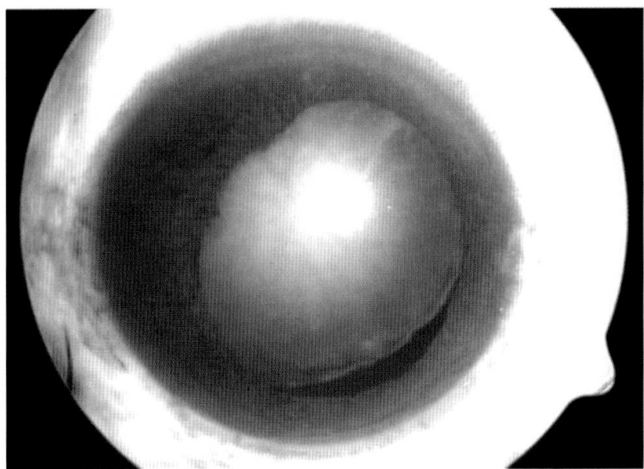

**Figure 111-10** Slit lamp photograph showing subluxation of the cataractous lens following trauma.

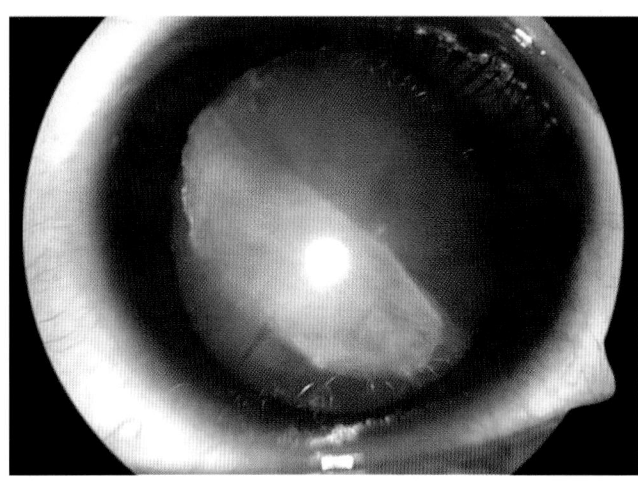

**Figure 111-11** Slit lamp photograph showing presence of posterior capsular dehiscence following trauma.

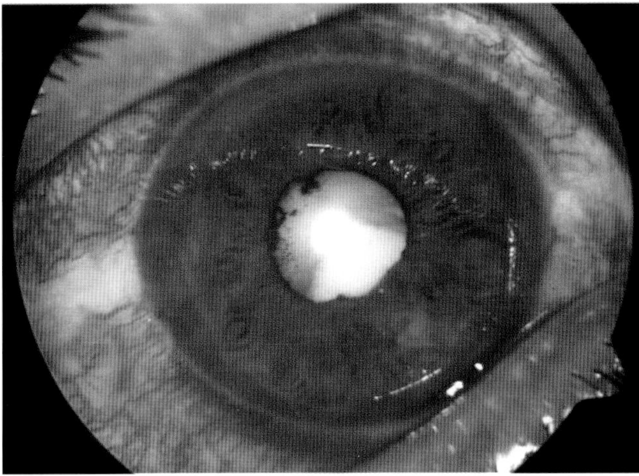

**Figure 111-12** Slit lamp photograph showing presence of partial lens abscess.

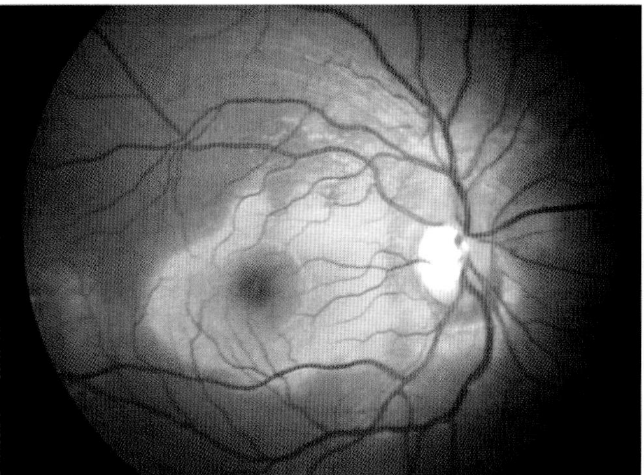

**Figure 111-13** Fundus photo of a patient with blunt ocular trauma showing presence of Berlin's edema at posterior pole.

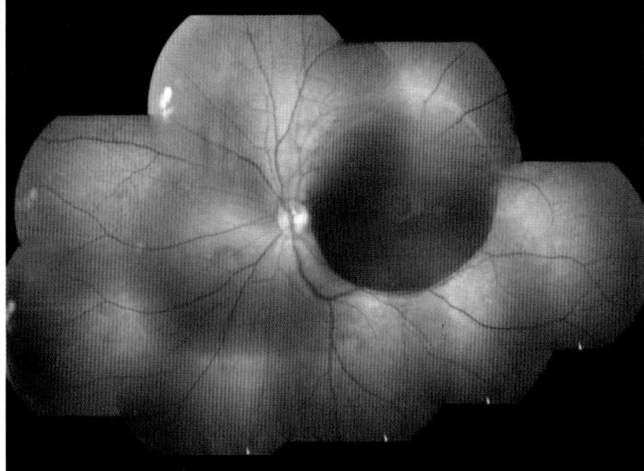

**Figure 111-14** Fundus photo of a patient with trauma showing subhyaloid hemorrhage.

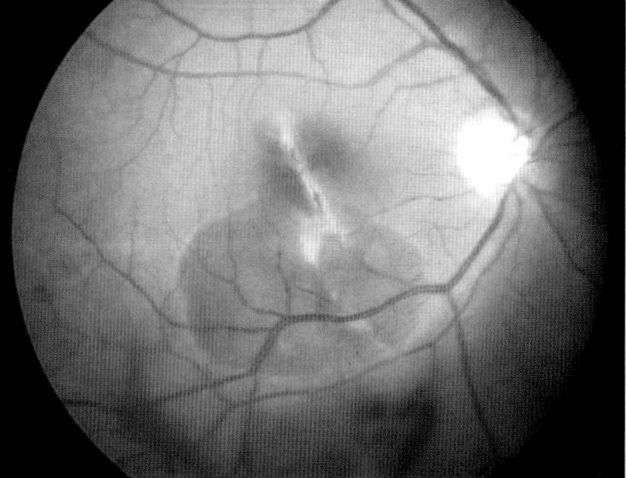

**Figure 111-15** Fundus photo of a patient with choroidal rupture with subretinal hemorrhage suggestive of retinitis sclopetria.

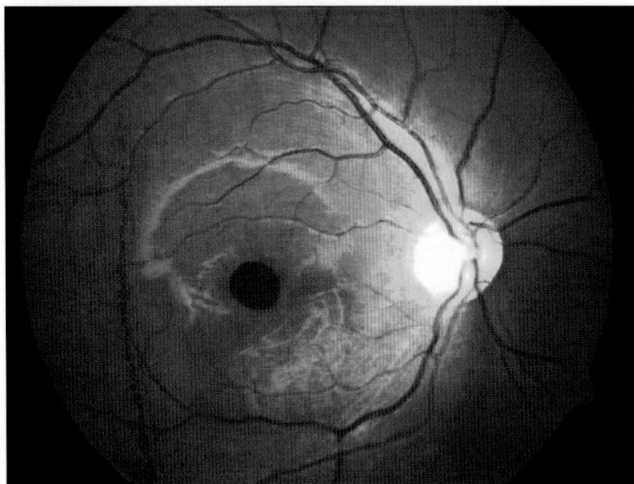

**Figure 111-16** Fundus photo of a patient with blunt ocular trauma showing presence of full thickness macular hole.

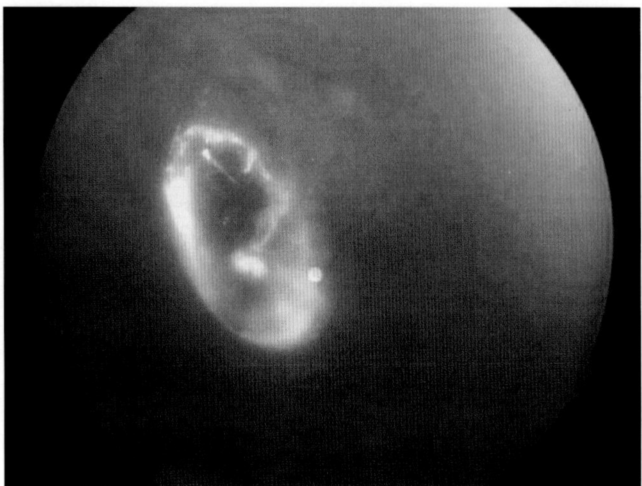

**Figure 111-17** Fundus photo of a patient with trauma showing presence of intraocular foreign body.

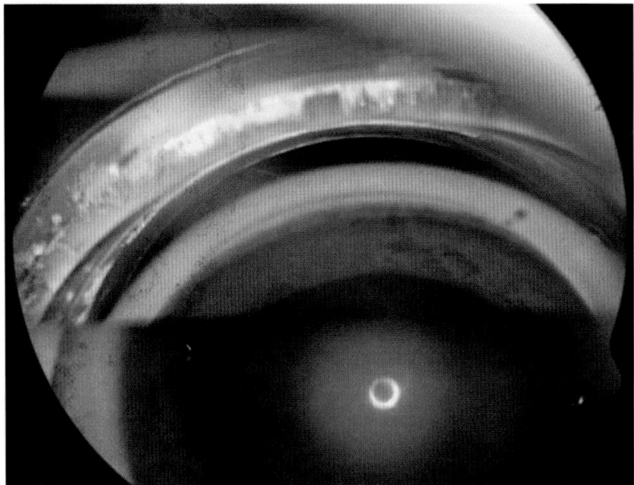

**Figure 111-18** Gonio photo showing presence of angle recession following blunt ocular trauma.

(Fig. 111-17). Inflammation and exudation in a previously non-inflamed vitreous indicates development of endophthalmitis.

*Gonioscopy*: Status of the angle needs to be assessed in cases with blunt ocular trauma. However, gonioscopy needs to be deferred for obvious reasons in open globe injury. In cases with hyphema, gonioscopy should be done after the hyphema has subsided completely as doing goniscopy in cases with active hyphema may cause rebleed in the anterior chamber. While performing gonioscopy, one should look for damage to the angle, presence of angle recession (Fig. 111-18) and intraocular foreign bodies in angle in suspected cases.

*Ancillary Testing as Necessary*: Ultrasound examination of the eye with gentle standoff technique can be employed to assess the posterior segment status and to localize both radiodense and radiolucent foreign bodies in suspected cases. It is however contraindicated in patients with open globe injury but can be selectively used in some patients with relatively small wound to rule out traumatic endophthalmitis. If any posterior segment intervention in the form of intravitreal antibiotics is planned with repair of open globe injury, it is always good to rule out suprachoroidal or retinal detachment.

Computed tomography (CT) imaging with thin overlapping cuts (1.5–3.0 mm) can be employed in patients with history suggestive of retained intraocular foreign body to rule out and localize radiodense intraocular foreign body. In patients with suspected orbital fracture or direct optic neuropathy, it can be used to assess the bone status of the orbit walls/optic canal.

Magnetic resonance imaging (MRI) can be used to identify vegetative matter and wood foreign bodies but is contraindicated when a metallic foreign body is suspected, as the magnetron may cause shifting of the metallic foreign body, causing further damage.

*Identification of any factors that could confound the management*: Infection: To be suspected in patients with delayed presentation. Wound margins have to be examined for evidence of infection. In case of disproportionate pain, inflammation and anterior chamber exudates, superadded infection should be suspected. All patients with hypopyon should be treated as traumatic endophthalmitis unless until proven otherwise. Corroboration with ultrasound to look for vitreous exudates may not be definitive in cases of associated vitreous hemorrhage, but an important clue would be associated sclera edema and "T sign" on ultrasound. In suspected cases, wound

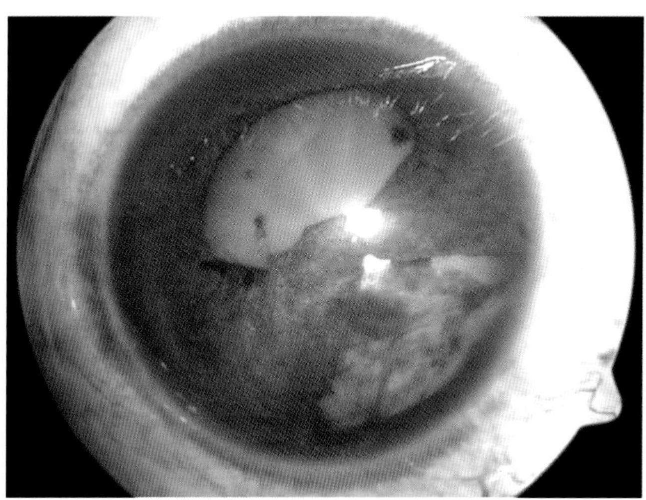

Figure 111-19 Slit lamp photograph of iridodialysis with macerated iris and traumatic cataract.

TABLE 111-1: Ocular trauma score: head to head—our study and USEIR ocular trauma score calculation

| Initial visual factor | Raw points | |
|---|---|---|
| (A) Initial visual acuity category | NLP | = 60 |
| | LP to HM | = 70 |
| | 1/200 to 19/200 | = 80 |
| | 20/200 to 20/50 | = 90 |
| | ≥20/40 | = 100 |
| (B) Globe rupture | | - 23 |
| (C) Endophthalmitis | | - 17 |
| (D) Perforating injury | | - 14 |
| (E) Retinal detachment | | - 11 |
| (F) Afferent pupillary defect (Marcus Gunn pupil) | | - 10 |
| Raw score sum = sum of raw points | | |

margins should be scraped and, if possible, ocular fluid should be sent for microbiological evaluation for identification and better treatment of the pathogen. A word of caution is best to personally ensure communication with the microbiologist as the ocular samples, being small in amount, require immediate and special processing. This will help in reducing the possibility of false negatives.

*Sympathetic ophthalmia*: Can present within weeks to years after injury to the inciting eye. Excessive uveal trauma (Fig. 111-19), irregularly sutured wounds with prolapsed uveal contents and an open globe for more than 10–14 days can trigger sympathetic ophthalmia. Therefore, it is absolutely essential to follow the surgical objectives of primary wound repair as outlined below. One should not refrain from repairing a badly traumatized globe with no light perception on presentation.

*Ocular Trauma Score*: To prognosticate the outcome of a patient with open globe injury in 2002, Kuhn et al. developed a prognostic model, the OTS, to predict the visual outcome of patients after ocular trauma. Authors analyzed over 2,500 eye injuries from the United States and Hungarian Eye Injury registries and evaluated more than 100 variables to identify these predictors. Essentially it is calculated by assigning certain numerical raw points to six variables: initial visual acuity, globe rupture, endophthalmitis, perforating injury, retinal detachment and relative afferent pupillary defect (RAPD). The scores are subsequently stratified into five categories from one to five with one being the lowest score and five being the highest score. The patient with OTS of one will have a higher risk of poorer final visual outcome as against the patient with OTS of five who will have higher probability of better final vision outcome. An independent study was conducted by the Ophthalmologists at Tan Tock Seng Hospital in Singapore where we attempted to compare and stratify our study subjects into the same scoring system. The study score in our series was comparable to international OTS system (Tables 111-1 and 111-2). It is recommended that ophthalmic surgeons apply the OTS more frequently in clinical settings to assist in proactive counseling of trauma patients.

## INITIAL MANAGEMENT OF OPEN GLOBE INJURY

No two cases are alike, but irrespective of the configuration or etiology of ocular trauma, the following standardized protocol will help in optimizing anatomical and visual results in ocular trauma patients.

The four essential components in management of open globe injuries are:

1. Prevent further trauma to the eye:
   - Application of rigid eye shield over the traumatized eye at the time of initial evaluation
   - Minimal preoperative manipulation
   - Try and operate at the earliest possible.
2. Minimize risk of infection:
   - Instituting systemic broad spectrum antibiotics
   - Wound closure at the earliest possible
   - Tetanus prophylaxis according to the recommendations from the Center for Disease Control and Prevention
   - Postsurgical institution of topical or intraocular antibiotics in cases of suspected infection.

TABLE 111-2: Comparison of ocular trauma score and final visual outcome in our study with United States Eye Injury Registry

| Raw score | OTS | | NLP (%) | LP/HM (%) | 1/200-19/200 (%) | 20/200-20/50 (%) | >20/40 (%) |
|---|---|---|---|---|---|---|---|
| 0–44 | 1 | Study | 56 | 17 | 18 | 6 | 3 |
| | | USEIR | 73 | 17 | 7 | 2 | 1 |
| 45–65 | 2 | Study | 19 | 23 | 25 | 23 | 10 |
| | | USEIR | 28 | 26 | 18 | 13 | 15 |
| 66–80 | 3 | Study | 2 | 0 | 20 | 33 | 45 |
| | | USEIR | 2 | 11 | 15 | 28 | 44 |
| 81–91 | 4 | Study | 0 | 6 | 0 | 28 | 67 |
| | | USEIR | 1 | 2 | 2 | 21 | 74 |
| 92–100 | 5 | Study | 0 | 0 | 0 | 11 | 89 |
| | | USEIR | 0 | 1 | 2 | 5 | 92 |

(OTS: Ocular trauma score; USEIR: US Eye Inquiry Registry; VA: Visual acuity; NLP: No light perception; LP: Light perception; HM: Hand motion).

*Note*: Higher the OTS, more the chances that patient can get good final visual outcome. With OTS 5, final VA was better than 20/40 in 89% of our patients similar to 92% of patients in USEIR. Similarly, lower the score, poorer the final vision outcome. With OTS1, final VA was NLP in 56% of our patients and in 73% of patients in USEIR.

3. Prevent psychological trauma to the patient and his/her family:

   It is important that the patient and his or her family are an integral part of the decision making. With the outcome being so uncertain, the treating physician should mainly be a facilitator to help them with the current trends and evidence and risks involved with management of open globe injury. It is essential that the physician does not inflict more psychological trauma to the patient or family but at the same time not to give any false hopes about anatomical or visual outcome. It is necessary to discuss the immediate and late complications that may develop the possible need for more than one surgery to salvage the eye, and possible eventual poor visual prognosis. It is also important to obtain the written, not just verbal, consent of the patient and relatives, along with a high risk consent documenting the patient's understanding of the situation, as the outcomes and responses are unpredictable. OTS facilitates physician with some evidence based prognostication in patients with open globe injury to counsel patients and relatives with outcome of traumatized eyes.

4. Minimize legal problems to treating physician and institute:

   Proper meticulous documentation and good perioperative counseling are the key factors in avoiding any litigation. It is often improper communication or documentation which accounts for medicolegal litigations and can be easily prevented by having patient involved in informed decision making at all stages of management.

## SURGICAL REPAIR

### Objectives of Globe Repair

#### *Primary*

- Restoration of anatomical integrity
- Achieve watertight closure
- Prevent infection
- Smooth and optically effective refractive surface
- Consider globe repair as refractive surgery and not merely plain closure of the tissues
- Reduce scarring.

#### *Secondary*

- Removal of disrupted lens and vitreous
- Removal of intraocular foreign bodies (Fig. 111-20)
- Management of any associated intraocular pathology or injury.

### Strategic Planning for Primary Globe Repair

*The objective of globe repair should be Primum non nocere, the universal truth of surgery: "first, do no harm".*

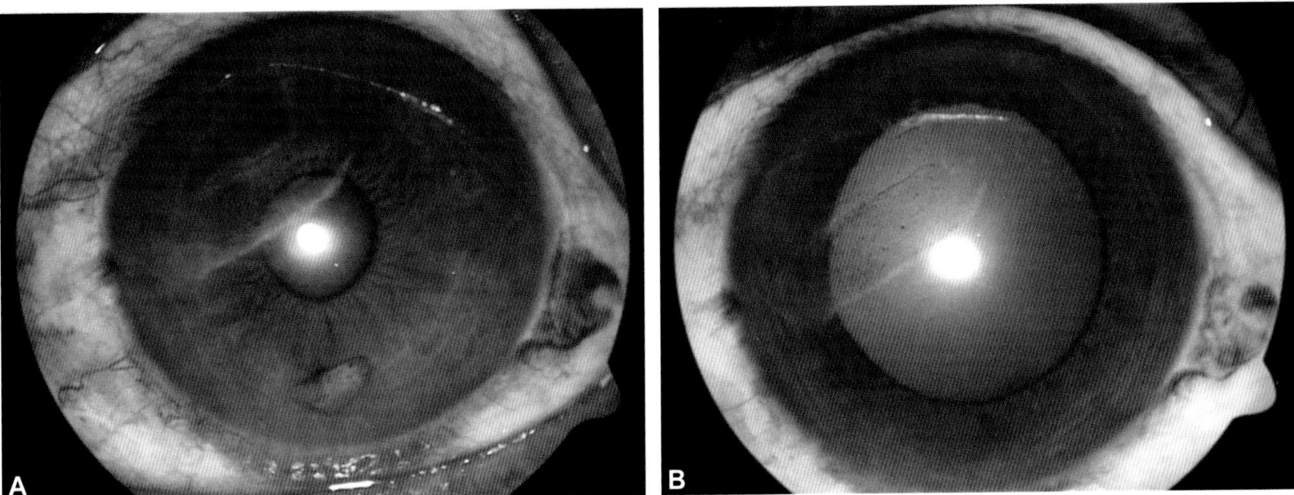

Figures 111-20A and B Composite photograph of wooden foreign body in anterior chamber and postoperative after removal of foreign body.

Depending on extent of injury, the management can be nonsurgical or surgical.

### *Nonsurgical Management*

Can be considered in cases with small conjunctival lacerations and tiny self-sealed corneal laceration which, if need be, can further be reinforced with the help of tissue adhesives. Cyanoacrylate glue is the tissue adhesive which can provide support lasting for several days to several weeks.

- *Small beveled self-sealed corneal wounds*: Bandage Contact Lens (BCL).
- *Tiny full thickness corneal perforation*: Cyanoacrylate glue with BCL.

### *Surgical Management*

The management of these injuries is a thought out process, rather than a reflexive response to an obvious injury. Any extent of open globe injury has to be considered a priority and taken up for immediate wound repair, to improve the chances of a good prognosis for the eye. Prompt, secure wound closure is especially important in children who are at greater risk of inadvertently rubbing the eye with consequent reopening of a tissue adhesive or contact lens supported wound.

*Anesthesia*: The recommended anesthesia in all open globe injuries should be general anesthesia, but the cases with small lacerations can be managed under local anesthesia. The patient is prepared for surgery as soon as possible and should be medically and neurosurgically assessed. An important advisory while mobilizing for surgery would be to keep the patient nil oral to ensure a minimum of 6 hours of fasting for solid foods for general anesthesia fitness. Anesthesia should be achieved without any increase in intraocular pressure, which could occur during intubation, extubation or because of anesthetic agents. Although succinyl choline possesses several advantages, it contracts extraocular muscles and increases intraocular pressure. Hence, in open globe injuries, depolarizing agents are not used. External pressure from the mask can also increase intraocular pressure, so the rigid eye shield should remain on the eye while intubation and positioning the patient for surgery.

*Preparing the eye*: The eye should be prepared and draped with care. Pressure should not be applied to the globe. The eye is irrigated with a sterile balanced salt solution (BSS) to remove any superficial foreign bodies. The eye is gently examined to evaluate the extent of damage. In cases of unstable globes, speculum can be avoided and lid sutures taken gently.

## Surgical Repair

### *Corneal Lacerations*

Corneal lacerations are sutured using 10-0 monofilament nylon suture on a fine spatulated microsurgical needle. For wounds closer to the visual axis, 11-0 monofilament nylon can be used (Figs. 111-21 and 111-22). At all times, the suture line should be perpendicular to the wound edge at the point of suturing.

### *Small Corneal Laceration with Reasonably Formed Anterior Chamber*

Corneal wound can be sutured directly with 10-0 Nylon suture without disturbing the anterior chamber. Anterior chamber if flattens can be reformed with saline.

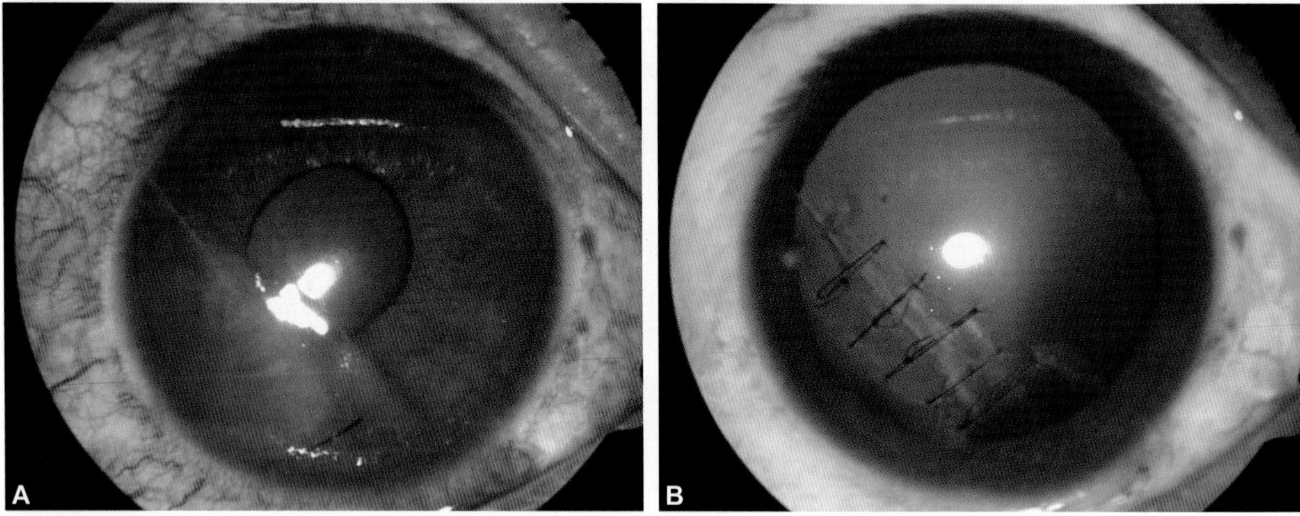


**Figures 111-21A and B** Composite photograph of preoperative and postoperative corneal laceration repair.

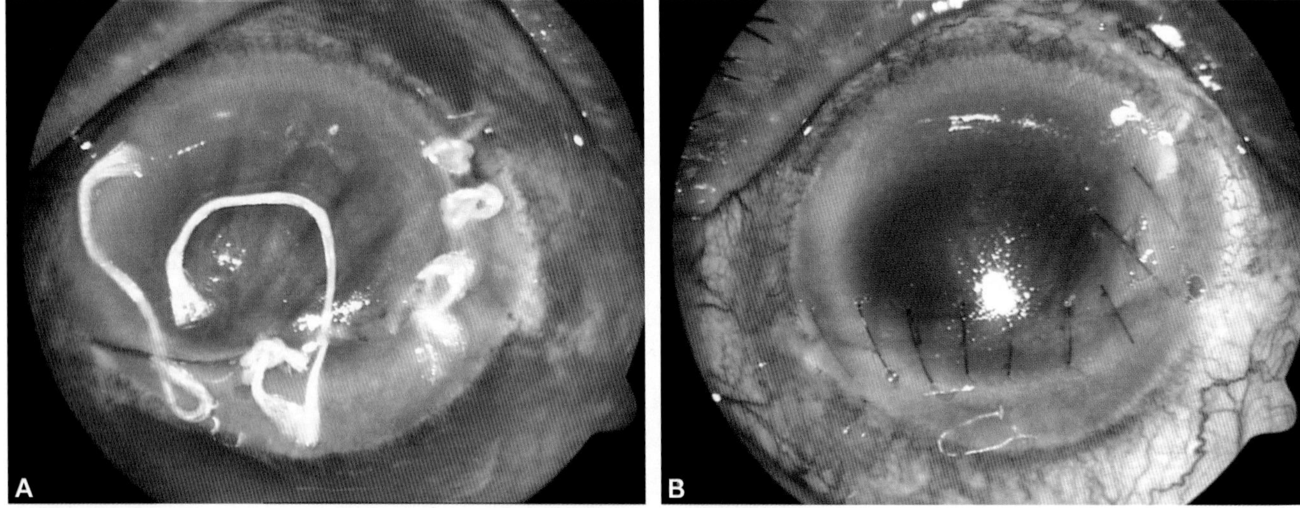


**Figures 111-22A and B** Composite photograph of corneal wound revision which was otherwise done without following standard surgical principles of open globe injury.

## *Less Stable Wound with Shallow or Flat Anterior Chamber*

- Wound should be cleaned with normal saline.
- *Formation of anterior chamber with viscoelastic*: Viscoelastic can be injected through a side port made with the help of micro vitreoretinal (MVR) blade. The side port should be made about 90–180° away from wound edge. But in cases of collapsed globe it might be difficult to make the side port and form the chamber with viscoelastic and hence only in such cases, viscoelastic can be injected directly through the corneal wound without distorting the wound and chamber can be completely or partly formed.
- Corneal wound should be divided in segments with interrupted sutures, each suture being perpendicular to the wound edge at that point. Perpendicular edges of the wound should be sutured before beveled edges to achieve a good approximation. The eventual aim in corneal laceration repair is definitive placement of corneal sutures to make the wound watertight, minimize scarring, and reconstruct the native nonastigmatic corneal contour.

*Corneal suturing*: A number of strategies for corneal suturing are available.

In corneal wound involving limbus, first suture should always be at limbus. It is imperative to identify limbus properly and approximate the limbal edges as accurately as possible as that will subsequently determine corneal contour. If limbus is not free, one may need to relax the limbal edges by doing conjunctival peritomy. Also, at every step one should ensure not to engage any part of iris tissue into the limbal or corneal wound suturing.

After approximating the limbus, one can start by taking superficial temporary interrupted sutures (halving) in order to approximate the wound edges and subsequently those sutures can be replaced with definite deep sutures at end of surgery. These definitive corneal sutures should be approximated 1.5 mm long, approximately 90% deep in the stroma, and of equal depth on both sides of the wound. Shallow sutures will cause internal wound gape; sutures that are asymmetric or of unequal depth will result in wound override. Full thickness sutures should be avoided as they can act as conduit for microbial invasion.

In shelved wounds, the placement of sutures should be equidistant with respect to internal aspect of the wound and tied without undue tension to optimize tissue apposition. On the other hand, wounds with macerated or edematous edges require longer sutures for security as once the edema resolves, there is always a chance that sutures will loosen up. Also, in edematous wound edges, there is always a possibility of cheesewiring of the corneal tissue while taking corneal sutures.

Suture bites through the visual axis should be avoided. It is best to try and straddle the visual axis. If suture needs to be taken through the visual axis, a number of techniques can be used to minimize scarring. Sutures near to visual axis should be shorter, superficial and relatively loose as against the peripheral sutures which should be longer, deeper and tighter. More importantly, No touch technique is employed with the corneal wound margin wherein the globe is stabilized away from the site of corneal wound and sutures are directly passed through the corneal wound without holding the corneal wound edges. This minimizes further tissue damage and resultant scarring in visual axis. This technique though requires considerable experience and if one is not comfortable with no touch technique, it is advisable to gently hold the edges of corneal wound with microforceps rather than putting undue pressure on the globe while attempting corneal suturing by no touch technique.

Stellate wounds have to be sutured in segments by first identifying each edge and ensuring a possible anatomical approximation, prior to suture placement. The suturing has to begin from base of wound toward the center. Bridging sutures can be used. A purse string suture can be taken near the wound center to ensure watertight closure of the apex. If the tissue is macerated, the center of the wound can be sealed with Cyanoacrylate glue with BCL. There may be situations where a corneal graft may have to be considered because of excessive macerated tissue, cheesewiring through tissue, or loss of tissue.

Suture knots are usually made by locked 3-1-1 suture loops, trimmed short and buried into the cornea on the side away from the visual axis.

Wound has to be checked for leaks using dry cellulose sponges or sterile 2% fluorescein.

## Corneoscleral Laceration

The first suture is applied to the limbus, to get the anatomical orientation of the globe and the wound. Limbus is sutured using 10-0 mono filament nylon and in some cases where it is long standing wound and limbal edges are further apart, it may be advisable to use 8-0 nylon sutures for limbal anchoring suture.

After the first suture is applied, any associated iris prolapse or vitreous prolapse is addressed. In the presence of prolapsed iris, depending on the viability of iris tissue it is either repositioned or abscised. The rule of thumb is any tissue prolapsed for longer than 24 hours should be abscised to avoid infection. Repositioning of iris can be done after forming the anterior chamber with viscoelastic. Using an iris repositor, the iris tissue can be sweeped back into the anterior chamber, making sure the instrument is at least 90°away from the prolapsed to allow for the fulcrum effect. Pushing in of the tissue should be avoided.

In the presence of a vitreous prolapse, a vitrectomy is performed with dry cellulose sponges and Vanna's scissors or an automated vitrector. During the process, any traction on the vitreous should be avoided. One should try and avoid any intraocular procedures during primary wound closure. But if the anterior chamber has a significant lens vitreous admixture, vitreous plugging the wound, or if there is significant hyphema, one should try and clean up the anterior chamber in the same sitting. It is advisable to control inflammation and let the wound stabilize before attempting subsequent intraocular interventions.

## Scleral Wound Suturing

Once the corneal wound is secured, the scleral wound is explored. This exploration is achieved by performing a limbal peritomy at the site of the limbal wound. Scleral wound is sutured using 8-0 nylon or 7-0 vicryl sutures. Exploration of extent of sclera wound should progress simultaneous with wound suturing to minimize repeated distortion of globe. A peritomy with tagging of rectus muscles can be done if posterior extension of the scleral wound is suspected. Gentle traction of the muscles can help reach the posterior edge of the wound. If required, the recti can be disinserted to gain access to the wound under them, and then reattached using 6-0 vicryl. But if the wound is too posterior, it is best left unsutured, as attempts to reach the wound could worsen the trauma.

The scleral wound is secured with the help of interrupted or continuous 7-0 vicryl suture or 8-0 nylon suture. Segments of scleral laceration are explored and repaired, direction of exploration being anterior to posterior. This method helps stabilize the eye prevent further uveal or vitreous prolapse. In the presence of uveal prolapse, the prolapsed tissue is reposited (Figs. 111-23A and B). The preferred method of sclera wound closure over prolapsed uveal tissue is a zippering technique wherein the sclera wound is closed from anterior end, i.e. limbal end with interrupted sutures placed successively proceeding posteriorly. Leaving the suture ends long will help by acting as successive traction sutures to help in viewing the posterior extent of the wound. One should never excise prolapsed uveal tissue unless it is necrotic because it causes excessive bleeding, and can damage retinal tissue. Vitreous prolapse is managed by performing a vitrectomy with cellulose sponges and scissors or by using an automated vitrector. At every step, care should be taken to prevent iatrogenic damage. The sutures are placed closely together and tied to achieve a watertight closure.

## Lens Matter Aspiration

Presence of loose lens matter in the anterior chamber necessitates its aspiration. In case of a small wound, a traumatic cataract can be removed in the same sitting.

Opinions differ over timing of traumatic cataract extraction and intraocular lens (IOL) implantation. Cataract extraction along with primary wound repair may have distinct advantages such as controlling inflammation and possibility of raised intraocular pressure due to soft lens matter in the anterior chamber. Secondary advantages are direct visualization of the posterior segment and optic nerve. Similarly, in pediatric patients, removal of media opacity may be crucial to prevent vision deprivation amblyopia. Lens vitreous admixture is a potent stimulator for proliferative vitreoretinopathy and can also result in traction on the retina; hence, primary extraction of lens and vitreous can be of benefit in such patients. Proponents of second-sitting cataract extraction recommend good control of intraocular inflammation, good media clarity and stable wound before planning for a traumatic cataract extraction. The injury is rarely limited to the lens alone, and may be associated with injuries to zonules, posterior capsule and posterior segment. Second staging the cataract extraction allows for time to assess the extent of internal damage and plan accordingly. Furthermore, if there is adequate control of inflammation then IOL implantation in second-stage cataract extraction may be associated with a better outcome. Second stage surgery also allows for a better IOL power calculation. Placing an IOL is best deferred in the primary sitting to allow

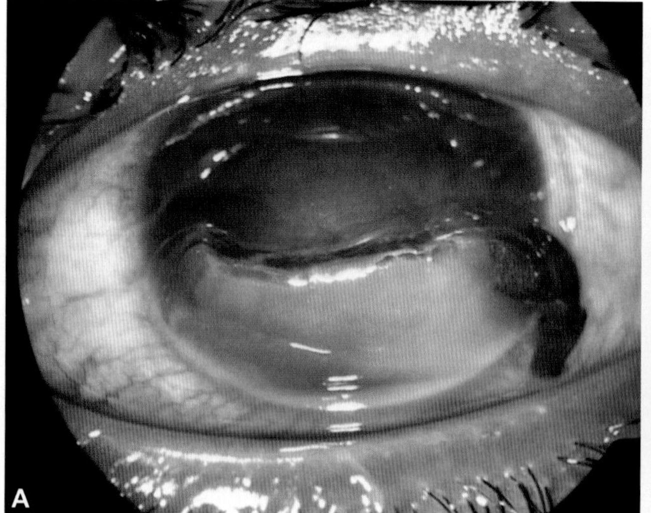


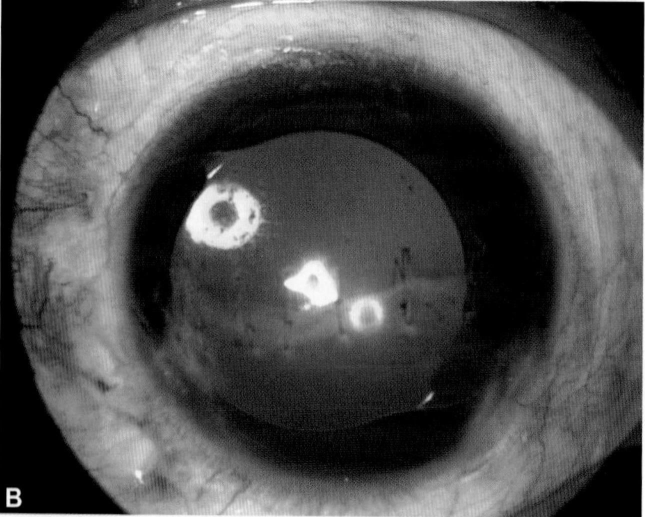


**Figures 111-23A and B** Composite photograph of corneal laceration with uveal tissue prolapse with inferior corneal edema. Final postoperative photograph after multistage visual rehabilitation and patient was happy with scleral fixated IOL.

for the internal post injury fibrosis of the eye, understanding that a traumatic cataract behaves differently than a senile cataract.

The ophthalmologist is therefore advised to make an independent planned decision after grading extent of injury and understanding the possible outcomes.

An advisory would be in adults, where amblyopia is not an issue; the choice of surgery is governed by the status of the cataractous lens.

If the anterior capsule is significantly disrupted and there is free-floating lens matter in the anterior chamber, there is a justification in primary cataract extraction usually without IOL implantation, and IOL implantation can always be done at later stage. Eyes with lens vitreous admixture should undergo combined cataract extraction with limited anterior vitrectomy and care should be taken to judiciously use a vitrector and not an aspirator while removing vitreous admixed in the ruptured lens matter. Any traction on the vitreous can result in inadvertent retinal breaks.

In the setting of additional injury to the posterior segment, early pars plana lensectomy and vitrectomy by a vitreoretinal surgeon is warranted.

In eyes with an intact anterior capsule and a total traumatic cataract, second-sitting cataract extraction with IOL implantation should be the best and safest approach for optimal visual outcome.

Wherever possible, a multi-step procedure should be adopted after control of inflammation and adequate corneal clarity and appropriate IOL power calculation.

### Closure

The conjunctiva is sutured using 8-0 or 9-0 vicryl. Suture knots should be buried or wing sutures should be taken to close the conjunctiva. In cases with larger peritomy, anchoring suture to episclera will prevent recession of the conjunctiva and avoid exposure of scleral wound. Anterior chamber is formed with saline. Air can be used as tamponade for minor bleeding in the anterior chamber. Once the wound is secured, antibiotic eye ointment, eye patch followed by a rigid eye shield are applied before attempting extubation.

### Postoperative Care

During immediate postoperative evaluation, patients should be carefully monitored for signs of infection. Pain, photophobia, redness, tearing or a deterioration of vision should alert the physician to look for signs of endophthalmitis. Conjunctival injection, chemosis, corneal edema and elevated intraocular pressure may be present but are not diagnostic of infection. A more than expected anterior chamber reaction and cells in the vitreous are most suggestive of endophthalmitis. Figure 111-20 illustrating preoperative and postoperative outcome suggests possible outcome in patients with open globe injury.

Patients of open globe injuries should be on long-term follow-up to ensure sequelae are picked up on time and treated accordingly. Patient should also be instructed to present on sudden onset of photophobia or red eye. They should be educated about possibilities of sympathetic ophthamia or infection. Visual rehabilitation is important aspect of any trauma repair and often it is the most neglected part in management of ocular trauma patients. These precautions will ensure the best possible outcome in traumatized eyes.

## SUMMARY

Corneal and scleral wounds commonly present to the emergency clinic and management of these cases should be prioritized to optimize visual potential in traumatized eyes. Management of corneal and scleral laceration requires careful evaluation and planning prior to closure. The globe must be closed so that it is watertight with the original anatomy restored and the original function as approximated as possible. Corneal wound is closed based on the principles explained whereas scleral wound should be carefully explored and should be addressed by doing atraumatic scleral laceration repair. An understanding by the primary care ophthalmologist that a traumatized eye is not a lost eye will lead to restoration of best possible function even in an eye with significant ocular trauma.

## BIBLIOGRAPHY

1. Agarwal R, Wei HS, Teoh S. Prognostic factors for open globe injuries and correlation of ocular trauma score at a tetiary referral eye care centre in Singapore. Indian J Ophthalmol. 2013;61(9):502-6.
2. Agrawal R, Rao G, Naigaonkar R, et al. Prognostic factors for vision outcome after surgical repair of open globe injuries. Indian J Ophthalmol. 2011;59:465-70.
3. Agrawal R, Shah M, Mireskandari K, et al. Controversies in ocular trauma classification and management: review. Int Ophthalmol. 2013;33:435-45.
4. Agrawal R, Wei HS, Teoh S. Predictive factors for final outcome of severely traumatized eyes with no light perception. BMC Ophthalmol. 2012;12:16.
5. Barkana Y, Belkin M, Kuhn F. Electromagnetic injuries. In: Kuhn F (Ed). Ocular Ocular Traumatology. Berlin: Springer; 2008. pp. 501-12.

6. Colby K. Management of open globe injuries. Int Ophthalmol Clin. 1999;39:59-69.
7. De Juan E, Sternberg P, Michels RG. Penetrating ocular injuries. Types of injuries and visual results. Ophthalmology. 1983;90:1318-22.
8. Desai P, MacEwen CJ, Baines P, et al. Incidence of cases of ocular trauma admitted to hospital and incidence of blinding outcome. Br J Ophthalmol. 1996;80:592-6.
9. Duke-Elder S, MacFaul PA. Injuries: Mechanical Injuries. In: CV Mosby (Ed). System of Ophthalmology. St. Louis; 1972.
10. Duke-Elder S, MacFaul PA. Injuries: Non Mechanical Injuries. In: CV Mosby (Ed). System of Ophthalmology. St Louis; 1972.
11. Freeman HM. Examination of the traumatized eye. In: Miller D, Stegman R (Eds). Treatment of Anterior Segment Ocular Trauma. Montreal: Medicopea; 1986. pp. 95-119.
12. Guly CM, Guly HR, Bouamra O, et al. Ocular injuries in patients with major trauma. Emerg Med J. 2006;23:915-7.
13. Kuhn F (Ed). Classification of mechanical eye injuries. Ocular Traumatology. Berlin: Springer; 2008. pp. 13-6.
14. Kuhn F, Maisiak R, Mann L, et al. The ocular trauma score (OTS) ophthalmology clinics of North America. 2002; 15(2):163-5.
15. Kuhn F, Maisiak R, Mann L. The OTS: predicting the final vision in the injured eye. In Kuhn F, Pieramici D (Eds). Ocular Trauma: Principles and Practice. New York: Thieme Medical Publishers; 2002. pp. 9-13.
16. Kuhn F, Mester V, Mann L, et al. Eye injury epidemiology and prevention of ophthalmic injuries. In: Kuhn F, Pieramici D (Eds). Ocular Trauma: Principles and Practice. New York: Thieme Medical Publishers; 2002. pp. 14-20.
17. Kuhn F, Morris R, Mester V, et al. Terminology of mechanical injuries: the Birmingham Eye Trauma Terminology (BETT). In: Kuhn F (Ed). Ocular traumatology. Berlin: Springer; 2008. pp. 3-12.
18. Kuhn F, Morris R, Mester V. Emergency management of ophthalmic injuries. Modern Management of Ophthalmology International. Panama City; 2006. pp. 35-48.
19. Kuhn F, Morris R, Witherspoon CD, et al. A standardized classification of ocular trauma. Ophthalmology. 1996;103:240-3.
20. Kuhn F, Morris R, Witherspoon CD, et al. Epidemiology of blinding trauma in the United States Eye Injury Registry. Ophthalmic Epidemiol. 2006;13:209-16.
21. Kuhn F. Clinical epidemiology, prevention and rehabilitation. In: Kuhn F (Ed). Ocular traumatology. Berlin: Springer; 2008. pp. 47-78.
22. Kuhn F. Evaluation. In: Kuhn F (Ed). Ocular Traumatology. Berlin: Springer; 2008. pp. 105-28.
23. Kuhn F. Open globe injury: a brief overview. Ocular Traumatology. Berlin: Springer; 2008. pp. 347-58.
24. Kuhn F. Strategic thinking in eye trauma managment. Ophthalmol Clin North Am. 2002;15:171-7.
25. McGwin G, Hall TA, Xie A, et al. Trends in eye injury in the United States, 1992-2001. Invest Ophthalmol Vis Sci. 2006; 47:521-7.
26. Pieramici DJ, Au Eong KG, Sternberg P, et al. The prognostic significance of a system for classifying mechanical injuries of the eye (globe) in open-globe injuries. J Trauma. 2003;54:750-4.
27. Pieramici DJ, MacCumber MW, Humayun MU, et al. Open-globe injury. Update on types of injuries and visual results. Ophthalmology. 1996;103:1798-803.
28. Rahman I, Maino A, Devadason D, et al. Open globe injuries: factors predictive of poor outcome. Eye (Lond). 2006;20:1336-41.
29. Schein OD, Hibberd PL, Shingleton BJ, et al. The spectrum and burden of ocular injury. Ophthalmology. 1988;95:300-5.
30. Thakker MM, Ray S. Vision-limiting complications in open-globe injuries. Can J Ophthalmol. 2006;41:86-92.
31. Vachon CA, Warner DO, Bacon DR. Succinylcholine and the open globe. Tracing the teaching. Anesthesiology. 2003;99: 220-3.

# Section 10

# The Practice of Ophthalmic Surgery

*Section Editor* George L Spaeth

CHAPTER

112

# Informed Choice Versus Informed Consent

George L Spaeth

## INTRODUCTION

*Principle of "informed consent"*: It has long been generally believed that damaging another person without a due cause is wrong. Phrased differently, each person is believed to have the right to protect his or her own body. The principle of "informed consent" grows out of this general belief. Specifically, as this relates to medical care, it is generally believed that no intellectually or emotionally competent person should have anything done to him or her that may cause unwanted damage, without that person giving others the permission to take the action that may cause the damage.

Need for an "informed consent":

- To respect the individual patient's autonomy[1-5]
- To protect the person initiating action. "Obtaining patients" consent... demonstrates respect for patient autonomy and should help prevent legal action against health professionals[6]
- To help patients to be proactive in preserving their own health.

Many studies have shown that involving patients in their own care leads to better outcomes,[7-10] and that such outcomes will be better when patients are knowledgeable and participate in their own care. Physicians, through their actions, may further the patient's well-being by giving advice, entering in a dialog, or transferring their enthusiasm for life. Administrative procedures, however, such as obtaining "informed consent" in the way it is usually presented may actually contribute to poorer health. This chapter will discuss the importance of informed consent, but will make a slight change, suggesting that what we are really interested in is informed choice.

## CONSENT VERSUS CHOICE

Consent and choice are not exactly the same. In fact, obtaining an informed consent in the way it is usually presented may actually contribute to an increase in the potential good health of the patient.

### Case Scenarios

*Case I*: Take as an example a patient who has trouble reading and thinks he needs new glasses. The doctor finds advanced cataracts and explains the benefits and risks of surgery, emphasizing that complications are rare and far outweighed by its benefits. The doctor then asks the patient for his consent to proceed with cataract extraction in conjunction with implantation of an intraocular lens. The patient acquiesces or demurs, troubled in a way because he had only wanted to improve his reading ability. Having a cataract extraction may not be at all he expected or wanted. At this point some patients will simply comply with the doctor's advice. Others may hesitate, wondering if their reading is really bad enough to risk the operation, this not even having been in the menu of expectations that brought them to the doctor's office. To ask the patient to "consent" to a cataract extraction places the initiation of the healing process squarely in the physician's hands; it is the physician's idea and the physician will "do" the job. This unequal power relationship is enhanced by the word "consent."

*Case II*: In a somewhat different case, a highly knowledgeable patient has a uveitis and already knows from her Internet searches that the treatment is cortisone. The doctor tells her she should also be tested for syphilis, sarcoidosis, and several other diseases that can cause uveitis. After further discussion, the patient "consents" to use the cortisone eye drops but "refuses" to have the tests for syphilis and the other diseases. Here, the patient is highly knowledgeable about her eye condition, but is asked to do something she does not wish to do – to be tested for "frightening" diseases. She resists the doctor's advice, and he wisely obtains an informed consent and informed refusal. Should her uveitis be caused by syphilis and should the doctor miss this diagnosis because appropriate tests were not done, he would be at risk of being held negligent. The doctor also wants the record to show that the patient was informed that she could get cataracts and glaucoma as a result of the cortisone treatment.

In the first case, the patient was surprised to learn he needed surgery. In the second, the patient has come to the doctor pumped with information, but still uses the doctor as a powerful authority to whom she will either accede or against whom she will resist. In neither case is there a partnership. In neither case is there a transfer of power from the caregiver to the patient. In both cases, different as they are, the doctor's words lead to consent or refusal. Probably, one of the reasons the second patient did not follow the doctor's advice is that the doctor presented himself as an authority figure, not as a caring source of information. He came across as a "caregiver" attempting to dispense health rather than an expert trying to help a staunchly independent person make up her own mind in a way that would allow her to feel autonomous and in control.

*Conversation model of informed consent*: Brody cogently discusses the inevitable inequality between physician and patient, even in what he calls the "conversation model of informed consent,"[11] a matter also discussed in detail by Wear.[12] Even if the doctor's request or proposal (here, to proceed with a cataract extraction or treatment for uveitis) is welcome in that it suggests a way to achieve the patient's goal of getting better, an element of concern is evoked in the consenter's mind, simply because the solution has been proposed by somebody else, who inevitably has some conflict of interest, while that "somebody else" presumably has the patient's interests in mind, but that is a presumption, not a demonstrated certainty.

Consent implies a relationship based on power. There is a difference in the power of patients and health professionals. But it is not solely the professionals who are in possession of all the power. They are presumably more powerful because they know more about the pathophysiology of disease and the methods of treatment; but the patient is more powerful in that he has the option of acting on the advice of the professionals. Ideally the attitudes and actions of professionals should increase their patient's power. Patients who consent yield some power and control to the professionals, whereas patients given the option of "choosing" retain their power. No matter how beneficently professionals intend their suggestions, no matter how amicably patients acquiesce to their suggestions, if the word "consent" is used, the implication remains that professionals are operating from a position of controlling power.

## TOWARD A PARADIGM OF INFORMED CHOICE

"Choice",[13] unlike "consent" or "refusal", is not necessarily related to another person's proposal. A waiter describing a menu to a diner may recommend the beef and mutton entrees; he may even add that he prefers the beef. The diner then considers the waiter's remarks and makes a choice, perhaps to have the beef. We do not say that the diner has consented to have the beef. Some waiters are highly knowledgeable regarding the menu and may be viewed as an authority; nevertheless, the diner does not "consent to" or "refuse" the waiter's comments. In some cases the diner may ask the waiter to make a choice for him. But even in this situation, the diner is still acting autonomously and has chosen to have the waiter make the decision.

Health-care professionals might approach patients in a similar manner, asking patients to choose from a "menu of choices" rather than give consent to a particular suggestion. The health-care professional should not merely present "the menu", but should annotate it, adding that he would advise, perhaps strongly, a certain choice. When the patient chooses, the professional is perceived as an advisor, more knowledgeable about some things than the patient, a source of information to be used by the patient, but leaving the patient in charge, in control, even should the patient choose to have the professional make the decision.

## REVISITING THE CASE SCENARIOS

Reconsidering now the first case from the viewpoint of "choice" rather than "consent", the doctor would explain the nature of the cataract and of cataract extraction, answering questions regarding risks and benefits, and tailoring the discussion to the patient's needs and wants. He might then say something like, "Did I answer your questions; I want to make sure they are all answered". The doctor then says something like, "What would you like me to do? I don't think you want to choose to have new glasses, because it is very unlikely that they will help you. But you may choose to have the cataract extraction now. There is no urgency". The patient may respond, "What do you advise" enlisting the following response from the doctor? "You came to see me because you were unhappy with your vision. You are in good health. Cataract surgery is usually successful and there is a great likelihood that such surgery would make you happier with your vision. As such, you may choose to have such surgery. If so, we will plan to proceed with that".

In the case of the woman with uveitis, the doctor would offer a detailed explanation and advise that she has a variety of choices. Studies can be done to try to determine the cause of the uveitis; because such a cause is often not found, the studies may not show anything. However, for some of the conditions that can cause uveitis, such as sarcoid and syphilis, there are effective treatments, and she may choose to have tests for those conditions. Because of her Internet searches, the woman already knows that the usual treatment for uveitis is cortisone, but knowing that cortisone can cause cataracts and glaucoma, she challenges her eye doctor, asking him which poses the greater risk, the cortisone treatment or the uveitis. The eye doctor answers that in his opinion the uveitis poses the greater risk, and then explains the risk of missing a treatable condition such as syphilis or sarcoid. What he is trying to do is to help the patient prioritize her choices in a way that will allow her to be most likely to choose her highest priority. The patient, thus, is helped to use the doctor to direct the treatment as she chooses.

## HEALTH-CARE PROFESSIONAL'S PERSPECTIVE

No matter how well intentioned, professionals are not highly reliable judges as to the choices their patients will make.[14] When physicians have in their minds the action to which they want their patients to consent in a formal, legalistic proposal, often in writing, then the physician becomes the power figure to whom the patient must submit (consent) or against whom the patient feels forced to rebel (refuse), and who often is requesting an action that the patient does not want.

Professionals are routinely instructed that they must have a discussion with the patient in order "to obtain an informed consent", and that this must be in writing. But when a written informed consent is required, the health professional is in some way saying to the patient, "I know I have explained things to you and that you have consented, but I do not trust you, so I will require that you sign an informed consent."

Health-care professionals are also advised to obtain an informed consent to protect themselves,[15-17] to prove that a discussion was held, and that the patient consented to the professional's recommendation. Obtaining written permission is understandable and prudent, especially in a litigious society. Fear of being sued is so deep that a major purpose of obtaining written consents is the belief that it protects the health professionals or the administrators. In this regard, hospital nurses are firmly instructed to delay any surgery until a signed informed consent is on the chart. This is clearly not done to protect the patient, and patients sense that. Furthermore, this method of obtaining an informed consent does not discourage suits and has little protective effect. While the written informed consent may be of some help in the courtroom, it does not engender trust or make the patient feel cared for.

Unless the underlying purpose has been fulfilled, specifically, helping the patient move toward an informed decision that the patient believes is in his or her best interest, protection is rarely advanced by the form itself. Some patients in signing such forms recognize the perfunctory nature of the form and, if they are content that they know what they need to know, they will sign the form without reading it. Some manifest mild irritation about the waste of everybody's time involved with the "record treating". Other patients are seriously put off by the global "truth dumping" of some forms, which mention the potential for serious problems without putting them into perspective. A few patients are frankly upset and see the forms as something behind which the health-care professionals hope to hide. When professionals notice this response in the patient, they are foolish to proceed; something is very wrong, and even if the patients were to sign the form, it would not achieve its purposes of providing the patients the knowledge they need or want and of protecting the professional. Requiring a written informed choice would serve the same "protective purpose" and yet make clear to the patient that it was the patient who was electing to have the treatment, not the surgeon.

Patients may choose not to follow their physicians' recommendations. At present this is recorded on the chart as a refusal to follow advice. The antonym of "consent" is "refuse". "To refuse" means "to decline to submit". The person who "refuses" is stating that he will not do what another has suggested. For example, some patients may refuse to stay in the hospital, even against the advice of their physician. Some patients, as in the second case presented here, may refuse a certain test, such as having blood drawn. "Refuse" connotes acting contrary to a proposal, even if the action is merely "not consenting to" the proposal. When patients decide not to follow a health-care professional's advice, it is preferable to say that they "choose" not to follow a recommendation rather than that they "refuse." Again, the word "choose" suggests that the power balance favors the patient, who is directing his/her own course, rather than being directed into that course by the more powerful physician.

## CONCLUSION

In health care, the difference between "choice" and "consent" is important; choice encourages autonomy while the other discourages it. Fundamental to proper patient care is enhancing the patient's autonomy, helping the patient take charge of his own life, especially as it relates to health. This is fundamental not only for philosophical and legal reasons but also because self-care is essential for achieving a state of health, which is, after all, the goal of therapy. To speak of informed choice rather than informed consent would help eliminate paternalism in medicine without detracting from the intent of health-care professionals to be helpful or in any way decreasing their ability to be beneficial. To speak of informed choice rather than informed consent will emphasize that people need to be in charge of their own health and that they themselves must make those decisions that affect their own health.

## REFERENCES

1. Mayer KF. The process of obtaining informed patient consent. Nurs Times. 2002;98(31):30-31.
2. Jenna JK. Toward the patient-driven hospital. Health Forum. 1986;29(4):52-9.
3. Shendell-Falik N. Creating self-care units in the acute care setting: a case study. Patient Educ Couns. 1990;15(1):39-45.
4. Lott TF, Blazey ME, West MG. Patient participation in health care: an underused resource. Nurs Clin North Am. 1992; 27(1):61-76.
5. Meyer MJ. Patients' duties. J Med Philos. 1992;17(5):541-55.
6. Furlong S. Self-care: the application of a ward philosophy. J Clin Nurs. 1996;5(2):85-90.
7. McMurray MH. Seniors and self-care hemodialysis. J CANNT. 1995;5(1):13-14.
8. Brody BL, Roch-Levecq AC, Gamst AC, et al. Self-management of age-related macular degeneration and quality of life: a randomized controlled trial. Arch Ophthalmol. 2002;120(11): 1477-83.
9. Shoor S, Lorig KR. Self-care and the doctor-patient relationship. Med Care. 2002;40(4 Suppl):II 40-44.
10. Benson H. Timeless Healing: The Power and Biology of Belief. New York: Simon & Shuster, Inc.; 1997.
11. Brody S. The Healer's Power. New Haven: Yale U. Press; 1993.
12. Wear SE. Informed Consent: Patient Autonomy and Clinician Beneficence in Clinical Medicine, 2nd edn. Washington, DC: Georgetown University Press; 1998.
13. Webster's New World Collegiate Dictionary. 4th edition. Eds: Agnes M, Guralnik DB. Foster City, Calif: IDG Book Worldwide, Inc., 2001.p 1205.
14. Zweibel NR, Cassel CK. Treatment choices at the end of life: a comparison of decisions by older patients and their physician-selected proxies. Gerontologist. 1989;29:615-21.
15. O'Connor RJ. Informed consent: legal, behavioral, and educational issues. Patient Couns Health Educ. 1981;3:49-57.
16. Woody KJ. Legal and ethical concepts involved in informed consent to human research. Cal W L Rev. 1981;18:50-79.
17. Lee S. Medical paternalism: informed consent. In: Lee S (ed.), Law and Morals: Warnock, Gillick and Beyond. New York: Oxford University Press; 1986. pp. 63-67, 95.

CHAPTER

113

# Medicolegal Issues

George L Spaeth

## INTRODUCTION

*Medical malpractice is an important subject*: The fear of being sued affects what physicians do, most practicing so-called "defensive medicine"; being sued is an unpleasant, even life-changing event; malpractice insurance is expensive; institutes design their relationships with patients and physicians so as to minimize legal problems; and, literally, many millions of dollars are spent annually trying to avoid, manage, and settle legal issues related to patient care.

In United States, the already bad situation has been made more complex by increasing regulations, such as those related to the Health Insurance Portability and Accountability Act (HIPAA). The new omnibus rule greatly enhances a patient's privacy protections, provides individuals new rights to their health information, and strengthens the government's ability to enforce the law. Patients can ask for a copy of their electronic medical record in an electronic form. When individuals pay by cash they can instruct their provider not to share information about their treatment with their health plan. The final omnibus rule sets new limits on how information is used and disclosed for marketing and fundraising purposes and prohibits the sale of an individuals' health information without their permission.

Further, any physician interested in performing research must spend many hours being "certified" and then must work with institutional review boards in a careful way. While it would be nice to believe that our job as physicians is simply to take care of patients, there are individuals eager for physicians to act in ways that will bring a large sum of money to the patients, lawyers, and legal firms. While the intent of the law is clearly not to be something that enriches people inappropriately or causes so many administrative and regulatory hurdles that patient care is made worse, in actuality that can be the case. Nevertheless, it is also important to recall that the very unfortunate situation that now exists is largely the result of what physicians have done. Not all physicians are either conscientious or competent. Furthermore, and ironically, in trying to be excessively careful, physicians set a standard of care that is inappropriate.

*This chapter will consider two quite separate issues*: (1) how to decrease the likelihood of being sued; and (2) how to decrease the likelihood of being held liable, if sued. Much of what is written about medical/legal considerations is directed toward the latter issue,[1-3] but merely being named in a suit has unpleasant consequences. The emotional stress is obvious.[4-7] A reputation can be lost even after a trial has exonerated the physician.

## PREVENTING AN ACTION FROM BEING BROUGHT

The presence of a trusting relationship between the caregiver and the patient is the most important factor in avoiding the caregiver being named in an action.[8] Trusting relationships are the result of being honest, caring, realistic, and cumulative. A second, essential way to avoid being sued for medical malpractice is to make sure that the patient has realistic expectations.

The initiation of a suit, then, is often the result of lack of trust combined with unfulfilled expectations. These expectations may be "natural" or acquired. It is natural for a person to expect a good outcome from a routine event, such as childbirth. When the outcome is not what was anticipated, the result is often anger, hurt, and confusion, all of which instinctively trigger actions against the apparent source of the anger, hurt, or confusion. Few people recognize that outcomes, even from routine events, are not able to be predicted with accuracy. Everybody, perhaps most of all the actors—the physician, the surgeon, the nurse, the herbalist—need to remember that there is no truly safe medication, no truly safe procedure, and no truly surgery. Even tests carry inherent risks that are inevitable. The admonition, "First, do no harm", is unfortunate, even bad advice. Harm cannot be avoided. What makes harm tolerable is that the potential benefit of the action leading to the harm justifies the potential harm. The intent of "First, do no harm," is clearly good, but it leads to unrealistic expectations. Every act has within it the kernel of harm.

Clearly a patient cannot make a reasoned decision without a reasonable understanding of the risks and the benefits. The caregiver should not under- or overestimate either the risks or the benefits, acknowledging, however, that both the risks and the benefits are approximations. Merely mentioning the major issues is usually adequate when there is a trusting relationship to start with. Giving the patient an extensive legalistic form to explain the risks and benefits is either useless or even counterproductive, as it may be interpreted as a move designed primarily to protect the caregiver, not the patient. In actuality, this interpretation is usually correct. Reasonable, intuitive expectations should be reinforced when they are appropriate, as gently, but clearly explained as not applicable when inappropriate.

Poor outcomes may trigger suits, but most often when they are unexpected. A bad result from a routine cataract extraction is likely to lead to a dissatisfied patient. Considering these thoughts, a second way to decrease the likelihood of being named in a legal action is to do a good job. Numerous examples prove that caregivers—like everyone else—vary in their ability to assess accurately their knowledge, skills, and judgment. Every caregiver should periodically request an evaluation from an individual competent to make such an assessment. This system only works, however, when the judge is able and free to evaluate meaningfully. In actual practice this system rarely works because those most likely to be acting inappropriately are those least likely to want a realistic, honest evaluation. Institutions are usually required by law to perform periodic evaluations. More often than not, these are "window dressing" and are not likely to identify those who will need remediation or removal from practice. Nevertheless, required "credentialing" serves the important purpose of defining what is considered necessary to practice, and providing a legal basis for taking action. Such credentialing, however, is not an adequate substitute for honest, critical self-evaluation followed by decisive action, depending on the results of such an evaluation. To repeat, however, the "catch-22" is that those needing the evaluations are not likely to request them or may falsify information, whereas those not needing the evaluations are the ones most likely to make sure they get evaluated.

Many expectations are acquired. That understanding may come from a personal experience, from a friend, a brochure, an advertisement, the Internet, or from a caregiver. Of these, the first and last are most telling, that is the personal experience and the caregiver. The person who has had a bad result is likely—often with reason—to expect a second bad result, and vice versa. Explaining convincingly and honestly what are reasonable expectations for the second (or tenth) episode requires knowing the risks and benefits for that new episode and, additionally, being able to communicate those considerations despite the barriers raised by the previous experience.

What the caregiver communicates through words and body language is critically important. Inappropriately minimizing potential problems is unwise. Exaggerating concerns is an equal disservice, as it may dissuade the patient from choosing a needed next step.

## AVOIDING BEING HELD NEGLIGENT IF NAMED IN AN ACTION

The best way—by far!—to avoid having a legal judgment of medical negligence brought against one is to act so that an action is not brought. Once the suit has been brought, permanent damage has already been done: expenses increased, reputation lost, relationships strained or broken, and life disrupted. The unpleasantnesses of dealing with a legal action do not simply go away even if the suit is withdrawn or thrown out, much less settled or decided in the defendant's favor. Should the case come to trial, the desire of the plaintiff to win leads the prosecuting attorney to build a case that is as damning as possible. The defendant should be prepared to be characterized as dishonest, uncaring, heartless, and incompetent, as a result of which the plaintiff's life, as well as the lives of others, has been permanently ruined. The lawyer's

**TABLE 113-1** Factors predisposing to initiation of a suit

| *Suits are usually initiated by unhappy patients. Patients are unhappy because:* |
|---|
| • They believe they have been demeaned, misled, ignored, not heard, or discouraged |
| • They believe they have had an unexpected result, or their expectations are unfulfilled, or they have a different follow-up than expected |
| • They believe their physician has been incompetent |
| • They have heard critical comments from others – other physicians, patients, friends or relatives, unhappy members of the physician's staff, or lawyers |
| • Because they are unhappy people to start with |

**TABLE 113-2** Factors that decrease the likelihood of a malpractice suit being brought

| An environment and experiences that engender trust |
|---|
| A physician who is able validly to evaluate his or her own abilities and limitations |
| Physicians and staff who listen, hear, and treat their patients respectfully |
| Physicians and staff who sincerely care for patients |
| *Clear and adequate communication between patients, staff, and physicians:* |
| • Accurate, appropriate, complete, and legible medical records |
| • Written, dated instructions to patients regarding tests and treatments |
| • Letters to patients summarizing the results of their visits, with copies to other interested parties to whom the patient wants letters sent |

fee is likely to be based on the amount of the judgment. One $5 million judgment every 5 years will assure that the prosecuting attorney has a very comfortable income.

Factors predisposing to initiation of suit are listed in Table 113-1. Factors that decrease the likelihood of a malpractice suit being initiated are shown in Table 113-2.

## STEPS THAT HELP PROTECT A PHYSICIAN FROM BEING HELD NEGLIGENT IF A SUIT IS BROUGHT AGAINST HIM OR HER

The defendants' lawyers, that is lawyers who work for insurance companies or work for physicians, are primarily interested in their client not getting "convicted" if a suit is brought. After all, it is not in their best interest for physicians never to be sued. What they are, then, primarily interested in is what happens after the suit is brought. This is important to remember, because the advice of lawyers, law firms, and insurance companies who are involved in protecting physicians from having judgments brought against them, may not be appropriate to help prevent a suit from being brought and may not represent good medicine. For example, many defendants' lawyers will say something like, "If you think of a test, order it". That is bad advice. Tests should only be ordered when there is a reasonable likelihood that the result of a test is necessary in order to decide what is appropriate treatment.

Some lawyers make themselves readily available and encourage unhappy patients to bring legal action. Some even try to make patients unhappy in order to encourage them to bring a legal action. When lawyers believe that they have a reasonable chance of winning a case in which there will be a large judgment, they become increasingly interested in representing the client.

No matter how competently caregivers practice, and no matter how sincerely physicians care for patients, there is a reasonable chance that they will be sued sometime during their career. It is, then, prudent to be prepared for such a situation and to act in a way that will lessen the likelihood of being held liable or culpable. These protective issues are the ones that are most frequently discussed when medical malpractice is considered. They are important; however, it cannot be said too frequently that the major effort should be directed at avoiding a suit being initiated.

Practices that can help prevent being held liable should a suit be brought are shown in Table 113-3. These are really self-explanatory and need not be discussed in detail, though they are often forgotten and frequently not followed. In summary, and in the simplest terms, the best way to avoid being held liable for medical malpractice is to avoid being sued, and the best way to avoid being sued is to be a good caregiver—trustworthy, competent, respectful—recognizing, however, that even competent and compassionate physicians sometimes get sued, it is prudent to take reasonable steps, such as making sure the documentation is adequate and the communications with patients are clear and thorough.

**TABLE 113-3** Practices that will help prevent being held liable if a suit is brought

| |
|---|
| *Document records well:* |
| • Thoroughly, appropriately, and legibly |
| • If not following standard procedure, discuss with the patient, note in the chart that the patient has agreed, and, ideally, have the patient sign the note |
| Be sure that communications are clear and accurate. If errors are made, they should be corrected promptly and properly (the old entry should neither be erased nor made illegible) and the date of the correction indicated with the initials of who made the correction |
| Make sure that notes are placed in the chart regarding the dates, subject matter, and recommendations that relate to telephone calls or other oral communications |
| Make sure that copies of all authorizations, including suggested diagnostic procedures and treatments, are noted accurately and legibly in the chart |
| Indicate in the record when a patient does not keep an appointment, notify the patient, and document that the patient was informed of the missed appointment and that an attempt was made to schedule a new appointment |
| When a patient initiates a contact through a letter, e-mail, or telephone call, make sure the record indicates who responded, when the response was made and the outcome of the response. If the patient cannot be reached, indicate clearly the efforts that were made in order to try to reach the patient |
| Retain records for the length of time required by law |
| Obtain truly informed consents customized for the individual patient. Make sure that it is clear to the patient that the intent is to help the patient make a decision, and that the obtaining of the informed consent is not primarily for the purpose of protecting the physician |
| Do not make comments that would be easily misinterpreted, or, worse, properly interpreted, as indicating disrespect for the patient. This applies to whether or not the patient is apparently able or unable to appreciate the comment |
| *Make sure every person in the office – the physicians and every member of the staff – acts respectfully toward every patient:* |
| • Never "makes fun" of a patient |
| • Never demeans a patient even when such comments are thought to be being made "in private" |
| • Never criticizes other caregivers |

## REFERENCES


1. Levinson W. Physician-patient communication. A key to malpractice prevention. JAMA. 1994;27:1619-20.
2. Glabman M. The top ten malpractice claims [and how to minimize them]. Hosp Health Netw. 2004;78:60-2, 64-6.
3. Pawlson LG, O'Kane ME. Malpractice prevention, patient safety, and quality of care: a critical linkage. Am J Manag Care. 2004;10:281-4.
4. Couch CE, Thiebaud S. Who supports physicians in malpractice cases? Physician Exec. 2002;28:30-3.
5. Wenokur B, Campbell L. Malpractice suit emotional trauma. JAMA. 1991;266:2834.
6. Martin CA, Wilson JF, Fiebelman ND 3rd, et al. Physicians' psychologic reactions to malpractice litigation. South Med J. 1991;84:1300-4.
7. Martin CA, Wilson JF, Fiebelman ND 3rd, et al. Physicians' psychologic reactions to malpractice litigation. South Med J. 1991;84:1300-4.
8. Levinson W. Physician-patient communication. A key to malpractice prevention. JAMA. 1994;27:1619-20.

CHAPTER

# 114

# Ethics of Surgery

George L Spaeth, Parul Ichhpujani

## INTRODUCTION

Ethics comes from the Greek word ethikos, which means "character".[1] It is the branch of philosophy that deals with values relating to human conduct, with respect to the actions and the motives and ends of such actions. When we talk of ethics in ophthalmology, we are actually talking of "Applied Ethics".

## HOW TO DETERMINE WHAT IS "ETHICAL"?

To determine whether a surgical procedure is ethical is, at first glance, an easy task. What we need to do is ask the following questions.

### Is the surgery in the best interest of the patient?

If it is, presumably the surgery is ethical. However, while there is truth in that tautology, such a way of thinking about whether surgery is ethical is not is so simplistic as to be meaningless. For example, in truth new surgical procedures are never performed (if the surgeon is honest) because they are known to be in the best interest of the patient.[2] They cannot be known to be in the best interest of the patient, because the outcomes of such surgery have not been established. How do you define "the best interest of the patient?"

### Is it better (more ethical) to have surgery performed locally by a barely adequate surgeon or to have the patient travel at major inconvenience to have surgery performed by the acknowledged leader in the field?

Surgeons are like baseball players, and everybody else; some are better than others. Not all surgeons perform adequately, much less excellently.

When surgeons are performing procedures with which they are familiar, but they make a modification they hope will result in a better surgical outcome, is that really "in the best interest of the patient?" Perhaps yes; perhaps no. The surgeon, however, does not know that it is in the best interest of the patient. He or she hopes it may be, but whether he or she is right is unknown.

### Is it ethical to perform a long surgical procedure in hope of giving one patient "The Best Care" when others who need surgery would not be able to have the needed surgery because they cannot get put on the Operating Schedule?

This is a matter of doing justice. In such a situation, is it better to perform adequately or even marginally inadequate surgery in order to be able to try to help more people? Is it ethical to spend money and effort on a procedure designed to have an outcome that is the best possible, when that time and effort means that others would not have the chance to have surgery at all?

### Is it ethical to have inexperienced surgeons performing surgery simply because if they do not there will be no way that they can learn how to do surgery in order to take care of patients in the future?

All of these issues make it readily apparent that determining whether a surgical procedure is "ethical" cannot be answered by the simple litmus test, "Is it in the best interest of the patient?" Complicating the matter further is the fact that all surgeons are biased. While it is likely that few surgeons perform surgery unless they think they are competent to do so, the history of medicine is rife with evidence that physicians are not good judges of their own competency.[3] Additionally, the reality of the situation is that surgeons want to support themselves and their families and realize that performing surgery is a good way to do that. However, surgeons also know that making somebody "worse" is one of the quickest ways to be sued, to develop a bad reputation, and to lose patients. Consequently, there is a built in reluctance to perform surgery on patients in whom the results are likely to be bad, regardless of whether or not the patient really needs that surgery. Add to that the fact that some surgeons really love the challenge of a difficult procedure; such individuals are not at all risk averse, but, rather, enjoy putting themselves in situations of high procedural and emotional intensity. The more impossible the case, the more obsessed they are with being the person to solve the problem.

## IS THERE A SOLUTION TO ADDRESS THE ETHICAL DILEMMAS?

Despite these complexities, determining whether a surgical procedure is needed, which procedure to do, and who should do it, is not an impossibly difficult task. The key to the appropriate solution is to remember that each person is unique, that each situation is unique, and that the only appropriate approach is:

- To recognize that uniqueness
- To be thorough in considering the risks and benefits in a way that the patient can really understand them both,
- To be honest, and
- To acknowledge as best one can one's own biases.

## PRINCIPLES OF MEDICAL ETHICS

The three fundamental principles of medical ethics provide strong guidance,[4] as long as they are considered in a way that is truly honest:

1. Will the surgery increase the patient's autonomy?
2. Is the surgery likely to benefit or to harm?
3. Is the surgery fair, fair to the patient under consideration, and to all patients?

## DETERMINATION OF NECESSITY OF A PROCEDURE

For a surgical procedure to be ethical it must be necessary. To be necessary it means that without it the patient would develop a disability. Consequently, this development requires estimating risk—but what risks? The standard risk factors are virtually useless unless they are in a range that is always abnormal. Means and standard deviations do not help when considering individuals. There is no way to estimate with accuracy the likelihood that a person without visual field loss and an intraocular pressure will develop a disability. It is simply as simple and disturbing as that. Therefore, if no disability is present, it is necessary to establish the presence of damage and the rate of change of that damage, and match that against the duration the damage is likely to continue. This is still an estimate. Without taking all those considerations into play, one cannot even approximate with any certainty the likelihood that a person will develop a disability. Current risk calculators are useless in this regard.

What findings are always abnormal? An intraocular pressure of 35 mm Hg will almost always be associated with progressive glaucomatous nerve damage. Intraocular pressure that can be fairly well ascertained to be typical for the patient in question and is in a range where it has been documented that the patient has gotten worse at that level of pressure is almost certain to cause a continuing worsening of glaucoma, and highly asymmetric intraocular pressures (>5 mm Hg difference between the two eyes). Other than those three considerations, the role of intraocular pressure is extraordinarily difficult to predict with accuracy.

Patients who have not yet developed definite glaucoma damage can be assumed to be unlikely to develop glaucoma damage. Paradoxically, the longer such individuals have had pressures above normal limits and the longer their optic nerves have remained normal, the less likely they are to develop damage. Their disks have demonstrated that they are not likely to become damaged.

Cup/disk ratios are of little use in determining whether or not progressive damage is likely to occur. Unless the cup/disk ratio is >.8, it cannot be considered a reliable indication of glaucoma damage, and even those with cup/disk ratios of .9 cannot be normal if they have large disks and no areas of rim absence. Disk Damage Likelihood Scale scores of 6, 7, 8, 9, or 10 are always pathologic and as such indicate that the disk has definitely become damaged, and presumably, therefore, unless there is some change, the disk will continue to be damaged.

Rate of change can only be established by accumulating valid markers. Visual fields can be valid, but they are difficult, highly variable, and must be interpreted with great caution. Structural changes tend to be more reliable, but the value of such structural changes depends on the value of the documentation of the structure. Of the presently available techniques, disk photographs probably provide the most cost affordable and reliable help in this regard.

The duration with which the disease will continue to progress varies with the type of disease. For the primary glaucomas, such as the angle closure and the open angle glaucomas, this usually means the duration of the patient's life. It is possible to estimate life expectancy for a period of 5 years with considerable accuracy by taking into account patient general health, lifestyle, and family history. Age is obviously a consideration, but becomes increasingly less valuable as the person ages. A healthy 90-year-old woman, e.g. has a 97% chance of living to be 94 and an 85% chance of living to be 98. In contrast, a 50-year-old man who is overweight, smokes, has a strong family history of males dying in their 50s, has had a heart attack, and is in congestive failure has about a 50% chance of living for the same 4 years than the 90-year-old woman has to live and a far smaller chance of living for 8 years than the 90-year-old woman has to live. However, a 25-year-old healthy woman, while not having as great a chance of living to be 94 as the 90-year-old woman, has an estimated years remaining of around 60 years. Clearly it is much wiser to base treatment on the estimated number of years remaining rather than on an anticipated age at the time of death.

The Glaucoma Graph can be of considerable help in plotting the stage of disease, the rate of change, and the estimated years remaining. Unless there is a reasonable certainty that the individual is already in the red zone, or will reach the red zone prior to death, it is hard to justify the risks of the surgery (Fig. 114-1).

*Autonomy*: This ethical belief has its origins in Greek and Roman culture, and the Latin translation is *Voluntas aegroti suprema lex*, which means that there is a supreme agreement to voluntarily accept treatment for illness.

For surgery to be ethical it should enhance the patient's ability to be in control of his or her own health. Some patients are meticulous about learning what they need to learn to do to care for themselves and then acting on that knowledge. Some patients do not learn what they need to know and others may learn what they need to know but then do not act on it. A surgical procedure will not educate the patient,

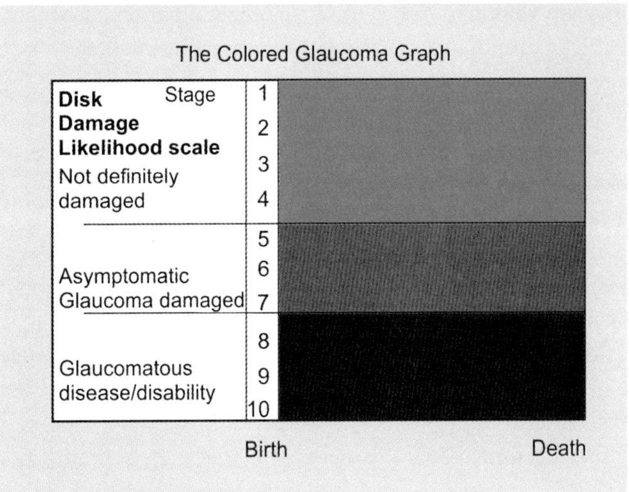


**Figure 114-1** The Glaucoma Graph.

and is not likely to result in a change in behavior. However, if patients understand that they will become disabled without a surgical procedure, they may develop the motivation to learn or to change behavior. When patients do not learn or do not behave appropriately, performing surgery can enhance their autonomy by helping preserve their vision.

*Beneficence/nonmaleficence*: The concept of the beneficence is embodied by the phrase, "the well-being of the patient is the most important law" or *Salus aegroti suprema lex* while nonmaleficence is best described by the phrase, "first, do no harm", or the Latin, *primum non nocere*. In surgical practice, however, many times treatments carry some risk of harm. In some circumstances, if the outcome without the treatment will be grave, then it is wiser to undertake a risk, as the risk of not treating is also very likely to do harm. Hence, the principle of nonmaleficence is not absolute. It is upon the treating physician to balance against the principle of beneficence (doing good). The effects of the two principles together often give rise to a double effect.

Surgical procedures can be of benefit to patients. They may preserve vision by lowering intraocular pressure to a safe level. They may protect the surface of the eye or improve quality of life by minimizing or eliminating the need for medications. However, surgical procedures always cause some harm. Even in the best hands and in the best circumstances, complications cannot be completely avoided. Outcomes cannot be predicted accurately with total certainty. Eyes that have had surgery may be improved in certain ways, but they are never the same as before the surgery. It is essential for both the patient and the surgeon to be honest about this reality and to acknowledge that it is impossible to perform surgery without doing some harm. Patients have the right to decide how much harm they are willing to risk in order to obtain a particular benefit. Patients cannot make that decision rationally unless they have a realistic idea of the harms and the benefits and the likelihood of the harms and the benefits.

There are always a variety of options and it is the physician's responsibility to make sure that the patients are aware of what options are open to them. For example, a patient whose glaucoma is getting worse despite maximal medicinal treatment, but who is obsessively concerned about appearance, needs to know that a tube shunt procedure may cause the muscles of the eye to work incorrectly and change her appearance, and that there is a great likelihood of some type of droopy lid following a filtering procedure such as a trabeculectomy. For a patient who desperately wants not to have a change in cosmetic appearance, it may be that a cyclodestructive procedure would be a procedure of choice, because such procedures are slightly less likely than a trabeculectomy or tube shunt procedure to be associated with visible change of appearance.

*Justice*: Providing care for patients in the future demands passing knowledge and skills onto those who do not have them. There is no way that can be done without some concerns. An ophthalmic surgeon performing his first trabeculectomy, even under supervision, is not likely to perform it as well as his fifth or fiftieth. Just as some surgeons are more competent than others, some are better supervisors than others. It has been shown that the complication rate with learning surgeons is more related to the supervisor than to the learning surgeon.

Health resources are not unlimited. Dollars or time spent on X are not available for Y. The medical profession has been reluctant to acknowledge the truth of Thoreau's comment that the enemy of the good is the perfect. Effort and funds are expended today in hopes that the operating time to perform a cataract extraction can be reduced and that the visual result improved. It is extremely hard to justify this as an ethical use of resources. Visual results today with standard phacoemulsification or small incision extracapsular cataract extraction are excellent, most patients achieving a visual acuity of 20/20 unless there is some other cause for visual reduction. That's good enough! The responsible investigator would be trying to determine how to make those results more accessible and affordable, not trying to get vision to 20/15!

## SUMMARY

For a surgical procedure to be ethical it must satisfy the tenets of medical ethics: (1) Does it enhance the patient's autonomy in a way the patient wants? (2) Is it more likely to benefit than harm, again in ways that are important to the patient?, and (3) Is it fair, fair to the patient, and fair to society?

## REFERENCES

1. Veatch RM. A Theory of Medical Ethics. New York: Basic Books; 1981.
2. Ethics Committee, American Academy of Ophthalmology. The Ethical Ophthalmologist: A Primer. San Francisco, CA: American Academy of Ophthalmology; 1993.
3. Day SH. A structured curriculum on ethics for ophthalmology residents is valuable. Arch Ophthalmol. 2002;120(7):963-4.
4. Engelhardt HT Jr. The Foundations of Bioethics. New York: Oxford University Press; 1986.

## SUGGESTED READING

1. Shaarawy T, Sherwood MB, Grehn F. Guidelines on Design and Reporting of Glaucoma Surgical Trials. The Hague, Amsterdam, The Netherlands: World Glaucoma Association. Kugler Publications; 2009.

# Index

*Note: Page numbers followed by f and t indicate figures and tables, respectively. Those followed by b indicate boxes.*

## C

## D



## E

## F

## G



## H



## I

## J



## K



## L



## M

## N



## O

## P

## T



## U